# Toxicology and Risk Assessment

# Toxicology and Risk Assessment

## Principles, Methods, and Applications

edited by

## Anna M. Fan
**California Environmental Protection Agency**
**Berkeley, California**

## Louis W. Chang
**University of Arkansas for Medical Sciences**
**Little Rock, Arkansas**

**Marcel Dekker, Inc.**                    **New York•Basel•Hong Kong**

**Library of Congress Cataloging-in-Publication Data**

Toxicology and risk assessment : principles, methods, and applications
/ [edited by] Anna M. Fan, Louis W. Chang.
    p.  cm.
    Includes index.
    ISBN 0-8247-9490-7 (hardcover : alk. paper)
    1. Toxicology. 2. Health risk assessment.  I. Fan, Anna M.
II. Chang, Louis W.
    [DNLM: 1. Toxicology. 2. Risk Assessment.  QV 600 T75565 1996]
RA1211.T635  1996
615.9—dc20
DNLM/DLC
for Library of Congress

95-39860
CIP

The publisher offers discounts on this book when ordered in bulk quantities.  For more information, write to Special Sales/Professional Marketing at the address below.

This book is printed on acid-free paper.

MARCEL DEKKER, INC.
270 Madison Avenue, New York, New York  10016

Current printing (last digit):
10  9  8  7  6  5  4  3  2  1

**PRINTED IN THE UNITED STATES OF AMERICA**

*To*
*Rocky Cheuk*
*and*
*Jane C. Wang-Chang*

*our spouses, for they are like the wind beneath our wings,*
*giving us constant and much needed support.*

*Anna M. Fan*
*Louis W. Chang*

# Foreword

*The problem with toxicology is not the practicing toxicologists, but chemists who can detect precisely toxicologically insignificant amounts of chemicals.*
(René Truhaut, Late Professor of Toxicology, University of Paris, 1909–1994)

*Our theories are the mirrors in which we see ourselves.* (Unknown)

There have been monographs dealing with toxicology in which risk assessment played an incidental role. There have been other books and reviews on risk assessment in which the question of the underlying toxicological phenomena was not the main emphasis. The current monograph, to be published toward the end of this century, combines—rightfully so—the essentials in toxicology logically extending into risk assessment.

Although the concept of toxicology is ancient, in practice, the field of toxicology was a specialty within the discipline of pharmacology. It was only about 1960 that toxicology began to establish itself as a field in its own right.

Overall, toxicology attempts to define possible adverse effects in humans through laboratory research, or to review and explore in the field observations of certain toxic or adverse effects in humans. These can be quite varied, from the occurrence of poisoning from overdosages of drugs, of alcoholic beverages, or from exposure to certain products at the place of work, or combinations thereof. A major early concern, therefore, was in occupational toxicology.

Professional pursuits, and also widespread media attention, in recent decades, have singled out the observation and evaluation of chronic chemical exposures leading to cancer, allergies, neurotoxicity, or to effects on the immune system. In many instances, it is the question of cancer that has caught the imagination of the public, with no discrimination of whether justified, or scientifically unjustified, allegations were raised of cancer risks from environmental chemicals. That chemicals could cause cancer was first observed at the workplace, especially at the end of the last century and in the first half of this century. Such observations, involving relatively few cases, were made in many of the industrialized countries, and public attention was fostered by extensive publicity. In turn, this public knowledge led to the generalization, in the 1940s, that the existing cancer burden, affecting several 100,000s patients per year, was related to exposures to chemicals. The obvious candidates for suspicion in the general population were chemicals in the food chain as additives or contaminants. After relatively brief hearings, the Congress of the United States amended the existing food and drug laws by addition of the Delaney Clause in 1958, which stipulated that carcinogens, as documented in humans or in animals, could not be added to foods. One might say that this clause was justified, based on knowledge existing at the time. This understanding was meager indeed in the area of the mechanisms of carcinogenesis, or that of causes of major types of cancer in humans.

Beginning with that period, concern with health in general, and cancer in particular, has dramatically enlarged research funding through the National Institutes of Health and other public health service agencies, and also other voluntary societies, such as the American Cancer Society, the American Heart Association, and other disease-related groups.

These funds have been a splendid investment. The base of knowledge on causes of major chronic diseases, heart disease, stroke, diabetes, many types of cancer and, importantly, the underlying mechanisms have increased dramatically. Even more relevant are the substantial advances in fundamental knowledge in the basic sciences, including those associated with toxicology. The genetic apparatus and DNA were virtually unknown 50 years ago, whereas currently studies on the gene are common and, in fact, are the basis of a new exciting industry that is based on biotechnology.

On the other hand, legislation and regulatory actions by varied agencies in the United States have not taken advantage of the factual knowledge and mechanistic understanding achieved. Yet, the time is opportune to consider mechanisms in evaluating and defining environmental problems, especially those relating to cancer, allergies, the immune system, or the nervous system. We have introduced the term *genotoxic* to denote a reactive form or metabolite of a chemical that can act as an electrophilic reactant, or can generate reactive oxygen compounds. Such specific reactive chemicals can interact with the genetic apparatus to yield somatic mutations, the fundamental change eventuating in cancer, or those that can modify DNA or proteins, including specific receptor proteins, that would eventually be expressed in virtually all other adverse effects. In many instances, cells carrying abnormal DNA, or others with abnormal proteins, need to duplicate to express the initial changes. Thus, any activity affecting cell duplication rates necessarily will be reflected in the ultimate outcome.

A number of nongenotoxic chemicals play a major role in controlling DNA synthesis and cell duplication. However, for nongenotoxic mechanisms, dose–response action must be considered in applying any results to public health activities. In fact, high dose levels of nongenotoxic chemicals have displayed a variety of adverse effects, including cancer, in laboratory animals. For that reason, such chemicals were labeled carcinogens. In turn, this evaluation has led to regulatory actions, or even public pressures, that given an understanding of the underlying science, are not well justified, in my opinion. For example, there is widespread fear of environmental contamination with a group of chlorinated chemicals known as dioxins. At high dosages in animals, dioxins have induced cancer. However, in studies involving a number of dosages, a low level was found that failed to induce a significant number of specific cancers under the conditions of the test. After high-level human exposure during industrial accidents in the United States and in Italy, the affected individuals displayed chloracne, but observation of the individuals affected has not produced evidence of cancer, except a few select cases, for whom other factors may have been involved. On the other hand, dioxin is a potent enzyme inducer, even at low levels. The enzymes induced are not only those of the cytochrome P-450 system, but also phase II detoxification enzymes. Studies in animal models with low level dioxins and a carcinogen show inhibition of the action of the carcinogen through such mechanisms. The data from the extensive contamination of people in Seveso, Italy, begin to show that the breast cancer rate in the exposed population may be lower than in uncontaminated control groups. Chemical procedures can accurately measure tiny amounts of environmental dioxins. The question arises of whether these are really health risks, or perhaps, might even be beneficial. Recently, it was proposed that hospital incinerators be shut down because of emissions of dioxins. This raises the key problem of the safety to ship and bury hospital waste, which contains hazardous bacterial and viral contaminants, including HIV. I believe that traditional high-temperature destruction of any wastes by local incineration is the safest, most effective, and most economic means. This also applies to solid waste incineration by energy plants, which is occasionally not supported by lay groups with a different interpretation and understanding of the toxicology and objectives, and who often emphasize the potential risks from dioxins. Overall, experienced toxicologists should serve as a sound, objective, information resource on such questions.

Pharmacokinetic parameters are important controlling elements in the disposition and metabolism of xenobiotics and endogenous products. One reason dioxin displays prolonged activity is the slow elimination of this chemical and, in addition, it binds to the Ah receptor, extending its action on several physiological and pharmacological effectors. In contrast, ethanol is metabolized rapidly and its effect at several target sites evanescent. Metabolic and other pharmacological elements are frequently modified quantitatively by chemicals. Thus, it is important to consider not only the action of individual chemicals, but also of realistic mixtures of chemicals. Furthermore, it is clear that chemicals usually do not act in a qualitative, absolute way, but that quantitation is most important. One can state that an individual who smokes 40 cigarettes per day is at a high risk of heart disease or of specific cancers. In contrast, the effect in individuals smoking three to five cigarettes per day is hard to define. The question of risk assessment in relation to evaluation of toxicological data is critical. This is especially so for chemicals forming DNA-reactive metabolites that are labeled, thus, genotoxic. In the past, many scientists and regulatory agencies commonly used the linear extrapolation without threshold for all chemicals. Yet, other scientists hold that mechanistic considerations would suggest that the linear extrapolation should be applied only to DNA-reactive chemicals. Even in this instance, there may be deviations from linearity at low doses or exposures, and consideration needs to be given to practical thresholds for this class of chemicals. Indeed, there are mechanisms for removal of damaged DNA through processes such as DNA repair. Damaged cells can be eliminated through cell death or through the phenomenon of apoptosis. The mycotoxin aflatoxin $B_1$ is a powerful genotoxic chemical in the human dietary environment. It was discovered to be a carcinogen in 1962, and the FDA and USDA established regulations on the maximal amount of aflatoxin in foods for human consumption. The action level selected, 20 ppb, was appropriate, based on practical considerations of ensuring an adequate food supply, even though in rats, this dose level displays active carcinogenicity. In all species tested, aflatoxin $B_1$ causes liver cancer. This disease has a low incidence in the United States, but a high incidence in equatorial Africa, where the level of food contamination is 100–500 times higher, and the people are more likely to carry the hepatitis antigen. This might suggest that there is a no-effect level for this powerful genotoxic carcinogen. The regulatory action reflected the proper decision, displaying reasoning and approaches based on sound toxicological considerations.

There are also many nongenotoxic carcinogens, and we emphasize carcinogens mainly because, in the context of environment and health, the question of cancer causation and prevention is a field of general broad interest. Early developments in risk assessments for such chemicals assumed that they were no different from genotoxic chemicals. Such cases have not considered that nongenotoxic chemicals function by totally different mechanisms from those applicable to genotoxic carcinogens. Increased support is given to the operation of nongenotoxic mechanism, as evidenced by sound laboratory research and considerations of human epidemio-logical studies, establishing that these agents present a nonlinear dose–response, with a threshold. Thus, prevailing environmental concentrations below the threshold should have no adverse effects. Furthermore, it has been demonstrated that mixtures of such chemicals affecting distinct target organs would act independently. Yet, failure to consider these facts can lead to costly proposals to completely eliminate such chemicals, for example, from drinking water. Parts per billion of chloroform and similar halogenated compounds stem from the chlorination of water, an important and, in fact, essential health-preserving process. Chloroform can be measured very precisely through accurate chemical techniques. Nonetheless, the amounts usually present in water have no toxicological significance, given their mechanism of action. However, debate still continues over the adequacy of existing or needed evidence to support a threshold phenomenon for nongenotoxic carcinogens.

Risk assessment, thus, needs well-informed individuals to consider its use for risk manage-ment decision making. One noteworthy point is that risk management is often performed by scientifically lay people, and it often involves social, economic, legal, and political considera-tions, sometimes responding to public pressures, and cannot be totally oriented to health promotion. A more efficient use of public and private funds would be to develop more scientifically sound approaches to risk reduction and disease prevention, that are understood and accepted by everybody. Risk managers can best use the toxicological data base to inform and educate the public, so that options are clearly understood, and decisions can be made by all concerned that conform to a reasonable and sound toxicological evaluation and risk assessment. For example, relative to concerns with hazards attached to exposure to electro-magnetic radiation from electric wiring, different opinions are held among some toxicologists, and thus the general public, concerning the associated resource priority.

Much has been learned through research about the causes of major diseases affecting people worldwide. In contrast with the views prevailing at the beginning of this century, current evidence, although not totally conclusive, shows that environmental contamination by chemicals play a smaller role than previously thought, at least in North America. In any event, environ-mental contamination should be avoided through risk reduction and pollution prevention.

Importantly, the locally prevailing lifestyle is associated with major public health prob-lems. This includes the use of tobacco and, particularly, smoking of cigarettes, associated with a high risk of cardiovascular diseases and specific types of cancer. Excessive drinking of alcoholic beverages, meaning more than two glasses per day, is hazardous in some spe-cific way, either as such or through interaction with other factors such as cigarette use. Traditional nutritional habits—high in fat and salt and too low in vegetables and fruits—account for a large fraction of heart disease, cancer, stroke, diabetes, and even premature aging, as well as obesity. Greater efforts are needed to inform people of the need to change their lifestyles, and to educate the younger generations toward health-promoting personal habits. Those controlling public opinion and political actions need to be aware that legislation and regulations on toxic materials and ensuing risk control will have little influence on the current high expenditures associated with the burden of chronic disease diagnosis and treatment. Active health promotion related to proper, low-risk lifestyles needs to be implemented, to ensure a healthy public through disease prevention.

Humans are entitled to clean water, clean air, and clean foods, and sociable personal interactions make life worth living. Great progress has been made to ensure clean air and water that in the 1990s is better, in many instances, than it was in the 1930s. The public has to understand the differences between theoretical and predicted risk, or the perceived and the real risk. Unfortunately, the media often seem to emphasize the few cases of criminal activities and play up the low, uncertain risk of disease stemming from exposure to trace amounts of chemicals in the environment. It is important that the public be informed and educated about the major, proved, definitive risks of lifestyle-associated premature killing or maiming diseases.

The current volume illustrates a number of these points with reports on chemicals and mixtures with varied toxic actions, the underlying mechanisms, and, eventually, the quantitative aspects expressed as risk assessment. It is a relevant and contemporary standard for teaching and research. At the same time, it is hoped that those utilizing this volume would incorporate in their educational approaches some thoughts on interactions of toxicological processes and personal lifestyles in disease causation and prevention.

*John H. Weisburger*

# Preface

Recent advances in toxicology have brought us from the period of qualitative evaluation of toxicological effects of hazardous substances to the new era of quantitative assessment and prediction of the health risk from exposure to these agents. Classical toxicology has progressed from trying to answer the question, "Is it toxic?" to modern toxicology that attempts to address the concern, "How toxic is it?" The emphasis on the quantitative assessment of the probability of health risk, supported by qualitative evaluation, provides the basis for logical risk assessment. This information is useful to characterize the health risk and provide guidance for regulators and decision makers to develop regulatory and risk management options, especially those relating to setting priorities for managing environmental health problems.

In the 1960s, the book *Silent Spring* by Rachel Carson brought to our attention the toxic properties of pesticides. Other major environmental contaminants identified include: polychlorinated biphenyls (PCBs) and methylmercury in fish, dioxins in various environmental media, arsenic in drinking water, and lead in old homes from leaded paint. Occupational exposures of various agents related mesothelioma from asbestos, male reproductive toxicity from dibromochloropropane, and angiosarcoma of the liver from vinyl chloride. Identification of the agents in association with human disease conditions has led to the attempts to control and regulate environmental chemicals in order to reduce exposure drastically to these agents, and to eliminate or minimize the diseases resulting from exposure.

Efforts to control and regulate chemicals to prevent excessive human exposure have led to the perplexing question "How safe is safe?" Typical actions include developing drinking water and air standards and issuing health advisories for toxic chemicals in fish. These actions are based on risk assessment approaches leading to decisions on the levels of restrictive chemical intake. But the process involved and the considerations included are not simple or straightforward. We have gone through concerns and debates relating to the benzene ruling and the Delaney Clause, and arguments regarding insignificant risk level and voluntary versus involuntary risk. Development of more sensitive analytical methods has led to the capability of detecting lower and lower levels of chemicals and, at times, corresponding lower chemical standards. The concepts of threshold and no threshold for chemicals, especially carcinogens, have generated debates and different approaches for risk assessment. Mathematical models and statistical approaches are continuing to be developed to address the need to analyze data and conduct high to low dose extrapolation in order to support assessment of human health risk.

In the 1980s, we saw risk assessments receiving national attention. Ethylene dibromide, a fumigant originally thought not to leave a residue because of its high volatility, was found in cereal grains and bakery products. A mathematical model that incorporated exposure early in life was used to address the concern of infant or childhood exposure in the risk assessment. Following was the growth regulator daminozide used on apples. The risk assessments focused on the potential carcinogenicity of 1,1-dimethyl hydrazine, resulting from hydrolysis of daminozide. This product concentrated in apple juice following food processing, and again the major concern was the health effects in young children who consume apple juice. The development of the regulatory decisions in these two cases was the subject of intensive debate and discussions. Dietary exposure to pesticides has been brought to public attention in two recent reports by the National Academy of Sciences, and the related concerns are receiving programmatic attention at the federal level. Decisions for effective control measures for naturally occurring (versus intentionally used) substances or environmental byproducts are also difficult to make. Examples are arsenic, disinfectant byproducts and nitrate in drinking water, and methylmercury in fish.

Not all agencies that need the results of risk assessment to support their activities have the capability or resources to conduct risk assessment. In this regard, the U.S. Environmental Protection Agency has made available to the public and other agencies results of their chemical-specific risk assessment for applications in local programs. The need for more trained toxicologists is recognized, and educational programs for such purposes have steadily increased. Risk assessment is now often included as an important aspect of a modern toxicology training program, but availability of educational and training materials to meet the training needs has not been encouraging.

We have frequently been approached by professors, instructors, students, environmental consultants, attorneys, environmental health scientists, risk managers and those interested in risk assessment to help identify a specific useful reference source on risk assessment. We soon came to realize that very useful information was available in journal articles, independent publications, and books on special topics. There was not a single publication, however, that readily integrated all the useful, related information into one independent volume, and one was desperately needed. It became apparent to us that this was the opportunity to develop one. An outline for the book on principles and methods was developed, plus aspects to be considered for practical applications that, from practical experience, one would need to know and explore to be a toxicologist and to perform risk assessment. This book is our first attempt to provide an answer to all those who had asked for a textbook or reference book, all in one volume, eliminating the need to go to a diversity of resources to get an overall view and perspective. Much effort was made to make this a comprehensive compilation; however, due to the vast knowledge developed in the fields of toxicology and risk assessment, it is not possible to be exhaustive or complete in scope and coverage. In this regard, readers are encouraged to obtain more detailed information by using the references provided at the end of each chapter.

For those who intend to pursue professional development in toxicology and risk assessment, it is important to get a formal education in basic toxicology to understand the toxicological principles and not to just mechanistically follow the methodological steps in risk assessment. There are limitations and uncertainties attendant to the risk assessment methodology, and much is gained from understanding the principles and issues continuously being debated. Current debates or considerations include the issues surrounding the following: interspecies scaling for body surface area, maximum tolerated dose, bolus dose (overdosing) compared to continuous dosing, benchmark dose, pharmacokinetic modeling, uncertainty factors, mechanism of toxic actions of chemicals [particularly those of genotoxic versus nongenotoxic (epigenetic) carcinogens], threshold versus nonthreshold models for carcinogens, specific cancer sites such as male rat kidney tumors and mouse liver tumors, multiple chemical sensitivity, and toxicity equivalent factors (e.g., dioxins and dioxin-like PCB congeners), among others. Those who use risk assessment for making risk management decisions often need to include social, economic, and technical feasibility considerations; above all expert advice from the toxicologists and risk assessors, or regulatory toxicologists, would be required.

The future of toxicological risk assessment is likely to include emphasis on special sensitive populations (e.g., infants and children, the elderly, ethnic groups), multiple chemical exposures, reducing uncertainties, multimedia exposure, exposure distribution analysis, and default assumptions. Reproductive/developmental toxicity and carcinogenicity are critical endpoints currently considered for environmental regulation. Immunotoxicity, neurotoxicity, and behavioral/developmental toxicity are getting increasing attention. Endocrine effects and ocular toxicity demand more information. Improved data bases on human activities (often termed lifestyle), chemical occurrence and monitoring, and overall exposure and toxicological data for chemicals are needed to adequately conduct risk assessments. Harmonization of risk assessment is an objective among different agencies and countries, and refinement of techniques is a goal among scientists. Coordination between researchers generating data and risk assessors using the data is important for the further advancement of risk assessment. Related areas with increasing attention are risk communication, ecological risk assessment, and environmental justice.

As is clear from the presentations in this volume, toxicological risk assessment is a complex and important science that will continue to guide and have an impact on future health risk prediction, public health protection, pollution prevention, and environmental regulations. In the twilight of the 20th century, we are proud of all the advancements made in the past decades. Looking into a new century, we can also see the dawn of new excitements and challenges ahead of us. The present volume, we hope, serves as a treatise reflecting the development, accomplishments, and current status in the science of toxicological risk assessment. We further hope that it will also serve as the stepping stone for a new generation of toxicologists to carry the torch into a new era of excellence.

Admittedly this accomplishment would not be possible without the refinement of the organization of the outline for the book and the diligent planning and coordination of the leading scientist(s) for each part of Parts I through VIII of the book, and the dedication of each author. Each is an eminent scientist in his or her area of expertise. Readers are strongly urged to refer to other publications and references provided by these authors in order to gain a better understanding of the relevant subject matters and issues described in their work. The review comments provided by peer reviewers, who are themselves authoritative experts, were invaluable to ensure the quality of this book. We acknowledge the important contributions of these individuals that made this book possible.

*Anna M. Fan*
*Louis W. Chang*

# Contents

# Contributors

**Charles O. Abernathy**   United States Environmental Protection Agency, Washington, D.C.

**Richard G. Ames**   California Environmental Protection Agency, Berkeley, California

**Linda A. Baldwin**   University of Massachusetts, Amherst, Massachusetts

**D. Blakey**   Health Canada, Ottawa, Ontario, Canada

**P. Michael Bolger**   United States Food and Drug Administration, Washington, D.C.

**Joseph P. Brown**   California Environmental Protection Agency, Berkeley, California

**Edward J. Calabrese**   University of Massachusetts, Amherst, Massachusetts

**Clark D. Carrington**   United States Food and Drug Administration, Washington, D.C.

**Louis W. Chang**   University of Arkansas for Medical Sciences, Little Rock, Arkansas

**James J. Chen**   National Center for Toxicological Research, Food and Drug Administration, Jefferson, Arkansas

**Wai Nang Choy**   Schering-Plough Research Institute, Lafayette, New Jersey

**I. Chu**   Health Canada, Ottawa, Ontario, Canada

**John L. Cicmanec**   United States Environmental Protection Agency, Cincinnati, Ohio

**Ellie F. Clark**   United States Environmental Protection Agency, Washington, D.C.

**Vincent J. Cogliano**   United States Environmental Protection Agency, Washington, D.C.

**David B. Couch**   University of Mississippi Medical Center, Jackson, Mississippi

**Roger A. Coulombe, Jr.** Utah State University, Logan, Utah

**Carl F. Cranor** University of California at Riverside, Riverside, California

**Brian K. Davis** California Department of Toxic Substances Control, Sacramento, California

**J. Denes** Health Canada, Ottawa, Ontario, Canada

**Ann de Peyster** San Diego State University, San Diego, California

**John M. DeSesso** The MITRE Corporation, McLean, Virginia

**Michael J. DiBartolomeis** California Environmental Protection Agency, Berkeley, California

**Gregg E. Dinse** National Institute of Environmental Health Sciences, Research Triangle Park, North Carolina

**Michael L. Dourson** Toxicology Excellence for Risk Assessment, Cincinnati, Ohio

**Anna M. Fan** California Environmental Protection Agency, Berkeley, California

**Denise D. Fort** University of New Mexico, Albuquerque, New Mexico

**Karen Fung** University of Windsor, Windsor, Ontario, Canada

**Arthur Furst** University of San Francisco, San Francisco, California

**James A. Garreffi** University of Massachusetts, Amherst, Massachusetts

**David W. Gaylor** National Center for Toxicological Research, Food and Drug Administration, Jefferson, Arkansas

**Lynn Goldman** United States Environmental Protection Agency, Washington, D.C.

**Stephen B. Harris** Stephen B. Harris Group, San Diego, California

**Sara Hale Henry** United States Food and Drug Administration, Washington, D.C.

**Richard C. Hertzberg** United States Environmental Protection Agency, Atlanta, Georgia

**I. K. Ho** University of Mississippi Medical Center, Jackson, Mississippi

**Virginia Stewart Houk** United States Environmental Protection Agency, Research Triangle Park, North Carolina

**Lubow Jowa** California Environmental Protection Agency, Sacramento, California

**A. K. Klein** California Department of Toxic Substances Control, Sacramento, California

**Ralph L. Kodell** National Center for Toxicological Research, Food and Drug Administration, Jefferson, Arkansas

**D. Krewski** Health Canada, Ottawa, Ontario, Canada

**Lung-fa Ku** Health Canada, Ottawa, Ontario, Canada

**Charleen Kubota** University of California at Berkeley, Berkeley, California

**Cynthia J. Langlois** University of Massachusetts, Amherst, Massachusetts

**Po-Yung Lu** Oak Ridge National Laboratory, Oak Ridge, Tennessee

**E. Georg Luebeck**   Fred Hutchinson Cancer Research Center, Seattle, Washington

**Mary Ann Mahoney**   University of California at Berkeley, Berkeley, California

**Todd Miller**   California Environmental Protection Agency, Berkeley, California

**Richard A. Minard, Jr.**   Vermont Law School, South Royalton, Vermont

**Suresh H. Moolgavkar**   Fred Hutchinson Cancer Research Center, Seattle, Washington

**Kenneth A. Mundt**   University of Massachusetts, Amherst, Massachusetts

**Walter W. Piegorsch**   University of South Carolina, Columbia, South Carolina

**Glenn E. Rice**   United States Environmental Protection Agency, Cincinnati, Ohio

**Welford C. Roberts***   United States Army Materiel Command, Alexandria, Virginia

**Kathleen Rodgers**   University of Southern California, Los Angeles, California

**Hanafi Russell**   California Environmental Protection Agency, Berkeley, California

**Andrew G. Salmon**   California Environmental Protection Agency, Berkeley, California

**Rita Schoeny**   United States Environmental Protection Agency, Cincinnati, Ohio

**Raghubir P. Sharma**   University of Georgia, Athens, Georgia

**Carl M. Shy**   University of North Carolina, Chapel Hill, North Carolina

**Barton P. Simmons**   California Environmental Protection Agency, Berkeley, California

**Katherine S. Squibb**   University of Maryland at Baltimore, Baltimore, Maryland

**James Stewart**   Harvard University, Cambridge, Massachusetts

**Moira A. Sullivan**   San Diego State University, San Diego, California

**Stella M. Swain**   San Diego State University, San Diego, California

**Susan F. Velazquez**   Toxicology Excellence for Risk Assessment, Cincinnati, Ohio

**Yi Y. Wang**   California Environmental Protection Agency, Berkeley, California

**John S. Wassom**   Oak Ridge National Laboratory, Oak Ridge, Tennessee

**Michael D. Waters**   United States Environmental Protection Agency, Research Triangle Park, North Carolina

**John H. Weisburger**   American Health Foundation, Valhalla, New York

**J. A. Wisniewski**   California Environmental Protection Agency, Sacramento, California

**J. R. Withey**   Health Canada, Ottawa, Ontario, Canada

**Amy L. Yorks**   University of Maryland at Baltimore, Baltimore, Maryland

**Jerry J. Zarriello**   Consultant, Tahoe City, California

**Yiliang Zhu**   University of South Florida, Tampa, Florida

---

*\*Current affiliation:* Uniformed Services University of the Health Sciences, Bethesda, Maryland

# PART I
## GENERAL TOXICOLOGY

### I. K. Ho
*University of Mississippi Medical Center*
*Jackson, Mississippi*

### Anna M. Fan
*California Environmental Protection Agency*
*Berkeley, California*

Fundamental to the conduct of risk assessment of environmental chemicals is the need to understand the principles of toxicology to provide a scientific basis for the use of toxicological data, whether derived from animal or human studies, for such an assessment. This section provides a discussion of the basic principles and modern concepts of toxicology, with a state-of-the-art coverage on specific disciplines, including general acute, subchronic, and chronic toxicity, carcinogenicity, genotoxicity, reproductive and developmental toxicity, neurotoxicity, and immunotoxicity. The mechanisms of action of specific chemicals and their toxic effects on specific organs are not explicitly discussed here, but examples are presented in other sections. Neurotoxicity and immunotoxicity are receiving increasing attention, and there are emerging concerns on endocrine effects and ocular toxicity. Readers are referred to Part II for discussions on toxicological testing to gain a more comprehensive understanding of the study of the toxic effects of chemicals and the types of effects that may result from chemical exposures. The pharmacokinetic principles, including the concepts of absorption, distribution, metabolism, and excretion, are presented. The importance of the dose–response relationship and cumulative effects are pointed out. All the toxicological principles form the basic foundation of knowledge for toxicologists who perform risk assessment, which would require sound judgments that are based on an ability to evaluate toxicological data, rather than a straightforward application of the methods used for risk assessment. It is this fundamental knowledge, coupled with a pertinent understanding of other related principles, issues, and perspectives described throughout this book, that enables toxicologists to become distinguished risk assessors.

All the factors and issues to be considered in toxicological risk assessment are not specified in any guidebooks or manuals, and the ability to interpret toxicological data for assessing human health implications is based on the education, training, and experience of the toxicologists who are the risk assessors. Considerable variations often exist in the interpretation of data and, for this reason, there are continuing debates on issues such as the significance of male rat kidney tumors, mouse liver tumors, contact carcinogens, threshold versus nonthreshold phenomenon, blood cholinesterase inhibition, and the finding of teratogenicity in the presence of maternal toxicity. In the area of immunotoxicity, in spite of well-documented immunomodulative effects of some known chemicals, such as tetrachlorodibenzodioxin (TCDD) and its congeners and some pesticides, it has been difficult to relate these changes to a more definitive health risk or a disease process.

Acute toxicity has been evaluated under conditions of occupational exposures to toxic gases and solvents (chlorine), dietary ingestion of pesticides (aldicarb), and accidental releases of toxic chemicals (metam). Chronic health risks have been the focus of risk assessments for regulatory purposes, such as these for metals, pesticides, organic chemicals, and inorganic chemicals, in air, water, food, hazardous waste sites, and consumer products. Potential cumulative effects from long-term, low-level exposures and irreversible effects, such as neurotoxicity and carcinogenicity, are of great concern. Reproductive and developmental toxicity receive priority evaluation because of the possibility of a lifelong effect in offspring, especially when teratogenic effects can occur after a single exposure during a sensitive period of organogenesis during gestation. As the regulatory guidance for evaluating reproductive toxicity (effects on function or structure of male and female reproductive systems, fetotoxicity) is still undergoing review, the authors have focused on developmental effects (birth effects) in the present chapter. Hypersensitivity and multiple chemical sensitivity are often complaints received from the public. Often the cause-and-effect relationship is difficult to establish, and toxicology risk assessment is used to predict potential health outcomes. An understanding of the disposition and chemical reactivity of a chemical and its metabolites is necessary, and pharmacokinetic information is important in this prediction.

# 1

# Principles and Highlights of Toxicology

**Arthur Furst**
*University of San Francisco*
*San Francisco, California*

**Anna M. Fan**
*California Environmental Protection Agency*
*Berkeley, California*

## I. INTRODUCTION

Toxicology as an established science is relatively new, but poisons have been known since antiquity. Perhaps one of the earliest attempts to describe the field was in 1198 by the Spanish physician and philosopher, Maimonides, who published a book entitled, *Poisons and Their Antidotes.*

*Toxicology* is now defined as the study of the toxic properties, or adverse health effects, of agents or substances. In essence, modern toxicology encompasses two facets: qualitative evaluation, and quantitative assessment of toxicity. Qualitative evaluation here is the study of an agent, either chemical or physical, that can cause or have the potential to cause an adverse or harmful effect in living organisms, be it an intact human or animal, or some subcomponents of it. The quantitative assessment aspect is described by Philippus T.A.B. von Holenheim (1493–1541), who called himself Paracelsus and enunciated a dictum: *All substances are poisons; there is none which is not a poison. The right dose differentiates a poison and a remedy.* In a more modern parlance, the statement is *the dose makes the poison.* In other words, not only is the "toxic culprit" with the capability of inducing harm of concern, but the amount of that agent needed that can cause the harm is equally important. This provides the basis for the concept of *dose–response* that is an integral part in understanding the principles of toxicology, and for the concept of *exposure,* an integral part of risk assessment.

Practically all phases of our culture is within the realm of the toxicologist who studies the adverse health effects of agents or substances. In the medical field, toxicity, diagnosis, treatment, and prevention are considered. In industries, workers are exposed to various agents in the form of gases, mists, or vapors; or particles such as metals, fibers, or dusts; or liquids such as organic solvents. In the food supply are fertilizers, pesticides, preservatives, and additives. In the ambient environment are criteria pollutants in air and contaminants in drinking water.

Following Paracelsus was the Italian physician, Bernardin Ramazzini (1633–1714), who was concerned with the plight of the workers; he convinced the medical profession at that time of the importance of exposure of the workers to toxic chemicals in their occupation. He first described silicosis, and is considered to be the founder of occupational/industrial medicine; this is another important contribution to modern toxicology. In most cases, much higher levels of exposure occur in the workplace compared with those in the general environment (e.g., ambient air and water).

## II.  TOXICOLOGIST AS A PROFESSION

The variety of potential harmful effects that can be caused by a diversity of agents in our environment is legion. Some chemicals produce a general toxic action, whereas others appear to be organ-specific. These effects range from subtle, almost imperceptible effects, to gross pathology and even death of the exposed subject. Scientists in this field of endeavor must be conversant (but not necessarily an expert) in a broad range of related disciplines; this group of scientists who study and evaluate chemical toxicity are designated toxicologists. Being in a relatively new field, the toxicologists often come from a variety of scientific disciplines. Until the last few decades, there were no specific courses in toxicology per se offered in universities, nor was there a separate department within an academic institution devoted to this field. It is now possible to obtain formal training and a degree in toxicology from a university department, or training and a degree in a related subject area with an emphasis on toxicology. Previously, toxicologists were trained in a related or ancillary field. Many physicians specialize in toxicology; others come from fields of chemistry, biology, physiology, biochemistry, or pathology. Other scientists, such as some statisticians and mathematicians, are interested in applying statistical techniques and mathematical models to the toxicological data generated by toxicologists.

The field of toxicology encompasses such a vast variety of disciplines that, as a result, many toxicologists are very knowledgeable not only in toxicology, but serve as specialists in a particular subject area, such as reproductive and development toxicity (teratology), carcinogenesis, genotoxicity, immunotoxicity, and neurotoxicity. Each of these is discussed in more detail throughout Chapters 2–6 in this section. In addition to having opportunities in conducting laboratory research or experiments, toxicologists can apply their training to major practical applications of the science that will have an effect in environmental health protection; they may work in a poison control center or forensic laboratory, engage in regulatory functions, or serve as a consultant to the legal profession or to other industries or organizations. Thus, there are specialties in basic research and in environmental and applied toxicology that provide a variety of opportunities for professional development.

## III.  TOXICOLOGICAL INVESTIGATIONS

### A.  Acute, Subchronic, and Chronic Studies

Traditionally, the first measurements made by the toxicologists are the general *acute, subchronic, and chronic effects* of the agent under investigation in experimental animals. Human data are preferred, but these studies are difficult to conduct. Use of human data is discussed in a chapter that follows in Part VI. General toxic effects are of great and continued interest, but they do not dominate the field. Acute toxic effects are generally measured or noted as effects occurring within a few hours after a single exposure (or dose) or after short-term exposure to the agent. The observation period would depend on the type of endpoint evaluated. Often in experimental animal studies, the observation of the percentage of mortality in the exposed population is the main object of the study. For these studies, the observation period is generally 2 weeks. By the graphic or statistical techniques, the relative (not absolute) values of the medium lethal dose or concentration ($LD_{50}$ or $LC_{50}$) after oral, dermal, or inhalation exposure are among the first measurements made. Other studies include eye irritation, skin irritation, and sensitization studies.

From the studies of acute toxicological action the initial concept of dose–response emerges. The *dose–response* relationship is an expression of the graded magnitude of response (or an effect) corresponding to the incremental increase in intensity of the dose and frequency of dosing (or exposure). This relationship is actually evaluated in more extensive longer-term studies, with refinements in the dosing regimen that incorporate a range of dose levels. In acute studies, however, a high-dose level of the test chemical is usually given, and the major target organ(s) of toxicity identified. The data generated help provide guidance on selecting dose levels and focusing on special toxicological endpoints for further toxicological evaluations. The various health effects that may result from acute exposures are evaluated in acute studies. From the information obtained from acute animal toxicity studies, the appropriate dose range is derived for further toxicity studies.

Subchronic studies are usually conducted for a duration of 30, 60, or 90 days. For these studies, more detailed pathological changes in organs or tissues, and other physiological and biochemical changes are evaluated. The results of these studies provide better insight into the toxic properties of the agent under study, and more information for conducting long-term or chronic studies, which could have a duration of longer than 90 days, or last the lifetime of the test animals. Detailed pathological, biochemical, or physiological effects are then determined in a chronic study. Toxicokinetics play an important role in the design of the chronic study. A chronic study can be combined with a carcinogenicity study (further described in Chapter 9 on carcinogenicity testing).

A detailed discussion of the potential health effects of substances to be predicted from animal studies is provided in Part II, *Toxicological Testing,* which describes the tests specifically designed to evaluate these effects. The mechanism of toxic action of chemicals can vary and for many chemicals it is not clearly understood. The biological basis of toxicity for specific chemicals is reflected in other chapters throughout this book. The use of testing data for risk assessment is discussed in Part III, *Risk Assessment.*

## B.  Experimental Systems

The nature of the investigations conducted by modern toxicologists encompasses a wide spectrum. Some studies involve the intact subject (in vivo), be it a human or animal, or a member of an alternative species. Others may study a specific and isolated tissue or organ (in vitro), such as lungs, brain, liver, or muscle. Assays or systems are developed with organ or cell culture, or with components of the cell, such as mitochondria or enzymes. Attention has been given to the interaction of agents with the ultimate genetic information found in nucleic acids, the DNA or RNA, and the proteins elaborated by them. There is no limit to the interests of toxicologists in the study of some living or near-living systems. The in vivo and in vitro testing and the associated assay systems are discussed in Part II, *Toxicological Testing.*

## C.  Factors Affecting Toxicity

The investigation of the adverse health effects of chemical in exposed biological systems is extremely complicated. Both absorption mechanisms and rates must be considered. The effects resulting from exposure to a substance is more closely related to the "effective dose" than the administered dose. Once in the bloodstream, the agent is usually carried by some component of the blood, be it a protein or the red blood cells. After passing through the liver, the agent can be metabolized to a product that can be more toxic than the original parent chemical, or the agent can be metabolized (detoxified) to a less active or toxic agent. The mode, rate, and route of distribution and excretion, all may play a role in the final evaluation of the effects of the material on the subject exposed. These natural biological events are lacking in in vitro test systems, to which experimentally derived metabolism activation is sometimes added. *Cumulative effects* may result in toxicity being seen in chronic studies that is not seen in acute and subchronic studies. More details relating to the interplay of these aspects are provided in Chapter 7 on pharmacokinetics and in related aspects in later chapters on pharmacokinetic modeling.

In the study and evaluation of chemical toxicity, emphasis has been placed on the use of data relevant to human exposure, as the route of exposure can affect the final toxicity. These data would involve major exposure routes such as ingestion, inhalation, or dermal absorption, or combinations thereof (see Part III, *Risk Assessment*). However, data have also been generated from studies in which the route of administration is not of major importance to humans. For intact animals, every conceivable route has been employed; just about every organ in the body has been injected and the agent under investigation has been deposited at the site. Thus, information is now available on chemicals following implantation in the brain, the lungs, the eye, the liver, the kidney, the spleen, the muscle, the testes, the ovary, and the subcutaneous tissue.

Toxicological endpoints from the various studies constitute a wide spectrum of observable effects, such as behavior modification, alterations in respiration, change of color of the eyes of rodents or the condition of the fur, and quantitative recordings of activities and other physiological events. Pathological and biochemical changes are often measured. Endpoints can range from the most subtle changes, to total oblivion, death. Many toxicologists are mostly involved with the observational part of the science, others are mainly engaged in elucidating the mechanism of action of the chemical producing the effects observed with the "toxic" agent or studying the toxicokinetics of the agent. Factors such as sex, age, species, or strain differences; nutritional status; and multiple chemical interactions, among others, may affect the toxicity observation following chemical exposure. More details on these considerations are provided in Part VI on issues concerning the use of human data and on extrapolating data from animals to humans.

## IV.  THE MANY USES OF TOXICOLOGY

By understanding how an agent produces its toxic effects, it may be possible to predict the potential toxicity of other related compounds based on the *structure–activity relationships*. This can lead to developing alternate agents that can have the same beneficial or pharmacological effect, but with much less detrimental side effects on the exposed population. Some materials that appear innocuous because of their low acute toxicity can have surprisingly profound pathological consequences; the thalidomide tragedy is a case in point. The understanding of the types of potential health effects and mechanism of action can also help identify potential chemicals of health concern so actions can be taken to prevent unnecessary exposure.

Data generated by the toxicological investigations also can result in a great variety of social actions (or even inactions). Some experiments result in pure academic exercises; it is never possible, however, to predict when esoteric results find a "practical" application. Information can be used to suggest further research, or can result in practical applications such as decisions to clean up a toxic waste site, development of testing requirements to ensure safe use of chemicals or establishment of environmental standards to limit chemical exposure (see Part VIII, *Risk Assessment and Risk Management*). Some research results in identifying logical antidotes for some toxic materials.

An entire group of toxicologists is concerned with the application of data generated by various toxicological investigations to make judgments about the risk to an individual or a population who may be exposed to toxic chemicals; these are the risk assessors. One major objective of a subgroup of these toxicologists is to protect the exposed individual or population from harmful effects of agents in the environment by minimizing exposure to the agents through technical support for the formulation of logical environmental regulations. At all times it is necessary to make educated judgments based on high-quality toxicological and exposure data. To this end, increasing attempts are made to quantitate, through the process of risk assessment, the potential or actual harmful effects of chemicals to those exposed or potentially exposed. Special considerations are now being given to protecting the more sensitive fraction of the population: infants, the elderly, and those in the population who are exquisitely sensitive. Mathematical and biological models and statistical approaches are being developed for data analysis and manipulation. Some formulas and computer-generated models are useful in attempting to examine high-dose exposures, and to extrapolate information from one or more data points, or from high doses (from experimental studies) to low doses, such as those found in the human ambient environment. These are discussed in Parts IV and V in this book in more detail. The specialty of risk assessment has evolved to evaluate toxicity and characterize the associated health risk of chemicals, or to predict the potential health risk and the associated probability that harm will result from such chemical exposure. Finally, of interest is that the science of toxicology is one of the very few disciplines that are concerned with protection of the general public from harmful substances. Increased use of risk assessment is also evident for management of health issues in the occupational environment.

As yet to be completely evaluated are the toxic effects of chemical mixtures; in such mixtures, the resulting toxicity can be additive, antagonistic, or synergistic. Every living organism in the universe is exposed to various complex mixtures of chemicals; this field still needs many more intensive investigations. Exposure to chemicals from multiple media also deserves increased attention. These are discussed in Part III and Part IV.

The key to performing adequate risk assessment is the availability of the needed information. More data are needed on toxicology of chemicals, exposure patterns in humans, and data on the issues receiving increasing attention, as noted in the foregoing. The regulatory basis for risk assessment and resources for providing existing available information is discussed in Part VII. Examples of the use of this information in risk assessment and risk management are discussed in Parts III and VIII.

## V. SUMMARY

Following the basic principles and highlights presented in this chapter on general toxicology, the remaining chapters of Part 1 present in-depth details of the various disciplines of toxicology. Each chapter discusses the principles and concepts with a state-of-the-art coverage of the current knowledge and status of research development, combined with excellent, pertinent references to that subject. Each of the following chapters has provided excellent references, including those relating to all aspects discussed in this chapter; the compilation is comprehensive and the topics specific. Therefore, readers are referred to the references found in all these chapters, as they will serve as a complete compilation for this chapter.

# 2
# Carcinogenesis: Basic Principles

**David B. Couch**
*University of Mississippi Medical Center*
*Jackson, Mississippi*

## I. INTRODUCTION

In multicellular organisms, cell growth is generally a well-regulated process that responds to specific needs of the organism. Occasionally, however, normal regulation of cellular proliferation is lost, and a cell can replicate in excess of those needs. If daughter cells retain the property of unregulated growth, a clone of cells with unlimited growth potential, or neoplasm, can be formed. This chapter concerns malignant transformation of normal cells and the ability of chemicals to participate in that process.

## II. DISTURBANCES OF NORMAL CELL GROWTH

Normal cell replication and cancerous growth represent the two extremes of a continuum of growth patterns (reviewed in Lieberman and Lebovitz, 1990). In the adult, cell replication is generally limited to replacing cells lost through normal turnover. In addition, some tissues can regenerate an approximately normal structure through replication, which ceases after replacement of lost cells. *Hyperplasia,* an increase in a tissue or organ cell number, may increase the risk of neoplasia in an organ, especially if a chronic stimulus of cell division exists. Replacement of one cell type in a tissue with another is referred to as *metaplasia,* which can occur in response to different stimuli, including irritation. Since the replacement cells are morphologically normal, metaplasia is not usually considered a precancerous lesion, although occasionally, it may precede neoplasia. *Dysplasia* is characterized by morphologically atypical cells and a disorganized growth pattern. In dysplasia, cells are often pleiotropic and show an increase in the ratio of nucleus to cytoplasm, and severe dysplasia can be difficult to distinguish from carcinoma in situ, or preinvasive malignancy. A *neoplasm* (new growth) is defined as an abnormal mass of cells that exhibits uncontrolled proliferation and that persists after cessation of the stimulus (most often unknown) that produced it. Cells with proliferative capacity can give rise to neoplasms, which, although they express varying states of differentiation, usually have sufficient normal characteristics that they can be classified according to the tissue and cell type from which they were derived. If a cause of neoplastic change can be identified, there is almost always a long delay, or latent period, between the causal event and the clinical manifestation of disease. *Benign* tumors remain localized in the area in which they arise, whereas *malignant* tumors, or cancers, have the ability to invade contiguous tissue and metastasize to distant sites where a subpopulation of cells can take up residence and continue unregulated growth. Cancerous cells, then, are characterized by lack of normal growth control, invasiveness, and metastasis, the underlying mechanisms of which are not yet completely understood.

## A.  Cellular Growth Control

Cell growth involves duplication of cellular contents, including DNA, and physical division of the cell into two daughter cells (reviewed in Murray and Hunt, 1993). These events can be used to describe a cell cycle, the ordered set of processes by which cells grow and divide. The cell cycle is divided into two fundamental parts, interphase and mitosis (M). Cells in mitosis, which includes the various stages of nuclear and cytoplasmic division, are easily recognized, as the replicated chromosomes condense and can be identified by light microscopy. Two types of processes occur during interphase: (1) continuous processes, such as ribosome, membrane, organelle, and (most) protein synthesis, which are collectively referred to as growth; and (2) stepwise processes, which occur once per cell cycle. DNA replication is an example of a stepwise process, and it is restricted to a specific part of interphase called S (synthesis) phase. Cells in S phase are readily visualized by a variety of techniques, including the use of radiolabeled DNA precursors and autoradiography. The remainder of interphase consists of $G_1$ phase, a gap between the previous cell division and S, and $G_2$ phase, a gap between DNA replication and mitosis. Cells in $G_1$ not yet committed to DNA replication can enter a resting state, referred to as $G_0$, distinct from proliferating cells in any stage.

The cell cycle is controlled by proteins that interact to induce and coordinate processes that duplicate and divide the cell contents (reviewed in Alberts et al., 1994). These proteins are regulated by signals from within the cell or from the environment that can stop or delay the cycle at multiple specific checkpoints. The cell cycle control system is primarily based on two families of proteins: the cyclin-dependent protein kinases (CDK) and the cyclins. Cyclin-dependent kinases are serine–threonine kinases capable of inducing downstream events. Cyclins, which build up during interphase and are degraded in mitosis by an ubiquitin-dependent pathway, are subunits that bind CDK molecules and regulate their catalytic activity. Animal cells have at least two CDK genes and multiple cyclins, referred to as $G_1$, S, and $G_2$, or mitotic, cyclins. Environmental signals generally act at one of two major check points, one in $G_1$ and the other in $G_2$. Mitotic induction, or passing the $G_2$ checkpoint, depends on $Cdk_2$ protein binding to cyclin B to produce a complex analogous to the yeast M–phase-promoting factor (MPF). When activated by phosphorylation, this complex triggers events that culminate in cell division. The $G_1$ checkpoint is the point at which the cell cycle control system can initiate DNA replication; when conditions are not favorable for cell division, cells may accumulate at this point. Formation of a CDK–$G_1$ cyclin (possibly a cyclin D) complex similar to MPF is thought to stimulate the events that lead to DNA replication. In addition to intracellular processes, positive signals, including protein growth factors, from other cells are generally required for cell growth and division in multicellular organisms. In the absence of these signals, which trigger intracellular signaling cascades to stimulate proliferation, cells can enter the $G_0$ phase. Negative-feedback signals are also important in ensuring that the cell cycle control system does not proceed until downstream events are completed. Another regulatory subunit family of CDK, the CDK inhibitory proteins (CKI), play a role in stopping progression of the cell cycle (reviewed in Peter and Herskowitz, 1994). An example of feedback control is the system that operates to prevent cells with damaged DNA from entering S phase; a protein, *p53*, accumulates in cells with damaged DNA and seems to block progress of the cell cycle in $G_1$ by inducing transcription of the *p21* gene, which encodes a CKI protein.

Many genes implicated in neoplastic transformation encode proteins that are involved in regulating cell proliferation, either positively, by helping to promote growth and drive the cell past the $G_1$ checkpoint, or negatively, by stopping progression through the cell cycle and dismantling the control system. If a gene's product promotes proliferation and is expressed inappropriately, the altered gene is termed an *oncogene,* and the normal cellular counterpart is referred to as a *protooncogene.* If the genes' products restrain proliferation, they are referred to as *tumor suppressor genes,* as changes that inactivate these genes may also accelerate neoplastic transformation. In addition to cell proliferation, oncogenes and tumor suppressor genes have been implicated in the regulation of *apoptosis,* or programmed cell death (reviewed in Harrington et al., 1994), the inhibition of which may be involved in the growth of some malignant tumors. The role of oncogenes and tumor suppressor genes in carcinogenesis is discussed further later in the chapter.

## B.  Alterations in Cell-to-Cell Interactions

Invasiveness and metastasis confer the property of malignancy on a cell. To create a metastatic colony, cells must be able to leave the primary tumor, first enter the circulation, then leave it at some distant site, invade local tissue, and proliferate. Angiogenesis is also essential for both primary tumor and metastatic growth. These events appear to require a cascade of linked steps involving poorly understood multiple host–tumor cell interactions dependent on activation of several genes, some of which are distinct from those that regulate proliferation (reviewed in Liotta and Stetler-Stevenson, 1991).

The restriction of a normal cell type to a given tissue or organ is maintained by cell-to-cell recognition and by physical barriers, including the basal lamina that underlies layers of epithelial cells. Tumor cell binding to the basement membrane through both integrin- and nonintegrin-type cell surface receptors is an important step in invasion and metastasis, which also depend, in part, on the ability of tumor cells to digest their way through cell barriers. Several proteinases, which can disrupt the basal laminae, have been associated with the metastatic phenotype, including a plasminogen activator and metalloproteinases. Host proteinase inhibitors, including tissue metalloproteinase inhibitors, exist and may act to block metastasis; loss of genes encoding these proteins may favor tumor progression to metastasis. After disruption of the basal lamina, tumor cells must move into the interstitial stroma, a process that may be regulated by tumor cell cytokines and influenced by host chemoattractants. Invasion and metastasis, therefore, are facilitated by proteins that enhance binding of tumor cells to extracellular matrices and tumor cell proteolysis and locomotion. Other factors exist that act to block the production or activity of these proteins, and an imbalance in positive- and negative-control elements can result in acquisition of metastatic potential.

Other properties of malignant cells that may be due to alteration in cell-to-cell interactions are the ability of malignant cells to grow surrounded by cells with which they do not normally interact and the ability to elude the immune system. Reduced immunosurveillance may also be due to production of immunosuppressive agents by the cancer. It is evident that tumor cells can produce cytokines with immunosuppressive activity, but the extent to which immunosuppression might be responsible for the growth and spread of the tumors is unclear (reviewed in Sulitzeanu, 1993).

## III.  CARCINOGENESIS AS A MULTISTAGE PROCESS

Because all cancers share the properties of uncontrolled growth, invasion, and metastasis, a common mechanism for their origin has often been suggested. Various theories of carcinogenesis have been postulated to address a particular feature of the morphological, biochemical, or molecular aspects of the disease, but these have usually lacked general applicability. Among the suggested bases for cancer are selective deletion of certain protein species; failure of the immune system to recognize transformed cells; alterations in cellular membranes, including those of mitochondria, or of signal transducing pathways; and disruption of hierarchical relations within and among tissues. An early explanation of malignancy, still widely held, is the *somatic mutation theory,* which states that a tumor can arise by clonal proliferation from a somatic cell that has been transformed by acquired modification of its DNA base sequence (discussed in Crawford, 1985). Currently, the most commonly held view of carcinogenesis is that virtually all malignant tumors arise from single cells that retain proliferative capacity by a complex, multistage process, in which both genetic and epigenetic alterations are important (see, e.g., IARC, 1992). This view of cancer has evolved over many years, based on both pathological and epidemiological observations, as well as experimental studies of chemical carcinogenesis. As a result of these studies, the process of neoplastic development has been divided into operationally defined stages of initiation, promotion, and progression, each of which may also consist of multiple steps.

### A.  Initiation

Skin cancer studies provide support for the concept of carcinogenesis as a multistage process (reviewed in Hennings et al., 1993). Mouse skin tumors can be induced by applying initiators, that is, mutagenic agents, such as polycyclic aromatic hydrocarbons, directly to the skin. A single treatment of these agents does not typically give rise to a tumor, but may produce latent damage that can result in tumor formation following subsequent insult. The correlation between the ability to induce mutations and tumorigenesis is good for most chemical initiating agents, as well as ionizing radiation and viruses.

### B.  Promotion

Following initiation, subsequent application of certain substances, referred to as tumor promoters, to the skin can result in development of numerous benign papillomas. Tumor promoters have, in general, properties quite different from those of initiators (Pitot et al., 1992). First, promoters are not themselves mutagenic, that is, promotion is commonly an epigenetic phenomenon, which, like differentiation, involves changes in gene expression, not gene structure. Although promoting agents are incapable of directly inducing structural genetic changes, they may induce metabolic changes that lead to mutation. Specifically, the formation of active oxygen radicals that occurs as a consequence of exposure to various promoters can produce base modifications, DNA strand breaks, and chromosomal alterations. These secondary effects may accelerate the transition of cells from promotion to progression. Second, unlike most initiating agents, many promoters do not require metabolic activation, and several act through specific target cell receptors to enhance gene transcription. Whereas initiation is generally considered to be an irreversible process, promotion is not, so repeated exposure to promoters may be required for tumorigenesis. Possible mechanisms of tumor promotion, which need not be mutually exclusive, include induction of cell proliferation; inhibition of intercellular communication, which relieves initiated cells from restraint normally exerted by surrounding normal tissue; and immunosuppression.

## C. Progression

The rate of conversion of papillomas to carcinomas, termed progression or malignant conversion, can be increased by treatment with some agents. Similar to initiation, progression is thought to have a genetic basis and be essentially irreversible. As aneuploidy (an abnormal number of chromosomes) is a common feature of cancer cells, it has been suggested that genomic instability itself could contribute to tumor progression (see, e.g., Nowell, 1991). A great number of genes code for proteins involved in maintaining genomic stability, including those involved in DNA replication and repair, mitosis, and control of the cell cycle. Mutations in these genes, which could decrease stability, would not necessarily produce the malignant phenotype directly, but would increase the likelihood of mutation throughout the genome, which could contribute to the evolution toward malignant behavior and heterogeneity characteristic of tumors.

## D. Molecular Targets in Multistage Carcinogenesis

Heritable alterations that lead to altered expression or function of genes involved in regulation of proliferation and differentiation are important in carcinogenesis. Protooncogenes and tumor suppressor genes are two such gene classes. Protooncogenes are normal cellular genes that, when inappropriately activated by mutational events to oncogenes, alter regulation of growth and differentiation (reviewed in Cooper, 1990). Mutations of this sort have a dominant effect (i.e., only one affected allele confers the mutant phenotype on the cell). Many oncogenes have been identified through their presence in transforming retroviruses or by their association with chromosomal abnormalities. Protooncogene products include molecules implicated in all phases of cell signaling. Signaling elements encoded by oncogenes, with a representative gene given in parentheses, include growth factors (*sis*), membrane-associated tyrosine-specific kinases (*src*), GTP-binding proteins (*ras*), growth factor receptors (*erb* B), cytoplasmic tyrosine kinases (*fes*), steroidlike growth factor receptors (*erb* A), serine/threonine-specific protein kinases (*raf*), and nuclear proteins associated with gene expression (*myc*). Genetic mechanisms by which protooncogenes can become activated include insertional mutagenesis (proviral insertion or transposition into a defined host genomic locus), gene amplification, point mutation (base-pair substitutions, insertions, and deletions), and chromosomal rearrangement (deletions, inversions, and translocations). Alterations in protooncogene expression are not associated with all tumors, however, and it has been argued that generation of cancer genes by genetic transpositions, or recombination between largely nonhomogenous regions, may also be important in human disease (Cairns, 1981; Duesberg et al., 1991). Translocations can, if the breaks occur within genes on each involved chromosome, also result in creation of chimeric, or fusion proteins, which, like oncogene proteins, are often transcription factors and are commonly associated with tumors (Rabbitts, 1994).

Genetic alterations that inactivate tumor suppressor genes may also lead to loss of control of proliferative and differentiation processes and increase the likelihood of neoplastic transformation (reviewed in Knudson, 1993). As both alleles must usually be affected to alter phenotype, mutations in tumor suppressor genes have recessive effects on the cell. The best-studied tumor suppressor genes are the *Rb* gene and the *p53* gene. The *Rb* gene, associated with retinoblastoma, a rare human cancer, codes for a protein that, when not phosphorylated, appears to block passage from $G_1$ to S, apparently by complexing with a transcription factor. Individuals predisposed to the disease have experienced germline mutations inactivating one allele of the *Rb* gene, and cancers can develop if the remaining gene function is lost. Most genetic mechanisms that lead to inactivation of the second allele usually involve loss of flanking regions of the chromosome as well, and the resulting loss of heterozygosity of restriction fragment length polymorphisms is indicative of a cancer-dependent loss of function of a tumor suppressor gene (reviewed in

Dunlop, 1991). In addition, inactivation of one tumor suppressor gene allele through genomic imprinting, or differential expression of paternal and maternal genes, may be a relatively common phenomenon (Hochberg et al., 1994).

Mutations of the *p53* gene are the most common genetic lesions associated with human cancer. As with the *Rb* gene, people who inherit only one functional copy of the *p53* gene are predisposed to cancer development (the Li-Fraumeni syndrome) and, like the *Rb* gene product, the p53 protein acts to block cell replication. The p53 protein binds DNA and induces expression of a gene the product of which inhibits protein kinase activity of a CDK–cyclin complex. As previously noted, *p53* may function to halt proliferation in cells with damaged DNA, allowing the cells to repair damage before replication. Loss or inactivation of *p53,* then, may not only allow proliferation of initiated cells, but also generate further mutations when damaged DNA is replicated, contributing to the genomic instability that characterizes cancer cells. It has been technically easier to identify protooncogenes than tumor suppressor genes, so many more of the former (about 60) are currently known, whereas there are about 15 known or suspected tumor suppressor genes. The multiple tumor suppressor gene (*MTS-1*), that encodes the cell cycle regulatory protein, p16, and the *BRCA1* gene, implicated in some human breast cancers have been recently described, however, and it is likely that more genes of this type will soon be identified.

Many lines of evidence suggest that a single alteration is not sufficient to convert a normal cell into a malignant one, and it seems apparent that neoplastic disease development involves loss or inactivation of multiple tumor suppressor genes, or activation of protooncogenes, or a combination thereof, throughout the carcinogenic process. In addition to protooncogenes and tumor suppressor genes, other targets important for neoplastic transformation may exist. For example, transformation effector and suppressor genes have been described that are normal cellular genes which encode proteins that cooperate with, or oppose, oncogene functions, respectively (Boylan and Zarbl, 1991). Many other cancer-related gene targets have been proposed, including migration genes, metastasis and metastasis suppressor genes, genomic instability genes, immune tolerance genes, and epigenetic regulation genes (Cheng and Loeb, 1993), and cooperative interactions between various genes seems to be involved in acquisition of malignant properties.

## E. Epigenetic Changes

Heritable alterations that are not genetic, that is, due to alterations in DNA sequence, or mutations, are referred to as *epigenetic*. Epigenetic changes involved in regulating gene expression include alterations in DNA methylation, transcription activation, translational control, and posttranslational modifications. These changes, which may be heritable and stable (Holliday, 1987), are not unique to carcinogenesis, but also occur during normal development and differentiation. It is also possible that mutations can result from interactions of xenobiotics with targets other than DNA, as shown, for example, by the ability of manganese ion to reduce the fidelity of DNA polymerase (Beckman et al., 1985). Nonheritable epigenetic changes, such as stimulation of cell proliferation through cytotoxicity or hormonal effects, may also contribute to neoplastic transformation (see, e.g., Melnick et al., 1993 and references cited therein). Cell division is essential for converting DNA damage into mutations and for selection of cells with altered phenotype. If an initiating event has occurred in a cell, clonal expansion also increases the likelihood of further genetic or epigenetic changes, and agents that induce cell division may influence each stage of carcinogenesis involving genetic change. An agent's ability to induce proliferation in a given tissue does not, however, unequivocally demonstrate its potential carcinogenicity, as the only relevant population to carcinogenesis is the initiated cell(s). Finally, some investigators believe the somatic mutation theory may place undue emphasis on only one element of a multifaceted, dynamic process (see, e.g., Vasiliev, 1983; Farber, 1984; Epstein, 1986). One alternate view is that a hierarchy of morphogenic fields or tissue organizers are of primary importance in maintaining control of growth and differentiation (Rubin, 1985). This concept identifies epigenetic changes that alter tissue organization as the principal determinants of malignant transformation, and the chromosomal and other genetic modifications that occur are regarded as epiphenomena, or adaptive changes secondary to the primary events.

## IV. CHEMICAL CARCINOGENESIS

The term *chemical carcinogenesis* is usually defined as the induction or enhancement of neoplastic disease, including both benign and malignant tumors, by xenobiotics. Chemical carcinogenicity can be manifested by (1) an increased frequency of tumors also seen in controls, (2) appearance of a type of tumor not seen in controls, (3) a decreased latent period before appearance of tumors, or (4) an increase in the number of tumors produced per animal (Lu, 1991). Epidemiological evidence for chemical carcinogenesis existed before animal models were developed, and both animal and human data are now used to classify compounds according to their carcinogenicity. Different risk assessment methodologies and regulatory approaches have been developed for environmental chemicals classified as carcinogens and those considered noncarcinogenic.

In evaluation of chemicals for carcinogenic potential by the International Agency for Research on Cancer (IARC), human data, usually from occupational or medical exposures, are given more weight than animal data, and evidence for carcinogenicity is considered stronger when malignant tumors are induced, when carcinogenicity can be demonstrated at low dose, in several species and strains, and if the chemical under consideration reacts with DNA. On the basis of these considerations, chemicals are placed in one of four categories: *group 1* includes those agents for which there is sufficient evidence to conclude they are carcinogenic to humans; agents in *group 2* are considered either probably (group 2a) or possibly (2b) carcinogenic to humans, depending on the strength of the supporting data; agents in *group 3* are not classifiable as to carcinogenicity; and agents in *group 4* are considered to be unlikely to be carcinogenic to humans. Presently, over 50 agents, mixtures, and occupational settings are considered to be carcinogenic to humans, and about 200 more are classified in group 2 (IARC, 1987). The compounds that have been identified as carcinogens are not believed to account for most human neoplastic disease, however, which appears to be associated with lifestyle, particularly diet, the use of tobacco products, and alcohol consumption (see, e.g., Weisburger, 1994b).

## A. Mode of Action

### 1. Initiators

In the multistage paradigm of carcinogenesis, chemicals may act to increase the likelihood of cancers by initiating neoplastic transformation in a cell, promoting tumor formation, or conferring malignant properties on a neoplasm. Chemicals that can, by themselves, induce cancer are called *complete carcinogens,* which exhibit properties of all three (initiating, promoting, and progressor) agents (reviewed in Lu, 1991). Few agents are known that are pure initiators, without promoter or progressor capability, but many carcinogens act as initiators at low doses. Most initiating agents are genotoxic (i.e., they, or their metabolites, can react with DNA to produce adducts or other genetic lesions). Initiator-induced damage may be unrepaired, reversed through error-free DNA repair, or, if the DNA sequence is not exactly restored, misrepaired before S phase DNA replication, which may be blocked by some nonrepaired lesions, but that can proceed past others. Following replication, then, misrepaired lesions would be expected to result in a high, and repaired lesions in a low, probability of mutation, whereas unrepaired lesions would be expected to lead to cytotoxicity or mutation with high probability. Carcinogenic initiation becomes essentially irreversible after the cell undergoes replication.

### 2. Promoters

Tumor promoters are known to produce a variety of effects on cells, ultimately leading to cellular proliferation. In skin cancer models, promoters increase the frequency of tumor formation markedly only when given after exposure to initiators and if sufficient exposure to promoter occurs. Phorbol esters, especially tetradecanoylphorbol acetate (TPA), are the best-studied tumor promoters (reviewed in Castagna, 1987). Cytosolic and membrane-bound protein kinase C (PKC) is a receptor for the phorbol esters, and their biological effects are probably produced by modulating PKC activity and the subsequent activation or inhibition by PKC of enzymes involved in cell proliferation. Other promoters that are structurally dissimilar to TPA, such as teleocidin and aplysiatoxins, may also produce their effects by interacting with PKC. Some cytotoxicants, such as nitriloacetic acid, and hormones, such as estradiol, do not interact with PKC, but act by increasing cell proliferation. If cell antioxidant defenses are overwhelmed, oxygen radicals can induce DNA damage and alter membrane-associated activities, such as signal transduction, and generation of free radicals may be involved in promoting effects of compounds such as chrysarobin, palytoxin, and peroxides. In contrast with promoters, co-carcinogens, such as ethanol, increase the carcinogenicity of simultaneously administered initiators. These compounds may increase the effective concentration of the ultimate carcinogen, for example, through effects on absorption or metabolism, but the agents alone are not considered to be genotoxicants.

### 3. Progressor Agents

Chemicals capable of inducing transition from the stage of promotion to that of progression are progressor agents. Since karyotypic alterations are a distinctive trait associated with progression, genotoxicants, especially clastogens, are potential progressor agents. The human carcinogens arsenic, asbestos, and benzene can induce chromosomal aberrations and may have progressor activity as well (Pitot et al., 1992), and it is possible that more progressor agents without significant initiating or promoting activities are yet to be discovered.

## B.  Chemical Classes of Carcinogens

A wide variety of chemical compounds, often with no obvious structural similarities, are carcinogenic (reviewed in Williams and Weisburger, 1991). A common mechanism for many diverse chemical agents has been proposed; namely, that compounds that are not themselves electrophilic reactants (*direct,* or *ultimate carcinogens*) must be metabolized to an electrophilic form that can react with nucleophilic moieties of cellular macromolecules (reviewed in Miller and Miller, 1981). Direct carcinogens are sometimes classified as genotoxic (DNA-reactive), whereas chemicals classified as nongenotoxic or epigenetic carcinogens do not damage DNA, but enhance the growth of tumors induced by genotoxic carcinogens. Chemicals may work through both genotoxic and nongenotoxic mechanisms, however, and it is not often easy to assign a chemical to a given category (Barrett, 1992). As most known chemical carcinogens are *procarcinogens,* which require metabolic intervention to become ultimate carcinogens either directly or through an intermediate stage, the *proximate carcinogens,* biotransformation is an important process in initiating chemical carcinogenesis and in determining the site of tumor formation. Xenobiotic metabolism, including that of carcinogens, is generally divided into *phase I* reactions, which include oxidations, especially those mediated by the cytochrome P-450 group of enzymes, reductions, and hydrolyses, and *phase II* reactions, which involve conjugation of a number of substrates with the xenobiotic. Many agents require more than one enzymatic step for activation (i.e., they are converted first to proximate carcinogens then to ultimate carcinogens). The amount of ultimate carcinogen produced depends on the relative activities of the activation and detoxification pathways.

### 1. Polycyclic Aromatic Hydrocarbons

It is beyond the scope of this chapter to describe all known carcinogens and their metabolism, but some representative classes will be discussed. Some carcinogens, including *polycyclic aromatic hydrocarbons* (PAH) can be produced by incomplete combustion of organic matter, including fossil fuels, and are widely distributed in the environment. A common source of human exposure to these agents is tobacco smoke. Many PAH, including benzo[*a*]pyrene, 7, 12-dimethylbenz[*a*]anthracene, and 3-methylcholanthrene, have been carcinogenic in animal studies. The metabolic activation of PAH requires a sequence of three reactions, catalyzed by enzymes of the cytochrome P-450 system, specifically CYP1A1, leading to generation of a dihydrodiol epoxide. Initially, it was felt that carcinogenicity was associated with K-region (i.e., the 9–10 phenanthrene-like double bond) epoxides, but it has since been shown that metabolites with epoxides adjacent to a bay region of the molecule are the active compounds. In vitro, dihydrodiol epoxides do not appear to be substrates for epoxide hydrolase, which may be important to their carcinogenicity. A class of sterically hindered bay region derivatives termed *fjord region* diol epoxides display marked genotoxic properties, together with resistance to hydrolysis, and may be important carcinogens, as well (see, e.g., Hecht et al., 1994). *Heterocyclic aromatic compounds* are a related group of carcinogens, which also can arise from combustion, and some members of this class, the heterocyclic aromatic amines, are pyrolysis products of amino acids and proteins and are found in cooked foods (reviewed in Sugimura and Wakabayashi, 1990). Representative members of this group include IQ, MeIQ, Glu-P-1, and Trp-P-1. Polycyclic aromatic heterocyclic agents undergo oxidation by another member of the cytochrome P-450 family, CYP1A2. Prostaglandin H synthase can, in the presence of arachidonic acid, generate free radical intermediates that also can bioactivate many chemical carcinogens, such as PAH and aromatic amines (reviewed in Eling et al., 1990). This pathway is probably of most significance in extrahepatic tissues with low monooxygenase activities.

### 2. Aromatic Amines and Azo Dyes

Unlike PAH, aromatic amines and azo dyes are not widely encountered in the environment, but individuals are exposed to these synthetic agents in certain occupational settings. Indeed, the initial observation that led to the discovery of this group of carcinogens was the finding of bladder cancer in aniline dye workers. The metabolism of the prototype aromatic amine, 2-naphthylamine, also involves oxidation by cytochrome P-450 monooxygenases. One product, 2-naphthylhydroxylamine, rapidly undergoes conjugation with glucuronic acid in the liver, and the unreactive conjugate is excreted in the urine. In the urinary bladder, however, low pH and the presence of a soluble β-glucuronidase regenerate the hydroxylamine, which can form the ultimate carcinogen. Other aromatic amine carcinogens, such as 2-acetylaminofluorene (AAF), also are converted to active *N*-hydroxyl compounds. Azo dyes undergo both reductive and oxidative metabolism, the latter catalyzed by both cytochrome P-450 and flavin-containing monooxygenases. Like aromatic amines, azo dyes are converted to *N*-hydroxyl derivatives that can be further metabolized to esters that serve as proximate carcinogens.

### 3. N-Nitroso Compounds

Many *N*-nitroso compounds are carcinogenic, producing tumors at a wide variety of sites. The prototype agent is *N*-nitrosodimethylamine, a symmetrical *N*-nitrosamine reported to be carcinogenic in all animal species tested. Other nitrosamines, including asymmetrical compounds, such as *N*-nitrosomethyl-*n*-propylamine, and cyclic compounds, such as 4-(methylnitrosamino)-1-(3-pyridyl)-1-butanone (NNK), a tobacco-specific compound, are also animal carcinogens. Humans can be exposed to certain of these agents (e.g., NNK) in the environment, and other compounds in this class may be generated in vivo through the reaction of nitrite ion with amines and amides. Nitrosamines undergo oxidation by several enzymes, including the cytochrome P-450 monooxygenases CYP1A2, CYP2A6, and CYP2D6. The resulting metabolites are converted nonenzymatically to the ultimate carcinogens, which may be diazonium compounds or carbonium ions. A subgroup of *N*-nitroso compounds, including alkylnitrosoureas, introso-urethanes, and nitrosoguanidines, give rise to reactive intermediates without the intervention of cellular metabolism. The symmetrical hydrazines may be converted through a series of reactions to the same ultimate carcinogens that are produced from nitrosamines.

### 4. Other Carcinogens

Carcinogenic properties are also associated with some natural products, including aflatoxin $B_1$, formed by certain strains of *Aspergillus flavus,* safrole, cycasin, and isatidine. Halogenated aliphatic hydrocarbons, such as carbon tetrachloride, ethylene dibromide, and vinyl chloride are another class of carcinogens, and urethane and related compounds make up another small group. Inorganic chemicals, including some metals and metalloids (e.g., beryllium, chromium, nickel, and asbestos), and miscellaneous organics, including thiourea and thioacetamide, have also been implicated as carcinogens. Agents that increase the number of peroxisomes in tissues, although not considered genotoxic themselves, can produce tumors in rodents (reviewed in Gibson, 1993). These agents damage DNA through increased production in the cell of active oxygen species and can induce proliferation, oncogene activation, CYP4504A1 induction, and hepatomegaly. Examples of peroxisome proliferators include clofibrate, di(2-ethylhexyl)phthalate and 1,1,2-trichlorethane.

## C. Anticarcinogens

Dietary constituents are known that inhibit carcinogenesis (reviewed in Weisburger, 1994a). Several antipromoters have been identified that are analogues of vitamin A, a retinoid essential for normal epithelial cell differentiation. Retinoids and other carotenoids appear to block the promotion–progression phase of carcinogenesis, as they are ineffective when given before or together with an initiating carcinogen, but can block the promoting effects of phorbol esters. Anticancer activity has also been demonstrated in some models with other antioxidants, such as vitamin E, selenium, and the polyphenol, epigallocatechin gallate. Sphingolipids, which are hydrolyzed to PKC inhibitors, and some fatty acids, such as conjugated linoleic acid and the $\omega$-3 fatty acids, especially eicosapentaenoic acid and docosahexaenoic acid, which modify the conversion of arachidonic acid to prostaglandins, also show anticarcinogenic activity in some circumstances (Borek, 1993). Components of cruciferous vegetables, such as phenethyl isothiocyanate, inhibit production of lung cancer by a nitroso compound found in tobacco smoke; and ellagic acid, which inhibits CYP1A1 activity and reduces the incidence of PAH-induced carcinomas, are other examples of this group. Both synthetic and naturally occurring compounds with the ability to inhibit preneoplastic events of carcinogenesis have been employed in cancer chemoprevention studies (see, e.g., El-Bayoumy, 1994).

## V. VARIABLES IN MULTISTAGE CARCINOGENESIS

Variation, both in number and site of tumors, has been noted in the response of different animal species and strains to the same chemical carcinogens. This variability may be related to endogenous factors, such as extent of metabolic activation and detoxification reactions, DNA repair capability, and capacity for cell proliferation.

### A. Animal Studies

Over 400 long-term chemical carcinogenesis studies using rats and mice have recently been reviewed (Huff et al., 1991), and some similarities in incidence and site of tumor development were found. For example, in both species of rodents, liver is the most common tumor site, and, although mice are more likely to experience liver tumors, there is an 80% interspecies concordance for hepatocarcinogenicity. Other organ sites, such as lung, forestomach, and the hematopoetic system, also show a high interspecies correlation. Differences were also noted in response of the two rodent species. For example, female rats had the most chemically associated mammary tumors, whereas the male rat was most prone to chemically induced tumors of the kidney and pancreas. Furthermore, tumors at some sites were far more common in a particular species: for example, urinary bladder cancers occur more frequently in the rat, but harderian gland neoplasms are found mainly in the mouse.

Sites of tumor formation in humans show some similarities to those produced in rodent carcinogenicity bioassays (Huff et al., 1991). The lung, hematopoetic system, mammary gland, urinary bladder, and uterus are among the ten most frequent sites of tumor development in both the United States population and in rodent bioassays. Moreover, all agents for which there is evidence of carcinogenicity in humans cause cancer at a common site in at least one animal species. In contrast, the data for induction of human tumors by known animal carcinogens are much less consistent, perhaps because human data are lacking for some chemicals, or because of the difference between genotoxic and nongenotoxic carcinogens. Most known human carcinogens are genotoxicants, whereas about half known rodent carcinogens are of the nongenotoxic variety, which usually require long exposures to relatively high doses to cause their effect. The mechanism of tumorigenesis by these agents may thus be so different from that of genotoxic carcinogens that extrapolation to the low doses to which humans are exposed is questionable. Some chemicals, however, also produce tumors in humans in the same organs as found in rats or mice. Examples are aflatoxin and diethylstilbesterol, which were first shown to be carcinogenic in rodents.

### B. Biotransformation

Many carcinogens must undergo biotransformation to produce the ultimate carcinogen, and some observed species differences in susceptibility to carcinogenesis have a metabolic basis. Many of the reactions that convert chemically stable procarcinogens to electrophilic, reactive agents are carried out by cytochrome P-450 enzymes. Multiple P-450 isozymes exist with different substrate specificities or differences in their distribution among organs, species, and individuals (Harris, 1991). The differential sensitivity of rodents and humans to vinyl chloride-induced liver tumors is one example of metabolic capacity determining tumor incidence (cited in IARC, 1992). Rats and mice oxidize vinyl chloride 12 and 15 times faster (normalized by body weight), respectively, than do humans, and the rodent sensitivity to vinyl chloride-induced liver cancer is greater by approximately the same degree. There are also many instances in which species differences in carcinogenicity cannot be explained by metabolism: Cotton rats, for example, are resistant to the carcinogenic effects of AAF, although the compound is readily metabolized in vivo to genotoxic products.

In addition to species differences, xenobiotic-metabolizing activity can be modified by other variables, such as pharmacokinetic factors. The relatively high doses employed in testing regimens may saturate some metabolic reactions, whereas, at the lower doses to which humans are exposed, rates and pathways of metabolic processes may be qualitatively and quantitatively different. Nutritional factors, hormonal influences, or exposure to carcinogens or other drugs can also alter drug-metabolizing enzymatic activity. In animal studies that use reasonably homogenous populations, these factors can be controlled, and metabolic differences between individual animals are generally small. In humans, however, there can be considerable interindividual differences, which may be reflected in different risk of neoplastic disease. In addition to environmental or nutritional factors, genetic polymorphisms exist in several enzymes that catalyze carcinogen activation or detoxification (reviewed in Idle et al., 1992). Polymorphisms that may modulate chemical carcinogenesis are known for both phase I reactions, including those catalyzed by members of the cytochrome P-450 family—CYP1A1, CYP1A2, CYP2A6, CYP2D6, and CYP3A4—and phase II reactions, including UDP-glucuronosyltransferases, *N*-acetyltransferases, sulfotransferases, and glutathione *S*-transferases. Although these polymorphisms are well-established, epidemiological data linking a particular phenotype to increased or decreased cancer risk are often lacking. An association between the extensive metabolizer phenotype of debrisoquine-4-hydroxylase (CYP2D6) and increased lung cancer risk has been reported, and the tobacco-specific nitrosamine, NNK, is a substrate for this enzyme. Associations between arylhydrocarbon hydroxylase inducibility (CYP1A1) and lung and laryngeal cancer and between the slow-acetylator phenotype (*N*-acetyltransferase) and bladder cancer and the fast-acetylator phenotype and colon cancer have also been reported.

## C.  DNA Repair

The DNA molecules undergo frequent, potentially mutagenic alterations, including spontaneous deaminations, depurinations, and oxidative damage, as well as damage from xenobiotic exposure. Most alterations are quickly corrected by a variety of DNA repair processes, most of which depend on the existence of double-stranded DNA in the region of the damage (reviewed in Barnes et al., 1993; Sancar and Tang, 1993). Animal cells have pathways for direct reversal of DNA damage in a single enzymatic step, such as repair of alkylated bases or strand breaks, for both base and nucleotide excision repair and for mismatch repair. Recombinational repair of daughter strand gaps and inducible SOS repair response to severely damaged DNA exist in prokaryotes, and analogous processes are thought to operate in animal cells as well. The enzymes involved in DNA repair interact to form a network of reactions, such that alterations in a single component of the system might have a marked influence in overall repair capacity. In addition, some proteins involved in DNA repair processes are also involved in other cellular activities relevant to carcinogenesis, such as gene regulation and DNA replication (Hanawalt et al., 1994). The carcinogenicity of some chemical agents, such as arsenicals, may, at least partly, be due to inhibition of DNA repair processes.

Human mutagen–hypersensitivity syndromes provide evidence that defective DNA repair systems can increase the risk of cancer (reviewed in Heddle et al., 1983). Individuals with xeroderma pigmentosum develop skin cancer as a result of accumulated sunlight (UV)-induced DNA damage and are defective in the incision step of nucleotide excision repair. At least seven different gene products are associated with the disorder, which may reflect the need for chromosomal structural modification before incision. Other rare genetic disorders characterized by DNA repair deficiencies that render individuals more susceptible to neoplastic disease are Bloom's syndrome, Fanconi's anemia, and ataxia-telangiectasia. The basis of a more common condition, hereditary nonpolyposis colorectal cancer, is a defect in repair of mismatched sequences on the two DNA strands, which leads to intrinsic instability in genomic microsatellite repeat sequences characteristic of the disease (reviewed in Cleaver, 1994). In addition to these severe defects in DNA repair, relatively large differences in the ability to repair DNA, as measured by unscheduled DNA synthesis or $O^6$-alkyltransferase activity, exist in the general population. These genetic polymorphisms influencing the rate and fidelity of DNA repair may contribute to interindividual differences in cancer risk (Shields and Harris, 1991). Repair capacity also varies between different organs and species, which may be relevant to observed differences in patterns of tumor formation.

## D. Cell Proliferation

Responses to tumor promoters in skin carcinogenesis models also varies markedly with species and strain of animal used, and in some well-established cases, differences in cell proliferation are responsible for species-specificity of carcinogenesis (reviewed in Swenberg et al., 1992). For example, $\alpha$-2$\mu$-globulin nephropathy, is a disease that occurs only in male rats. Chemicals known to cause the disease all bind $\alpha$-2$\mu$-globulin, leading to toxic accumulation of this protein, specific to male rats, in the nephron. Cell proliferation restores the resulting necrosis, and chronic exposure to the agents results in appearance of renal cell tumors. Furthermore, chemicals that produce rodent thyroid neoplasia, secondary to hypothyroidism caused by induction of hormonal imbalance, can also be considered to be species-specific, as the phenomenon does not occur in primates. Finally, although variation in drug-metabolizing enzymes can result in some differences in species specificity of genotoxic urinary bladder carcinogens, such as aromatic amines, considerably greater species differences are found with nongenotoxic carcinogens, such as melamine. At high doses, these agents induce sustained urothelial proliferation and, eventually, urinary bladder carcinomas. Rats seem more susceptible to this form of carcinogenesis than mice and humans.

## VI. DOSE–RESPONSE RELATIONSHIPS IN CHEMICAL CARCINOGENESIS

There is general agreement that a knowledge of the mechanism of their action is necessary to evaluate risks of exposure to potential chemical carcinogens. Interpretation of dose–response relationships is complicated by whether or not (1) changes at the molecule or cellular levels are reversible, (2) carcinogenic effects can persist or accumulate, and (3) thresholds exist for carcinogenic effects. Time– and dose–response relationships can be demonstrated for chemical carcinogenesis, but the existence of thresholds (i.e., doses below which there is no carcinogenic response) remains uncertain. Some issues concerning dose–response relationships can be addressed in animal experiments in which there is little variation in the tested population; furthermore, the dose and other experimental conditions can be controlled and the production of tumors can be monitored from the beginning of the exposure throughout the animals' lives. Reliably detecting relative rare events, such as induction of tumors at low exposure levels, however, requires too many animals to be practical. Estimation of risk to low doses, then, involves extrapolation based on a model, and different models that fit the experimental (high-dose) data equally well may predict low-dose responses that differ greatly. One view of threshold phenomena in carcinogenesis is that for genotoxic chemicals, it may be correct to assume, in theory, that no threshold (or a very low one) exists, but for agents that work through epigenetic mechanisms, (larger) thresholds are to be expected (Cohen and Ellwein, 1991). For some carcinogens, there might not be a threshold for initiation, but the observed dose–response could be modified considerably by thresholds for effects on promotion. For example, in some studies, the time required for appearance of tumors, or latent period, appears to be dose-related; even if irreversible genetic changes occur, at low doses the latent period would exceed the life of the animal and no evidence for tumorigenicity would be seen.

Threshold phenomena have also been examined in mutational assays, in which a very large number of treated individuals can be analyzed, particularly when single-celled organisms are used (reviewed in Ehrenberg et al., 1983). In some such experiments that used low doses of ionizing radiation or ethylene oxide, no deviations from linearity in the dose–response curves were observed, even at doses corresponding to the "one-hit" level. According to this concept, although the average dose per cell can be infinitesimally small, an individual cell either is hit by an ionizing particle, for example, or is not, and that particle imparts a fixed quantum of energy. At average doses that are lower than those which correspond to the one-hit dose, fewer cells are hit, but those that are can still experience one critical lesion; under these circumstances, the observed linear dose–response curve is consistent with lack of a threshold. There does not appear to be any reason, however, why true or apparent thresholds should not exist for some mutagens. For example, the requirement for metabolic activation or the existence of saturable DNA repair processes might lead to an apparent no-effect level of exposure, and experimental data exist that support this notion, as well.

## VII.  SUMMARY

Many steps are required to convert a normal cell into a cancerous one. The cancer cell must be able to multiply under conditions that a normal cell would not and to invade surrounding tissue and spread throughout the body. Both genetic changes, such as activation of oncogenes or inactivation of tumor suppressor genes, and epigenetic changes, such as stimulation of cell proliferation, contribute to the development of cancers. Chemical agents can increase the probability of malignant transformation by inducing mutations that can ultimately lead to tumor formation, by promoting the development of tumors in cells with preexisting genetic damage, or by increasing the rate of acquisition of malignant traits by benign tumors. Chemical carcinogens are structurally diverse, but all initiating agents are either already electrophiles or can be converted to electrophilic reactants through metabolic activation. Genetic and environmental factors can alter an individual's ability to metabolize carcinogens, to repair DNA damage, and to respond to mitogenic stimuli, all of which can alter susceptibility to chemical carcinogenesis. The incidence and time required for appearance of tumors appear to be dose-related, but the existence of no-effect doses of carcinogens remains controversial.

## REFERENCES

Alberts, B., Bray, D., Lewis, J., Raff, M., Roberts, K., and Watson, J. D. (1994). *Molecular Biology of the Cell,* 3rd ed., Garland Publishing, New York, pp. 863–910.

Barnes, D. E., Lindahl, T., and Sedgwick, B. (1993). DNA repair, *Curr. Opinion Cell Biol.,* 5, 424–433.

Barrett, J. C. (1992). Mechanism of action of known human carcinogens. In *Mechanisms of Carcinogenesis in Risk Identification* (H. Vainio, et al., eds.), IARC, Lyon, France, pp. 115–134.

Beckman, R. A., Mildvan, A. S., and Loeb, L. A. (1985). On the fidelity of DNA replication: Manganese mutagenesis in vitro, *Biochemistry,* 24, 5810–5817.

Borek, C. (1993). Molecular mechanisms in cancer induction and prevention, *Environ. Health Perspect.*, 101 (Suppl. 3), 237–245.

Boylan, M. O. and Zarbl, H. (1991). Transformation effector and suppressor genes, *J. Cell. Biochem.*, 46, 199–205.

Cairns, J. (1981). The origin of human cancers, *Nature*, 289, 353–357.

Castagna, M. (1987). Phorbol esters as signal transducers and tumor promoters, *Biol. Cell*, 59, 3–13.

Cheng, K. C. and Loeb, L. A. (1993). Genomic instability and tumor progression: mechanistic considerations, *Adv. Cancer Res.*, 60, 121–156.

Cleaver, J. E. (1994). It was a very good year for DNA repair, *Cell*, 76, 1–4.

Cohen, S. M. and Ellwein, L. B. (1991). Genetic errors, cell proliferation, and carcinogenesis, *Cancer Res.*, 51, 6493–6505.

Cooper, G. M. (1990). *Oncogenes,* Jones and Bartlett, Boston.

Crawford, B. D. (1985). Perspectives on the somatic mutation model of carcinogenesis. In *Advances in Modern Environmental Toxicology,* Vol. 12 (M.A. Mehlman, ed.), Princeton Scientific Publishing, Princeton, pp. 13–59.

Duesberg, P. H., Goodrich, D., and Zhou, R.-P. (1991). Cancer genes by non-homologous recombination. In *Boundaries between Promotion and Progression During Carcinogenesis* (O. Sudilovsky, et al., eds.), Plenum Press, New York, pp. 197–211.

Dunlop, M. G. (1991). Allele losses and onco-suppressor genes, *J. Pathol.*, 163, 1–5.

Ehrenberg, L., Moustacchi, E., and Osterman-Golkar, S. (1983). Dosimetry of genotoxic agents and dose–response relationship of their effects, *Mutat. Res.*, 123, 121–182.

El-Bayoumy, K. (1994). Evaluation of chemopreventive against breast cancer and proposed strategies for future clinical intervention trials, *Carcinogenesis*, 15, 2395–2420.

Eling, T. E., Thompson, D. C., Foureman, G. L., Curtis, J. F., and Hughes, M. F. (1990). Prostaglandin H synthase and xenobiotic oxidation, *Annu. Rev. Pharmacol. Toxicol.*, 30, 1–45.

Epstein, R. J. (1986). Is your initiator really necessary? *J. Theor. Biol.*, 122, 359–374.

Farber, E. (1984). The multistep nature of cancer development, *Cancer Res.*, 44, 4217–4223.

Gibson, G. G. (1993). Peroxisome proliferators: Paradigms and prospects, *Toxicol. Lett.*, 68, 193–201.

Hanawalt, P. C., Donahue, B. A., and Sweder, K. S. (1994). Repair and transcription: collision or collusion? *Curr. Biol.*, 4, 518–521.

Harrington, E. A., Fanidi, A., and Evan, G. I. (1994). Oncogenes and cell death, *Curr. Opinion Genet. Dev.*, 4, 120–129.

Harris, C. C. (1991). Chemical and physical carcinogenesis: Advances and perspectives for the 1990s, *Cancer Res.*, 51 (Suppl.), 5023s–5044s.

Hecht, S. S., el-Bayoumy, K., Rivenson, A., and Amin, S. (1994). Potent mammary carcinogenicity in female CD rats of a fjord region diol-epoxide of benzo[*c*]phenanthrene compared to a bay region diol-epoxide of benzo[*a*]pyrene, Cancer Res., 54, 21–24.

Heddle, J. A., Krepinsky, A. B., and Marshall, R. R. (1983). Cellular sensitivity of mutagens and carcinogens in the chromosome-breakage and other cancer-prone syndromes. In *Chromosome Mutation and Neoplasia,* Alan R. Liss, New York, pp. 203–234.

Hennings, H., Glick, A. B., Greenhalgh, D. A., Morgan, D. L., Strickland, J. E., Tennenbaum, T., and Yuspa, S. H. (1993). Critical aspects of initiation, promotion, and progression in multistage epidermal carcinogenesis, *Proc. Soc. Exp. Biol. Med.*, 202, 1–8.

Hochberg, A., Gonik, B., Goshen, R., and de Groot, N. (1994). A growing relationship between genomic imprinting and tumorigenesis, *Cancer Genet. Cytogenet.*, 73, 82–83.

Holliday, R. (1987). The inheritance of epigenetic defects, *Science*, 238, 163–170.

Huff, J., Cirvello, J., Haseman, J., and Bucher, J. (1991). Chemicals associated with site-specific neoplasia in 1394 long-term carcinogenesis experiments in laboratory rodents, *Environ. Health Perspect.*, 93, 247–270.

[IARC] International Agency for Cancer Research (1987). *IARC Monographs on the Evaluation of Carcinogenic Risks to Humans,* Supplement 7, *Overall Evaluation of Carcinogenicity: An Updating of IARC Monographs Vols. 1–48*, IARC, Lyon, France.

[IARC] International Agency for Research on Cancer (1992). Consensus report. In *Mechanisms of Carcinogenesis in Risk Identification* (H. Vainio, et al., eds.), IARC, Lyon, France, pp. 9–54.

Idle, J. R., Armstrong, M., Boddy, A. V., Boustead, C., Cholerton, S., Cooper, J., Daly, A. K., Ellis, J., Gregory, W., Hadidi, H., Hofer, C., Holt, J., Leathart, J., McCracken, N., Monkman, S. C., Painter, J. E., Taber, H., Walker, D., and Yule, M. (1992). The pharmacogenetics of chemical carcinogenesis, *Pharmacogenetics, 2*, 246–258.

Knudson, A. G. (1993). Antioncogenes and human cancer, *Proc. Natl. Acad. Sci. USA, 90*, 10914–10921.

Lieberman, M. W. and Lebovitz, R. M. (1990). Neoplasia. In *Anderson's Pathology,* Vol. 1 (J. M. Kissane, Ed.), C. V. Mosby, St. Louis, MO, pp. 566–614.

Liotta, L. A. and Stetler-Stevenson, W. G. (1991). Tumor invasion and metastasis: An imbalance of positive and negative regulation, *Cancer Res., 51*(Suppl.), 5054s–5059s.

Lu, F. C. 1991). Carcinogenesis. In *Basic Toxicology: Fundamentals, Target Organs, and Risk Assessment,* Hemisphere Publishing, Washington, DC, pp. 93–115.

Melnick R. L., Huff, J., Barrett, J. C., Maronpot, R. R., Lucier, G., and Portier, C. F. (1993). Cell proliferation and chemical carcinogenesis: Symposium overview, *Environ. Health Perspect., 101*(Suppl. 5), 3–7.

Miller, E. C. and Miller, J. A. (1981). Mechanisms of chemical carcinogenesis, *Cancer, 47*, 1005–1064.

Murray, A. and Hunt, T. (1993). *The Cell Cycle: An Introduction,* W. H. Freeman, New York.

Nowell, P. C. (1991). Genetic instability and tumor development. In *Boundaries Between Promotion and Progression During Carcinogenesis* (O. Sudilovsky, et al., eds.), Plenum Press, New York, pp. 221–231.

Peter, M. and Herskowitz, I. (1994). Joining the complex: cyclin-dependent kinase inhibitory proteins and the cell cycle, *Cell, 79*, 181–184.

Pitot, H. C., Dragan, Y., Xu, Y.-H., Peterson, J., Hully, J., and Campbell, H. (1992). Pathways of carcinogenesis—genetic and epigenetic. In *Multistage Carcinogenesis* (C. C. Harris, et al., eds.), CRC Press, Boca Raton, FL, pp. 21–33.

Rabbitts, T. H. (1994). Chromosome translocations in human cancer, *Nature, 372*, 143–149.

Rubin, H. (1985). Cancer as a dynamic developmental disorder, *Cancer Res., 45*, 2935–2942.

Sancar, A. and Tang, M.-S. (1993). Nucleotide excision repair, *Photochem. Photobiol., 57*, 905–921.

Shields, P. G. and Harris, C. C. (1991). Molecular epidemiology and the genetics of environmental cancer, *JAMA, 266*, 681–687.

Sugimura, T. and Wakabayashi, K. (1990). Mutagens and carcinogens in food. In *Mutagens and Carcinogens in the Diet* (M. W. Pariza, et al., eds.), Wiley–Liss, New York, pp. 1–18.

Sulitzeanu, D. (1993). Immunosuppressive factors in human cancer, *Adv. Cancer Res., 60*, 247–267.

Swenberg, J. A., Dietrich, D. R., McClain, R. M., and Cohen, S. M. (1992). Species-specific mechanisms of carcinogenesis. In *Mechanisms of Carcinogenesis in Risk Identification* (H. Vainio, et al., eds.), IARC, Lyon, France, pp. 477–500.

Vasiliev, J. M. (1983). Cell microenvironment and carcinogenesis in vivo and in vitro, *IARC Sci. Publ., 51*, 247–256.

Weisburger, J. H. (1994a). Practical approaches to chemoprevention of cancer, *Drug Metab. Rev., 26*, 253–260.

Weisburger, J. H. (1994b). Environmental hazards, lifestyle and disease prevention, *J. Hazard. Mater., 39*, 129–133.

Williams, G. M. and Weisburger, J. H. (1991). Chemical carcinogenesis. In *Casarett and Doull's Toxicology. The Basic Science of Poisons* (M. O. Amdur, et al., eds.), McGraw-Hill, New York, pp. 127–200.

# 3
# Principles of Genetic Toxicology

**Wai Nang Choy**
*Schering-Plough Research Institute*
*Lafayette, New Jersey*

## I. INTRODUCTION

Genetic toxicology is the study of damages to the genes by chemical or physical agents. Damages to the genes (i.e., to DNA) if not repaired timely and correctly, change the DNA sequence and cause mutations. Mutations often result in the elimination or alteration of gene functions, and if the damages are not lethal, will lead to inheritable changes. *Genotoxicity* is thus customarily defined as the ability to damage DNA and to change DNA sequence. DNA sequence changes can be single nucleotide changes that result in point mutations, or multiple nucleotide changes that result in visible chromosomal aberrations. The adverse effect of a mutation is dependent on the gene and the tissue affected. The most serious effects of mutations in somatic cells are neoplasms, and in germ cells, inheritable neoplasms or birth defects.

The development of genetic toxicology, both for testing and research, has been closely associated with advances in genetics. Early genetic toxicology tests were developed based on classic microbial, *Drosophila,* and somatic cell genetics and cytogenetics. In vivo mammalian tests were developed from rodent reproductive studies (Brusick, 1987; Li and Heflich, 1991). Many tests were validated in the past 20 years, and those judged reliable for the detection of mutagens have become standardized routine tests. The tests that are commonly used by regulatory agencies for the determination of genotoxicity of chemicals are listed in Table 1. Recent advances in recombinant DNA and transgenic animal technologies have initiated developments of new tests for changes at the molecular level (Glickman and Gorelick, 1993), and for gene mutations in vivo (Tennant et al., 1994). Since many validated tests can reliably detect mutagens, the usefulness of these new tests is dependent on their ability to identify carcinogens. The routine genetic toxicology tests are described in Chapter 10. This chapter is focused on the role of genetic toxicology in cancer and genetic risk assessment.

Among the four components of risk assessment: hazard identification, dose–response relationship, exposure assessment, and risk characterization, genetic toxicology has been mostly

**Table 1**   Common Genetic Toxicology Tests

| *In Vitro* | | |
| --- | --- | --- |
| Gene Mutation | Bacteria | *Salmonella typhimurium* (Ames test) |
| | Mammalian cells | Chinese hamster ovary cells (CHO/HGPRT) |
| | | Mouse lymphoma cells (L5178Y/TK) |
| Cytogenetics | | |
|   Chromosome aberration | Mammalian cells | Human peripheral blood lymphocytes (HPBL) |
| | | Chinese hamster lung fibroblasts (CHL) |
| | | Chinese hamster ovary cells (CHO) |
| *In Vivo* | | |
| Gene mutation | Transgenic mice (Muta™Mouse and Big Blue™) | |
| Cytogenetics | | |
|   Micronucleus | Mouse bone marrow erythrocytes | |
|   Chromosome aberration | Rat bone marrow cells | |
| DNA repair | Rat hepatocyte unscheduled DNA synthesis (UDS) | |

confined to hazard identification. Since almost all genetic toxicology studies, both in vitro and in vivo, are conducted at high doses and for short durations, the dose–response data are not suitable for risk extrapolation to low doses and long-term exposures to humans. Recent developments in molecular epidemiology have extended the application of genetic toxicology to exposure assessments using quantifiable biomarkers, such as protein and DNA adducts (Groopman and Skipper, 1991). Genetic toxicology is important for cancer risk characterization as it distinguishes genotoxic from nongenotoxic carcinogens, which affects the selection of a cancer risk assessment model.

## II.  GENOTOXICITY AND CARCINOGENICITY

The "somatic cell mutation theory of carcinogenesis" (Boveri, 1929) postulates that cancer can be caused by mutations. This theory was first supported by early studies in childhood cancers

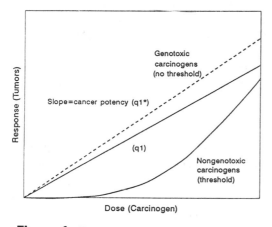

**Figure 1**   Dose-response curves of tumor induction by genotoxic and nongenotoxic carcinogens at the low dose region. Genotoxic carcinogens are not assumed to have threshold doses below which carcinogenesis does not occur. *Cancer potency* is the slope of the dose-response curve, designated as (q1), and its upper 95% confidence level is (q1*). Nongenotoxic carcinogens are assumed to have threshold doses.

which showed that the incidences of retinoblastomas is dependent on the number of defective genes (Knudson et al., 1975). Approximately 100 human cancer genes were estimated based on the occurrence of inheritable tumors (Knudson, 1986). Recent developments in molecular cancer genetics further showed that carcinogenesis is often associated with mutations in oncogenes and antioncogenes (tumor suppressor genes) (Knudson, 1993). In fact, multiple mutations and genetic alternations have been demonstrated to be required for human tumor development (Vogelstein et al., 1988; Kern and Vogelstein, 1991). The association of mutations to neoplasms supports the somatic cell mutation theory. Accordingly, it seems reasonable to use mutagenicity tests to identify carcinogens. The limitation of which is that these tests cannot detect non-genotoxic carcinogens.

Carcinogenesis not associated with genetic alternations, at least at its early stages, has recently become an important issue in cancer risk assessment (Butterworth and Slaga, 1987). Studies in rodent cancer bioassays have identified several chemicals that are carcinogenic, but are not mutagenic in standard routine toxicology tests. Nongenotoxic carcinogenesis is often species-, sex- and tissue-specific, and its mechanisms are diverse. A common mechanism of nongenotoxic carcinogenesis is believed to be enhanced cell proliferation (Cohen and Ellwein, 1990). Cell proliferation is an attractive hypothesis because it resembles the loss of growth control at early stages of neoplastic transformation. Direct evidence that cell proliferation alone can lead to neoplasms, however, is still lacking.

Since neoplastic progression is a multistep process (Barrett, 1987) and cancer phenotypes are inheritable in cancer cells, there must be a step during progression at which genetic alternation occurs (Littlefield, 1976). Genotoxic carcinogens may induce genetic changes at an initial step, whereas nongenotoxic carcinogens may create conditions favorable for genetic changes at a later step. The implications of these two mechanism of carcinogenesis for quantitative cancer risk assessment will be discussed later.

## III. GENOTOXICITY AND GERM CELL MUTATIONS

Germ cell mutations are inheritable, and genetic alternations are transmissible to the offsprings (Allen et al., 1990). Genetic risk assessment is the risk assessment of germ cell mutations. In fact, the United States Environmental Protection Agency (USEPA) guidelines on risk assessment of mutagenicity was addressed primarily for heritable mutagenic risk (USEPA, 1986), although study of germ cell mutations is a confined area in genetic toxicology. All somatic cell mutagens are potential germ cell mutagens, and the susceptibility of germ cells to these mutagens is dependent on the ability of these mutagens to cross the blood–germ cell barrier (Setchell and Main, 1978), and the DNA replicative stages of the germ cells (Russell et al., 1992). Reports on germ cell mutagenesis in rodents and in humans showed that male animals are more sensitive to germ cell mutagens, especially at the stem cell spermatogonia and poststem-cell stages (Russell, 1994; Brewen et al., 1975). The resting oocytes in females are not dividing cells, and they are less susceptible to mutagens (Russell, 1994). In a recent study, many chemotherapeutic agents were identified as rodent germ cell mutagens, and a ranking system of mutagens was proposed (Shelby et al., 1993; Shelby, 1994). Human germ cell mutagens, however, are difficult to identify (Shelby, 1994).

## IV. GENETIC TOXICOLOGY AND REGULATORY RISK ASSESSMENT

### A. Hazard Identification

The most recognized role of genetic toxicology in risk assessment is the identification of mutagens. Mutagens are usually identified by test results from a battery of standard genetic toxicology tests. These tests are validated for their ability in detecting mutagens, but their reliability in detecting carcinogens vary. Among the common in vitro and in vivo genetic toxicology tests that have been validated, only four major types of tests are routinely performed for mutagen identification. They are the bacterial mutagenicity assays, the mammalian cell mutagenicity assays, the in vitro cytogenetic assays, and the in vivo cytogenetic assays (see Table 1). These tests are briefly described in the following, and they are described in greater detail in Chapter 10.

For bacterial mutagenicity, the most popular test by far is the *Salmonella* reverse gene mutation test, which is also known as the Ames test (Ames, 1975; Maron and Ames, 1983). This test uses several (usually five) genetically altered tester strains of *Salmonella typhimurium* to detect two types of mutations—DNA base-pair substitution and frameshift—as monitored by reverse mutations of the histidine gene, from autotropic for histidine (*his–*) to prototrophic for histidine (*his+*). Several genetic alternations were introduced into the bacteria to increase their sensitivity to mutagenesis. These are mutations to enhance permeability of chemicals to the cells (*rfa* mutation), to eliminate DNA repair (*uvrA* mutation), and to enhance sensitivity by introducing multiple copies of the *his–* gene into the bacteria by plasmids.

For the mammalian cell mutagenicity assays, the most widely used tests are the Chinese hamster ovary cell (CHO) mutagenicity assay (Hsie et al., 1981) and the mouse lymphoma cell mutagenicity assays (Clive et al., 1983, 1987). The CHO assay detects mutations at the hypoxanthine–guanine phosphoribosyltransferase (*HGPRT*) gene located on the X chromosome, and the mouse lymphoma assay, thymidine kinase (*TK*) gene on chromosome 11. The mouse lymphoma assay has been considered to be more sensitive because of its ability to detect mutations caused by large DNA deletions, and presumably, it can also detect cytogenetic changes based on the occurrence of mutant colonies of smaller diameter (USFDA, 1993). The mouse lymphoma assay, however, often produces false-positive results for the prediction of carcinogenicity.

The in vitro cytogenetic assay is to detect chromosomal aberrations in cultured cells. The commonly used cells are the Chinese hamster ovary cells (CHO, Galloway et al., 1985, 1987), Chinese hamster lung cells (CHL; Ishidate et al., 1988), or human peripheral blood lymphocytes (HPBL; Evens, 1962). The testing procedures are often complicated, with multiple treatment durations and multiple harvests. Chromosomal aberrations examined in the assay are chromosomal breaks, gaps, rearrangement, endoreduplication, and aneuploidy.

The most commonly conducted in vivo cytogenetic assays are the mouse bone marrow micronucleus assay (Schmid, 1976; MacGregor et al., 1987) and the rat bone marrow chromosomal aberration assay (Preston et al., 1981). The mouse bone marrow micronucleus assay is to detect the induction of micronuclei (small nuclei) by the test article as a result of chromosomal breaks and abnormal chromosomal segregations in mouse bone marrow polychromatic erythrocytes (young RNA-containing erythrocytes). The rat bone marrow chromosomal aberration assay detects chromosomal aberrations, and it is often performed to confirm findings in the in vitro chromosomal aberration assay.

As evidenced by validation studies, all potent mutagens are detectable by this battery of four tests. However, for weak mutagens, or for resolution of inconclusive results, additional tests are often performed. The most common additional tests are the in vitro and the in vivo–in vitro unscheduled DNA synthesis (UDS) for DNA damages in rat liver cells (Mirsalis and Butterworth, 1980; Steinmetz et al., 1988). For definitive demonstration of DNA reactivity, DNA adduct induction studies using [32]P postlabeling technique (Randerath et al., 1981) are usually performed.

Chemical or physical agents are classified as "genotoxic" or "nongenotoxic," based on the results of these tests, although interpretation of equivocal results can sometimes be controversial. A chemical identified as genotoxic is generally considered to associate with high health risks, simply because cancer and birth defects are serious diseases.

The use of genetic toxicology tests for identification of carcinogens was initiated with the development of the *Salmonella* bacterial mutagenicity assay (Ames et al., 1973; Ames, 1979). Early correlation studies showed that the Ames test was reliable in detecting carcinogens, reportedly up to 90% accuracy (Ames et al., 1975; McCann et al., 1975; Purchase et al., 1978). This level of accuracy, however, diminishes in subsequent validation studies using different genotoxicity databases. In a correlation study of 222 National Cancer Institute–National Toxicology Program (NCI/NTP) bioassays with *Salmonella* test results and chemical structure (potential electrophilic sites), only 73% of rodent carcinogens (rats and mice; tumors at single or multiple sites) were positive in the *Salmonella* test. A strong concordance of 92% was observed between positive *Salmonella* test results and chemicals containing potential DNA-reactive functional groups (Ashby and Tennant, 1988). This finding is similar to a recent correlation study of 251 chemicals in the Carcinogen Potency Database (CPDB) that 81% of carcinogens (rats and mice, multiple sites) and 60% of carcinogens (rats and mice, single site) were positive in the *Salmonella* assay (Gold et al., 1993).

When the test results of a battery of genetic toxicology tests were compared with the results of rodent cancer bioassays, the correlations were not as good as those for the *Salmonella* assay alone (Shelby and Stasiewicz, 1984; Auletta and Ashby, 1988). In a NTP study, test results of four genetic toxicology tests were compared with carcinogenicity data of 114 NTP rodent cancer bioassays (Tennant et al., 1987; Zeiger et al., 1990). The four tests evaluated were the *Salmonella* bacterial mutagenicity assay (SAL), the mouse lymphoma assay (MLA), the CHO chromosomal aberration assay (ABS), and the CHO sister chromatid-exchange assay (SCE) [*Note:* The SCE assay is a cytogenetic assay for chromosomal breakage and reunion between sister chromatids. This assay is no longer a routine assay, partly because the biological consequences of SCE are unknown]. The *positive predictivity,* defined as the proportion of chemicals positive in a mutagenicity assay that are also carcinogenic in rodents, was 89% for SAL, 73% for ABS, 64% for SCE, and 63% for MLA. The *concordance,* defined as the overall proportion of carcinogens and noncarcinogens that are correctly identified, was 66% for SAL, 61% for ABS, 59% for SCE, and 59% for MLA. A combination of four tests improved neither the positive predictivity nor the concordance for carcinogenicity (Zeiger et al., 1990). For human carcinogens, a correlation study was performed on the 39 International Agency for Research on Cancer (IARC) group I human carcinogens (IARC, 1987a,b) with the *Salmonella* assay and the rodent cytogenetic assay (chromosomal aberration or micronucleus) (Shelby and Zeiger, 1990). Except for 6 hormones and 3 fibers, which were not tested or negative in these two mutagenicity assays, 2 of 3 metals; 4 of 5 soots, tars, and oils; and all 21 organic compounds showed positive responses in one or both assays. This led to the conclusion that a combination of the *Salmonella* assay and a rodent in vivo cytogenetic assay can predict most genotoxic human carcinogens (Shelby and Zeiger, 1990).

Although not as intensively studied, genetic toxicology tests are also used for the identification of germ cell mutagens. The significance of germ cell mutation in risk assessment, however, has been overshadowed by routine animal reproductive toxicology studies. A variety of germ cell mutation assays were developed (Allen et al., 1990), and the common in vivo germ cell mutation assays were the *Drosophila* sex-linked recessive lethal (SLRL) test (Auerbach and Robson, 1946; Lee et al., 1983), the mouse specific-locus (MSL) test (Russell, 1951), and the dominant lethal test (Green et al., 1985). The *Drosophila* assay is to examine the susceptibility of male flies to germ cell mutagens at various stages of sperm maturation using a recessive genetic marker. The mouse specific-locus tests detects the occurrence of a variety of recessive traits, such as coat color, eye color, ear morphology, or hair structure as results of mutations in the exposed parent. A modification of this assay was developed to measure the changes of mobility of proteins by electrophoresis (Johnson and Lewis, 1981). The dominant lethal test is to detect mutations that cause embryo death (Green et al., 1985). Recent developments in assays that use transgenic mice permit concomitant screening of mutations in somatic and germ cells in the same animal. In vitro assays of DNA damage in germ cells were also developed, and the most widely used assays are germ cell unscheduled DNA synthesis (UDS; Sega, 1982; Working and Butterworth, 1984; Bentley and Working, 1988), and DNA strand breaks by alkaline elution (AE; Bradley and Dysart, 1985; Skare and Schrotel, 1985).

In a recent correlation study of the *Drosophila* SLRL, the UDS, and AE assays with the MSL assay, the overall concordance of SLRL with the MLS was only 59%, which is lower than that of the 92%, and 100% for UDS and AE in postspermatogonia cells, respectively. This finding has prompted the USEPA to favor UDS and AE over SLRL in the development of the agency testing scheme (Bentley et al., 1994).

## B.  Dose–Response Relationship

Dose–response studies are essential for the identification of genotoxic chemicals and the estimation of their "mutagenic potency." Although dose–response analyses are often included in genetic toxicology tests, the data are seldom, if ever, used beyond hazard identification. One reason is that regulatory risk assessment is based on low-dose chronic exposure, which is the usual condition for human exposure to chemicals. The doses used for genetic toxicology studies, especially for in vitro assays, are always very high, with the endpoint being the highest dose that causes severe cytotoxicity or creates an unphysiological condition (Brusick, 1986; Scott et al., 1991). For in vivo genetic toxicology tests, the doses are lower, but the high doses are still doses approaching lethal doses (greater than the median lethal dose [LD50] because of the shorter duration of the test). These high doses are not expected to be encountered in vivo in animals or humans before severe systemic toxicity or death occurs; however, response at the low doses in in vivo studies may be useful for dose–response assessment.

Correlation studies of mutagenicity between in vitro and in vivo assays, or between species, are possible if pharmacokinetic data are available. Simple pharmacokinetic parameters, such as chemical concentrations in the blood or in the target tissue, can be used as effective doses for extrapolation of mutagenicity to different test systems.

A second reason is that, although genotoxicity may lead to cancer or reproductive toxicity, the adverse effects of genotoxicity cannot be readily identified as clinical signs. The genotoxic data, in practice, are not used for cancer or reproductive risk assessment. Carcinogenicity and reproductive toxicity data are obtained from animal bioassays. Recent developments in germ cell mutation assays may provide a basis to justify germ cell mutation as a discrete endpoint for quantitative risk assessment (Waters and Nolan, 1994).

## C.  Exposure Assessment

The toxicity chemicals and their levels of exposure determine their hazard to public health. Current exposure assessment is based on the amount of chemicals in the environment, such as air, water, food, soil, and the amount of intake from such sources, based on human physiological parameters. Accurate measurements of exposures are not always possible. Genetic toxicology had not been used for exposure assessment until the development of molecular epidemiology. Most epidemiology studies use chemically modified cellular macromolecules, also known as biomarkers, to quantify chemical exposure. The most widely used biomarkers are DNA and protein adducts. These adducts can be detected by radioactive labeling, immunoassays, or high-performance liquid chromatographic (HPLC) methods. Quantification of adducts in exposed animals provides direct information on the amount of chemical, or its metabolites, in the target tissues.

DNA adducts have been used in molecular dosimetry studies of many carcinogens, including aflatoxin $B_1$ (Groopman et al., 1985), PAH (Perera et al., 1988), cisplatin (Reed et al., 1986),

8-methoxypsoralin (Santella, 1988), and styrene oxide (Liu et al., 1988). The reliability of adduct estimation is dependent on the sensitivity of the assay.

Molecular epidemiology studies also include conventional genotoxicity endpoints. Chromosomal aberrations have been studied in lymphocytes and in other cell types in workers exposed to industrial chemicals (Evans, 1982; Carrano and Moore, 1982). Micronuclei in lymphocytes were also studied in workers exposed to organic chemicals and metals (Hogstedt et al., 1983; Stich and Dunn, 1988). More recently, mutations at the *HGPRT* gene in human lymphocytes (Messing et al., 1986; O'Neill et al., 1987) and glycophorin A gene in human red blood cells (Jensen et al., 1986; Langlois et al., 1987) were studied in humans exposed to chemotherapeutic agents or radiation. Other markers, such as DNA breaks (Walles et al., 1988), unscheduled DNA synthesis (Pero et al., 1982), and oncogene activations have also been studied (Brandt-Rauf, 1988).

## D. Risk Characterization

Genetic toxicology has a major role in risk characterization of carcinogens for the estimation of cancer potency. *Cancer potency* is the slope of the dose–response curve of tumor induction. Since the dose–response of tumor induction at low doses cannot be demonstrated experimentally, a variety of mathematical models were proposed for high-dose to low-dose extrapolations (Crump et al., 1977; Moolgavkar and Venzon, 1979; Crump, 1981; Moolgavkar and Knudson, 1981; Anderson et al., 1982; Bogen, 1989). For genotoxic carcinogens, the linearized multistage model (Crump et al., 1977; Crump, 1981) is customarily used by regulatory agencies for the calculation of cancer potency and, in turn, the regulatory exposure levels (Anderson et al., 1983; CDHS, 1985). This model was constructed from the assumptions that carcinogenesis is a multistep process, and that the dose–response does not have a threshold dose below which carcinogenesis does not occur (see Figure 1). Limited DNA adduct dosimetry studies have shown that a linear dose–response may exist at low doses for aflatoxin $B_1$ (Buss et al., 1990; Choy, 1993), but similar data for most genotoxic carcinogens are not available.

As discussed earlier, a variety of mechanisms have been proposed for nongenotoxic carcinogenesis (Butterworth and Slaga, 1987). The dose–response for nongenotoxic carcinogens is considered to have a threshold dose below which carcinogenesis does not occur (see Figure 1). Risk assessment of nongenotoxic carcinogens, therefore, may be performed by the safety factor method, with an extra safety factor to account for carcinogenicity (CDHS, 1990). Risk analysis using the linearized multistage model always generates a more conservative estimate of carcinogenicity than the safety factor method which, in turn, results in more stringent regulatory standards. These regulatory standards have major implications to society, relative to public health and the economy for regulatory compliance.

## V. CONCLUSIONS

This chapter described the roles of genetic toxicology as related to regulatory risk assessment. Genetic toxicology is mostly used for hazard identification of mutagens and carcinogens. The validity of this approach is based on evidence that mutations are often associated with neoplastic transformation, and many carcinogens are mutagens. Once a carcinogen is identified, genetic toxicology is used to distinguish if the carcinogen is genotoxic or nongenotoxic, which in turn, determines the cancer risk assessment method for risk characterization.

As for the future, genetic toxicology is expected to develop along several directions. Continued developments of new test technology, such as the transgenic mouse assays, will undoubtedly provide new insight into the dose–response of in vivo mutagenesis and for comparative mutagenesis in target tissues. Incorporation of genetic toxicology tests into routine toxicology testes and pharmacokinetic studies will permit meaningful interpretation of genetic toxicological results related to metabolism, systemic toxicity, and carcinogenicity. Molecular studies on mutant DNA, DNA adducts, and DNA repair should provide new insights into the mechanism of chemical-specific mutagenesis and carcinogenesis. Finally, harmonization of regulatory guidelines will eliminate inconsistence in testing requirements, testing procedures, and data interpretations. Progress in these areas will increase the reliability of genetic toxicology in the assessment of genetic and cancer risks.

## REFERENCES

Allen, J. W., Bridges, B. A., Lyon, M. F., Moses, M. J., and Russell, L. B., eds. (1990). *Biology of Mammalian Germ Cell Mutagenesis,* Cold Spring Harbor Laboratory Press, Cold Spring Harbor, New York.

Ames, B.N. (1979). Identifying environmental chemicals causing mutations and cancer. *Science,* 204, 587–593.

Ames, B. N., Durston, W. E., Yamasaki, E., and Lee, F. D. (1973). Carcinogens are mutagens: A simple test system combining liver homogenates for activation and bacteria for detection. *Proc. Natl. Acad. Sci. USA,* 70, 2281–2285.

Ames, B. N., McCann, J., and Yamasaki, E. (1975). Methods for detecting carcinogens and mutagens with the *salmonella*/mammalian-microsome mutagenicity test. *Mutat. Res.,* 31, 347–364.

Anderson, E. L. and U.S. Environmental Protection Agency Carcinogen Assessment Group. (1983). Quantitative approaches in use to assess cancer risk. *Risk Anal.,* 3, 277–295.

Ashby, J. and Tennant, R. W. (1988). Chemical structure, salmonella mutagenicity and extent of carcinogenicity as indicators of genotoxic carcinogenesis among 222 chemicals tested in rodents by the U. S. NCI/NTP. *Mutat. Res.,* 204, 17–115.

Auletta, A. and Ashby, J. (1988). Workshop on the relationship between short-term test information and carcinogenicity; Williamsburg, Virginia, January 20–23, 1987. *Environ. Mol. Mutagen.,* 11, 135–145.

Auerbach, C. and Robson, J. M. (1946). Chemical production of mutations. *Nature,* 157, 302.

Barrett, J. C. (1987). A multistep model for neoplastic development: Role of genetic and epigenetic changes. In *Mechanisms of Environmental Carcinogenesis,* Vol. 2 (J. C. Barrett, ed.), CRC Press, Boca Raton, FL, pp. 117–126.

Bentley, K. S. and Working, P. K. (1988). Activity of germ-cell mutagens and nonmutagens in the rat spermatocyte UDS assay, *Mutat. Res.,* 203, 135–132.

Bentley, K. S., Sarrif, A. M., Cimino, M. C., and Auletta, A. E. (1994). Assessing the risk of heritable gene mutation in mammals: *Drosophila* sex-linked recessive lethal test and tests measuring DNA damage and repair in mammalian germ cells, *Environ. Mol. Mutagen.,* 23, 3–11.

Bogen, K. T. (1989). Cell proliferation kinetics and multistage cancer risk models, *JNCI,* 81, 267–277.

Boveri, T. H. (1929). *The Origin of Malignant Tumors,* Williams & Wilkins, Baltimore, MD.

Bradley, M. O. and Dysart, G. (1985). DNA single-strand breaks, double-strand breaks, and crosslinks in rat testicular germ cells: Measurement of their formation and repair by alkaline and neutral filter elution, *Cell. Biol. Toxicol.,* 1, 181–195.

Brandt-Rauf, P. W. (1988). New markers for monitoring occupational cancer: The example of oncogene proteins, *J. Occup. Med.,* 30, 399–404.

Brewen, J. G., Preston, R. J., and Gengozian, N. (1975). Analysis of x-ray-induced chromosomal translocation in human and marmoset spermatogonial stem cells, *Nature,* 253, 468–470.

Brusick, D. (1986). Genotoxicity effects in cultured mammalian cells produced by low pH treatment conditions and increased ion concentration, *Environ. Mutagen.,* 8, 879–886.

Brusick, D. (1987). *Principles of Genetic Toxicology,* 2nd ed., Plenum Press, New York.

Buss, P., Caviezel M., and Lutz, W. K. (1990). Linear dose–response relationship for DNA adducts in rat liver from chronic exposure to aflatoxin $B_1$, *Carcinogenesis,* 11, 2133–2135.

Butterworth, B. E. and Slaga, T. J. (1987). *Nongenotoxic Mechanisms of Carcinogenesis,* Cold Spring Harbor Laboratory Press, Cold Spring Harbor, New York.

Butterworth, B. E., Ashby, J., Bermudez, E., Casciano, D., Miralis, J., Probst, G., and Williams, G. M. (1987). A protocol and guide for the in vitro rat hepatocyte DNA-repair assay, *Mutat. Res.*, 189, 113–121.

Carrano, A. V. and Moore, D. H. (1982). The rationale and methodology for quantifying sister chromatic exchange frequency in humans. In *Mutagenicity: New Horizons in Genetic Toxicology* (J. A. Heddle, ed.), Academic Press, New York, pp. 267–304.

[CDHS] California Department of Health Services, (1985). *Guidelines for Chemical Carcinogen Risk Assessment and Their Scientific Rationale.* CDHS, Health and Welfare Agency, State of California.

[CDHS] California Department of Health Services, (1990). Intake level for butylated hydroxyanisole (BHA) for the purpose of Proposition 65. CDHS, Health and Welfare Agency, State of California.

Choy, W. N. (1993). A review of the dose–response induction of DNA adducts by aflatoxin $B_1$ and its implications to quantitative cancer risk assessment, *Mutat. Res.*, 296, 181–198.

Clive, D., McCuen, R., Spector, J. F. S., Piper C., and Mavournin, K. H. (1983). Specific gene mutations in L5178Y cells in culture: A report of the U. S. Environmental Protection Agency Gene-Tox Program, *Mutat Res.*, 115, 225–256.

Clive, D., Caspery, W., Kirby, P. E., Krehl, R., Moore, M., Mayo, J., and Oberly, T. J. (1987). Guide for performing the mouse lymphoma assay for mammalian cell mutagenicity, *Mutat. Res.*, 189, 143–156.

Cohen, S. M. and Ellwein L. (1990). Cell proliferation in carcinogenesis, *Science*, 249, 1007–1011.

Crump, K. S. (1981). An improved procedure for low-dose carcinogenic risk assessment from animal data, *J. Environ. Pathol. Toxicol.*, 52, 675–684.

Crump, K. S., Guess, H. A., and Deal, L. L. (1977). Confidence intervals and test of hypotheses concerning dose–response relations inferred from animal carcinogenicity data, *Biometrics*, 33, 436–451.

Evans, H. J. (1962). Chromosomal aberrations produced by ionizing radiation, *Int. Rev. Cytol.*, 13, 221–321.

Evans, H. J. (1982). Cytogenetic studies on industrial populations exposed to mutagens. In *Indicators of Genotoxic Exposure* (B. A. Bridge, B. E. Butterworth, and I. B. Weinstein, eds.), Banbury Report 19, Cold Spring Harbor Laboratory Press, Cold Spring Harbor, New York, pp. 325–340.

Galloway, S. M., Bloom, A. D., Resnick, M., Margolin, B. H., Nakamura, F., Archer, P., and Zeiger, E. (1985). Development of a standard protocol for in vitro cytogenetic testing with Chinese hamster ovary cells: Comparison of results for 22 compounds in two laboratories, *Environ. Mutagen.*, 7, 1–51.

Galloway, S. M., Armstrong, M. J., Reuben, C., Colman, S., Brown, B., Cannon, C., Bloom, A. D., Nakamura, F., Ahmed, M., Duk, S., Rimpo, J., Margolin, B. H., Resnick, M. A., Anderson, B., and Zeiger, E. (1987). Chromosome aberration and sister chromatid exchanges in Chinese hamster ovary cells: Evaluation of 108 chemicals, *Environ. Mol. Mutagen.*, 10, 1–109.

Glickman, B. W. and Gorelick, N. J., eds. (1993). Advanced technology. *Mutat. Res.*, 288, 181.

Gold, L. S., Slone, T. H., Stern, B. R., and Bernstein L. (1993). Comparison of target organs of carcinogenicity for mutagenic and non-mutagenic chemicals, *Mutat. Res.*, 286, 75–100.

Green, S., Auletta, A., Fabricant, J., Kapp, R., Manandhar, M., Sheu, C., Springer, J., and Whitfield, B. (1985). Current status of bioassays in genetic toxicology—the dominant lethal assay: A report of the U. S. Environmental Protection Agency Gene-Tox Program, *Mutat. Res.*, 154, 49–67.

Groopman, J. D. and Skipper, P. L. (1991). *Molecular Dosimetry and Human Cancer,* CRC Press, Boca Raton, FL.

Groopman, J. D., Donahue, P. R., Zhu, J., Chen, J., and Wogan, G. N. (1985). Aflatoxin metabolism in humans: Detection of metabolites and nucleic acid adducts in urine by affinity chromatography, *Proc. Natl. Acad. Sci. USA*, 82, 6492–6497.

Hogstedt, B., Akesson, B., Axell, K., Gullberg, B., Mitelman, F., Pero, R. W., Skerving, S., and Welinder, H. (1983). Increased frequency of lymphocyte micronuclei in workers producing reinforced polyester resin with low exposure to styrene, *Scand. J. Work Environ. Health*, 49, 271–276.

Hsie, A. W., Casciano, D. A., Couch, D. B., Krahn, D. F., O'Neill, J. P., and Whitfield, B. L. (1981). The use of Chinese hamster ovary cells to quantify specific locus mutation and to determine mutagenicity of chemicals: A report of the U. S. Environmental Protection Agency Gene-Tox Program, *Mutat. Res.*, 86, 193–214.

Ishidate, M., Jr., Harnois, M. C., and Sofuni, T. (1988). A comparative analysis of data on the clastogenicity of 951 chemical substances tested in mammalian cell cultures, *Mutat. Res.*, 195, 151–213.

[IARC] International Agency for Research on Cancer (1987a). *IARC Monographs on the Evaluation of Carcinogenic Risks to Humans, Genetic and Related Effects: An Updating of Selected IARC Monographs from Vols. 1–42.* Supplement 6. IARC, Lyon, France.

[IARC] International Agency for Research on Cancer (1987b). *IARC Monographs on the Evaluation of Carcinogenic Risks to Humans, Overall Evaluations of Carcinogenicity, An Updating of Selected IARC Monographs from Vols. 1–42.* Supplement 7, IARC, Lyon, France.

Jensen, R. H., Langlois, R. G., and Bigbee, W. L. (1987). Determination of somatic mutations in human erythrocytes by flow cytometry. In *Genetic Toxicology of Environmental Chemicals,* Part B: *Genetic Effects and Applied Mutagenesis* (C. Ramel, B. Lambert, and J. Magnusson, eds.), Alan R. Liss, New York, pp. 177–184.

Johnson, F. M. and Lewis, S. E. (1981). Electrophoretically detected germinal mutations induced in the mouse by ethylnitrosourea, *Proc. Natl. Acad. Sci. USA,* 78, 3138–3141.

Kern, S. E. and Vogelstein, B. (1991). Genetic alternations in colorectal tumors. In *Origins of Human Cancer* (J. Brugge, T. Curran, E. Harlow, and F. McCormick eds.), Cold Spring Harbor Laboratory Press, Cold Spring Harbor, New York, pp. 577–585.

Knudson, A. J. (1986). Genetics of human cancer. *Annu. Rev. Genet.,* 20, 231–251.

Knudson, A. G. (1993). Antioncogenes and human cancer, *Proc. Natl. Acad. Sci. USA,* 90, 11914–11921.

Knudson, A. G., Hethcote, H. W., and Brown, B. W. (1975). Mutation and childhood cancer. A probabilistic model for the incidence of retinoblastoma, *Proc. Natl. Acad. Sci. USA,* 72, 5116–5120.

Langlois, R. G., Bigbee, W. L., Kgoizumi, S., Nakamura, N., Bean, M. A., Akiyama, M., and Jensen, R. H. (1987). Evidence for increased somatic cell mutations at the glycophorin A locus in atom bomb survivors, *Science,* 236, 445–448.

Lee, W. R., Abrahamson, S., Valencia, R., von Halle, E. S., Wurgler, F. E., and Zimmering, S. (1983). The sex-linked recessive lethal test for mutagenesis in *Drosophila melanogaster, Mutat. Res.,* 123, 183–279.

Li, A. P. and Heflich, R. H. (1991). *Genetic Toxicology,* CRC Press, Boca Raton, FL. Liu, S. F., Rappaport, S. M., Pongracz, K., and Bodell, W. J. (1988). Detection of styrene oxide–DNA adducts in lymphocytes of a worker exposed to styrene. In *IARC, Method for Detecting DNA Damaging Agents in Humans: Applications in Cancer Epidemiology and Prevention* (H. Bartsch, K. Hemminki, and I. K. O'Neill, eds.), *IARC Sci. Publ.* 89, Lyon, France, pp. 217–222.

Littlefield, J. W. (1976). *Variation, Senescence, and Neoplasia in Culture Somatic Cells,* Harvard University Press, Cambridge, MA.

MacGregor, J. T., Heddle, J. A., Hite, M., Margolin, B. H., Ramel, C., Salamone, M. F., Tice, R. R., and Wild, D. (1987). Guidelines for the conduct of micronucleus assays in mammalian bone marrow erythrocytes, *Mutat. Res.,* 189, 103–112.

Maron, D. M. and Ames, B. N. (1983). Revised methods for the salmonella mutagenicity tests, *Mutat. Res.,* 113, 173–215.

McCann J., Choi, E., Yamasaki, E., and Ames, B. N. (1975). Detection of carcinogens as mutagens in the salmonella/microsome test: Assay of 300 chemicals, *Proc. Natl. Acad. Sci. USA,* 72, 5135–5139.

Messing, K., Siefert, A. M., and Bradley, W. E. C. (1986). In vivo mutant frequency of technicians professionally exposed to ionizing radiation. In *Monitoring of Occupational Genotoxicants* (M. Sorsa and H. Norppa, eds.), Alan R. Liss, New York, pp 87–97.

Mirsalis, J. C. and Butterworth, B. E. (1980). Detection of unschedule DNA synthesis in hepatocytes isolated from rats treated with genotoxic agents: An in vivo–in vitro assay for potential carcinogens and mutagens, *Carcinogenesis,* 1, 621–625.

Moolgavkar, S. and Venzon, D. (1979). Two-event models for carcinogenesis: Incidence curves for childhood and adult tumors, *Math. Biosci.,* 47, 55–77.

Moolgavkar, S. and Knudson, A. (1981). Mutation and cancer: A model for human carcinogenesis. *JNCI,* 66, 1037–1052.

O'Neill, J. P., McGinniss, M. J., Berman, J. K., Sullivan, L. M., Nicklas, J. A., and Albertini, R. J. (1987). Refinement of a T-lymphocyte cloning assay to quantify the in vivo thioguanine-resistant mutant frequency in humans, *Mutagenesis,* 2, 87–94.

Perera, F. P., Hemminki, K., Young, T. L., Brenner, D., Kelley, G., and Santella, R. M. (1988). Detection of polycyclic aromatic hydrocarbon–DNA adducts in white blood cells of foundry workers, *Cancer Res.,* 48, 2288–2291.

Pero, R. W., Bryngelsson, T., Widegren, B., Hogstedt, B., and Welinder, H. (1982). A reduced capacity for unscheduled DNA synthesis in lymphocytes from individuals exposed to propylene oxide and ethylene oxide, *Mutat. Res.,* 104, 193–200.

Preston, R. J., Au, W., Bender, M. A., Brewen, J. G., Carrano, A. V., Heddle, J. A., McFee, A. F., Wolff, S., and Wassom, J. A. (1981). Mammalian in vivo and in vitro cytogenetics assays: A report of the U. S. EPA Gene-Tox Program, *Mutat. Res.,* 87, 143–188.

Purchase, I. F. H., Longstaff, E., Ashby, J., Styles, J. A., Anderson, D., Lefevre, P. A., and Westwood, F. R. (1978). An evaluation of 6 short-term tests for detecting organic chemical carcinogens, *Br. J. Cancer,* 37, 873–903.

Randerath, K., Reddy, M. V., and Gupta, R. C. (1981). $^{32}$P-postlabeling test for DNA damage, *Proc. Natl. Acad. Sci. USA,* 78, 6126–6129.

Reed, E., Yuspa, S., Zwelling, L. A., Ozols, R. F., and Poirier, M. C. (1986). Quantitation of *cis*-diamminedichloroplatinum (II) (cisplatin)–DNA–intrastrand adducts in testicular and ovarian cancer patients receiving cisplatin chemotherapy, *J. Clin. Invest.,* 77, 545–550.

Russell, L. B., Hunsicker, P. R., Cacheiro, N. L. A., and Rinchik, E. M. (1992). Genetic, cytogenetic, and molecular analyses of mutations induced by melphalan demonstrate high frequencies of heritable deletions and other rearrangements from exposure of post spermatogonial stages of the mouse, *Proc. Natl. Acad. Sci. USA,* 89, 6182–6186.

Russell, L. B. (1994). Role of mouse germ-cell mutagenesis in understanding genetic risk and in generating mutations that are prime tools for studies in modern biology, *Environ. Mol. Mutagen,* 23 (Suppl. 24), 23–29.

Russell, W. L. (1951). X-ray-induced mutation in mice, *Cold Spring Harbor Symp. Quantit. Biol.,* 16, 327–336.

Santella, M., Yang, X. Y., De Leo, V., and Gasparro, F. P. (1988). Detection and quantification of 8-methoxypsoralen–DNA adducts. In *IARC Method for Detecting DNA Damaging Agents in Humans: Applications in Cancer Epidemiology and Prevention* (H. Bartsch, K. Hemminki, and I. K. O'Neill, eds.), *IARC Sci. Publ.* 89, Lyon, France, pp. 333–340.

Schmid, W. (1976). The micronucleus test for cytogenetic analysis. In *Chemical Mutagens: Principles and Methods for Their Detection,* Vol. 4 (A. Hollander, ed.), Plenum Press, New York, pp. 31–53.

Scott, D., Galloway, S. M., Marshall, R. R., Ishidate, M., Jr., Brusick, D., Ashby, J., and Myhr, B. C. (1991). Genotoxicity under extreme culture conditions. A report for ICPEMC task group 9, *Mutat. Res.,* 257, 147–204.

Sega, G. A. (1982). DNA repair in spermatocytes and spermatids of the mouse. In *Indicators of Genotoxic Exposure* (B. A. Bridge, B. E. Butterworth, and I. B. Weinstein, eds.), Cold Spring Harbor Laboratory Press, Cold Spring Harbor, New York, pp. 503–513.

Setchell, B. P. and Main, S. F. (1978). Drugs and the blood–testis barrier, *Environ. Health Prospect.,* 24, 61–64.

Shelby, M. D. (1994). Human germ cell mutagens, *Environ. Mol. Mutagen.,* 23 (Suppl. 24), 30–34.

Shelby, M. D. and Stasiewicz, S. (1984). Chemicals showing no evidence of carcinogenicity in long-term, two species rodent studies: The need for short-term test data, *Environ. Mutagen.,* 6, 871–878.

Shelby, M. D. and Zeiger, E. (1990). Activity of human carcinogens in the salmonella and rodent bone marrow cytogenetics test, *Mutat. Res.,* 234, 257–261.

Shelby, M. D., Bishop, J. B., Mason, J. M., and Tindall, K. R. (1993). Fertility, reproduction and genetic disease: Studies on the mutagenic effects of environmental agents on mammalian germ cells, *Environ. Health Perspect.,* 100, 283–291.

Skare, J. A. and Schrotel, K. R. (1985). Validation of an in vivo alkaline elution assay to detect DNA damage in rat testicular cells, *Environ. Mutgen.,* 7, 563–576.

Steinmetz, K. L., Green, C. E., Bakke, J. P., Spak, D. K., and Mirsalis, J. C. (1988). Induction of unscheduled DNA synthesis in primary cultures or rat, mouse, hamster, monkey, and human hepatocytes, *Mutat. Res.,* 206, 91–102.

Stich, H. F. and Dunn, B. P. (1988). DNA adducts, micronuclei and leukoplakias as intermediate endpoints in intervention trials. In *IARC, Method for Detecting DNA Damaging Agents in Humans: Applications in Cancer Epidemiology and Prevention* (H. Bartsch, K. Hemminki, and I. K. O'Neill, eds.), *IARC Sci. Publ.* 89, Lyon, France, pp. 137–145.

Tennant, R. W., Spalding, J. W., Stasiewicz, S., Caspary, W. D., Mason, J. M., and Resnick, M. A. (1987). Comparative evaluation of genetic toxicity patterns of carcinogens and noncarcinogens: Strategies for predictive use of short-term assays, *Environ. Health Perspect.,* 75, 87–95.

Tennant, R. W., Hansen, L., and Spalding, J. (1994). Gene manipulation and genetic toxicology, *Mutagenesis,* 9, 171–174.

[USEPA] United States Environmental Protection Agency (1986). *Guidelines for Mutagenic Risk Assessment, Fed. Reg.,* 51, 34006–34012.

[USFDA] United States Food and Drug Administration (1993). *Toxicological Principles for the Safety Assessment of Direct Food Additives and Color Additives Used in Food. "Redbook II."* Center for Food Safety and Applied Nutrition, Draft.

Volgelstein, B., Fearson, E. R., Hamilton, S. R., Kern, S. E., Preisinger, A. C., Leppert, M., Nakamura, Y., White, R., Smits, A. M. M., and Bos, J. L. (1988). Genetic alterations during colorectal-tumor development, *N. Engl. J. Med.,* 319, 525–529.

Walles, S. A. S., Norppa, H., Osterman-Golkar, S., and Maki-Paakkanen, J. (1988). Single-strand breaks in DNA of peripheral lymphocytes of styrene-exposed workers. In *IARC, Method for Detecting DNA Damaging Agents in Humans: Applications in Cancer Epidemiology and Prevention* (H. Bartsch, K. Hemminki, and I. K. O'Neill, eds.), *IARC Sci. Publ.* 89, Lyon, France, pp. 223–226.

Waters, M. D. and Nolan, C. (1994). Meeting report on the EC/US workshop on genetic risk assessment: Human genetic risks from exposure to chemicals focusing on the feasibility of a parallelogram approach, *Mutat. Res.,* 307, 411–424.

Working, P. K. and Butterworth, B. E. (1984). An assay to detect chemically induced DNA repair in rat spermatocytes, *Environ. Mutagen.,* 6, 273–286.

Zeiger, E., Haseman, J. K., Shelby, M. D., Margolin, B. H., and Tennant R. W. (1990). Evaluation of four in vitro genetic toxicity tests for predicting rodent carcinogenicity: Confirmation of earlier results with 41 additional chemicals, *Environ. Mol. Mutagen.,* 16, 1–14.

# 4

# Principles Underlying Developmental Toxicity

**John M. DeSesso**
*The MITRE Corporation*
*McLean, Virginia*

**Stephen B. Harris**
*Stephen B. Harris Group*
*San Diego, California*

## I. INTRODUCTION

Developmental toxicity in humans is a widespread problem. Approximately 250,000 infants (~7% of births) are born with birth defects in the United States each year (National Foundation, 1979). In addition, more than 560,000 pregnancies annually terminate in miscarriage, stillbirth, or infant death because of maldevelopment. Among liveborn infants who die by the age of four, 20% die as a result of congenital defects (Department of Health and Human Services, 1981). This makes birth defects the leading cause of death among children.

The causes of some birth defects have been traced to genetic transmission, chromosomal aberrations, and environmental factors, including ionizing irradiation, infections, maternal metabolic disease, and chemical substances (Table 1). Although drugs and chemicals account for no more than about 6% of birth defects some 18 chemical substances or classes of substances have been identified as proved human teratogens, (Table 2; Koren and Nulman, 1994), and approximately 1000 chemicals (out of ~2800 tested) have elicited some measure of developmental toxicity in at least one species of laboratory animal (Schardein et al., 1985). Since (1) the etiology of more than two-thirds of all congenital defects is unknown, and (2) humans are exposed to more than 65,000 chemicals for which there are some toxicity data (National Research Council, 1984), it behooves us to perform developmental toxicity testing on chemicals that are likely to come into broad contact with women of reproductive years.

## II. BRIEF HISTORICAL PERSPECTIVE

Despite the foregoing statistics, the problems of birth defects and other adverse outcomes of pregnancy are not new to the industrial era. Congenital malformations have fascinated and awed man for centuries, stretching back before the brief span of recorded history. Neolithic statues found in Turkey (Warkany, 1971), Stone Age rock drawings discovered in Oceania (Brodsky,

**Table 1**   Causes of Congenital Defects in
Humans (Estimates as a Percentage of Total)

| | |
|---|---|
| Genetic transmission | 20% |
| Chromosomal aberrations | 3–5% |
| Environmental agents | |
|     Ionizing Radiation | 1% |
|     Infections | 2–3% |
|     Maternal metabolic imbalance | 1–2% |
|     Drugs and chemicals | 4–6% |
| Combinations and interactions | ? |
| Unknown | 65–70% |

*Source:* Wilson (1977a).

**Table 2**   Drugs and Chemicals: Proved Human Teratogens

| Drug, chemical, or chemical class | Selected adverse effects in offspring |
|---|---|
| Alcohol | Fetal alcohol syndrome: mental retardation, microcephaly, short up-turned nose, micrognathia, hypoplastic philtrum |
| Alkylating agents (e.g., busulfan, chlorambucil, cyclophosphamide, mechlorethamine) | Growth retardation, cleft palate, agenesis of kidney, malformations of digits, cardiac defects |
| Antimetabolite agents (e.g., aminopterin, azauridine, cytarabine, 5-FU, 6-MP, methotrexate) | Hydrocephalus, meningoencephalocele, growth retardation, eye and ear malformations, cleft palate, micrognathia |
| Carbamazepine | Increased risk for neural tube defects (NTDs) |
| Carbon monoxide | Mental retardation, microcephaly |
| Coumadins | Fetal warfarin syndrome: brachydactyly, malformed eyes and ears, microcephaly, hydrocephalus, mental retardation |
| Diethylstilbestrol (DES) | Female offspring: vaginal or cervical adenocarcinoma |
| | Male offspring: hypogonadism, diminished spermatogenesis |
| Lead | Lower scores in developmental tests |
| Lithium carbonate | Ebstein's anomaly of tricuspid valve |
| Methylmercury, mercuric sulfide | Microcephaly, eye malformations, mental retardation |
| PCBs | Stillbirth; irritated/swollen gums, hyperpigmentation ("cola" staining); delayed postnatal development |
| Penicillamine | Hyperelastosis of skin |
| Phenytoin | Fetal hydantoin syndrome: inner epicanthal folds, hypertelorism, low set or abnormal ears, microcephaly and mental retardation, growth deficiency |
| Systemic retinoids (isotretinoin, etretinate) | Spontaneous abortions; deformities of face, limbs; heart defects |
| Trimethadione | Growth retardation, cardiac anomalies, cleft palate and lip |
| Thalidomide | Phocomelia, amelia, heart defects, deafness, microtia, anotia |
| Tetracycline | Staining of deciduous teeth, destruction of enamel |
| Valproic acid | Spina bifida with meningomyelocele, microcephaly |

*Source:* Koren and Nulman (1994).

1943), and prehistoric Peruvian pottery (Saxen and Rapola, 1969) attest to primitive man's interests in these phenomena all over the world. Early written records of congenital malformations both described them and conjectured as to their significance. The Chaldeans of ancient Babylon believed they could augur the future from celestial and terrestrial omens, including oddities seen at birth (Leix, 1940). In 1894, Ballantyne published the translation of a Chaldean tablet that catalogued 62 human malformations and the appropriate prophecy for each. In contrast to the Chaldeans' belief that malformations could help foretell the future, the ancient Hebrews believed that congenital malformations were manifestations of God's wrath and were sent as a punishment for evil deeds committed in the past (Landauer, 1962).

Early scientific theories concerning the etiology of congenital malformations were grouped into 13 categories by Ambrose Paré in 1573. Paré included hereditary influences, the mechanical effects of a narrow uterus, the will of God, the work of the devil, and hybridization between animals and humans among the possible causes (Persaud, 1970; Clegg, 1971). Although the consideration of animal–human hybridization may seem unlikely today, it was both considered plausible and dealt with seriously by the public and legal communities of Europe and America. As late as 1643 in Copenhagen, a young woman who had delivered a child "with the head of a cat" (probable anencephaly) was burned alive after being convicted of having had bestial relations (Bartholin, 1661). In 1642 in New Haven Colony (Connecticut), George Spencer, a common farm worker "of lewd spirit" was similarly convicted of having allegedly indulged himself in the pleasure of a sow who subsequently gave birth to a cyclopic piglet (Hoadly, 1857). The description of the piglet included the likening of its proboscis to "a man's instrument of generation." The evidence against Spencer, who had a cataract in one eye, was (1) that he had worked on the farm from which the sow had been obtained (although not at the critical period of her pregnancy), and (2) the piglet's sole eye was cataractous. The court found Spencer guilty of bestiality, which it declared to be a capital offense, and both Spencer and the sow were executed.

Even though nonscientific explanations for congenital malformation continued to circulate among the rather naive lay public, serious scientists persevered in their search for credible causes. In 1651, William Harvey offered a new scientific explanation for congenital malformations based upon experimental observation: the arrest of embryonic development at specific loci. Unfortunately, Harvey's theory did not gain ascendancy for another 150 years (Warkany, 1959).

The basis for the modern study of teratology was laid by Geoffrey St. Hilaire, the Elder, who described and classified most of the known human abnormalities during the 1820s (Barrow, 1971). Between 1855 and 1891, Dareste performed early experimental studies. He demonstrated that influences such as hyperthermia, hypothermia, or anoxia could cause congenital malformations in chicken embryos (Hickey, 1953). Because the mammalian prenatal maternal–offspring relationship is so different from that of avian and reptilian animal models, many of Dareste's contemporaries did not consider his experiments to be relevant to the human condition. Rather, they believed that mammalian embryos were protected from untoward environmental effects.

During the period from 1920 to 1940, it was demonstrated that mammalian teratogenesis could be induced environmentally by x-irradiation (Goldstein and Murphy, 1929; Job et al., 1935) and by dietary deficiency (Hale, 1933, 1935; Warkany and Nelson, 1940). In 1941, Gregg identified the rubella virus as a human teratogen. These significant observations established the susceptibility of mammalian embryos, including humans, to environmental influences. In spite of these scientific advances, most of the medical community and virtually the entire lay public remained apathetic about the possible susceptibility of humans to environmentally induced birth defects. They firmly believed that human embryos existed in a privileged site that was safeguarded by the uterus and the "placental barrier" (Fig. 1). It took the thalidomide tragedy of

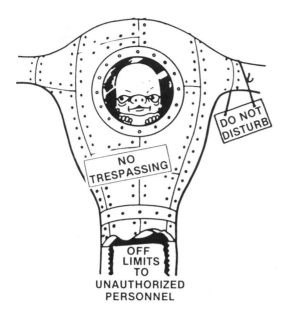

**Figure 1**  A conceptualization of the protected environment of the human embryo. Until the occurrence of the thalidomide tragedy, many scientists and most of the public believed that the human uterine contents were protected from environmental insults. (After a cartoon designed by Dr. James G. Wilson.)

the late 1950s and early 1960s (Lenz, 1961; McBride, 1961) to shatter their complacency. Thalidomide was a seemingly harmless sedative–hypnotic drug that, when taken during early pregnancy, caused the severe malformation of an estimated 10,000 babies. The results of this painful experience were to arouse the awareness of the public to the human embryos' vulnerability to environmental insult, to amplify research efforts into the causes of birth defects, and to prompt the design of developmental toxicity safety tests for substances with which humans were expected to come into contact.

## III.  PRINCIPLES OF DEVELOPMENTAL TOXICOLOGY

During the ensuing decades, considerable headway has been made in identifying agents that cause birth defects in experimental animals and in understanding the scientific principles that govern how environmental agents adversely impinge on mammalian embryos. These scientific principles were first enunciated by Wilson (1959, 1965, 1973, 1977b) and have been discussed, augmented, and modified by others (Langman, 1969; Saxen and Rapola, 1969; Brent, 1976; Poswillo, 1976; Harbison, 1980; Beckman and Brent, 1994).

### A.  Definitions

*1.  Teratology (Developmental Toxicology)*

The science that emerged from these principles is teratology or, more inclusively, developmental toxicology. *Teratology* is concerned with the study of the causes, mechanisms, and manifestations of adverse outcomes of pregnancy. The four major manifestations of developmental toxicology include the death, structural malformation, altered growth, or functional deficits of offspring. A biologically significant increase in any one of the four manifestations of developmental toxicity caused by the environmental exposure to a test substance is a reason for concern, because it indicates that the test agent may impair development, giving rise to a developmental hazard.

### 2. Mechanism

The means by which developmental toxicants interact with the affected embryo is termed its mechanism of action. *Mechanisms* have been defined at many levels of biological organization (e.g., cellular, subcellular, biochemical, and molecular). All levels of organization in an embryo are important for its continued development and are potentially vulnerable to teratogenic attack. However, not all agent-induced changes in embryos result in developmental toxicity. Thus, we believe a working definition of a teratogenic mechanism is necessary. An agent's mechanism of developmental toxicity is the fundamental physical or chemical process that sets in motion a perturbed sequence of developmental events that result in one of the four manifestations of developmental toxicity. Because an agent may interact with an embryo in more than one way, it is possible for an agent to have more than a single mechanism of developmental toxicity. This has been shown for even simple molecules, such as hydroxyurea, which interferes with uterine bloodflow, initiates free radical reactions in embryonic cells, and inhibits embryonic DNA synthesis (Millicovsky et al., 1980a,b, 1981; DeSesso et al., 1979, 1990, 1994; Scott et al., 1971).

Embryonic development is an intricate phenomenon that involves numerous simultaneous processes that must occur in specific sequences and at particular times in gestation. For instance, the information required to direct differentiation (e.g., manufacture of cellular structural proteins, receptor molecules, and extracellular matrix molecules) is contained within the genetic material of the cell's nucleus, whereas the information required to maintain developmental schedules is usually from environmental stimuli (e.g., inducer molecules, as well as permissive and instructive signal molecules). Since both the embryo's genetic material and its environment are instrumental in successful development, it should not be surprising that abnormalities in either an embryo's genetic material (i.e., mutations) or its environment can lead to developmental toxicity. Although the thrust of the remainder of this chapter will be primarily with adverse environmental influences that can alter development, a few brief comments about normal variations in the genome of developing organisms are in order.

## B. Embryonic Genome

### 1. Embryonic Susceptibility

In simplest terms, the genome of the conceptus is important because it controls the development of the organism. It is the genome that ultimately determines what tissues are being laid down, their metabolic enzyme complements, and therefore, the overall inherent susceptibility of the embryo to any exogenous agent at any given time of development. Because healthy development of an organism requires timely interactions between (normal) environmental factors and genes as they are expressed and repressed throughout development (Edelman, 1988), it is not surprising that if exogenous agents gain access to the embryo, they may disrupt the appropriate environmental factor–gene interactions resulting in developmental errors. Thus, the susceptibility of an embryo to an adverse environmental factor depends both on the expressed genome at the time of the exposure and the manner in which the genome interacts with the adverse environmental factor. Moreover, because the commonly used laboratory animals produce more than one offspring per litter, each with its own genome and developmental schedule, it is not unusual to observe intralitter variation in response to a teratogen. Typically, offspring in an affected litter may be malformed, dead (resorbed), growth retarded, or normal.

### 2. Species Differences

*Species* are groups of related and physically similar individuals that share common attributes and nearly identical genomes. Just as the genome of an individual embryo controls its development and determines its susceptibility to environmental agents, so too the genotypic makeup of a given species determines the likelihood of an agent to adversely affect the development of embryos of that species. It can be inferred that embryos of some species may be unaffected by environmental agents that induce predictable, consistent developmental toxicity in others. For example, mice are usually more susceptible to cleft palate induced by steroid hormones (i.e., cortisone and progesterone) than are rats. Another example is that humans and other higher primates are more susceptible to limb malformations caused by thalidomide exposure than are rats or mice.

Within a given species, there are subsets (strains) of that species that are genetically more homogeneous relative to other groups of the same species. That these strains may react differently to environmental agents should not be surprising. Thus, there are strain differences in susceptibility to environmental factors, such that different strains of mice exposed to cortisone exhibit different frequencies of cleft palate (Fraser, 1965).

## C. Embryonic (Gestational) Stage

The age of the embryo at the time of exposure to the environmental agent is an important determinant of whether the agent will induce developmental toxicity and which manifestation is produced. Embryonic susceptibility to developmental toxicants varies greatly during the course of gestation (Fig. 2). During the period between fertilization of the ovum, but before implantation

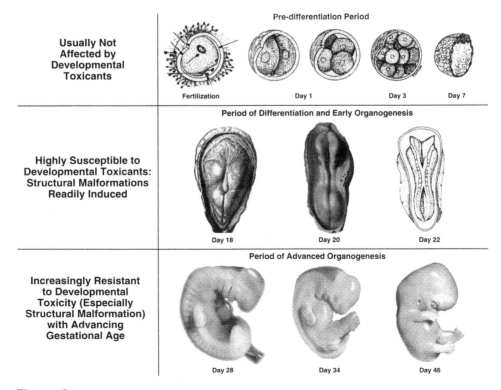

**Figure 2** A schematic illustration of various stages of human embryonic development to depict the embryo's changes in sensitivity to developmental toxicants at different times in gestation. (After Wilson, 1965.)

of the blastocyst into the uterine wall, the embryo is usually resistant to the induction of malformations by environmental agents. Embryos at this stage are small, comprising no more than 100 cells or so. In addition, the cells are morphologically similar, having the same susceptibilities and metabolic needs, but not yet having begun differentiation into specific tissues. Insults to the early embryo during this period would be likely to affect all cells uniformly. Severe effects that could kill cells are likely to kill all of the cells, or to kill so many that an embryolethal effect is produced. In the event that some cells survived, the insult is likely to retard growth, rather than cause malformations, because the cells of the embryo at this early stage are all able to differentiate into any embryonic tissue, although recent experiments exposing females to mutagens within hours of mating have produced malformed young in a few instances (Generoso et al., 1988).

During the early embryonic period, the germ layers form, cells begin to differentiate, and early organ development begins. This period is characterized by maximal susceptibility to teratogenic insult. During the time when organs are first laid down (*organogenesis*), most organs undergo their "critical period," during which they are most susceptible to damage by environmental agents. Differentiation and early organogenesis begin near the time of implantation. Their total duration differs from species to species, but it is positively correlated with the length of the gestational period for the particular species (Table 3). Although a developmentally toxic insult may cause a malformation during this time, if the insult is great enough, embryonic death may also occur.

To help understand the effect of embryonic age on developmental toxicity, two concepts related to embryonic development will be explained. The two concepts relate to the potential fate of a given cell (embryonic cellular potency) and its state of differentiation. Briefly, *embryonic cellular potency* is the total range of developmental possibilities (i.e., all possible adult tissues) that an embryonic cell is capable of becoming under any conditions. In contrast, *cellular differentiation* is a progressive, continuous process whereby an embryonic cell attains the intrinsic properties and functions that characterize a particular adult tissue. As depicted in Figure 3, an embryonic cell's potency and its state of differentiation are reciprocal. Cells in the early stages of development, such as those of the morula, are not differentiated; they are

**Table 3** Comparative Gestational Milestones and Developmental Toxicity Testing Schedules for Mammals

| Species | Gestational milestones[a] | | | | Developmental toxicity-testing schedules[a] | |
|---|---|---|---|---|---|---|
| | A[b] Implantation ends | B Differentiation ends | C Organogenesis ends | D Parturition | Exposure period | Cesarean section |
| Hamster | 4.5–5 | 8 | 13 | 16 | 5–14 | 16 |
| Mouse | 7 | 9 | 15 | 19–20 | 6–15 | 18 |
| Rat | 5–6 | 10 | 15 | 21–22 | 6–15 | 21 |
| Rabbit | 7.5 | 9 | 18 | 31–33 | 6–18 or 7–19 | 29 |
| Guinea Pig | 6 | 14.5 | ~29 | 64–68 | 6–30 | 60 |
| Monkey | 9 | 21 | ~44–45 | 166 | 9–45 or 10–50 | 100 |
| Human | 6–7 | 21 | ~50–56 | 266 | NA[c] | NA |

[a]In gestational days; day of confirmed mating = gestational day 0.
[b]Capital letters refer to milestones on the time line shown in Figure 4.
[c]NA, not applicable.

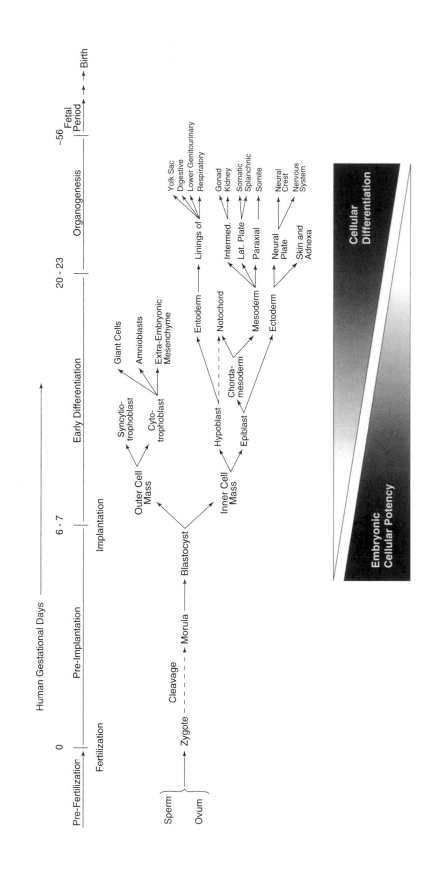

morphologically similar and have the potential to become nearly any type of embryonic cell. As development proceeds, however, developmental decisions are made concerning the fate of each cell. Thus, at later periods of gestation, the cells have become dissimilar from one another; one cell may have become an endoderm cell that will give rise to an alveolar cell lining the lung, the other may be a mesoderm cell that will give rise to a cell in the proximal convoluted tubule of the kidney. The possible ultimate fates available to the endoderm cell are not the same as those of the mesoderm cell. Thus, potency of the cells have declined; but their state of differentiation has increased, as they now look different from one another and perform different cellular functions.

Developmental toxicants generally affect only a percentage of the cells in an embryo. A single developmentally toxic insult early in gestation (when cells have higher potency) has the opportunity to affect cells that can eventually give rise to more adult tissues than a similar dose administered to an older embryo the cells of which (1) are more differentiated, (2) have made more developmental decisions, and (3) therefore, can contribute to fewer adult tissues. In general, the more developmental decisions that have been made, the less severe the effect of the developmental toxicant. Thus, from the end of the early embryonic period (when the embryo undergoes advanced organogenesis and the rudiments of the organ systems have been formed) continuing throughout the fetal period, the incidence of fetal deaths and malformations decline. However, malformations of late-developing organ systems and functional deficits can occur. For example, the central nervous and urogenital systems do not develop completely until after birth. Thus, it is possible to cause damage to these systems, particularly cellular and functional maturational impairment. Figure 4 is a generalized depiction of the extent of offspring sensitivity to developmental toxicants with advancing gestational age.

In human development, the period of organogenesis, with its maximum susceptibility to teratogenesis, occurs from day 20 to 55 of gestation (see Table 3). In the rat and mouse, differentiation and organogenesis occur from day 6 to 15 of gestation, and in the rabbit they occur from day 6 to 18 of gestation. In animal teratogenesis studies, knowing the period of organogenesis of the test species is crucial so that test agents may be administered during the time of maximum teratogenic susceptibility.

Usually, experimental administration of test substances in developmental toxicity safety tests begins after embryos have implanted into the uterine wall and development of early placentae have commenced. Depending on the test species, as many as 8 days may elapse between fertilization of ova in the upper female reproductive tract and implantation of the zygote (see Table 3). If the test species is either a mouse or a rabbit, exposure to the test substance is initiated before implantation is completed, because mouse and rabbit embryos begin differentiation before they implant.

The foregoing discussion notwithstanding, the developmental stage of an embryo at the time an agent is given to the pregnant female does not always determine the time of exposure to the embryo. Ritter et al., (1973) showed that cytosine arabinoside palmitate (a slow-release form of cytarabine [cytosine arabinoside]) implanted intraperitoneally on gestational day 12, exerted its

---

**Figure 3** A diagram of a conceptualized synopsis of development. The flow of time is from left to right. The developmental decisions of tissues as they differentiate are designated by diverging arrows. Note that early differentiation coincides with the time of implantation. Susceptibility to developmentally toxic agents is greatest during the periods of early differentiation and organogenesis. Note that as time elapses, developmental decisions are made, and early tissues differentiate. Early cells (e.g., cells of the inner cell mass) are morphologically similar and have the potential to become nearly any type of embryonic tissue. As the cells increase in differentiation, their embryonic cellular potency decreases.

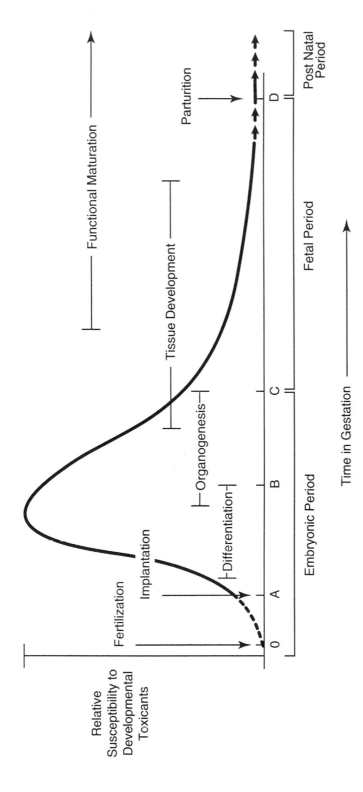

**Figure 4** A diagram that illustrates the relationship between the relative teratogenic sensitivity of embryos and increasing gestational age. The dashed line between fertilization and implantation represents the limited number of agents that have been reported to cause effects in term offspring when administered at this time. Susceptibility increases rapidly after implantation and peaks during the period of organogenesis. While susceptibility declines during the late embryonic and fetal periods, alterations in late-forming organs and tissues (e.g., the brain) can occur during these periods. Letters designate times in gestation that correlate with the gestational milestones for individual species listed in Table 3. (After Wilson, 1973.)

developmentally toxic effect 48–72 h after exposure, whereas intraperitoneal administration of cytarabine produced the same embryonic effects within 23–29 h. These results led them to conclude that the susceptibility of an embryo depends on its developmental stage at the time when an agent is effective. Later studies showed that much longer intervals could transpire between the time of administration of a test compound and its effect. In humans, women whose exposure to lipid-soluble substances had been terminated for an extended period before impregnation have given birth to malformed infants (Lammer, 1988). Presumably, this is due to the sequestering of the compound in the body's lipid stores and its prolonged elimination half-life leading to (1) sustained low concentrations in maternal blood and (2) a delayed time of exposure to the embryo that coincided with release of the material from her lipid stores.

## D. Dose or Embryonic Exposure

### 1. *Dose–Response*

Functional deficits are usually not manifested until some time after weaning. Consequently, the endpoints that are monitored in most developmental toxicity safety tests are fetal death, malformation, and growth retardation. In addition, not all embryos will respond identically to a given dose of a test agent, because there are differences between embryos within litters relative to stage of development, genetic makeup, and position related to uterine blood flow. Within a given litter, there are typically some dead fetuses, some malformed fetuses, some growth-retarded fetuses, in addition to some normal individuals. Because the different endpoints (death, malformation, or growth retardation) may be caused by different mechanisms of the test agent, graphs of the dose–response curves for each endpoint frequently do not overlap (Neubert et al., 1980). If, however, all of the endpoints of developmental toxicity are combined as a positive response, then the quantitative relationship between increasing embryonic dose and the manifestations of developmental toxicity increase in frequency and severity from no-effect doses to a maximally effective (often totally a lethal) dose. The graph of the relationship exhibits the shape of a typical dose–response curve (Fig. 5). Typically, the slope of the dose–response curve is steep. It lies between lower doses that fail to elicit fetal effects and higher doses that kill the embryos.

The purpose of performing a developmental toxicity safety test is to establish a no-observable adverse effect level (NOAEL). Figure 5 depicts a hypothetical dose–response curve constructed from data for five dose groups (designated by triangles). The NOAEL is the higher of the two doses that produced no effects in offspring. The lowest dose that caused a significant effect is the lowest-observable adverse effect level (LOAEL). Because the dose–response curve intersects the abscissa (dose scale) at a point greater than zero, it is said to exhibit a threshold (see next section), and there is a safe level of exposure to developmental toxicants. This is in contrast with genotoxic carcinogens, which have dose–response curves that intersect the dose–response curve at the origin, and for which there is some probability of risk at any dose.

Infectious agents (e.g., viruses) do not exhibit typical dose–response relationships. Even a small "exposure" to a virus can result in symptoms of disease in the female and developmental toxicity in offspring. The reason for this is that such agents can reproduce within the pregnant animal, placenta, or embryo, thereby increasing the exposure of the offspring.

### 2. *Threshold*

For developmentally toxic effects (including functional deficits, growth retardation, structural malformation, and death) an embryonic dose exists below which the incidence among treated litters is neither statistically nor biologically different from incidence in untreated litters. This dose is termed the *threshold dose*. Wilson (1973) has asserted that every developmental toxicant

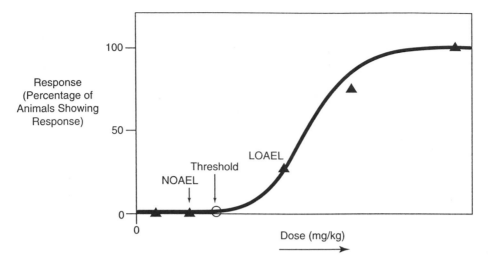

**Figure 5**  Depiction of a hypothetical dose–response curve. Data points are represented by triangles. The no-observable adverse effect level (NOAEL) is the highest dose that caused no significant effects (over background) in offspring. The lowest-observable adverse effect level (LOAEL) is the lowest dose that caused significant effects (over background) in offspring. The threshold is the *calculated* lowest point on the dose–response curve at which a dose of test agent would elicit changes in offspring; doses below the threshold will not cause deleterious effects in offspring and should be considered safe.

that has been examined under well-designed test conditions has demonstrated a threshold. That developmental toxicants exhibit a threshold is an extremely important concept from the stand-point of risk assessment, because it means that a safe exposure level exists for the agent in question. This stands in stark contrast with the situation presented by genotoxic cancer-causing agents, which are thought to possess the risk of initiating tumorigenesis at extremely low doses and for which an absolutely safe exposure level does not exist (see discussions in Brent, 1986a; Johnson, 1986).

It must be stressed that determining a NOAEL does not identify the threshold for develop-mental toxicity. On the dose–response curve for the agent tested (see Fig. 5), the threshold is higher than the NOAEL, but lower than the LOAEL. Determining a NOAEL simply establishes that, under the conditions of the study, no adverse effects were detected at the dose level(s) used. Depending on the spacing between the doses selected for testing, the NOAEL may be an order of magnitude smaller than the LOAEL and, therefore, is often a poor estimate of the true threshold dose. Because the use of point estimates, like the NOAEL, as surrogates for the developmental toxicity threshold has limitations for human health risk assessment, the U.S. Environmental Protection Agency (EPA, 1991a) is presently evaluating other techniques for quantifying dose–response relationships, such as the benchmark dose method (Crump, 1984; Kimmel and Zenick, 1993).

One of the challenges that faces the real-world interpretation of developmental toxicity results occurs when an embryo is exposed to two or more agents that, when acting together, have a greater effect than either agent acting alone. This situation exemplifies the notion of *synergism.* As noted by Fraser (1977), the existence of threshold doses in developmental toxicity can lead to difficulties when interpreting the results of a situation wherein two substances are applied at a low dose during the embryo's critical period. If both agents are given at high subthreshold doses (i.e., doses approaching the threshold), and if the agents share the same mechanism or biochemical site of action, they may appear to be acting synergistically when they are not. The reason that the agents appear to act synergistically is that if they are given separately, neither exerts a deleterious effect (because they are both below their respective thresholds). However, when given together, their threshold is exceeded, but it is merely by an additive mechanism. Consequently, situations involving exposure to multiple agents must be interpreted with caution.

### 3. Modifiers of Embryonic Dose

*Pharmacokinetics.* The pregnant mammal is a unique experimental system that differs greatly from the usual biological systems studied in toxicology experiments because the pregnant mammal is composed of three interdependent, functional units: the pregnant dam, the placenta, and the embryo. From a pharmacokinetic perspective, the pregnant female is not the same organism as a somewhat heavy nonpregnant female. Numerous changes occur in the pregnant female with time over the course of gestation (see Page et al., 1976; Koren, 1994). These include increases in renal function (resulting in augmented clearance rates for substances excreted by the kidney), decreased gastrointestinal transit time (leading to increased likelihood of absorption of poorly absorbed agents), increased total body water (affecting the concentration-dependent transfer of agents), and decreased serum protein binding (altering the kinetics of substances that are usually bound to albumin).

In animals that produce multiple young, each individual embryo has its own placenta attached to the uterine wall of the dam. Therefore, any test substance that is administered to the pregnant dam must traverse not only her vascular system, but also one of several placentae to reach the vascular system of a particular embryo. This means that all embryos of a given litter share a common maternal environment, but each embryo maintains its own placenta and internal (embryonic) milieu. Each of these functional units (pregnant female, placentae, or embryos) may be affected by the test agents that traverse it, and each functional unit has the opportunity to alter the distribution of substances that pass through it. Depending on the metabolic activities of individual placentae and embryos and the position of these relative to uterine blood flow, the embryos of a given litter may not be exposed to the same substances or similar amounts of those substances.

*Placental Transport.* The apposition of maternal to embryonic tissues for the purpose of physiological exchange is the placenta. In primates (including humans), this transient organ comprises tissues and vasculature from the chorion and allantois and, therefore, is termed the chorioallantoic placenta (Ramsey, 1982). The placenta acts as a lung, kidney, and digestive tract for the embryo. It is the site of transfer for nutrients, gases, metabolic waste, and foreign substances.

Since the placenta is the interface between the embryo and the maternal environment, it is the site of absorption, transfer, and metabolism of nutrients and foreign compounds. As recently as the 1950s, many scientists believed that the placenta was a barrier that prevented the movement of all unwanted, foreign xenobiotic substances into the embryo. The mammalian embryo (especially the human embryo) was believed to exist in a "privileged" environment that was protected from unwanted environmental assaults. More recently, the placenta has been conceptualized as a sieve that retards or blocks the transfer of molecules that weigh more than 1000 D, are highly charged or polar, are hydrophilic, or are strongly bound to (serum) proteins. Currently, however, it is recognized that a wide diversity of mechanisms exist for the transport of molecules through the placenta (Miller et al., 1976, 1983; Miller, 1986; Wild, 1981). The transport mechanisms include both simple diffusion for smaller molecules (relative molecular mass [$M_v$] of less than 1000 D, but especially those under 600 D such as urea, oxygen, carbon dioxide) and carrier-mediated transport (Mirkin, 1973; Miller, 1986). The carrier-mediated mechanisms include active transport (e.g., sodium and potassium, calcium, amino acids) facilitated diffusion (e.g., D-glucose), and receptor-mediated endocytosis (e.g., immunoglobulins, vitamin $B_{12}$, transferrin). Under some situations, depending on the amount of agent presented to the placenta, more than one mechanism may be available to the agent (Miller et al., 1983). Thus, given the multiplicity of available transport mechanisms, when any substance is presented to the placenta, the question concerning entry into the embryo should not be whether or not placental transfer occurs, but rather, by which mechanism(s) and at what rate transfer will occur.

Rodents and lagomorphs (e.g., rabbit and guinea pig), with their relatively short gestational periods, differ from primates in that an early placenta develops from the yolk sac (the inverted yolk sac placenta) and is later replaced by the chorioallantoic placenta. Although the yolk sac placenta experiences reduced importance after the establishment of the chorioallantoic placenta, it does continue to function until relatively late in gestation. Consequently, there remain distinct differences in placental structure and function between humans and typical laboratory species. These differences complicate the interspecies extrapolation of developmental toxicology data.

*Biotransformation.* When compounds that are foreign to an organism enter its body, the foreign substances (xenobiotics) are chemically transformed by various enzymes that are present in the organism to prepare the xenobiotic for excretion (Neal, 1980). Xenobiotics that are lipophilic (more soluble in lipidlike materials than in aqueous media) tend to accumulate in the body and may perturb cellular functions, leading to a toxic effect. A subset of biotransformation enzymes metabolizes the xenobiotic substance (e.g., the test agent) to make it more water-soluble and, hence, more readily excreted. This situation becomes considerably more complicated in pregnant mammals, because each part of the maternal–placental–embryonic unit is capable of metabolizing xenobiotics that enter it. Consequently, each of the three units may be exposed not only to the test agent, but also to biotransformation products of the other units. This means that the proximate developmental toxicant may not actually be the agent that was administered to the pregnant female, and the dose–response curve using the maternally administered dose of test agent, is only a surrogate for the true dose–response curve of the embryonic dose of the proximate developmental toxicant versus developmentally toxic effect. It is assumed that the true dose–response curve is proportional to the one based on maternal exposure.

Maternal Metabolism. As an adult organism, the pregnant female is capable of biotransforming test agents according to any of the appropriate detoxification mechanisms available to her species (see the following for discussions: Williams, 1959; Testa and Jenner, 1976; Jakoby et al., 1982). The time of exposure during her gestation will also affect her ability to biotransform or excrete the test agent. For instance, as mentioned in Sec. III.D.3 on pharmacokinetics, normal physiological changes of pregnancy will increase plasma and extracellular volumes, increase gastrointestinal absorption, and enhance renal excretion. These changes will affect the kinetics of biotransformation. In addition, the maternal liver demonstrates increased clearance rates of some drugs during early and middle pregnancy (see Page et al., 1976; Koren, 1994). Consequently, the pregnant female differs metabolically from the nonpregnant female adult and, depending on the time in gestation, from other pregnant females as well.

Placental Metabolism. In addition to transferring molecules to the embryo, the placenta may also metabolize substances, whether they are xenobiotic compounds or nutrients. In the cow and sheep, the trophoblast of the placenta converts maternally delivered glucose to fructose which, in turn, is transferred to the embryo. In those species, an intravenous dose of glucose to the pregnant animal causes a dramatic rise in fetal blood levels of fructose, rather than fetal blood levels of glucose. This illustrates both species differences among placentae and that the placentae are not merely sieves.

Placentae also contain various enzymes (at low concentrations that change with gestational age) that are capable of metabolizing xenobiotics (Battaglia, 1981; Juchau, 1972, 1980, 1982;

Juchau and Rettie, 1986). These enzymes include reductases, epoxide hydrases, cytochrome P-450 monooxygenases, glucuronidases, and others. The enzymes are not present at all times during gestation, but make their appearances at different times. The presence (or absence) of these enzymes reflects the genome of the embryo, rather than that of the mother. Placental enzymes can be induced by inducers of monooxygenases, such as phenobarbitol, benzo[a]pyrene, and 3-methylcholanthrene. In addition, the formation of reactive intermediates from xenobiotic compounds by placental enzyme preparations has been demonstrated in vitro.

Embryonic Metabolism. Throughout gestation, developing embryos continually change morphologically, biochemically, and metabolically. The response of a younger embryo (e.g., gestational day 9) to a given dose of a test agent may differ from the response of an older embryo (e.g., gestational day 14) to an identical dose, because the metabolic and biochemical capabilities (i.e., the detoxification as well as catabolic and anabolic enzyme complements) of the two ages of the same embryo are not the same. Thus, different ages of the same embryo may handle and react to the same amount of test substance as if they were different organisms.

## E. Risk Assessment

### 1. Maternal Toxicity

The pregnant female provides her developing embryo(s) with a physical environment, nutrients, and a mechanism for eliminating metabolic waste. In as much as the physiological status of the dam affects her ability to provide those requirements for the embryo(s), it should be no surprise that factors that compromise her physiological state can affect the well-being of the embryo(s). Thus, the health status of the pregnant dam (see discussion in DeSesso, 1987) as well as environmental stress (Chernoff et al., 1987; Schardein, 1987) may affect her offspring. Test agent-induced toxicity in the dam may cause indirect effects in her offspring. This means that, although developmental toxicity is often described as an independent effect, it can be intimately tied to maternal toxicity. When there is significant maternal toxicity, it is often difficult to distinguish effects mediated through toxicity in the mother from those caused by direct action of the test agent within the embryo itself (Khera, 1985, 1987). Therefore, it is important to (1) minimize extraneous environmental factors that could affect the health of the dams and possibly compromise the healthy outcome of pregnancy; and (2) utilize a range of doses that includes a high dose that causes maternal toxicity.

Given a knowledge of the physiology of the maternal–placental–embryonic complex, it should not be surprising that for compounds that are toxic to adults, there is a likelihood that it could also be toxic to embryos. Consequently, if a dose of a compound is high enough to elicit toxicity in a pregnant female, then it is biologically plausible that the compound will also produce effects in offspring. This may mean that the compound itself simultaneously exerts effects in both the maternal organism and her offspring. Because maternal toxicity also exerts nonspecific effects on developing offspring, it is important to identify a NOAEL for developmental toxicity safety tests in the absence of maternal toxicity, if possible.

Those agents of greatest concern are those that cause severe developmental effects in offspring, but no adverse effects in the pregnant female. Methylmercury and thalidomide are examples of this type of dangerous human developmental toxicant.

### 2. Predictive Value of Animal Findings

The four major developmental toxicity endpoints do not necessarily share the same underlying mechanism. This means that their dose–response curves are often nonlinear. Moreover, as the dose of test agent increases, one endpoint (e.g., death of the offspring) may preclude the manifestation of the others.

The predictive value of teratogenicity tests in animals for inferring human risk is not clear-cut (Kalter, 1965). The induction of a particular developmentally adverse effect in one animal species does not predict the same effect in another species (including humans). Whereas virtually every known human teratogen is teratogenic in at least one laboratory species, roughly 71% of substances that have been correlated with human no-adverse developmental effects are positive in at least one test animal (Frankos, 1985). Even though the amount of human data is generally limited and the shape of the human dose–response curve for developmental toxicity is unknown, the lack of concordance between animal and human studies means that the predictability of a single animal study is unknown. Thus, although an adequately designed, positive animal teratology study *suggests* the possibility of risk to humans, it cannot *predict* whether or not that substance will cause developmental toxicity in humans. Nevertheless, because animals do respond to known human teratogens, a biologically significant increase in any of the major endpoints in a developmental toxicity study is a concern for risk assessment purposes, and that concern is heightened when a given test agent causes developmentally adverse effects in more than one test species.

### 3. Establishment of Human Teratogenicity

Determination of whether an environmental agent causes developmental toxicity in humans is a difficult task. Animal studies are useful in elucidating the mechanism of action for known human developmental toxicants and for alerting regulators and the public to suspect agents that might have the potential to cause human developmental toxicity. Animal studies, however, are not able to predict human effects because interspecies extrapolations cannot be performed with certainty. Consequently, most human developmental toxicants have been discovered by vigilant physicians and biomedical scientists. The process involves the tentative identification of a relationship between exposure to an environmental agent and an adverse outcome of pregnancy, usually in a case report. Subsequent epidemiological studies are used to analyze the incidence and trends of the particular adverse outcome to understand whether a causal relationship is plausible. Brent (1986b) has established several criteria that strengthen the causal relationship between human exposure to an environmental agent and developmental toxicity. The criteria are summarized below:

1.  Well-designed epidemiology studies consistently demonstrate that exposure to a given agent is associated with increased incidence of a particular developmentally toxic effect or set of developmentally toxic effects.
2.  For widespread exposures, secular trend data support the relationship between the exposures in humans and the incidence of the developmentally toxic effect or set of developmentally toxic effects.
3.  An animal model is (or can be) developed that mimics the human findings at doses that cause neither maternal toxicity nor reduced consumption of food or water.
4.  The developmentally toxic effects increase with increasing doses of the environmental agent.
5.  The mechanism(s) underlying the developmentally toxic effects are plausible and do not contradict the scientific principles of biology.

Note that none of the criteria individually prove the human teratogenesis of an agent, but the more of the criteria that apply to the situation, the stronger is the argument for a causal relationship.

## IV. CONCLUSIONS

Teratology or, more broadly, developmental toxicology, investigates the causes, mechanisms, and effects of adverse pregnancy outcomes including congenital malformations, growth perturbations, functional deficits, or death of offspring. Environmental agents are estimated to cause 8–12% of human congenital defects, although only 18 drugs, chemicals, or chemical classes have been positively identified as human teratogens. In experimental animals, over 1000 test agents have elicited developmental toxicity in at least one laboratory species. Environmental agents that induce aberrant development follow several basic principles that determine the extent and type of adverse effect. The concepts that are important to developing the principles include the embryonic genome; embryonic (gestational) stage; and embryonic exposure or dose, including the existence of a threshold and modifiers of embryonic dose (pharmacokinetics, placental transport, and biotransformation by mother, placenta or embryo). Continued investigation of environmental developmental toxicants is important because it will lead us to an understanding of the mechanisms of developmental toxicity that may enable us to prevent, ameliorate, or perhaps reverse developmental toxicities from all causes.

## ACKNOWLEDGMENT

Supported in part by MITRE Sponsored Research Project 9587C.

## REFERENCES

Ballantyne, J. W. (1894). The teratological records of Chaldea, *Teratologia,* 1, 127.

Bartholin, T. (1661). *Thomae Bartholini Historarium Anatomicarum et Medicarum Raiorum Centuria V et VI,* Hafniae (sumptibus P. Hauboldi) (cited in Landauer, 1962).

Barrow, M. V. (1971). A brief history of teratology to the early 20th century, *Teratology,* 4, 119–130.

Battaglia, F. (1981). Metabolism of the placenta: Its physiologic applications. In *Placental Transport,* Mead Johnson Symposium on Perinatal Medicine and Developmental Medicine, No. 18, Mead Johnson & Co., Evansville, IN, pp. 9–13.

Beckman, D. A. and Brent, R. L. (1994). Basic principles of teratology. In *Medicine of the Fetus and Mother* (E. A. Reece, J. C. Hobbins, M. J. Mahoney, and R. H. Petrie, eds.), J. B. Lippincott, Philadelphia, pp. 293–299.

Brent, R. L. (1976). Environmental factors: Miscellaneous. In *Prevention of Embryonic, Fetal and Perinatal Disease* (R. L. Brent and M. I. Harris, eds.), DHEW Publication NIH 76, Bethesda, MD, pp. 211–220.

Brent, R. L. (1986a). Definition of a teratogen and the relationship of teratogenicity to carcinogenicity, *Teratology,* 34, 359–360.

Brent, R. L. (1986b). Evaluating the alleged teratogenicity of environmental agents, *Clin. Perinatol.,* 13, 615–648.

Brodsky, I. (1943). Congenital abnormalities, teratology and embryology: Some evidence of primitive man's knowledge as expressed in art and lore in Oceania, *Med. J. Aust.,* 1, 417–420.

Chernoff, N., Kavlock, R. J., Beyer, P. E., and Miller, D. (1987). The potential relationship of maternal toxicity, general stress, and fetal outcome, *Teratogenesis Carcinog. Mutagen.,* 7, 241–253.

Clegg, D. J. (1971). Teratology, *Annu. Rev. Pharmacol.,* 11, 409–424.

Crump, K. S. (1984). A new method for determining allowable daily intakes, *Fundam. Appl. Toxicol.,* 4, 854–871.

Department of Health and Human Services (1981). *Child Health and Human Development: An Overview and Strategy for a Five Year Plan,* NIH Publication 82-2303, Bethesda, MD.

DeSesso, J. M. (1979). Cell death and free radicals: A mechanism for hydroxyurea teratogenesis, *Med. Hypotheses,* 5, 937–951.

DeSesso, J. M. (1987). Maternal factors in developmental toxicity, *Teratogenesis Carcinog. Mutagen.,* 7, 225–240.

DeSesso, J. M. and Goeringer, G. C. (1990). The nature of the embryo–protective interaction of propyl gallate with hydroxyurea, *Reprod. Toxicol.,* 4, 145–152.

DeSesso, J. M., Scialli, A. R., and Goeringer, G. C. (1994), D-Mannitol, a specific hydroxyl free radical scavenger, reduces the developmental toxicity of hydroxyurea in rabbits, *Teratology,* 49, 248–259.

Edelman, G. (1988). *Topobiology: An Introduction to Molecular Embryology,* Basic Books, New York.

Frankos, V. H. (1985). FDA perspectives on the use of teratology data for human risk assessment. *Fundam. Appl. Toxicol.,* 5, 615–625.

Fraser, F. C. (1965). Some genetic aspects of teratology. In *Teratology: Principles and Techniques* (J. G. Wilson and J. Warkany, eds.), University of Chicago Press, Chicago, pp. 21–38.

Fraser, F. C. (1977). Interactions and multiple causes. In *Handbook of Teratology,* Vol. I (J. G. Wilson and F. C. Fraser, eds.), Plenum Press, New York, pp. 445–459.

Generoso, W. M., Rutledge, J. C., Cain, K. T., Hughes, L. A., and Downing, D. J. (1988). Mutagen-induced fetal anomalies and death following treatment of females within hours after mating, *Mutat. Res.,* 199, 175–181.

Goldstein, L. and Murphy, D. P. (1929). Etiology of the ill-health in children born after maternal pelvic irradiation, *Am. J. Roentgenol. Radiat. Ther.,* 22, 322–331.

Gregg, N. M. (1941). Congenital cataract following German measles in mothers, *Trans. Ophth. Soc. Austr.,* 3, 35–46.

Hale, F. (1933). Pigs born without eyeballs, *J. Heredit,* 24, 105–106.

Hale, F. (1935). The relation of vitamin A to anophthalmos in pigs, *Am. J. Ophthalmol.,* 18, 1087–1093.

Harbison, R. D. (1980). Teratogens. In *Casarett and Doull's Toxicology,* 2nd ed. (J. Doull, C. D. Klaassen, and M. O. Amdur, eds.), Macmillan Publishing, New York, pp. 158–175.

Hickey, M. F. (1953). Genes and mermaids: Changing theories of the causation of congenital abnormalities, *Med. J. Aust.,* 1, 649–667.

Hoadly, C. J. (1857). *Records of the Colony and Plantation of New Haven from 1638 to 1649,* Case Tiffany & Co., (cited in Landauer, 1962).

Jakoby, W. B., Bend, J. R., and Caldwell, J. (1982). *Metabolic Basis of Detoxication,* Academic Press, New York.

Job, T. T., Leibold, G. L., and Fitzmaurice, H. A. (1935). Biological effects of roentgen rays. The determination of critical periods in mammalian development with X-rays, *Am. J. Anat.,* 56, 97–117.

Johnson, E. M. (1986). False positive/false negatives in developmental toxicology and teratology, *Teratology,* 34, 361–362.

Juchau, M. R. (1972). Mechanisms of drug biotransformation reactions in the placenta, *Fed. Proc.,* 31, 48–51.

Juchau, M. R. (1972). Drug biotransformation in the placenta, *Pharmacol. Ther.,* 8, 501–524.

Juchau, M. R. (1982). The role of the placenta in developmental toxicology. In *Developmental Toxicology* (K. Snell, ed.), Praeger, New York, pp. 187–210.

Juchau, M. R. and Rettie, A. E. (1986). The metabolic role of the placenta. In *Drug and Chemical Action in Pregnancy: Pharmacologic and Toxicologic Principles* (S. Fabro and A. R. Scialli, eds.), Marcel Dekker, New York, pp. 153–182.

Kalter, H. (1965). Experimental investigation of teratogenic action, *Ann. N. Y. Acad. Sci.,* 123, 287–294.

Khera, K. S. (1985). Maternal toxicity: A possible etiological factor in embryo-fetal deaths and fetal malformations of rodent–rabbit species, *Teratology,* 31, 129–153.

Khera, K. S. (1987). Maternal toxicity in humans and animals: Effects on fetal development and criteria for detection, *Teratogenesis Carcinog. Mutagen.,* 7, 287–295.

Kimmel, C. A. and Zenick, H. (1993). Alternatives to the NOAEL/uncertainty factors (UF) approach for quantitative noncancer risk assessment, *Fundam. Appl. Toxicol.,* 20, 7–9.

Koren, G. (1994). Changes in drug disposition in pregnancy and their clinical implications. In *Maternal–Fetal Toxicology,* 2nd ed. (G. Koren, ed.), Marcel Dekker, New York, pp. 3–13.

Koren, G. and Nulman, I. (1994). Teratogenic drugs and chemicals in humans. In *Maternal–Fetal Toxicology,* 2nd ed. (G. Koren, ed.), Marcel Dekker, New York, pp. 33–48.

Lammer, E. J. (1988). A phenocopy of the retinoic acid embryopathy following maternal use of etretinate that ended one year before conception, *Teratology,* 37, 472.

Landauer, W. (1962). Hybridization between animals and man as a cause of congenital malformations, *Arch. Anat.,* 44, 155–164.

Langman, J. (1969). Congenital malformations and their causes. In *Medical Embryology,* 2nd ed. (J. Langman), Williams & Wilkins, Baltimore, pp. 84–106.

Leix, A. (1940). Babylonian medicine, *Ciba Symp.,* 2, 663–690.

Lenz, W. (1961). Kindliche missbildungen nach medikament wahrend der Draviditat? *Deutsch. Med. Wochenschr.,* 86, 2555–2586.

McBride, W. G. (1961). Thalidomide and congenital abnormalities, *Lancet,* 2, 1358.

Miller, R. K. (1986). Placental transfer and function: The interface for drugs and chemicals in the conceptus. In *Drug and Chemical Action in Pregnancy: Pharmacologic and Toxicologic Principles* (S. Fabro and A. R. Scialli, eds.), Marcel Dekker, New York, pp. 123–152.

Miller, R. K., Koszalka, T. R., and Brent, R. L. (1976). Transport mechanisms for molecules across placental membranes. In *Cell Surface Reviews* (G. Poste and G. Nicholson, eds.), Elsevier/North Holland, Amsterdam, pp. 145–332.

Miller, R. K., Ng, W. W., and Levin, A. A. (1983). The placenta: Relevance to toxicology. In *Reproductive and Developmental Toxicity of Metals* (T. Clarkson, G. Nordberg, and P. Sager, eds.), Plenum Press, New York, pp. 569–605.

Millicovsky, G. and DeSesso, J. M. (1980). Cardiovascular alterations in rabbit embryos in situ after a teratogenic dose of hydroxyurea: An in vitro microscopic study, *Teratology,* 22, 115–124.

Millicovsky, G. and DeSesso, J. M. (1980). Uterine versus umbilical vascular clamping: Differential effects on the developing embryo, *Teratology,* 22, 335–343.

Millicovksy, G., DeSesso, J. M., Clark, K. E., and Kleinman, L. I. (1981). Effects of hydroxyurea on maternal hemodynamics during pregnancy. A maternally mediated mechanism of embryotoxicity, *Am. J. Obstet. Gynecol.,* 140, 747–752.

Mirkin, B. L. (1973). Maternal and fetal distribution of drugs in pregnancy, *Clin. Pharmacol. Ther.,* 14, 643–647.

National Foundation (1979). Facts 1979, National Foundation/March of Dimes, White Plains, New York.

National Research Council (1984). *Toxicity Testing: Strategies to Determine Needs and Priorities,* National Academy of Science, Washington, DC.

Neal, R. A. (1980). Metabolism of toxic substances. In *Casarett and Doull's Toxicology, 2nd ed.* (J. Doull, C. D. Klaassen, and M. O. Amdur, eds.), Macmillan Publishing, New York, pp. 56–69.

Neubert, D., Barrach, H. J., and Merker, H. J. (1980). Drug-induced damage to the embryo or fetus: Molecular and multilateral approach to prenatal toxicology, *Curr. Top. Pathol.,* 69, 241–331.

Page, E. W., Villee, C. A., and Villee, D. B. (1976). Physiologic adjustments in pregnancy. In *Human Reproduction, 2nd ed.,* W. B. Saunders, Philadelphia, pp. 251–268.

Persaud, T. V. N. (1970). Congenital malformations: From Hippocrates to thalidomide, *West Indian Med. J.,* 19, 240–246.

Poswillo, D. (1976). Mechanisms and pathogenesis of malformation, *Br. Med. J.,* 32, 59–64.

Ramsey, E. M. (1982). *The Placenta: Human and Animal,* Praeger, New York.

Ritter, E. J., Scott, W. J., and Wilson, J. G. (1973). Relationship of temporal patterns of cell death and development to malformations in the rat limb. Possible mechanisms of teratogenesis with inhibitors of DNA synthesis, *Teratology,* 7, 219–226.

Saxen, L. and Rapola, J. (1969). *Congenital Defects,* Holt, Rinehart and Winston, New York.

Schardein, J. L., Schwartz, B. B., and Kenel, M. F. (1985). Species sensitivity and prediction of teratogenic potential, *Environ. Health Perspect.,* 61, 55–62.

Schardein, J. L. (1987). Approaches to defining the relationship of maternal and developmental toxicity, *Teratogenesis Carcinog. Mutagen.*, 7, 255–271.

Scott, W. J., Ritter, E. J., and Wilson, J. G. (1971). DNA synthesis inhibition and cell death associated with hydroxyurea teratogenesis in rat embryos, *Dev. Biol.*, 26, 306–315.

Testa, B. and Jenner, P. (1976). *Drug Metabolism: Chemical and Biochemical Aspects*, Marcel Dekker, New York.

Warkany, J. (1959). Congenital malformations in the past, *J. Chronic Dis.*, 10, 84–96.

Warkany, J. (1971). *Congenital Malformations: Notes and Comments*, Year Book Medical Publishers, Chicago.

Warkany, J. and Nelson, R. C. (1940). Appearance of skeletal abnormalities in the offspring of rats reared on a deficient diet, *Science*, 92, 383–384.

Wild, A. E. (1981). Endocytic mechanisms of protein transfer across the placenta, *Placenta*, 1, 165–186.

Williams, R. T. (1959). *Detoxication Mechanisms, 2nd ed.*, Chapman & Hall, London.

Wilson, J. G. (1959). Experimental studies on congenital malformations. *J. Chronic Dis.*, 10, 111–130.

Wilson, J. G. (1965). Embryologic considerations in teratology, *Ann. N. Y. Acad. Sci.*, 123, 219–227.

Wilson, J. G. (1973). *Environment and Birth Defects*, Academic Press, New York.

Wilson, J. G. (1977a). Teratogenic effects of environmental chemicals, *Fed. Proc.*, 36, 1698–1703.

Wilson, J. G. (1977b). Current status of teratology: General principles and mechanisms derived from animal studies. In *Handbook of Teratology*, Vol. 1 (J. G. Wilson and, F. C. Fraser, eds.), Plenum Press, New York, pp. 47–75.

# 5
# Principles of Neurotoxicity

**I. K. Ho**
*University of Mississippi Medical Center*
*Jackson, Mississippi*

**Anna M. Fan**
*California Environmental Protection Agency*
*Berkeley, California*

## I. INTRODUCTION

*Neurotoxicity* is defined as "any adverse effect on the structure or function of the central and/or peripheral nervous system related to exposure to a chemical substance" (USEPA, 1987; U. S. Congress, Office of Technology Assessment, 1990). Any chemical substance that exerts neurotoxicity is a neurotoxicant. It is estimated that among the 70,000 chemicals being used in commerce (National Research Council, 1992), a large number are known to be neurotoxicants. These do not include chemicals used as therapeutic drugs or found in natural sources. Twenty-eight percent of the chemicals that have been substantially used in American industries were indicated to be potential neurotoxicants (Anger, 1984).

Neurotoxic effects of a chemical in vivo are usually produced when the target site within the nervous system is exposed to a sufficient amount of the chemical or its toxic metabolite for a duration of time that is sufficient to induce biological changes. These may be seen as changes in behavior, biochemistry, physiology, morphology, and pharmacology.

There are several special considerations that should be given to the assessment of adverse effects on the nervous system, compared with other body organs or systems. First, the nervous system controls all physiological functions of the body, including those of the cardiovascular, digestive, or respiratory systems. Second, neurons in the brain are formed before birth and cannot be regenerated, as can other cellular components. Third, the interconnections among neurons within a nervous pathway or among different pathways and other organs are very complex and sophisticated. All these contribute to the difficulties in predicting the nature of neurotoxicity that may be induced by a neurotoxicant and in delineating the site and mechanisms of action of a neurotoxicant.

The Congress of the United States has designated the 1990s as the "Decade of the Brain" (U. S. Congress, Office of Technology Assessment, 1990). Neurological disorders are among the most frequently encountered diseases (U. S. Congress, Office of Technology Assessment, 1990).

Neurotoxicity from exposure to chemicals is emerging as an endpoint for risk assessment of potentially toxic substances (USEPA, 1993). This chapter provides general background on how neurotoxicity may be induced when humans or animals are exposed to neurotoxicants.

## II. CLASSIFICATION OF NEUROTOXICANTS

There is currently no unified system established for classifying neurotoxicants, although several classifications have been proposed (Biereley et al., 1971; Brucher, 1967; Malamud, 1963; Norton, 1986; Scholz, 1953; Windle, 1963). Most textbooks of toxicology or neurotoxicology usually classify neurotoxicants based on multiple considerations, such as functional use and chemical structure (pesticides: inorganic compounds, pyrethroids, chlorinated hydrocarbons, organophosphates, and carbamates, among others), chemical property (heavy metals, solvents), physical property (gases, vapors, corrosives), effects or neurotoxic endpoints (convulsants, depressants, substances of abuse), and source (natural, semisynthetic, and synthetic products). Table 1 gives examples of neurotoxicants classified under some of these categories.

## III. SPECIFICITY OF NEUROTOXICANTS

*Neurotoxicants* are considered to be agents that produce neurotoxicity by direct actions on the structure or function of the central nervous system or peripheral nervous system, or both. A chemical that exerts indirect consequence secondary to the effect induced by acting on other organs should not be considered a neurotoxicant. For example, carcinogens, such as benzo[*a*]pyrene, aflatoxins, and dimethylnitrosamine induced cancers that could make patients exhibit some degree of behavioral abnormality because of severe sickness. However, these compounds themselves are not considered to be neurotoxicants.

Environmental chemicals, such as organophosphates and carbamate pesticides, alcohols, lead, and mercury, are neurotoxicants as listed in Table 1. They are known to directly affect the structure or function of the nervous system. However, the effects of neurotoxic agents are not specific only to the nervous system and, depending on the extent of exposure, neurotoxicants can also affect other organs or systems. Even for neurotoxicants with relatively well-known mechanisms of action, there is still a lack of specificity. For example, chlorpromazine, an antipsychotic agent, is believed to be a dopamine receptor antagonist, for which the therapeutic rationale is based. This compound also acts on $\alpha_1$- and $\alpha_2$-adrenergic receptors, histamine $1(H_1)$ receptors, serotonin $2(5\text{-}HT_2)$ receptors, and muscarinic cholinergic receptors. This is why significant adverse reactions and toxic side effects always accompany the use of this agent. Central nervous system stimulants, such as amphetamines and cocaine, are known to interfere with monoamines (norepinephrine, dopamine, and serotonin). Methylmercury also produces renal toxicity at exposures higher than those associated with neurotoxicity (WHO, 1990). Benzene causes leukemia in addition to CNS depression (Hume and Ho, 1994). Cholinersterase-inhibiting pesticides are often known to produce other biological responses (Hayes and Laws, 1991). The complexity of the nervous system, the many potential endpoints that may be affected, the sensitivity of some neurological endpoints, the difficulties in detecting them methodologically, and the potential for masking such effects by other toxicological responses, all make the identification of neurotoxicity of chemicals a complicated task.

## IV. STRUCTURE AND FUNCTION OF THE NERVOUS SYSTEM

The nervous system comprises the central nervous system (CNS) and peripheral nervous system (PNS). The CNS consists of the brain and spinal cord, whereas the PNS consists of the autonomic, sympathetic, and parasympathetic nervous systems. The PNS communicates neuronal transmission between the spinal cord and peripheral organs, such as the heart, muscles, and glands.

A simplified diagram of neuronal structures is illustrated in Figure 1. The major function of the nervous system is to handle neuronal transmissions. This function is carried out by two major types of cells in the nervous systems: neurons and glial cells. Neurons are responsible for neuronal transmissions. The glial cells support and protect neurons by providing nutrition, structural support, and protection and insulation (such as myelin sheath). It is obvious that any chemical agent that interferes with nonneuronal processes, such as maintaining integrity of the cell structures, may indirectly affect neuronal processes and produce neurotoxicity. Examples are the chemicals that disturb neuronal energy metabolism and the synthetic and degradative pathways, such as carbohydrates, lipids, nucleic acids, and proteins. These processes are essential for maintaining the primary functions of the cells and their suborganelles (nucleus, mitochondria, endoplastic reticulum, Golgi apparatus, among others).

The information transfer and processing by neurons are achieved by electrical currents flowing across neuronal membranes, and chemical transmission occurs at the synaptic junctions between neurons. Although there are different morphologically distinctive types of neurons (e.g., unipolar, pyramidal, bipolar, and multipolar), a neuron generally consists of the cell body, axon, dendrites, and nerve endings (terminals). The cell body contains the organelles responsible for the synthesis of macromolecules necessary for the metabolism of chemicals called neurotransmitters, which are essential for neuronal transmission and cellular maintenance. The axon is mainly responsible for transport of macromolecules and precursors from the cell body to the nerve endings for the synthesis and maintenance of neurotransmitters. Another major function of the axon is transporting action potentials down toward the nerve endings for the initiation of chemical transmission. The output of information takes place at nerve endings. The synthesis of small molecular weight neurotransmitters (e.g., acetylcholine, biogenic amines, amino acid neurotransmitters) also occurs at the nerve endings. A specialized contact zone with a gap of 300–400 Å, called synapse, connects a presynaptic nerve ending and the postsynaptic site of another neuron. The synapse consists of pre- and postsynaptic membranes, and the gap is called the synaptic cleft. Dendrites usually receive and integrate information, but some also function similarly to the nerve endings that contain mitochondria and neurotransmitters.

In general, neurotransmitters are synthesized at the presynaptic sites of the nerve endings. The precursor and synthetic machinery of a neurotransmitter would travel down to the ending from the cell body through microtubules in the axon. After synthesis is completed, the neurotransmitter is stored in synaptic vesicles. On stimulation of the nerve, the neurotransmitter is released. When it is released into the synaptic cleft, it can bind to postsynaptic receptors. After the interaction of the neurotransmitter with the receptors, the reuptake process into the presynaptic site, or degradation at the postsynaptic site of the neurotransmitter will occur to inactivate the action of the released neurotransmitter. The neurotransmitter that is taken back to the presynaptic site can be either metabolized or restored in vesicles. When receptors recognize the neurotransmitter, a conformational change of the receptor protein occurs, which results in transmembrane signaling and the induction of intracellular responses. For more detailed knowledge on structure and function of the nervous system, refer to the book, *Biochemical Basis of Neuropharmacology,* by Cooper et al. (1991).

## V. SITES OF NEUROTOXICANT ACTION

It is clear that neurotoxicants could act on presynaptic sites of neurotransmitters, such as those for synthesis, storage, release, reuptake, autoreceptors, and metabolism. They could also act on

**Table 1** Examples of Various Classes of Neurotoxicants

| Classes | Neurotoxic signs and symptoms | Possible biochemical actions |
|---|---|---|
| Insecticides (according to chemical structures) | | |
| Organophosphorus compounds | | |
| Malathion Parathion Fenthion Dimpylate Paraoxon | Headache, dizziness, weakness, incoordination, muscle twitching, tremor, nausea, abdominal cramps, diarrhea and sweating, salivation, tearing, blurred vision, pulmonary edema, incontinence, unconsciousness, convulsion, and respiratory depression. Chronic exposure may cause weakness, anorexia, and malaise. | Irreversible inhibition of cholinesterases |
| Carbamates | | |
| Aldicarb Benthiocarb Carbofuran Ethiofencarb Formetanate | Similar to those of organophosphorus compounds cited above. | Reversible inhibition of cholinesterases |
| Organochlorines | | |
| Aldrin Chlordane Chlordecone DDT Dieldrin Endrin Lindane | Convulsions, hyperesthesia and paresthesia of the face and extremities, headache, dizziness, nausea, vomiting, incoordination, tremor, and mental confusion | Affecting $Na^+$ channels? or inhibiting $Na^+$, $K^+$–ATPase? |
| Pyrethroids, type II | | |
| Allethrin Permethrin | Tremor and behavioral hyperexcitability | Blocking $Na^+$ channels Antagonists of $GABA_A$ receptors. |

| | | |
|---|---|---|
| Additive for gasoline<br>Trio-o-cresyl phosphate (TOCP) | Polyneuritis | Inhibition of neuropathy target enzyme (neurotoxic esterase, NTE)<br>Peripheral neuropathy |
| Organic solvents<br>Benzene | CNS depression characterized by headache, nausea, insomnia, agitation, stupor, coma, and convulsions. Chronic exposure may cause hematotoxicity, fatal aplastic anemia, leukemia, etc. | Unknown |
| Methanol | CNS depression characterized by headache, vertigo, severe upper abdominal pain, blurred vision, slow shallow breathing, coma, and death. It may cause optic neuritis and permanent blindness. | Unknown |
| Natural products<br>Stimulants or convulsants<br>Strychnine | Convulsions | Antagonist of glycine receptors |
| Picrotoxin<br>Bicuculline | Convulsions | Antagonists of GABA$_A$ receptors |
| Marine toxins<br>Tetrodotoxin | Weakness; dizziness; paresthesia of the lips, tongue, and throat; and paralysis | Blocking Na$^+$ ions passing through the channel |
| Saxitoxin | Paralysis | |
| Heavy metals<br>Aluminum | Dementia, facial seizures, asterixis, tremulousness, myoclonus, excephalopathy, incoordination and cognitive deficits | Unknown |
| Lead | Hyperactivity, learning deficiency, irritability, headache, facial pallor, lead palsy, hypertension (adults) | Unknown |
| Mercury | Cough, dyspnea, weakness, salivation, nausea, vomiting | Binding to sulfhydryl groups |

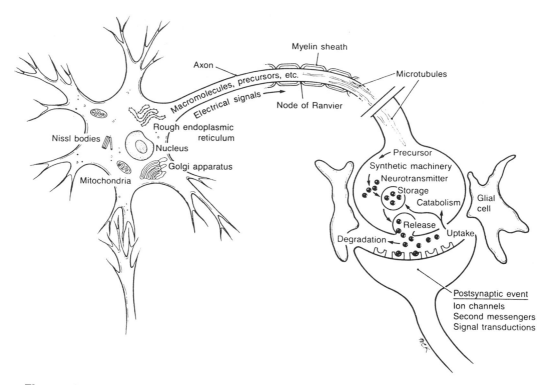

**Figure 1** Diagrammatic presentation of a neuron. The simplified diagram shows a neuron with organelles (nucleus, Golgi apparatus, endoplastic reticulum, Nissl bodies, mitochondria), dendrites, axon, myelin sheath, nerve ending, and synaptic connection (synapse) with other neurons. A neuron may be surrounded by glial cells.

postsynaptic sites of the neurotransmitters, such as those of receptors, degradation, and signal transduction. Any of these sites affected by a neurotoxicant could potentially result in neurotoxicity. With the complexity of the nervous systems, it is difficult to pinpoint where the exact sites of action of neurotoxicants are. Neurotoxicity induced by neurotoxicants can be by direct or indirect actions on the nervous systems. For example, the CNS is protected by the blood–brain barrier (BBB), formed by endothelial cells surrounding capillaries that supply the brain and interact with astrocytes. The BBB allows only certain smaller–molecular-sized substances, such as lipophilic compounds or certain nutrients, amino acids, hormones, fatty acids, peptides, and carbohydrates, that require active transport systems to reach the brain (Pardridge, 1988). However, not all areas of the brain are equally protected by the BBB. Certain regions, such as the postrema area and circumventricular area, lack the protection of the BBB. Furthermore, in the young, the BBB is not well developed. Chemicals that affect the BBB can lead to neurotoxicity by itself or to other substances as a result of entry to the brain. Table 2 summarizes the sites of possible neurotoxicant action on the nervous systems.

## VI. NEUROTRANSMITTERS IN NEUROTOXICITY

With the complexity of the nervous system, the most well-understood sites at which neurotoxicants might act are the synapses. The great majority of synaptic contacts involve processes of chemical transmission in which the arrival of an action potential at the terminal region from

**Table 2** Sites of Neurotoxicant Action

| Site of the nervous system | Affected process |
|---|---|
| The central nervous system (CNS) and the peripheral nervous system (PNS) | |
|    Neurons (cell body, axon, nerve endings, and dendrites) | Electrical properties through ionic events |
| |    Pumps |
| |    Channels |
| | Chemical actions (neurotransmitters) through synaptic transmission |
| |    Presynaptic |
| |       Transportation |
| |       Synthesis |
| |       Storage |
| |       Release |
| |       Autoreceptors |
| |       Reuptake |
| |       Metabolism |
| |    Postsynaptic |
| |       Receptors |
| |       Metabolism |
| |       Second messengers |
| |       Signal transduction |
|    Glia (astrocytes, oligodendrocytes and microglial cells) | Reuptake |
| | Metabolism |
|    Other nonneuronal processes related to the functions of neurons and glia | Synthesis and degradation of |
| |    Carbohydrates |
| |    Lipids and fatty acids |
| |    Nucleic acids |
| |    Proteins |
| Blood–brain barrier (BBB) | Modified entry to the brain |

the axon initiates the release of the neurotransmitter (see Fig. 1). This chemical transmitter diffuses across the synaptic cleft and then interacts with specialized receptor sites on the surface of the postsynaptic cell to trigger a rapid and short-lasting change in the permeability of the cell membrane. Depending on which neurotransmitter and which type of receptor sites are involved, the change in membrane permeability may either excite or inhibit the firing of action potentials by the postsynaptic cells. When an excitatory pathway is stimulated, a depolarization or excitatory postsynaptic potential (EPSP) is recorded. When an inhibitory pathway is stimulated, the postsynaptic membrane is hyperpolarized and an inhibitory postsynaptic potential (IPSP) is recorded.

The neurotransmitter may be a small molecule that is synthesized at the nerve endings (e.g., acetylcholine, monoamines, histamine, γ-aminobutyric acid, glycine, glutamate), or a larger peptide (e.g., β-endorphin, substance P, neurotensin, cholecystokinin) which is synthesized at the cell body. Table 3 lists most of the widely recognized small molecular weight nonpeptide neurotransmitters and their subtypes of receptors.

These neurotransmitters have demonstrated electrophysiological activity and an effect on human behaviors. These substances are also unevenly distributed throughout the nervous

**Table 3** Nonneuropeptide Neurotransmitters and Their Receptor Subtypes

| Neurotransmitter | Receptor subtypes |
|---|---|
| Acetylcholine (ACh) | Nicotinic: muscle-type and neuronal-type |
| | Muscarinic: $M_1$, $M_2$, $M_3$, and $M_4$ |
| Adenosine | $A_1$, $A_{2A}$, and $A_{2B}$ |
| γ-Aminobutyric acid (GABA) | $GABA_A$ and $GABA_B$ |
| Aspartic acid | |
| Dopamine (DA) | $D_1$, $D_2$, $D_3$, $D_4$, and $D_5$ |
| Glutamic acid (Glu) | Inotropic: NMDA, AMPA, and kainate |
| | Metabotropic: $mGluR_1$, $mGluR_2$, $mGluR_3$, $mGluR_4$, and $mGluR_5$ |
| Glycine (Gly) | |
| Histamine (His) | $H_1$, $H_2$, and $H_3$ |
| Norepinephrine (NE) | $\alpha_1$: $\alpha_{1A}$, $\alpha_{1B}$, $\alpha_{1C}$, and $\alpha_{1D}$ |
| | $\alpha_2$: $\alpha_{2A}$, $\alpha_{2B}$, and $\alpha_{2C}$ |
| | $\beta$: $\beta_1$, $\beta_2$, $\beta_3$ |
| Serotonin (5-HT) | $5\text{-HT}_1$: $5\text{-HT}_{1A}$, $5\text{-HT}_{1B}$, $5\text{-HT}_{1D}$, $5\text{-HT}_{1E}$, and $5\text{-HT}_{1F}$ |
| | $5\text{-HT}_2$: $5\text{-HT}_{2A}$, $5\text{-HT}_{2B}$, and $5\text{-HT}_{2C}$ |
| | $5\text{-HT}_3$ |
| | $5\text{-HT}_4$ |

systems. For instance, most of the cell bodies of the norepinephrine-containing neurons are located in the locus ceruleus and other nuclei in the pons and medulla. Some of the axons descend in the spinal cord, innervating the dorsal and ventral horns and lateral gray columns. Some enter the cerebellum. Some ascend in the ventral bundle to innervate the hypothalamus, and some ascend in the dorsal bundle to innervate the dorsal hypothalamus, limbic system, and neocortex. Serotonin-containing neurons have their cell bodies in the raphe nuclei of the brain stem and project to the hypothalamus, the limbic system, and the neocortex. Distributions of norepinephrine and serotonin in the brain appear to be parallel. Both serotonin and norepinephrine are related to mental function. On the other hand, dopamine, another monoamine, has a distribution pattern quite different from those of norepinephrine and serotonin. Many dopaminergic neurons have their cell bodies in the midbrain. They project from the substantia nigra to the striatal region (nigrostriatal pathway) and from ventral tegmental area to the olfactory tubercle, nucleus accumbens, and related areas (mesolimbic pathway). There is also a separate intrahypothalamic system of dopaminergic neurons that project from cell bodies in the arcuate nucleus to the external layer of the median eminence of the hypothalamus (tuberoinfundibular pathway). It is evident that dopamine in the CNS is involved in the endocrine, motor, and mental functions. The amino acid neurotransmitters (γ-aminobutyric acid [GABA] and glutamate), are much more abundant than those of monoamines. They are detected at levels of micromoles per gram of brain, instead of nanomoles per gram of brain, as with monoamines. However, their distribution in the CNS is much more ubiquitous and less defined. More detailed information on neurotransmitters can be found in the book, *The Biochemical Basis of Neuropharmacology,* by Cooper et al. (1991).

Neurotransmitters, after being released from presynaptic terminals, can activate their receptors at the postsynaptic and presynaptic (autoreceptor) sites. It is well established that a general class of receptors can be classified into subtypes of receptors. Subtypes of receptors for different neurotransmitters, as listed in a recent reference (TIPS, 1993) are also summarized in Table 3. Furthermore, many receptors are multimeric proteins consisting of multiple subunits. For example, the $GABA_A$ receptor complex is a heterooligomeric protein consisting of several distinct protein subunits. At least five types of $GABA_A$ receptor subunits exist, $\alpha$, $\beta$, $\gamma$, $\delta$, and $\rho$. Evidence indicates that the $GABA_A$ receptors are highly heterogeneous, not only in terms of anatomical structure, but also vulnerability in response to toxicological challenges.

## VII. TOXICOKINETICS OF NEUROTOXICANTS

Neurotoxicity induced by neurotoxicants would be evident when a certain amount of the agent reached the target site. The fraction of neurotoxicant that enters the CNS after a subject is exposed to the agent is determined by how much of it is in a free or unbound state. Therefore, the plasma concentration of free or unbound chemical or its biologically active metabolite is the primary factor that determines the intensity of biological actions. The study of toxicokinetics of a neurotoxicant has become one of the most important means of determining the toxicity of suspected toxic compound. It includes absorption from the administration site; distribution into body compartments, including tissue depots, such as adipose tissue; biotransformation or metabolism to active or inactive metabolites; and excretion of parent compounds or metabolites from the body. Excellent textbooks (Abou-Donia, 1992; Amdur et al., 1993) are available on these topics. These parameters also determine the onset and duration of the actions of a neurotoxicant.

One of the best examples to illustrate the importance of toxicokinetic factors that influence the action of compounds with similar structure is the action of barbiturates. As shown in Figure 2, thiopental, pentobarbital, phenobarbital, and barbital share a similar chemical formula, barbituric acid (2, 4, 6-trioxohexahydropyrimidine). However, different functional groups are attached to the basic structure, and differences in lipid solubility make significant differences in the rate of absorption, distribution, biotransformation, and excretion of these chemicals. For example, the

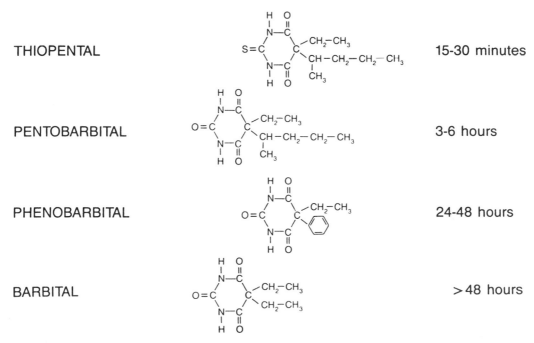

**Figure 2** Representative structures of barbiturates and their duration of action (sedative–hypnotic property).

**Table 4** Examples of Neurotoxicants That Might Be Metabolized to Form Active Toxic Metabolites

| Parent compound | Metabolite(s) |
| --- | --- |
| Phenacetin | Phenetidin |
| Acetanilid | Aniline |
| Acetaminophen | N-Acetyl-P-benzoquinone |
| Parathion | Paraoxon |
| Malathion | Malaoxon |
| Meperidine | Normeperidine |
| Cocaine | Norcocaine |
| 1-Methyl-4-phenyl-1,2,3,6-tetrahydropyridine (MPTP) | 1-methyl-4-phenylpyridinium ion ($MPP^+$) |
| Chloral hydrate | Trichloroethanol |
| Methanol | Formaldehyde, formic acid |
| Benzene | Phenol, dihydrodiol |
| Codeine | Morphine |
| Ethanol | Acetaldehyde |
| Ephedrine | Norephedrine |
| Primidone | Phenobarbitol |

lipid solubility of thiopental is about 600, 200, and 15 times higher than that of barbital, phenobarbital, or pentobarbital, respectively. Thiopental can reach peak concentration in the brain in seconds. It will also distribute to other tissues and fluids rapidly. Therefore, the rapid rate of distribution of thiopental is the determining factor for the rapid onset and short duration of action of this compound, although its rate of metabolism is comparable with that of pentobarbital. Although pentobarbital administered intravenously produces rapid onset of effects, the duration of action is determined entirely by the rate of metabolism of the compound by the liver. In contrast, barbital and phenobarbital, with their low lipid solubility, slowly penetrate the BBB. Therefore, even if they are being administered intravenously, about 15–30 min are required to initiate the peak effect of these compounds. The central action of barbitol is mainly determined by the rate of renal excretion, since nearly 100% of barbital administered is excreted intact in the urine. For phenobarbital, 70% is metabolized in the liver and 30% is excreted unchanged from the kidney.

The biotransformation of a neurotoxicant is usually the primary mechanism for its detoxification. Most of the neurotoxicants would be metabolized to more polar metabolite(s) that can be readily excreted by the kidneys. For example, pentobarbital alcohol, a major metabolite of pentobarbital, has no obvious toxicological property. However, there are always exceptions. For the examples cited in Table 4, some neurotoxicants are biotransformed to metabolite(s) that can be more active, or equally as active, as the parent compounds.

## VIII. FACTORS THAT MIGHT INFLUENCE NEUROTOXICITY OF NEUROTOXICANTS

Exposure of humans or animals to the same dose of a neurotoxicant under the same environmental conditions can induce varying degrees of neurotoxicity in different individuals. Numerous factors are known to influence the severity of neurotoxicity in different subjects. For a neurotoxicant, the physicochemical property, forms of preparation, dose and concentration, routes of administration, and metabolic rate of the agent would significantly affect the degree of neurotoxicity after the subjects have been exposed to the agent. Variations of biological systems, such as age, sex, genetics, state of health, nutritional or dietary factors, are also important parameters to be considered for the occurrence of neurotoxicity induced by neurotoxicants. Environmental factors, such as physical location, temperature, and occupation, also deserve consideration.

Examples of neurotoxicity influenced by various factors are cited in the following. Accidental exposure to neurotoxicants is usually by the inhalation, oral, or dermal route. In general, the order of severity is inhalation > oral > dermal. Different routes of administration with certain compounds will also influence the degree of neurotoxicity. Francis (1985) illustrated routes of administration on organophosphorus ester-induced delayed neurotoxicity in experimental animals. Tri-*o*-cresyl phosphate (TOCP) induced delayed neuropathy in monkeys and dogs by subcutaneous injection but not by oral administration. Mipafox, an organophosphorus insecticide, also produced delayed neurotoxicity in rats by the subcutaneous route, but only marginal effect when it was given in the diet. The difference could be due to the difference in metabolism of these organophosphorus compounds with different routes of administration. The first pass through the liver may be why oral administration causes much less delayed neurotoxicity of these compounds. Differences in species are also obvious. Excellent examples in comparisons of the susceptibility of humans and animals to various insecticides are summarized by Hayes (1991). More examples on age, sex, strain differences, and so on, can also be found in the *Handbook of Pesticide Toxicology* (Hayes and Laws, 1991).

Species differences in metabolism of neurotoxicants can also influence neurotoxicity. Parathion is activated to paraoxon, a cholinesterase inhibitor, by the microsomal enzyme, desulfurase. The rank order of microsomal parathion desulfurase activity in vitro in the animals tested is guinea pig > hamster > mouse > rat > rabbit (Hodgson and Guthrie, 1980). Sex variation in enzyme activity is also evident. Parathion is metabolically activated to paraoxon faster by female rats than by the male. Therefore, it is more toxic to the female rats (Hodgson, 1987).

## IX.  ACUTE AND CHRONIC EXPOSURES TO NEUROTOXICANTS

Acute exposures to neurotoxicants usually are related to accident or intentional exposures. Symptoms of acute neurotoxicity are obvious or are easier to be detected. However, slowly developing neurotoxicity by chronic exposures to low doses or subtoxic doses of neurotoxicants is difficult to detect. Chronic exposure is a long-term process that can also be complicated by numerous factors. Symptoms induced by a neurotoxicant following acute or chronic exposure are not always identical. Most often, they can be completely different. For example, the neurotoxicity of organophophorous cholinesterase inhibitors is due to their irreversible inhibition of acetylcholinesterase. They produce acute symptoms such as anxiety, restlessness, insomnia, confusion, slurred speech, ataxia, tremor, or convulsion. However, these symptoms can disappear, even when the cholinesterase activities have not appreciably recovered. In cases of long-term exposure to organophosphorus pesticides such as parathion, octamethyl pyrophosphoramide, Syston, EPN, Di-Syston, and Delnav, tolerance to these agents has been well recognized (Barnes and Denz, 1951, 1954; Bombinski and DuBois, 1958; Cooper, 1962; Hodge, et al., 1954; Oliver and Funnell, 1961; Rider et al., 1952). Sumerford et al. (1953) reported that farm workers in Wenatchee, Washington, had erythrocyte and plasma cholinesterase activity as low as 15% of the normal level without complaints of any symptoms throughout the spray season. This suggested that they had developed tolerance to organophosphorus insecticides. Chronic exposure to organophosphorus insecticides can also lead to delayed peripheral neuropathy.

The solvent, *n*-hexane, which is a CNS depressant, can cause headache and anoxia at acute low-dose exposures. At higher concentrations, it can cause severe CNS toxicity, such as confusion, stupor, and coma. However, chronic exposure to this solvent in workers exposed to ambient air containing high concentration of *n*-hexane produces a polyneuropathy believed to be due to the metabolite, 2, 5-hexanedione (Goto et al., 1974).

## X. GOALS AND TRENDS FOR STUDYING NEUROTOXICITY INDUCED BY TOXICANTS

With the increasing knowledge of neurotoxicology and the need to evaluate the public health significance of the presence of chemicals in our environment, it is essential to investigate the potential neurotoxicity that may be induced by these chemicals. The goals for the study of chemically induced neurotoxicities include the following:

1. Identification of toxicants that are potentially neurotoxicants
2. Detection of the nature of neurotoxicity induced by neurotoxicants
3. Determination of specific mechanisms of action involved
4. Correlation of neurotoxicity with possible mechanisms of action
5. Development of predictive testing techniques
6. Design suitable regimens for the prevention and treatment of neurotoxicity potentially induced by neurotoxicants
7. Provide a reliable database for risk assessment and risk management

Current testing data requirements for regulation of chemicals in the environment, such as those specified under the Federal Insecticide, Fungicide, and Rodenticide Act (FIFRA) and Toxic Substances Control Act (TSCA), are minimal. Neurotoxicity testing guidelines for pesticide assessment have been revised in 1991 by the USEPA. Regulatory agencies and scientific bodies are developing risk assessment guidelines for neurotoxicity evaluation of chemicals (USEPA, 1993). The National Academy of Sciences (NAS, 1993), in its recent report, *The Pesticides in the Diet of Infants and Children,* also recommended neurotoxicity evaluation as part of the overall safety evaluation for pesticides. Expanded neurotoxicity testing and risk assessment will help better characterize the public health implications of the presence of environmental chemicals and provide a basis for improve regulations to minimize unnecessary human exposure.

Finally, for an up to date understanding of the principles and methods of neurotoxicology and risk assessment of neurotoxicity, readers are referred to the books by Chang and Dyer (1995), Chang and Slikker (1995), and Chang (1995).

## REFERENCES

Abou-Donia, M. B. (1992). *Neurotoxicology,* CRC Press, Boca Raton, FL.

Amdur, M. O., Doull, J., and Klaassen, C. D. (1993). *Casarett and Doull's Toxicology: The Basic Science of Poisons,* 4th ed., McGraw-Hill, New York.

Anger, K. W. (1984). Neurobehavioral testing of chemicals: Impact on recommended standards, *Neurobehav. Toxicol. Teratol.,* 6, 147–153.

Barnes, J. M. and Denz, F. A. (1951). The chronic toxicity of *p*-nitrophenyl diethyl thiophosphate (E. 605); a long term feeding experiment with rats, *J. Hyg.,* 49, 430–441.

Barnes, J. M. and Denz, F. A. (1954). The reaction of rats to diets containing octamethyl pyrophosphoramide

(Schraden) and *O, O*-diethyl-*S*-ethylmercaptoethanol thiophosphate ("Systox"), *Br. J. Ind. Med.*, 11, 11–19.

Biereley, J. R., Brown, A. W., and Meldrum, B. S. (1971). The nature and time course of the neuronal alterations resulting from oligaemia and hypoglycaemia in the brain of *Macaca mulatta, Brain Res.*, 25, 483–499.

Bombinski, T. J. and DuBois, K. P. (1958). Toxicity and mechanism of action of Di-Syston, *AMA Arch. Ind. Health,* 17, 192–199.

Brucher, J. M. (1967). Neuropathological problems posed by carbon monoxide poisoning and anoxia, *Prog. Brain Res., 24,* 75–100.

Chang, L. W., and Dyer, R. S. (1995). *Handbook of Neurotoxicology,* Marcel Dekker, Inc., New York.

Chang, L. W., and Slikker, W., Jr. (1995). Neurotoxicology, Academic Press, San Diego, CA.

Chang, L. W. (1995). *Principles of Neurotoxicology,* Marcel Dekker, Inc., New York.

Cooper, F. A. (1962). Delnav [2:3 *p*-dioxane *S*-bis-(*O, O*-diethyl dithiophosphate)] as an ixodicide, *Vet. Rec.,* 74, 103–112.

Cooper, J. R., Floom, F. E., and Roth, R. H. (1991). *The Biochemical Basis of Neuropharmacology,* 6th ed., Oxford University Press, New York.

Francis, B. M. (1985). Effects of dosing regimens and routes of administration on organophosphorus ester induced delayed neurotoxicity, *Neurotoxicology,* 4, 139–146.

Goto, I., Matsumura, I., Inoue, N., Murai, Y., Shida, K., Santa, T., and Kuroiwa, Y. (1974). Toxic polyneuropathy due to glue sniffing, *J. Neurol. Neurosurg. Psychiatry,* 37, 848–873.

Hayes, W. J., Jr. (1991). Dosage and other factors influencing toxicity. In *Handbook of Pesticide Toxicology,* Vol. 1 (W. J. Hayes, Jr. and J. R. Laws, eds.), Academic Press, San Diego, CA, pp. 39–105.

Hayes, W. J., Jr., and Laws, J. R. (1991). *Handbook of Pesticide Toxicology.* Academic Press, San Diego.

Hodge, H. C., Maynard, E. A., Hurwitz, L., DiStefano, V., Downs, W. L., Jones, C. K., and Blanchet, H. J., Jr. (1954). Studies of the toxicity and of the enzyme kinetics of ethyl *p*-nitrophenyl thionobenzene phosphonate (EPN), *J. Pharmacol. Exp. Ther.,* 112, 29–39.

Hodgson, E. (1987). Modification of metabolism. In *A Textbook of Modern Toxicology.* (E. Hodgson and P. E. Levi, eds.), Elsevier, New York, pp. 85–121.

Hodgson, E., and Guthrie, F. E. (1980). *Introduction to Biochemical Toxicology,* Elsevier, New York.

Hume, A. S. and Ho, I. K. (1994). Toxicity of solvents. In *Basic Environmental Toxicology* (L. G. Cockerham and B. S. Shane, eds.), CRC Press, Boca Raton, FL, pp. 157–184.

Malamud, N. (1963). Patterns of CNS vulnerability in neonatal hypermia. In *Selective Vulnerability of the Central Nervous System in Hypoxaemia* (J. F. Schade and W. H. McMenemy eds.), F. A. Davis, Philadelphia.

[NAS] National Academy of Science (1993). *Pesticides in the Diets of Infants and Children,* National Academy of Sciences, Washington, DC.

National Research Council Committee on Neurotoxicology and Models for Assessing Risk (1992). *Environmental Neurotoxicology,* National Academy Press, Washington, DC.

Norton, S. (1986). Toxic response of the central nervous system. In *Casarett and Doull's Toxicology: The Basic Science of Poisons,* 3rd ed. (C. D. Klaasen, M. O. Amdur, J. Doull, eds.), Macmillan Publishing, New York, pp. 359–386.

Oliver, W. T. and Funnell, H. S. (1961). Correlation of the effects of parathion on erythrocyte cholinesterase with symptomatology in pigs, *Am. J. Vet. Res.,* 22, 80–84.

Pardridge, W. M. (1988). Recent advances in blood–brain barrier transport. *Annu. Rev. Pharmacol. Toxicol.,* 49, 219–225.

Rider, J. A., Ellinwood, L. Z., and Coon, J. M. (1952). Production of tolerance in the rat to octamethyl pyrophosphoramide (OMPA), *Proc. Soc. Exp. Biol. Med.,* 81, 455–459.

Scholz, W. (1953). Selective neuronal necrosis and its topistic patterns in hypoxemia and oligenia, *J. Neuropathol. Exp. Neurol.,* 12, 249–261.

Sumerford, W. T., Hayes, W. J., Johnston, J. M., Walker, K., and Spillane, J. (1953). Cholinesterase response and symptomatology from exposure to organic phosphorus insecticies, *AMA Arch. Ind. Hyg. Occup. Med.,* 7, 383–398.

[TIPS] *Trends in Pharmacological Sciences* (1993). *1993 Receptor Nomenclature Supplement,* Elsevier, Amsterdam.

U.S. Congress, Office of Technology Assessment (1990). *Neurotoxicity: Identifying and Controlling Poisons of the Nervous System,* (OTA-BA-436): U.S. Government Printing Office.

[USEPA] United States Environmental Protection Agency (1987). Health effects testing guidelines, CFR 798, 52 FR 26150, July 13, *Chem. Reg. Rep.,* 31, 7001–7872.

[USEPA] United States Environmental Protection Agency (1991). Neurotoxicity testing guidelines, National Technical Information Service, Springfield, VA.

[USEPA] United States Environmental Protection Agency (1993). Draft report: Principles of neurotoxicity risk assessment, *Fed. Reg.,* 58, 41556–41599.

[WHO] World Health Organization (1990). Methylmercury, Environmental Health Sciences No. 59, Geneva.

Windle, W. F. (1963). Selective vulnerability of the central nervous system of rhesus monkeys to asphyhyxia during birth. In *Selective Vulnerability of the Central Nervous System in Hypoxaemia* (J. F. Shade and W. H. McMenemy, eds.), F. A. Davis, Philadelphia.

# 6
# Biology of the Immune System and Immunotoxicity

**Kathleen Rodgers**
*University of Southern California*
*Los Angeles, California*

## I. INTRODUCTION

The immune system is the body's defense against foreign materials (called antigens), which include transformed cells, transplanted tissues, viruses, bacteria, and parasites. Immunology is the study of immunity. *Immunity* means "protection from," here, protection from infectious disease or neoplasia. The body has both innate and adaptive immunity. Innate immunity is the nonspecific defense against disease, such as the skin or polymorphonuclear cells (PMNs), and is constitutive. The adaptive immune response is specific and requires antigenic stimulation and the interaction and cooperation of several different cell types in the immune system (Katz and Benacerraf, 1972).

*Immunotoxicology* is the study of the toxic effects of xenobiotics, such as therapeutic drugs, narcotics, and environmental pollutants, on the immune system. The immune system is influenced by stress and alterations in the homeostasis of other physiological systems (Folch and Waksman, 1974; Heiss and Palmer, 1978; Jose and Good, 1973; Monjan and Collector, 1977; Purtilo et al., 1972). Therefore, the study of the immunotoxic potential of a chemical must be conducted at doses that are below that which produces other toxic reactions. Immunotoxicity can be the result of either (1) the suppression of the ability of the immune system to respond to a foreign antigen, or (2) nonspecific or antigen-specific enhancement of an immune response. Immune suppression can result in an increase in the incidence or duration of an infectious disease or neoplasia. Immune enhancement may result in allergic responses (respiratory, gastric, or dermal), autoimmune disease, or exacerbation of these processes.

## II. LYMPHOID TISSUES

The tissues in which the immune system resides are dispersed throughout the body and include the lymphatic vessels, spleen, liver, thymus, lymph nodes, appendix, skin, and bone marrow

(Virella et al., 1990). The lymphatic vessels retrieve lymph from the extracellular space and return white blood cells to lymphoid organs. Lymphoid organs act as sites for the differentiation of cells involved in the immune response and the generation of immune responses. Lymphoid organs are situated at locations where foreign material might enter the body. For example, gastrointestinal lymphoid organs (i.e., Peyers patches and appendix) are located along the absorptive areas of the gastrointestinal tract.

## III.  INNATE IMMUNITY

Innate immunity includes mechanical barriers, secreted products, and inflammatory cells (Sell, 1987a). Innate resistance is modulated only by physiological conditions, such as age and nutrition, and does not distinguish between different microorganisms. Mechanical barriers include the skin, mucous membranes, and the epithelial lining of the lungs. Stomach acid, saliva, lysozyme, and mucous or waxy secretions, all are secretory products of the innate defense systems. Macrophages and PMNs are nonspecific inflammatory cells that are the first line of defense against invading organisms that breach epithelial barriers. The adaptive immune system is a backup to this first line of defense.

## IV.  INFLAMMATORY RESPONSE

Inflammation is a primary response to infection or trauma and involves both innate and adaptive defense mechanisms (Sell, 1987b). Following an initial vasoconstriction, increased blood flow (vasodilation) occurs, which causes redness and increases temperature. In turn, an influx of blood proteins, fluids, and blood cells occurs at this site of increased blood flow. Secondarily, there is a chemotaxis of white blood cells or leukocytes (first PMNs then macrophages) into the site of inflammation. Leukocytes ingest and dispose of invading organisms or tissue debris. These cells also release proteolytic enzymes and inflammatory mediators during the course of the inflammatory response. Some of these mediators, such as interleukin-1 (IL-1) and IL-6 and prostaglandins, are also involved in the regulation of an immune response, as will be discussed later.

## V.  ADAPTIVE OR SPECIFIC IMMUNITY

The functioning of the adaptive immune system is highly regulated and requires the interaction and communication of multiple cell types, including macrophages, lymphocytes, and granulocytes (Erb and Feldman, 1975; Gorczynski et al., 1971; Miller et al., 1971). Each cell type of the immune system has distinct functions that are unique to that cell type (Goust, 1990; Virella, 1990). However, the functional capability of many of these cell types can overlap.

### A.  Lymphocytes

The lymphocytes are small, mononuclear cells (6–15 μm) that originate in the bone marrow and are differentiated either in the "bursa equivalent" (B cells) or thymus (T cells) (Stobo et al., 1987). Lymphocytes constitute the component of the immune system that responds to and neutralizes antigen in a specific manner. Each lymphocyte bears on its cell surface a receptor that is capable of recognizing a specific and distinct portion of the antigen. For the B cell, the antigen-specific receptor is a membrane form of an antibody. For the T cell, the receptor that confers recognition of antigen and specificity for self, termed *T-cell receptor,* is a molecule with immunoglobulin like domains, but is much more complex in its design (Arden et al., 1985). The T-cell receptor complex consists of (1) the T-cell receptor, which has two disulfide-linked glycoproteins ($\alpha$ and $\beta$ or $\delta$ and $\gamma$), and (2) CD3, an invariant complex of proteins ($\xi$, $\delta$, $\varepsilon$, and $\gamma$) that transduces the signal generated by antigen binding to the receptor. The portion of the antigen recognized by the T-cell receptor or membrane-bound antibody is called an *epitope*. An epitope is a small portion of the antigenic molecule, such as a protein or carbohydrate, that can fit into the binding site of the antigen receptor, termed a *paratope*. On exposure to this epitope, the immature lymphocyte, which is capable of responding to the antigen, is stimulated to differentiate and proliferate. This proliferation, termed *clonal expansion,* allows the formation of many cells that are capable of eliminating the antigen. After the initial immune response to an antigen is completed, some of these lymphocytes become *memory cells* and generate a stronger and more rapid response to antigen with subsequent exposures. This latter feature of the immune response is the basis of immunizations against pathogens such as tetanus.

Each individual lymphocyte is able to recognize and respond to a single epitope. The uniqueness of each lymphocyte is determined by a genetic rearrangement event in the DNA coding for the antigen receptor, which occurs before an encounter with the antigen (Tonegawa, 1983). For example, the germline DNA for immunoglobulin molecule, which is present in each non-B cell and the stem B cell, contains multiple copies of regions termed variable region genes (V), joining chain genes (J), diversity genes (D), and constant region genes (C, which determines the class of antibody). During B-cell maturation, the intervening sequences between V and J or V and D and J is removed, such that the antibody-secreting cell contains DNA with the VJ or VDJ genomic regions in juxtaposition. This rearrangement deletes the unnecessary genomic material and creates a unique immunoglobulin gene for that individual B cell. It also brings together the V region promoter site and the J region enhancing site, which action allows transcription of this immunoglobulin gene. This mechanism permits the generation of millions of unique lymphocytes that are ready to respond to millions of antigenic epitopes when needed.

## 1. T Cells

T-cell maturation involves stem cells that are produced in the bone marrow and circulate to and mature in the thymus (Sell, 1987c). In the thymus, these cells acquire cell surface proteins that are specific for T cells (to which monoclonal antibodies are available such that these cells can be phenotyped by flow cytometry). In addition to the antigen-specific receptor (discussed earlier), thymocytes express receptors for the tissue transplantation antigens from the gene family called the major histocompatibility complex (*MHC*), which is responsible for self-recognition. Self-recognition is required for T-cell response to antigen and for T-cell help to B cells in the generation of humoral response. After differentiation in the thymus, the T cells migrate from the thymus and settle in other lymphoid organs.

T cells are the effector cells of the cell-mediated immune response and the regulatory cells of the adaptive immune response (Goust, 1990). The cell-mediated immune response clears antigen through direct cell–cell interaction. Cytotoxic T cells destroy cells that are recognized by their T-cell receptor. Other T cells, called Td cells, mediate delayed hypersensitivity. Another subset of T cells, which are identified by function and distinct patterns of cell surface proteins, are able to regulate the immune response. These include helper T cells, which function to augment an immune response through the release of cytokines, and suppressor T cells, which suppress the generation of an immune response.

## 2. B Cells

Bone marrow cells also differentiate into B cells under the influence of many possible lymphoid organs in the mammal (Sell, 1987c). In the chicken, the differentiation of B cells occurs in the bursa of Fabricus (hence, B cells); it is unclear where this occurs in mammals. After the B cells develop, they migrate to lymphoid organs to await antigenic stimulation.

The B cells are the effector cells of the humoral immune response. The humoral immune response is mediated through soluble factors such as immunoglobulins (Virella, 1990). Although B cells can aid in the initial generation of an immune response through the presentation of antigen, the function of B cells is to differentiate into plasma cells, which secrete immunoglobulin molecules or antibodies. Antibodies can agglutinate or neutralize an antigen, or they can opsonize an antigen for subsequent lysis, by complement fixation or antibody-dependent cytotoxicity (ADCC), or by phagocytosis. There are five classes of antibodies. The class of antibody is determined by the constant region of the molecule and is changed during B-cell differentiation through a gene-splicing event in the immunoglobulin heavy chain gene. The IgM, IgG, and IgA antibodies aid in the neutralization or elimination of the antigen (Goodman, 1987). Antibodies of the IgE class bind to a receptor on mast cells or basophils and mediate the degranulation of these cells following exposure to polyvalent forms of their antigen. The IgD antibody is found on the surface of immature B cells and may act as the cellular receptor for antigen.

### 3. Natural Killer Cells

Natural killer (NK) cells (i.e., cells that can lyse selected tumors without previous contact with the antigen) are nonadherent lymphocytes that share some properties with T cells (e.g., the lytic mechanism) and macrophages (e.g., size and nuclear shape). The NK cells appear to have a receptor for their tumor target, but the nature of this receptor is unclear, and the lysis is not restricted by self-MHC proteins.

## B.  Macrophages

The macrophage is the largest cell in the lymphoid system (12–15 μm) (diZerega and Rodgers, 1992). The myeloid stem cell differentiates in the bone marrow to the promyelocyte (the common precursor to granulocytes and macrophages), then to the megakaryocyte. The megakaryocyte differentiates into a monocyte, which is the blood-borne precursor to the macrophage or histiocyte, the tissue macrophage. The macrophage is the terminal cell in the differentiative schema.

Macrophages are multifunctional cells (in that they mediate both inflammatory and immune responses), the activity of which depends on their differentiative status. In the generation of an immune response, macrophages phagocytose and process antigen as well as secrete monokines that regulate immune responsiveness. Antigen processing includes ingestion of the molecule and degradation of the antigen into fragments in phagolysosomes that can be recognized by the T cell. Following processing, the antigenic fragments are placed on the surface of the macrophage in conjunction with the MHC class II protein, termed Ia, which mediates the interaction between macrophages and lymphocytes bearing a cell surface protein called CD4.

## VI.  GENERATION OF AN IMMUNE RESPONSE

### A.  Cellular Interactions in Immune Responses

To generate a humoral immune response (i.e., production of specific antibody by plasma cells), the interaction of at least T and B cells and macrophages is required (Erb and Feldman, 1975; Gorczynski et al., 1971; Miller et al., 1971). Macrophages, or antigen-presenting cells, are required for the stimulation of helper T cells, which, in turn, produce growth and differentiative factors for B cells. B cells are then stimulated to proliferate and differentiate into antibody-secreting plasma cells. Certain antigens are called "thymus-independent," which means that

T cells are not required for the B cell to respond to this molecule. Such antigens can stimulate B cells directly, perhaps through direct interaction with the antigen receptor on the B cell.

Helper and suppressor T cells also have a regulatory role in the generation of mature effector T cells (Miller et al., 1971). Some of these regulatory processes may occur through direct cell–cell interaction through the release of soluble factors.

## B. Cytokines

Cytokines, more specifically interleukins, interferons, and colony-stimulating factors are produced by cells activated during an immune response and are critical in the induction, maintenance, and control of this response (Oppenheim et al., 1987). Interleukin (IL)-1 is released by macrophages and stimulates helper/inducer T cells in conjunction with antigen to produce IL-2 and express IL-2 receptors. Interleukin-2 can act in an autocrine fashion to stimulate activated T cells to proliferate and produce various growth and differentiative factors for B and T cells and macrophages, such as IL-4 and interferon gamma. Current knowledge indicates that different types of helper T cells, called TH1 and TH2, secrete a different set of cytokines, depending on the type of immune response they are inducing.

## VII. IMMUNOSUPPRESSION

Suppression of the immune response can occur through many avenues and can have devastating consequences. The occurrence of repeated infections in an individual may result from suppression of host defense mechanisms (Ammann, 1987). Immune deficiency may be due to primary or secondary diseases. Primary immune deficiencies block the acquisition of immune maturity and may result from genetic or developmental abnormalities. Secondary immune deficiencies result from diseases and interfere with the expression of an immune response.

Primary immune deficiencies result in the permanent loss of immune cells at specific sites. Three major primary immune deficits can occur: combined antibody and cellular, antibody alone, and cellular alone. Combined immune deficiencies include reticular dysgenesis, severe combined immune deficiencies (Swiss type agammaglobulinemia, ataxia telangiectasia, and others), dysgammaglobulinemias, and DiGeorge syndrome. Primary immune deficiencies also result from defects in the complement system, phagocytic dysfunction, and deficiencies in cytokine production.

Secondary immune deficiencies may result from naturally occurring disease processes or subsequent to the administration of suppressive agents. These processes affect the expression of established defense mechanisms. Diseases affecting the cellular immune system include leprosy, measles and other viral infections, diabetes, and cancer. The clinical manifestations of immune deficiency diseases include infection with organisms that are not usually pathogenic (opportunistic infections).

As stated, exposure to immunosuppressive agents may also cause secondary immune deficiencies. The study of this phenomenon is one aspect of field of immunotoxicology and immunopharmacology. The mechanisms of action of immunosuppressive agents are extremely varied and include (1) direct destruction of lymphoid cells, (2) interference with DNA synthesis, (3) interference with the production of cytokines, and (4) interference with the functional capabilities of immunocytes. The result of exposure to immunosuppressive agents, either in a therapeutic situation or through environmental exposure, may be increased in the incidence or duration of infections or neoplasia. Several studies have shown this to occur following the administration of immunosuppressive agents following tissue transplantation (Penn, 1985).

## VIII.  IMMUNOPATHOLOGY

### A.  Introduction

*Immunopathology* is the study of tissue damage and disease that is the result of immune effector mechanisms (Rose and MacKay, 1992). In the study of diseases caused by immune mechanisms, many organ systems may be involved; therefore, the lesions are best described by the effector mechanism used. Because these effector mechanisms also act as protective immune mechanisms, the immune response can be a two-edged sword. The five effector mechanisms that are involved in both the protective and destructive functions of the immune system are as follows: (1) neutralization, (2) cytotoxicity, (3) immune complex reaction, (4) allergic reaction, and (5) cell-mediated immunity (Table 1). For example, specific antibodies to antigens, such as diphtheria, lead to neutralization and clearance of the bacteria. However, when specific antibodies are made to molecules necessary for physiological homeostasis (such as insulin or parts of the nervous system), diseases (such as insulin resistance or myasthenia gravis) occur.

### B.  Neutralization

Formation of antibodies specific for enzymes, hormones, or cell surface receptors may inactivate the function of the molecule or, in the latter case, may activate the function of the receptor (Sell, 1987d). The resultant disease depends on the biological function of the molecule affected. Inactivation can result from (1) direct inactivation (i.e., steric hindrance of an active site or alteration in the tertiary structure of the molecule), (2) indirect inactivation (i.e., aggregation and enhanced clearance by the reticuloendothelial system), or (3) receptor loss (i.e., steric hindrance or down-regulation of the receptor).

Many diseases are the result of specific antibodies to biologically active molecules. Diabetes mellitus is a group of diseases in which carbohydrate metabolism is abnormal owing to the inability of insulin to act. Type I diabetes mellitus may result from antibodies to insulin, insulin receptors, or islet cells. The antibody can neutralize insulin, block the availability of the receptor to the insulin, or mediate the lysis of insulin-producing cells. Myasthenia gravis, which is characterized by muscle weakness and fatigue, is a functional abnormality in the conduction of nerve impulses from the motor nerve to the muscle fiber owing to antibody formation, with subsequent binding to the acetylcholine receptor. Thyroid disease can also result from auto-antibody formation; antibodies can neutralize thyroid hormones or block receptor access.

**Table 1**   Effector Mechanisms of the Immune System and Their Functions

| Effector mechanism | Protective function | Destructive function |
|---|---|---|
| Neutralization | Diphtheria, tetanus | Insulin resistance, myasthenia gravis |
| Cytotoxicity | Bacteriolysis | Hemolysis, leukopenia |
| Immune complex reaction | Acute inflammation | Vasculitis, arthritis |
| Allergic reaction | Focal inflammation Parasite expulsion | Asthma, uticaria, hay fever |
| Cell-mediated reaction | | |
| DHR | Destruction of virus-infected cell, cancer surveillance | Contact dermatitis, auto-immunity |
| GR | Leprosy, tuberculosis | Beryllosis |

Additionally, other diseases that can result from autoantibody formation include pernicious anemia, polyendocrinopathy, infertility, and hemophilia.

## C. Cytolytic Reaction

A cytolytic reaction can occur when an antibody or an immunized cell binds to an antigen present on a cell (Sell, 1987e). Cytolysis resulting from antibody binding can occur through the activation of complement (a series of blood proteins, the activation of which by IgM or some subtypes of IgG results in the insertion of a pore into the membrane of the coated cell), or ADCC, which is mediated by macrophages or ADCC cells. The diseases that result from lysis of cells that are hematopoietic in origin, including hemolytic anemia, thrombocytopenia, agranulocytosis, and vascular purpura, can be called immunohematological diseases. Other diseases that result from cytolytic reactions include autoimmune diseases, such as allergic thyroiditis and acute endocarditis.

## D. Immune Complex Reactions

An immune complex reaction is the result of the interaction of an antibody with an antigen, followed by the deposition of this complex in tissues (Sell, 1987f). The aggregated antigen–antibody complexes cause the activation of complement and the production of anaphylatoxic and chemotactic fragments of complement, C4a, C3a, and C5a. Following this initial event, an inflammatory response ensues that leads to tissue destruction. Examples of disease states that result from this tissue damage are serum sickness, Arthus reaction, glomerulonephritis.

Serum sickness, symptoms of which include glomerulonephritis, arthritis, and vasculitis, was first noted in 1905 in patients who had been injected with immune horse serum to tetanus toxin 10–14 days previously. In this instance, the patient who received the horse serum recognized these proteins as foreign, made a specific antibody response to these proteins, and the antigen–antibody complexes precipitated in the glomeruli of the kidneys, the walls of the small arteries, and the joints. The ensuing inflammatory response led to the symptoms that characterized the disease. Glomerulonephritis is inflammation of the glomeruli of the kidney and is a common manifestation of immune complex disease. This phenomenon is due to interference with the structure and function of the glomeruli in their concentration of excreted metabolites into urine.

Skin reactions are also common manifestations of immune reactions. One example of this is the Arthus reaction. An Arthus reaction is a dermal inflammatory response of a precipitating antibody with its antigen, characterized by edema, erythema, and hemorrhage, and usually occurs within a few hours. Many other skin diseases are the result of immune complex deposition, including erythema nodosum, erythema multiforme, and dermatitis herpeformis.

## E. Atopic or Anaphylactic Reactions (Allergy)

An allergic reaction occurs following the release of inflammatory mediators by the crosslinking of specific IgE antibodies (termed reagins), which passively bind to basophilic granulocytes through cell surface receptors in the constant region of the antibody, by multivalent antigens (termed allergins) (Terr, 1987). The inflammatory response has two phases: (1) the early phase is initiated by the release of histamine, heparin, and serotonin by basophilic granulocytes and is characterized by smooth-muscle constriction (by $H_1$ receptors on the smooth muscles of the pulmonary bronchi, gastrointestinal tract, and others) or dilation of arterioles (by $H_2$ receptors on the vascular smooth muscles); and (2) the late phase is initiated by arachidonic acid metabolites (prostaglandins and leukotrienes), characterized by infiltration of PMNs, lymphocytes, and macrophages. This later phase causes the painful, indurated responses in the skin and the prolonged decrease in airflow to the lung.

Manifestation of allergic reactions include anaphylaxis, urticaria, asthma, and hay fever. For example, asthma is a reversible acute respiratory disease caused mainly by constriction of the smooth muscles of the small bronchi. There are at least two forms of asthma: (1) the allergic form, mediated by mast cell activation through IgE antibody and allergin, and (2) the nonallergic form, although not well understood, may be due to an imbalance of smooth-muscle tone.

## F.  Cell-Mediated Immune Disease

The immune-mediated diseases just discussed, which involve hyper-reactivity or inappropriate responsiveness of the humoral immune system and the specificity of the reaction, were based on the presence of an antibody specific for the antigen (Sell, 1987g). In this section, the immunopathology that results from inappropriate expression of, or as the side effect of, the cell-mediated immune response is discussed. These reactions are called delayed hypersensitivity and granulomatous reactions.

### 1.  Delayed Hypersensitivity Reactions

A delayed hypersensitivity reaction (DHR) is an immune-mediated inflammatory reaction initiated by immune T cells. This response is characterized by a perivascular accumulation of mononuclear cells at the site of antigen localization. The inflammatory response is induced and maintained by the release of inflammatory cytokines and enzymes, such as IL-1, lymphotoxin, interferon, and lysosomal hydrolases. The reaction is termed delayed because it occurs over a period of days or weeks, rather than minutes or hours, as in the Arthus reaction. This response is mediated by cytotoxic T lymphocytes (which directly destroy antigen-bearing cells), Td cells (which release inflammatory lymphokines), and macrophages (which infiltrate in response to chemotactic factors released by sensitized lymphocytes).

The DHR results in contact dermatitis, graft rejection, graft-versus-host reactions, and many of the lesions characteristic of viral infections. Contact dermatitis is mediated mainly by cytotoxic T lymphocytes that cross the epidermis and kill epithelial cells. The classic contact dermatitis reaction is observed with poison ivy or poison oak and is characterized by redness, induration, and vesiculation. Graft rejection is also the result of target cell death (recognized as foreign by the expression of nonself-MHC class I proteins) and lymphokine release by sensitized T cells. A DHR to viral antigens expressed on host cells may be either protective, by limiting viral infection, or destructive, by destroying functioning host cells. The DHR mediates the fever and eruptive skin lesions observed with some viral infections.

### 2.  Granulomatous Reactions

Granulomatous reactions (GR) are also cell-mediated and are identified by a focal collection of mononuclear cells (Sell, 1987h). Granulomatous reactions are cellular responses to irritating, persistent, and poorly soluble substances that may be initiated by sensitized lymphocytes with the deposition of immune complexes. Granulomas may progress from highly cellular reactions to fibrous scars or central necrosis surrounded by fibrous scars. Granulomatous hypersensitivity diseases include infectious disease (e.g., tuberculosis), antigenic responses (e.g., zirconium granuloma, berylliosis), and diseases of unknown etiology (e.g., sarcoidosis).

## G.  Autoimmune Disease

Most diseases discussed in the foregoing were placed in the context of an immune response to an exogenous agent, such as a heavy metal or virus, which, in turn, has debilitating consequences

(Druet et al., 1982). However, as was described in the section on antibody-mediated disease, an immune response can occur to one's own antigens, termed *autoimmunity,* through loss of tolerance to self. Acquired hemolytic anemia, idiopathic thrombocytopenia, and lupus erythematosus are examples of autoimmune disease that are the result of a humoral immune response. There are many other autoimmune diseases that are the result of cell-mediated immune responses. One disease, encephalomyelitis, can be experimentally induced in animals by immunization with tissues from the central nervous system. The resulting disease is very similar to acute hemorrhagic and acute disseminated encephalomyelitis in the acute phase and to multiple sclerosis in the chronic phase. Many other diseases, including uveitis, peripheral neuritis, thyroiditis, orchitis, and Sjogren's syndrome, fall into this category of autoimmunity. However, most diseases in which the immune system attacks self (i.e., autoimmunity) are a mixture of all of the effector mechanisms discussed earlier and are the result of many interacting factors.

## H. Immunostimulation

Immunostimulation may occur in a therapeutic setting, such as during vaccination to a pathogen or stimulation of the immune system of patients with immunodeficiencies or neoplasia, or as the result of exposure to environmental toxicants capable of stimulating immune responsiveness. Therefore, exposure to environmental toxicants can result in immune-mediated disease. It is also conceivable that exposure to an agent that causes nonspecific immune stimulation can exacerbate preexisting immune-mediated diseases.

## IX. SUMMARY

The immune system is in constant flux and responds to our environment to protect us from foreign invaders. Modulation of the immune system, either through disease or exposure to xenobiotics, can result in the inability to rid ourselves of foreign invaders (suppression) or inappropriate immune responses and subsequent immune-mediated disease (stimulation).

## REFERENCES

Ammann, A. J. (1987). Immunodeficiency disease. In *Basic and Clinical Immunology* (D. P. Stites, J. D. Stobo, and J. V. Wells, eds.), Appleton & Lange, Norwalk, CT, pp. 317–355.

Arden, C. J., et al. (1985). Diversity and structure of genes of the alpha family of mouse T cell antigen receptor, *Nature,* 316, 783–788.

diZerega, G. S. and Rodgers, K. E. (1992). Peritoneal macrophages. In *The Peritoneum,* Springer-Verlag, New York, pp. 136–154.

Druet, P., Bernard, A., Hirsch, F., Weening, J. J., Gengoux, P., Mahieu, P., and Birkeland, S. (1982). Immunologically mediated glomerulonephritis induced by heavy metals, *Arch. Toxicol.* 50, 197–194.

Erb, P. and Feldmann, M. (1975). The role of macrophages in the generation of T helper cells. III. Influence of macrophage-derived factors in helper cell induction, *Eur. J. Immunol.,* 5, 759–766.

Folch, H. and Waksman, B. H. (1974). The splenic suppressor cell. I. Activity of thymus dependent adherent cells: Changes with age and stress, *J. Immunol.,* 113, 127–139.

Goodman, J. W. (1987). Immunoglobulin I: Structure and function. In *Basic and Clinical Immunology* (D. P. Stites, J. D. Stobo, and J. V. Wells, eds.), Appleton & Lange, Norwalk, CT, pp. 27–36.

Gorczynski, R. M., Miller, R. G., and Phillips, R. A. (1971). In vivo requirement for radiation resistent cell in the immune response to sheep erythrocytes, *J. Exp. Med.,* 134, 1201–1221.

Goust, J. M. (1990). Cell-mediated immunity. In *Introduction to Medical Immunology* (G. Virella, J. M. Goust, H. H. Fudenberg, and G. G. Patrick, eds.), Marcel Dekker, New York, pp. 195–216.

Heiss, L. E. and Palmer, D. L. (1978). Anergy in patients with leukocytosis. *Am. J. Med.,* 56, 323–333.

Jose, D. J. and Good, R. A. (1973). Quantitative effects of nutritional essential amino acid deficiency upon immune responses to tumors in mice, *J. Exp. Med.,* 137, 1–9.

Katz, D. H. and Benacerraf, B. (1972). The regulatory influence of activated T cells on B cell responses to antigen, *Adv. Immunol.,* 15, 1–24.

Miller, J. F. A. P., Sprent, F. R. S., Basten, R. S., et al. (1971). Cell to cell interaction in the immune response. VII. Requirement for differentiation of thymus-derived cells, *J. Exp. Med.,* 134, 1266–1284.

Monjan, A. A. and Collector, M. I. (1977). Stress induced modulation of the immune response, *Science,* 196, 307–308.

Oppenheim, J. J., Ruscetti, F. W., and Faltynek, C. R. (1987). Interleukins and interferons. In *Basic and Clinical Immunology* (D. P. Stites, J. D. Stobo, and J. V. Wells, eds.), Appleton & Lange, Norwalk, CT, pp. 82–95.

Penn, I. (1985). Neoplastic consequences of immunosuppression. In *Immunotoxicology and Immunopharmacology* (J. H. Dean, M. I. Luster, A. E. Munson, et al., eds.), Raven Press, New York, pp. 79–89.

Purtilo, D. T., Halgrew, M., and Yunis, E. J. (1972). Depressed maternal lymphocyte responses to phytohemagglutinin in human pregnancy, Lancet, 1, 769–771.

Rose, N. R. and Mackay, I. R. (1992). *The Autoimmune Diseases,* Academic Press, San Diego, CA.

Sell, S. (1987a). Introduction to immunology. In *Immunology, Immunopathology and Immunity,* Elsevier Science, New York, pp. 3–14.

Sell S. (1987b). Inflammation. In *Immunology, Immunopathology and Immunity,* Elsevier Science, New York, pp. 261–306.

Sell, S. (1987c). The immune system III: Development of lymphoid organs (ontogeny). In *Immunology, Immunopathology and Immunity,* Elsevier Science, New York, pp. 57–68.

Sell, S. (1987d). Inactivation or activation of biologically active molecules. In *Immunology, Immunopathology, and Immunity,* Elsevier Science, New York, pp. 323–348.

Sell, S. (1987e). Cytotoxic or cytolytic reactions. In *Immunology, Immunopathology and Immunity,* Elsevier Science, New York, pp. 349–372.

Sell, S. (1987f). Immune complex reactions. In *Immunology, Immunopathology and Immunity.* Elsevier Science, New York, pp. 373–412.

Sell, S. (1987g). Delayed hypersensitivity reactions (cell-mediated immunity). In *Immunology, Immunopathology and Immunity,* Elsevier Science, New York, pp. 471–510.

Sell, S. (1987h). Granulomatous reactions. In *Immunology, Immunopathology and Immunity,* Elsevier Science, New York, pp. 529–544.

Stobo, J. D., Levitt, D., and Cooper, M. D. (1987). Lymphocytes. In *Basic and Clinical Immunology* (D. P. Stites, J. D. Stobo, and J. V. Wells, eds.), Appleton & Lange, Norwalk, CT, pp. 65–81.

Terr, A. I. (1987). Allergic diseases. In *Basic and Clinical Immunology* (D. P. Stites, J. D. Stobo, and J. V. Wells, eds.), Appleton & Lange, Norwalk, CT, pp. 435–456.

Tonegawa, S. (1983). Somatic generation of antibody diversity, *Nature,* 302, 575–579.

Virella, G., Patrick, C. C., and Goust, J. M. (1990). Tissues and cells in the immune response. In *Introduction to Medical Immunology* (G. Virella, J. M. Goust, H. H. Fudenberg, and G. G. Patrick, eds.), Marcel Dekker, New York, pp. 11–30.

Virella, G. (1990). Humoral immune response. In *Introduction to Medical Immunology* (G. Virella, J. M. Goust, H. H. Fudenberg, and G. G. Patrick, eds.), Marcel Dekker, New York, pp. 217–238.

# 7
# Pharmacokinetics and Risk Assessment

**Raghubir P. Sharma**
*University of Georgia*
*Athens, Georgia*

**Roger A. Coulombe, Jr.**
*Utah State University*
*Logan, Utah*

## I. INTRODUCTION

The exposure of an animal to a foreign chemical initiates a series of events in which the compound is absorbed, distributed, altered, and eliminated. When the chemical reaches the blood from the site of administration, it is quickly diffused into nearly every tissue of the body, until an equilibrium occurs. The study of these processes is called *pharmacokinetics*. More accurately, pharmacokinetics is the study of the behavior (i.e., absorption, distribution, and elimination) of foreign (and endogenous) chemicals in the body. The term pharmacokinetics is derived from the Greek words *pharmacon* (medicine or poison) and *kineticos* (movement). In describing and quantitating the behavior of chemicals in the body, pharmacokinetics makes wide use of words, symbols, or equations derived from animal data. Because classic pharmacokinetic studies all rely on determinations of the plasma or blood concentration of the chemical, the analysis is only as good as the accuracy of these determinations. Within the context of the present discussion, an ultimate goal of pharmacokinetics is to predict the risk posed to various tissues and to the individual from chemical exposure. Pharmacokinetic data generated from animal and human studies are an important component in the overall assessment of human health risk.

## II. GENERAL PHARMACOKINETIC PRINCIPLES

### A. The Compartment Concept

In an effort to simplify the description of chemical behavior in the body, pharmacokineticists make use of the term *compartment* to include any tissue, or more accurately, any group of tissues that have rates of uptake and elimination of the chemical in question. In this sense, the body is composed of countless compartments, because each cell can be considered a small compartment. In practice, however, only a few compartments, generally up to three, can be discerned from conventional plasma chemical concentration determinations. The blood serves as the common conduit that conducts chemicals into and out of various compartments and is often called the *central compartment,* this compartment actually includes all organs and tissues in which the chemical is in rapid equilibrium. Conversely, peripheral compartments would include those tissues and organs in which the chemical equilibration occurs more slowly than in the central compartment.

Whether the chemical is said to be in equilibrium with one or more compartments, is determined by analyzing the time course of the log plasma concentration of a chemical in an animal. Since most chemicals enter cells by diffusion, the rate of transport is first-order relative to the concentration of the chemical. In the simplest case following a single bolus injection, a chemical's behavior is best described by one-compartment pharmacokinetics; the log plasma concentration versus time curve yields a straight line when plotted on a semi-logarithmic scale (Fig. 1).

Here, the data depict the body as one unit relative to drug movement (i.e., the chemical partitions into the various tissues, such as the blood, liver, and kidneys, at an equal rate). This can be illustrated by a one-compartment model in which $k_{ab}$ and $k_{el}$ are constants that describe the rate of entry and elimination, respectively, of the chemical from the central compartment (Fig. 2).

The movement (appearance and disappearance) of the chemical in the plasma over time can be described by the first-order expression

$$C = C_0 \, e^{-k_{el} \, t}$$

where $C$ is the concentration of the chemical at any time $t$ and $C_0$ is the concentration of the chemical when time $= 0$, and $k_{el}$ the first-order elimination rate constant. The plasma concentration at time 0 can be obtained as the $y$-intercept of the straight line. A plot of the log $C$ against time is linear with a slope of $k_{el}/2.303$.

From this data, we can determine an important measure of the residence time of the chemical in the body, or *half-life* ($t_{1/2}$). The half-life is the time required to eliminate one-half of the chemical from the blood or plasma (where the drug is usually sampled) and is calculated by the equation:

$$t_{1/2} = \frac{0.693}{k_{el}}$$

Note that $t_{1/2}$ is *independent* of dose and is affected only by the rate of elimination. Plasma

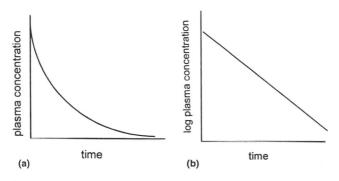

**Figure 1**   (a) Plasma concentration vs. time; (b) curve is linear when log plasma concentration vs. time is plotted.

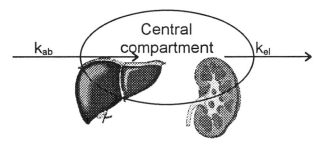

**Figure 2** Illustration of a one-compartment model.

half-life can also be easily obtained by inspecting the curve of this relationship, as can $C_0$, $k_{el}$, and $t_{1/2}$.

The $k_{el}$ is a first-order elimination rate constant with units of reciprocal time (such as min$^{-1}$ or hr$^{-1}$) and is defined as the proportion of the drug eliminated to the total amount remaining at any one time. Therefore, a $k_{el}$ of 0.05 min$^{-1}$ means that 5% of the total amount of chemical present at any time is eliminated in 1 min. Although the absolute amount of the chemical being eliminated declines over time, the *fraction* of the total amount present in the body that is eliminated remains constant.

The idealized curve in Figure 3, with instantaneous absorption approximates the events following a single intravenous administration of a chemical. When a chemical is administered to an animal other than intravenously, such as orally, dermally, or subcutaneously, absorption is not instantaneous, and a distinct lag period before peak concentration of the chemical in the plasma is seen. This lag period is due to the time necessary for the chemical to reach the plasma from the site of administration. Following administration of a single oral dose of a chemical, the plot is similar to that seen after an intravenous dose, except for the lag period (Fig. 4). The curve is the result of two exponential processes, one describing the "absorptive phase," the other describing the "postabsorptive" or "elimination phase." The equation describing this plot is similar to that for instantaneous administration, except for the addition of an exponential expression describing absorption of the chemical into the central compartment.

The plasma chemical concentration at time 0 ($C_0$) can be determined by extrapolating the linear portion of the elimination curve to the y-axis. A is the y-intercept of the absorptive rate curve created using the method of *residuals*. This entails plotting the points obtained by

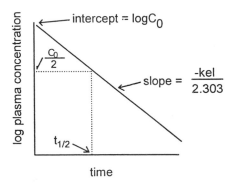

**Figure 3** Plasma concentration vs. time plot illustrating one-compartment pharmacokinetics following a single intravascular bolus dose.

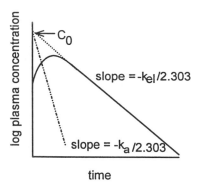

**Figure 4**   Plasma concentration vs. time plot illustrating one-compartment pharmacokinetics following a single oral dose.

subtracting the experimentally determined plasma concentration values from the extrapolated plasma chemical concentration values at the early time intervals. The absorptive rate constant $k_a$ is determined from the slope of this line.

This extrapolated line can be used to obtain a quantitative measurement of the rate of chemical absorption. In this example, two opposite influences, absorption and elimination, simultaneously determine the time course of the concentration of the chemical in the plasma. The plasma concentration will continue to rise until the rate of absorption equals the elimination rate. At the early time periods, the absorption dominates drug behavior, but the elimination term eventually characterizes plasma concentration of the chemical.

The behavior of a chemical in the body is frequently too complex to be described by a one-compartment model. In this instance, the chemical is distributed more slowly into a second group of tissues, as is evident from the log plasma concentration versus time plot which may show a multiexponential character, with more than one linear region. The equilibrium of a chemical about the central and peripheral tissue compartments is illustrated by Figure 5.

Movement of the chemical into and out of the central and peripheral compartment(s) can be measured by various pharmacokinetic relationships described later. In addition to the absorption and elimination rate constants, the kinetics for the chemical is described by the intermediate constants $k_{1,2}$ and $k_{2,1}$. The first number of the subscript designates the originating compartment and the second number designates the receiving compartment. Figure 6 shows an idealized plot of the distribution of a chemical in the plasma following a bolus injection in which the time course of chemical in the plasma is a composite of two distinct exponential functions, one representing a rapidly equilibrating group of tissues (central compartment) and a second, more slowly equilibrating compartment (peripheral compartment). These two exponential phases can be described by the equation.

$$C = Ae^{-\alpha t} + Be^{-\beta t}$$

in which the first exponential term represents the distributive phase, whereas the second represents the postdistributive or elimination phase. In the two-compartment model, $A$ and $B$ are the intercepts of the extrapolated lines for the elimination and absorption rate processes, respectively. The slope of the elimination phase of the curve is used to determine $\beta$, the overall elimination rate constant, whereas the slope of the absorptive phase curve is $\alpha$. The overall or hybrid elimination rate constant $\beta$ is a composite of several individual constants and can be used

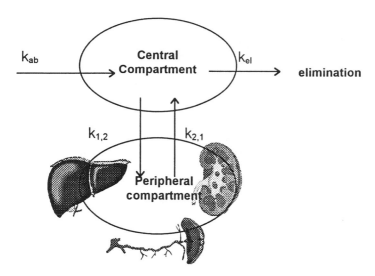

**Figure 5** Illustration of a two-compartment model.

to calculate the biological half-life of the compound as $0.693/\beta$. Likewise, $\alpha$ is the hybrid value for absorption into the second compartment.

Other useful parameters describing chemical fate in the body, such as volume of distribution and area-under-the-curve (AUC), can be determined, and the reader is referred to a more definitive source for their derivations (Gibaldi and Perrier, 1982).

## B. The Plateau Principle

Human exposures to environmental contaminants in water, air, and food, do not usually occur as a single bolus, but usually occur on a regular basis and at a constant rate. Thus, the rate of exposure to environmental toxins is *zero-order* (i.e., exposure is independent of other factors). However, as with single exposures, the rate of chemical elimination is always a first-order process relative to the amount of chemical in the body, unless the exposure is very high and elimination is governed by saturation kinetics.

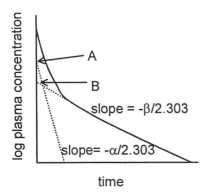

**Figure 6** Plasma concentration vs. time plot illustrating two-compartment pharmacokinetics following a single intravenous bolus dose.

In such multiple-dose situations, in which the rate of input of chemical in the body is constant and the rate of output or elimination of the chemical in the body is first-order relative to the amount present in the body, the body burden of chemical can be predicted from the ratio of the regular, zero-order intake rate of a chemical ($k_a$ with units of amount per time) to the overall elimination rate constant ($k_e$ with units of reciprocal time) according to the equation

$$X = \frac{k_a}{k_e}$$

Over time, the body burden of chemical ($X$) will increase in a zigzag pattern until a plateau ($X_{max}$) is reached, which represents an equilibrium between intake and elimination. Although the proportion of chemical eliminated ($k_e$) always remains constant, at plateau, the absorption and elimination of the chemical are equal (Fig. 7). Accumulation of chemical to the plateau is 50% complete when $t = t_{1/2}$ for that chemical. Thus, for any chemical, half-plateau is reached according to the equation

$$t_{1/2} = \frac{0.693}{k_e}$$

and $X_{max}$ is reached in approximately five to seven half-lives.

Accumulation of chemicals in the body resulting from constant exposures can be compared with a bank account in which there are regular deposits and regular withdrawals, when the amount of money withdrawn is based on some constant proportion of the available balance. Assume that you opened an account with $1 and deposited an additional dollar each day (i.e., $k_a = \$1$ $day^{-1}$), and withdrew half of the total balance available each day (i.e., $k_e = 0.5$ $day^{-1}$), your account would reach a maximum balance or "plateau" (i.e., $X_{max}$) of $1.99 (about $2) in approximately 7 days at which time the amount of money deposited would be in near equilibrium with the amount withdrawn. The balance would rise and fall in a zigzag pattern identical with that seen with zero-order chemical intake and first-order chemical elimination.

The elimination rate constant for most chemicals is significantly less than 0.5 $day^{-1}$, but the principles underlying chemical accumulation in the body are identical. This phenomenon is called the *plateau principle,* and for a more in-depth description as well as mathematical derivations, the reader is encouraged to consult a more definitive source (Neubig, 1990).

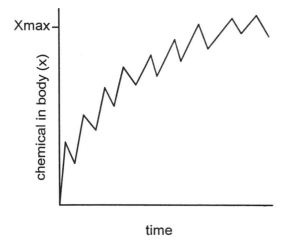

**Figure 7** Plasma concentration vs. time plot following multiple doses of a chemical.

## III. LINEAR VERSUS NONLINEAR KINETICS

The pharmacokinetics of chemicals in the body are generally linear if the dose of chemical is small and processes, such as metabolism and excretion, are not saturated. The kinetics is considered linear if the decline (or various phases of decline) is linear when the logarithm of plasma concentration of a chemical is a straight line when plotted against time. As indicated earlier, there may be more than one phase of decline yielding several corresponding half-life values ($t_{1/2}$); each successive $t_{1/2}$ is larger than the preceding value. Therefore, the pharmacokinetics of a chemical with multiple compartments (multiexponential), representing phases of distribution (or distribution in several compartments), excretion, and metabolism, is essentially linear. Here, the $t_{1/2}$ values, composition of metabolites, and route of excretion are independent of dose, whereas AUC value is proportional to dose (Levy, 1968).

In many toxicology studies, however, relatively large doses are used. Many long-term studies are conducted at the so-called maximum-tolerated dose (MTD) level, and the experiments involving pharmacokinetics may also involve doses that are several orders of magnitude larger than the intended or inadvertent exposure levels. Use of large doses facilitates the quantitative characterization of transformation products or, in some cases, simplifies analytical methods. Large-dose pharmacokinetics helps determine the large-dose exposures in long-term experiments. It has now been well recognized that pharmacokinetic parameters may be dose-dependent, and for the purpose of risk-assessment, pharmacokinetic values at exposure levels closest to real-life situations are extremely important.

It is not unusual to saturate the metabolism or excretion when evaluating xenobiotics of relatively low toxicity. Metabolic pathways are easy to saturate with chemicals that have low $K_m$ values. Excretory processes are saturated for substances that are eliminated by active transport mechanisms. For example, many organic acids and quaternary amines follow active secretary pathways in renal tubules or in bile. The decline of chemicals in plasma at these levels will, therefore, not be log-linear, but should follow a Michaelis-Menten type kinetics. The $t_{1/2}$ pattern of excretory products, and even the route of excretion can be altered by increasing the dose.

Ethanol is a good example of such nonlinear pharmacokinetics. The $K_m$ of ethanol in humans is estimated to be 82 mg/L (Holford, 1987), and since the toxic and euphoric effects of alcohol begin at blood alcohol levels of 800 mg/L (legal basis of intoxication in many states), the plasma decline of alcohol is largely linear with time, rather than exponential. The disappearance rates become linear when blood levels are close to the $K_m$ value and the metabolism reverts to a first-order process, rather than a zero-order at high-alcohol levels. An approximated blood concentration of ethanol after a large dose of 96 ml of ethanol (roughly equivalent to five drinks of 80 proof liquor) is illustrated in Figure 8.

The process is similar for 1,4-dioxane, a widely used organic solvent (Young et al., 1978). When rats were injected with an intravenous dose ranging between 3 and 1000 mg/kg (the median lethal dose [$LD_{50}$] of 1,4-dioxane in rats is 5600 mg/kg), the plasma decline for this chemical was linear between 3- and 30-mg/kg doses (Fig. 9). A saturation phenomenon was obvious at doses of 100 mg/kg and above, at which the decline in plasma for 1,4-dioxane levels was linear when concentrations declined below 30 μg/ml. 1,4-Dioxane is carcinogenic in rats at high levels of exposure, particularly when organ pathology is also associated with the treatment (Kociba et al., 1974), suggesting that biotransformation of 1,4-dioxane to a toxic metabolite in the body occurs only at levels at which saturation of its normal metabolism (which is observed at relatively lower concentrations) has occurred. Since the rate of elimination of 1,4-dioxane at low-level exposure (e.g., 50 ppm in air for 6 h) in humans (Young et al., 1977) is similar to that observed in the rat (Young et al., 1978), it was predicted that the metabolism of this chemical

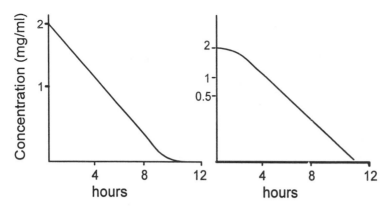

**Figure 8** Simulated decline of ethanol in adult human blood. The model is based on estimated values as $K_m$ of 82 mg/L and $V_{max}$ of 125 mg/kg$^{-1}$hr$^{-1}$. Nonlinearity at the exponential scale (right) suggests a saturation phenomenon and a nonlinear pharmacokinetics.

will probably not be saturated in occupational exposures, and 50 ppm may be considered a safe exposure value.

## IV. PHARMACOKINETICS AND EXTRAPOLATION OF TOXICITY DATA FROM ANIMALS TO HUMANS

Toxicology is largely a predictive science. A thorough testing of chemicals for their untoward effects is neither feasible nor desirable in people. Laboratory animals, particularly rodents, therefore, are largely used for routine toxicity evaluation. For new chemicals and chemicals with low toxicity, or for carcinogen evaluations, large doses are administered to test animals and various toxicity parameters are observed. Models to extrapolate the large-dose effects to probability of effect at low doses in animals and humans are described, many of these are considered in detail elsewhere in this monograph. In several instances, however, these extrapolations are not corroborated with observations in humans, for whom accidental or occupational exposures have provided a reasonable amount of data.

Toxicity of a chemical is a net effect of large numbers of processes. Besides the dose, other major factors that need to be considered are variations in absorption, distribution, metabolism, and excretion, among others. These are commonly referred to as pharmacokinetic parameters and are generally species-dependent. These are not the only considerations, however; differences in species sensitivity can be determined by other genetic factors (e.g., variation in specific receptors, ability of certain species to repair the damage, or other). But when all factors are considered, pharmacokinetic variables are of major importance and should be considered in extrapolation of laboratory data to humans, since changes in various parameters of pharmacokinetics are either easily determined experimentally or can be predicted with a reasonable accuracy.

An illustration of high-dose to low-dose extrapolation has been indicated in the forgoing, in which 1,4-dioxane is characterized by a saturation kinetics at relatively higher doses, but shows a linear one-compartment model at doses of less than 30 mg/kg in rats. In addition to a saturation phenomenon observed at high doses, differences in pharmacokinetics at relatively similar levels can also be seen. An example of that is the insecticide, 2,4-dinitrophenol.

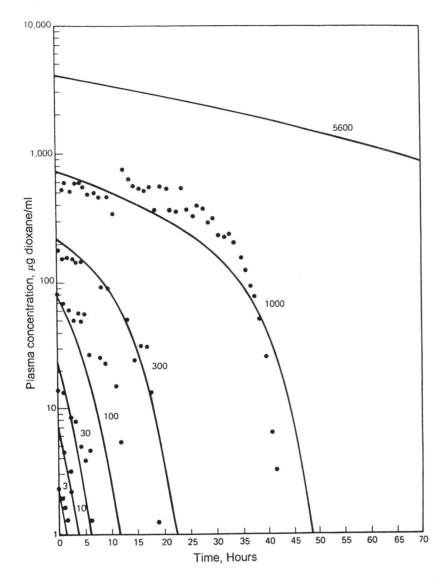

**Figure 9** Concentration of dioxane in plasma of rats given various intravenous doses of 1,4-dioxane. The values close to graphs depict milligram per kilogram of dioxane. (From Young et al., 1978.)

Dinitrophenol is highly toxic, and in low doses, it produced corneal opacity in ducklings and young rabbits (Gehring and Buerge, 1969). A close examination of pharmacokinetic parameters suggested that the first-order elimination of dinitrophenol in young versus mature rabbits was 0.15 and 0.82 hr$^{-1}$, respectively. Ducklings are also very susceptible to cataractogenic effects of dinitrophenol, and its kinetics are compatible with a two-compartment open model with elimination constants of 0.25 and 0.11 hr$^{-1}$ for the rapid and slow phases, respectively.

Differences in pathways of metabolism can also play a major role in determining toxicity of a given chemical. Some of the examples indicated here will illustrate this point; however, important consideration should be given to the information available for each chemical.

## V.  DOSE-DEPENDENT METABOLIC FATE OF CHEMICALS

Although biotransformation of chemicals is usually a first-order process, deviation of this general rule often occurs when the chemical in question is present in large amounts and saturates the metabolic systems. Examples of saturated metabolism (i.e., that of ethanol and 1,4-dioxane) have been indicated earlier. If a chemical is toxic, or is converted to toxic products in vivo, the fraction of chemical or its toxic metabolite observed in the body or tissues at usual test doses may not necessarily reflect the proportions that would be expected at the low levels of exposure that are relevant. Detoxification processes can be saturated when large doses of chemicals are employed, thereby providing larger fractions of toxic intermediates or of the parent compound.

The problem can be further complicated when certain metabolic processes appear only when large concentrations of the chemical are available in tissues. If an enzyme has a high $K_m$ value, its product will not be found at low concentration when other enzymes of relatively low $K_m$ values may be more operative. This phenomenon was elegantly illustrated by Gehring et al. (1976) for chemicals that are eliminated or metabolized by more than one process. Figure 10 provides a diagrammatic representation of such processes, the secondary pathway appears and magnifies as the dose or exposure increases. The phenomenon is apparently more prevalent when nonlinear pharmacokinetics is apparent at high-dose levels. Repeated exposures can also build a high body burden and may saturate the primary pathways of metabolism; therefore, results obtained from pharmacokinetic studies at a high-dose level should be carefully considered in extrapolating the information to small-dose conditions.

This point can be adequately illustrated by the dose-related toxicity of *o*-phenylphenol. This chemical caused bladder tumors in F344 rats when diets contained 1% or more of *o*-phenylphenol for 13–91 weeks (Hiraga and Fujii, 1981). Reitz et al. (1983) investigated the dose-related toxicity of this chemical and its sodium salt. At low levels in rats, the primary

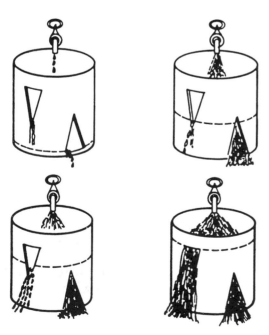

**Figure 10**  Diagrammatic representation of elimination of a chemical by a primary saturable pathway and by a secondary pathway, the significance of which increases with saturation of the primary pathway. (From Gehring et al., 1976.)

metabolites of *o*-phenylphenol were water-soluble glucuronides or sulfate esters. The chemical can also be activated to a dihydroquinone derivative by the liver microsomal mixed function oxidase system, the activated molecule that can produce macromolecular adducts in the urinary bladder. The presence of dihydroquinone metabolite was not detected when *o*-phenylphenol was administered as 5 or 50 mg/kg, but when doses were increased to 500 mg/kg, nearly a quarter of the total radioactivity was in the form of this metabolite. The dose-related tissue binding and toxicity were also confirmed in subchronic studies. *o*-Phenylphenol, therefore, can be considered a carcinogen only at doses that saturate the conjugation pathways, thereby allowing production of a toxic metabolite that is capable of DNA-binding.

# VI. SPECIES DIFFERENCES IN FATE OF CHEMICALS AND EFFECT ON PHARMACOKINETICS AND BIOLOGICAL EFFECTS

## A. Differences in Metabolism

There are major differences in the rates of metabolism between species (Williams, 1971). Differences have been found in both phase I and phase II reactions. For example, when aniline is hydroxylated by microsomal enzymes, it produces both *p*-hydroxyaniline and *o*-hydroxyaniline. The ratio of para/ortho derivatives is close to or less than 1 in dog, cat, and ferret, 4–6 in mouse, rats, and rabbit, whereas it is 15 in the gerbil. Cats are deficient in glucuronic acid conjugation, whereas the pig is relatively poor in sulfate conjugation, compared with the dog. These differences not only alter the nature of biotransformation products, but also affect the rates of metabolism of xenobiotics and can have profound effects on pharmacokinetic behavior of chemicals.

An illustration of the role of metabolism and its effect on pharmacokinetics is apparent from the species variability for the metabolism of thiopental. Thiopental is a sulfur-containing barbiturate used for the induction of short-term surgical anesthesia. After an intravenous dose, it produces anesthesia in humans for only 5–15 min; its short-term effect has been attributed to a rapid redistribution of the chemical from central nervous system to rest of the organs. Thiobarbiturates are relatively more lipid-soluble and, hence, able to enter the brain without an apparent blood–brain barrier. As the levels decline in plasma owing to rapid distribution in other organs of the body, brain levels also decline rapidly, causing a termination of anesthetic effects. In some species, however (e.g. in cattle), the anesthetic effect of a single intravenous dose of thiopental persists for more than an hour. Sharma et al. (1970a) determined the role of metabolism on the kinetics of this drug in various large animal species. Thiopental is metabolized by cattle liver at a rate that is two to three times lower than in sheep, goat, or swine, species that have an anesthesia lasting for only 5–20 min. When the pharmacokinetics of thiopental was evaluated in all these species, the initial or delayed rates of distribution were similar in all species, the final elimination rate from plasma was three to five times slower in cattle than in other farm animals. Even in cattle, when the rate of thiopental and metabolism was increased by pretreatment of animals with phenobarbital, a known inducer of microsomal metabolism, the terminal plasma rate was increased by 2.5 times over untreated animals; accordingly, the liver metabolism was also increased to the same extent (Sharma et al., 1970b). The duration of anesthesia was not altered after phenobarbital pretreatment because the distribution phase for thiopental lasts for 2 h in most animal species; the recovery from depression was reduced by nearly fivefold, as it was determined by the final elimination phase, and it was considerably altered.

## B. Renal Elimination and Species or Sex Differences

The differences in renal elimination in different species are expected and well known, largely owing to relative kidney size and blood flow. Even considerable sex differences in elimination have been noticed for some chemicals. Braun and Sauerhoff (1976) measured urinary excretion of pentachlorophenol in both sexes of monkeys. Although the extent of renal excretion was similar in male and female monkeys, the total elimination was completed twice as fast in males as in females. The corresponding plasma disappearance half-life values were 72 and 83.5 h for males and females, respectively. The importance of sex differences on pharmacokinetics can be emphasized by such an example.

## VII. PHYSIOLOGICAL MODELING IN PHARMACOKINETICS

Risk assessment is largely extrapolation of experimental data either from a high-dose scenario to environmental levels, or from animal experimentation to human situations. Indeed much of this is done by using various models. However, the use of modeling is nowhere greater in risk assessment of chemicals than it is in defining pharmacokinetics. Pharmacokinetic parameters are largely result of various processes, such as absorption, distribution, accumulation, metabolism, and elimination. Many of these processes are defined by known rate orders, and variations are understood both in dose-related differences or in species variations. Modeling of pharmacokinetics thus provides an excellent opportunity for incorporating these differences into refinement of risk assessment.

Pharmacokinetic modeling based on physiological behavior of chemicals is relatively new, at least in its present form. Currently, there is a great interest in physiologically based models, partly because much experimental data has been accumulated so these models can be verified, and also because of the popularity of computers and available software. Modeling that is based on physiological processes has been performed for a long time; however, most toxicologists either did not want to undertake difficult computational problems, or did not appreciate the far-reaching consequences that such models can provide. Much of the earlier models were based on the fit of available experimental data, rather than on predicting the experimental variables based on known physicochemical values for the chemical.

Briefly, a physiologically based pharmacokinetic (PBPK) model is a prediction of pharmacokinetic behavior of a given chemical, given the distribution and elimination of the chemical. Rates of distribution can be accurately predicted by total mass and blood flow to various organs, provided the transport is essentially by diffusion. Parameters such as octanol/water partition coefficient to describe the lipid solubility, and thus the rate of transport or tissue/blood ratio of the drug, can be incorporated in the function. The elimination process is predicted by the rate of metabolism, and a Michaelis-Menten type of kinetics can be incorporated to describe a saturable phenomenon. Renal elimination rates, or loss by other routes, are either known experimentally or predicted from chemicals with similar physicochemical characteristics. A set of simultaneous differential equations is thus derived and solved by using a computer. The reader is referred to other publications for details of such equations (Andersen et al., 1987; Gerlowski and Jain, 1983). The principle has been applied to a variety of chemicals and models, then verified (Leung et al., 1988; Andersen et al., 1991). The role of specific-binding receptors, generation and distribution of metabolites, and resulting toxicological effects are incorporated in these models that have been described. A general kinetic model is provided in Figure 11.

Such a model was predicted after an intravenous injection of 20 mg/kg of thiopental in swine using parameters described earlier (Sharma et al., 1970a). The differential equations were approached using an analog computer and the model shown in Figure 11. The resulting predicted and experimentally derived plasma concentrations are shown in Figure 12.

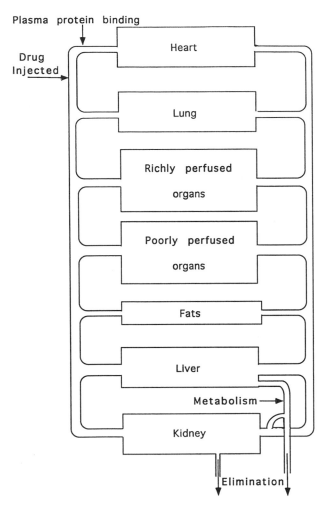

**Figure 11** A simplified general presentation of physiologically based pharmacokinetic model after intravenous injection of a drug. The main differential equation will be: $\frac{dQ_u}{dt} = (k_{ux}Q_u + k_{uy}Q_u) + \frac{dQ_a}{dt}$ $+ \frac{dQ_b}{dt} + \cdots$, where $Q_u$ is the quantity of unbound (free) drug is plasma, $t$ is time, $k_{ux}$ and $k_{uy}$ represent rates of metabolism and excretion, respectively, and $dQ_{a \to e}/dt$ represents the change in the amount of drug in a given organ. This last function $dQ_{a \to e}/dt$ can be predicted by a set of simultaneous equations (e.g., $dQ_a/dt = k_{au}Q_a - k_{ua}Q_u$ and so on, where $k_{au}$ and $k_{ua}$ refer to rate constants that indicate transport rates of drug from plasma (unbound) to the organ "a" and vice versa, and $Q_a$ is the amount of the drug in the organ. Richly perfused organs include liver and kidney uptake of the drug. Parameters $Q_{au}$ and $Q_{ua}$ may be approximately the same if there are no factors such as ion trapping or protein binding in tissues influencing the transport.

## VIII. PHARMACOKINETICS AND DEVELOPMENTAL RISK

One of the advantages of pharmacokinetics is prediction or experimental determination of chemical concentration in altered tissue states. Models have been applied to accumulation of anticancer drugs in cancerous tissue, for example, where it may be possible to determine the optimum differences in drug levels between the target cancerous tissue and blood or normal tissues and, therefore, increase the therapeutic ratio. These approaches are particularly useful in

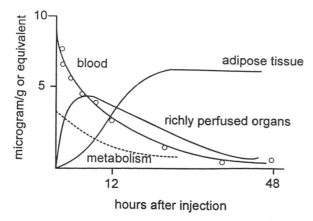

**Figure 12**  Predicted model of thiopental distribution after an intravenous injection in swine. The parameters used were those described by Sharma et al. (1970) and a set of differential equations indicated in Figure 11. The solid lines are the computer estimated curves, whereas the open circles are experimentally determined values. (Sharma, R. P., unpublished observations.)

development of drugs for which targeted drug delivery is the primary goal. Similar approaches are also important in providing therapeutic drug concentrations in other pathological tissues or organs. The role of pharmacokinetics, however, is highly evident in expression of developmental toxicity or for protection of the developing fetus from harmful agents.

To understand the risk of a developing human fetus to tetracycline, physiological models were developed (Olanoff and Anderson, 1980). These models are similar to the PBPK models (see Sec. VII), an extra function of placental blood flow and the resulting pharmacokinetics in various fetal tissues were added. These simulations can be modified to account for changing fetal mass and maternal blood flow to the uterus. However, it should be recognized that a difference in fetal pharmacokinetic parameters does not necessarily explain differences in the teratogenic potential of chemicals.

Several retinoids (derivatives of vitamin A) are teratogenic, and birth defects have been noticed in newborns after therapeutic use of these drugs by mothers. In the case of one such retinoid, etretinate (a methoxy derivative and acetate ester of retinoic acid), teratogenicity occurred even when the pregnancy started more than 1 year after the therapy had ceased (Lammer et al., 1987). The teratogenic potential of various retinoids varies over several orders of magnitude and pharmacokinetic differences have been investigated to describe some of these differences. Creech-Kraft et al. (1987) investigated the embryo concentrations of 13-*cis*-retinoic acid and suggested that its relatively low teratogenicity compared with its all-*trans* isomer can be described by low accumulation in the embryo. Similar findings were later reported for other metabolites of retinoic acid (Creech-Kraft et al., 1989). These workers suggested that pharmacokinetic parameters may be partly responsible for the observed differences in teratogenic potential (Kochhar et al., 1987). After further investigations with other retinoids (Howard et al., 1989a,b), it became apparent that pharmacokinetic differences do not explain the teratogenic potential of retinoids. New information suggests that a large contribution in retinoid teratogenesis comes from these compound's nuclear receptor interactions and perhaps their chemical stability to metabolic biotransformation, rather than to pharmacokinetic differences (Kim et al., 1994).

## IX. CANCER RISK ASSESSMENT AND PHARMACOKINETICS

Pharmacokinetic data have been critical in assessing the cancer risk associated with environmental and industrial exposures to many chemicals. Pharmacokinetics of a chemical is an important consideration because "real-world" exposures generally are much less than those that are used in long-term tumor studies to establish the carcinogenic activity of a chemical. It is often assumed that large doses are handled by the body in the same manner as smaller, more environmentally relevant doses, when in fact, high doses are known to often saturate enzymatic processes that activate or detoxify the chemical. Although the use of higher doses in long-term tumor studies is generally scientifically valid, pharmacokinetic analysis can be of great value in reconciling high-dose tumor studies with the risk expected at exposures to much lower doses. One of the best examples in which pharmacokinetic data contributed to an understanding of low-dose cancer risk estimates is vinyl chloride.

Vinyl chloride is an important monomeric starting material for the polymer polyvinyl chloride. Vinyl chloride is a volatile gas, and occupational inhalation of vinyl chloride is especially high in workers who clean reactor vessels used in the polymerization process. Vinyl chloride is a recognized human carcinogen, and it is these workers who are at the greatest risk for developing liver angiosarcomas (Maltoni and Selikoff, 1988). The carcinogenic action of vinyl chloride is presumably owing to cytochrome P-450-dependent activation to a reactive epoxide intermediate.

The pharmacokinetic fate of vinyl chloride appears to be affected primarily by the amount of vinyl chloride metabolized by an animal, rather than the dose. In a series of studies to determine the dose effects on the pharmacokinetics of vinyl chloride, Watanabe and Gehring (1976) noted that, as the oral doses were increased from 0.05 to 100 mg/kg, the amount of unmetabolized vinyl chloride in expired air increased, whereas the amount of vinyl chloride metabolites (as fraction of dose) found in urine, feces, and tissues, decreased. Thus, as the dose of vinyl chloride is increased, pulmonary expiration of vinyl chloride per se becomes the most important route of excretion. However, because the slopes of urinary vinyl chloride excretion over time were similar among these doses, the authors concluded that urinary excretion of nonvolatile vinyl chloride metabolites is independent of dose. Likewise, when rats are exposed for 6 hr to various concentrations of vinyl chloride in inhalation chambers, metabolism did not increase proportionately in response to increasing concentrations of vinyl chloride, but rather, obeyed Michaelis-Menten, or saturation kinetics (Gehring et al., 1978). If one uses a linear transformation of the Michaelis-Menten equation where $v$ and $V_m$ are the velocity and maximum velocity, respectively, for the biotransformation of vinyl chloride in microgram ($\mu$g) equivalents of vinyl chloride metabolized per 6 hr,

$$v = -K_m \frac{v}{S} + V_m$$

and $S$ and $K_m$ are the concentration of vinyl chloride inhaled and the Michaelis constant in micrograms per liter ($\mu$g/L) air, respectively, one can see that vinyl chloride kinetics follows saturation kinetics from the linearity of the data plot (Fig. 13).

When this nonlinear pharmacokinetic model was considered in light of the published tumor incidence in rats that were exposed to concentrations from 50 to 10,000 ppm vinyl chloride for 4 hr/day 5 days/week for 12 months (Maltoni and Lefemine, 1975), a probit plot for the incidence of hepatic angiosarcomas versus the amount of vinyl chloride metabolized, $v$, over the exposure concentration, $S$, yielded a straight line (Fig. 14). Assuming no threshold for the response (angiosarcomas) the authors calculated the lowest amount of vinyl chloride to produce

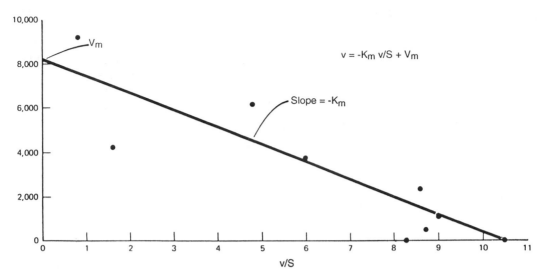

**Figure 13**  Metabolism of vinyl chloride analyzed in accordance with the Wolf-Augustinson-Hofstee form of the Michaelis-Menten equation. The line was fit by linear regression analysis with a regression coefficient of 0.88. (From Gehring et al. 1978.)

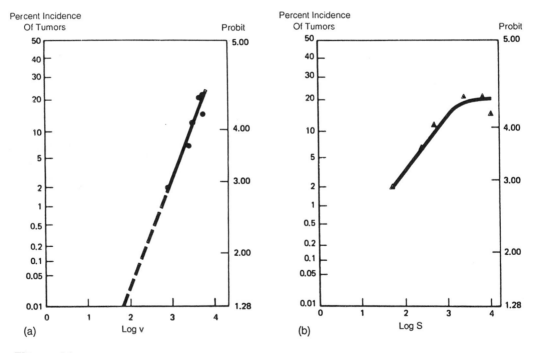

**Figure 14**  (a) Metabolism of vinyl chloride expressed as log $v$ (micrograms vinyl chloride metabolized every 4 hr) versus percentage incidence of hepatic angiosarcoma (probability scale). (b) Exposure concentration expressed as log $S$ (ppm vinyl chloride) versus the percentage incidence of hepatic angiosarcoma. The probit equivalents of the percentage incidence are shown on the right-hand ordinate. The solid line is the best fit for experimentally observed responses, and the dashed line represents extrapolation below those doses producing an observable response, assuming no threshold (Gehring et al. 1978.)

one angiosarcoma in 10,000 rats (an incidence of 0.01%), to be 4.6 ppm given an exposure of 4 h/day, 5 days/week for 1 year.

If the overall goal of pharmacokinetic analysis is to develop risk assessment models, how then does this data apply to human exposures? When corrected for body surface area and assuming no-response threshold, the theoretical extrapolation for persons exposed to 1 ppm vinyl chloride for 8 h/day, was calculated to be 1.5:100 million, which is less than the expected incidence of spontaneous angiosarcomas in humans (Gehring et al., 1978).

From this example, it is obvious that the pharmacokinetics of a chemical is an important consideration when assessing the risk posed by human exposure. Other examples for which pharmacokinetics has been used in risk assessment and low-dose extrapolation include, 1,3-butadiene, chloroform, and styrene.

## X. PROBLEMS AND FUTURE PERSPECTIVES

It is apparent that the principles of pharmacokinetics are indispensable in risk assessment. Variations in rates of distribution, excretion, and metabolism are very important when data are extrapolated from high-dose levels to low-dose levels and also from experimental animals to humans. A clear understanding of how different processes may vary in different situations is very important in predicting the health effects at exposure levels of practical importance in industrial or environmental situations. By using pharmacokinetic principles, it is possible to estimate the total body burden after a constant or repeated exposure for a certain time and how much time would be needed to completely eliminate the chemical from the body. This is particularly important in assessing a safe level of chemical exposure in special circumstances (e.g., extended shifts, pregnancy, or disease state).

It should be remembered, however, that pharmacokinetics is not a substitute for a better understanding of the mechanism of action of toxic compounds. Occasionally, a single parameter (e.g., peak plasma concentration) may be of greater importance than the clearance rates or half-life values in determining toxicity. In other instances, molecular mechanisms of chemicals need to be understood before a full assessment of their toxicity is possible.

Physiology-based pharmacokinetic models are extremely useful in evaluating the risk of chemicals. Several software programs have been developed to simplify this approach (Menzel et al., 1987). The greatest usefulness of these models is their flexibility. If a situation changes (e.g., because of disease, pregnancy, physical activity), the parameters can be easily rearranged to accommodate such alterations. The models can take account of saturable phenomena, such as high-dose kinetics for metabolism and elimination. If a chemical induces or inhibits its own metabolism, appropriate consideration for the same can be incorporated. The models are also flexible enough to include toxicological effects; for example, production of blood carboxy-hemoglobin after dichloromethane was modeled by Andersen et al. (1991). Extrapolation between species is easily done if differences in physiological processes related to them in these species are understood. Data are now available on relative mass and blood flow to different organs and tissues in many species, including humans (Gerlowski and Jain, 1983).

One of the challenges in pharmacokinetics is validation of these models for chemicals for which no experimental data are available. In most instances the models were constructed after a large volume of data on various parameters were experimentally derived, to check if these data fit a predictive model. Although validation is an important task in model development, it does little for prospective modeling for new chemicals. If physicochemical properties of the new chemical are known, and factors such as its metabolism and excretion can be adequately predicted, reasonably accurate models can be constructed. However, it is necessary to carry out more extensive studies with a series of chemicals to ascertain structure–activity relationships in pharmacokinetics. A better prediction of models for new chemicals will then be possible.

So far very little has been done in evaluating pharmacokinetics or modeling for special compartments. Only a handful of examples exist for which the kinetics of fetal or tumor uptake has been attempted. This is especially true for newer biotechnology products. Macromolecules, such as small peptides, are being proposed for specific targeting of drug delivery. Not much information is available in defining the kinetics of such products. The possible increasing use of gene therapy may provide additional opportunities for evaluating pharmacokinetics of such therapeutic agents.

In conclusion, in spite of large advances made in the field of pharmacokinetics, much more needs to be done in the future. A better prediction of risk is possible only after all necessary underlying processes are well understood and a rational extrapolation based on factual data can be made. It is likely that we will have a greater involvement of pharmacokinetics in future directions of risk assessment.

## ACKNOWLEDGMENTS

The authors wish to acknowledge the support of National Institutes of Health Grants, HD28259 and ES04813, and the Utah State University Agricultural Experiment Station. This publication has been approved as Utah Agricultural Experiment Station Journal Paper No. 4650.

## REFERENCES

Andersen, M. E., Clewell, H. J., Garages, M. L., Macnaughton, M. G., Reitz, R. H., Nolan, R. J., and McKenna, M. J. (1991). Physiologically based pharmacokinetic modeling with dichloromethane, its metabolite, carbon monoxide and blood carboxyhemoglobin in rats and humans, *Toxicol. Appl. Pharmacol.,* 108, 14–27.

Anderson, M.E., Clewell, H. J., Gargas, M. L., Smith, F. A., and Reitz, R. H. (1987). Physiologically based pharmacokinetics and the risk assessment process for methylene chloride, *Toxicol. Appl. Pharmacol.,* 87, 185–205.

Braun, W. H. and Sauerhoff, M. W. (1976). The pharmacokinetic profile of pentachlorophenol in monkeys, *Toxicol. Appl. Pharmacol.,* 38, 525–533.

Creech-Kraft, J., Kochhar, D. M., Scott, W. J., and Nau, H. (1987). Low teratogenicity of 13-*cis*-retinoic acid (isotretenoin) in mouse corresponds to low embryo concentrations during organogenesis: Comparison to the all-*trans* isomer, *Toxicol. Appl. Pharmacol.,* 87, 474–482.

Creech-Kraft, J., Lofberg, B., Chahoud, I., Bochert, G., and Nau, H. (1989). Teratogenicity and placental transfer of all-*trans*-, 13-*cis*-, 4-oxo-all-*trans*-, and 4-oxo-13-*cis*-retinoic acid after administration of a low oral dose during organogenesis in mice, *Toxicol. Appl. Pharmacol.,* 100, 162–176.

Gehring, P. J. and Buerge, J. (1969). The distribution of 2,4-dinitrophenol relative to its cataractogenic activity in ducklings and rabbits, *Toxicol. Appl. Pharmacol.,* 15, 574–592.

Gehring, P. J., Watanabe, P. G., and Blau, G. E. (1976). Pharmacokinetic studies in evaluation of the toxicological and environmental hazard of chemicals. In *Advances in Modern Toxicology, New Concepts in Safety Evaluation,* Vol. I, Part 1 (M. A. Mehlman, R. E. Shapiro, and H. Blumenthal, eds.), Halstead Press, New York, pp. 195–270.

Gehring, P. J., Watanabe, P. G., and Park, C. N. (1978). Resolution of dose–response toxicity data for chemicals requiring metabolic activation: Example—vinyl chloride, *Toxicol. Appl. Pharmacol.,* 44, 581–591.

Gerlowski, L. E. and Jain, R. K. (1983). Physiologically based pharmacokinetic modeling: Principles and applications, *J. Pharm. Sci.,* 72, 1103–1127.

Gibaldi, M. and Perrier, D. (1982). *Pharmacokinetics,* 2nd ed., Marcel Dekker, New York.

Hiraga, K. and Fujii, T. (1981). Induction of tumors of the urinary system in F344 rats by dietary administration of *o*-phenylphenate, *Food Cosmet. Toxicol.*, 19, 303–310.

Holford, N. H. G. (1987). Clinical pharmacokinetics of ethanol, *Clin. Pharmacokinet.*, 13, 273–292.

Howard, W. B., Willhite, C. C., Omaye, S. T., and Sharma, R. P. (1989a). Comparative distribution, pharmacokinetics and placental permeabilities of all-*trans*-retinoic acid, 13-*cis*-retinoic acid, all-*trans*-4-oxo-retinoic acid, retinyl acetate and 9-*cis*-retinal in hamsters, *Arch. Toxicol.*, 63, 112–120.

Howard, W. B., Willhite, C. C., Omaye, S. T., and Sharma, R. P. (1989b). Pharmacokinetics, tissue distribution and placental permeability of all-*trans*- and 13-*cis*-N-ethyl retinamides in pregnant hamsters, *Fundam. Appl. Toxicol.*, 12, 621–627.

Kim, Y. W., Sharma, R. P., and Li, J. K. K. (1994). Characterization of heterologously expressed recombinant retinoic acid receptors with natural or synthetic retinoids. *J. Biochem. Toxicol.*, 9, 225–234.

Kochhar, D. M., Kraft, J., and Nau, H. (1987). Teratogenicity and disposition of various retinoids in vivo and in vitro. In *Pharmacokinetics in Teratogenesis*, Vol. 2 (H. Nau, and W. J. Scott, eds.), CRC Press, Boca Raton, FL, pp. 173–186.

Kociba, R. J., McCollister, S. B., Park, C., Torkelson, T. R., and Gehring, P. J. (1974). 1,4-Dioxane. I. Results of a 2-year ingestion study in rats, *Toxicol. Appl. Pharmacol.*, 30, 275–286.

Lammer, E. J. (1987). A phenocopy of the retinoic acid embryopathy following maternal use of etretinate that ended one year before conception, *Teratology*, 37, 472.

Leung, H.-W., Ku, R. H., Paustenbach, D. J., and Andersen, M. E. (1988). A physiologically based pharmacokinetic model for 2,3,7,8-tetrachlorodibenzo-*p*-dioxin in C57Bl/6J and DBA/2J mice, *Toxicol. Lett.*, 42, 15–28.

Levy, G. (1968). Dose dependent effects in pharmacokinetics. In *Importance of Fundamental Principles in Drug Evaluation* (D. H. Tedeschi, and R. E. Tedeschi, eds.), Raven Press, New York, pp. 141–172.

Maltoni, C. and Lefemine, G. (1975). Carcinogenicity assays of vinyl chloride: Current results, *Ann. N. Y. Acad. Sci.*, 246, 195–224.

Maltoni, C. and Selikoff, I. J., eds. (1988). Living in a chemical world: Occupational and environmental significance of industrial carcinogens, *Ann. N. Y. Acad. Sci.*, 534, 1–1045, 1988.

Menzel, D. B., Wolpert, R. L., Boger, J. R., and Kootsey, J. M. )1987). Resources available for simulation in toxicology: Specialized computers, general software and communication networks. In *Pharmacokinetics and Risk Assessment: Drinking Water and Health*, Vol. 8, National Academy Press, Washington, DC, pp. 229–250.

Neubig, R. R. (1990). The time course of drug action. In *Principles of Drug Action* (W. B. Pratt, and P. Taylor, eds.), Churchill Livingston, New York, pp. 308–326.

Olanoff, L. S. and Anderson, J. M. (1980). Controlled release of tetracycline—III. A physiological pharmacokinetic model of the pregnant rat, *J. Pharmacokinet. Biopharm.*, 8, 599–620.

Reitz, R. H., Fox, T. R., Quast, J. F., Hermann, E. A., and Watanabe, P. G. (1983). Molecular mechanisms involved in the toxicity of *ortho*phenylphenol and its sodium salt, *Chem. Biol. Interact.*, 43, 99–119.

Sharma, R. P., Stowe, C. M., and Good, A. L. (1970a). Studies on the distribution and metabolism of thiopental in cattle, sheep, goats and swine, *J. Pharmacol. Exp. Ther.*, 172, 128–137.

Sharma, R. P., Stowe, C. M., and Good, A. L. (1970b). Alteration of thiopental metabolism in phenobarbital-treated calves, *Toxicol. Appl. Pharmacol.*, 17, 400–405.

Watanabe, P. G. and Gehring, P. J. (1976). Dose-dependent fate of vinyl chloride and its possible relationship to oncogenicity in rats, *Environ. Health Perspect.*, 17, 145–152.

Williams, R. T. (1971). Species variation in drug biotransformations. In *Fundamentals of Drug Metabolism and Drug Disposition* (B. N. LaDu, H. G. Mandel, and E. L. Way, eds.), Williams & Wilkins, Baltimore, pp. 187–205.

Young, J. D., Braun, W. H., and Gehring, P. J. (1978). Dose-dependent fate of 1,4-dioxane in rats, *J. Toxicol. Environ. Health*, 4, 709–726.

Young, J. D., Braun, W. H., Rampy, L. W., Chenoweth, M. B., and Blau, G. E. (1977). Pharmacokinetics of 1,4-dioxane in humans, *J. Toxicol. Environ. Health*, 3, 507–520.

# PART II
## TOXICOLOGICAL TESTING

**Arthur Furst**
*University of San Francisco*
*San Francisco, California*

**Anna M. Fan**
*California Environmental Protection Agency*
*Berkeley, California*

Risk assessments are performed based on either experimental animal data or human data that are used to extrapolate to real-life human situations. Although human data are preferred and such data are available for some of the environmental chemicals of major concern, overall the availability of such data is limited, and most of the assessments have been performed using animal data. Relevant animal data are generated by toxicological research studies to address specific interests, or by laboratory testing to meet regulatory requirements. The data most useful for risk assessment are those obtained from well-designed and well-conducted studies, following Good Laboratory Practice guidelines, which generate data suitable for quantitative assessment. There are toxicological study or testing guidelines provided by various scientific bodies or regulatory agencies, the latter of which may specify data requirements for chemicals that are intended to be used, and for which human exposure is anticipated and, accordingly, need to be regulated to prevent harmful exposures. There are existing efforts to achieve consistency in testing guidelines and requirements, and coordination among different agencies and countries is needed to accomplish this goal. To address the need for toxicological data, this section provides a discussion of the principles and methods in toxicological testing in areas of acute, subchronic, and chronic toxicity, carcinogenicity, reproductive and developmental toxicity, genotoxicity, immunotoxicity, and neurotoxicity. It must be emphasized that as new techniques are developed and as new questions or concerns arise that relate to environmental chemicals and toxicology, the toxicological testing of chemicals will continue to evolve with new guidelines and requirements. One hopes that, at the same time, they will generate more and more data that will be useful for risk assessment.

In experimental animal acute, subchronic, and chronic studies, observations are made on general appearance and behavior, food consumption, and survival rate. Acute studies provide information on target organ toxicity and dose for designing longer-term studies. Eye and skin irritation studies and skin sensitization studies are also conducted. In subchronic and chronic studies, observations are made on biochemical, physiological, and pathological changes. Testing guidelines have been developed for most of the toxicological studies in specialized areas; those for neurotoxicity have undergone recent development, and those for immunotoxicity need further development. Genotoxicity testing has involved using a batter of tests, including microbial and plant systems, in addition to the animal model. The evaluation of developmental effects, particularly in relation to birth defects in the offspring, has been a subject of considerable discussion. The regulatory guidance for developmental toxicity has recently undergone review and revision, and the present discussion is current and informative. For reproductive toxicity, the same authors feel that regulatory guidance is still undergoing review and comments, and decided that discussion on reproductive toxicity testing should wait until such guidance becomes finalized in the future. Carcinogenicity studies have received the most attention, as carcinogens are of great concern to the general public and a subject of focused regulatory control.

Animal studies have successfully identified or demonstrated health effects that can be or are found in humans. Examples are dibromochloropropane (male reproductive effect), aldicarb (cholinergic symptoms), mercury (neurotoxicity), and vinyl chloride (liver cancer). But others, such as arsenic (carcinogenicity), are not as successful. In the absence of human data, animal data continue to be a reasonable source of information for studying the potential health effects of chemicals and for prediction in the human population. Continued progress and development are being made in the design and conduct of these studies to generate quality data.

# 8
# Acute, Subchronic, and Chronic Toxicity Testing

**Ann de Peyster and Moira A. Sullivan**
*San Diego State University*
*San Diego, California*

## I.  INTRODUCTION

The terms *acute, subchronic,* and *chronic* refer to both the types of effects seen after defined periods of exposure to chemicals and the experimental protocols used to test for these effects. This chapter describes the basic components of acute, subchronic, and chronic toxicity tests, including specific tests for the ability of a chemical to cause death (e.g., median lethal dose [LD$_{50}$] or median lethal concentration [LC$_{50}$]), eye irritation, skin irritation, or sensitization (allergic) reactions, and studies of metabolism. In addition to describing the basic toxicity test components, this chapter discusses how information obtained from each type of study is used. For example, data from general acute studies, as well as eye and dermal toxicity studies, are often used to communicate health risks by warning statements on product labels. Data from subchronic and chronic studies are often suitable for establishing reference doses (RfD) or regulatory standards, such as maximum contaminant levels (MCLs) or permissible exposure levels (PELs). Readers are also referred to other chapters for more detailed coverage of applications of toxicity test data. Other specialized tests performed to study specific toxic effects, such as cancer, reproductive toxicity, genotoxicity, immunotoxicity, and neurotoxicity, are discussed elsewhere in this book. Another good reference text that discusses both the general principles and technical aspects of toxicity testing in detail and provides additional references is *Principles and Methods of Toxicology* edited by A. Wallace Hayes (Hayes, 1994).

   This chapter focuses on standardized guidelines for human health effects testing established by the U. S. Environmental Protection Agency (USEPA) for evaluating chemicals to meet requirements of the Toxic Substances Control Act (TSCA) and the Federal Insecticide, Fungicide, and Rodenticide Act (FIFRA) (USEPA, 1984a,b). It is important to understand that the procedures described in this chapter are guidelines, not rigid laws imposed on testing facilities. The need for some flexibility in interpreting these guidelines when performing toxicity tests is recognized by the agencies requiring the data, provided that the basic principles and foundation of the study design are followed, the deviations proposed can be justified, and the scientific validity of the results is not compromised. For example, FIFRA policy guidelines acknowledge that a toxicity test that combines two different protocols to reduce the use of laboratory animals and other resources, but still fulfills the necessary data requirements, may be acceptable if good scientific practices are not compromised. Thus, health professionals, such as risk assessors, may encounter circumstances under which toxicology studies used to assess health risk and set safe levels of environmental contaminants do not necessarily follow standardized test protocols to the letter.

The guidelines described in this chapter were developed specifically for testing chemicals to generate data that will meet regulatory data requirements and will permit informed decisions about whether production of specific chemical products should be allowed, and whether they can be released to consumers. Although individual chemicals are most often tested, the same approaches can also sometimes be used to examine the toxicity associated with exposure to environmental samples containing one or more chemicals as complex mixtures. These procedures were not developed expressly for providing data for human health risk assessments, as they are now conducted; however, many studies that follow these protocols are suitable for this purpose. On the other hand, the best study available for a risk assessment may not have been performed for the express purpose of meeting TSCA, FIFRA, or other regulatory requirements, and may depart significantly from these standard TSCA and FIFRA guidelines. The best available study data also may have been collected at a time when scientific practices in toxicology were slightly different or less stringent. Thus, although standardized guidelines have helped promote uniformity in toxicity testing procedures, not all studies used for risk assessments can necessarily be expected to strictly follow the protocols described here.

Standardized toxicity test protocols have also been adopted by the U. S. Food and Drug Administration (USFDA) for foods, drugs, and cosmetics. Other countries, including Canada, Japan, and the United Kingdom, have established their own requirements for chemical product toxicity testing. These test protocols vary, as do the types of tests required by the United States and certain other countries. A comparison of current USEPA, TSCA, and FIFRA guidelines and requirements with those adopted by other agencies and organizations is beyond the scope of this chapter. Consultation with the agencies and organizations promulgating the guidelines is advised if it is necessary to know the most current guidelines and data requirements in a given situation.

Efforts are currently underway to develop more of a consensus worldwide on procedures used in toxicity testing and on product safety requirements, a process commonly referred to as harmonization. Toxicity-testing guidelines issued by the Organization for Economic Cooperation and Development deserve special recognition here (OECD, 1981). The 24 OCED member nations include the United States, Canada, Japan, New Zealand, and Australia, with the balance from Europe. Although the OECD is not a regulatory agency like the USEPA, the OECD guidelines serve as a widely acknowledged basis for establishing common principles and methods for testing the health effects of chemicals. In recent years, industry and regulatory toxicologists, other scientists, and policymakers from around the world have been meeting to work toward an agreement on chemical product safety assessment protocols and data requirements, as well as how human health risk assessments should be conducted. Ideally, properly conducted studies and health risk assessments generated by one country could then be acceptable anywhere in the world. Worldwide harmonization of toxicity-testing approaches may soon eliminate some tests and result in substantial revision of others. For example, certain procedures may become optional, or the numbers of animals or species recommended may be reduced. Many, although not all, of the tests described in the OECD guidelines are now very similar to the USEPA guidelines described in this chapter. However, harmonization may lead to some changes in these study protocols.

In summary, it is important to realize at the outset that deviations from standardized test protocols do not necessarily invalidate data from a toxicity study, and that different agencies and organizations may require different information. In addition, modifications in the standard toxicity test protocols described in this chapter can be expected.

## II. TOXICITY TEST OBJECTIVES AND GENERAL APPROACHES

## A. Protocol Selection

Selection of a protocol for a toxicity study depends on the kind of information needed about the substance or sample of interest. The objective of an acute study is to determine short-term effects of relatively high exposures, a situation analogous to an abnormally high or accidental exposure for a human. Examples might be a single, high exposure to a toxic gas following an explosion, or an accidental acute pesticide poisoning by ingestion or by contact with unprotected skin. Accordingly, testing for acute effects involves single or multiple doses administered within a 24-hr period and observation of effects soon thereafter and up to a period of 14 days. Effects observed include general behavior and appearance, lethality, and macroscopic pathological changes. Subchronic and chronic exposures are more common than single, acute exposures. Subchronic toxicity refers to effects observed after multiple exposures and observation for a longer period, generally up to 90 days. Repeated doses are given that may or may not produce immediate effects. In the context of animal studies, a subchronic study is one that lasts up to approximately 10% of the lifespan of the organism. Thus, an objective of a subchronic study is to determine the consequences of more prolonged, repeated exposures. Examples of situations most likely to result in subchronic chemical exposures in the human population might be an occupational exposure to a solvent over an extended, but limited, time while a new process was being used, or repeated ingestion of a medication for a limited time to cure an illness. Chronic toxicity tests involve multiple, low-dose exposures for long time periods, possibly for the lifetime of the individual. A chronic toxicity test would be appropriate for studying effects of daily exposure to low levels of a pollutant in water or air, or regular daily intake of a toxic component found in a popular beverage consumed on a regular basis.

The term *subacute* toxicity is sometimes used to refer to dosing periods lying between the single acute dose and 10% lifespan. Protocols for these short-term, repeated-dose studies, lasting 14, 21, and 28 days, are not included among the standard test guidelines recommended by the USEPA and, therefore, are not discussed here. The Organization for Economic Cooperation and Development can be consulted for more information on the subacute toxicity test guidelines (OECD, 1981).

Some specialized tests focusing on the skin and eye as target organs or other specific endpoints are also discussed in this chapter. The skin has the largest surface area of any organ in the human body, with the average adult having about 1.86 $m^2$ (20 $ft^2$) of skin surface. There are two principal categories of toxicants that affect the skin: sensitizers and irritants. Chemicals that are irritants are especially destructive to the eyes and mucous membranes. Because of the likelihood of contact of unprotected skin and eyes with toxicants, information on dermal and ocular irritation has been used to support warning statements on product labels. Although some information can be obtained from general acute and subchronic studies, specialized protocols for eye and skin irritation are used to generate data for this purpose. Skin sensitization tests are used to evaluate the sensitizing potential of a chemical on an individual with repeated exposure to the same chemical. Similarly, a separate study is usually performed to study metabolism. In toxicity testing, acute, subchronic, and other short-term studies generally precede chronic toxicity testing.

## B.  Exposure Routes

With recognition that the effects occurring with different exposure scenarios can vary with the route of exposure, standardized protocols have been developed for the most common routes of chemical exposure which are dermal (skin) absorption, oral ingestion, and inhalation. Doses are typically expressed in units of grams per kilogram (g/kg) or milligrams per kilogram (mg/kg), interpreted as weight of substance administered per kilogram of the animal body weight. A group of animals, designated as controls, is usually given any vehicle used to dissolve the test substance, such as water or corn oil, and are otherwise handled in a manner identical with that of animals treated with the test substance to observe any effects caused by the experimental procedures themselves.

The dermal route is a primary route of human exposure to many chemicals, particularly those to which persons are exposed occupationally. In dermal studies, the substance is applied on the back of the animal on an area of unabraded skin that has been clipped of fur or shaved 24 hr before the test. This area must comprise roughly 10% of the total body surface area. Suitable dressings are applied to retain the test substance, and residual, unabsorbed test substance is removed with water or other appropriate solvent at the end of the 24-hr exposure period. In oral exposure studies, the test substance is often given by gavage, placing the substance directly into the gastrointestinal tract of the animal with a blunt-ended gavage needle or stomach tube, rather than adding it to the animal's food or water. This ensures that the dose of the substance to each animal is known and also reduces the dispersion of toxic substances in uneaten food. Guidelines are provided for supplying food and water during these studies to minimize the confounding effects of diet. Inhalation is also a common route of exposure to toxicants found in both ambient and workplace air. Inhalation toxicity test experiments are conducted in inhalation test chambers. These experiments require specialized facilities and additional personnel with specialized training to operate and maintain the test chambers. Test guidelines also specify how the inhalation test exposure should be created and monitored.

When conducting a health risk assessment or setting a standard, the desired data for specific exposure route(s) of concern may not yet be available. It may then be necessary to use studies employing other routes of exposure. This may be appropriate if reliable information is available on the toxicokinetics of the chemical to determine whether or not route-to-route extrapolation and adjustments may be done with some degree of confidence. Although sometimes used in risk assessment when no other data exist for a chemical, short-term exposure studies in laboratory animals provide very limited information for predicting effects of long-term exposure in humans.

## C.  Laboratory Models

All of the standardized toxicity study protocols specify that common laboratory animal species and strains should be used to enable comparison with existing data. Justification must be provided for the use of alternatives. There is now a serious effort to minimize the unnecessary use of experimental animals in toxicity testing. For example, there have been changes proposed recently in acute pesticide toxicity testing under FIFRA that result in the use of fewer animals. These changes include (1) elimination of the requirement for a concurrent vehicle control group; (2) limiting studies to the more sensitive sex, using previous history on the chemical class to make the determination, and testing of only a few animals of the other sex; and (3) whenever possible, the use of test protocols employing the lowest feasible number of animals, rather than routinely requiring at least ten animals (five of each sex) at each dose level.

## D. Use of Structure–Activity Relationships

Regulatory agencies currently recommend review and use of existing information on structurally related chemicals before initiating tests, particularly acute toxicity tests. If all other chemicals tested with similar structures show similar toxicity, then certain tests may not be required. Structure–activity relationship (SAR) data may also be used in risk assessments of chemicals for which no test data are available. Intelligent use of the concept of SARs can eliminate unnecessary testing.

## E. Limit Tests

Performance of a limit test is recommended in general acute and subchronic toxicity testing. Initially, a single group of animals receives a large dose of the test substance. If no compound-related mortality occurs with this high dose, then additional acute toxicity tests, using multiple doses as described in Secs. III and IV, are not required, particularly if toxicity would not be expected based on data of structurally related compounds. If the limit test indicates that further acute toxicity studies are needed, then three different doses must be used to reveal how responses vary over a wide dose range. Figure 1 illustrates the use of the limit test to decide whether additional acute and subchronic tests need to be conducted.

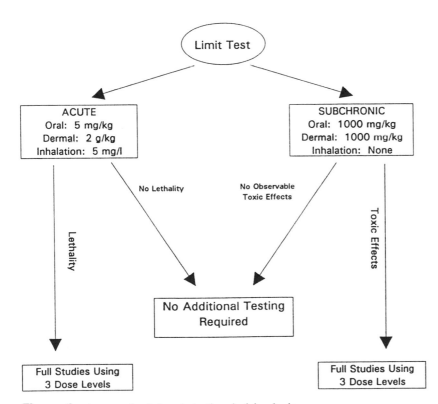

**Figure 1** Acute and subchronic testing decision logic.

## F. Satellite Groups

A satellite group is a group of animals that is treated with the high dose of the substance of interest and observed after treatment ceases. For example, in subchronic studies lasting 90 days, observation of the animals in the satellite group are made for a period of appropriate duration after treatment stops, normally for not less than 28 days. The satellite group provides additional information about the reversibility, persistence or delayed toxicity of the substance, all of which are important for a thorough evaluation of the health risks associated with exposure.

## III.  ACUTE TOXICITY

## A.  Objectives

Acute toxicity tests provide information on the harmful health effects associated with short-term exposure. Although human health risk estimates and regulatory standards are not usually based directly on data from acute studies, under FIFRA the USEPA can issue a rebuttable presumption against registration (RPAR), or classify a pesticide for general use, or restrict it for use only by certified applicators on the basis of acute toxicity data. Acute toxicity data may also serve as the basis for classifying and labeling a chemical.

It is important to appreciate the value of acute toxicity test data in the overall toxicity testing sequence. Acute toxicity tests are generally performed first, and the information from these studies is used to design protocols for longer-term studies, including subchronic and chronic toxicity tests and others described elsewhere in this book in chapters devoted to reproductive, developmental, carcinogenicity, and neurotoxicity testing. If designed appropriately, these studies may also provide initial information on toxicokinetics and mechanisms of action.

## B.  Median Lethal Dose Test Versus the General Acute Toxicity Test

Many in the general public have become familiar with the term $LD_{50}$ (lethal dose 50, or median lethal dose), a statistically derived dose of a substance that can be expected to cause death in 50% of a given test population exposed for a specified time. Familiarity with this term may stem from the fact that common expressions of potency are sometimes based on the $LD_{50}$ (Tables 1 and 2). Materials can also be classified as hazardous waste on the basis of the $LD_{50}$ of the material (Table 3). A number of protocols exist for conducting $LD_{50}$ studies (Litchfield and Wilcoxon, 1949; Weil, 1958; Bruce, 1985). The majority of $LD_{50}$ studies con-

**Table 1** Commonly Used Acute Toxicity Classifications

| Commonly used term | $LD_{50}$ <br> Single oral dose for rats (g/kg) | 4-hr vapor causing 2–4 deaths in 6-rat groups (ppm) | $LD_{50}$ <br> Skin for rabbits (g/kg) | Probable lethal dose for humans |
|---|---|---|---|---|
| Extremely toxic | 0.001 or less | Less than 10 | 0.005 or less | Taste (1 grain) |
| Highly toxic | 0.001–0.05 | 10–100 | 0.005–0.043 | 1 tsp (4 ml) |
| Moderately toxic | 0.05–0.50 | 100–1,000 | 0.044–0.340 | 1 Tblsp (30 g) |
| Slightly toxic | 0.50–5.0 | 1,000–10,000 | 0.35–2.81 | 1 pt (250 g) |
| Practically nontoxic | 5.0–15.0 | 10,000–100,000 | 2.82–22.6 | 1 qt |
| Relatively harmless | > 15.00 | > 100,000 | > 22.6 | > 1 qt (946 ml) |

**Table 2** Categories of Toxicity and Signal Words for Pesticides

| Hazard category<br>Signal words | Category I<br>"Danger" | Category II<br>"Warning" | Category III<br>"Caution" | Category IV<br>"Caution" |
|---|---|---|---|---|
| Oral $LD_{50}$ | Up to and including 50 mg/kg | > 50–500 mg/kg | > 500–5000 mg/kg | > 5000 mg/kg |
| Dermal $LD_{50}$ | Up to and including 200 mg/kg | > 200–2000 mg/kg | > 2000–5000 mg/kg | > 5000 mg/kg |
| Inhalation of $LC_{50}$ (actual chamber concentration measured for a 4-hr exposure) | Up to and including 0.2 mg/L | > 0.2–2.0 mg/L | > 2–20 mg/L | > 20 mg/L |
| Eye effects | Corrosive (irreversible destruction of ocular tissue) or corneal involvement or irritation persisting for more than 21 days | Corneal involvement or irritation clearing in 8–21 days | Corneal involvement or irritation clearing in 7 days or less | Minimal effects clearing in less than 24 hr |
| Skin effects | Corrosive (tissue destruction into the dermis and/or scarring) | Severe irritation at 72 hr (severe erythema or edema) | Moderate irritation at 72 hr (moderate erythema) | Mild or slight irritation (no irritation or slight erythema) |

*Source:* USEPA (1984c).

ducted in recent years employ protocols calling for the fewest numbers of animals possible while still retaining statistical significance.

The $LD_{50}$ values are often used to compare the potency of different chemicals. Strictly speaking, this is most appropriate when the acute toxicity dose–response curves of the chemicals being compared have the same slope. This can occur if the chemicals have the same effects and mechanisms of action: for example, for a group of organophosphorus insecticides that all reversibly inhibit acetylcholinesterase. A common misconception is that the $LD_{50}$ is an absolute number. In reality this number may vary from one study to the next depending on species, sex, diet, and other biological and environmental factors. Nevertheless, the $LD_{50}$ can be a useful piece of information contributing to the total toxicity profile of a chemical if its significance and limitations are fully understood and appreciated.

**Table 3** Toxicity Criteria for Hazardous Waste

A waste is considered to be hazardous on the basis of toxicity if it has:
>    an oral $LD_{50}$ in rats of < 5000 mg/kg (single administration)
>    or
>    a dermal $LD_{50}$ in rabbits of < 4300 mg/kg at 24 hr
>    or
>    an inhalation $LC_{50}$ in rats of < 10,000 ppm (gas or vapor)
>    or
>    a 96-hr $LC_{50}$ in fish of < 500 mg/L (in fathead minnows, golden shiners, or rainbow trout)

*Source:* USEPA (1984d).

Acute toxicity tests are sometimes mistakenly equated with tests performed specifically to determine an $LD_{50}$. In fact, lethality is just one of many measures of toxicity evaluated in general acute toxicity studies. The focus of the general acute toxicity-testing guidelines described here is to identify sublethal effects and target organs, with emphasis on behavioral, gross anatomical, hematological, biochemical, and histopathological changes. The requirement for determining $LD_{50}$ with precise information on statistical limits and slope has been relaxed by many regulatory agencies. Instead, dose selection in acute toxicity tests should aim to produce a dose–response curve that will enable an "acceptable estimation" of the median lethal dose, usually defined as that which occurs within 24 hr after initiation of exposure.

## C. Test Species

Most agency guidelines specify that dermal acute toxicity tests may use adult rats, rabbits, or guinea pigs. The albino rabbit is preferred in USEPA guidelines because of size, ease of handling, skin permeability characteristics, and the extensive existing data base. For acute inhalation and oral exposure studies, rats are the preferred species. Ten adult animals are exposed at each dose level in acute toxicity tests, five males and five nulliparous, nonpregnant females per group. In acute studies, concurrent untreated controls are unnecessary, and concurrent vehicle controls are necessary only when historical data are unavailable to indicate whether there is any acute toxicity associated with the vehicle.

## D. Exposures

The doses used in the acute toxicity limit tests are 2 g/kg dermal, 5 mg/L for 4 hr by inhalation, or 5 g/kg given orally. If toxicity is evident, then the full test is performed with at least three doses of the test substance (see Fig. 1). As noted earlier, dose selection in these tests should aim to produce a dose–response curve that will enable an acceptable estimation of the median lethal dose, in addition to providing much information about sublethal effects. In the acute dermal and inhalation studies, the test substance is administered over a period of up to 24 hr. If possible, all of the desired oral dosages are given by single-gavage administration, although divided doses are permitted.

## E. Observations

Test and control animals are observed at least daily for a minimum of 14 days in studies involving all of these routes. Observations made routinely in acute toxicity tests are listed in Table 4. The condition of the fur, skin, eyes, and mucous membranes is noted daily, as well as unusual behaviors, such as lethargy, tremors, seizures, or hyperactivity. Abnormal physiological responses indicating damage to any of the major organ systems (e.g., gastrointestinal, nervous, respiratory, or cardiovascular) are also noted. Animals found dead are necropsied, and those that are weak or sick are isolated for closer observation. At the end of the test, surviving animals are sacrificed. Time of death and body weight at death or sacrifice are noted. Necropsy procedures consist of gross pathology examinations of all test animals. As indicated in Table 4, acute toxicity study protocols recommend that clinical chemistry and microscopic examination of slides prepared from organs showing gross pathology should be considered for animals surviving over 24 hr because this may yield additional useful information about mechanisms of action and the design of future studies.

## F. Applications of Acute Toxicity Data

Potential for causing death and other manifestations of acute toxicity only partly describe the toxicity of a chemical. However, because information on acute toxicity is most often available,

**Table 4** General Acute, Subchronic, and Chronic Toxicity Study Observations and Frequency

| Observation | Acute | Subchronic | Chronic |
|---|---|---|---|
| Cage-side appearance<br>Fur, skin, eyes, mucous membranes; behavior;<br>gastrointestinal function; nervous system function;<br>somatomotor activity;<br>respiratory and circulatory function | Daily | Daily | Weekly |
| Other periodic observations<br>Weight, food consumption, death, time of death | Daily | Weekly | Weekly |
| Gross necropsy | Yes | Yes | Yes |
| Clinical | Surviving animals | All | All |
| Hematology: Hct, Hb, erythrocyte count, total and differential leukocyte count, clotting potential (e.g., clotting time, prothrombin time, thromboplastin time, or platelet count) | | | |
| Blood biochemistry: electrolyte balance, carbohydrate metabolism, liver and kidney function (suggested: calcium, phosphorus, chloride, sodium, potassium, fasting glucose, ALT, AST, ornithine decarboxylase, GGT, urea nitrogen, albumin, blood creatinine, total bilirubin, total serum protein) | | | |
| Additional: lipids, hormones, acid–base balance, methemoglobin, cholinesterase, and more, where necessary | | | |
| Opthalmological: before exposure and at termination of study. If changes seen in the few (5/dose) examined, examine all | | | |
| Urinalysis: Not suggested routinely; only if indicated | | | |
| Histopathology | Only if indicated | All | All |

*Source:* USEPA (1984a,b).

and also probably because death and other acute toxic responses are best understood and appreciated by the general public, acute toxicity properties often serve as the basis for classifying chemicals and communicating risks to the public. For example, variations of Table 1, which relates an acute toxicity endpoint (death) to expressions of toxicity that are more familiar to the lay public, are found in many toxicology textbooks. This table is useful for understanding relative potency of chemicals causing acute effects, but can be misleading. Some chemicals that are currently the focus of great regulatory interest owing to their potential for causing harmful health effects actually have very low acute toxicity. They are of great concern because of their persistence in the environment, ability to bioaccumulate, and adverse health effects, especially following chronic exposures. These chemicals would be classified as relatively harmless according to Table 1 because their $LD_{50}$s are very high.

Many pesticides produce toxicity in humans and other mammals, even after a single, acute exposure. Warning labels applied to pesticide containers must carry specific, signal words indicating the level of acute toxicity (see Table 2). For example, a pesticide causing severe eye or skin injury, or producing severe acute toxicity in another vital organ and thus having a low $LD_{50}$, may be classified in toxicity category I and carry the signal word "Danger."

## IV. SUBCHRONIC TOXICITY

### A. Objectives

The extended exposure period and more extensive observations made during repeated subchronic dose experiments permit the study of cumulative effects from bioaccumulation potential of the toxicant and, also, clearer identification of specific target organs. Data from subchronic studies are used to choose dose levels for general chronic toxicity or carcinogenesis studies, such as the maximum tolerated dose (MTD). They are also used to establish safety criteria or reference values for human exposures, such as the RfDs developed by the USEPA based on no-observed effect levels (NOEL) or no-observed adverse effect levels (NOAEL) in animal studies.

## B.  Test Species

Recommendations for selection of species and numbers of test animals are currently similar to those for acute toxicity tests discussed earlier, with the following exceptions. More animals are included in each dose group; that is, 20 adult animals per group versus 10 in acute studies, with equal numbers of each sex. In addition, dogs of defined breeds, such as beagles, can be used for subchronic inhalation studies involving nonrodent species. If dogs are used, then each exposure level should include at least eight animals, four per sex.

## C.  Exposures

Doses recommended for the subchronic limit test are 1000 mg/kg for dermal or oral studies. If no toxic effects are observed, and chemicals with similar structure have low toxicity, then full studies using three dose levels may not be necessary (see Fig. 1).

A minimum of three different dose groups and a control group should be used in subchronic toxicity tests. Whereas an acute study aims for some lethality at the highest dose to enable an approximation of an $LD_{50}$, the highest dose in rodent subchronic studies should produce toxic effects, but not fatalities to the extent that prevents meaningful analysis of sublethal effects. There should be no fatalities at the high dose in experiments involving nonrodent species. The lowest dose in a subchronic study should exceed the estimate of human exposure, but not produce any evidence of toxicity. Ideally, the intermediate dose(s) should produce minimal observable toxic effects.

Dose frequency is as follows: For dermal and inhalation studies, dosing should occur 6 hr/day, 7 days/week for 90 days, although 5 days/week is acceptable. In subchronic oral studies, the test substance may be administered in the diet or in capsules, or for rodents, by gavage or in drinking water. The treatment period is typically 90 days.

## D.  Observations

For some chemicals, subchronic studies are the first, and sometimes the only, repeated-dose studies. Thus, the data collected are more extensive than those required for acute studies, and are generally similar to those required in chronic studies, as illustrated in Table 4. In addition to the required cage-side observations made in acute studies, clinical chemistry and histopathology data should be collected routinely on all animals involved in subchronic studies. The physical condition, behavior, and other overt signs of altered physiological function should be recorded at least daily during the 90-day observation period. Any test animals dying before the conclusion of the 90-day observation period are necropsied. Body weights and food consumption are recorded weekly in subchronic studies. At the end of the study, extensive clinical chemistry, gross pathology, and histopathological examination of tissues is performed on all animals. Ophthalmic examinations are also completed, and results are compared with pretreatment observations for each animal.

## E.  Application

If there is no evidence that the test substance causes cancer, and the establishment of a reference value for comparison with actual or expected human exposures in a given situation is the desired goal, then a NOEL (no-observed effect level) can sometimes be determined from a subchronic study if human exposures are likely to be subchronic. An uncertainty factor is applied to the NOEL to derive the reference value (see Part IV for details). In the absence of adequate chronic toxicity data, the reference value can be derived from subchronic toxicity data with the incorporation of an additional uncertainty factor. However, it is important to note that toxicity data used in establishing reference values should be carefully evaluated for biological significance and interpreted according to sound scientific principles. The data should not be viewed simply as numbers that can be manipulated mathematically in a mechanical way to achieve the desired end result.

## V. CHRONIC TOXICITY

### A. Objectives

Chronic toxicity tests are designed to examine the effects of a substance following prolonged and repeated exposure. Many chemicals are not acutely toxic at the concentrations found in the environment. However, latent and cumulative effects can become apparent through chronic toxic studies, which are designed to reveal long-term dose–response relationships. There are many examples of this. For example, dioxin and polychlorinated biphenyls (PCBs) cause skin chloracne, but are not acutely toxic to internal organs. When they accumulate in the body they can cause liver damage and other types of adverse effects. Similarly, concentrations of lead may be low enough not to cause frank adverse health effects, but long-term exposures to such levels may result in blood, neurological, and reproductive disorders.

The chronic toxicity study guidelines discussed in this section are designed to reveal general toxic effects, including some basic neurotoxicity, and physiological, biochemical, hematological, and pathological effects other than cancer. Chronic studies with a main objective of testing specifically for cancer-causing potential, referred to as oncogenicity studies, involve specialized protocols and are discussed elsewhere. Sometimes the general chronic study is combined with an oncogenicity study to save time and resources.

### B. Test Species

The USEPA requires that two mammalian species, one rodent and one nonrodent, be used to evaluate the chronic toxicity of a substance. The rat is the preferred rodent species; the dog is the preferred nonrodent species. The minimum numbers of animals currently recommended per dose group are 40 rats or 8 dogs, half males and half females. If additional interim sacrifices are planned before the end of the study, then these numbers should be increased to provide enough animals for meaningful statistical evaluation of data from the last sacrifice.

### C. Exposures

Dosing of test and control animals begins at an early age in chronic studies to mimic near lifetime exposures. (See also Chapter 11 on reproductive and developmental toxicity tests that study effects on newborn and perinatal periods.) For rats, dosing begins as soon as possible after weaning, and for dogs between 4 and 6 months of age. At least three dose levels should be administered in addition to a concurrent control. Selection of doses is based on several considerations, including results from 90-day subchronic toxicity studies and doses or concentrations expected in human populations. Ideally, chronic toxicity study results should reveal (1) a dose–response relationship for the toxic substance, (2) a no-observed toxic effect level, and (3) some evidence of toxicity at the highest dose level. If inappropriate doses are selected, it may take many months to discover this. Needless to say, final selection of dosages for a long-term study is one of the more difficult challenges faced by toxicologists. Dosing frequency for chronic studies is the same as for subchronic studies, but treatment should last at least 12 months to constitute a chronic study. It is unusual to subject a given test substance to chronic studies using all possible routes of exposure. This is partly because of the expense and time involved, and also because it is likely that the chemical will find its way to sensitive target tissues with prolonged exposure, regardless of the route of administration. The route(s) chosen should typify human exposures that are most likely to occur.

## D. Observations

The condition of each animal should be observed at least daily during chronic exposure studies. As illustrated in Table 4, the information collected in chronic and subchronic toxicity studies is similar. The longer exposure time and larger number of animals involved in the chronic study increases the likelihood that adverse effects will be detected if they are to occur.

## E. Application

Chronic studies are often used as the basis for setting regulatory standards for specific chemicals in environmental media that involve long-term human exposure. When properly designed and conducted, a chronic study can generate data for use in a human health risk assessment for noncancer endpoints. Only chronic studies designed to study cancer-causing potential should be used for cancer risk assessments.

## VI. DERMAL SENSITIZATION

## A. Objectives

Sensitization tests are used to identify substances with significant sensitization potential. A sensitization reaction is typically one that results from repeated exposure to a substance. Sensitizers differ from irritants in that sensitizers initiate an immunologically mediated reaction, whereas irritants cause localized tissue destruction, without initially involving the immune system. Prior exposure to a sensitizer, or a similar chemical that cross-reacts with it, is necessary to see its effects. The effects of irritants can be seen on first contact. In humans, the hypersensitive state that develops after recurrent exposure to a sensitizer may be characterized by dermatitis or hives. Examples of substances that are sensitizers arc nickel, chromium salts, formaldehyde, and hexamethylenediisocyanate.

The dermal sensitization test method consists of two repeated applications of the test substance, an induction exposure, followed by a challenge exposure, separated by a period of at least 1 week. Sensitization is determined by comparing the challenged state with the induced state. Chemicals that are sensitizers are expected to produce significantly greater reactions after the challenge exposure.

## B. Test Species and Exposures

Under most guidelines, the preferred species for dermal sensitization tests is the young adult guinea pig. There are seven acceptable test protocols specified in both USEPA and OECD guidelines: Freund's complete adjuvant test, guinea-pig maximization test, split adjuvant technique, Buehler test, open eqicutaneous test, Mauer optimization test, and footpad technique in guinea pig. The number of test animals and dose levels used depends on which method is chosen. Females should be nulliparous and nonpregnant. Animals may serve as their own controls; alternatively, induced animals may be compared with animals that received only the challenge dose. Intermittent use of positive control substances with an acceptable level of reliability for the chosen test system is recommended.

## C. Observations

Two endpoints, erythema (redness) and edema (swelling) are graded according to the extent of response (none, slight, moderate, severe). Reactions are observed at specific times after the challenge exposure, according to the protocol selected, usually at 24, 48 and 72 hr after exposure.

## VII. DERMAL IRRITATION AND PRIMARY EYE IRRITATION

## A. Objectives

Dermal and eye irritation tests provide information on the irritant or corrosive properties of a test substance. *Irritation* is defined as reversible inflammatory changes in skin following exposure to a substance, whereas *dermal corrosion* is the production of irreversible tissue damage in the skin. Substances known to be highly toxic by the dermal route, that is, with an $LD_{50}$ less than 200 mg/kg, and substances that are strongly acidic (pH of 2 or less) or alkaline (pH equal to or greater than 11.5) need not be tested by this protocol. Likewise, strongly acidic or alkaline substances and materials that have demonstrated severe irritant or corrosive properties in the skin irritation test do not require further testing for eye irritation. Figure 2 illustrates the decision logic used for dermal and eye irritation testing.

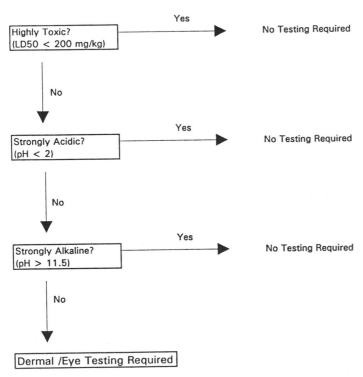

**Figure 2** Dermal and eye irritation testing logic.

## B.  Test Species and Exposures

The albino rabbit is the preferred species for both of these tests. At least six animals should be used, unless fewer can be justified.

Twenty-four hours before the start of the dermal irritation test, fur is shaven from the back of the animal without abrading the skin. The use of untreated control animals is not recommended. Instead, untreated areas of skin of the test animal that are adjacent to the test site are used as a control for the dermal test. The untreated eye of the test animal is used as a control in the primary eye irritancy test.

In the dermal test a single dose of 0.5 ml of liquid or 500 mg of solid or semisolid is applied to an area of approximately 6 cm². Solids may require use of a vehicle to ensure good contact with the skin. A dosage level of 0.1 ml is recommended for liquids in the eye irritant test. For solids, pastes, or particulate substances, the amount used should have a volume of 0.1 ml or a weight not greater than 100 mg. Solids should be ground to a fine dust. The irritant effect of the vehicle, if any, must be taken into account. Liquids should be applied undiluted. In the skin test, the area is then covered with a semiocclusive dressing, generally for 4 hr. Longer exposures may be required under certain conditions. At the end of the exposure period, residual test substance should be removed.

## C.  Observations

In the dermal test the dressing is removed and the animals are examined for erythema and edema at least 72 hr and no more than 14 days after application. Responses are scored within 30–60 min after patch removal and then again at 24, 48, and 72 hr. The scoring system for dermal irritation consists of a 4-point scale for degree of erythema and edema observed, where 0 = no response; 1 = very slight, 2 = slight/well-defined, 3 = moderate, and 4 = severe. In addition to irritation, any other lesions or toxic effects should be fully described. Reactions are also observed in the eye irritancy test at 1, 24, 48, and 72 hr after exposure using a slit-lamp microscope. Damage to the cornea, iris, and conjunctivae should be exposed according to a standardized ocular lesion-grading system.

## VIII.  METABOLISM

## A.  Objectives

Although acute, subchronic, and chronic toxicity tests are valuable for determining the harmful effects of a substance and levels at which the substance may be used safely, these tests are not designed to provide detailed information on absorption, distribution, biotransformation, and excretion (ADME). From a toxicologist's perspective, this information is of critical importance for a complete understanding of the toxicity of a chemical. Information from metabolic studies is used to aid in the initial design of toxicology studies. For example, metabolic studies are often performed in various species to aid in selection of appropriate test species to use in toxicity studies to increase the predictive value of this information when used for human health risk assessment. Metabolic studies are also performed to identify appropriate dose levels to use to achieve internal concentrations expected under different routes of human exposure.

When selecting species and routes of exposure for metabolic studies, consideration is given to the intended use of the substance under study and the conditions of anticipated human exposure. Current TSCA and FIFRA guidelines stipulate that the test compound be administered by the oral route, either in single or repeated doses, and that the rat is the preferred species to use. However, dermal and inhalation exposure studies are also encouraged if these are clearly more likely routes of human exposure, or if marked differences in the behavior of a chemical in the body are suspected depending on route of exposure. In some instances little-used routes of exposure may be employed. For example, when chronic low-level exposure to a compound is anticipated, continuous infusion may provide the most accurate prediction of how the compound is handled by the body over time.

Similarly, known species differences between rats and humans suggest that the rat may not always be the best model for human exposures. As an example, rats are obligate nose breathers; that is, they inhale primarily through the nose, not the mouth, whereas humans inhale through either the nose or the mouth. Additionally, the nasal passages of rats are more complex than human nasal passages. Consequently, airborne substances inhaled by rats are subject to more filtration and absorption in their nasal passages than they might be in humans. Hence, a species that breathes through both nose and mouth, such as a dog, may be a better one to use in inhalation toxicity and metabolism studies.

## B.  Species

Under TSCA and FIFRA guidelines, the preferred species to use in metabolic studies is the young adult rat if no information is available suggesting that another species would be better to evaluate human exposures. Equal numbers of males and females should be used at each dose levels. Females should be nulliparous and nonpregnant. The minimum number of animals to use at each dose level is eight under TSCA or ten under FIFRA, with equal numbers of each sex.

## C.  Exposures

A minimum of two test doses should be used. The highest should produce toxic effects, but not fatalities to such an extent as to prevent meaningful analysis of sublethal effects. The lowest dose should be approximately equivalent to the NOEL. The test substance should be administered by the oral route by capsule or gavage, either as a single or as a repeated dose. If an alternative route of administration is chosen, then the basis for its selection should be provided. Single-dose testing should be performed with a radioactively labeled compound that can be detected easily in body fluids and tissues.

Four groups of animals, designated A through D, should be studied. These groups differ in terms of route of administration of the test substance, use of labeled versus unlabeled compound, single versus repeated doses, and dose level. This format maximizes the data yield per number of animals used. Animals in groups A, B, and D receive a labeled substance, whereas group C animals receive the nonlabeled version. Group A receives a single low dose by the intravenous route, group B a single low dose by the oral route, and group D a single high dose by the oral route. Group C animals receive a series of daily oral doses of unlabeled substance for a 14-day period at the low dose. Twenty-four hours after the last dose, the animals receive a single oral dose of labeled compound.

## C.  Observations

The concentration and quantity of the test substance and major metabolites should be measured in organs, urine, and fecal extracts of all animals, using suitable analytical techniques. Tissues should be analyzed at the time of sacrifice. When rats are used, quantities of test chemical and major metabolites in urine, feces, and expired air should be measured at several hourly time points following the exposure (i.e., 4, 8, 12, and 24 hr) and daily thereafter, until 95% of the administered dose is excreted or until 7 days after dosing. If dogs are used, then these measurements should be taken at regular intervals for the first 2 days after dosing and then every

12 hr for the remaining 5 days. If a preliminary study shows that no volatile, labeled materials are being excreted in exhaled air within the 24-hr period after dosing, then expired air measurements are not required.

## IX. GOOD LABORATORY PRACTICES AND OTHER METHODOLOGICAL CONSIDERATIONS

In an effort to minimize the potential for misrepresentation of toxicity study results and other unlawful or otherwise undesirable practices that could jeopardize the health of the public, the USFDA and USEPA both adopted Good Laboratory Practices (GLP) standards for health effects testing of chemicals and other products undergoing review for human or veterinary use (USFDA, 1989; USEPA, 1983). These standards were adopted first by the USFDA in 1979 and later in 1983 by the USEPA and have undergone subsequent revisions. They address such issues as proper recordkeeping practices, the requirement for an internal quality assurance unit and regular inspections, and control in all important aspects of toxicity testing. Data submitted to these agencies in support of product development, manufacturing, and use is now routinely scrutinized for adherence to GLP standards of quality. Not all data used for calculating risks and setting standards were collected after the GLPs were adopted. These data may be the only available information, however, and may be entirely suitable for this purpose.

As was stated in the Introduction to this chapter, it is important to remember that deviations from standardized test protocols do not necessarily invalidate data from a study, and that modifications in the current guidelines can be expected. Conversely, a toxicity test that seems on the surface to meet the basic criteria outlined in these guidelines may have other problems that raise serious concerns about the validity of the data. The testing approaches and protocols summarized in the previous sections do not necessarily address all of the important issues in toxicity testing that should be considered carefully when evaluating the suitability and quality of toxicity test data and applying it for a specific purpose. Highlighted in the following are a few of these considerations that are equally important to those outlined in the test guidelines described earlier.

It could easily be argued that the two most important components of a toxicity test are the test animal and the test substance. Maintaining the overall health and welfare of the animal before and during a study should be a main concern. If the requirements of the animal to maintain good health are not understood and attended to, and all animals are not cared for in the same manner, aside from the doses of test substance administered, then toxicity test results are likely to be invalid. Evidence of inappropriate or contaminated feed or bedding, unnecessary stress owing to neglect or improper handling, or inadequately controlled lighting or other climatic conditions in the animal quarters also raise questions about external factors that could be affecting the toxicity response. Likewise, if the purity or composition of the test substance administered is not known or is not consistent, then the results of a toxicity study are virtually impossible to interpret. Laboratories conducting experiments following GLPs should be able to provide thorough documentation of the health of the animals and the composition of the substances being tested.

The GLPs emphasize the importance of standard operating procedures and specify the extensive documentation expected. An audit of a study of adherence to GLPs may reveal observations that were made inconsistently, or clinical chemistry and pathology specimens that were not collected, preserved, analyzed, or interpreted in a consistent way. Conversely, even though a study may have been done before the adoption of GLPs, good laboratory records may be available and may contain sufficient detail about how toxicity test data were collected, reference standards used for comparison, precision, accuracy, and service records of the analytical equipment used, and other important information to allow evaluation of the quality of the study.

The ultimate responsibility for the conduct and interpretation of study data rests with an individual identified as the study director. However, a toxicology study is rarely conducted by a single person, but rather by a team of scientists, technicians, and other specialists. No one person can claim expertise and experience in all of the many aspects of toxicity testing discussed in this volume. For example, a person with the specialized expertise in pathology necessary to interpret histology slides may have limited experience with recognizing abnormal animal behavior or relating abnormal clinical chemistry data to altered functions in internal organs. Additional expertise in risk assessment and regulatory policy are also necessary in the interpretation and application of toxicity study data in risk assessment. As with any complex process, the design, conduct, evaluation, and interpretation of toxicity studies and application of the results to risk assessment requires a team of professionals with broad expertise and experience. The qualifications and training of clinical and other analytical personnel should be documented according to GLPs.

## X. MODIFICATION OF TOXICITY TEST GUIDELINES

Changes in standard test protocols can be expected to occur as a result of harmonization of test guidelines, as was discussed at the beginning of this chapter. Modifications have also been adopted over the years because of scientific advances, such as new knowledge about how the body handles chemical insults. Introduction of new technologies has made certain diagnostic procedures easier to perform and appropriate routes and types of exposure easier to achieve. For example, many laboratories now have the analytical capability to measure dozens of parameters simultaneously in a single small sample of blood, urine, or other body fluid. The use of tiny minipumps implanted beneath the skin and continuous infusion pumps used to administer low levels of a substance to mimic continuous exposures over extended time periods has become more widespread as this technology has improved. These procedures for delivering test substances may eventually be incorporated into standard test guidelines. Toxicity test protocol modifications typically are usually adopted only after a period of discussion, with opportunities for public comments.

## XI. RESPONSIBILITY AND COSTS OF TESTING

In the United States, the responsibility for establishing the safety of chemical products typically falls to the manufacturer of the product, who also pays for the costs of the testing. Most studies of health effects of new drugs, household and industrial solvents, pesticides, or other chemicals, are conducted either by toxicologists or other scientists working directly for the manufacturer, or by outside testing laboratories under contract to the manufacturer. Some toxicity studies are conducted and financed by the federal government. For example, when a chemical of concern is a naturally occurring substance (e.g., asbestos, aflatoxin), or a process used by numerous industries results in a potentially toxic mixture of chemicals (e.g., coke oven emissions, trihalomethanes resulting from chlorination of drinking water).

Most of the studies discussed in this chapter are now required routinely by regulatory agencies. Some knowledge of the costs of routine acute, subchronic, and chronic toxicity tests is important for a full appreciation of the effort involved in conducting these tests according to GLPs. Acute toxicity studies currently cost anywhere from 1,000 to 30,000 in U. S. dollars. The low-end figure might apply to a simple mouse $LD_{50}$ study or an eye or skin irritation or sensitization test, whereas higher costs are incurred, for example, in general acute toxicity studies that involve more animals per sex and observation of multiple endpoints. Costs of a 90-day repeat-dose rodent study climb to 100,000 dollars or more. Expenses are even higher for inhalation studies because of the additional facilities, equipment, and specialized personnel involved in maintaining an inhalation test atmosphere during these studies. In general, the longer the study, the greater the cost, although direct proportionality to length of study cannot be assumed (i.e., costs for a year-long study are not necessarily four times the cost of a 90-day study). A 1-year general chronic toxicity study in rodents costs up to 500,000 dollars and in dogs between 500,000 and 800,000 dollars. A lifetime chronic toxicity study in rodents can cost over a million U. S. dollars. Costs of testing thus depend largely on species, duration, exposure route, and number of endpoints measured, as well as whether the testing is done by the manufacturer in an in-house testing facility or by an outside contract laboratory (Amdur et al., 1991; and personal communications). The public is often surprised to learn how little information exists about the toxic effects of some chemicals. Although the cost of toxicology studies is not the only factor that discourages exhaustive testing of a chemical, given the relatively high cost of testing, it is not surprising that product manufacturers concerned about profits will typically conduct only those studies that are required by the regulatory agencies involved in approving the manufacture and sale of their products.

Readers of this chapter should have developed an appreciation for the effort involved in conducting toxicology studies, as well as some of the subtleties that lie beneath the surface of what might, at first glance, appear to be fairly straightforward standard test protocols. Experience and good judgment, in addition to knowledge of how toxicology studies should be conducted, are needed to collect and interpret toxicity study data in a meaningful way. Likewise, health risk assessments and interpretation of regulatory standards should be undertaken in consultation with individuals having this specialized knowledge and experience.

## REFERENCES

Amdur, M. O., Doull, J., and Klaassen, C. D. (1991). *Casarett and Doull's Toxicology: The Basic Science of Poisons,* 4th ed., Pergamon Press, New York.

Bruce, R. D. (1985). An up-and-down procedure for acute toxicity testing. *Fundam. Appl. Toxicol.,* 5, 151–157.

Hayes, A. W. (1994). *Principles and Methods of Toxicology,* 3rd ed., Raven Press, New York.

Litchfield, J. T. and Wilcoxon, F. (1949). Simplified method of evaluating dose–effect experiments, *J. Pharmacol. Exp. Ther.,* 96, 99–113.

[OECD] Organization for Economic Cooperation and Development (1981). *Guidelines for the Testing of Chemicals.* Section 4: *Health Effects,* 1981 and subsequent addenda (1984, 1987, 1993). Environmental Health and Safety Division, Paris, France.

[USEPA] United States Environmental Protection Agency (1983). Toxic substance control: Good Laboratory Practice standards; final rule (and subsequent revisions), *Fed. Reg.,* 48(230), 53921–53944, November 29.

[USEPA] United States Environmental Protection Agency (1984a). New and revised health effects test guidelines, Office of Pesticides and Toxic Substances, USEPA, *Fed. Reg.* 49(198), October 11, 1984.

[USEPA] United States Environmental Protection Agency (1984b). *Pesticide Assessment Guidelines,* Subdivision F, *Hazard Evaluation: Human and Domestic Animals,* PB86-108958, Office of Pesticide Programs, EPA 540/9-84-014.

[USEPA] United States Environmental Protection Agency (1984c). *Labeling Requirements for Pesticides and Devices,* 40 CFR Part 156.

[USEPA] United States Environmental Protection Agency (1984d). Resource Conservation and Recovery Act, 40 CFR Parts 240–271.

[USFDA] United States Food and Drug Administration (1989). *Good Laboratory Practice Standards for Nonclinical Laboratory Studies,* 21 CFR Part 58.

Weil, C. S. (1956). Tables for convenient calculation of median-effective dose ($LC_{50}$ or $EC_{50}$) and instructions in their use, *Biometrics,* 8, 249.

# 9
# Carcinogenicity-Testing Methods

**J. A. Wisniewski**
*California Environmental Protection Agency*
*Sacramento, California*

## I. INTRODUCTION

Epidemiological studies suggest a causal relationship between exposure to a chemical and the occurrence of cancer in a population. However, most suggestive evidence for human carcinogenicity comes from experimental studies performed on animals. Although the production of neoplasia in animals is not definitive evidence of human carcinogenicity, we assume that a chemical that induces cancer in animals has the potential to behave similarly in humans (NTP, 1984). This provides a conservative approach to risk assessment for public health purposes. Extrapolations from rodents to humans are based on the best scientific evidence available at that time, and these estimates are subject to change when newer scientific evidence becomes available.

The primary goal of carcinogen-testing methods is to provide data for evaluating carcinogenic risk to humans (Williams and Weisburger, 1991). Current testing methods for long-term studies in rodents have improved over those first initiated during the 1960s by the U. S. Food and Drug Administration (USFDA) and the National Cancer Institute (NCI). The same basic procedures are used today, but with multiple species and sufficient numbers of animals to assure statistically significant results and with proper quality control to ensure the validity and integrity of study results.

Lifetime cancer bioassays in animals are an essential component of estimating chemical carcinogenicity. They are, however, extremely expensive and time-consuming to perform. Short-term genotoxicity tests provide much information on the potential of a chemical to bind to deoxyribonucleic acid (DNA), but they provide little insight on whether this actually induces neoplastic lesions in the body. A need for testing methods to bridge the gap between short-term genotoxicity tests and conventional long-term testing led to the development of several medium-term in vivo bioassays (Ito et al., 1992). These assays are based on the two-stage or multiple-stage theory of carcinogenesis, and they involve induction of specific steps in the carcinogenic process. One of the most promising is the rat liver-altered foci assay.

The purpose of this chapter is to present an overview of in vivo carcinogen-testing methods, including both medium-term and long-term bioassays, that are accepted or have been proposed for use in human health risk assessment. For more detailed discussion of particular aspects of carcinogenicity testing, readers are directed to Arnold et al. (1990a), IARC (1980), Milman and Weisburger (1985), NTP (1984), Robens et al. (1989), and Sontag et al. (1976). Other topics I present include a synopsis of the decision point approach to carcinogenicity testing proposed by Weisburger and Williams (1984) and an overview of the National Toxicology Program (NTP). Short-term genotoxicity tests are not discussed here, but are treated in Chapter 10 of this book.

## II.  THE MULTISTEP CARCINOGENIC PROCESS

Carcinogenesis is a multistage process, which is initiated when a genotoxic or DNA-reactive agent produces an irreversible genetic alteration in the cell (Barrett, 1993; Goldberg and Diamandis, 1993). Initiated cells undergo clonal expansion to a preneoplastic lesion or benign tumor after exposure to a "promoting" agent. Promotion is a reversible change that is believed to result from a nongenetic alteration, such as defects in terminal differentiation or growth control, or resistance to cytotoxicity (Harris, 1992). Conversion of the benign tumor to a malignant tumor involves additional genetic changes, such as activation of protooncogenes and inactivation of tumor suppressor genes. The final event of the carcinogenic process is the progression of malignant tumors to metastases and clinical cancer. [Detailed treatment of the principles of carcinogenicity can be found in Chapter 2 of this volume.]

Weisburger and Williams (1981) have grouped chemical carcinogens into two broad categories based on their mechanism of action—genotoxic carcinogens and epigenetic agents. Genotoxic carcinogens interact with DNA or genetic material, either directly or after undergoing metabolic conversion to a reactive molecule. The term *genotoxic* has now been replaced with *DNA-reactive* (Barrett, 1993). Agents that act through mechanisms other than DNA interactions are termed *epigenetic,* and are further grouped into the following classes: solid-state carcinogens, hormones, immunosuppressors, cocarcinogens, and promoters (Weisburger and Williams, 1981). A problem with this classification scheme is that carcinogenic agents may not act exclusively by one mechanism or the other. Furthermore, the classification may not accurately describe the mechanism by which the cellular phenotype is altered, even though it describes the action of the chemical. For example, an agent may not be directly reactive with DNA, but it may indirectly elicit a genetic change, such as chromosomal rearrangement or aneuploidy, through an epigenetic mechanism (Barrett, 1993). Such a chemical could not strictly be called an epigenetic carcinogen.

Regardless of the chemical classification, most known human carcinogens are active in a variety of genetic toxicology tests. Subsequently, much current research has focused on molecular genetics, in particular, the identification of genes and gene mutations involved in the carcinogenic process. In general, the genetic damage found in cancer cells is of two types: dominant, with protooncogenes as targets; and recessive, with tumor suppressor genes or antioncogenes as targets (Bishop, 1991). The dominant lesions normally result in a gain of function, whereas the recessive damage results in a loss of function. More specifically, protooncogenes are involved in the regulation of normal cellular growth and differentiation. Oncogenes are the mutated forms of the protooncogenes; they act by subverting the normal-signaling pathways governing entry into the $G_1$ phase of the cell cycle (Schmandt and Mills, 1993). This generally results in gene overexpression, inappropriate gene expression, or expression of an abnormal gene product, which leads to increased cellular proliferation and malignancy. Tumor suppressor genes, on the other hand, are growth-inhibitory genes that provide a second level of regulation of the cell cycle and cellular differentiation (Schmandt and Mills, 1993). They must be inactivated or lost in tumor cells. Multiple tumor suppressor genes frequently are affected in common human tumors, such as lung, colon, and breast, indicating that malignant growth is subject to several levels of negative control (Barrett, 1993). As many as ten or more mutational events have been proposed to occur in adult human cancers. These include point mutations, deletion mutations, chromosomal rearrangements, gene amplification, and chromosomal losses and gains (Barrett, 1993; Schmandt and Mills, 1993).

Several oncogenes have been identified in human cancers, including *neu, ras, myc, fos, src, sis,* and *erb B* (Bishop, 1991; Hunter, 1991; Schmandt and Mills, 1993). Some of the tumor suppressor genes that have been incriminated in human tumors include: *p53, Rb1* (retinoblastoma), *WT1* (Wilms' tumor), *DCC, NF1, FAP,* and *MEN*-1 (Bishop, 1991; Harris, 1992; Jones et al., 1991; Levine et al., 1991; Marshall, 1991). The *p53* gene is the most frequently altered gene in human cancers, including astrocytoma, carcinoma of the breast, colon, liver, esophagus, and lung, and osteosarcoma.

Recent advances in molecular genetics have provided much insight into the mutational (and nonmutational) basis of chemical carcinogenesis, but have had minimal influence on methods' development for human health risk assessment. Nevertheless, the techniques employed in studies of molecular carcinogenesis show promise for application as carcinogen-screening tests. Measurement of endpoints associated with promotion or progression, such as inhibition of gap–junction and cell–cell communication, formation of radicals and clastogenic factors, increased DNA synthesis and cell proliferation, and inflammatory effects, may be useful in identifying nongenotoxic carcinogens (Ramel, 1992). Analysis of mutational spectra provides a method by which the action of specific chemicals can be fingerprinted (Harris, 1992, 1993; Jones et al., 1991). Immunohistochemical detection of oncogene products, such as p21-*ras,* has been used to identify and characterize preneoplastic and neoplastic lesions in human tissues (Gulbis and Galand, 1993). Although these and other methods for detecting molecular targets of carcinogens will undoubtedly be incorporated into a battery of short-term tests for screening carcinogens in the future, they are still in the developmental phase and have not been validated for use in risk assessment. Therefore, they will not be treated further in this chapter.

## III. TESTING PROCEDURES

## A. Medium-Term Assays

### 1. Introduction

The evaluation of potential human carcinogens typically is based on the results of long-term carcinogenicity bioassays with rodents. These assays are performed over the lifetime of the animal, generally 2 years, and many animals are used to obtain statistically relevant results. Detailed histopathological examinations must be performed on numerous tissue samples to detect any neoplastic changes resulting from exposure to the test chemical. Consequently, the long-term cancer bioassay is extremely expensive and takes years to complete. With the ever-increasing numbers of chemicals that have been introduced into the environment in recent years, it is not practical to test all of them for carcinogenesis by the current comprehensive testing methods. Therefore, a need arose for more rapid, convenient, and economical bioassays capable of predicting the carcinogenic potential of chemicals.

Several short-term bioassays have been developed to screen chemicals for potential genotoxicity. Examples include the tests for mutations in *Salmonella typhimurium* and for sister chromatid exchanges and chromosomal aberrations in Chinese hamster ovary cells. Although these tests are quite useful, some recent evidence suggests that mutagenicity and genotoxicity do not always correlate with carcinogenicity (McGregor, 1992; Zeiger, 1987). Moreover, these short-term assays are limited in that they cannot determine organ-specific carcinogenicity or promoting activity of chemicals.

Various medium-term bioassays have been developed in rodents that use liver, skin, lung, mammary gland, and other organs as targets to test the carcinogenic potential of chemicals. The most promising methods are based on the two-stage or multiple-stage theory of carcinogenesis, such as the mouse skin tumor assay and the rat liver altered-foci assay. Another more recent development is the multiorgan model, in which neoplastic lesions are initiated in rats by the sequential administration of three or more carcinogens, and then enhanced by various test agents. I present five medium-term bioassays in this chapter. They are the mouse skin tumor assay, the rat liver altered-foci assay, the strain A mouse lung tumor assay, the rat mammary gland tumor assay, and the multiple-organ model.

## 2. *Mouse Skin Tumor Assay*

Chemical carcinogenesis in skin is a multistage process, consisting of initiation, promotion, and progression, or malignant conversion (Hennings et al., 1993a; Warren et al., 1993). Initiation can result from single exposure to a genotoxic agent, which produces a mutation in a critical gene. Initiation is generally considered an irreversible genetic change. The initiated cells remain in a repressed state owing to interactions from surrounding normal cells. During promotion, these cells lose their ability to respond to the repressive signals from adjacent cells, and they begin a clonal expansion to form a benign papilloma. This step is thought to be a reversible, epigenetic change. Malignant conversion of papillomas to carcinomas occurs spontaneously at a low rate, but can be enhanced by exposure of papilloma-bearing mice to a gentoxic agent. These "progressor" agents appear to act by a second genetic change in the papilloma (Hennings et al., 1993a; Warren et al., 1993). Like initiation, progression is irreversible.

Bioassays for the induction of mouse skin tumors are based on this multistage process. Chemicals can be tested for activity as initiator, promoter, and progressor agents. There are three standard protocols for induction of mouse skin tumors: (1) the complete carcinogenesis protocol, (2) the two-stage model, and (3) the multistage model. In the following I will present the standard procedures for all three protocols and then specific details for each.

The standard skin tumor protocol uses the SENCAR strain mouse, which has been selectively bred for sensitivity to skin tumor induction (Slaga et al., 1982; Slaga and Nesnow, 1985). Other strains that have been used are CD-1, C57BL/6, BALB/c, ICR/Ha Swiss, and NMRI, which generally are less sensitive than the SENCAR strain (Slaga et al., 1982; Slaga and Nesnow, 1985; Edler et al., 1991). Another strain used recently, the FVB/N mouse, had a higher rate of malignant conversion of papillomas to squamous cell carcinomas than did SENCAR and other mouse strains after treatment with 7,12-dimethylbenz[*a*]anthracene (DMBA) or 12-*O*-tetradecanoylphorbol-13-acetate (TPA), or both (Hennings et al., 1993b). The FVB/N mice are widely used to establish transgenic lines containing active oncogenes.

Female mice generally are used, since they are more docile than males when housed five or more in cages. The age of the mice at the beginning of treatment ranges from 3 to 9 weeks. Mice that are 3 weeks old or between 7 and 9 weeks old are in the resting phase (telogen) of the hair growth cycle. Whereas earlier studies by Borum (1954) and Berenblum et al. (1958) suggested that mouse skin in the resting phase was more susceptible to tumor induction, a recent study showed that mice in the sustained hair growth phase (anagen) were more sensitive to tumor initiation by DMBA, with or without TPA (Miller et al., 1993). The effect of the hair cycle on tumor growth, however, appears to be time-dependent. That is, the anagen-treated animals yielded significantly more tumors than the telogen-treated animals after 20 weeks posttreatment, but differences were not significant at 10 weeks posttreatment. These results should be confirmed, since the increase in cellular proliferation accompanying the hair growth phase could affect not only the induction of tumors, but possibly even the type of tumor formed (benign vs. malignant).

A minimum of 15 mice per treatment group should be used to obtain statistically significant results (Edler et al., 1991), but 20–40 mice per group is typical (Pereira, 1982a).

The usual route of administration is topical application or subcutaneous injection. If a topical treatment is chosen, the backs of the animals should be shaved 2 days before treatment. Other routes of administration include oral, intraperitoneal (IP) injection, and transplacental transmission (Pereira, 1982a).

During the study, body weights should be recorded at least once a month, but as often as weekly. The presence of tumors is recorded weekly. This includes papillomas larger than 1 mm that persist for 1 or 2 consecutive weeks, and carcinomas (Slaga and Nesnow, 1985; Hennings et al., 1993b; Miller et al., 1993; Chen et al., 1994). Other general data that should be recorded or calculated are presented in Table 1.

A complete carcinogen induces tumors in the absence of other treatments, provided the dose and the frequency of administration are sufficient. The protocol involves the administration of either a single large dose or smaller weekly doses of the test chemical to each animal. Multiple doses typically are given once a week for 20 weeks (Hennings et al., 1993b; Chen et al., 1994), but treatment periods have extended to 52 weeks or more (Slaga and Nesnow, 1985). There should be a minimum of three dose groups of the test chemical to establish a dose–response relationship. A negative control (for example, acetone) and a positive control (for example, DMBA in acetone) are also included.

The two-stage protocol consists of the administration of a subthreshold dose of a carcinogen, *initiation*, followed by repeated doses of a noncarcinogenic promoting agent, *promotion*. A subthreshold dose is one that will not produce tumors in the animals's lifetime without other treatments. A chemical with unknown carcinogenic activity can be tested for both initiating and promoting properties. For initiating activity, a single dose of the test chemical is applied topically. Treatment groups should include a negative control, that is, the carrier solvent, usually acetone; a positive control, such as DMBA or 3-methylcholanthrene (3-MC) in acetone; and at

**Table 1**  Mouse Skin Tumor Assay: Data to Be Collected or Calculated

| Data | Definition |
| --- | --- |
| Papilloma incidence | Percentage of mice with one or more papilloma |
| Papilloma multiplicity (yield) | Average number of papillomas per surviving mouse |
| Papilloma latent period | Number of weeks until 50% of the mice had one or more papilloma |
| Carcinoma incidence | Cumulative percentage of mice with one or more carcinoma among the mice alive when the first carcinoma appeared |
| Carcinoma multiplicity (yield) | Cumulative number of carcinomas per number of mice alive when the first carcinoma appeared in all animals |
| Carcinoma latent period | Number of weeks required for development of the first carcinoma, or the average time for carcinoma development $\pm$ S.E |
| Conversion frequency | Percentage conversion, for each group is (total carcinomas divided by total papillomas) $\times$ 100 |

*Source:* Hennings et al. (1993b) and Chen et al. (1994).

least two dose groups (low- and high-dose) (Hennings et al., 1993b; Möller et al., 1993; Slaga and Nesnow, 1985). Weekly or twice-weekly doses of the promoting chemical are applied topically 1–2 weeks after initiation, usually for a minimum of 20 weeks. If testing for promoting activity, treatment groups should include a control and at least two dose groups. Although TPA is used most often as the promoting agent in two-stage protocols, benzoyl peroxide, chrysarobin, and mezerein also have been effective (DiGiovanni et al., 1993). Slaga and Nesnow (1985) recommended that either benzoyl peroxide or chrysarobin be used, since TPA is subject to degradation by esterases.

With the standard DMBA–TPA protocol, papillomas become visible at 6–8 weeks and reach a plateau at about 20 weeks. Carcinomas develop at about 30 weeks and reach a maximal number at about 50 weeks. Most carcinomas develop from existing papillomas. The maximum number of carcinomas that a mouse can support is three to four (Warren et al., 1993).

The multistage model further employs the administration of a progressor agent to papilloma-bearing mice to increase the frequency of conversion to malignant carcinoma. The progressor agent typically is a direct-acting carcinogen, such as ethylnitrosourea (ETU) or $N$-methyl-$N'$-nitro-$N$-nitrosoguanidine (MNNG), which affects existing papillomas, rather than producing new tumors (Hennings et al., 1993a; Warren et al., 1993). Therefore, it is administered to mice after the 20-week promotion period, when the formation of papillomas has reached a plateau.

The following protocol for tumor progression was described by Warren et al. (1993). Subsequent to initiation with DMBA and promotion with TPA (as just described), the progressor agents are administered topically to mice twice a week for 2 weeks. The number of agents tested may vary, but Warren and colleagues used three groups: a control (1 μg TPA), 10 μmol ETU, and 1 μmol MNNG. (The progressor agents also may be administered as a single dose, either topically or IP, or they may be given once or twice weekly for up to 30 weeks.) After these treatments, TPA is again administered twice a week until week 40 of the study. The investigators found that animals treated with ETU and MNNG formed carcinomas earlier and in greater numbers than those treated with TPA alone.

Approximately 15–20% of squamous cell carcinomas undergo further progression to metastatic lesions; however, a specific protocol for this activity has not been reported (Hennings et al., 1993a).

Over 500 chemicals have been assayed for carcinogenic activity in mouse skin. The predominant class of chemicals that has tested positive as initiators and complete carcinogens is the polycyclic aromatic hydrocarbons (PAHs), their metabolites, and environmental samples containing mixtures of PAHs. Of the non-PAH chemicals, most are direct or indirect alkylating agents. An extensive listing of these chemicals can be found in Pereira (1982a) and Slaga and Nesnow (1985). These two references also provide a list of chemicals tested for promoting activity.

Several agents, along with ETU and MNNG, have increased papilloma progression in mouse skin. They include benzo[$a$]pyrene (B[$a$]P) diol epoxide, cisplatin, urethane, 4-nitroquinoline-$N$-oxide, benzoyl peroxide, hydrogen peroxide, acetic acid, diethyl maleate, and ionizing radiation (Hennings et al., 1993a; Warren et al., 1993). Although most progressor agents do not produce papillomas, benzoyl peroxide is active as both a tumor promoter and progressor agent (Hennings et al., 1993a; Warren et al., 1993). It possesses genotoxic activity, but does not have activity as a complete carcinogen or tumor initiator. Benzoyl peroxide possesses clastogenic activity, that is, it produces single-strand DNA breaks. Hennings et al. (1993a) and Warren et al. (1993) suggested this activity as the mechanism by which benzoyl peroxide enhances progression of papillomas to carcinoma.

A favorable characteristic of the mouse skin tumor assay is that tumors are formed on the exterior of the animals, which permits easy detection and monitoring of tumor size and type.

Therefore, fewer animals are needed for the study because necropsies scheduled midstudy can be limited or omitted altogether. The assay also has an extensive database for skin carcinogens, and good dose–response data have been obtained for several chemicals (Slaga et al., 1982; Slaga and Nesnow, 1985). Additionally, the assay allows investigators to distinguish among initiators, promoters, and progressors.

A limitation of this assay is that the topical route may prevent systemic absorption of chemicals that require metabolic activation in other organ systems for carcinogenic activity to occur. Also, the protocol requires frequent application and sometimes large doses of the test chemical to be effective. Moreover, most of the data obtained have been on PAHs, and limited numbers of chemical classes have been tested.

Data are not yet adequate to correlate the results of the mouse skin tumor assay with results of lifetime cancer studies in animals and humans. However, five chemicals that tested positive in the mouse skin tumor assay also had positive activity as animal or human respiratory carcinogens. They included the chemical classes of carbamates, PAHs, chloromethyl ethers, quinolines, and coke oven emissions (Slaga and Nesnow, 1985). There also appears to be some correlation between the mouse skin tumor assay and the mouse lung adenoma assay. That is, the lowest dose administered systemically that elicits a positive carcinogenic response appears to be similar with both assays, but this requires further study (Pereira, 1982a).

The mouse skin tumor assay has limited application as a replacement for the long-term cancer bioassay, but it would be an integral test in a decision scheme for evaluating carcinogenic agents. It also is an important tool for determining mechanisms of tumor formation and progression, especially for pharmacological research on chemotherapeutic agents.

### 3. Rat Liver Altered-Foci Assay

As with skin, carcinogenesis in the liver apparently is a multistage process, consisting of initiation, promotion, and progression. Initiated cells with altered DNA undergo clonal expansion during promotion. Focal changes in the phenotype, or altered hepatic foci, are recognized as aggregates of cells that display altered enzymatic activity or other cellular constituents (Pereira, 1982b). For example, the altered foci have excessive storage of glycogen, a change in enzymes involved in carbohydrate and drug metabolism, and an increase in proliferation rate (Bannasch and Zerban, 1992; Ito et al., 1992). It is generally accepted that altered foci are the earliest detectable preneoplastic lesion, and that they progress either directly into hepatocarcinoma, or first to hyperplastic nodules and then to carcinoma (Bannasch and Zerban, 1992; Goldfarb and Pugh, 1982; Ito et al., 1992; Pereira, 1982b, 1985). Hence, the altered hepatic foci are an especially sensitive indicator of a chemical's carcinogenic potential.

Numerous histochemical markers have been used to detect altered foci, including changes in γ-glutamyl transpeptidase (GGT), basophilia, DT-diaphorase, glycogen storage, glucose-6-phosphate dehydrogenase, adenosine triphosphatase (ATPase), glucose-6-phosphatase (G6Pase), and iron storage (Bannasch and Zerban, 1992; Ito et al., 1992; Pereira, 1982b, 1985). The most widely used marker is GGT because it has strong activity in preneoplastic lesions and very low activity in background parenchymal cells. It is present in approximately 90% of the foci, and also is associated with most liver cancer, including rat and human hyperplastic nodules and hepatocellular carcinomas (Pereira, 1982b). A limitation of using GGT activity as a biomarker is that numerous chemicals, such as phenobarbital, butylated hydroxytoluene (BHT), and ethanol, can induce the enzyme in the periportal region of the liver lobule (Ito et al., 1992; Pereira, 1985). Therefore, any increase in GGT activity in the periportal region must be differentiated from the actual induction of GGT-positive foci. Another limitation is that not all initiators or promoters produce GGT-positive foci. For example, altered foci induced in F344 rats after administration of clofibrate, di(2)ethylhexylphthalate, and Wy-14,643, all of which are peroxisome proliferators, were negative for GGT activity (Ito et al., 1992; Rao et al., 1982). The best approach may be to select at least two biomarkers that differ in sensitivity to the test chemical.

Glutathione-*S*-transferase placental form (GST-P) activity also has been used to detect altered foci, and it was a more reliable marker than GGT for diethylnitrosamine (DEN)-initiated lesions (Ito et al., 1992). There was a slight induction of GST-P in the periportal region after BHT administration, but to a much lesser extent than GGT. A reported advantage of this marker is the ease of immunohistochemical staining and the clearly distinguishable foci that are produced (Ito et al., 1992).

Most studies of carcinogenesis in rat liver have focused on the initiation–promotion (IP) model. This model predicts neoplastic effects from administration of a nonnecrogenic, sub-carcinogenic dose of an initiating agent, such as DEN, coupled with administration of the test chemical (i.e., putative promoting agent) for a specified time period. Alternatively, a test chemical can be given followed by administration of a promoter, such as phenobarbital. A "stimulus" of hepatocyte proliferation may be employed to increase the interaction of the test chemical with initiated cells. This is accomplished either by treating immature animals with DEN or by performing a two-thirds (70%) partial hepatectomy (PH), on adult animals. Apparently with both practices, the resulting regenerative cell proliferation "fixes" DNA alterations (Bannasch and Zerban, 1992). Numerous variations of the IP assay are presented in the literature. I refer readers to the reviews of Bannasch and Zerban (1992), Goldsworthy et al. (1986), Osterle and Deml (1990), and Pereira (1982b, 1985) for details of additional protocols.

With the initiation–promotion–progression (IPP) assay, administration of the promoter is followed by treatment with a known or putative progressor agent, depending on which stage of carcinogenesis is being examined. Another method, referred to as "stop protocol" by Bannasch and Zerban (1992), is similar to the complete carcinogenesis protocol described in mouse skin. It employs administration of a carcinogen either in a single dose or in multiple doses over a specified time period. This protocol is useful for investigating mechanisms of carcinogenic action, but the lag period to formation of altered foci is quite lengthy without additional experimental manipulations. Therefore, only protocols for the IP and the IPP models in the rat liver will be presented.

Rats are the species of choice for the altered liver foci assay, but other species, such as mice (Vesselinovitch et al., 1985), hamsters (Stenbäck et al., 1986), and fish (Hinton et al., 1988), have been used to study foci induction after chemical exposure. Male or female F344 or Sprague-Dawley rats are the most commonly used strains. Depending on the protocol, ages of animals range from 5 days to 6 weeks.

One of the most straightforward procedures for the IP model is described by Ito and colleagues (Cabral et al., 1991; Hakoi et al., 1992; Ito et al., 1992). Male F344 rats, 6 weeks old, are divided into three groups, using 15 or 16 animals per group. Group 1 is the treatment group. Animals receive an IP injection of 200 mg/kg DEN in 0.9% NaCl on day 0 of the study. Two weeks later, administration of the test compound begins. It typically is added to the diet, but may be administered in the drinking water or by injection (IP or IV). Treatment continues for 6 weeks. Group 2, the control, also is initiated with DEN, but only receives basal diet without the test compound for 6 weeks. Group 3 receives saline (vehicle control) without DEN and the test compound in the diet; it is used to assess the ability of the test compound to induce altered foci without initiation. The PH is performed in all three groups at week 3, and the experiment is terminated at week 8.

Animals are sacrificed and body weights are recorded. The livers are removed, weighed, sectioned, and fixed in ice-cold acetone for immunohistochemical examination of GST-P activity. Additional sections are fixed in 10% phosphate-buffered formalin solution for routine staining with hematoxylin and eosin.

The numbers per square centimeters (no./cm$^2$ of liver) and areas [millimeter per square centimeter (mm$^2$/cm$^2$) of liver] of GST-P-positive foci that are larger than 0.2 mm in diameter are measured using a color video image processor. Statistical analyses are performed by comparing the differences between groups 1 and 2. Results are considered positive when both the numbers and areas of foci are increased significantly.

Another IP protocol described by Pereira (1982b) has been used by the Health Effects Research Laboratory in Cincinnati, Ohio as part of their Carcinogenesis Testing Matrix. In one method, rats are given a two-thirds PH 18–24 hr before administration of the test compound. Then, the animals receive 500 ppm phenobarbital in their drinking water ad libitum starting 6 days after the test chemical is administered and continuing for 7 weeks. Alternatively, initiation begins on day 0 with the test chemical. Starting with day 7, phenobarbital (500 ppm) is administered in the animals' drinking water for 7 weeks (to day 56). The PH is performed during phenobarbital promotion on day 14. From day 7 to day 14, the phenobarbital concentration is decreased to 100 ppm because of increased toxicity after PH. A favorable characteristic of this protocol, as well as that described by Ito and colleagues, is that both have a relatively short study duration of 8 weeks.

Dragan et al. (1991) described still another variation of the IP protocol. A 70% PH is performed on male and female Fischer 344 rats weighing 130–200 g. Four to 11 animals are used per treatment group. Twenty-four hours later, DEN at 10 mg/kg is administered by gastric intubation, and the animals are allowed a 2-week recovery period. Then a promoter, either the test chemical or phenobarbital (positive control), is given to animals that have or have not been initiated with DEN. Animals are sacrificed after 6 months of promotion. Tissues are prepared as described earlier, except that staining is performed for GGT, ATPase, and G6Pase activities, in addition to GST-P activities. The number of altered foci per cubic centimeter of liver, liver weight, and the number of foci per liver are recorded for each rat.

Ito et al. (1992) tested 179 chemicals in the altered liver foci assay using the initiation–promotion protocol described earlier. These chemicals were classified into four categories: (1) liver carcinogens, (2) nonliver carcinogens, (3) noncarcinogens, and (4) unknown carcinogenicity. Of the 41 known liver carcinogens, 38 tested positive. Two of the three negative chemicals, that is, di(2)ethylhexylphthalate and clofibrate, were peroxisome proliferators, which appear to produce preneoplastic lesions that are phenotypically different from foci produced by most hepatocarcinogens. Consequently, the most commonly used markers (i.e., GGT and GST-P activity) are not effective in predicting carcinogenic activity from this class of compounds. Eight of the 33 nonliver carcinogens showed positive, and all of the noncarcinogens gave negative results in the altered liver foci assay. Of the 68 chemicals with unknown carcinogenic activity, 18 tested positive. The 84 chemicals that gave positive results belong to a range of chemical classes, including

Aromatic amines and azo dyes [e.g., 2-acetylaminofluorene (2-AAF) and 3′-methyl-4-dimethylaminoazobenzene (3′-Me-DAB)]

Nitrosamines (e.g., DEN)

PAHs, (e.g., B[*a*]P)

Hormones (e.g., diethylstilbestrol)

Pesticides (e.g., captan, *p,p*′-DDT, trifluralin)

Drugs and dyes (e.g., doxorubicin, phenobarbital)

Miscellaneous compounds (e.g., aflatoxin B$_1$, safrole, and urethane)

Similar results have been reported in Pereira (1982b) in which alternative protocols were used for the altered foci assay. These results indicated that the IP protocol can be used to predict the carcinogenicity of a variety of chemicals, both liver and nonliver carcinogens.

Dragan et al. (1993) described a protocol for the IPP model similar to Pereira's IP protocol except that administration of a progressor agent is incorporated. Additionally, this protocol measures the formation of foci-in-foci (FIF), which are smaller (presumably more recent) lesions observed within larger (presumably older) lesions. The FIF are indicative of the progressive development of initiated cells to preneoplastic foci and further to malignant neoplasms. Carcinoma incidence is monitored, too, since the study duration is about 12 months. The protocol is described in the following:

Neonatal (5-day old) male and female Sprague-Dawley rats (7–12 animals per group) are initiated with a single IP injection of DEN (10 mg/kg body weight). Promotion begins at weaning (about 3 weeks of age) with administration of 0.05% phenobarbital in the diet for 6 months. Six months after weaning, 70% PH is performed on the animals, followed by administration of the progressor agent 24 hr later. A control group does not receive the progressor agent. At this point, promotion by phenobarbitol either is maintained for another 6 months or is discontinued and basal diet is fed. Discontinuation allows the detection of foci that develop independently of exposure to a promoting agent.

Animals are sacrificed 10–14 months after weaning and livers are removed. Sections are taken and frozen on dry ice and stained for GST-P, GGT, ATPase, or G6Pase activity. Additional sections are fixed in formalin, embedded in paraffin, and stained with hematoxylin and eosin for histological examination. The number of altered foci per cubic centimeter of liver, the liver weight, and the number of foci per liver are recorded for each animal. The FIF are measured qualitatively by visual inspection of overlays of the four phenotypic markers. That is, serial sections of liver are stained for the four different enzymes, and the tracings from each of these are overlaid to show the presence of heterogeneous foci.

Dragan et al. (1993) tested the progressor activity of hydroxyurea (HU; 150 mg/kg) or *N*-nitroso-*n*-ethylurea (ENU; 100 mg/kg) after administering DEN as an initiating agent and phenobarbital as a promoting agent to rats. Phenobarbital treatment was discontinued after administration of the progressor agents. They observed a significant increase in FIF per liver and in FIF per altered foci compared with animals without progressor treatment. Additionally, promoter-independent foci were significantly increased in the treatment groups compared with the control, but ENU was a more potent progressor than HU. However, the hepatocarcinoma incidence was low in all groups. In the groups in which phenobarbital promotion continued after treatment with HU and ENU, hepatocarcinoma incidence was increased markedly. These results provide evidence that the IPP model mimics cancer development in liver. Furthermore, the protocol appears to be useful in classifying chemicals as having initiator, promoter, or progressor activities.

A major limitation of the rat liver foci assay, as with other single-organ models, is that negative results cannot rule our carcinogenic activity in target organs other than the liver. Additionally, a large discrepancy exists between the number of foci that appear early during hepatocarcinogenesis and the final tumor yield. Estimates of carcinoma formation from altered liver foci range from 1:1,300 to 1:12,000 (Bannasch and Zerban, 1992), but about 2% of hyperplastic nodules develop to carcinoma (Ito et al., 1992). The reason for this discrepancy is unknown. Other problems include strain and species differences in sensitivity to foci induction and to choice of biomarker for measuring foci (Deml et al., 1981; Ito et al., 1992).

Several advantages of the altered foci assay in rat are as follows: (1) It requires fewer animals, and it takes less time for preneoplastic and neoplastic lesions to appear compared with the conventional 2-year bioassay; (2) it is accepted that the altered foci represent an early response of liver cells to hepatocarcinogens, and that they precede the appearance of hepatic carcinomas; and (3) it appears to offer a good correlation with results from the 2-year bioassay.

In summary, the rat liver altered foci assay appears to be a reliable method for identifying chemicals with carcinogenic potential. Because more than 60% of the carcinogens listed by International Agency for Research on Cancer (IARC) as having sufficient evidence for carcinogenicity in humans are hepatocarcinogens in animals (Hakoi et al., 1992), and because the altered foci is accepted as a preneoplastic lesion, this assay is particularly relevant as a tool for screening carcinogens. Whether the altered foci can be used in addition to hepatic neoplasms as a toxicological endpoint in 2-year carcinogenicity studies is still under debate (Bannasch and Zerban, 1992).

### 4. Strain A Mice Lung Tumor Assay

When compared with other inbred strains, strain A mice develop a higher incidence of age-related, spontaneous lung neoplasms during their lifetime (Stoner, 1991; Stoner and Shimkin, 1982, 1985). The tumors, usually adenomas, are located at or near the pleural surface and are distributed throughout both lungs, but more frequently in the right lung (Dixon et al., 1991). They can be observed either by gross examination or with the use of a dissecting microscope. Treatment of strain A mice with certain chemicals increases the average number of lung tumors per mouse when compared with control animals (Stoner, 1991; Stoner and Shimkin, 1982, 1985). This is the basis for using the mouse lung tumor assay to assess the carcinogenic potential of specific chemicals. The protocol for the bioassay, which was developed by Dr. Michael Shimkin, follows.

The animals used in the lung tumor assay should be healthy and free of pneumonia and other diseases. If possible, endogenous murine viruses, such as Reo-3, Sendai, lactate dehydrogenase virus, and Moloney-sarcoma virus, should be identified in the mouse colony, since these have been shown to influence the chemical induction of lung adenomas in strain A mice (Stoner, 1991; Stoner and Shimkin, 1985).

Male and female strain A mice, 6–8 weeks old with an average weight of 18–20 g, are distributed randomly among control and treatment groups. It is recommended that corncob bedding be used in place of cedar shavings, which contain terpene compounds that may induce drug-metabolizing enzymes (Stoner, 1991; Stoner and Shimkin, 1985).

Before performing the bioassay, the maximum tolerated dose (MTD) must be determined for each test chemical. Serial twofold dilutions of the chemical are injected IP into groups of five mice; the MTD is the maximum single dose that all five mice survive for 2 weeks after receiving six IP injections (three injections per week) (Stoner and Shimkin, 1985). Animals should be observed for at least 2 months following treatment, since some test chemicals may be immunosuppressant and likely to produce delayed toxicity.

For the bioassay, the test agent can be administered by several different routes, although IP injection is the most common. For each test, three dose levels are used: the MTD, one-half the MTD, and one-fifth the MTD. At least 30 mice, 15 of each sex, are used per dose for a total of 90 animals per test chemical. For highly toxic chemicals, the number can be increased to 50 mice per dose. Animals are dosed three times per week for 8 weeks. A positive control group (10 animals per dose, 5 each of males and females) is treated with urethane, using a single injection of 10 or 20 mg/mouse. Two other control groups are included: (1) untreated control (30 mice, 15 males and 15 females), for incidence of spontaneous tumors; and (2) vehicle control (30 mice, 15 males and 15 females). The bioassays are terminated 16 weeks after the last injection, for a total period of 24 weeks. For weak carcinogens, the animals may need to be maintained until 36 weeks to demonstrate carcinogenicity. Animals are sacrificed, and the lungs are removed and fixed in Tellyesniczky's fluid (20 parts 70% alcohol:2 parts formaldehyde:1

part acetic acid) or 10% buffered formalin for 24 hr. The tumors, which appear as pearly white or yellowish nodules on the lung surface, are counted and the numbers recorded. A few tumors from test animals and controls should be removed for histological examination to confirm the morphological appearance of adenoma (Stoner, 1991; Stoner and Shimkin, 1985).

Unlike the long-term cancer bioassay, significant evidence of carcinogenicity can be obtained in 30–35 weeks with the mouse lung tumor assay. However, extending the test longer than 36 weeks is not desirable because the incidence of pulmonary tumors in control animals increases rapidly after 35 weeks; consequently, the test loses sensitivity (Williams and Weisburger, 1991). The rate of spontaneously occurring tumors in untreated mice after 24 weeks varies from 0.2 to 0.4 tumors per mouse. The minimum carcinogenic response in treated animals considered to be statistically significant is 0.8–1 tumor per mouse, when 30 mice are used per dose level (Stoner, 1991).

A similar bioassay was described by Wang and Busby (1993), who used newborn CD-1 mice instead of strain A mice. Animals were treated with a potential carcinogen, in this case fluoranthene, and maintained for 6 and 9 months. An average of 44 pups (about half males and half females) were used for each control and the three treatment groups. A dose-dependent increase in fluoranthene-induced lung tumors (predominantly adenomas) was observed in both the 6-month and 9-month groups. Tumor multiplicity in the highest fluoranthene treatment group (17.3 µmol/mouse) was significantly different from the control group (0.6–0.7 vs. 0–0.05, respectively).

Nearly 400 chemicals have been tested for carcinogenic activity in the lung tumor assay (Stoner, 1991). Positive responses have been produced with compounds within the following chemical classes: PAHs, *N*-nitroso compounds, nitrogen mustards, carbamates, hydrazines, and chemotherapeutic agents (Stoner, 1991; Stoner and Shimkin, 1982, 1985). However, the assay was relatively insensitive to aromatic amines, metal salts, and organohalides. These results indicate that the assay is somewhat chemical-specific, which may decrease its usefulness as a screening test for carcinogens.

An advantage of this assay is that it can measure both the percentage of animals with neoplasms compared with controls and the multiplicity or yield of tumors, which indicates carcinogenic potency (Williams and Weisburger, 1991; Stoner, 1991). The potency, or *carcinogenic index* is the dose of the test chemical that is required to produce a minimum response of 0.8–1 tumor per mouse. This can be obtained by plotting the average number of lung tumors versus the log of the molar dose of the chemical (Stoner, 1991). The most potent carcinogen tested in strain A mice is DMBA. The dose required to produce one lung tumor was 0.6 µmol/kg (Stoner, 1991).

A limitation of the assay is the poor correlation of results from the strain A mouse assay with the long-term rodent bioassay. Maronpot and colleagues (Maronpot et al., 1986; Maronpot, 1991) compared the results of the lung tumor assay performed in two different laboratories, using 59 chemicals, with the results of 2-year carcinogenicity test previously performed by the National Cancer Institute for the same 59 chemicals. Laboratory A tested 53 of the 59 chemicals and laboratory B tested 30 of the 59 chemicals. Twenty-four of the 59 were tested in both laboratories. Among the 59 chemicals, 32 were aromatic amines, 5 were aromatic nitro-containing compounds, 4 were ureas, 5 were aliphatic halides, and 13 were classified into a miscellaneous category. Genotoxicity test data from GENETOX and CHEMTRACK databases were also compared with the results of the lung tumor assay.

Although most chemicals that tested positive in the lung tumor assay were carcinogenic in the long-term cancer bioassay, the converse was not true. For example, of the 16 chemicals that were positive in the lung tumor assay, 11 were positive in the 2-year bioassay (Maronpot, 1991). But, of the 40 chemicals that were positive in the 2-year bioassay, only 11 were positive in the lung tumor assay. There also was poor agreement of the gentoxicity tests with the strain A assay results (Maronpot et al., 1986). Of the 61 chemicals with genotoxicity data, 50 had positive results for genotoxicity in one or more tests. However, there were no clear differences in genotoxicity between the chemicals that were positive in the strain A assay and those that were negative. Therefore, the selection of carcinogens with a nongenotoxic or epigenetic mechanism of action for testing does not appear to be a plausible explanation for the lack of concordance between the lung tumor assay and the 2-year cancer bioassay. The investigators (Maronpot et al., 1986; Maronpot, 1991) suggested that differences in pharmacokinetics and metabolism, duration of treatment, total dose given, and target organ and species specificity might explain the discrepancies in results. In addition, the lung tumor assay is relatively insensitive to aromatic amines, and the majority of the chemicals used in this comparison were aromatic amines.

In summary, the strain A mouse lung tumor assay has limited applicability as a short-term screening tool for carcinogens, but it might be useful in a decision point approach to carcinogen testing (described in Sec. IV). Moreover, this assay would be useful in studies of mechanisms of pulmonary carcinogenesis (Maronpot, 1991).

### 5. Rat Mammary Gland Tumor Assay

During the 1940s, Bielschowsky and Shay independently studied the carcinogenic effects of subchronic or chronic exposures of 2-AAF and 3-MC on the rat mammary gland. Their work was extended by Huggins, who reported that single intragastric or IV doses of several PAHs could induce mammary cancer in rats (McCormick and Moon, 1985; Weisburger and Williams, 1984). The current rat mammary gland tumor assay is based on the work of Huggins (1959, 1961), and this single-dose model is described in the following.

Mammary tumors have been induced in many strains of rats, including Wistar, F-344, Long-Evans, and Lewis, but the Sprague-Dawley appears to be the most sensitive and, therefore, the animal of choice. Two limitations of using this strain, however, are (1) dose–response relationships may vary substantially among Sprague-Dawley rats obtained from different sources, and (2) the Sprague-Dawley rat develops a high incidence of age-related spontaneous mammary tumors, although they are primarily benign fibroadenomas (McCormick and Moon, 1985). These limitations should be taken into consideration when choosing a rat strain.

Sensitivity to tumor induction in the mammary gland peaks in 50- to 70-day-old rats. This appears to result from age-related changes in the mammary gland, including maximal cell division at 50 days of age, when female rats undergo puberty. Additionally, morphological changes occur in parenchymal tissue at this age. These changes include differentiation of tissues with a high level of cellular proliferation (terminal end buds) to those that have less proliferative capacity (acini and lobules) (McCormick and Moon, 1985). Therefore, animals used in the assay should be 50-day-old females. Additionally, virgin rats should be used, since they are significantly more sensitive to mammary tumor induction than are animals that have undergone one or more full-term pregnancies. That is, the nonpregnant animals have many more terminal end buds, which are sensitive to mammary carcinogenesis (McCormick and Moon, 1985). A minimum of 20 animals per dose group is used (Berger et al., 1983).

The test compound can be administered by several routes, including oral gavage, IV injection, subcutaneous injection, or direct application to the mammary fat pad (McCormick and Moon, 1985). With gavage, the test compound is dissolved in a vehicle carrier, such as corn oil, sesame oil, or trioctanoin, and 1.0 ml of the test compound is administered to animals that have been fasted overnight. With IV administration, the test compound is dissolved in sterile phosphate-buffered saline, or other suitable carrier, and the solution is injected at a volume of 0.4 ml/100 g body weight (McCormick and Moon, 1985). The IV route is used primarily with water-soluble compounds.

Animals are weighed and palpated weekly or semiweekly to monitor appearance of mammary tumors beginning 4–6 weeks after administration of the test compound (Berger et al., 1983; McCormick and Moon, 1985; Sobottka et al., 1993). Since most tumors develop in the cervical–thoracic chains of the mammary glands surrounding the forepaws, rather than in the abdominal–inguinal glands, the former should be examined more thoroughly (McCormick and Moon, 1985). Careful palpation can detect tumors at a diameter of 2 mm or smaller. The presence of any tumors or masses should be mapped for later confirmation with necropsy and histological findings, especially since some tumors may regress. These data are valuable for time-to-tumor appearance as well.

Depending on the carcinogenic potency of the test compound, tumors can become palpable as early as 4–6 weeks after administration of the test compound, as with DMBA, or as long as 9 months following exposure to B[*a*]P (McCormick and Moon, 1985). Thus, depending on the test compound, as well as the dose, the assay period may extend to 6–9 months. Beyond this time, however, spontaneous tumor induction increases, which may influence interpretation of the results. Nevertheless, this should have a minimal effect, since most spontaneous tumors are fibroadenomas or fibrosarcomas, rather than adenocarcinomas. Furthermore, histopathological diagnosis is essential to differentiate between these tumor types.

At the termination of the study, tissue samples are collected from all palpable and nonpalpable mammary tumors and stained with hematoxylin and eosin for histological examination and classification. A positive response is indicated by an increase in the incidence and multiplicity of mammary gland tumors. The preponderant tumor type is the adenocarcinoma, with or without papillary characteristics (McCormick and Moon, 1985). Mixed adenocarcinoma–fibroadenomas also may be found.

Various PAHs have been tested for carcinogenic activity in the rat mammary tumor assay: DMBA was the most potent; 3-MC and B[*a*]P were much less potent than DMBA; however, both benz[*a*]anthracene and phenanthrene were inactive in this system (McCormick and Moon, 1985). Other active chemicals include 2-AAF, arylamines, heterocyclic amines, nitrosoureas, especially *N*-methyl-*N*-nitrosourea (MNU), ethyl methanesulfonate, and 1,2-dichloroethane (Berger et al., 1983; McCormick and Moon, 1985; Williams and Weisburger, 1991). Single exposures to radiation (neutrons, x-rays, or gamma rays) also induce mammary tumors in Sprague-Dawley rats, although differences have been noted between tumor induction by radiation versus chemical agents in site of tumor formation, age-dependency, and reproductive status (McCormick and Moon, 1985).

The rat mammary gland tumor assay has many favorable characteristics for a short-term carcinogen screening test. As mentioned previously, data can be obtained on tumor incidence as well as multiplicity or yield, which is an indicator of carcinogenic potency. Strong carcinogens will produce positive responses in 9 months or less, and tumors can be detected in the animals by palpation over the course of the study without performing interim sacrifices. This provides data on tumor latency period and reduces the numbers of animals needed for significant results. More importantly, the mammary tumors produced in the rat model are similar to those produced in humans; that is, tissues are of epithelial origin and histologically similar.

Although the rat mammary tumor assay has many positive attributes as a screening test, it also has some disadvantages. As mentioned previously, spontaneous tumor production increases in older Sprague-Dawley strains. This problem can be circumvented by limiting the assay period to 9 months or less. Chemicals that induce rat mammary tumors may be inactive in other test systems, which is a general problem with many single-organ screening tests. Furthermore, little information was available on whether results from the mammary tumor assay correlated with results of long-term cancer studies. These disadvantages limit the applicability of the rat mammary gland tumor assay as a carcinogen-screening test. This bioassay has been used, however, in initiation–promotion systems to explore the relationship among dietary fat, hormones, and breast cancer incidence (Williams and Weisburger, 1991). Additionally, it has been used to study the effects of various anticancer treatments on MNU-induced mammary tumors in rats (Berger et al., 1983; Sobottka et al., 1993).

### 6. Multiple-Organ Carcinogenesis Model

Ito and colleagues (Ito et al., 1992; Hasegawa et al., 1993; Hirose et al., 1993a,b) developed a multiorgan carcinogenesis system in rats that utilizes treatment with multiple potent carcinogens and either concurrent or sequential administration of a test compound. It has a relatively short duration of 36 weeks or less. By using multiple carcinogens, neoplastic changes can be initiated in a wide variety of organs in each animal, which eliminates the need to perform several assays, each targeting a separate system. A protocol is described in the following.

Male Fischer 344 rats, 5–6 weeks old, are divided into at least three treatment groups, each containing 15–16 animals. Group 1 is treated with the "DMD" regimen (see later) and the test chemical; group 2 with the DMD regimen, but without the test chemical (control); and group 3 with the test chemical, but without the DMD regimen (vehicle only) (Ito et al., 1992; Hasegawa et al., 1993).

The DMD regimen is administered as follows: animals are injected IP at day 0 with a single dose of DEN at 100 mg/kg body weight; DEN is a potent hepatocarcinogen. A wide-spectrum carcinogen, MNU, is administered IP in four consecutive doses (20 mg/kg body weight) 3 days apart, beginning 2 days after DEN administration (i.e., days 2, 5, 8, and 11). On day 14, rats are given 2,2′-dihydroxy-di-*n*-propylnitrosamine (DHPN) in their drinking water at a dose level of 0.1% for 2 weeks; DHPN induces tumors in the kidney, lung, thyroid, and urinary bladder in rats. An alternative treatment regimen, which is designed to target the upper digestive tract, includes two or more additional carcinogens, such as dimethylhydrazine (Hirose et al., 1993a,b).

Test chemicals are administered either in the drinking water or the diet for 16–20 weeks (Ito et al., 1992; Hasegawa et al., 1993). Animals are then killed and organs removed. Livers and kidneys are weighed, and liver slices are fixed in ice-cold acetone and immunohistochemically stained for quantitative assessment GST-P-positive foci. Stomachs are inflated with sublimated formaldehyde, cut into strips, and immunohistochemically stained for quantitative assessment of pepsinogen-1-altered pyloric glands (PAPG). The GST-P-positive foci and PAPG are biomarkers for preneoplastic lesions in the liver and glandular stomach, respectively (Ito et al., 1992). The other main organs (i.e., thyroid, lung, forestomach, intestines, kidney, and urinary bladder) and the remainder of the liver are fixed in buffered formalin, stained with hematoxylin and eosin, imbedded in paraffin, and sections are made for histopathological examination. Statistical analyses are performed by comparing the results in group 1 (test group) with group 2 (control).

Ito et al. (1992) examined the ability of several carcinogens and noncarcinogens to enhance the neoplastic changes in various organs induced by the DEN–MNU–DHPN treatment. Phenobarbital, 2-AAF, DL-ethionine, and 3′-Me-DAB, which are liver carcinogens, caused a significant increase in the GST-P-positive area ($mm^2/cm^2$). Catechol targets the stomach, and it enhanced hyperplasia and papilloma of the forestomach and submucosal growth of the glandular stomach. Benzo[*a*]pyrene, a lung and skin carcinogen, was inactive in this system. In another study, five pesticides were examined for their carcinogenic potential (Hasegawa et al., 1993). Folpet, a B2 carcinogen based on duodenal cancer (IRIS, 1993), produced a significant increase in PAPG in the glandular stomach and hyperplasia of the forestomach. Similar effects were seen in captan-treated animals, but to a much greater extent. The carcinogenicity of captan is currently under review by the U. S. Environmental Protection Agency (USEPA) (IRIS, 1992). However, neoplasia has been reported in the duodenum and other regions of the digestive tract of mice after exposure to captan (Ito et al., 1992).

The multiple-organ assay shows promise for detecting the carcinogenic potential of some chemicals. Those that target the liver or the gastrointestinal tract appear to be the most sensitive in this assay, possibly because the biomarkers that are used in these organs are very sensitive toxicity endpoints. The development of more specific markers in other organs should enhance the usefulness of this model as a carcinogen-screening tool. This model is also quite useful in determining the chemopreventive and other modifying effects of chemicals on neoplastic lesions in different organs (Hirose et al., 1993a,b).

## B.  Long-Term Cancer Bioassay

Procedures for the lifetime cancer bioassay in animals were first standardized in the early 1960s by the USFDA, who were concerned with safety assessment of food- and drug-related chemicals and pesticides (Weisburger and Williams, 1984; Robens et al., 1989). The NCI published guidelines for their bioassay program in the mid 1970s (Sontag et al., 1976), and these were adopted and modified by the NTP after its establishment in 1978 (Moore et al., 1981; NTP, 1984). Other cancer-testing procedures have been published by the IARC (1980) and the USEPA (Jaeger, 1984).

The goals of the animal bioassay are (1) to determine if exposure to a test substance increases the incidence of tumor production over the background rate, and (2) to provide some information, such as time-to-tumor, dose–response, and mechanistic data, that can be used in human health risk assessment (NTP, 1984; Hamm, 1985). The cancer bioassay, as the final step in a decision point approach, also can be used to confirm questionable results from more limited testing, such as short-term mutagenicity assays, and the medium-term in vivo tests described earlier (Weisburger and Williams, 1984). The conventional protocol is presented in the following.

### 1.  Test Chemicals

*Test Chemical.*  Selecting a chemical to test is the first and certainly an important step in the carcinogen bioassay process. For chemical manufacturers or processors that are mandated under federal or state laws to provide carcinogenicity data, the selection of chemicals is clear-cut. For example, the Federal Insecticide, Fungicide, and Rodenticide Act (FIFRA; USEPA, 1991a) requires that oncogenicity tests be conducted to support the registration of each manufacturing-use product or end-use product that meets specific criteria (Jaeger, 1984). For other agencies or institutes performing studies, such as the NTP or the Chemical Industry Institute of Toxicology (CIIT), selection is based on the potential for human exposure, production levels, chemical structure, and available toxicological data (Hamm, 1985; NTP, 1984, 1989). Chemicals may be nominated by other agencies for testing by the NTP; for example, the USFDA nominated acetaminophen because of its increasing over-the-counter use and lack of information on the health risks associated with long-term exposure (NTP, 1993).

A thorough literature review is performed to obtain all information available on the chemical's toxicity and to determine if there are data gaps to be filled. Other relevant information includes chemical class, synonyms and trade names, structural and molecular formula and molecular weight, melting point, boiling point, solubility, stability and reactivity, and analytical methods for identifying and quantitating the test chemical, both in its pure form and in the vehicle used to administer it (Feron et al., 1980; NTP, 1984; Robens et al., 1989).

The test substance is a highly purified chemical, or an actual product, including the impurities, to which humans are exposed. The chemical typically is administered to animals in a vehicle, such as water, corn oil, or feed. It is critical that analytical methods are developed for the dosage formulation before testing to confirm the stability of the test compound and the presence of impurities over the duration of the study (Feron et al., 1980; Sontag et al., 1976).

Special handling should be given to chemicals that are hygroscopic, or are altered in the presence of water (Robens et al., 1989). Because impurities or contaminants may enhance or diminish the toxicity or carcinogenicity of a test chemical, identifying these compounds is crucial. Additionally, a misdosage because of inaccurate analysis or other errors could cause inadequate exposure to the test chemical, unexpected toxicity, or possibly animal death (Robens et al., 1989).

*Dosage.* At least two (Jaeger, 1984), but preferably three, dose levels (NTP, 1984) should be used, in addition to the control group. Although two doses may provide positive evidence for carcinogenicity, they may be inadequate for providing dose–response data or no-effect levels. The doses should be chosen so that there are no statistically significant differences in survivability among the test groups, except for a carcinogenic or tumorigenic response (Arnold, 1990a). The highest dose, the MTD, is that dose level sufficient to elicit signs of minimal toxicity without causing a significant decrease in survival (Feron et al., 1980; Hamm, 1985; Jaeger, 1984; Sontag et al., 1976). It is chosen based on acute, 14-day, 90-day, and metabolic studies performed in the same species, strain, and sex of animal, and using the same exposure route as for the chronic bioassay. A 10% decrease in body weight gain, in the absence of other signs of toxicity, usually defines the MTD (Weisburger and Williams, 1984). The lowest dose is near the threshold limit value, if one is available (Hamm, 1985). It should not be lower than 10% of the highest dose used. The intermediate dose is between the lowest dose and the MTD, on a log scale (Hamm, 1985).

For feeding studies, the highest dose should not exceed 5% of the diet, except for nutrients, to maintain the nutritional balance of the diet (Arnold, 1990a; Weisburger and Williams, 1984). For inhalation studies, the limiting factor for dosage is the available oxygen. This should not drop below 18% by volume under standard atmospheric pressure, or the test compound may cause asphyxiation (Hamm, 1985).

### 2. Animals and Their Environment

*Species and Strain.* Long-term carcinogenicity studies are performed in two mammalian species over the greater portion of the animals' lifetime (Sontag et al., 1976; Jaeger, 1984; NTP, 1984). Because many animals are required to detect a statistically significant increase in tumor incidence, the species used should be relatively inexpensive to maintain, yet have a relatively short life span. Rats and mice meet these criteria. They are well adapted to the laboratory environment and are used widely in pharmacological and toxicological studies. Other species, such as guinea pigs, dogs, or monkeys, may be considered if the bioavailability or the metabolism of the test chemical is similar to that in humans, and the added costs for these animals can be rationalized (Robens et al., 1989). The particular animal strain chosen should be susceptible, but not hypersensitive, to tumor induction by the chemical being tested (Robens et al., 1989). F-344 rats and B6C3F1 mice are the rodents used most commonly. Consequently, there is a considerable historical database for these strains.

*Age and Weight.* Rodents used in a long-term carcinogenicity study should be weaned and between 6 and 8 weeks old at the start of the study (Sontag et al., 1976; Jaeger, 1984; Weisburger and Williams, 1984). Animal weights should vary no more than ±20% of the mean weight of each sex at the beginning of the study. Studies using prenatal or neonatal animals may be recommended under special conditions, such as when the test agent is suspected of having reproductive or teratogenic activity (Jaeger, 1984; NTP, 1984).

*Sex.* Males and females are used at each dose level (Sontag et al., 1976; Feron et al., 1980; NTP, 1984; Jaeger, 1984). Females should be nulliparous and nonpregnant (Jaeger, 1984).

*Numbers.* For rodents, a minimum of 50 animals per sex is used at each dose level and concurrent control (Sontag et al., 1976; Feron et al., 1980; Jaeger, 1984; NTP, 1984). If interim sacrifices are planned midstudy, another 10 animals should be added per sex per dose group.

Additional animals may be used per dose group as disease sentinels. The CIIT uses 74 animals per sex per species per dose group to provide 10 animals for a 15-month necropsy, 4 sentinel animals for animal health studies throughout the bioassay, and 60 animals for a 24-month necropsy (Hamm, 1985).

A minimum number of animals in each group must survive to the end of the study to permit pathological and statistical evaluation. Survival rate at 15 months for mice and 18 months for rats should be at least 50%. At 18 months for mice and 24 months for rats, survival rate should be at least 25% in any group (Jaeger, 1984).

*Controls.* A concurrent control is required. This would include an untreated or sham-treated control or a vehicle control which is the same vehicle used in administering the test substance (Sontag et al., 1976; Feron et al., 1980; Jaeger, 1984). Both are recommended if the toxicity of the vehicle is unknown. Additionally, a concurrent negative control may be needed under certain conditions (e.g., inhalation studies using aerosols). This group is treated in the same manner as all other test animals, except that it is not exposed to the test substance or any vehicle.

*Animal Husbandry.* The major sources of information for animal husbandry requirements are the U.S. Department of Health, Education, and Welfare (USDHEW, 1978) and the Institute of Laboratory Animals Resources (ILAR, 1976, 1978). The important aspects for the animal bioassay are summarized.

Animals typically are purchased from commercial stocks. They should be of high quality, disease-free, genetically stable, and adequately identified as to colony source (Sontag et al., 1976). Animals must be housed in a sanitary environment; the facilities must be properly ventilated, and the air adequately filtered. A "clean–dirty" corridor flow will minimize the inadvertent transfer of contaminants between the animal rooms and the remaining facilities (Sontag, 1976). This not only protects the animals, but also protects laboratory personnel from exposure to hazardous materials. Also, a slightly positive air pressure in the animal room will minimize air contamination from the "dirty" corridor. There should be 10–15 fresh air exchanges per hour, and the temperature and relative humidity should be maintained within the ranges of $23.3° \pm 1.1°C$ and $40 \pm 5\%$, respectively (Sontag et al., 1976; Robens et al., 1989). The lighting mimics natural circadian rhythm and is placed on timers with a 12-hr light–dark cycle (Hamm, 1985; Weisburger and Williams, 1984). These environmental parameters are automatically controlled and recorded. An emergency power supply should be available, especially for the lighting and air-conditioning systems.

Animals are housed in plastic or stainless steel cages, with no more than five per cage. Each is given an identification number using standard methods, such as ear notching, toe clipping, or tagging (Sontag et al., 1976). The animals are randomly distributed to treatment and control groups before initiating the experiment. A typical randomization procedure stratifies the animals by initial body weight (Hamm, 1985; Robens et al., 1989). This is done after the animals have been allowed to acclimate to their environment for a couple of weeks, to avoid changes in body weight from stress (Hamm, 1985).

Fresh, suitably treated water and a standard, nutritionally balanced laboratory feed are provided ad libitum. (Sontag et al., 1976; Robens et al., 1989; Weisburger and Williams, 1984). The bedding material is either ground corncob or hardwood chips and is sterilized.

## 3. Exposure to Test Substance

*Route.* The route of administration of the test substance either should be the same as in humans, if a potential human hazard is being evaluated, or it should be one that provides for adequate absorption and distribution of the test chemical in the animal (Feron et al., 1980; Hamm, 1985; Jaeger, 1984; NTP, 1984; Sontag et al., 1976). The physical and chemical characteristics of the test substance must be considered, as well. The three main routes of administration are oral, dermal, and respiratory (inhalation), which are described in the following paragraphs. Intraperitoneal and subcutaneous injection are used also, but much less frequently.

The oral route is preferred over respiratory and dermal, providing that the test chemical is absorbed from the gastrointestinal tract. The test substance is either administered in the diet, dissolved in drinking water, or given by gavage or capsule (Feron et al., 1980; Jaeger, 1984; Weisburger and Williams, 1984).

With the dermal route, animals are administered the test chemical by topical application, ideally for at least 6 hr day (Jaeger, 1984). An area approximately 10% of the total body surface area is clipped or shaved, and the test substance is applied uniformly over the prepared surface. When highly toxic substances are applied, less surface area is covered, but with as thin and uniform a film as possible. The test substance may be held in place with a porous gauze dressing and nonirritating tape. The test site should be protected further with a suitable covering to ensure that the animals cannot ingest the test substance (Jaeger, 1984).

For respiratory exposure, animals are exposed to the test substance in a dynamic inhalation chamber with a suitable analytical system to control air concentrations (Jaeger, 1984). The airflow rate should be adjusted so that conditions are essentially the same throughout the exposure chamber. Maintenance of slight negative pressure inside the chamber will prevent leakage of the test substance into the surrounding area (Jaeger, 1984). Temperature should be maintained at $22° \pm 2°C$, and relative humidity should be maintained between 40 and 60%. Food and water are withheld during exposure. For details on inhalation exposure chambers and aerosol generation, see Snellings and Dodd (1990).

*Duration.*   The duration of exposure should comprise most of the life span of the test animals (NTP, 1984; Sontag et al., 1976; Weisburger and Williams, 1984). Treatment usually is started after weaning, although it may be started in the neonatal period or even during fetal development, since some organ systems may be more susceptible to certain carcinogens at this time. The exposure period is typically 24–30 months for rats and 18–24 months for mice. Ideally, animals are dosed with the test substance 7 days/week, but for practical reasons, dosing 5 days/week is acceptable (Jaeger, 1984). Exposure is continuous if the test chemical is administered in the drinking water or the diet. For inhalation studies, either intermittent (6 hr/day, 5 days/week) or continuous (22–24 hr/day, 7 days/week) exposures are used (Feron et al., 1980).

## 4.  *Observation of Animals*

Body weights and measurements of food and water consumption should be recorded for each animal once a week during the first 12–13 weeks of the test period and once a month thereafter (Feron et al., 1980; Hamm, 1985; Jaeger, 1984). A detailed clinical examination of each animal is made at least twice each week. In addition, animals are observed once or twice daily, and observations are recorded for changes in skin and fur; eyes and mucous membranes; respiratory, circulatory, autonomic and central nervous systems; somatomotor activity and behavior pattern; and for development of tissue masses (Feron et al., 1980; Hamm, 1985; Jaeger, 1984; Sontag et al., 1976). The following information should be recorded on each visible or palpable mass: time of onset, location, size, appearance, and progression (Jaeger, 1984). Weak or moribund animals should be removed to individual cages to avoid loss by cannibalism or tissue autolysis, or should be sacrificed to minimize suffering. Losses such as these can be prevented or minimized with good management practices, and should not exceed 10% of the animals in any test group (Arnold, 1990a).

## 5.  *Clinical Pathology*

A blood smear should be obtained from ten animals per sex per dosage group at 12 months, 18 months, and at sacrifice (Jaeger, 1984). Differential blood counts are performed on blood smears from the highest-dose group and the controls only, unless these data or data from the pathological examination show a major discrepancy between these two groups. Then blood counts should be done on the lower-dose group(s) at 12 and 18 months. In addition, a differential blood count should be performed on all animals in which health deteriorated during the study. Zawidzka (1990) provides a detailed discussion of the hematological evaluation performed as part of a toxicological study. Other clinical chemistry parameters are described by Basel et al. (1990).

## 6. Gross Necropsy

A complete postmortem examination is performed of all animals, including those that died during the experiment or were killed in moribund conditions (Jaeger, 1984; NTP, 1984). The liver, kidneys, brain, and testes (males) are weighed from at least ten rodents per sex per group, and the wet weights are recorded. Other organs are selected based on the expected effects of the test chemical. The information obtained from any clinical examinations should be available to the pathologist before microscopic examination, as the results may alert the pathologist to a significant effect.

## 7. Histopathology

The most important component of the histopathological examination is the proper collection and preservation of abnormal tissues during the postmortem examination. It is the responsibility of the pathologist to recognize any abnormalities immediately; if a tissue is not saved during the initial necropsy, it cannot be recovered at a later date. Table 2 lists the tissues that are collected and preserved in a suitable medium. Specific methods are described in Sontag et al. (1976). Rather than examine all tissues from all animals in the study, full histopathology is performed only on tissues from the following groups (NTP, 1984; Jaeger, 1984; Hamm, 1985):

1. All animals in which gross abnormalities were found
2. The high-dose and control animals that died or were killed before study termination
3. The lower-dose animals in which chemically related lesions (neoplastic or nonneoplastic) were identified in the high-dose group
4. The next highest dose (and the high dose) if survival in the high-dose group was reduced because of toxicity unrelated to neoplasia

An alternative approach proposed by NTP (1984) is to perform examination only on "core" tissues or organs (see Table 2) that have previously been associated with spontaneous neoplasms (> 1%) in control animals. Although this "selected inverse pyramid" approach would reduce the pathology workload, it would also diminish the database over time for noncore tissues. Opponents of this approach understandably are concerned that certain chemical-specific neoplasia, occurring at distinct tissue and organ sites, can be missed completely by examiners looking only for increased numbers of spontaneous tumors.

## 8. Data Acquisition and Management

Computers are used in toxicological studies for protocol design, data acquisition, data management, and data analysis. Where data once were transcribed manually from laboratory records and entered into the computer, today analytical results can be transferred directly to the computer from instruments, such as balances, clinical chemistry or hematology analyzers, and colony counters. Automated data collection systems record experimental data on an on-going basis, providing current information on dosing regimens, body weights, and clinical status of experimental subjects throughout the in-life phase of the study (Krewski et al., 1990). Bar codes may be used to identify each experimental animal and facilitate data collection. Use of codes to describe daily observations, clinical pathology, necropsy, histopathology, and other experimental

**Table 2** Tissues Collected for Possible Histopathological Examination[a]

|  | Tissue/Organ | |
| --- | --- | --- |
| Adrenals[b] | Large intestine | Skeletal muscle (thigh) |
| Aorta | Cecum | Skin |
| Bone | Colon | Small intestine |
|    Sternum and/or | Rectum |    Duodenum |
|      femur | Larynx[b] |    Jejunum |
| Bone marrow | Liver[b] |    Ileum |
|    Sternum and/or | Lungs[b] and bronchi | Spinal cord |
|      femur | Lymph node |    Cervical |
| Brain[b] |    Mandibular[b] |    Midthoracic |
|    Medulla/pons |    Mesenteric |    Lumbar |
|    Cerebellar cortex | Nasal passages[b] | Spleen[b] |
|    Cerebral cortex | Nerves | Stomach[b] |
| Cervix |    Peripheral | Testes/epididymis[b] |
| Costochondral junction, |    Sciatic | Thymus |
|    rib | Ovaries/uterus[b] | Thyroid/parathyroids[b] |
| Esophagus | Pancreas[b] | Trachea |
| Eyes and optic nerve | Pharynx | Urinary bladder[b] |
| Gallbladder (when | Pituitary[b] | Vagina |
|    present) | Prostate/seminal | |
| Harderian glands |    vesicles[b] | Gross lesions |
| Heart[b] | Salivary glands | Masses or suspect tumors |
| Kidneys[b] | |    and associated tissues |

[a]Tissues that are collected and preserved during necropsy for possible future histopathological examination.
[b]Core tissues proposed by the National Toxicology Program (1984) for the selected inverse pyramid approach to histopathological examination.
*Source:* NTP (1984); Hamm (1985); Jaeger (1984); Robins et al. (1989).

results allows standardized terminology for identifying toxicological effects and helps to assure collection of consistent and error-free results by study personnel. Some data collection and management systems are able to examine data entries and detect obvious discrepancies in results before they are stored. Examples of commercial toxicology data management systems include Toxicology Data Management Systems (TDMS), developed by the National Center for Toxicological Research, LABCAT, XYBION Path/Tox System, and ARTEMIS Toxicology Data System (Krewski et al., 1990; Updike, K. A., personal communication).

## 9. Data Evaluation and Reporting

All observed results should be evaluated by an appropriate statistical method, which should be selected during the design of the study. I refer readers to Goddard et al. (1990), NTP (1984), Park and Kociba (1985), and Peto et al. (1980), for guidance on choosing significance tests appropriate for the long-term cancer bioassay. Many of the commercially available computer data management systems listed in the previous paragraph include statistical functions that perform data analyses and automatically generate reports.

The results of the study should first be evaluated for their scientific adequacy (Feron et al., 1980). For example, if the animal survival rate was low, because the highest dose was too toxic or an outbreak of an infectious disease occurred, then there may be insufficient numbers of live animals remaining to perform meaningful statistical evaluations. Next, the results are evaluated in terms of the relationship between the dose of the test chemical and the response, such as the presence or absence, the incidence, and the severity of abnormalities, including effects on survival rate, body weight changes, behavioral and clinical abnormalities, gross lesions, identified target organs, and any other general or specific toxic effects (Jaeger, 1984). Additionally, historical control data may be used to assess the significance of rare tumors or marginal increases of tumor incidence in treated animals compared with concurrent controls. However, these data should be carefully scrutinized, because there are many sources of variability in the database, such as laboratory differences, species or strain differences in tumor susceptibility over time, and differences in pathological techniques and diagnoses (NTP, 1984; Robens et al., 1990).

In animal bioassays, a chemical is considered to have a positive carcinogenic effect if (1) it produces types of neoplasms not seen in control animals, (2) it increases the incidence of tumors compared with controls, (3) it decreases the time to development of malignant tumors compared with controls, or (4) it increases the number of tumors per individual animal compared with controls (Weisburger and Williams, 1984).

Carcinogenicity studies performed under the NTP are classified according to their strength of experimental evidence using the following guidelines (NTP, 1994):

1. *Clear evidence of carcinogenic activity* is demonstrated by studies that are interpreted as showing a dose-related (1) increase of malignant neoplasms; (2) increase of a combination of malignant and benign neoplasms; or (3) marked increase of benign neoplasms if there is an indication from this or other studies of the ability of such tumors to progress to malignancy.

2. *Some evidence of carcinogenic activity* is demonstrated by studies that are interpreted as showing a chemically related increased incidence of neoplasms (malignant, benign, or combined) in which the strength of the response is less than that required for clear evidence.

3. *Equivocal evidence of carcinogenic activity* is demonstrated by studies that are interpreted as showing a marginal increase of neoplasms that may be chemically related.

4. *No evidence of carcinogenic activity* is demonstrated by studies that are interpreted as showing no chemically related increases in malignant or benign neoplasms.

5. *Inadequate study of carcinogenic activity* is demonstrated by studies that because of major qualitative or quantitative limitations cannot be interpreted as valid for showing either the presence or absence of a carcinogenic effect.

Each individual study or experiment—that is, male rats, female rats, male mice, female mice—is given a strength of evidence classification. The NTP levels of evidence refer only to the individual study, and not to the overall weight-of-evidence classification of the chemical as a human carcinogen. Other organizations, such as the IARC or the USEPA, use the strength of evidence ranking, along with other available data, such as structure–activity relationships, pharmacokinetic data, and results of genotoxicity and other toxicity studies, to classify carcinogens according to a weight-of-evidence scheme, such as USEPA classification A, B1, B2, C, D, or E; or IARC group 1, 2A, 2B, or 3. For more information on the weight-of-evidence classification, I refer readers to IARC (1982) and USEPA (1989).

*Study Report.*    The technical report is composed of the study protocol (see Arnold et al., 1990b for a list of information included in the protocol), conduct of the study, individual animal data and data summary tables, pathology results, statistical analyses, standard operating procedures and other quality control information, results of any quality assurance inspections or audits, discussion, and conclusions (Sontag et al., 1976). The raw data and corresponding summary tables should include toxic response and other effects data by dose and sex, and individual animal data for (1) time of death during the study or whether animals survived to termination; (2) time of observation of each mass and subsequent course; (3) food or water consumption, if appropriate; (4) body weight; (5) hematological tests and results; (6) necropsy findings; and (7) detailed description of all histopathological findings (Jaeger, 1984). The discussion should include limitations or inadequacies in the study design and conduct of the experiment (Feron et al., 1980).

*10. Quality Assurance and Control*

Quality assurance and control must be applied through each stage of the toxicological study, including experimental design, choice and care of animals to be used, procurement and use of the test agent, animal observations, necropsy and histopathological examinations, data collection, management, analyses, and preparation of the final report.

Toxicological studies submitted to regulatory agencies, such as the USFDA or USEPA, must comply with Good Laboratory Practices (GLPs). These were first introduced by the USFDA in 1976, and subsequently were developed by the European Chemical Industry Ecology and Toxicology Center, the Organization for Economic Cooperation and Development, and the USEPA (Arnold, 1990b). These regulations arose as a result of inspections conducted in the toxicological testing facilities of pharmaceutical companies and contract laboratories, and internal review of USFDA's own laboratories. Problems encountered during these inspections raised serious concerns about the integrity and validity of data collected for human health safety assessment (Arnold, 1990b). The GLPs were designed to minimize the opportunity for significant error in toxicity testing. They cover personnel, including responsibilities of the study director; testing facilities; equipment; test, control and reference substances; protocols and study conduct; animal care and handling; control animals; analytical methods; and records and reports, including data collection and management (Arnold, 1990b; Boorman et al., 1985; Robens et al., 1989; USEPA, 1991b). The GLPs developed by the USFDA include a component for use of computer technology in nonclinical laboratory studies. Standard operating procedures (SOPs) are required in written form under GLPs for all laboratory practices and should be available to the laboratory technicians and other personnel. The SOPs are a stepwise listing of how each routine or repetitive procedure is to be performed. Any changes in these procedures are made only with written authorization by the study director. A quality assurance unit (QAU) is responsible for monitoring each study to ensure compliance with GLPs (Arnold, 1990b; Arnold et al., 1990b). The QAU personnel are not associated with planning or conduct of the study to maintain objectivity. Compliance with GLPs will facilitate the complete reconstruction of a study in the absence of all principal study personnel for the purpose of a study audit or a reevaluation of results in light of future findings (Arnold 1990b). There are two types of inspections that can be performed under GLPs. The first is a routine surveillance inspection to determine compliance with GLPs. The second is a study audit, which is performed if the regulatory agency has some concerns about the quality of data submitted. In this instance, a detailed investigation is conducted of the study, from the time of conception through the completed report. Depending on the type of problem revealed, GLPs allow for legal action to be taken against the study director or other testing facility personnel. The regulatory agency subsequently may refuse to accept any data from the study director or testing facility (Arnold, 1990b).

## IV. DECISION POINT APPROACH TO EVALUATE CARCINOGENICITY

The public demands that chemicals to which they are exposed are proved "safe." These chemicals are found in food, drugs, consumer products, pesticides, the workplace, and elsewhere. Toxicity testing requirements have increased over the years, in part because the public has demanded it, but also because our knowledge of mechanisms of toxic action has expanded. This knowledge has lead to the development of numerous in vitro and in vivo bioassays to study the effects of chemicals. Many of these tests have been designed to detect or evaluate the potential carcinogenicity of chemicals.

As mentioned previously, most evidence for chemical carcinogenicity in humans comes from animal studies, in particular, the conventional long-term cancer bioassay. However, these tests require a considerable investment of time and funding, as well as animals. Unnecessary testing could be reduced by using a systematic approach–progressively rigorous tests are carried out in stages that allow evaluation of the results before proceeding to the next level. Chemicals that test positive early in the testing scheme can be eliminated from further testing, whereas those that test negative advance to the next stage. This "decision point approach" (Table 3) has been suggested by Weisburger and Williams as a guide for the elimination of unnecessary procedures, and provides a logical step approach in performing testing for potentially carcinogenic chemicals. Similar decision processes for evaluating carcinogens have been proposed by Bull and Pereira (1982) and Ito et al. (1992). A description of the decision process can be found in Williams and Weisburger (1991) and Weisburger and Williams (1981, 1984).

Briefly, the decision point approach consists of a series of sequential steps, beginning with an evaluation of structure–activity relationships of the test chemical. Then, a variety of tests, designed to identify genotoxic or epigenetic agents, are conducted in stages, and the data obtained at each stage are evaluated. Both qualitative (yes or no) and quantitative (low, medium, high) effects are considered. A decision is made at each point indicated (see Table 3) on whether the data are sufficient to reach a definitive conclusion about the genotoxicity or potential carcinogenicity, or whether further, more-advanced testing is required (Weisburger and Williams,

**Table 3**   Decision Point Approach to Carcinogen Testing

| | |
|---|---|
| Stage A: | Structure of chemical |
| Stage B: | Short-term in vitro tests |
| |     Mammalian cell DNA repair |
| |     Bacterial mutagenesis |
| |     Mammalian mutagenesis |
| |     Chromosome integrity |
| |     Cell transformation |
| *Decision Point 1:* | *Evaluation of all tests conducted in stages A and B* |
| Stage C: | Tests for promoters |
| |     In vitro |
| |     In vivo |
| *Decision Point 2:* | *Evaluation of results from stages A through C* |
| Stage D: | Limited in vivo bioassays |
| |     Altered foci induction in rodent liver |
| |     Skin neoplasm induction in mice |
| |     Pulmonary neoplasm induction in mice |
| |     Breast cancer induction in female Sprague-Dawley rats |
| *Decision Point 3:* | *Evaluation of results from stages A through C, and the appropriate tests in stage D* |
| Stage E: | Long-term bioassay |
| *Decision Point 4:* | *Final evaluation of all the results and application to health risk analysis. This evaluation must include data from stages A through C to provide a basis for mechanistic considerations* |

*Source:* Weisburger and Williams (1984); Williams and Weisburger (1991).

1981, 1984; Williams and Weisburger, 1991). The final decision on carcinogenic potential and classification, such as DNA-reactive or epigenetic mechanism, of the test chemical is based on all of the preceding evaluations. The information then is applied to human health risk assessment.

This approach is particularly beneficial to pharmaceutical, industrial, agricultural, or other production-type companies that develop new products for consumer use. By detecting potential carcinogens early in the developmental process, the companies can halt or suspend further development of that chemical and invest in another potentially safer product.

## V. NATIONAL TOXICOLOGY PROGRAM

## A. The Program

The National Toxicology Program (NTP) was established in 1978 as a cooperative effort with the U. S. Department of Health and Human Services (USDHHS) to coordinate toxicology research and testing activities within the department, including methods development and validation; to provide information about potentially toxic chemicals to research and regulatory agencies, and the public; and to strengthen the science base in toxicology (Moore et al., 1981; NTP, 1994). Since its inception, the NTP has been a leader in designing, conducting, and interpreting animals assays for toxicity (NTP, 1994).

The participating agencies within the USDHHS are (1) the National Institute of Environmental Health Sciences (NIEHS), National Institutes of Health (NIH); (2) the National Center for Toxicological Research (NCTR), Food and Drug Administration (USFDA); and (3) the National Institute for Occupational Safety and Health (NIOSH), Centers for Disease Control and Prevention (CDC) (NTP, 1994; Moore et al., 1981). The NIH's National Cancer Institute (NCI) was a charter member of the NTP, but its carcinogenesis bioassay program was transferred to the NIEHS in July 1981. Still, the NCI remains active in the NTP through membership on the executive committee, which provides oversight of the program. Other members of the NTP Executive Committee include the lead persons of the NIEHS, NIH, NIOSH, FDA, EPA, Consumer Product Safety Commission (CPSC), Occupational Safety and Health Administration (OSHA), and the Agency for Toxic Substances and Disease Registry (ATSDR) (NTP, 1994).

The programs within the NTP are grouped into two broad categories: toxicological research and testing, and coordinative management activities (Moore et al., 1981; NTP, 1994). The former includes carcinogenesis (short-term test development and tumor pathology), chemical disposition, general toxicology (toxicopathology), genetic toxicology, immunotoxicology, neurotoxicology, respiratory toxicology, and reproductive and developmental toxicology (Moore et al., 1981). The NTP also is seeking alternative methods to replace, reduce, and refine the use of animals in its testing programs. Coordinate management activities include bioassay coordination, chemical nomination, chemical repository, data management and analysis (carcinogenesis, mutagenesis, toxicology, and Toxicology Data Management System (TDMS) development), information dissemination, laboratory animal quality control, and laboratory health and safety technical information (Moore et al., 1981).

Chemicals selected for study by the NTP are nominated by various groups, such as academia, industry, labor, public, NTP research and regulatory agencies, for example, USFDA and NIOSH, and other federal agencies, such as CPSC. Many more chemicals are nominated than can be tested, so the NTP developed eight criteria for selecting chemicals for study. Operating under the principle that "industry will test chemicals for health and environmental effects as intended and mandated by Congress under legislative authorities," NTP will nominate chemicals from the following categories (Moore et al., 1981; NTP, 1994):

1. Environmental chemicals that are not closely associated with commercial activities
2. Potential substitutes for existing chemicals, particularly therapeutic agents, that might not be developed or tested without federal involvement
3. Chemicals that should be tested to improve scientific understanding of structure–activity relationships and, thereby, limit the numbers of chemicals requiring extensive evaluations
4. Biological or physical agents that may not be adequately evaluated without federal involvement
5. Chemicals or agents that will aid our understanding of chemical toxicities, or our understanding of the use of test systems to evaluate potential toxicities
6. Substances that occur as mixtures for which evaluation cannot be required of industry
7. Chemicals that have the potential for large-scale or intense human exposure, which were marketed before current testing requirements, or those that generate too little revenue to support further evaluations by industry
8. Emergencies or other events that warrant immediate government evaluation of a chemical or agent

Most chemicals are selected on the basis of human exposure, production levels, chemical structure, availability or lack of toxicological data, potential biological activity, and metabolic pathways (NTP, 1989; 1994). The majority of the NTP carcinogenesis studies are managed by the NIEHS component. The NCTR studies usually involve chemicals relevant to the USFDA, whereas NIOSH studies are frequently performed on substances and route of administration associated with occupational exposures (NTP, 1994).

## B. Interaction with Federal Agencies

Over 600,000 chemicals are used commercially in America (NTP, 1994). The public is exposed to these chemicals in the workplace, in their residences, or in the environment. The responsibility for demonstrating whether a chemical is safe or hazardous, that is, the "burden of proof," may fall on the producer or user of the chemical, or may lie with the appropriate regulatory agency. This all depends on how the law governing the regulatory agencies was written. For example, the USFDA has the authority under the 1958 Amendment to the Food, Drug, and Cosmetics Act to require that safety of food additives be demonstrated before marketing (Merrill, 1991). This places the burden for testing food additives on industry. Likewise, the USEPA has the authority under FIFRA to require toxicological studies, including long-term cancer bioassays, for the registration of new pesticides and for those undergoing reevaluation (Merrill, 1991; USEPA, 1991a). A similar authority is provided under the Toxic Substances Control Act (TSCA). This act covers all chemicals manufactured or processed in or imported into the United States, except for those already regulated under other laws. It allows the USEPA to collect scientific data or to require testing to develop the necessary data on chemicals suspected of posing an unreasonable health risk to the public or environment (Merrill, 1991). It also requires manufacturers to inform USEPA if adverse health or environmental effects are indicated in animal or human studies.

Some agencies, however, do not have the authority to require toxicity testing, and must rely on other sources for data. The NTP is a primary source of toxicology data, particularly on carcinogens. For example, OSHA, under the Occupational Safety and Health Act of 1970, was not empowered with the authority to mandate employer testing of suspected occupational hazards, or to do its own research (Beliles, 1985). OSHA relies on NIOSH, also established under the OSH Act, for research support in setting workplace standards. Additionally, it may nominate chemicals for testing by the NTP that are found in the workplace and appear to be carcinogens or other health hazards.

The Consumer Products Safety Commission (CPSC) regulates an assortment of chemical-containing products, such as paints, aerosol products, cleaners, dyes, textile products, pressed wood products, and plastics (Ulsamer et al., 1985). Its jurisdiction excludes foods, drugs, cosmetics, pesticides, fungicides, and rodenticides. Under the Consumer Products Safety Act (CPSA), the CPSC can require manufacturers to provide technical and performance data about products (Ulsamer et al., 1985). Under the Federal Hazardous Substances Act (FHSA), the CPSC also has jurisdiction over products that are toxic, corrosive, combustible, radioactive, or that generate pressure (Merrill, 1991). However, neither the CPSA nor the FHSA requires manufacturers to notify the CPSC of plans to market a new product or to obtain approval for any design or material (Merrill, 1991). Sources of information on chemical hazards are obtained mostly from other programs, such as the NTP and the IARC monographs. For data on carcinogens, the CPSC relies on bioassays performed by the NTP.

## VI.  CONCLUDING REMARKS

Cancer is one of the leading causes of death in the United States. It is not surprising that the public is concerned about this disease and how to prevent it or reduce its incidence. Scientists estimate that 30–60% of cancers are caused by environmental chemicals, such as air, soil, and water contaminants; naturally occurring substances, such as aflatoxin and radiation; drugs; and lifestyle factors, such as diet, smoking, and alcohol consumption. In response to the public's concern over environmental chemicals, regulatory agencies, private industries, and other research groups have increased carcinogenicity testing of chemicals to which the public is exposed.

Since most suggestive evidence for human carcinogenicity comes from experimental studies performed in animals, the conventional 2-year cancer bioassay remains the accepted method for testing the carcinogenic potential of chemicals. Nevertheless, in vivo and in vitro carcinogen testing methods continue to be developed and refined as the need for more rapid and economical methods increases and our knowledge of carcinogenic mechanisms expands. We expect as this important research area continues to progress that the capacity for rapid selective screening of potentially carcinogenic chemicals will grow, as will the confidence of the scientific community and the general public in these methods.

## REFERENCES

Arnold, D. L. (1990a). Oral ingestion studies. In *Handbook of In Vivo Toxicity Testing* (D. L. Arnold, H. C. Grice, and D. R. Krewski, eds.) Academic Press, San Diego, CA, pp. 167–188.

Arnold, D. L. (1990b). Compliance with good laboratory practice. In *Handbook of In Vivo Toxicity Testing* (D. L. Arnold, H. C. Grice, and D. R. Krewski, eds.), Academic Press, San Diego, CA, pp. 581–587.

Arnold, D. L., Grice, H. C., and Krewski, D. R. (1990a). *Handbook of In Vivo Toxicity Testing.* Academic Press, San Diego, CA, 678 pp.

Arnold, D. L., McGuire, P. F., and Nera, E. A. (1990b). The conduct of a chronic bioassay and the use of an interactive-integrated toxicology data system. In *Handbook of In Vivo Toxicity Testing* (D. L. Arnold, H. C. Grice, and D. R. Krewski, eds.), Academic Press, San Diego, CA, pp. 589–607.

Bannasch, P. and Zerban, H. (1992). Predictive value of hepatic preneoplastic lesions as indicators of carcinogenic response. In *Mechanisms of Carcinogenesis in Risk Identification* (H. Vainio, P. N. Magee, D. B. McGregor, and A. J. McMichael, eds.), International Agency for Research on Cancer, Lyon, France, pp. 389–427.

Barrett, J. C. (1993). Mechanisms of multistep carcinogenesis and carcinogen risk assessment, *Environ. Health Perspect.,* 100, 9–20.

Basel, D. L., Villeneuve, D. C. and Yagminas, A. P. (1990). Clinical chemistry. In *Handbook of In Vivo Toxicity Testing* (D. L. Arnold, H. C. Grice, and D. R. Krewski, eds.), Academic Press, San Diego, CA, pp. 509–534.

Beliles, R. P. (1985). Workplace carcinogens: Regulatory implications of investigations. In *Handbook of*

*Carcinogen Testing* (H. A. Milman and E. K. Weisburger, eds.), Noyes Publications, Park Ridge, NJ, pp. 345–357.

Berenblum, I., Haran-Ghera, N., and Trainin, N. (1958). An experimental analysis of the "hair cycle effect" in mouse skin carcinogenesis, *Br. J. Cancer,* 12, 402–413.

Berger, M., Habs, M., and Schmähl, D. (1983). Noncarcinogenic chemotherapy with a combination of vincristine, methotrexate and 5-fluorouracil (VMF) in rats, *Int. J. Cancer,* 32, 231–236.

Bishop, J. M. (1991). Molecular themes in oncogenesis, *Cell,* 64, 235–248.

Boorman, G. A., Montgomery, C. A. Jr., Eustis, S. L., Wolfe, M. J., McConnell, E. E., and Hardisty, J. F. (1985). Quality assurance in pathology for rodent carcinogenicity studies. In *Handbook of Carcinogen Testing* (H. A. Milman and E. K. Weisburger, eds.), Noyes Publications, Park Ridge, NJ, pp. 345–357.

Borum, K. (1954). The role of the mouse hair cycle in epidermal carcinogenesis, *Acta Pathol. Microbiol. Scand.,* 34, 542–553.

Bull, R. J. and Pereira, M. A. (1982). Development of short-term testing matrix for estimating relative carcinogenic risk, *J. Am. Coll. Toxicol.,* 1, 1–15.

Cabral, R., Hoshiya, T., Hakoi, K., Hasegawa, R., Fukushima, S., and Ito, N. (1991). A rapid in vivo bioassay for the carcinogenicity of pesticides, *Tumori,* 77, 184–188.

Chen, L.-C., Kirchhoff, S., and De Luca, L. M. (1994). Effect of excess dietary retinoic acid on skin papilloma and carcinoma formation induced by a complete carcinogenesis protocol in female Sencar mice, *Cancer Lett.,* 78, 63–67.

Deml, E., Oesterle, D., Wolff, T., and Greim, H. (1981). Age-, sex-, and strain-dependent differences in the induction of enzyme-altered island in rat liver by diethylnitrosamine, *J. Cancer Res. Clin. Oncol.,* 100, 125–134.

DiGiovanni, J., Walker, S. E., Aldaz, C. M., Slaga, T. J., and Conti, C. J. (1993). Further studies on the influence of initiation dose on papilloma growth and progression during two-stage carcinogenesis in SENCAR mice, *Carcinogenesis,* 14, 1831–1836.

Dixon, D., Horton, J., Haseman, J. K., Talley, F., Greenwell, A., Nettesheim, P., Hook, G. E., and Maronpot, R.R. (1991). Histomorphology and ultrastructure of spontaneous pulmonary neoplasms in strain A mice, *Exp. Lung Res.,* 17, 131–155.

Dragan, Y. P., Rizvi, T., Xu, Y.-H., Hully, J. R., Bawa, N., Campbell, H. A., Maronpot, R. R., and Pitot, H. C. (1991). An initiation–promotion assay in rat liver as a potential complement to the 2-year carcinogenesis bioassay, *Fundam. Appl. Toxicol.,* 16, 525–547.

Dragan, Y. P., Sargent, L., Xu, Y.-D., Xu, Y.-H., and Pitot, H. C. (1993). The initiation–promotion–progression model of rat hepatocarcinogenesis, *Proc. Soc. Exp. Biol. Med.,* 202, 16–24.

Edler, L., Schmidt, R., Weber, E., Rippman, F., and Hecker, E. (1991). Biological assays for irritant, tumor-initiating and -promoting activities. III. Computer-assisted management and validation of biodata generated by standardized initiation/promotion protocols in skin of mice, *J. Cancer Res. Clin. Oncol.,* 117, 205–216.

Feron, V. J., Grice, H. C., Griesemer, R., et al. (1980). Report 1. Basic requirements for long-term assays for carcinogenicity. *IARC Monogr.,* Suppl. 2, 21–83.

Goddard, M. J., Burnett, R. T., Collins, B. T., and Murdoch, D. J. (1990). Statistical analysis. In *Handbook of In Vivo Toxicity Testing* (D. L. Arnold, H. C. Grice, and D. R. Krewski, eds.), Academic Press, San Diego, CA, pp. 611–642.

Goldberg, D. M. and Diamandis, E. P. (1993). Models of neoplasia and their diagnostic implications: A historical perspective, *Clin. Chem.,* 39, 2360–2374.

Goldfarb, S. and Pugh, T. D. (1982). The origin and significance of hyperplastic hepatocellular islands and nodules in hepatic carcinogenesis, *J. Am. Coll. Toxicol.,* 1, 119–144.

Goldsworthy, H. P., Hanigan, H. M., and Pitot, H. C. (1986). Models of hepatocarcinogenesis in the rat–contrasts and comparisons, *CRC Crit. Rev. Toxicol.,* 17, 61–89.

Gulbis, B. and Galand, P. (1993). Immunodetection of the p21-*ras* products in human normal and preneoplastic tissues and solid tumors: A review, *Hum. Pathol.,* 24, 1271–1285.

Hakoi, K., Cabral, R., Hoshiya, T., Hasegawa, R., Shirai, T., and Ito, N. (1992). Analysis of carcinogenic activity of some pesticides in a medium-term liver bioassay in the rat, *Teratogenesis Carcinogen. Mutagen.,*12, 269–276.

Hamm, T. E. Jr. (1985). Design of a long-term animal bioassay for carcinogenicity. In *Handbook of Carcinogen Testing* (H. A. Milman and E. K. Weisburger, eds.), Noyes Publications, Park Ridge, NJ, pp. 252–267.

Harris, C. C. (1992). Tumor suppressor genes, multistage carcinogenesis and molecular epidemiology. In *Mechanisms of Carcinogenesis in Risk Identification* (H. Vainio, P. N. Magee, D. B. McGregor, and A. J. McMichael, eds.), International Agency for Research on Cancer, Lyon, France, pp. 67–85.

Harris, C. C. (1993). p53: At the crossroads of molecular carcinogenesis and risk assessment, *Science,* 262, 1980–1981.

Hasegawa, R., Cabral, R., Hoshiya, T., Hakoi, K., Ogiso, T., Boonyaphiphat, P., Shirai, T., and Ito, N. (1993). Carcinogenic potential of some pesticides in a medium-term multi-organ bioassay in rats, *Int. J. Cancer,* 54, 489–493.

Hennings, H., Glick, A. B., Greenhalgh, D. A., Morgan, D. L., Strickland, J. E., Tennenbaum, T., and Yuspa, S. H. (1993a). Critical aspects of initiation, promotion, and progression in multistage epidermal carcinogenesis, *Proc. Soc. Exp. Biol. Med.,* 202, 1–18.

Hennings, H., Glick, A. B., Lowry, D. T., Krsmanovic, L. S., Sly, L. M., and Yuspa, S. H. (1993b). FVB/N mice: An inbred strain sensitive to the chemical induction of squamous cell carcinoma in the skin, *Carcinogenesis,* 14, 2353–2358.

Hill, R. N. (1985). Regulatory implications: Perspective of the U. S. Environmental Protection Agency. In *Handbook of Carcinogen Testing* (H. A. Milman and E. K. Weisburger, eds.), Noyes Publications, Park Ridge, NJ, pp. 548–555.

Hinton, D. E., Couch, J. A., Teh, S. J., and Courtney, L. A. (1988). Cytological changes during progression of neoplasia in selected fish species, *Aquat. Toxicol.,* 11, 77–112.

Hirose, M., Hoshiya, T., Akagi, K., Takahashi, S., Hara, Y., and Ito, N. (1993a). Effects of green tea catechins in a rat multi-organ carcinogenesis model, *Carcinogenesis,* 14, 1549–1553.

Hirose, M., Yada, H., Hakoi, K., Takahashi, S., and Ito, N. (1993b). Modification of carcinogenesis by α-tocopheral, *t*-butylhydroquinone, propyl gallate and butylated hydroxytoluene in a rat multi-organ carcinogenesis model, *Carcinogenesis,* 14, 2359–2364.

Huggins, C., Briziarelli, G., and Sutton, H., Jr. (1959). Rapid induction of mammary carcinoma in the rat and the influence of hormones on the tumors, *J. Exp. Med.,* 109, 25–41.

Huggins, C., Grand, L. C., and Brillantes, F. P. (1961). Mammary cancer induced by a single feeding of polynuclear hydrocarbons, and its suppression, *Nature,* 189, 204–207.

Hunter, T. (1991). Cooperation between oncogenes, *Cell,* 64, 249–270.

[IARC] International Agency for Research on Cancer (1980). *IARC Monographs on the Evaluation of the Carcinogenic Risk of Chemicals to Humans. Long-term and Short-term Screening Assays for Carcinogens: A Critical Appraisal,* Supplement 2, IARC, Lyon, France.

[IARC] International Agency for Research on Cancer (1982). *IARC Monographs on the Evaluation of the Carcinogenic Risk of Chemicals to Humans. Chemicals, Industrial Processes and Industries Associated with Cancer in Humans,* Supplement 4, IARC, Lyon, France.

[ILAR] Institute of Laboratory Animal Resources (1976). *Long-Term Holding of Laboratory Rodents,* National Research Council, Washington, DC.

[ILAR] Institute of Laboratory Animal Resources (1978). *Laboratory Animal Housing,* National Research Council, Washington, DC.

[IRIS] Integrated Risk Information System (1992). *Captan,* CASRN 133-06-2. Last revised on July 1, 1992.

[IRIS] Integrated Risk Information System (1993). *Folpet,* CASRN 133-07-3. Last revised on October 1, 1993.

Ito, N., Shirai, T., and Hasegawa, R. (1992). Medium-term bioassays for carcinogens. In *Mechanisms of Carcinogenesis in Risk Identification* (H. Vainio, P. N. Magee, D. B. McGregor, and A. J. McMichael, eds.), International Agency for Research on Cancer, Lyon, France, pp. 353–388.

Jaeger, B. (1984). Chronic and long-term studies. Series 83. In *Pesticide Assessment Guidelines, Subdivision F. Hazard Evaluation: Human and Domestic Animals,* rev. ed., Health Effects Division, Office of Pesticide Programs, U.S. Environmental Protection Agency, Washington, DC.

Jones, P. A., Buckley, J. D., Henderson, B. E., Ross, R. K., and Pike, M. C. (1991). From gene to carcinogen: A rapidly evolving field in molecular epidemiology, *Cancer Res.,* 51, 3617–3620.

Krewski, D. R., Carr, P. L., Anderson, R., and Gilbert, S. G. (1990). Computer applications in toxicological research. In *Handbook of In Vivo Toxicity Testing* (D. L. Arnold, H. C. Grice, and D. R. Krewski, eds.), Academic Press, San Diego, CA, pp. 555–579.

Levine, A. J., Momand, J., and Finlay, C. A. (1991). The p53 tumour suppressor gene, *Nature,* 351, 453–456.

Maronpot, R. R. (1991). Correlation of data from the strain A mouse bioassay with long-term bioassays, *Exp. Lung Res.,* 17, 425–431.

Maronpot, R. R., Shimkin, M. B., Witschi, H. P., Smith, L. H., and Cline, J. M. (1986). Strain A mouse pulmonary tumor test results for chemicals previously tested in the National Cancer Institute carcinogenicity tests, *JNCI,* 76, 1101–1112.

Marshall, C. J. (1991). Tumor suppressor genes, *Cell,* 64, 313–326.

McCormick, D. L. and Moon, R. C. (1985). Tumorigenesis of the rat mammary gland. In *Handbook of Carcinogen Testing* (H. A. Milman and E. K. Weisburger, eds.), Noyes Publications, Park Ridge, NJ, pp. 215–229.

McGregor, D. B. (1992). Chemicals classified by IARC: Their potency in tests for carcinogenicity in rodents and their genotoxicity and acute toxicity. In *Mechanisms of Carcinogenesis in Risk Identification* (H. Vainio, P. N. Magee, D. B., McGregor, and A. J. McMichael, eds.), IARC, Lyon, France, pp. 323–352.

Merrill, R. A. (1991). Regulatory toxicology. In *Casarett and Doull's Toxicology, The Basic Science of Poisons,* 4th ed. (M. O. Amdur, J. Doull, and C. D. Klaassen, eds.), Pergamon Press, New York, pp. 970–984.

Miller, S. J., Wei, Z-G., Wilson, C., Dzubow, L., Sun, T-T., and Lavker, R. M. (1993). Mouse skin is particularly susceptible to tumor initiation during early anagen of the hair cycle: Possible involvement of hair follicle stem cells, *J. Invest. Dermatol.,* 101, 591–594.

Milman, H. A. and Weisburger, E. K. (1985). *Handbook of Carcinogen Testing,* Noyes Publications, Park Ridge, NJ, 637 pp.

Möller, L., Zeisig, M., and Toftgård, R. (1993). Lack of initiating capacity of the genotoxic air pollutant 2-nitrofluorene in the mouse skin two-stage carcinogenesis system, *Carcinogenesis,* 14, 1723–1725.

Moore, J. A., Huff, J. E., Hart, L., and Walters, D. B. (1981). Overview of the National Toxicology Program. In *Environmental Health Chemistry. The Chemistry of Environmental Agents as Potential Human Hazards* (J. D.. McKinney, ed.), Ann Arbor Science Publishers, Ann Arbor, MI, pp. 555–574.

[NTP] National Toxicology Program (1984). *Report of the NTP Ad Hoc Panel on Chemical Carcinogenesis Testing and Evaluation,* Department of Health and Human Services, National Toxicology Program, Research Triangle Park, NC.

[NTP] National Toxicology Program (1989). Chemical status report. 21 pp. Produced from NTP CHEMTRACK System, February 7, 1989. Department of Health and Human Services, National Toxicology Program, Research Triangle Park, NC.

[NTP] National Toxicology Program (1991). *Sixth Annual Report on Carcinogens 1991 Summary,* Department of Health and Human Services, National Toxicology Program, Research Triangle Park, NC.

[NTP] National Toxicology Program (1993). *NTP Technical Report on the Toxicology and Carcinogenesis Studies of Acetaminophen (CAS No. 103-90-2) in F344/N Rats and B6C3F1 Mice (Feed Studies),* NIH Publication No. 93-2849. Department of Health and Human Services, National Toxicology Program, Research Triangle Park, NC.

[NTP] National Toxicology Program (1994). *National Toxicology Program Annual Report for Fiscal Year 1993.* Department of Health and Human Services, National Toxicology Program, Research Triangle Park, NC.

Osterle, D. and Deml, E. (1990). Detection of chemical carcinogens by means of the "rat liver foci bioassay," *Exp. Pathol.,* 39, 197–206.

Park, C. N. and Kociba, R. J. (1985). Statistical evaluation of long-term animal bioassays for carcinogenicity. In *Handbook of Carcinogen Testing* (H. A. Milman and E. K. Weisburger, eds.), Noyes Publications, Park Ridge, NJ, pp. 358–371.

Pereira, M. A. (1982a). Mouse skin bioassay for chemical carcinogens, *J. Am. Coll. Toxicol.,* 1, 47–82.

Pereira, M. A. (1982b). Rat liver foci bioassay, *J. Am. Coll. Toxicol.,* 1, 101–117.

Pereira, M. A. (1985). Rat liver foci assay. In *Handbook of Carcinogen Testing* (H. A. Milman and E. K. Weisburger, eds.), Noyes Publications, Park Ridge, NJ, pp. 152–178.

Peto, R., Pike, M. C., Day, N. E., Gray, R. G., et al. (1980). Guidelines for simple, sensitive significance tests for carcinogenic effects in long-term animal experiments, *IARC Monogr.,* Suppl. 2, 311–426.

Ramel, C. (1992). Genotoxic and nongenotoxic carcinogens: Mechanisms of action and testing strategies. In *Mechanisms of Carcinogenesis in Risk Identification* (H. Vainio, P. N. Magee, D. B. McGregor, and A. J. McMichael, eds.), IARC, Lyon, France, pp. 195–209.

Rao, M. S., Lalwani, N. D., Scarpelli, D. G., and Reddy, J. K. (1982). The absence of $\gamma$-glutamyl-transpeptidase activity in putative preneoplastic lesions and in hepatocellular carcinomas induced in rats by hypolipidemic peroxisome proliferator Wy-14,643, *Carcinogenesis,* 3, 1231–1233.

Robens, J. F., Piegorsch, W. W., and Schueler, R. L. (1989). Methods of testing for carcinogenicity. In *Principles and Methods of Toxicology,* 2nd ed. (A. W. Hayes, ed.), Raven Press, New York, pp. 251–273.

Schmandt, R. and Mills, G. B. (1993). Genomic components of carcinogenesis, *Clin. Chem.,* 39, 2375–2385.

Slaga, T. J., Fischer, S. M., Triplett, L. L., and Nesnow, S. (1982). Comparison of complete carcinogenesis and tumor initiation and promotion in mouse skin: The induction of papillomas by tumor initiation–promotion a reliable short term assay. *J Am. Coll. Toxicol.,* 1, 83–99.

Slaga, T. J., and Nesnow, S. (1985). SENCAR mouse skin tumorigenesis. In *Handbook of Carcinogen Testing* (H. A. Milman and E. K. Weisburger, eds.), Noyes Publications, Park Ridge, NJ, pp. 230–250.

Snellings, W. M. and Dodd, D. E. (1990). Inhalation studies. In *Handbook of In Vivo Toxicity Testing* (D. L. Arnold, H. C. Grice, and D. R. Krewski, eds.), Academic Press, San Diego, CA, pp. 189–246.

Sobottka, S. B., Berger, M. R., and Eibl, H. (1993). Structure–activity relationships of four anti-cancer alkylphosphocholine derivatives in vitro and in vivo, *Int. J. Cancer,* 53, 418–425.

Sontag, J. M., Page, N. P., and Saffiotti, U. (1976). *Guidelines for Carcinogen Bioassay in Small Rodents.* NCI Carcinogenesis Technical Report Series No. 1, DHEW Publication No. (NIH) 76-801. National Cancer Institute, Bethesda, MD.

Stenbäck, F., Mori, H., Furuya, K., and Williams, G. M. (1986). Pathogenesis of dimethylnitrosamine-induced hepatocellular cancer in hamster liver and lack of enhancement by phenobarbital, *JNCI,* 76, 327–333.

Stoner, G. D. (1991). Lung tumors in strain A mice as a bioassay for carcinogenicity of environmental chemicals, *Exp. Lung Res.,* 17, 405–423.

Stoner, G. D. and Shimkin, M. B. (1982). Strain A mouse lung tumor bioassay, *J. Am. Coll. Toxicol.,* 1, 145–169.

Stoner, G. D. and Shimkin, M. B. (1985). Lung tumors in strain A mice as a bioassay for carcinogenicity. In *Handbook of Carcinogen Testing* (H. A. Milman and E. K. Weisburger, eds.), Noyes Publications, Park Ridge, NJ, pp. 179–214.

Ulsamer, A. G., White, P. D., and Preuss, P. W. (1985). Evaluation of carcinogens: Perspective of the Consumer Product Safety Commission. In *Handbook of Carcinogen Testing* (H. A. Milman and E. K. Weisburger, eds.), Noyes Publications, Park Ridge, NJ, pp. 587–602.

Updike, K. A., Personal communication. Director, Marketing, LABCAT Products, Innovative Programming Associates, Inc., Princeton, NJ.

[USDHEW] U. S. Department of Health, Education and Welfare (1978). *Guide for the Care and Use of Laboratory Animals,* Publication No. (NIH) 78-23, ILAR, National Research Council, Washington, DC.

[USEPA] U. S. Environmental Protection Agency (1989). *Risk Assessment Guidance for Superfund, Vol. 1. Human Health Evaluation Manual (Part A). Interim Final.* Office of Emergency and Remedial Response, U. S. Environmental Protection Agency, Washington, DC.

[USEPA] U. S. Environmental Protection Agency (1991a). Data requirements for registration. *40 CFR Ch. 1 Part 158 (7-1-91 ed.).* U. S. Government Printing Office, Washington, DC.

[USEPA] U. S. Environmental Protection Agency (1991b). Good laboratory practice standards. *40 CFR Ch. I Part 160 (7-1-91 ed.)*. U. S. Government Printing Office, Washington, DC.

Vesselinovitch, S. D., Hacker, H. J., and Bannasch, P. (1985). Histochemical characterization of focal hepatic lesions induced by single diethylnitrosamine treatment in infant mice, *Cancer Res.,* 45, 2774–2780.

Wang, J-S. and Busby, W. F., Jr. (1993). Induction of lung and liver tumors by fluoranthene in a preweanling CD-1 mouse bioassay, *Carcinogenesis,* 14, 1871–1874.

Warren, B. S., Naylor, M. F., Winberg, L. D., Yoshimi, N., Volpe, J. P. G., Gimenez-Conti, I., and Slaga, T. J.(1993). Induction and inhibition of tumor progression, *Proc. Soc. Exp. Biol. Med.,* 202, 9–15.

Weisburger, J. H. and Williams, G. M. (1981). The decision-point approach for systematic carcinogen testing, *Food Cosmet. Toxicol.,* 19, 561–566.

Weisburger, J. H. and Williams, G. M. (1984). Bioassay of carcinogens: In vitro and in vivo tests. In *Chemical Carcinogens,* Vol. 2, (C. E. Searle, ed.), ACS Monograph 182. American Chemical Society, Washington, DC, pp. 1323–1373.

Williams, G. M. and Weisburger, J. H. (1991). Chemical carcinogenesis. In *Casarett and Doull's Toxicology, The Basic Science of Poisons,* 4th ed. (M. O. Amdur, J. Doull, and C. D. Klaassen, eds.), Pergamon Press, New York, pp. 127–200.

Zawidzka, Z. Z. (1990). Hematological evaluation. In *Handbook of In Vivo Toxicity Testing* (D. L. Arnold, H. C. Grice, and D. R. Krewski, eds.), Academic Press, San Diego, CA, pp. 463–508.

Zeiger, E. (1987). Carcinogenicity of mutagens: Predictive capability of the salmonella mutagenesis assay for rodent carcinogenicity, *Cancer Res.,* 47, 1287–1296.

# 10
# Genetic Toxicology Testing

**Wai Nang Choy**
*Schering-Plough Research Institute*
*Lafayette, New Jersey*

## I. INTRODUCTION

The development of genetic toxicology began in the 1960s in the midst of increasing awareness of human exposure to toxic chemicals in the environment. Early genetic toxicology studies were designed to detect reproductive toxicants. It was not until the 1970s that most of the current routine genetic toxicology tests were developed, and test results were used for identification of carcinogens and risk characterization for cancer risk assessment (for review, see Brusick, 1987a; Li and Heflich, 1991).

## II. GENETIC TOXICOLOGY TESTS

Genetic toxicology tests are designed to detect mutations. The diversity and specificity of these tests, as related to test species and genetic endpoints, may seem bewildering. The reason for this diversity is that most test methods were adopted directly from existing genetic research systems by researchers of mutagen screening. The validity of these tests is based on the assumption that the DNAs in different organisms are similarly susceptible to chemical or physical damages. An estimate of about 100 test systems has been proposed, but fewer than 10 tests are routinely performed in recent years.

The justification for the use of genetic toxicology tests to predict carcinogens is based on the somatic mutation theory of carcinogenesis (Boveri, 1929), which postulated that cancer is caused by mutations in somatic cells. Evidences for this theory are strong. It has been shown that many rodent carcinogens are mutagens (Gold et al., 1993), and most known human carcinogens are mutagens (Shelby, 1988; Shelby and Zeiger, 1990). Cytogenetic studies also showed that all cancer cells are heteroploid, with specific chromosomal changes in some tumor types (Mitelman, 1988). Molecular cancer genetic studies further demonstrated that oncogene activations and tumor suppressor gene (antioncogene) inactivations are mostly mediated by mutational events (Knudson, 1993).

Since each genetic toxicology test measures only mutations in a single species at a specific genetic marker, a battery of several genetic toxicology tests are necessary to assess the mutagenicity of a chemical. Indeed, all regulatory agencies require a battery of genetic toxicology tests for mutagen identification, but the tests that are required for each battery are different. The conduct of each "routine" test is also different among different testing facilities. An effort for the standardization of testing procedures of several routine tests has recently been completed (Galloway, 1994), and two programs on the harmonization of international testing requirement guidelines (ICH2; OECD) are in progress.

The major genetic toxicology tests have been repeatedly evaluated (Stich and San, 1981; de Serres and Ashby, 1981; Ashby et al., 1985, 1988; Brusick, 1987a; Li and Heflich, 1991). Early in vivo tests for the detection of germ cell mutagens in *Drosophilia* (Lee et al., 1983) or in rodents (Green et al., 1985; Russell and Shelby, 1985; Russell et al., 1981; Preston et al., 1981) are no longer routinely performed. The common tests conducted in recent years are listed in Tables 1 and 2. For regulatory compliance, there are four basic types of tests in a test battery: the bacterial mutagenicity assay, the mammalian cell mutagenicity assay, the in vitro chromosomal aberration assay, and the in vivo cytogenetic assay. The DNA repair assay is sometimes required to clarify questionable findings. These tests, together with the transgenic mouse assays, are briefly described in the following.

## 2. The Bacterial Mutagenicity Assays

The bacterial mutagenicity assays are performed in *Salmonella typhimurium* (Ames, 1979; Ames et al., 1973, 1975), and sometimes also in *Escherichia coli* (Green, 1984). The *Salmonella* assay is often referred to as the "Ames test" because it was developed by Dr. Bruce Ames at the University of California at Berkeley (Ames et al., 1975; Maron and Ames, 1983).

The *Salmonella* mutagenicity assay is to test the ability of a chemical to induce mutations in the genes for histidine biosynthesis. Several *Salmonella* tester strains each carries a mutation in one of the histidine genes (collectively designated as *his⁻*) are used in the assay. The tester strains are auxotrophic and require exogenous histidine to growth. The mutation assay is to detect the mutation of the histidine gene (*his⁻*) back to wild-type (*his⁺*), and the bacteria no longer require histidine to grow. Because this assay is to detect reverse mutations, it is also

**Table 1**   Common In Vitro Genetic Toxicology Tests

| | |
|---|---|
| Bacteria | *Salmonella typhimurium* (Ames test) |
| | *Escherichia coli* |
| Mammalian cells | |
|   Gene mutations | Chinese hamster ovary cells (CHO/HGPRT) |
| | Chinese hamster ovary AS52 cells (CHOAS52/XPRT) |
| | Mouse lymphoma cells (L5178Y/TK) |
|   Chromosomal aberrations | Human peripheral blood lymphocytes (HPBL) |
| | Chinese hamster lung fibroblasts (CHL) |
| | Chinese hamster ovary cells (CHO) |
|   DNA repair | Primary rat hepatocytes (unscheduled DNA synthesis; UDS) |
| | Primary human hepatocytes (unscheduled DNA synthesis; UDS) |
|   Neoplastic transformation | Syrian hamster embryo fibroblasts (SHE) |
| | BALB/C3T3 mouse fibroblasts |

**Table 2** Common In Vivo Genetic Toxicology Tests

| | |
|---|---|
| Cytogenetics | |
| Chromosomal aberrations | Rat bone marrow cells |
| Micronucleus | Mouse bone marrow erythrocytes |
| | Mouse peripheral blood erythrocytes |
| | Rat bone marrow erythrocytes |
| Gene mutations | |
| Somatic cells | Transgenic mice (Muta™ Mouse and Big Blue™) |
| | Human lymphocytes |
| Germ cells | Mouse dominant lethal test |
| | Mouse specific locus test |
| DNA repair | Rat hepatocytes (unscheduled DNA synthesis; UDS) |

referred to as the "reversion assay," and the mutants "revertants." Revertants are selected in agar medium deficient in histidine.

Since the *his*⁻ strains are genetically characterized, the specificity of reversion (i.e., base-pair substitution or frameshift) can be elucidated by the pattern of mutagenic response in a combination of tester strains. To enhance the sensitivity of this assay, several genetic changes were also introduced to these tester strains. They are a mutation in the DNA repair gene (*uvrB*), a mutation to increase cell permeability (*rfa*), and the addition of plasmids (pKM101, pAQ1) to the cells. Plasmid pKM101 enhances error-prone DNA repair and multicopy plasmid pAQ1 provides multiple copies of the *his*⁻ gene, which increase the target size and, thus, the sensitivity of the assay. Four *Salmonella* tester strains are commonly used for this assay: TA1535, TA100, TA1537, and TA98. Strains TA97a, TA97, and TA1537 are used interchangeably (Gatehouse et al., 1994). Strain TA102 detects A–T base-pair changes (Maron and Ames, 1983; Levin et al., 1982) and is often added as the fifth strain. Strains TA1535, TA100, and TA102 detect base-pair substitution mutations, and TA98, TA1537, TA97, and TA97a detect frameshift mutations. The genetic characteristics of *Salmonella* tester strains are shown in Table 3.

The *Escherichia* mutagenicity assay is a complementary assay to the *Salmonella* assay. This assay is currently required by regulatory agencies in Japan. The ability of this assay in detecting A–T base-pair changes is similar to that of *Salmonella* TA102 (Wilcox et al., 1990). The *Escherichia* assay is also a reversion assay, but the target gene is involved in tryptophan biosynthesis. Tester strains are auxotrophic mutants (*trp*⁻) that require tryptophan to growth. The assay is to test the ability of the test agent to mutate the tryptophan gene (*trp*⁻) back to wild-type (*trp*+). Mutants are selected in tryptophan-deficient agar medium. Two *Escherichia* tester strains are used for this assay: WP2*uvrA* and WP2*uvrA*(pKM101). Both strains are defective in the DNA repair gene (*uvrA*), and one strain carries plasmid pUM101. The genetic characteristics of these two strains are shown in Table 3.

A metabolic activation system is included in all in vitro tests to detect mutagens that require metabolic activation. A host-mediated in vivo activation assay using rodent hosts for metabolism was developed in the 1970s (Legator et al., 1982), but this assay was replaced by in vitro activation systems. At present, the metabolic activation system customarily used in routine tests is the supernatant of Aroclor 1254-induced rat liver homogenate after centrifugation at $9000 \times g$. This supernatant is commonly referred to as the S9 fraction (Maron and Ames, 1983).

A typical *Salmonella* mutagenicity assay consists of a dose range-finding assay and a mutagenicity assay (Kier et al., 1986; Gatehouse et al., 1994). The mutagenicity assay is

**Table 3**  Genotypes of Bacteria Tester Strains

| Bacterial strains | Genes affected | Additional mutations | | | Types of mutation detected |
| | | DNA repair | LPS | R Factor | |
| --- | --- | --- | --- | --- | --- |
| *Salmonella typhimurium* | | | | | |
| TA 1535 | *his* G46 | *uvrB* | *rfa* | – | Base-pair substitution |
| TA 100 | *his* G46 | *uvrB* | *rfa* | pKM101 | Base-pair substitution |
| TA 97 | *his* D6610 | *uvrB* | *rfa* | pKM101 | Frameshift |
| | *his* 01242 | | | | |
| TA 97a | *his* D6610 | *uvrB* | *rfa* | pKM101 | Frameshift |
| | *his* 01242 | | | | |
| TA 98 | *his* D3052 | *uvrB* | *rfa* | pKM101 | Frameshift |
| TA 1537 | *his* C3076 | *uvrB* | *rfa* | – | Frameshift |
| TA 102 | *his* G428 | + | *rfa* | pKM101 | Base-pair substitution |
| | | | | pAQ1 | |
| *Escherichia coli* | | | | | |
| WP2*uvrA* | *trp* | *uvrA* | + | – | Base-pair substitution |
| WP2*uvrA* (pKM101) | *trp* | *uvrA* | + | pKM101 | Base-pair substitution |

conducted in two independent trials, each with at least four tester strains and five dose levels, with or without S9 metabolic activation. For the plate incorporation assay, which is the most common one, bacteria are treated with the test agent and plated onto histidine-deficient agar plates. Mutant colonies are scored 2 days after cell growth on agar. The *Escherichia* mutagenicity assay is similar to the *Salmonella* assay, except that only two tester strains are used and the selection medium are tryptophan-deficient agar plates.

## B.  Mammalian Cell Mutagenicity Assays

The mammalian cell mutagenicity assays presumably are more reliable than the bacterial mutagenicity assays for the evaluation of chemical mutagenicity in mammals. The most common assays are the CHO/HGPRT assay (Chinese hamster ovary cells using the hypoxanthine-guanine phosphoribosyltransferase gene [*HGPRT*] as the genetic marker; Hsie et al., 1981; Li et al., 1987), the mouse lymphoma L5178Y TK$^{+/-}$ assay (mouse lymphoma cell L5178Y using the heterozygous thymidine kinase gene [*TK*$^{+/-}$] as the genetic marker; Clive et al., 1983, 1987; Caspary et al., 1988; Blazak et al., 1989), and the CHOAS52/XPRT assay (Chinese hamster ovary cells AS52 using the xanthine-guanine phosphoribosyltransferase gene [*XPRT*] as the genetic marker; Stankowski and Hsie, 1986; Stankowski and Tindall, 1987; Tindall and Stankowski, 1987). These assays are forward mutation assays.

All three genetic markers are enzymes involved in nuclei acid biosynthesis. The tester cells are wild-type cells and mutations are monitored at the *HGPRT, XPRT,* and *TK* genes for the CHO/HGPRT, CHOAS52/XPRT, and the mouse lymphoma TK$^{+/-}$ assays, respectively. Mutations at these genes abolish the respective enzymes to incorporate certain nucleotides to the cells. Because of this defect, mutants are also resistant to toxic nucleotide analogues that can be mistakenly incorporated by wild-type cells and cause cell death. In these assays, toxic nucleotide analogues, 6-thioguanine (6-TG) and trifluorothymidine (TFT), are used for mutant selections. Mutants defective in HGPRT and XPRT are resistent to 6-TG, and mutants defective in TK are resistant to TFT. Both the CHO/HGPRT and the mouse lymphoma assays are well-established assays. The CHOAS52/XPRT assay may require further validations.

The procedures of the mammalian cell mutagenicity assay, although they vary with different cell types, follow a basic plan (Nestmann et al., 1991; Aaron, et al., 1994). A typical assay consists of a dose range-finding assay and a mutagenicity assay in two independent trial. For each trial, cells are treated with the test agent for 3–6 hr in the presence or absence of S9 metabolic activation. Treated cells are allowed to grow for a few days for phenotypic expression before mutant selection. Phenotypic expression is required for selection of mutants of a recessive trait because the preexisting wild-type gene product has to be removed by cell division or protein turnover before the mutant phenotype can be expressed. Mutants are selected with the respective selection agents, 6-TG or TFT.

For the mouse lymphoma assay, the size of the mutant colonies are also measured and mutants are classified into small-colony mutants and large-colony mutants. Small-colony mutants often associate with chromosome aberrations (Blazak et al., 1989), which led to the proposal that the mouse lymphoma assay also detects cytogenetic changes.

The mouse lymphoma assay is generally considered to be a more sensitive assay than other mammalian cell mutagenicity assays, but it is also known to produce more false-positive results, as related to carcinogenicity. Some false-positive findings may be caused by test agent-induced changes in the culture conditions. Changes in pH and osmolality in cultures are known to affect the results of this assay (Brusick, 1986; Cifone et al., 1987).

Recently, the mouse lymphoma assay has become the favored mammalian cell mutagenicity assay by several regulatory agencies. One reason is that the mouse lymphoma assay is believed to detect cytogenetic changes, as demonstrated in the small-colony mutants. Another reason is that the mouse lymphoma assay is considered to be more sensitive than the CHO/HGPRT assay because of the location of the *TK* gene on an autosome. The *HGPRT* gene in the CHO cells is located on the X chromosome, but the *TK* gene in the mouse lymphoma cells is located on Chromosome 11 (Kozak and Ruddle, 1977), and the *XPRT* gene in the CHOAS52 cells, are located on chromosome 6 or 7 (Michaelis et al., 1994). Since there is only one active X chromosome in a cell, it is believed that chemicals that induce large DNA deletions cannot be detected in the CHO/HGPRT assay. A large deletion in the *HGPRT* gene extending to its neighboring "essential" genes in the X chromosome is expected to be lethal to the cell because of the absence of a complementary homologous chromosome, and dead cells do not form mutants. Although this theoretical assumption has not been demonstrated experimentally, the mouse lymphoma assay is expected to be the preferred assay in the near future.

## C. Cytogenetic Assays

Cytogenetic assays detect clastogens and chemicals that cause abnormal chromosomal segregations. All cancer cells are heteroploid, and heteroploid conversion is a prerequisite step for cancer development (Littlefield, 1976). Chromosomal aberrations appear to be a relevant marker for the prediction of carcinogenicity.

### 1. In Vitro Chromosomal Aberration Assays

The in vitro chromosomal aberration assays detect the ability of the test agent to induce chromosomal damage. The most common aberrations are chromosomal gaps and breaks, but complex chromosomal exchanges, endoreduplications, and polyploidy are also identified. The cells commonly used for this assay are Chinese hamster lung cells (CHL; Ishidate and Sofuni, 1985; Ishidate et al., 1988), Chinese hamster ovary cells (CHO; Galloway et al., 1985, 1987a), and human peripheral blood lymphocytes (HPBL; Preston et al., 1981, 1987).

The procedures of the chromosomal aberration assay vary for different cell types (Swierenga, et al., 1991b; Galloway et al., 1994). A typical assay consists of a dose range-finding assay and a chromosomal aberration assay, usually in two trials. For each trial, cells are treated with the test agent, with or without S9 metabolic activation, for 3–6 hr and harvested at approximately 1.5 times that of the cell cycle after treatment. Variations to this procedure include prolonged treatments, multiple harvests, or prolonged harvests for up to two cell cycles. These variations are known to increase the sensitivity of the assay, especially for certain classes of chemicals, such as nucleotides (Sofuni, 1993) and nitrosamides (Ishidate et al., 1988). Harvested cells are fixed on microscope slides, stained, and examined for chromosomal aberrations. The chromosomal aberration assays are sensitive to nonphysiological cell culture conditions. Changes in pH and osmolality, test agent precipitates, and severe cytotoxicity induced by the test article affect the test results (Brusick, 1987b; Galloway et al., 1987b; Scott et al., 1991; Armstrong et al., 1992; Morita et al., 1992).

## 2. *In Vivo Cytogenetic Assay: The Mouse Micronucleus Test*

The micronucleus test is an in vivo assay for the detection of both clastogens and agents that induce aneuploidy (abnormal chromosomal segregation; i.e., nondisjunction). This test was initially developed in mouse bone marrow erythrocytes (Schmid, 1976), but it also has been conducted in rats (George, et al., 1990), hamsters (Basler, 1986), and monkeys (Choy et al., 1993). The routine micronucleus test is conducted in mouse bone marrow erythrocytes (Heddle, et al., 1983; Mavournin et al., 1990).

Micronuclei are small nuclei that arise from chromosomal fragments resulting from chromosomal breaks (double-stranded DNA breaks), or detached chromosomes (microtubule malfunctions in cell division). In the mouse micronucleus test, the target cells are the bone marrow erythroblasts. Chemically induced micronuclei in the erythroblasts are retained in the erythrocytes after the extrusion of the main nuclei from the cells during maturation and can be scored in polychromatic erythrocytes (PCE; young erythrocytes). An increase of micronuclei in PCE indicates genotoxicity of the test agent.

The procedures of the micronucleus test vary by the number of dosings, the number of harvests, and the timing of the harvest(s) (Tinwell, 1990). As genotoxic responses are expected to be different for each test agent, multiple dosing and multiple harvests are required to capture the window of maximum micronuclei occurrence in bone marrow PCE (MacGregor, et al., 1987; Hayashi et al., 1994). All common mouse strains can be used for this assay. A typical micronucleus test consists of a dose range-finding assay and a micronucleus assay. Male and female mice are dosed with the test agent, usually by intraperitoneal injection, but other routes of dosing are also acceptable. Toxicity is monitored by animal death or by bone marrow suppression, or both. Bone marrow suppression is measured by the decrease of the ratio of PCE to normochromatic erythrocytes (NCE; mature erythrocytes), or to total erythrocytes (RBC, PCE + NCE), in the bone marrow which is commonly referred to as the PCE/NCE, or PCE/RBC ratio. Dosing can be a single dose, or daily doses for 2–3 days. Bone marrow cells are harvested from the femurs of the mice at 24, 48, and/or 72 hr after the last dosing, dependent on the protocol. In general, two harvests, 24 and 48 hr after the last dosing, are considered sufficient for multiple dosings, but three harvests, 24, 48, and 72 hr, are needed for single dosing. Bone marrow smears are prepared on microscope slides, stained with giemsa or acridine orange (Hayashi et al., 1983), and scored for micronucleated PCE.

Micronuclei can also be detected in PCE in mouse peripheral blood (MacGregor, et al., 1980, 1983). With a recent improvement in the acridine orange-staining technique (Hayashi et al., 1990), an interlaboratory study was conducted in Japan for the validation of the peripheral blood micronucleus test (for review, see CSGMT, 1992). The advantages of the peripheral blood assay are that easy sampling and multiple sampling from the same animal for kinetic studies are possible. The peripheral blood micronucleus test, however, can be performed only in mice, but not in any other species yet studied, because the mouse is the only species in which micronucleated erythrocytes are not removed by the spleen, but persistent in the circulating blood. This ability of accumulating micronucleated erythrocytes also permits the scoring of micronuclei in NCE obtained from routine blood smears in toxicological multidose studies. Indeed, retrospective evaluations of micronuclei in NCE of peripheral blood have been performed in several National Toxicology Program (NTP) cancer bioassays (Choy et al., 1985; MacGregor et al., 1990). Incorporation of the micronucleus test into chronic animal bioassays provides early information on the genotoxicity of the test agent in the same system for the carcinogenicity bioassays.

## D. Unscheduled DNA Synthesis Assays

The unscheduled DNA synthesis (UDS) assay measures repairable DNA damages induced by the test agent. The UDS assays are customarily conducted in hepatocytes, both for in vitro or in vivo studies, and no exogenous metabolic activation system is required. Metabolic activation inside the hepatocytes proximal to DNA is believed to enhance the sensitivity for the detection of DNA damages induced by short-lived genotoxic metabolites.

### 1. In Vitro Assay

Routine in vitro UDS assays are performed in primary cultures of rat hepatocytes (Williams, 1977; Mitchell et al., 1983; Williams et al., 1985; Butterworth, et al., 1987), but assays in mouse, hamster, monkey, and human hepatocytes were also reported (San and Stich, 1975; Martin et al., 1978; Steinmetz et al., 1988).

The procedures of the in vitro UDS assay in rat hepatocytes do not vary much (Swierenga, et al., 1991a, Madle, et al., 1994). In a typical assay, primary rat hepatocyte cultures are exposed to the test agent simultaneously with tritium-labeled thymidine ($[^3H]$thymidine), a radioactive precursor of DNA synthesis. DNA damaged by the test agent will undergo DNA repair, referred to as unscheduled DNA synthesis (as compared with DNA synthesis in cell division), and incorporate $[^3H]$thymidine into DNA, which is detected by autoradiography and appears as dark grains in the nuclei. An increase of grain counts in the nuclear region indicated DNA repair, and, thereby, DNA damage by the test agent.

### 2. In Vivo–In Vitro Assay

The in vivo–in vitro UDS assay is similar to the in vitro UDS assay, except that the test agent is administered to the animals. The assay is then conducted in cultured hepatocytes (Mirsalis and Butterworth, 1980; Mirsalis et al., 1982; Mirsalis, 1988). This assay is usually conducted in rats, but studies in mice have also been reported (Mirsalis et al., 1988b; Ashby et al., 1991).

There are few variations in the procedures of the in vivo–in vitro UDS assay (Madle et al., 1994). A typical assay is to treat male and female rats with the test agent, usually by a single oral gavage dose, and to isolate hepatocytes at two harvests, usually 2 hr and 16 hr after dosing. Hepatocyte cultures are exposed to $[^3H]$thymidine, and the amount of $[^3H]$thymidine incorporation is detected by autoradiography as grain counts. An increase of grain counts in the nuclear region indicates DNA repair.

Both the in vitro and in vivo–in vitro UDS assays are capable of detecting liver carcinogens, but not necessarily carcinogens that affect other tissues (Tennant et al., 1987; Mirsalis et al., 1989). The in vivo–in vitro UDS assay is considered to be more reliable than the in vitro UDS assay, as the in vitro UDS assay is known to produce false-positive results, relative to rodent carcinogenicity (Mirsalis, 1987; Mirsalis et al., 1982, 1986, 1988a).

## E.  In Vivo Gene Mutation Assays: The Transgenic Mouse Assays

The development of the in vivo mutagenicity assays has been slow and plagued by many diffi-culties associated with inefficient mutant selection systems. Only one human assay (Albertini et al., 1982; Moreley et al., 1983) and one mouse assay (Jones et al., 1985) have been reported so far. Both assays are limited to the selection of HGPRT mutants in lymphocyte cultures, and neither has been validated for prospective genotoxicity studies.

Recent advances in transgenic animal technology have generated a variety of transgenic animals for carcinogenicity and mutagenicity studies (for review, see Short, 1994; Tennant et al., 1994). For in vivo gene mutation assays, two transgenic mouse assays are currently under intensive validations for their possible adoption to routine assays. They are the Big Blue (*lacI*) assay (Kohler et al., 1991; Dycaico et al., 1994) and the Muta Mouse (*lacZ*) assay (Gossen et al., 1989, 1994). Both assay monitor mutations in the bacterial lactose operon genes introduced into the mouse by a bacteriophage-λ shuttle vector. The Big Blue assay detects mutations in the *lacI* gene (the β-galactosidase repressor gene), or mutations in the operator region (the repressor-binding site for the inhibition of expression of β-galactosidase). Mutations in the *lacI* gene, or the operator region, inactivate repressor function and allow the expression of β-galactosidase gene. In the Big Blue assay, a mutation is monitored as the induction of the β-galactosidase activity. The Muta Mouse assay, on the other hand, detects mutations in the *lacZ* gene (the β-galactosidase structural gene), and mutations in this gene diminish β-galactosidase activity. In the Muta Mouse assay, a mutation is monitored as the loss of the β-galactosidase activity. The Big Blue mice are available in C57BL/6 and B6C3F1 strains, and Muta Mouse mice, in the CD2 strain.

The basic procedures of these two assays are similar, although there is much flexibility in the route of test agent administration, the duration of dosing, and the selection of tissue(s) for mutation screening. In a typical assay, mice are dosed with the test agent and allowed to express the mutant phenotype. The duration of the expression time is dependent on the metabolism and distribution of the test agent, or its metabolites, to the target tissue(s), and it has to be optimized for each study. DNA from the tissue to be studied is isolated and packaged into λ-phages by in vitro phage assembly. The DNA containing the mutated genes is encapsulated into individual λ-phages which are used to infect *Escherichia coli*. Infected cells are grown on agar plates containing a chromogenic substrate X-gal(5-bromo-4-chloro-3-indolyl-β-D-galactoside). Phages expressing β-galactosidase appear as blue plaques in the indicator plate, and the phages that do not express β-galactosidase, as clear plaques. In the Big Blue assay, mutations in the *lacI* gene allow the expression of β-galactosidase, and phages containing this mutation are detected as blue plaques (mutant phenotype) among clear plaques (parental phenotype). In the Muta Mouse assay, mutations in the *lacZ* gene abolish β-galactosidase activity and phages containing this mutation appear as clear plaques (mutant phenotype) among blue plaques (parental phenotype). When a large number of plaques are screened, typically 50,000–100,000 per phage package, the Big Blue assay has the advantage of easy identification of mutant plaques.

To improve the efficiency of scoring, a positive mutant selection system was recently developed for the Muta Mouse assay that eliminates the use of the chromogenic reaction for mutation screening (Myhr et al., 1993; Dean and Myhr, 1994). This selection is to use an *E. coli* mutant strain, *galE⁻*, as the host for phage infection. The *E. coli* strain *galE⁻* cannot grow in the presence of galactose. The *E. coli galE⁻* infected with phages are grown in agar plates containing *phenylgalactose* (P-gal), a precursor of galactose. Phages containing the intact *lacZ* gene (parental phenotype) are able to convert P-gal to galactose, which inhibits growth of *E. coli galE⁻*, and the phage cannot form plaques. In contrast, phages containing the mutated *lacZ* gene, lacking the β-galactosidase activity (mutant phenotype), are unable to convert P-gal to galactose, and are able to form plaques. Mutations at the *lacZ* gene are identified by the occurrence of phage plaques. A positive selection system was also developed for the Big Blue assay, but it is not widely used (Kretz et al., 1992; Lundberg et al., 1993).

The greatest advantage of the transgenic mouse assay is its ability to detect mutations in almost all the tissues in the mouse. Such information is useful for dose–response studies of genotoxicity as related to target tissue doses and target tissue toxicity. Current validation studies are focused on standardization of testing protocols, correlation of test results with conventional genotoxicity endpoints, and with rodent cancer bioassays.

## III.  REGULATORY GENETIC TOXICOLOGY TESTING GUIDELINES

Regulatory agencies worldwide have established genetic toxicology testing guidelines for risk assessment of pharmaceutical, agricultural, and environmental chemicals. These guidelines vary according to regional expertise and scientific opinions of regulators. Most guidelines are revised periodically as new knowledge of technology develop. All studies for regulatory submissions are performed in compliance with the Good Laboratory Practice (GLP) guidelines, as specified by the respective agencies (e.g., USFDA, 21 CFR Part 58; USEPA-FIFRA 40 CFR, Part 160; USEPA-TSCA, 40 CFR, Part 792; EEC Council Directive, 90/18/EED; and JMHW (Japan) Notification No. 313). These GLP guidelines, similar to other regulatory guidelines, are also amended periodically.

Several regulatory genetic toxicology guidelines have been developed in the United States, Canada, Europe, United Kingdom, Australia, Japan, and the Nordic countries. The major guidelines are those of the U.S. Food and Drug Administration (USFDA, *Redbook I,.* 1982; *Redbook II,* revision in progress, 1993); the U. S. Environmental Protection Agency (USEPA; Toxic Substance Control Act [TSCA] and the Federal Insecticide, Fungicide, and Rodenticide Act [FIFRA]; USEPA, 1985, 1986, 1987; Dearfield et al., 1991; Auletta et al., 1993); the European Economic Community Council (CPMP, 1989, 1990), and the United Kingdom (DH, 1989; UKEMS, 1990; Kirkland, 1993); The Organization for Economic Cooperation and Development (OECD) Guidelines for Genetic Toxicology (OCED, 1983, 1984, 1986); and the Japan Ministry of Health and Welfare (MHW, 1990; Sofuni, 1993). These guidelines define the battery of genetic toxicology tests required by their respective agencies.

The current requirements and expected changes of four major regulatory guidelines (USFDA, USEPA, Europe, and Japan) are summarized in Table 4. The OECD guidelines are being revised, and their final form is expected to be very similar to the USEPA guidelines. All guidelines require the *Salmonella* bacteria mutagenicity assay in at least four *Salmonella* strains: TA1535, TA1537 (interchangeable with TA97a or TA97), TA98, and TA100. Strain TA102 should also be included when testing oxidizing agents, crosslinking agents and hydrazines. The Japanese guidelines specifically require an additional assay in one *Escherichia* strain, which can be WP2*urvA* or WP2*uvrA*(pKM101). At least four strains are generally required for the bacterial mutagenicity assay. Except for Japan and EEC, most guidelines require a mammalian cell mutagenicity test, preferably the mouse lymphoma assay. For the USEPA, the CHO/HGPRT assay is acceptable if it is accompanied by an in vitro cytogenetic assay. Both Europe and Japan require an in vitro cytogenetic test, preferably in Chinese hamster lung cells or human peripheral blood lymphocytes. All guidelines require the mouse bone marrow micronucleus test. The European guidelines also require an in vivo–in vitro UDS assay, if positive findings are observed in in vitro assays. The transgenic mouse assays are considered supplementary.

There are two major efforts for international harmonization of testing guidelines. The "International Conference on Harmonization of Technical Requirements for Registration of Pharmaceuticals for Human Use (ICH2)," and the update of the "OECD Genetic Toxicology Test

**Table 4** Regulatory Genetic Toxicology-Testing Guidelines

| | USFDA RedBook II | Europe UK and EEC | Japan MHW | USEPA TSCA, FIFRA |
|---|---|---|---|---|
| In vitro gene mutation Bacteria | *Salmonella* 4 strains | *Salmonella* 5 strains | *Salmonella* 5 strains *Escherichia* 1 strain | *Salmonella* 5 strains |
| Mammalian cells | Mouse lymphoma CHOAS52 | Mouse lymphoma (not required by EEC) | Not required | Mouse lymphoma, CHOAS52 CHO/HGPRT, and cytogenetics |
| In vitro cytogenetics | CHO, CHL, or human lymphocytes | CHO, CHL, or human lymphocytes | CHO, CHL, or human lymphocytes | |
| In vivo cytogenetics | Mouse micronucleus and chromosomal aberrations | Mouse micronucleus (male only, UK; both sex, EEC) | Mouse micronucleus | Mouse micronucleus or chromosomal aberrations |
| In vivo DNA repair | In vivo UDS: case-by-case | Required if in vitro test positive | | |
| In vivo gene mutation | Transgenic mice may be acceptable | Transgenic mice supplementary information | Transgenic mice supplementary information | Transgenic mice supplementary information |

Guideline." A major goal of ICH2 is to define a "core" test battery and to clarify specific test requirements. The update of the OECD guidelines provides an opportunity for the harmonization of the OECD and the USEPA guidelines (Auletta, et al., 1993).

## IV. CONCLUSIONS

All current routine genetic toxicology tests for regulatory compliances are mutation tests for DNA sequence changes. The most common tests are described in this chapter. New testing methodologies are always being developed, and recombinant DNA technologies are often employed in new tests. Extensive validations of new tests are required before they are adopted for regulatory purposes.

Results of genetic toxicology tests are customarily used for hazard identification and for the classification of *genotoxic* and *nongenotoxic* carcinogens. The use of genetic toxicology tests for risk assessment of reproductive risk, often referred to as genetic risk, is not yet common.

The success of international harmonization of testing procedures and regulatory testing guidelines will be major achievements for genetic toxicity testing. Harmonization of data interpretation will further improve its consistence among various regulatory agencies.

## REFERENCES

Aaron, C. S., Bolcsfoldi, G., Glatt, H. R., Moore, M., Nishi, Y., Stankowski, L., Theiss, J., and Thompson, E. (1994). Mammalian cell gene mutation assays working group report, *Mutat. Res.,* 312, 235–239.

Albertini, R. J., Castle, K. L., and Borcherding, W. R. (1982). T-cell cloning to detect the mutant 6-thioguanine-resistant lymphocytes present in human periphcral bloud, *Proc. Natl. Acad. Sci. USA,* 79, 6617–6621.

Ames, B. N. (1979). Identifying environmental chemicals causing mutations and cancer, *Science,* 204, 587–593.

Ames, B. N., Durston, W. E., Yamasaki, E., and Lee, F.D. (1973). Carcinogens are mutagens: A simple test system combining liver homogenates for activation and bacteria for detection, *Proc. Natl. Acad. Sci. USA,* 70, 2281–2285.

Ames, B. N., McCann, J., and Yamasaki, E. (1975). Methods for detecting carcinogens and mutagens with the *Salmonella*/mammalian-microsome mutagenicity test, *Mutat. Res.,* 31, 347–364.

Armstrong, M. J., Bean, C. L., and Galloway, S. M. (1992). A quantitative assessment of the cytotoxicity associated with chromosomal aberration detection in Chinese hamster ovary cells, *Mutat. Res.,* 265, 45–60.

Ashby, J., de Serres, F. J., Draper, M., Ishidate, M., Jr., Margolin, B. H., Matter, B. E., and Shelby, M. D. (1985). *Evaluation of Short-Term Tests for Carcinogens.* Report of the International Programme on Chemical Safety's Collaborative Study on In Vitro Assays. Elsevier, Amsterdam.

Ashby, J., de Serres, F. J., Shelby, M. D., Margolin, B. H., Ishidate, M., Jr., and Becking, G. C. (1988). *Evaluation of Short-Term Tests for Carcinogens.* Report of the International Programme on Chemical Safety's Collaborative Study on In Vivo Assays. Cambridge University Press, Cambridge, UK.

Ashby, J., Lefevre, P. A., Shank, T., Lewtas, J., and Gallagher, J. E. (1991). Relative sensitivity of [32]P-postlabelling of DNA and the autoradiographic UDS assay in the liver of mice exposed to 2-acetylaminofluorene (2AAF), *Mutat. Res.,* 252, 259–268.

Auletta, A. E., Dearfield, K. L., and Cimino, M. C. (1993). Mutagenicity test schemes and guidelines: U. S. EPA Office of Pollution Prevention and Toxics and Office of Pesticide Programs, *Environ. Mol. Mutagen.,* 21, 38–45.

Basler, A. (1986). Aneuploid-inducing chemicals in yeast evaluated by the micronucleus test, *Mutat. Res.,* 174, 11–13.

Blazak, W. F., Los, F. J., Rudd, C. J., and Caspary, W. J. (1989). Chromosome analysis of small and large

L5178Y mouse lymphoma cell colonies: Comparison of trifluorothymidine-resistant and unselected cell colonies from mutagen-treated and control cultures, *Mutat. Res.*, 224, 197–208.

Boveri, T. H. (1929). *The Origin of Malignant Tumors*, Williams & Wilkins, Baltimore.

Brusick, D. (1986). Genotoxicity effects in cultured mammalian cells produced by low pH treatment conditions and increased ion concentration, *Environ. Mutagen.*, 8, 879–886.

Brusick, D. (1987a). *Principles of Genetic Toxicology*, 2nd ed., Plenum Press, New York.

Brusick, D., ed. (1987b). Genotoxicity produced in cultured mammalian cell assays by treatment conditions, *Mutat. Res.*, 189, 71–179.

Buss, P., Caviezel M., and Lutz, W. K. (1990). Linear dose–response relationship for DNA adducts in rat liver from chronic exposure to aflatoxin $B_1$, *Carcinogenesis*, 11, 2133–2135.

Butterworth, B. E., Ashby, J., Bermudez, E., Casciano, D., Mirsalis, J., Probst, G., and Williams, G. M. (1987). A protocol and guide for the in vitro rat hepatocyte DNA-repair assay, *Mutat. Res.*, 189, 113–121.

Butterworth, B. E. and Slaga T. J. (1987). *Nongenotoxic Mechanisms of Carcinogenesis*, Cold Spring Harbor Laboratory Press, Cold Spring Harbor, NY.

Caspary , W. J., Lee, Y. J., Poulton, S., Myhr, B. C., Mitchell, A. D., and Rudd, C. J. (1988). Evaluation of the L5178Y mouse lymphoma cell mutagenesis assay: Quality-control guidelines and response categories, *Environ. Mol. Mutagen.*, 12, 19–36.

Choy, W. N. (1993). A review of the dose-response induction of DNA adducts by aflatoxin $B_1$ and its implications to quantitative cancer risk assessment, *Mutat. Res.*, 296, 181–198.

Choy, W. N., MacGregor, J. T., Shelby, M. D., and Maronpot, R. R. (1985). Induction of micronuclei by benzene in B6C3F1 mice: Retrospective analysis of peripheral blood smears from the NTP carcinogenesis bioassay, *Mutat. Res.*, 143, 55–59.

Choy, W. N., Henika, P. R., Willhite, C. C., and Tarantal, A. F. (1993). Incorporation of a micronucleus study into a developmental toxicology and pharmacokinetic study of L-selenomethionine in nonhuman primates, *Environ. Mol. Mutagen.*, 21, 73–80.

Cifone, M. A., Myhr, B., Eiche, A., and Bolcsfoldi, G. (1987). Effect of pH shifts on the mutant frequency at the thymidine kinase locus in mouse lymphoma L5178Y TA$^{+/-}$ cells, *Mutat. Res.*, 189, 39–46.

Clive, D., Caspery, W., Kirby, P. E., Krehl, R., Moore, M., Mayo, J., and Oberly, T. J. (1987). Guide for performing the mouse lymphoma assay for mammalian cell mutagenicity, *Mutat. Res.*, 189, 143–156.

Clive, D., McCuen, R., Spector, J. F. S., Piper C., and Mavournin, K. H. (1983). Specific gene mutations in L5178Y cells in culture: A report of the U. S. Environmental Protection Agency Gene-Tox Program, *Mutat. Res.*, 115, 225–256.

CPMP (1989). *Commission of the European Communities: The Rules Governing Medicinal Products in the European Community*, Vol. III. Guidelines on the quality safety and efficacy of medicinal products for human use, January 1989, pp. 103.

CPMP (1990). *CPMP Working Party on Safety of Medicinal Products*. Note for guidance. Recommendations for the development of nonclinical testing strategies, III/58/89-EN. Draft No. 7, July 5, 1990.

[CSGMT] The Collaborative Study Group for the Micronucleus Test of the Mammalian Mutagenesis Study subgroup of the Environmental Mutagen Society of Japan, ed. (1992). Micronucleus test with rodent peripheral blood reticulocytes by acridine orange supravital staining, *Mutat. Res.*, 278, 81–213.

Dean, S. W. and Myhr, B. (1994). Measurement of gene mutation in vivo using Muta Mouse and positive selection of *LacZ* phage, *Mutagenesis*, 9, 183–185.

de Serres, F. J. and Ashby, J. (1981). *Evaluation of Short-Term Tests for Carcinogens*. Report of the International Collaborative Program, Elsevier/North-Holland, New York.

Dearfield, K. L., Auletta, A. E., Cimino, M. C., and Moore, M. M. (1991). Considerations in the U. S. Environmental Protection Agency's testing approach for mutagenicity, *Mutat. Res.*, 258, 259–283.

[DH] Department of Health, United Kingdom. (1989). *Guidelines for the Testing of Chemicals for Mutagenicity*. Department of Health report on health and social subjects, No. 35, HMSO, London, UK.

Dycaico, M. J., Provost, G. S., Kretz, P. L., Ransom, S. L., Moores, J. C., and Short, J. M. (1994). The use of shuttle vectors for mutation analysis in transgenic mice and rats, *Mutat. Res.*, 307, 461–478.

Galloway, S. M., ed. (1994). Report of the international workshop on standardization of genotoxicity test procedures, *Mutat. Res.*, 312, 195–322.

Galloway, S. M., Bloom, A. D., Resnick, M., Margolin, B. H., Nakamura, F., Archer, P., and Zeigler, E. (1985). Development of a standard protocol for in vitro cytogenetic testing with Chinese hamster ovary cells: Comparison of results for 22 compounds in two laboratories, *Environ. Mutagen.,* 7, 1–51.

Galloway, S. M., Armstrong, M. J., Reuben, C., Colman, S., Brown, B., Cannon, C., Bloom, A. D., Nakamura, F., Ahmed, M., Duk, S., Rimpo, J., Margolin, B. H., Resnick, M. A., Anderson, B., and Zeigler, E. (1987a). Chromosome aberration and sister chromatid exchanges in Chinese hamster ovary cells: Evaluation of 108 chemicals, *Environ. Mol. Mutagen.,* 10, 1–109.

Galloway, S. M., Deasy, D. A., Bean, C. L., Kraynak, A. R., Armstrong, M. J., and Bradley, M. O. (1987b). Effects of high osmotic strength on chromosome aberration, sister-chromatid exchanges and DNA strand breaks, and the relation to toxicity, *Mutat. Res.,* 189, 15–25.

Galloway, S. M., Aardema, M. J., Ishidate, M., Jr., Ivett, J. L., Kirkland, D. J., Morita, T., Mosesso, P., and Sofuni, T. (1994). Report from working group on in vitro tests for chromosomal aberrations, *Mutat. Res.,* 312, 241–261.

Gatehouse, D., Haworth S., Cebula, T., Gocke, E., Kier, L., Matsushima, T., Melcion, C., Nohmi, T., Ohta, T., Venitt, S., and Zeiger, E. (1994). Recommendations for the performance of bacterial mutation assays, *Mutat. Res.,* 312, 217–233.

George, E., Wootton, A. K., and Gatehouse, D. G. (1990). Micronucleus induction by azobenzene and 1,2-dibromo-3-chloropropane in the rat: Evaluation of a triple-dose protocol, *Mutat. Res.,* 234, 129–134.

Gold, L. S., Slone, T. H., Stern, B. R., and Bernstein L. (1993). Comparison of target organs of carcinogenicity for mutagenic and non-mutagenic chemicals, *Mutat. Res.,* 286, 75–100.

Gossen, J. A., de Leeuw, W. J. F., Tan, C. H. T., Zwarthoff, E. C., Berends, F., Lohman, P. H. M., Knook, D. L., and Vijg, J. (1989). Efficient rescue of integrated shuttle vectors from transgenic mice: A model for studying mutations in vivo, *Proc. Natl. Acad. Sci. USA,* 86, 7971–7975.

Gossen, J. A., de Leeuw, W. J. F., and Vijg, J. (1994). *LacZ* transgenic mouse models: Their application in genetic toxicology, *Mutat. Res.,* 307, 451–459.

Green, M. H. L. (1984). Mutation testing using $Trp^+$ reversion in *Escherichia coli*. In *Handbook of Mutagenicity Test Procedures*, 2nd ed. (B. J. Kilbey, M. Legator, W. Nichols, and C. Ramel, eds.), Elsevier, Amsterdam, pp. 161–187.

Green, S., Auletta, A., Fabricant, J., Kapp, R., Manandhar, M., Sheu, C., Springer, J., and Whitfield, B. (1985). Current status of bioassays in genetic toxicology—the dominant lethal assay: A report of the U. S. Environmental Protection Agency Gene-Tox Program, *Mutat. Res.,* 154, 49–67.

Hayashi, M., Sofuni, T., and Ishidate M., Jr. (1983). An application of acridine orange fluorescent staining to the micronucleus test, *Mutat. Res.,* 120, 241–247.

Hayashi, M., Morita, T., Kodama, Y., Sofuni, T., and Ishidate M., Jr. (1990). The micronucleus assay with mouse peripheral blood reticulocytes using acridine orange-coated slides, *Mutat. Res.,* 245, 245–249.

Hayashi, M., Tice, R. R., MacGregor, J. T., Anderson, D., Blakey, D. H., Kirsh-Volders, M., Oleson, F. B., Jr., Pacchierotti, F., Romagna, F., Shimada, H., Sutou, S., and Vannier, B. (1994). In vivo rodent erythrocyte micronucleus assay, *Mutat. Res.,* 312, 293–304.

Heddle, J. A., Hite, M., Kirkhart, B., Mavournin K., MacGregor, J. T., Newell, G. W., and Salamone, M. F. (1983). The induction of micronuclei as a measure of genotoxicity: A report of the U. S. Environmental Protection Agency Gene-Tox Program, *Mutat. Res.,* 123, 61–118.

Hsie, A. W., Casciano, D. A., Couch, D. B., Krahn, D. F., O'Neill, J. P., and Whitfield, B. L. (1981). The use of Chinese hamster ovary cells to quantify specific locus mutation and to determine mutagenicity of chemicals: A report of the U. S. Environmental Protection Agency Gene-Tox Program, *Mutat. Res.,* 86, 193–214.

Ishidate, M., Jr., Harnois, M. C., and Sofuni, T. (1988). A comparative analysis of data on the clastogenicity of 951 chemical substances tested in mammalian cell cultures, *Mutat. Res.,* 195, 151–213.

Ishidate, M., Jr. and Sofuni, T. (1985). The in vitro chromosomal aberration test using Chinese hamster lung (CHL) fibroblast cells in culture. In *Evaluation of Short-Term Tests for Carcinogens*. Report of the International Programme on Chemical Safety's Collaborative Study on in vitro Assays (J. Ashby, F. J. de Serres, M. Draper, M. Ishidate, Jr., B. H. Margolin, B. E. Matter, and M. D. Shelby, eds.), Elsevier, Amsterdam, pp. 427–432.

Jones, I. M., Burkhart-Schultz, K., and Carrano, A. V. (1985). A method to quantify spontaneous and in vivo induced thioguanine-resistant mouse lymphocytes, *Mutat. Res.,* 147, 97–105.

Kirkland, D. J. (1993). Genetic toxicology testing requirements: Official and unofficial views from Europe, *Environ. Mol. Mutagen.,* 21, 8–14.

Kier, L. E., Brusick, D. J., Auletta, A. E., von Halle, E. S., Brown, M. M., Simmon, V. F., Dunkel, V., McCann J., Montelmans, K., Prival, M., Rao, T. K. and Ray, V. (1986). The *Salmonella typhimurium*/mammalian microsomal assay: A report of the U. S. Environmental Protection Agency Gene-Tox Program, *Mutat. Res.,* 168, 69–240.

Knudson, A. G. (1993). Antioncogenes and human cancer, *Proc. Natl. Acad. Sci. USA,* 90, 11914–11921.

Kohler, S. W., Provost, G. S., Fiek, A., Kretz, P. L., Bulock, W. O., Sorge, J. A., Putman, D. L., and Short, J. M. (1991). Spectra of spontaneous and mutagen-induced mutations in the *lacl* gene in transgenic mice, *Proc. Natl. Acad. Sci. USA,* 88, 7958–7962.

Kozak, C. A., and Ruddle, F. H. (1977). Assignment of the genes for thymidine kinase and galactokinase to *Mus musculus* chromosome 11 and the preferential segregation of this chromosome in Chinese hamster/mouse somatic cell hybrids, *Somatic Cell Genet.,* 3, 121–133.

Kretz, P. L., Lundberg, K. S., Provost, G. S., and Short, J. M. (1992). The lamda/*lacl* transgenic mutagenesis systems: Comparisons between a selectable and a non-selectable system, *Environ. Mol. Mutagen.,* 19 (Suppl. 20), 31.

Lee, W. R., Abrahamson, S., Valencia, R., von Halle, E., Wurgler, F. E., and Zimmering S. (1983). The sex-linked recessive lethal test for mutagenesis in *Drosophila melanogaster:* A report of the U. S. Environmental Protection Agency Gene-Tox Program, *Mutat. Res.,* 123, 183–279.

Legator, M. S., Bueding, E., Batzinger, R., Connor, T. H., Eisenstadt, E., and Farrow, M. G. (1982). An evaluation of the host-mediated assay and body fluid analysis: A report of the U. S. Environmental Protection Agency Gene-Tox Program, *Mutat. Res.,* 98, 319–374.

Levin, D. E. I., Hollstein, M., Charistman, M. F., Schwiers, E. A., and Ames, B. N. (1982). A new *Salmonella* tester strain (TA102) with A–T base pairs at the site of mutation detects oxidative mutagens, *Proc. Natl. Acad. Sci. USA,* 79, 7445–7449.

Li, A. P. and Heflich, R. H. (1991). *Genetic Toxicology,* CRC Press, Boca Raton, FL.

Li, A. P., Carver, J. H., Choy, W. N., Hsie, A. W., Gupta, R. S., Loveday, K. S., O'Neill, J. P., Riddle, J. C., Stankowski, L. F., and Yang, L. L. (1987). A guide for the performance of the Chinese hamster ovary cell/hypoxanthine guanine phosphoribosyltransferase gene mutation assay, *Mutat. Res.,* 189, 135–141.

Littlefield, J. W. (1976). *Variation, Senescence, and Neoplasia in Culture Somatic Cells,* Harvard University Press, Cambridge, MA.

Lundberg, K. S., Kretz, P. L., Provost, G. S., and Short, J. M. (1993). The use of selection in recovery of transgenic targets for mutation analysis, *Mutat. Res.,* 301, 99–105.

MacGregor, J. T., Wehr, C. M., and Gould, D. H. (1980). Clastogen-induced micronuclei in peripheral blood erythrocytes: The basis of an improved micronucleus tests, *Environ. Mutagen.,* 2, 509–514.

MacGregor, J. T., Schlegel, R., Choy, W. N., and Wehr, C. M. (1983). Micronuclei in circulating erythrocytes: A rapid screen for chromosomal damage during routine toxicity testing in mice. In *Developments in the Science and Practice of Toxicology* (A. W. Hayes, R. C. Schnell, and T. S. Miya, eds.), Elseveir, Amsterdam, pp. 555–558.

MacGregor, J. T., Heddle, J. A., Hite, M., Margolin, B. H., Ramel, C., Salamone, M. F., Tice, R. R., and Wild, D. (1987). Guidelines for the conduct of micronucleus assays in mammalian bone marrow erythrocytes, *Mutat. Res.,* 189, 103–112.

MacGregor, J. T., Wehr, C. M., Henika, P. R., and Shelby, M. D. (1990). The in vivo erythrocyte micronucleus test: Measurement as steady state increases assay efficacy and permits integration with toxicity studies, *Fundam. Appl., Toxicol.,* 14, 513–522.

Madle, S., Dean, S. W., Andrae, U., Brambilla, C., Burlinson, B., Doolittle, D. J., Furihata, C., Hertner, T., McQueen, C. A., and Mori, H.(1994). Recommendations for the performance of UDS tests in vitro and in vivo, *Mutat. Res.,* 312, 263–285.

Maron, D. M. and Ames, B. N. (1983). Revised methods for the *Salmonella* mutagenicity tests, *Mutat. Res.,* 113, 173–215.

Martin, C.N., McDermid, A. C., and Garner, R. C. (1978). Testing of known carcinogens and noncarcinogens for their ability to induce unscheduled DNA synthesis in HeLa cells, *Cancer Res.,* 38, 2621–2627.

Mavournin, K. H., Blakey, D. H., Cimino, M. C., Salamone, M. F., and Heddle, J. A. (1990). The in vivo micronucleus assay in mammalian bone marrow and peripheral blood: A report of the U. S. Environmental Protection Agency Gene-Tox Program, *Mutat. Res.,* 239, 29–80.

[MHW] Ministry of Health and Welfare, Japan (1990). *1990 Guidelines for Toxicity Studies of Drugs Manual,* MHW, Japan, Yakuji Nippo, Tokyo, Japan.

Michaelis, K. C., Helvering, L. M., Kindig, D. E., Garriott, M. L., and Richardson, K. K. (1994). Localization of xanthine guanine phosphoribosyl transferase gene (gpt) of *E. coli* in AS52 metaphase cells by fluorescence in situ hybridization. *Environ. Mol. Mutagen.,* 24, 176–180.

Mirsalis, J. C. (1987). In vivo measurement of unscheduled DNA synthesis and hepatic cell proliferation as an indicator of hepatocarcinogenesis in rodents, *Cell Biol. Genet. Toxicol.,* 3, 165–173.

Mirsalis, J. C. (1988). Summary report on the performance of the in vivo DNA repair assays. In *Evaluation of Short-Term Tests for Carcinogens.* Report of the International Programme on Chemical Safety's Collaborative Study on In Vivo Assays (J. Ashby, F. J. de Serres, M. D. Shelby, B. H. Margolin, M. Ishidate, Jr., and G. C. Becking, eds.), Cambridge University Press, Cambridge, UK, pp. 1.345–1.351.

Mirsalis, J. C. and Butterworth, B. E. (1980). Detection of unscheduled DNA synthesis in hepatocytes isolated from rats treated with genotoxic agents: An in vivo–in vitro assay for potential carcinogens and mutagens, *Carcinogenesis,* 1, 621–625.

Mirsalis, J. C., Tyson, C. K., and Butterworth, B. E. (1982). Induction of DNA repair in hepatocytes from rats treated in vivo with genotoxic agents, *Environ. Mutagen.,* 4, 553–562.

Mirsalis, J. C., Steinmetz, K. L., Bakke, J. P., Tyson, C. K., Loh, E. K. N., Hamilton, C. M., Ramsey, M. J., and Spalding, J. (1986). Genotoxicity and tumor promoting capabilities of blue hair dyes in rodent and primate liver, *Environ. Mutagen.,* 8(Suppl. 6), 55–56.

Mirsalis, J. C., Tyson, C. K., Loh, E. N., Bakke, J. P., Hamilton, C. M., and Steinmetz, K. L. (1988a). An evaluation of the ability of benzo[a]pyrene, pyrene, 2- and 4-acetylaminofluorene to induce unscheduled DNA synthesis and cell proliferation in the livers of male rats and mice treated in vivo. In *Evaluation of Short-Term Tests for Carcinogens.* Report of the International Programme on Chemical Safety's Collaborative Study on in vivo Assays (J. Ashby, F. J. de Serres, M. D. Shelby, B. H. Margolin, M. Ishidate, Jr., and G. C. Becking, eds.), Cambridge University Press, Cambridge, UK, pp. 1.361–1.366.

Mirsalis, J. C., Tyson, C. K., Loh, E. N., Steinmetz, K. L., Bakke, J. P., Spalding, C. M., Deahl, J. T., and Spalding, J. W. (1988b). Induction of hepatic cell proliferation and unscheduled DNA synthesis in mouse hepatocytes following in vivo treatment, *Carcinogenesis,* 6, 1521–1524.

Mirsalis, J. C., Tyson, C. K., Steinmetz, K. L., Loh, E. N., Hamilton, C. M., Bakke, J. P., and Spalding, J. W. (1989). Measurement of unscheduled DNA synthesis and S-phase synthesis in rodent hepatocytes following in vivo treatment: Testing of 24 compounds, *Environ. Mutagen.,* 14, 155–164.

Mitchell, A. D., Casciano, D. A., Meltz, M. L., Robinson, D. F., San, R. H. C., Williams, G. M., and Von Halle, E. S. (1983). Unscheduled DNA synthesis test: A report of the U. S. Environmental Protection Agency Gene-Tox Program, *Mutat. Res.,* 123, 363–410.

Mitelman, F. (1988). *Catalog of Chromosome Aberrations in Cancer,* Alan R. Liss, New York.

Morita, T., Nagaki, T., Fukuda, I., and Okumura, K. (1992). Clastogenicity of low pH to various cultured mammalian cells, *Mutat. Res.,* 268, 297–305.

Morley, A. A., Trainor, K. J., Seshadri, R., and Ryall, R. G. (1983). Measurement of in vivo mutations in human lymphocytes, *Nature,* 302, 155–156.

Myhr, B. C., Custer, L., Khouri, H., Gesswein, G., Haworth, S., Brusick, D., Gossen, J., and Vijg, J. (1993). Positive selection for *lacZ*⁻ mutations in Muta Mouse tissues, *Environ. Mol. Mutagen.,* 21(Suppl. 22), 50.

Nestmann, E. R., Brillinger, R. L., Gilman, J. P. W., Rudd, C. J., and Swierenga, S. H. H. (1991). Recommended protocols based on a survey of current practice in genotoxicity testing laboratories: II. Mutation in Chinese hamster ovary, V79 Chinese hamster lung and L5178Y mouse lymphoma cells, *Mutat. Res.,* 246, 255–284.

[OECD] Organization for Economic Cooperation and Development (1983, 1984, 1986). *Guidelines for Genetic Toxicology,* OECD, Paris, France.

Preston, R. J., Au, W., Bender, M. A., Brewen, J. G., Carrano, A. V., Heddle, J. A., McFee, A., Wolff, S., and Wassom, J. S. (1981). Mammalian in vivo and in vitro cytogenetic assays: A report of the U. S. Environmental Protection Agency Gene-Tox Program, *Mutat. Res.,* 87, 143–188.

Preston, R. J., San Sebastian, J. R., and McFee, A. F. (1987). The in vitro human lymphocyte assay for assessing the clastogenicity of chemical agents, *Mutat. Res.,* 189, 175–183.

Russell, L. B. and Shelby, M. D. (1985). Tests for heritable genetic damage and for evidence of gonadal exposure in mammals, *Mutat. Res.,* 154, 69–84.

Russell, L. B., Selby, P. B., van Halle, E., Sheridan, W., and Valcovic, L. (1981). The mouse specific locus test with agents other than radiations: Interpretation of data and recommendations for future work, *Mutat. Res.,* 86, 329–354.

San, R. H. C. and Stich, H. G. (1975). DNA repair synthesis in cultured human cells as a rapid bioassay for chemical carcinogens, *Int. J. Cancer,* 16, 284–291.

Schmid, W. (1976). The micronucleus test for cytogenetic analysis. In *Chemical Mutagens: Principles and Methods for Their Detection,* Vol. 4 (A. Hollander, ed.), Plenum Press, New York, pp. 31–53.

Scott, D., Galloway, S. M., Marshall, R. R., Ishidate, M., Jr., Brusick, D., Ashby, J., and Myhr, B. C. (1991). Genotoxicity under extreme culture conditions. A report from ICPEMC Task Group, *Mutat. Res.,* 257, 147–204.

Shelby, M. D. (1988). The genetic toxicity of human carcinogens and its implications, *Mutat. Res.,* 204, 3–15.

Shelby, M. D. and Zeiger, E. (1990). Activity of human carcinogens in the *Salmonella* and rodent bone marrow cytogenetics test, *Mutat. Res.,* 234, 257–261.

Short, J. M., ed. (1994). Transgenic systems in mutagenesis and carcinogenesis, *Mutat. Res.,* 307, 247–595.

Sofuni, T. (1993). Japanese guidelines for mutagenicity testing, *Environ. Mol. Mutagen.,* 21, 2–7.

Stankwoski, L. F., and Hsie, A. W. (1986). Quantitative and molecular analyses of radiation-induced mutation in AS52 cells, *Radiat. Res.,* 105, 37–48.

Stankowski, L. F., Jr. and Tindall, K. R. (1987). Characterization of the AS52 cell line for use in mammalian cell mutagenesis studies. In *Mammalian Cell Mutagenesis, Banbury Report 28* (M. M. Moore, D. M. DeMarini, F. J. de Serres, and K. R. Tindall, eds.), Cold Spring Harbor Laboratory Press, Cold Spring Harbor, NY, pp. 71–79.

Steinmetz, K. L., Green, C. E., Bakke, J. P., Spak, D. K., and Mirsalis, J. C. (1988). Induction of unscheduled DNA synthesis in primary cultures of rat, mouse, hamster, monkey and human hepatocytes, *Mutat. Res.,* 206, 91–102.

Stich, H. F. and San, R. H. C. (1981). *Short-Term Tests for Chemical Carcinogens,* Springer-Verlag, New York.

Swierenga, S. H. H., Bradlaw, J. A., Brillinger, R. L., Gilman, J. P. W., Nestmann, E. R., and San, R. C. (1991a). Recommended protocols based on a survey of current practice in genotoxicity testing laboratories: I. Unscheduled DNA synthesis assay in rat hepatocyte cultures, *Mutat. Res.,* 246, 235–253.

Swierenga, S. H. H., Heddle, J. A., Sigal, E. A., Gilman, J. P. W., Brillinger, R. L., Douglas, G. R., and Nestmann, E. R. (1991b). Recommended protocols based on a survey of current practice in genotoxicity testing laboratories. IV. Chromosome aberration and sister-chromatid exchange in Chinese hamster ovary, V79 chinese hamster lung and human lymphocyte cultures, *Mutat. Res.,* 246, 301–322.

Tennant, R. W., Spalding, J. W., Stasiewicz, S., Caspary, W. D., Mason, J. M., and Resnick, M. A. (1987). Comparative evaluation of genetic toxicity patterns of carcinogens and noncarcinogens: Strategies for predictive use of short-term assays, *Environ. Health Perspect.,* 75, 87–95.

Tennant, R. W., Hansen, L., and Spalding, J. (1994). Gene manipulation and genetic toxicology, *Mutagenesis,* 9, 171–174.

Tinwell, H., ed. (1990). Serial versus single dosing protocols for the rodent bone marrow micronucleus assay, *Mutat. Res.,* 234, 111–261.

Tindall, K. R. and Stankowski, L. F., Jr. (1987). Deletion mutations are associated with the differential induced mutant frequency response of the AS52 and CHO-K1-BH4 cell lines. In *Mammalian Cell*

*Mutagenesis, Banbury Report 28* (M. M. Moore, D. M. DeMarini, F. J. de Serres, and K. R. Tindall, eds.), Cold Spring Harbor Laboratory Press, Cold Spring Harbor, NY, pp. 283–292.

UKEMS. (1990). *Basic Mutagenicity Tests: UKEMS Recommended Procedures* (D. J. Kirkland, ed.), Cambridge University Press, Cambridge, UK.

[USEPA] U. S. Environmental Protection Agency (1985). *Health Effects Testing Guidelines,* Part 798, Subpart F-Genetic Toxicity, *Fed. Reg.,* 50, 39435–39458.

[USEPA] U. S. Environmental Protection Agency (1986). *Guidelines for Mutagenicity Risk Assessment, Fed. Reg.,* 51, 34006–34012.

[USEPA] U. S. Environmental Protection Agency (1987). *Revision of TSCA Test Guidelines, Fed. Reg.,* 52, 19078–19081.

[USFDA] U. S. Food and Drug Administration (1982). *Toxicological Principles for the Safety Assessment of Direct Food Additives and Color Additives Used in Food, "Redbook I."* Bureau of Foods.

[USFDA] U. S. Food and Drug Administration (1983). *Toxicological Principles for the Safety Assessment of Direct Food Additives and Color Additives Used in Foods, "Redbook II."* Center for Food Safety and Applied Nutrition. Draft.

Wilcox, P., Naidoo, A., Wedd, D. J., and Gatehouse, D. G. (1990). Comparison of *Salmonella typhimurium* TA102 with *Escherichia coli* WP2 tester strains, *Mutagenesis,* 5, 285–291.

Williams, G. M. (1977). Detection of chemical carcinogens by unscheduled DNA synthesis in rat liver primary cell cultures, *Cancer Res.,* 37, 1845–1851.

Williams, G. M., Tong, C., and Brat, S. V. (1985). Tests with the rat hepatocyte primary culture/DNA repair test. In *Evaluation of Short-Term Tests for Carcinogens.* Report of the International Programme on Chemical Safety's Collaborative Study on In Vitro Assays (J. Ashby, F. J. de Serres, M. Draper, M. Ishidate, Jr., B. H. Margolin, B. E. Matter, and M. D. Shelby, eds.), Elsevier, Amsterdam, pp. 341–345.

# 11
# The Design, Evaluation, and Interpretation of Developmental Toxicity Tests

**John M. DeSesso**
*The MITRE Corporation*
*McLean, Virginia*

**Stephen B. Harris**
*Stephen B. Harris Group*
*San Diego, California*

**Stella M. Swain**
*San Diego State University*
*San Diego, California*

## I. INTRODUCTION

Mammalian reproduction and embryonic development are complicated and carefully controlled phenomena at all levels of biological organization. Although a knowledge of reproductive physiology and embryology are helpful for understanding the mechanisms whereby environmental toxicants interfere with these processes, many individuals who are responsible for the review of developmental toxicity safety test reports have not had significant experience in these areas. Consequently, the present chapter will briefly summarize the essentials of the science underlying regulatory developmental toxicology.

The reasons for performing reproductive and developmental toxicology safety tests are to identify substances that are potentially hazardous to development and to establish a no-observable adverse effect level (NOAEL). Hence, these findings should be the focus of the developmental toxicity reports, which are the first steps in the assessment of human developmental risk.

Since many reviewers of developmental toxicology reports are not trained in these specialized areas of toxicology, we have included brief descriptions of, and commentaries on, the underlying assumptions, basic experimental design, kinds of data that are collected, and interpretation of conventional developmental toxicity studies. More detailed information about the regulatory requirements and the theory underlying developmental toxicity testing have been published elsewhere (USFDA, 1966; USEPA, 1982, 1985, 1991a; Ministry of Health and Welfare, 1973; OECD, 1981; IRLG, 1981; Wilson, 1973; Schardein, 1985; Manson and Kang, 1989).

## II.  GENERAL CONSIDERATIONS

## A.  Animals

### 1.  Appropriate Test Animals

Disease-free animals of similar reproductive age and parity and possessing uniform genetic background should be used. Females should be nulliparous (virgin) because the confirmation of pregnancy in previously gravid females is not easily resolved. Animal husbandry practices are a necessity in the laboratory (NIH, 1985) and should comply with guidance issued by the U. S. Department of Agriculture (USDA, 1970, 1990).

### 2.  Choice of Species

Registration of products that are intended for use in foods (i.e., when tolerances or exemptions from tolerances are to be considered) and for nonfood uses, when women of reproductive age are likely to be exposed to significant amounts of the product, requires developmental toxicity testing in two species. The usual test species are one rodent (rat or mouse) and one nonrodent (rabbit). Although the use of different species may be acceptable, a clear justification of the selection of the species will be required. The species that responds to the test agent most like humans (i.e., the "most appropriate" animal species) should be used to estimate risk. When a particular species is not known to react to the test substance like humans, the most sensitive species is used for risk estimation. The rationale for this, is that, for those agents that are known to be human developmental toxicants, humans are at least as sensitive as the most sensitive animal species (Kimmel and Price, 1990).

## B.  Test Material and Exposure

### 1.  Purity of the Test Substance

Impurities in the test material may play an important role in the potential reproductive or developmental toxicity of a compound. In some cases, the impurities may be responsible for any observed adverse effects. For this reason, the purity of the test compound and the identity of all impurities should be disclosed in the final report. Usually, it is the active ingredient (i.e., the technical material intended for commercial use) that is tested; consequently, testing of the product formulation is not required.

### 2.  Dosing Formulations

Test substances are rarely administered neat, but rather are mixed with either vehicle, drinking water, or feed for administration to the test animals. Obviously, it is essential that the concentration of test material in the exposure formulation be accurate. Predosing and postdosing chemical analyses of the exposure formulations should be performed to confirm the accuracy of the calculated concentration. A major problem in reproductive and developmental toxicology studies arises when the administered dose of test agent is not the intended dose. This most commonly occurs when the analyzed concentration of test agent in the exposure formulation is not the same as the nominal, or target, concentration specified in the protocol. The analytical concentrations of the exposure formulations should fall within $\pm 10\%$ of the target concentration. If the analytical exposure concentrations are outside the target range, the study should be rejected.

### 3.  Vehicle

When a vehicle is used to administer the test agent, a control group of animals should be administered an equal volume of the vehicle without the test substance. The vehicle should not cause either parental or developmental toxicity. If there is inadequate information concerning the potential toxicity of the vehicle, the rationale for the choice of that vehicle should be provided. A sham and an untreated control group may be required if the toxicity of the vehicle is unknown.

### 4. Route of Exposure

The route of exposure selected for reproductive and developmental toxicity studies should be the likely route of human exposure.

### 5. Concurrence of Test Groups

All treated and control groups should run concurrently. While staggering the induction of pregnancy within dose groups is acceptable, the mean time of induction of pregnancy should not differ significantly among the treated and control groups. Prolonged periods before achieving the mandated number of presumed pregnant females in the study suggest a mating problem that could be caused by such factors as poor health among the animals or a stressful environment in the animal facility.

## C. Documentation

### 1. Study Protocol

The protocol is a detailed description of all aspects for the planned study, including test species, dosage levels, mode of exposure, numbers of animals per group, and all observations that are to be made. The study protocol should clearly define the timing and types of all maternal and fetal observations, including all methods of fetal examination. If these methods are not adequately addressed in the protocol, they should be available in the standard operating procedures of the laboratory. It is imperative that these procedures are spelled-out.

Although the protocol must meet the requirements of the guidelines and testing requirements of the appropriate regulatory agencies, it must be understood that the testing requirements are minimum data needs. Additional testing or modification of routine study designs may be required to assess the developmental toxicity potential of a particular agent. For instance, deviations from basic protocols are acceptable with proper reasoning. An example of this would be a situation in which a postnatal phase may be necessary to distinguish dilated renal pelvis (which is a reversible condition) from true hydronephrosis (a kidney malformation).

All experimental data must be accurately recorded and quality-assured. This can be achieved by performing data inspections and audits according to the Good Laboratory Practices (GLPs) regulations promulgated by the U. S. Food and Drug Administration (USFDA; 1978) and guidance that was subsequently developed by the European Chemical Industry Ecology and Toxicology Center (1979), the Organization for Economic Cooperation and Development (OECD; 1982) and the U. S. Environmental Protection Agency (USEPA; 1983a,b). Compliance with GLPs provides a framework for the practice of good science and helps facilitate the reconstruction of a study in the event it becomes necessary. Although the purpose of these guidelines is to ensure the quality and integrity of the data, they were not intended to limit informed scientific judgment when the data are inconclusive.

### 2. Presentation of Findings

Well-organized, clear table formats should be used to present both individual animal and summary data because they facilitate both scientific and regulatory audit and review. It is imperative that all reported parental and fetal findings be readily traceable to individual animals from which they were derived. The data should be displayed such that the identity of any female presenting with any clinical sign on any gestational day can be readily accessed by the reviewer. Similarly, the complete identity of each fetus (including maternal parent) that exhibited a given variation or malformation should be easily traceable. All reported mean data should be carefully compared with the individual data from which the mean was calculated for possible inconsistencies. The appropriate use of statistical methods should be verified.

### 3.  Final Reports

All reports submitted as final must be signed and dated by both the Study Director and the Director of Quality Assurance. Any report that fails to be so signed and dated should be considered a draft report that may be changed. It should be assumed that unsigned reports do not represent the final conclusions of the laboratory. Draft reports cannot be used to fulfill regulatory requirements.

## III.  DEVELOPMENTAL TOXICITY STUDIES

## A.  Introduction

Developmental toxicity studies determine whether a test agent administered to a pregnant mammal causes adverse effects on her offspring. Although data from the pregnant dam are collected throughout the study and analyzed in the final report, the four major endpoints of developmental toxicity studies relate to the offspring. These endpoints include the death of developing offspring, structural abnormalities in offspring (congenital malformations), altered growth, and functional deficits. All four manifestations are considered important; a biologically significant increase in any of them suggests that the test agent disrupts development and poses a developmental hazard. Standard developmental toxicity tests are designed to examine the potential for test compounds to induce the first three manifestations. Although functional deficits have seldom been evaluated in routine testing, several recent developmental toxicity assessments have included functional evaluations (USEPA 1986, 1988, 1989, 1991b).

## B.  Testing Procedures

### 1.  Type of Study

The main types of developmental toxicity studies are the range-finding or pilot and the definitive developmental toxicity (segment II) studies. A range-finding study determines the dose levels to be used in the definitive developmental toxicity study. A range-finding study uses more dose levels with fewer animals per group than the definitive study. A typical range-finding study consists of four to six dose groups of eight to ten pregnant animals each. A successful range-finding study establishes the dose of test substance that causes minimal maternal toxicity (to be used as the high dose in the definitive study) and a dose that elicits no adverse effects in the offspring (to be used as the low dose). In-life maternal data collection requirements in the pilot study are virtually identical with those of the definitive study, but the data collected at term are usually limited to gross examination and weighing of fetuses.

The goal of a definitive developmental toxicity study is the determination of whether or not the test agent causes adverse effects in developing organisms and, if so, the establishment of the NOAEL. A copious amount of postmortem data is collected in the definitive developmental toxicity study.

## C.  Experimental Design

### 1.  Dose Selection

The doses that are used in the definitive developmental toxicity study are based on the results of the range-finding study. Except when the biological, physical, or chemical properties of the test agent limit the exposure amount, the highest dose should cause overt maternal toxicity (e.g., statistically significant reduction in maternal body weight or body weight gain). The dose is considered too high if more than 10% of the treated dams die. Dose levels that produce excessive, but nonlethal, maternal toxicity may produce an unexpected increase in fetal deaths or abortions. Studies that experience excessive maternal deaths or loss of the products of conception have limited usefulness in determining developmental toxicity potential and may have to be repeated. Although excessive maternal toxicity must be avoided, a study in which the high dose causes no maternal toxicity may also have to be repeated. Ideally, the range of doses in a developmental toxicity should be set such that the high dose causes mild maternal toxicity and the low dose should produce no adverse effects on the pregnant animal or her offspring.

## 2. Treatment Group

A sufficient number of treatment groups should be used to establish a dose–response relationship. At a minimum, three treatment groups at different dose levels and a concurrent vehicle-treated control group are required. The number of animals per group should be large enough to provide statistical power for the results. The number suggested in most regulatory guidance is 20 pregnant rodents (we recommend 30 pregnant mice or hamsters; 25 pregnant rats) and 12–16 pregnant rabbits (we recommend 20 pregnant rabbits). If body weight data are to be used as an indicator of potential toxicity, test animals must be randomized in a way that ensures that all dose groups (including the control group) start with similar mean maternal body weights and variances. Although a positive control is not required by regulators, a concurrent positive control group should be considered for inclusion in the study design if the laboratory performing the study is inexperienced.

## 3. Exposure Period

Adequate study designs for developmental toxicity studies (USFDA, 1966; USEPA, 1985; OECD, 1981; Kimmel and Price, 1990) require timed-mating of healthy laboratory animals. The usual reference point for timing of gestation defines gestational day 0 in one of the following ways, depending on the species used and method of breeding. Gestational day 0 is (1) the day that a vaginal plug is detected (in rats or mice), or (2) the day that sperm are found in the vaginal lavage (in rats), or (3) the day that mating was observed (rabbits), or (4) the day that artificial insemination was performed (rabbits). Exposure of assumed pregnant animals continues throughout the time of major organogenesis (days 6–15 for rats and mice; 6–18 or 7–19 for rabbits; and 5–14 for hamsters; see Table 3 in Chapter 4). In experiments wherein the test agent is not incorporated into drinking water or feed and the animals must be individually exposed by technicians (e.g., by gastric intubation), dosing should be performed at the same time each day with no longer than 2 hr elapsing between the dosing of the first and last animals, if possible. The timing of exposure is a critical consideration in developmental toxicology studies because embryological schedules operate during narrow periods of time during gestation. This is especially true in those species with short gestations, such as those that are routinely used in developmental toxicity studies.

## 4. Extended Exposure Regimens

Occasionally, a study design may require the exposure of pregnant animals to begin at the end of implantation and continue throughout the entire period of gestation. Such an extended exposure design may provide results that disclose developmental changes that would not be detected under the exposure conditions of a standard developmental toxicity study. For instance, continuous treatment of pregnant animals from the beginning of organogenesis to cesarean section often causes a higher incidence of growth retardation, characterized by decreased mean fetal body weights, than is seen under standard studies. An extended dosing regimen can cause structural alterations in organs, such as the heart, brain, lungs, and gonads, because these organs undergo significant functional and morphological development after the end of major organogenesis. Thus, the length of the exposure period may affect the findings of a study and must be carefully stated when interpreting the results of the study.

### 5. Study Termination

Pregnant females should be scheduled for cesarean section and sacrifice just before delivery to prevent cannibalization of malformed young (see Chapter 4, Table 3).

## D. In-Life Procedures and Data

As mentioned earlier, good animal husbandry practices (NIH, 1985; USDA, 1970, 1990) must be followed at all times. Animals should be observed at least once daily for mortality, moribundity, and clinical signs. This is usually accomplished at the time of weighing. Additional daily observation times may be scheduled if the test material is known to be toxic.

### 1. Maternal Deaths and Abortions

Factors other than the test agent can cause death of the pregnant animal or abortions. Possible causes of non–test agent-induced maternal death or abortion include maternal disease, environmental factors, and technical errors, such as misdosing of the animals. If a pregnant animal dies, the autopsy records should be inspected to ascertain the probable reason for the death. For instance, if the autopsy records reveal that dam exhibited inflamed (reddened) tracheal lining, pulmonary congestion, nasal discharge, and the presence of fluid in the lungs, then the likely cause of death was either accidental intratracheal intubation, a technician error, or respiratory disease. Another example would be the death of a pregnant rabbit in which the daily clinical signs included localized hair loss (alopecia), decreased or absent appetite (anorexia), and diarrhea. These signs are consistent with the presence of a hairball in the stomach, a common occurrence in rabbits. Therefore, maternal deaths cannot always be accurately interpreted as being due to test agent-induced toxicity, because the death may be caused by an event (whether spontaneous or iatrogenic) that is unrelated to the toxicity of the test agent.

In a similar fashion, abortions and total litter resorptions may be caused by factors that are unrelated to the toxicity of the test agent (Chernoff et al., 1987; Schardein, 1987). For instance, environmental stress from conditions, such as excessive noise in the animal room, deviations in light–dark cycles, and rough manipulation by technicians, may induce abortions, particularly in rabbits. Although total litter resorptions do happen in rabbits, they take place more regularly in rodents (e.g., mice, rats, or hamsters), which do not usually abort.

### 2. Maternal Body Weights and Maternal Body Weight Gains

Optimally, pregnant animals should be weighed daily. Alternatively, dams must be weighted on the following schedule: the day of mating; gestational day 5; each day of the exposure period; at 3- to 5-day intervals during the postdosing period; and at study termination. The maternal body weight gain during specific segments of gestation, especially during the exposure period or throughout major organogenesis, is ordinarily a more sensitive gauge of maternal adverse effect than either the final mean body weight at study termination or the mean body weight gain over the entire gestational period. The increased sensitivity of incremental body weight changes is due to their easy detection and the likelihood that they will not be masked by the "rebound" weight gain that often takes place among treated animals in the postdosing period, after exposure has ended.

### 3. Clinical Signs

Clinical observations are significant qualitative indicators of toxicity. They are objective observations (e.g., presence of tremors, excessive salivation, hunched posture in mice) that should be noted by well-trained technicians. The pilot (range-finding) and other toxicological studies should provide an awareness of the anticipated clinical signs of toxicity induced by the test agent. Such signs are probably among the most reliable criteria of maternal toxicity. In many cases, clinical sign data are a more sensitive indicator of maternal toxicity than changes in maternal body weight or maternal body weight gain.

Documentation of clinical sign data must comprise the identity of the observed effect, its time of onset, intensity, and duration. Examples of clinical observations include the presence of diarrhea, excessive salivation and mastication, discharges from the eyes or nose, hair loss (alopecia), listlessness, tremors, and convulsions. Likewise, changes in respiratory rate, alertness, posture, movement within the cage, consumption of food and water (see next section), color of mucous membranes, color of urine, and frequency of urination should be recorded.

Behavioral changes (e.g., animals that appear aggressive or depressed) reported during daily observations of animals are not as objective as clinical sign data. They are similar to symptoms reported by human patients. Both behavioral changes in animals and symptoms in patients require a subjective interpretation by the reporter. Although changes noted in animal behavior should be recorded, it is not possible to ascertain if behavioral changes are early signs of subclinical toxicity that may be manifested as "objective" clinical signs at higher doses.

### 4. Food and Water Contamination

When the test agent is administered in the feed or drinking water, food and water consumption must be measured daily to calculate the dose. Food and water consumption should also be monitored when the test agent is suspected of causing appetite or excretory effects. Altered food and water consumption after the start of test agent exposure are endpoints that can be used to assess possible maternal effects. It must be recalled, however, that test agents in either the diet or drinking water can cause reduced consumption owing to unpalatability.

## E. Necropsy Procedures and Data

Several detailed descriptions of methods for examining offspring in both pilot and definitive development toxicity studies have been published (Wilson, 1973; Manson and Kang, 1989). Briefly, after the female is humanely killed, her gravid uterus, with the ovaries intact, is removed and weighed. The number of corpora lutea on each ovary are recorded for both rats and rabbits; however, because of the difficulty of differentiating luteal tissue from that of the ovary, this is not necessary in mice. The contents of the uterus are examined by incising it along the antimesometrial border. The numbers and locations of implantation sites, resorptions, and viable and dead fetuses should be recorded. Viable fetuses are removed from the uterus, weighed, and examined to determine sex of each fetus and to discern the presence of any external malformations. Pilot studies require no further offspring analysis; in fact, it is minimally acceptable to record only the numbers of implantation sites, resorptions, and live and dead fetuses. In the definitive developmental toxicology study, further analysis of the offspring takes place. One half of the viable fetuses undergo visceral examination by either dissection (Manson and Kang, 1989; Staples, 1974; Stuckhardt and Poppe, 1984) or the Wilson free-hand razor blade-sectioning technique (Wilson, 1965); the remainder are prepared for the visualization of skeletal structures by staining with dyes specific for bone (alizarin red S) (Staples and Schnell, 1968) or bone and cartilage (alizarin red S–alcian blue) (Inouye, 1976). An alternative procedure subjects all fetuses to fresh, visceral dissections, after which either they are all prepared for skeletal visualization, as just outlined; or one half of the fetuses are decapitated to allow the heads to be prepared for free-hand razor blade sectioning, and the remaining intact fetuses and all bodies are stained for skeletal visualization.

### Maternal Data

Confirmation of Pregnancy.   When the uterus is examined at the time of laparotomy, the presence of offspring or resorption sites is considered evidence of pregnancy. The pregnancy (conception) index for each treatment group can be calculated by dividing the number of confirmed pregnancies in that group by the number of females mated. The pregnancy index is used in the assessment of reproductive performance. Depression of this index relative to that of the control group may indicate a possible reproductive toxic effect only if treatment began before mating and implantation. Since treatment in developmental toxicity studies usually begins after implantation is completed, a low pregnancy index suggests maternal health problems, poor animal husbandry, or that the time for initial dosing was miscalculated (i.e., begun too early).

Pregnancy indices in pregnant animals that are shipped from suppliers are generally lower than the pregnancy indices of animals bred in-house. This is especially true in mice. Developmental toxicity studies will usually have to be repeated if there are statistically significant differences in pregnancy indices among groups.

Number of Corpora Lutea.   Corpora lutea mark the sites on the ovary from which eggs were emitted during ovulation. Each corpus luteum contained a single ovum (egg). This means that the number of corpora lutea equals the number of ova that were available for fertilization. If the corpora lutea outnumber the total number of implantations (i.e., the number of fetuses plus resorption sites), then the litter experienced preimplantation loss. Increased preimplantation loss in a standard developmental toxicity study can *not* be a compound-induced effect because the loss of embryos occurred before the initiation of dosing. Thus, reviewers should examine individual data sheets to verify (1) that dosing did not begin prematurely (i.e., before completion of implantation), and (2) that there is no evidence of environmental stress in the animal facility.

Gravid Uterine Weight and Corrected Maternal Body Weight.   The pregnant uterus together with the ovaries are considered the "products of conception." They are excised by transecting the vagina just inferior to the union of the uterine horns and incising the mesentery connecting them to the posterior body wall. The weight of these organs is a useful measurement when an animal bearing few fetuses per litter is compared with other animals with many fetuses per litter. For instance, if a control animal were to have many more pups than usually expected in a litter, then the average fetal weight within that litter is likely to be less than the usual mean pup weight; conversely, animals that bear litters with only a few (e.g., two or three) fetuses (but not a high number of resorptions), the average pup weight is frequently much greater than the normal average fetal weight. Even though the mean pup weights in the two preceding examples may be significantly different from each other, oftentimes the gravid uterine weights will not differ. The gravid uterine weight can be used to determine how much weight the pregnant female gained as a result of being pregnant, regardless of the number of fetuses.

The corrected maternal body weight is calculated by subtracting the gravid uterine weight (as determined above) from the final body weight of the pregnant dam before sacrifice. Comparison of this measurement among groups allows the determination of whether compound-induced adverse body weight changes were caused primarily by toxic effects in the mother or in the fetal–placental unit (products of conception).

Numbers of Implantations, Resorptions, Living and Dead Fetuses.   In rodents, especially rats and mice, dead offspring may present as resorptions or dead fetuses. This type of finding is termed "fetal wastage." Rabbits either resorb or abort their litters. Together, these findings are considered postimplantation loss. They are expressed as a percentage of the total number of implantations per litter. The causes of fetal wastage include direct lethal effects of the test substance, lethal malformations of the offspring (whether spontaneous or compound-induced), maternal toxicity (whether compound-induced or because of disease), and environmental stress. The presence of a dose–response relationship for fetal wastage strengthens conclusions about the developmental toxicity of a test compound. When one type of postimplantation loss predominates, it may be possible to deduce the time or stage in development at which the test compound was toxic to the developing organism.

The number of live fetuses per litter is also recorded. This endpoint, when presented as the percentage of implantations per litter, provides a measure of a compound's developmental toxicity that includes its ability to kill offspring during all stages of development.

Organ Weights and Clinical Chemistry. Although current regulations do not require the collection of maternal organ weight and clinical chemistry data, dose-related effects on the absolute and relative (absolute organ weight divided by the corrected maternal body weight) maternal organ weights can be useful when assessing maternal toxicity. As an example, the liver often exhibits early signs of toxicity (e.g., induction of enzymes, fatty change, or hydropic change) that are generally associated with increased liver weights. Consequently, if a report provides maternal liver weights, they should not be ignored, but rather, should be carefully evaluated.

Occasionally, clinical chemistry data (e.g., hematology and enzyme markers) are reported in developmental toxicology studies. When they are reported and notable effects are seen, the data may be useful in assessing maternal toxicity, even in the absence of overt signs, such as decreased food consumption.

*Fetal Data*

Fetal Weights. Fetal body weight is a sensitive endpoint for assessing developmental toxicity. Because the sizes of fetuses vary within any litter, the parameter that is assessed is the mean fetal body weight. Reduced mean fetal body weight in treated groups compared with control values is evidence of growth retardation (one of the four major endpoints of developmental toxicity). When the number of fetuses per litter is similar between control and treated groups, decreased mean fetal body weight in a treated litter generally implies a compound-related, embryo–fetotoxic effect. Often, reduced mean fetal body weights may be the only sign of developmental toxicity. When evaluating the data it must be recalled, however, that male fetuses weigh more than females (so the similarity of sex distribution within groups should be verified) and that individual fetal body weights tend to be greater in litters with fewer fetuses (see foregoing section, *Gravid Uterine Weight*).

Little is known about the long-term health effects of fetal body weight reduction on test animal species. When reduced mean fetal body weights are the only findings in a developmental toxicity study, their interpretation is not clear-cut. Modest fetal weight reductions may be only temporary. That is to say, during the postnatal period, fetuses that were smaller at birth may increase in weight, size, and maturation, thereby abolishing any appreciable differences between treated and control pups. In other cases, the fetal weight reduction may be lasting (i.e., offspring fail to recover after birth). The possibility that fetal weight differences may disappear during the perinatal period can be assessed by considering available offspring growth and viability data from multigeneration reproduction studies (wherein the pups are allowed to mature).

Extremely small fetuses, described as "runts" or "stunted," are classified as malformed young. The criteria used to classify runts vary from laboratory to laboratory. Typical criteria are body weights that are two or three standard deviations less than the mean control fetal body weight or 25–30% below the historical mean control body weight.

Fetal Examinations.  Live offspring are usually inspected for the presence of external, soft-tissue and skeletal alterations. All morphological differences from the normal anatomical pattern should be recorded. The differences are classified as malformations, anomalies, or variations according to their severity (Palmer, 1977). Malformations are extreme anatomical changes that interfere with the viability, health, or quality of life of the fetus. Spina bifida, cleft palate, absence of digits, and cyclopia are examples of malformations. Anomalies are minor anatomical changes that cause only a slight amount of fetal impairment. Absence of nails on the digits is an example of an anomaly. Variations are structural alterations that commonly appear in control animals. Asymmetrical sternebrae in rabbits and rodents and bifurcated gallbladder in rabbits are examples of anatomical variations. The determination of whether a particular alteration should be classified as a malformation, an anomaly, or a variation is a subjective process that depends on the training, experience, and competence of the observer. Divergence in the classification of the same fetal alterations by different observers has led to significant disagreements in the conclusions reached by different laboratories studying the same compounds. The ensuing sections offer some guidance concerning the classification of findings during fetal examinations.

Gross structural changes.  At cesarean section, the gravid uterus and fetuses should be manipulated gently. Rough handling of these tissues before the external examination can induce artifactual subcutaneous hemorrhages. Reviewers should be especially wary of studies in which these are the only signs of developmental toxicity. A clue that should lead one to investigate possible technician-induced hemorrhages is their occurrence in both the experimental and control groups.

The fetuses should be recovered and examined quickly to avoid possible artifacts. For example, rodent and rabbit fetuses that remain in the uterus for prolonged times may present with flexed wrists and ankles that can be readily mistaken for arthrogryposis (clubpaws). Similarly, fetuses lingering on the examining table for prolonged intervals before being examined can develop hyperextended or stiff joints.

External fetal examination should include the determination of the sex of each fetus, as well as the presence of any structural alterations. The possibility that a compound may preferentially affect a particular sex should be analyzed, although verified agent-induced effects on sex ratio (number of females/number of males) are quite rare.

Skeletal changes.  Many differences among the skeletal structures of fetuses are so common that a variety of patterns are considered to be "normal." Examples of multiple normal skeletal patterns include the presence of either 13 or 14 pairs of ribs in rodents, either 12 or 13 pairs of ribs in rabbits, and retarded ossification of sternebra number 5 in rodents and rabbits.

Minor abnormal changes in skeletal patterns are called variations. Variations do not seem to adversely impinge on the health or longevity of affected fetuses. Presumably, variations are the consequence of transient delays in developmental schedules. Findings such as reduced ossification in phalanges or sternebrae; permanent supernumerary ribs in the lumbar region, and wavy ribs (which can repair themselves during postnatal development) are examples of variations. Although the biological significance of variations has not been determined, supernumerary ribs in mice and wavy ribs in rats have often been observed in fetuses borne by dams that exhibited nonspecific maternal toxicity. Thus, although skeletal variations such as wavy or supernumerary ribs are not themselves considered to be adverse developmental effects, they may be indicative of maternal toxicity or maternal stress. If a statistically significant, dose-related increase in the incidence of a particular variation (above the concurrent control incidence) is observed, the laboratory's historical control data should be evaluated to assess whether the findings of the study in question are outside the range of a larger population of controls.

If fetuses are removed by cesarean section 12–24 hr earlier than recommended (e.g., on gestational day 19 or 20, rather than on day 21 for rats), development (especially ossification) of some bony elements will not be complete. The bones, although normal for their gestational age, will appear to exhibit what would be described as reduced or absent ossification and are likely to be recorded as variations. Had the fetuses been examined at the recommended time, ossification would have appeared normal. This is because the bones of rodent fetuses ossify rapidly during the last 48 hr of gestation. Thus, scheduling mistakes for sacrifice times can lead to the reporting of spurious increases in developmental variations.

Visceral (soft-tissue) changes. The viscera (organs) of the body are also susceptible to developmental toxicity, although alterations in the viscera are not as readily observed as are those of the external body and skeleton. Visceral malformations commonly occur in the heart and great vessels (e.g., ventricular septal defects, tetralogy of Fallot, transposition of the great vessels), brain (e.g., hydrocephalus), kidneys (e.g., agenesis of kidneys, polycystic kidney), diaphragm (e.g., diaphragmatic hernia), and other organs. A knowledge of the normal anatomy of the test species provides an important context within which to evaluate visceral alterations. For instance, evaluators should know the normal shapes of organs, their usual relation to vessels, nerves, and each other, and the accepted range of normal patterns. Thus, they should know that the diaphragm exhibits both a muscular and a membranous region, and that the membranous region can be transparent. Fetuses can be erroneously reported to exhibit a diaphragmatic hernia if the technician can see through it, and surmises the appropriate portion of the diaphragm is missing without probing the area to discern the presence of a membrane.

The visceral anatomies of test species differ markedly in some respects. For instance, rabbits and mice possess gallbladders, but rats do not. Furthermore, changes in the organs of one species may qualify as a malformation, but the same change may not necessarily be a malformation when seen in others. As examples, presence of a ventral pancreas, accessory spleen, or retroesophageal subclavian artery are malformations when seen in rats, but are considered within the range of normal patterns when they are observed in rabbits.

As when performing cesarean sections and external fetal examinations, dissections should be performed gently and with care. Rough handling of fetuses can induce petechial hemorrhages on the surface of viscera. Improper cutting of the umbilical cord can result in backflow of blood from the placenta into the fetus, causing either intra-abdominal hemorrhage or an apparent hemorrhagic liver. Careless probing or pulling on delicate fetal organs can tear the tissues. The edges of *all* organs, whether malformed or normal, are smooth. Malformed organs do not present with jagged edges. Rather, the presence of jagged edges on organs is an indication that tissue damage occurred during the dissection.

A knowledge of the embryology of the structures being evaluated will aid in determining the classification of any observed alterations. For example, in rabbits, when a bifurcated or duplicated gallbladder is attached to a single bile duct, the finding is not considered to be a malformation. The reasoning behind this is that these alterations ensue from slight shifts in the branching pattern of the hepatic diverticulum during development. Similarly, abnormal lobulations of the liver or accessory renal arteries are not considered to be malformations because they also emanate from slight deviations in normal developmental processes.

## F. Interpretation of Results

### 1. Maternal Toxicity

The endpoints employed to assess maternal toxicity include maternal death, abortion or resorption of litters, reduced maternal body weights and body weight gains, and the presence of clinical signs. Because animals in the high-dose group of the definitive developmental toxicity study should exhibit mild maternal toxicity, the data collected daily during the in-life phase of the study must include the aforementioned signs of maternal toxicity.

Findings in animals of the high-dose group may include some maternal deaths as well as an increased incidence of total litter resorptions and abortions among surviving females, especially in rabbits. Although such findings clearly indicate maternal toxicity, dosages that produce a high proportion of maternal deaths or abortions or total litter resorptions are not desirable because there will be too few offspring for evaluation. Ideally, mild maternal toxicity should occur in only the high-dose group. With some test compounds, however, the dose–response curve for maternal toxicity is steep. In such cases, the difference between a dose that causes maternal death and abortion or total litter resorption and doses that induce less extreme endpoints of maternal toxicity (e.g., decreased body weight gain, tremors) may be small. When that happens, maternal deaths and abortions or total resorptions may be prominent findings even in the lowest-dose group.

Maternal body weight and body weight gain data are sensitive indicators of maternal toxicity. In most test species, these endpoints are frequently the basis for determining the NOAEL for maternal toxicity. Rabbits, however, are an exception because pregnant rabbits often lose weight during a normal pregnancy. Optimally, mean body weight gain (or percentage change in body weight) for all dose groups should be similar during the predosing period. Decreases in mean maternal body weights observed during the treatment period are usually the result of either toxicity of the test compound or decreased food consumption.

In general, test substance-induced reductions in maternal body weights or body weight gains are dose-related. Nevertheless, there may be some situations in which low-dose animals are affected, whereas animals in the high-dose group are not. Examples such as these occur when the high-dose group experienced excessive maternal mortality, eliminating sensitive animals and reducing the number of surviving animals for comparison. In such a situation, the absence of a dose–response in a maternal body weight parameter does *not* imply the absence of a compound-related effect. Likewise, maternal body weight parameters are not useful for determining the presence or absence of a treatment-related maternal effects if a high proportion of surviving females have experienced numerous resorptions per litter. To assess a possible compound-induced effect on the female alone, the starting body weight of the females should be compared with their corrected maternal body weight (terminal body weight minus gravid uterine weight). This removes the variability introduced by the differing uterine weights between those animals that experienced total litter resorptions (or a high proportion of resorptions) versus those that bore a litter to term.

Reduced food consumption is another indicator of possible maternal toxicity. This may be observed soon after the initial exposure, or it may require repeated exposures before becoming apparent. Frequently, when there has been reduced mean body weights during the exposure period, treated animals experience an increase in maternal body weight (adaptation or "rebound" effect) during the postexposure period. This is especially common when the animals reduced their food consumption during the exposure period. To determine whether the reduced food consumption is caused by a maternally toxic effect of the test substance or to unpalatability of the food, another experiment could be performed in which feed intake would be measured in groups of animals presented with either control or treated diet. Alternatively, a food efficiency index (FEI) could be determined for each group. The FEI is the grams of food consumed per gram of body weight gained. The FEI is considered to be a measure of how effectively food is used by the animal (e.g., body weight gain). If the FEIs for the treated and control groups are similar, then a maternally toxic effect is unlikely and unpalatability is the probable cause for reduced food consumption.

Rabbits provide several challenges to the determination of maternal toxicity. Because of their inherent erratic body weight gains and losses during gestation, maternal body weight changes in rabbits are difficult to interpret. During the last week of gestation, rabbits often reduce their food consumption while they attend to preparation of a nest, rather than eating. At the same time, rabbits often experience hair loss (alopecia) in the abdominal region because the hair is being used to construct the nest. Especially for rabbits, it is important to be cognizant of those changes that occur normally and to compare the data in the treated groups with both concurrent control and historical control data when evaluating maternal toxicity.

## 2. *Developmental Toxicity*

When exposure to a test substance is associated with a demonstrable increase in the incidence of any developmental toxicity endpoint, compared with the spontaneous incidence, the agent can be suspected of being a developmental toxicant. The spontaneous incidence is estimated primarily from concurrent control data, but historical control data may also be used (see below). If the increased endpoint is congenital malformations, the agent is a suspected teratogen. Because of the importance of developmental toxicity as a noncancer endpoint for human health risk assessment, determining the existence of a causal relationship between exposure to the test substance and the appearance of the endpoint is crucial.

The results of developmental toxicity tests can be confounded by the proclivity for the fetuses of a given litter to exhibit similar endpoints, thereby artificially increasing the apparent incidence of any given endpoint. This proclivity has been designated the "litter effect." The litter effect is thought to be caused by the fact that all fetuses in any given litter are exposed to the same maternal environment as their littermates (accounting for the similarity in outcomes of that litter), but the maternal environment differs from litter to litter within the same treatment group.

Another potential difficulty in the interpretation of results is that, owing to the large number of offspring that are evaluated, findings may too easily achieve statistical significance (1) if they are analyzed with the statistical methods routinely used in toxicology studies, and (2) if the fetus is the sampling unit. Several statistical procedures have been developed to address this problem (Weil, 1970; Gaylor, 1978; Gad and Weil, 1986). For regulatory purposes, the appropriate sampling unit for developmental toxicity safety tests is the number of treated females (USEPA, 1991a). To address the challenges of varying numbers of fetuses per litter and the litter effect, some statistical procedures express fetal endpoints as incidence per litter and analyze that value, whereas others analyze the number of litters with a fetus (or fetuses) that exhibit a particular endpoint. The choice of statistical methods should be clearly stated in both the protocol and the final report.

The results of statistical analyses alone are not sufficient to judge whether or not an agent should be considered a developmental toxicant. When the level of statistical significance is set at a probability of $p \leq 0.05$, 1 of every 20 (1:20) comparisons will be statistically significant by chance alone. Since so many observations are made and analyzed in developmental toxicity studies (e.g., all of the individual skeletal elements that are checked and all of the viscera that are examined), it should be expected that one to several observations per study will attain statistical significance by chance alone. Consequently, other considerations must be evaluated to resolve whether or not the statistically significant finding is cause for concern.

An important consideration in the determination of developmental toxicity is whether the finding at issue displays a dose–response. When the finding is statistically significant in the higher-dose group(s), a positive dose–response is strong evidence for developmental toxicity. Positive dose-related trends in the incidence of fetal effects, however, may appear without attaining statistical significance in the high-dose group. By way of illustration, a congenital malformation, such as spina bifida, may occur at a low, but dose-related, incidence in the treated groups with none of them being statistically different from control values. When such cases arise, it is important to know the spontaneous incidence of the observed finding in the test species. If the finding is one that rarely occurs in the test species, then the dose-related trend will be an important factor in determining the developmental toxicity of the agent. This is not true if the finding is seen regularly among controls (see following Sec. III F.3).

A second consideration is that the major endpoints (e.g., death, malformation, growth retardation) may be related to each other such that the presence of one precludes the presence of others. For instance, embryonic death obviously prevents growth retardation, functional deficits, and malformations in living fetuses. This helps explain situations in which increased malformation incidences may occur in the low- or mid-dose groups, but not in the high-dose group when the high dose produced a large amount of postimplantation loss. In other cases, when no adverse fetal effects are induced by the low and middle doses, but the high dose elicits extensive postimplantation loss, its teratogenic potential may have been masked. In such an event, a decrease in the magnitude of the high dose might cause fewer embryo or fetal deaths and an increased incidence of malformed surviving fetuses. The preceding discussion notwithstanding, the mechanisms that cause postimplantation loss are not always the same as those leading to malformations (see discussion in Manson and Kang, 1989). That is to say, it is possible for an agent to cause embryo or fetal deaths, but not malformations.

A third consideration is whether or not the dam experienced maternal toxicity during gestation. The developmentally toxic effects of a test agent are considered to be those produced in the absence of maternal toxicity. When adverse fetal effects occur in litters from females that experienced notable maternal toxicity, the fetal effects may have been produced either directly (by the test agent) or indirectly. As alluded to previously, maternal toxicity is associated with a low incidence of "nonspecific" alterations such as wavy ribs, retarded ossification of sternebrae and phalanges, or reduced fetal body weight. Occasionally, adverse fetal effects appear at doses that cause only minimal maternal toxicity. In such instances, the findings should not be interpreted to have been caused by the maternal toxicity. Rather, the findings suggest that both the embryo and the mother are susceptible to the same dose of test agent. Furthermore, the appearance of maternal toxicity in a pregnant dam does not guarantee that adverse fetal effects will occur, because some agents elicit profound maternal toxicity, but exert no apparent adverse effects on offspring.

The final consideration is to realize that *not all malformations are caused by test agents.* Not only can virtually all malformations appear spontaneously (Palmer, 1977), but also a particular malformation can be produced by multiple agents or conditions. Each test species has a background incidence of spontaneously occurring malformations. When malformations arise in the absence of a dose–response, they may be spontaneous in origin. When rare malformations do occur, examination of the laboratory's historical control data (see next discussion) is required to establish whether or not that malformation has been experienced previously.

### 3. Historical Control Data

Laboratories should collect and maintain a database of their control results to serve as the historical data. As discussed in the preceding section, the large amount of data analyzed in developmental toxicity studies increases the likelihood that statistically significant differences between data from treated and control groups will arise by chance alone. At times, even an apparent dose–response may be present. An example of this occurs when the control incidence of a particular effect is lower than usual, whereas its incidence in the high-dose group is slightly greater than normally observed. Knowing the range of incidence among control litters for the effect in question is helpful in the evaluation of the data. When the incidence of the effect in the treated groups is within the range of historical incidence, the finding is likely due to chance. Thus, a laboratory's historical control data may prevent evaluators from falsely concluding that an agent is a developmental toxicant based on statistical significance that arose by random chance. Over time, historical control data provide important information about changes in the incidence of various findings that may be due to such factors as genetic drift, modifications in the animals' diet, seasonal changes, or even differences in the proficiency of technicians in handling animals and recording observations.

## IV. CONCLUSION

The challenge for all subdisciplines of regulatory toxicology is to establish safe levels of exposure for environmental agents. This entails identifying both those exposure levels of test agents that cause adverse effects and those that do not. Developmental toxicity safety tests are a preliminary part of the assessment of a test agent's potential risk to human development. Because of (1) the complicated nature of the maternal–placental–embryonic relationships (see discussion in Chapter 4), (2) the necessity for multidisciplinary scientific knowledge, and (3) the numerous interrelated maternal and fetal parameters that are evaluated, the determination of the developmental toxicity of an agent can be a daunting task. This chapter has provided a concise introduction to the discipline from the perspective of the information that is routinely evaluated in developmental toxicity test reports. The chapter has focused on those aspects of regulatory developmental toxicology that are essential in the critical evaluation of developmental toxicity test results.

## ACKNOWLEDGMENT

Supported in part by MITRE Sponsored Research Project 9587C.

## REFERENCES

Chernoff, N. R., Kavlock, J., Beyer, P. E., and Miller, D. (1987). The potential relationship of maternal toxicity, general stress, and fetal outcome, *Teratogenesis Carcinog. Mutagen.*, 7, 241–253.

European Chemical Industry Ecology and Toxicologic Center (1979). *Good Laboratory Practice,* Monograph No. 1, Brussels, Belgium.

Gad, S. C. and Weil, C. S. (1986). Data analysis applications in toxicology. In *Statistics and Experimental Design for Toxicologists* (S. C. Gad and C. S. Weil, eds.), Telford Press, Caldwell, NJ, pp. 147–175.

Gaylor, D. W. (1978). Methods and concepts of biometrics applied to teratology. In *Handbook of Teratology,* Vol. 1, (J. G. Wilson and F. C. Fraser, eds.), Plenum Press, New York, pp. 429–444.

Inouye, M. (1976). Differential staining of cartilage and bone in fetal mouse skeleton by alcian blue and alizarin red S, *Congenital Anom.,* 16, 171–173.

[IRLG] Interagency Regulatory Liaison Group (1981). *Testing Standards and Guidelines Workgroup, Recommended Guidelines for Teratogenicity Studies in the Rat, Mouse, Hamster or Rabbit,* Publication No. PB-82-119 488, National Technical Information Services, Springfield, VA.

Kimmel, C. A. and Price, C. J. (1990). Developmental toxicity studies. In *Handbook of In Vivo Toxicity Testing* (D. L. Arnold, H. C. Grice, and D. R. Krewski, eds.), Academic Press, San Diego, CA, pp. 271–301.

Manson, J. M. and Kang, Y. J. (1989). Test methods for assessing female reproductive and developmental toxicology. In *Principles and Methods of Toxicology,* 2nd ed. (A. W. Hayes, ed.), Raven Press, New York, pp. 311–359.

Ministry of Health and Welfare, Canada (1973). *The Testing of Chemicals for Carcinogenicity, Mutagenicity and Teratogenicity,* Minister of Supply and Services, Canada, Ottawa.

[NIH] National Institutes of Health (1985). *Guide for the Care and Use of Laboratory Animals.* NIH Publ. No. 86-23 U. S. Department of Health and Human Services, Public Health Service, Washington, DC.

[OECD] Organization for Economic Cooperation and Development (1981). *Guideline for Testing of Chemicals' Teratogenicity,* Paris, France.

[OECD] Organization for Economic Cooperation and Development (1982). *Good Laboratory Practice in the Testing of Chemicals;* Final Report of the Group of Experts in Good Laboratory Practice, Paris, France.

Palmer, A. K. (1977). Incidence of sporadic malformations, anomalies and variations in random bred laboratory animals. In *Methods in Prenatal Toxicology* (D. Neubert, H. J. Merker, and T. E. Kwasigroch, eds.), PSG Publishing, Boston, pp. 52–71.

Schardein, J. L. (1985). *Chemically Induced Birth Defects,* Marcel Dekker, New York.

Schardein, J. L. (1987). Approaches to defining the relationship of maternal and developmental toxicity, *Teratogenesis Carcinog. Mutagen.,* 7, 255–271.

Staples, R. E. (1974). Detection of visceral alterations in mammalian fetuses, *Teratology,* 9, 37A–38A.

Stuckhardt, J. L. and Poppe, S. M. (1984). Fresh visceral examination of rat and rabbit fetuses used in teratogenicity testing, *Teratogenesis Carcinog. Mutagen.,* 4, 181–188.

[USDA] U. S. Department of Agriculture (1970). *Animal Welfare Act,* Public Law 39-544, Section 6, USDA, Washington, DC.

[USDA] U. S. Department of Agriculture (1990). Animal Welfare: Proposed rules, *Fed. Reg.,* 55, 33448–33531.

[USEPA] U. S. Environmental Protection Agency (1982). *Pesticides Assessment Guidelines. Subdivision F. Hazard Evaluation: Human and Domestic Animals,* EPA 450/98-2-025, National Technical Information Service, Springfield, VA.

[USEPA] U. S. Environmental Protection Agency (1983a). Toxic substance control: Good Laboratory Practice standards; final rule, *Fed. Reg.,* 48, 53922–53944.

[USEPA] U. S. Environmental Protection Agency (1983b). Pesticide programs: Good Laboratory Practice standards; final rule, *Fed. Reg.,* 48, 53946–53969.

[USEPA] U. S. Environmental Protection Agency (1985). Toxic Substances Control Act test guidelines. Final rules, *Fed. Reg.,* 50, 39252–39516.

[USEPA] U. S. Environmental Protection Agency (1986). Triethylene glycol monomethyl, monoethyl and monobutyl ethers: Proposed test rule, *Fed. Reg.,* 51, 17883–17894.

[USEPA] U. S. Environmental Protection Agency (1988). Diethylene glycol butyl ether and diethylene glycol butyl ether acetate: Final test rule, *Fed. Reg.,* 53, 5932–5953.

[USEPA] U. S. Environmental Protection Agency (1989). Triethylene glycol monomethyl ether: Final test rule, *Fed. Reg.,* 54, 13472–13477.

[USEPA] U. S. Environmental Protection Agency (1991a). Guidelines for developmental toxicity risk assessment, *Fed. Reg.,* 56, 63798–63824.

[USEPA] U. S. Environmental Protection Agency (1991b). Pesticide assessment guidelines. subdivision F. Hazard evaluation: Human and domestic animals, Addendum 10: Neurotoxicity, series 81, 82, and 83, EPA 540/09-91-123, Office of Pesticides and Toxic Substances, Washington, DC.

[USFDA] U. S. Food and Drug Administration (1966). *Guidelines for Reproduction Studies for Safety Evaluation of Drugs for Human Use,* Food and Drug Administration, Washington, DC.

[USFDA] U. S. Food and Drug Administration (1978). Good Laboratory Practice regulations for nonclinical laboratory studies, *Fed. Reg.,* 43, 59985–60025.

Weil, C. S. (1970). Selection of the valid number of sampling units and a consideration of their combination in toxicological studies involving reproduction, teratogenesis, and carcinogenesis, *Food Cosmet. Toxicol.,* 8, 177–182.

Wilson, J. G. (1965). Methods for administering agents and detecting malformations in animals. In *Teratology: Principles and Techniques* (J. G. Wilson and J. Warkany, eds.), University of Chicago Press, Chicago, pp. 262–277.

Wilson, J. G. (1973). *Environment and Birth Defects.* Academic Press, New York.

# 12
# Neurotoxicity Testing

**I. K. Ho**
*University of Mississippi Medical Center*
*Jackson, Mississippi*

**Anna M. Fan**
*California Environmental Protection Agency*
*Berkeley, California*

## I. INTRODUCTION

With the increasing awareness of neurotoxicity associated with environmental chemicals (Abou-Donia, 1992; National Research Council 1992; U. S. Congress, Office of Technology Assessment, 1990), data from neurotoxicity testing will provide important information for future risk assessment (USEPA, 1993) and for risk management of these chemicals to minimize expense and provide health protection. The previous chapter on neurotoxicity (Chapter 5) has presented background on neurotoxicity induced by neurotoxicants. This chapter presents the different disciplines used to detect neurotoxicity, and outline the U. S. Environmental Protection Agency's Neurotoxicity Testing Guidelines (USEPA, 1991), and future perspectives in neurotoxicology.

## II. ASSESSMENTS OF NEUROTOXICITY

Neurotoxicity induced by neurotoxicants, regardless of the sites of action (i.e., central nervous system or peripheral nervous system; CNS or PNS), direct or indirect actions on the nervous system, and specificity of action on target sites, can be detected in terms of changes in four areas: behavior, biochemistry (or neurochemistry), pathology, and physiology. These four different disciplines are described in the following.

### A. Behavioral Toxicology

Behavioral changes following acute or chronic exposure to neurotoxicants are sensitive and rapid indices of neurotoxicity (Annua and Cuomo, 1988; Gad, 1989; Kulig, 1989; Moser, 1989; Rice, 1990; Schaeppi and Fitzgerald, 1989; Tilson and Mitchell, 1984). A series of tests have been widely used by neurotoxicologists for screening of neurotoxicity. The methods designed for neurobehavioral testing are based on changes in motor function, sensory function, reactivity, learning and memory, and naturally occurring behaviors (Tilson and Mitchell, 1984). As detailed in Moser's study (Moser, 1989), the functional observational battery for characterizing neurotoxicants falls in three categories. These are as follows:

1.  Home cage and open field behaviors: posture, convulsions and tremors, palpebral closure, lacrimation, piloerection, salivation, vocalizations, tearing, urination, defecation, gait, arousal, mobility, stereotypy, and bizarre behavior
2.  Manipulative responses: ease of removal, ease of handling, approach response, click response, tail pinch response, righting reflex, landing foot splay, forelimb grip strength, hindlimb grip strength, and pupil response
3.  Physiologic measurements: body temperature and body weight

For evaluating cognitive functions, such as learning and memory, procedures designed are to determine acquisition using positive and negative reinforcing contingencies and to evaluate intermediate and long-term memory (Tilson and Mitchell, 1984).

## B.  Neurochemical Toxicology

Most of the chemicals that produce neurotoxicity act on the biochemical processes of the CNS and PNS, either through a general action or by specific mechanism at the molecular or cellular level. Although the biochemical mechanisms of most known neurotoxicants are not well understood, certain agents have been relatively extensively studied. One of the best examples is organophosphorus cholinesterase inhibitors (OP.ChEI). The well-known organophosphorus insecticides, such as parathion, chlorpyrifos, diazinon, disulfoton, malathion, phorate, and terbufos, are some of the examples. The major action of these insecticides is their potent irreversible inhibitory action of acetylcholinesterase (AChE) and other esterases. Their chemistry, fate, and effects have recently been reviewed (Chambers and Levi, 1992). Their mechanism of action is to inhibit AChE by the phosphorylation of a serine residue of the active site of this enzyme which, in turn, leads to the accumulation of acetylcholine and produces cholinergic overactivity. The carbamate type of insecticides also act on AChE, except in a reversible manner.

Some of the OP.ChEI also produce delayed neurotoxicity called organophosphate-induced delayed neuropathy (OPIDN; Johnson 1975, 1982, 1987, 1990; Lotti et al., 1984; Richardson, 1992). The target site for these compounds to induce OPIDN is a membrane-bound nerve cell protein called neurotoxic esterase or neuropathy target enzyme (NTE). The characteristics of OPIDN are a dying back of long myelinated nerve axons, especially in the sciatic nerve and within the spinal cord. Some organophosphorus compounds (e.g., tri-*o*-cresyl phosphate; TOCP) that are not insecticides are also potent inhibitors of NTE.

Other neurotransmitter systems have also been demonstrated to be affected by neurotoxicants. Bicuculline and picrotoxin, two alkaloids isolated from plants, are γ-aminobuteric acid A (GABA$_A$) receptor antagonists and are potent convulsants. However, they act at different sites of the GABA$_A$ receptors. Bicuculline is a direct competitive antagonist of the GABA-binding site (Cooper et al., 1991), and picrotoxin is a blocker of Cl$^-$ ionophores. Strychnine, another potent convulsant, exerts its effects by acting on glycine receptors, another amino acid inhibitory neurotransmitter (Cooper et al., 1991). 1-Methyl-4-phenyl-1,2,3,6-tetrahydropyridine (MPTP), a contaminant identified in a synthetic street opioid preparation, caused a Parkinson-like syndrome in some persons who were administered the preparation containing MPTP. It is a relatively selective neurotoxin that destroys nigrostriatal dopaminergic neurons through its metabolite (Langston et al., 1987; Zigmond and Stricker, 1989). It appears that some of the neurotoxicants, such as the examples just cited, have been demonstrated to act specifically on certain biochemical processes.

## C.  Electrophysiological Toxicology

An electrophysiological approach is one of several means to study neurotoxicity. Electrical signals that are generated by nerve and muscle cells are associated with ionic fluxes across the cell membranes. A variety of neurotoxins excite these cells. This excitation occurs by changing membrane potential caused by membrane permeability changes to different cations such as $Na^+$, $K^+$, and $Ca^{2+}$. Marine neurotoxins, such as tetrodotoxin and saxitoxin, have been well demonstrated to block $Na^+$ channels (Catterall, 1980; Narahashi, 1974; Richie, 1979). Brevetoxins, toxins isolated from *Ptychodiscus brevis,* which depolarize nerve and muscle membrane, also act on $Na^+$ channels as their target site (Wu and Narahashi, 1988). The insecticides, DDT and type I pyrethroids, cause repetitive discharges of the nervous system (Narahashi, 1992). Because of the easy access of peripheral neuromuscular junctions, isolated rat phrenic nerve hemidiaphragm, the frog sciatic nerve and sartorius muscle, the crayfish neuromuscular junctions, and electroplax of the electric eel are generally used for electrophysiological investigations of neurotoxicants.

## D.  Neuropathological Toxicology

Neuropathological investigation is one of the essential aspects of neurotoxicology. The objectives of neuropathology are to furnish information on the topography or location of the lesions and to define the nature and characteristics of the damage of the nervous systems caused by neurotoxicants (Chang, 1992). The observation in neuropathological findings may provide valuable correlation with the results obtained from behavioral, neurochemical, and electrophysical studies. For example, OPIDN is often seen in neuropathological changes in the sciatic, peroneal, and tibial nerves. The pathological findings can be correlated with the inhibition of NTE and neurological symptoms such as ataxia and paralysis.

## III.  OUTLINES OF UNITED STATES ENVIRONMENTAL PROTECTION AGENCY NEUROTOXICITY TESTING GUIDELINES

With the increasing importance of neurotoxicology, design of methods for neurotoxicity-testing of chemicals that have potential as neurotoxicants becomes crucial to the success of identifying and controlling poisons of the nervous systems. The following provides a brief description of neurotoxicity-testing guidelines published by the USEPA (1991). These tests include five different test procedures that encompass evaluation of changes in behavior, neuropathology, biochemistry, and electrophysiology.

## A.  Delayed Neurotoxicity of Organophosphorus Substances Following Acute and 28-Day Exposures

*1.  Purpose*

The test is intended to identify and characterize potential effects of organophosphorus substance-induced delayed neurotoxicity in adult hens. It includes behavioral observation of gait; histopathological assessment of brain, peripheral nerve, and spinal cord; and neurochemical assessment of inhibition of acetylcholinesterase (AChE) and neuropathy target esterase (or neurotoxic esterase; NTE).

## 2. Definitions

Organophosphorus-induced delayed neurotoxicity (OPIDN) is defined by

1.  Neurological syndromes: limb weakness and upper motor neuron spasticity
2.  Pathological signs: distal axonopathy of peripheral nerve and spinal cord
3.  Biochemical changes: inhibition and aging of NTW in neural tissues

Neuropathic target enzyme (NTE) is a membrane-bound enzyme that hydrolyzes phenyl valerate. It is resistant to paraoxon, but sensitive to mipafox or neuropathic organophosphorus ester inhibition.

## 3. Principle

Acute and 28-day exposure studies are used.

## 4. Test Procedure

*Species.*    Adult domestic laying hen (*Gallus gallues domesticus,* 8–14 months of age) are used for the test.

*Route of Administration.*    Administration is oral (preferably by gavage).

*Dose Levels.*    There are three types of dosage levels:

1.  Acute: 1 dose. Levels of test substances greater than 2g/kg need not be tested. Either a median lethal dose ($LD_{50}$) or an approximate lethal dose (ALD) in the hen may be used to determine the acute high dose.
2.  28-day study: Levels of test substances greater than 1g/kg need not be tested.
    High dose: sufficient to cause OPIDN or maximum tolerated dose based on the acute high dose
    Low dose: minimum effective level (e.g., $ED_{10}$) or a no-effect level
    Intermediate dose: equally spaced between the high and low doses
3.  Control groups
    Positive control: tri-*o*-cresyl phosphate (TOCP)-treated animals
    Vehicle control

*Group size.*    The group sizes include:

Exposure groups: at least nine survivors (six for behavioral observations/histopathology and at least three for NTE)
Positive control group: at least nine survivors (six for a concurrent or historical control and at least three for NTE)
Vehicle control group: at least nine survivors (six for histopathology and three for NTE)

*Study Conduct.*    The study will comprise the following features:

1.  Biochemical measurements: NTE and AChE. These studies will be conducted in brain and spinal cord of three hens from each group at 48 hr after the last dose. Other times may be chosen to optimize detection of effects.
2.  21-day observation: All remaining hens of each group will be observed at least once daily for at least 21 days. Observations of toxicity include: behavioral abnormality, locomotor ataxia, and paralysis.
3.  Necropsy and histopathological studies: Gross necropsies—the brain and spinal cord. Tissue sections for microscopic examination include medulla oblongata, spinal cord (the rostral cervical, the midthoracic, and the lumbosacral regions), and peripheral nerves.

*5. Data Reporting and Evaluation*

Test report
Treatment of results
Evaluation of results

## B. Neurotoxicity Screening Battery

*1. Purpose*

The test battery consists of the following:

1. Functional observational battery: noninvasive procedures designed to detect gross functional deficits in animals and to quantify behavioral or neurological effects detected in other studies;
2. Motor activity test using an automated device to measure the level of activity of individual animals; and
3. Neuropathology: providing data to detect and to characterize histopathological changes in the central and peripheral nervous system.

*2. Definitions*

*Neurotoxicity:* any adverse effect on the structure or function of the nervous system related to exposure to a chemical substance.

*Toxic effect:* an adverse change in a structure or function of an experimental animal as a result of exposure to a chemical substance.

*Motor activity:* any movement of the experimental animals.

*3. Principle*

Acute studies
Subchronic (and chronic) studies

*4. Test Procedure*

*Species.*   Both male and female (nulliparous and nonpregnant) young adult rats (at least 42 days old) are generally the choice. Other species (e.g., the mouse or the dog) under some circumstances, may be used.

*Route of Administration.*   Selection criteria are based on the most likely route of human exposure, bioavailability, the likelihood of observing effects, practical difficulties, and the likelihood of producing nonspecific effects. The route that best meets these criteria should be selected. Dietary feeding is generally acceptable for repeated exposure studies.

*Dose Levels.*   Dose levels are related to the type of study:

1. Acute studies: 3 doses
   High dose: highest nonlethal dose (< 2g/kg)
   Low dose: minimal effect or no-effect dose
   Middle dose: successive fraction of high dose
2. Subchronic (and chronic) studies: 3 doses
   High dose: dose producing significant neurotoxic or clearly toxic effects, but not lethal
       dose (accumulative)
   Low dose—middle dose: fractions of the high dose

3.  Control groups
    Positive control: The test laboratory should provide evidence of the ability of the observational methods used to detect major neurotoxic endpoints and includes limb weakness or paralysis (e.g., repeated exposure to acrylamide), tremor (e.g., ppDDT), and autonomic signs (e.g., carbaryl). Positive control data are also required to demonstrate the sensitivity and reliability of the activity measuring device and testing procedures.
    Concurrent (vehicle) control

*Group Size.*    At least 10 males and 10 females shall be used in each dose and control group for behavioral testing. At least five males and five females shall be used in each dose and control group for terminal neuropathology.

*Study Conduct.*    The studies will include the following:

1.  Time of testing (observations and activity testing)
    Acute studies: before the initiation of exposure, at the estimated time of peak effect within 8 hr of dosing, and at 7 and 14 days after dosing.
    Subchronic (and chronic) studies: before the initiation of exposure and before the daily exposure; or, for feeding studies, at the same time of day, during the 4th, 8th, and 13th weeks of exposure (every 3 months for chronic). All animals shall be weighed on each test day and at least weekly during the exposure period.
2.  Functional observational battery
    *General consideration*
        Blind test
        Minimize variations in the test conditions
        Observations in the home cage
    *List of measures*
        1.  Signs of autonomic function: lacrimation and salivation (ranking score from none to severe); piloerection and exophthalmus (presence or absence); urination and defecation, including polyuria and diarrhea (ranking); pupillary function; and degree of palpebral closure.
        2.  Description, incidence and severity of any convulsions, tremor, or abnormal motor movements (home cage and open field)
        3.  Reactivity to general stimuli
        4.  Arousal level
        5.  Posture and gait abnormalities (home cage and open field)
        6.  Forelimb and hindlimb grip strength
        7.  Landing foot splay
        8.  Sensorimotor responses to stimuli (pain or sound)
        9.  Body weight
        10. Unusual or abnormal behaviors, stereotypies, emaciation, dehydration, hypotonia or hypertonia, altered fur appearance, red or crusty deposits around the eyes, nose, or mouth, and so on.
    *Additional measures*
        1.  Count of rearing ability on the open field
        2.  Ranking of righting ability
        3.  Body temperature
        4.  Excessive or spontaneous vocalizations
        5.  Alterations in rate and ease of respiration (e.g., rales or dyspnea)

6. Sensorimotor responses to visual or proprioceptive stimuli
7. Others
3. Motor activity (by automated activity recording apparatus)
4. Neuropathology
   Fixation and processing of tissue: in situ fixation, paraffin/plastic embedding, hematoxylin and eosin (H&E) or comparable staining
   Quantitative examination
   Subjective diagnosis

5. *Data Reporting and Evaluation*
   Description of equipment and test methods
   Results
   Evaluation of data

## C. Appendix: Guideline for Assaying Glial Fibrillary Acidic Protein

This procedure is designed to be used in conjunction with behavioral and neuropathological investigations as part of the neurotoxicity screening battery described in the foregoing.

*1. Purpose*

Astrocyte hypertrophy has been demonstrated to be associated with chemically induced injury at the site of damage. Assay of glial fibrillary acid protein (GFAP), the major intermediate filament protein of astrocytes can document the existence and location of chemical-induced injury of the CNS.

*2. Test Procedure*

*Species.* These are usually laboratory young adult rats used in other tests for neurotoxicity.

*Group Size.* At least six animals for both the exposed and control groups will be studied.

*Tissue To Be Studied.* Six regions: cerebellum, cerebral cortex, hippocampus, striatum, thalamus/hypothalamus, and the rest of the brain are evaluated.

*3. Data Reporting and Evaluation*

Test report
Evaluation of results

## D. Developmental Neurotoxicity Study

*1. Purpose*

The test is intended to develop data on the potential functional and morphological hazards to the nervous system that may occur in the offspring from exposure of the mother during pregnancy and lactation.

*2. Principle*

Pregnant animals shall be administered test substance during gestation and early lactation. The test includes observations to detect gross neurological and behavioral abnormalities. Determination of motor activity, response to auditory startle, assessment of learning, neuropathological evaluation, and brain weights.

*3. Test Procedure.*

*Species.* Young, pregnant, adult female rats (nulliparous females) are used for the study.

*Route of Administration.*   Administration of the test agent is oral (although other routes may be acceptable).

*Dose Levels.*   The exposure groups have three dose levels.

Highest dose: (1) When the test substance is known to be developmentally toxic, the dose to be used is the maximum dose that will not induce in utero or neonatal death or malformations. (2) When it is unknown, the dose shall induce some overt maternal toxicity, but shall not reduce weight gain exceeding 29% during gestation and lactation.

Lowest dose: not to produce any grossly observable evidence of either maternal or developmental neurotoxicity.

Intermediate dose: equally spaced between the two.

(2) The control group includes concurrent control groups or vehicle–treated concurrent control groups.

*Dosing Period.*   The dosing period covers from day 6 of gestation through day 10 postnatally (but not on the day of parturition).

*Observation of Dams*

1.   Gross examination: once each day before daily treatment
2.   Functional observational battery: once each day before daily treatment

*Tests for the Offspring*

1.   Observation of offspring to include cage-side examination daily for gross signs of mortality or morbidity and gross signs of toxicity (functional observational battery).
2.   Developmental landmarks:
     Live pup counts
     Weight of each pup within a litter at birth and on postnatal days 4, 11, 17, 21, and at least once every 2 weeks thereafter
     Age of vaginal opening and preputial separation
3.   Motor activity is monitored on postnatal days 13, 17, 21, and 60 (±2 days).
4.   Auditory startle test is performed on the offspring on days 22 and 60± (2 days).
5.   Learning and memory tests are conducted as associative learning and memory tests at about the time of weaning (postnatal day 21–24) and at adulthood (postnatal day 60 ± 2).
6.   Neuropathology: A neuropathological evaluation is conducted on animals on postnatal day 11 and at the termination of the study. At day 11, one male or female pup from each litter (six male and six female) is evaluated, and also at the termination.

*4.   Data Collection, Reporting, and Evaluation*

Description of test system and test methods
Results
Evaluation of data

## E.   Schedule-Controlled Operant Behavior

*1.   Purpose*

The test is to evaluate the effects of acute and repeated exposures on the rate and pattern of responding under schedules of reinforcement. The test is intended to assess the effects of neurotoxicants on learning, memory, and behavioral performance.

*2. Definitions*

*Behavioral toxicity:* any adverse change in the functioning of the organism with respect to its environment in relation to exposure to a chemical substance

*Operant:* a class of behavioral responses that change or operate on the environment in the same way

*Operant behavior:* further distinguished as behavior that is modified by its consequences

*Operant condition:* the experimental procedure used to modify some class of behavior by reinforcement or punishment

*Schedule of reinforcement:* the relation between behavioral responses and the delivery of reinforcers (e.g., food or water)

*Fixed ratio* (FR) *schedule:* a fixed number of responses to produce a reinforcer (e.g., FR30)

*Fixed interval* (FI) *schedule:* the first response after a fixed period of time is reinforced (e.g., FI 5 min)

*3. Principle*

Animals are trained to perform under a schedule of reinforcement and measurements of their operant behavior are made. Testing substance is then administered according to the experimental design (between groups or within subjects) and the duration of exposure (acute and repeated).

*4. Test Procedures*

*Species.* Young laboratory male and female mice (6 weeks old) or rats (14 weeks old) are recommended.

*Route of Administration.* Selection of route is based on the most likely route of human exposure, bioavailability, the likelihood of observing effects, practical difficulties, and the likelihood of producing nonspecific effects. Dietary feeding is generally acceptable for repeated exposure studies.

*Dose Levels*

1. Acute studies: three doses
   High dose: a dose that produces significant neurotoxic effects or other clearly toxic effects ($< 2g/kg$).
   Low dose: fraction of a high dose that produces minimal effects (e.g., an $ED_{10}$) or no effects
   Middle dose: fraction of the high dose
2. Subchronic (and chronic) studies: three doses
   High dose: a dose that produces significant neurotoxic effects or other clearly toxic effects ($< 1g/kg$).
   Low dose: fraction of the high dose that produces minimal effects (e.g., an $ED_{10}$) or no effects
   Middle dose: fraction of the high dose
3. Control groups
   A concurrent control group or control session(s) are required.
   Positive control data that indicate the experimental procedures are sensitive to substances known to affect operant behavior are also required.

*Group Size.* Six to 12 animals shall be exposed to each dose of the test substance or to the control procedure.

*Study Conduct*

1. Apparatus: automated equipment
2. Chamber assignment: concurrent treatment group shall be balanced across chambers

3. Schedule of food availability
4. Time, frequency, and duration of testing
5. Schedule selection

*5. Data Reporting and Evaluation*

Description of equipment and test methods
Results
Evaluation of data

## F.  Peripheral Nerve Function

*1. Purpose*

The guideline defines procedures for evaluating aspects of the neurophysiological functioning of peripheral nerves. It is intended to evaluate the effects of exposures on the velocity and amplitude of conduction of peripheral nerves.

*2. Definition*

*Conduction velocity:* the speed at which the compound nerve action potential traverses a nerve
*Amplitude:* the voltage excursion recorded during the process of recording the compound nerve
    action potential (an indirect measure of the number of axons firing).

*3. Principle*

The peripheral nerve conduction velocity and amplitude are assessed by electrophysiological techniques in experimental and control animals.

*4. Test Procedures*

*Species.*   Young male and/or female rats (at least $60 \pm 15$ days) are generally the selection.

*Route of Administration.*   Selection criteria are the same as those cited under Sec. E on schedule-controlled operant behavior.

*Dose Levels*

1. Acute studies: three doses
2. Subchronic (and chronic) studies: three doses
    The criteria for selection of doses are the same as those listed under Sec. E on schedule-
        controlled operant behavior.
3. Control groups
    Concurrent control group.
    Positive control data shall also be provided.

*Group Size.*   Twenty animals per dose level or controls are required.

*Study Conduct*

1. Choice of nerve(s): both sensory and motor nerve axons: either a hind limb (e.g., tibial) or tail (e.g., ventral caudal) nerve.
2. Preparation for in vivo testing.
3. Monitoring both core and nerve temperature.
4. Testing shall be conducted on motor nerve and sensory nerve.

*5. Data Collection, Reporting, and Evaluation*

Description of equipment and test methods
Results
Evaluation of data

## IV. FUTURE PERSPECTIVES

As listed in the previous section, testing procedures are available for use in assessment of neurotoxicity of chemicals. These procedures encompass behavioral, functional, biochemical, pathological, and electrophysiological endpoints. However, neurotoxicants do not usually produce single specific endpoints; multiple systems are more likely to be involved. Therefore, neurotoxicity-testing procedures used to assess acute toxicity, subacute toxicity, and chronic toxicity of a given potential neurotoxicant should be able to evaluate chemically induced neurotoxicity as specifically as possible. Future perspectives on the importance of elucidating the mechanisms by which neurotoxic chemicals exert their effects on the nervous systems should be emphasized. Information obtained from such investigations can lead to the development of sensitive, reliable, and simple detecting methods, (e.g., in vitro testing) for the potential neurotoxicants. The problems associated with chemical–chemical interactions, which may exaggerate or potentiate neurotoxicity, and the potential hazards induced by low-dose chronic exposure should also be addressed. For developing a better neurotoxicity testing battery, several points listed in the following deserve serious attention to develop more specific-testing procedures for reliably detecting neurotoxicity induced by neurotoxicants.

### A. Investigations on the Mechanisms of Action of Neurotoxic Chemicals

As noticed from the previous section, the available guidelines for neurotoxicity testing have heavily relied on the existing knowledge of organophosphorus compounds. This class of compounds has been extensively studied and their mechanism of action has been demonstrated. However, the mechanisms of action of the majority of neurotoxicants are not yet available. For instance, mechanisms of action of some widely used insecticides (e.g., cyclodienes, hexachloro-cyclohexanes, lindane, toxaphene, and pyrethroids) are largely unknown. Use of the guidelines developed from organophosphorus compounds would not allow reliable detection of neurotoxicity induced by these chemicals. Evidence has accumulated suggesting that these insecticides may also inhibit other neurotransmitter systems. With [$^3$H]dihydropicrotoxinin as a ligand, Leeb-Lundberg and Olsen (1980) reported that cyanophenoxybenzyl pyrethroids (type 2) interacted with convulsant binding sites of GABA$_A$, receptor complex of rat brain synaptosomes. Studies of 37 pyrethroids by Lawrence and Casida (1983) indicated a correlation between inhibition of [$^{35}$S]TBPS binding to rat brain synaptic membranes and intracerebral neurotoxicity in the mouse. Their studies revealed that all toxic cyano compounds, but not their nontoxic stereoisomers, are [$^{35}$S]TBPS-binding inhibitors; *cis*-isomers were more potent than *trans*-isomers as both neurotoxicants and inhibitors; and noncyano pyrethroids (type 1) are much less potent or are inactive.

Further evidence has also indicated that the pyrethroid-binding site may be closely related to the convulsant benzodiazepine site of action (Lawrence et al., 1985). These studies showed that the most toxic type 2 pyrethroids are the most potent inhibitors of the specific binding of [$^3$H]Ro 5-4864, a convulsant benzodiazepine ligand, to rat brain membranes. Additional studies on the effects of pyrethorids on GABA-induced chloride influx into mouse brain vesicles

(Bloomquist et al., 1986) and rat brain microsacs (Abalis et al., 1986) further support the notion that type 2 pyrethroids interact with $GABA_A$ receptors.

Other insecticides (e.g., cyclodienes, hexachlorocyclohexane, toxaphene, and avermectin) have been suggested to act at $GABA_A$ receptors as well. Lawrence and Casida (1984) demonstrated that three major chlorinated hydrocarbon insecticides (lindane/hexachlorocyclohexane, toxaphene and aldrin/dieldrin) are potent, competitive, and stereospecific inhibitors of [$^{35}$S]TBPS binding to fresh rat brain synaptic membranes. Toxicity in the mouse has also been shown to be closely related to the potency for inhibition of TBPS binding (Lawrence and Casida, 1984; Abalis et al., 1985) or GABA-induced $^{36}Cl^-$ flux (Abalis et al., 1986; Ogata et al., 1988). Therefore, investigation on the mechanisms of action of neurotoxicants is essential for the future development of more specific-testing methods.

## B. Investigations on Multiple Systems Involved in the Action of Neurotoxic Chemicals

Because of the complex interconnections of the nervous systems, multiple systems are more likely affected by neurotoxic chemicals. For instance, the toxicities of organophosphorus cholinesterase inhibitors are due to their irreversible inactivation of acetylcholinesterase, thereby producing long-lasting inhibitory activity. Organophosphorus cholinesterase inhibitors exhibit behavioral, neurological, and biochemical effects in both animals and humans. On long-term exposure, these compounds are known to induce neurotoxic effects. However, tolerance also develops to the behavioral effects of these agents, and evidence suggests that this may result from subsensitivity to acetylcholine. It is not yet well established whether all of the toxic symptoms are due to the alterations of cholinergic function, or if other neurochemical changes might also be intimately involved. Recent evidence available has strongly indicated that noncholinergic systems (e.g., biogenic amines, glutamic acid, $\gamma$-aminobutyric acid, cyclic nucleotides, or others) may also play important roles in the initiation, continuation, and disappearance of organophosphorus cholinesterase inhibitor-induced neurotoxicity. Kar and Martin (1972) suggested that paraoxon convulsions are related to GABA levels in the CNS. Certain organophosphorus compounds cause convulsions and death, but do not inhibit AChE (Bellet and Casida, 1973) and are believed to produce their effects by altering central GABA function (Bowery et al., 1976). The study of diisopropylfluorophosphate (DFP; Sivam et al., 1983) revealed that the numbers of both GABA and dopamine (DA) receptors were significantly increased after acute treatment, but the increases were less prominent after chronic treatment. The evidence, therefore, seems to indicate that the $GABA_A$ and the DA receptor activation may play a part in the acute effects of organophosphorus compounds.

Evidence available also shows that not only $GABA_A$ receptor density, but also DA receptor density was increased after a single injection of DFP (Sivam et al., 1983). It has also been reported that DA levels are increased after acute DFP treatment (Glisson et al., 1974). On the other hand, mipafox decreased DA levels after chronic administration (Freed et al., 1976). The increased motor activity of parkinsonism is due to an imbalance of cholinergic and dopaminergic activity in the basal ganglia (i.e., increased cholinergic activity owing to DA deficiency; Helbronn and Bartfai, 1978; Weiss et al., 1976). It has been reported that striatal DA has an inhibitory effect on striatal neurons (Krnjevic and Phillis, 1963) and also reduces the spontaneous and cholinergic neuronal firing in the striatum (McGeer et al., 1975). It has been suggested that dopaminergic (inhibitory) and cholinergic (excitatory) mechanisms interact in a delicate way to maintain the normal function of striatum (Anden et al., 1966). The striatal increases in $GABA_A$ and DA receptor densities observed after acute treatments with DFP returned gradually to control levels after cessation of treatment. Thus, the neurochemical imbalance produced as a result of acute inhibition of AChE may be partially counteracted by an acute increase in dopaminergic activity supported by an increase in GABAergic activity.

These studies indicate an involvement of ACh, DA, and GABA receptors in the effects of organophosphorus cholinesterase inhibitors. It is suggested that the GABA and DA systems, singularly or in combination, counteract the enhanced cholinergic activity induced by organophosphorus compounds.

Almost all of the neurotoxins one encounters elicit toxicity that involves interactions of multiple complex systems. It is, therefore, important to focus more attention on interactions of neuronal systems by using multidisciplinary approaches.

## C. Alteration in Susceptibility After Repeated Exposure to Neurotoxic Chemicals

The nervous system changes its sensitivity to certain neurotoxic chemicals after being exposed to a neurotoxicant. For example, paraoxone and DFP are extremely potent inhibitors of acetylcholinesterase, with rapid enzyme-aging action (Holmstedt, 1959; Coult et al., 1966). They cause CNS cholinergic overstimulation, which includes tremors, convulsions, chewing movements, and hind-limb abduction (Fernando et al., 1984, 1985a). These effects usually disappear within a few hours after a single dose of these agents, whereas the acetylcholinesterase activity recovers from inhibition gradually over days (Fernando et al., 1985a). Muscarinic receptor antagonists, such as atropine, effectively block the cholinergic neurotoxicity produced by anticholinesterase agents, DFP being a common example (Fernando et al., 1985a). On the other hand, if an antimuscarinic agent is given several hours after the administration of DFP, a characteristic form of hyperactivity results (Fernando et al., 1985b). It appears that after repeated exposure to neurotoxic chemicals, the vulnerability (susceptibility) of a subject could be significantly modified.

## D. Investigation on Drug Interactions, Chemical–Drug, or Chemical–Chemical Interactions

Toxicities are often seen when different drugs are taken together. Adverse reactions or additive or synergistic toxicity owing to drug–drug, drug–chemical, or chemical–chemical interactions should be important areas of future research, since these are realities that occur daily. However, the knowledge of drugs or of chemical interactions is limited. For example, consumption of alcoholic beverages, such as wine, beer, or liquor, is considered to be one of social functions. If one takes certain medications, such as sedative–hypnotics, opioid analgesics, antianxiety agents, antipsychotics, antidepressants, or anticonvulsants, the actions of these drugs will be potentiated by alcohol. Furthermore, since alcohol is a potent CNS depressant, adverse reactions or toxicity from some substances (which would not be obvious under usual situations), could be significantly increased in a person who is under the influence of alcohol. These examples alone demonstrate that it is necessary to emphasize the importance of drug–chemical interactions in modern neurotoxicology evaluation.

## E. Development of In Vitro System for Neurotoxicity Testing

As mentioned under the earlier Sec. III.A, when the mechanism of action of a specific class of neurotoxicants is well understood, an in vitro system, which is effective, rapid, and relatively inexpensive, can be developed for neurotoxicity testing. For example, the acetylcholinesterase assay procedure has been used to screen organophosphate and carbamate analogues. The NTE assay has been used to detect possible OPIDN caused by agents similar to TOCP. Potential in vitro systems at molecular levels and target organs should be emphasized for the development of preliminary neurotoxicity testing. In the past 20 years, significant progress has been made in the development of in vitro procedures for research in neuroscience. For example, heavy metals produce their primary toxic effects on the nervous system (Aschner and Kimelberg, 1991). Cell culture techniques, which are relatively simple and yet easy to control, and in which experimental variables can be manipulated, are feasible for use as an in vitro model system for the initial step in developing neurotoxicity testing. For more information on neurotoxicity testing, see Chang and Slikker (1995).

## REFERENCES

Abalis, I. M., Eldefrawi, M. E., and Eldefrawi, A. T. (1985). High affinity stereospecific binding of cyclodiene insecticides and γ-hexachlorocyclohexane to γ-aminobutyric acid receptors of rat brain, *Pestic. Biochem. Physiol.*, 24, 95–102.

Abalis, I. M., Eldefrawi, M. E., and Eldefrawi, A. T. (1986). Effects of insecticides on GABA-induced chloride influx into rat brain microsacs, *J. Toxicol. Environ. Health*, 18, 13–23.

Abou-Donia, M. B. (1992). *Neurotoxicology*, CRC Press, Boca Raton, FL.

Anden, N. E., Dahlstrom, A. L., Fuxe, K., and Larsson, K. (1966). Functional role of the nigro-neostriatal dopamine neurons, *Acta Pharmacol.*, 24, 263–266.

Annua, Z. and Cuomo, V. (1988). Mechanisms of neurotoxicity and their relationship to behavioral changes, *Toxicology*, 49, 219–225.

Aschner, M. and Kimelberg, H. K. (1991). The use of astrocytes in culture as model systems for evaluating neurotoxic-induced injury, *Neurotoxicology*, 12, 505–517.

Bellet, E. M. and Casida, J. E. (1973). Bicyclic phosphorus esters: High toxicity without cholinesterase inhibition, *Science*, 182, 1135–1136.

Bloomquist, J. R., Adams, P. M., and Soderlund, D. M. (1986). Inhibition of γ-aminobutyric and stimulated chloride flux in mouse brain vesicles by polychlorocycloalkane and pyrethroid insecticides, *Neurotoxicology*, 7, 11–20.

Bowery, N. G., Collins, J. F., and Hill, R. G. (1976). Bicyclic phosphorus esters that are potent convulsants and GABA antagonists, *Nature*, 261, 601–603.

Catterall, W. A. (1980). Neurotoxins that act on voltage-sensitive sodium channels in excitable membranes, *Annu. Rev. Pharmacol. Toxicol.*, 20, 15–43.

Chambers, J. E. and Levi, P. E. (1992). *Organophosphates: Chemistry, Fate and Effects*, Academic Press, San Diego, CA.

Chang, L. W. (1992). Basic histopathological alterations in the central and peripheral nervous systems: Classification, identification, approaches, and techniques. In *Neurotoxicology* (M. B. Abou-Donia, ed.), CRC Press, Boca Raton, FL, pp. 223–252.

Chang, L. W. and Slikker, W. Jr. (1995). *Neurotoxicology: Approaches and Methods*, Academic Press, San Diego, CA.

Cooper, J. R., Floom, F. E., and Roth, R. H. (1991). Amino acid transmitters. In *The Biochemical Basis of Neuropharmacology*, 6th ed., Oxford University Press, New York, pp. 133–189.

Coult, D. B., Marsh, B. J., and Read, G. (1966). Dealkylation studies on inhibition of acetylcholinesterase, *Biochem. J.*, 98, 869–873.

Fernando, J. C. R., Hoskins, B., and Ho, I. K. (1984). Effect on striatal dopamine metabolism and differential motor behavioral tolerance following chronic cholinesterase inhibition with diisopropyl-fluorophosphate, *Pharmacol. Biochem. Behav.*, 20, 951–957.

Fernando, J. C. R., Hoskins, B., and Ho, I. K. (1985a). Variability of neurotoxicity of and lack of tolerance to the anticholinesterases Soman and Sarin, *Res. Commun. Pharmacol. Chem. Pathol.*, 48, 415–430.

Fernando, J. C. R., Hoskins, B., and Ho, I. K. (1985b). Rapid induction of supersensitivity to muscarinic antagonist-induced motor excitation by continuous stimulation of cholinergic receptors, *Life Sci.*, 37, 883–892.

Freed, V. H., Martin, M. A., Fang, S. C., and Kar, P. P. (1976). Role of striatal dopamine in delayed neurotoxic effects of organophosphorous compounds, *Eur. J. Pharmacol.,* 35, 229–232.

Gad, S. C. (1989). Neurotoxicity screening survey, *J. Am. Coll. Toxicol.,* 8, 5–11.

Glisson, S. N., Karczmar, A. G., and Barnes, L. (1974). Effects of diisopropylphosphofluoridate on acetylcholine, cholinesterase, and catecholamines of several parts of rabbit brain, *Neuropharmacology,* 13, 623–631.

Heilbronn, E. and Bartfai, T. (1978). Muscarinic acetylcholine receptor, *Prog. Neurobiol.,* 11, 171–188.

Holmstedt, B. (1959). Pharmacology of organophosphorus compounds, *Pharmacol. Rev.,* 11, 567–620.

Johnson, M. K. (1975). The delayed neuropathy caused by some organophosphorus esters: Mechanism and challenge, *Crit. Rev. Toxicol.,* 3, 289–316.

Johnson, M. K. (1982). The target for initiation of delayed neurotoxicity by organophosphorus esters: Biochemical studies and toxicology applications, *Rev. Biochem. Toxicol.,* 4, 141–212.

Johnson, M. K. (1987). Receptor or enzyme: The puzzle of NTE and organophosphate-induced delayed polyneuropathy, *Trends Pharmacol. Sci.,* 8, 174–179.

Johnson, M. K. (1990). Organophosphates and delayed neuropathy—is NTE alive and well? *Toxicol. Appl. Pharmacol.,* 102, 385–399.

Kar, P. O. and Martin, M. A. J. (1972). Possible role of γ-aminobutyric acid in paraoxon induced convulsions, *J. Pharm. Pharmacol.,* 24, 996–997.

Krnjevic, K. and Phillis, J. W. (1963). Iontophoretic studies of neurons in the mammalian cerebral cortex, *J. Physiol. (Lond.),* 165, 274–304.

Kulig, B. M. (1989). A neurofunctional test battery for evaluating the effects of long-term exposure to chemical, *J. Am. Coll. Toxicol.,* 8, 71–83.

Langston, J. W., Irwin, I., and Ricaurte, G. A. (1987). Neurotoxins, parkinsonism and Parkinson's disease, *Pharmacol. Ther.,* 32, 19–49.

Lawrence, L. J. and Casida, J. E. (1983). Stereospecific action of pyrethroid insecticides on the γ-aminobutyric acid receptor–ionophore complex, *Science,* 221, 1399–1401.

Lawrence, L.J. and Casida, J. E. (1984). Interactions of lindane, toxaphene and cyclodienes with brain-specific *t*-butyl-bicyclophosphorothionate receptor, *Life Sci.,* 35, 171–178.

Lawrence, L. J., Gee, K. W., and Yamamura, H. I. (1985). Interactions of pyrethroid insecticides with chloride ionophore-associated binding sites, *Neurotoxicology,* 6, 87–98.

Leeb-Lundberg, F. and Olsen, R. W. (1980). Picrotoxinin binding as a probe of the GABA postsynaptic membrane receptor–ionophore complex. In *Psychopharmacology and Biochemistry of Neurotransmitter Receptors* (H. I. Yamamura, R. W. Olsen, and E. Usdin, eds.), Elsevier, New York, pp. 593–606.

Lotti, M., Becker, C. E., and Aminoff, M. J. (1984). Organophosphtae polyneuropathy: Pathogenesis and prevention, *Neurology,* 34, 658–662.

McGeer, E. G., McGeer, P. L., Grewaal, D. S., and Singh, V. K. (1975). Striatal cholinergic interneurons and their relation to dopaminergic nerve endings, *J. Pharmacol.,* 6, 143–152.

Moser, V. C. (1989). Screening approaches to neurotoxicity: A functional observational battery, *J. Am. Coll. Toxicol.,* 8, 85–93.

Narahashi, T. (1974). Chemicals as tools in the study of excitable membranes. *Physiol. Rev.,* 54, 813–819.

Narahashi, T. (1992). Cellular electrophysiology. In *Neurotoxicology* (M. B. Abou-Donia, ed.), CRC Pres, Boca Raton, FL, pp. 155–189.

National Research Council, Committee on Neurotoxicology and Models for Assessing Risk (1992). *Environmental Neurotoxicology,* National Academy Press, Washington, DC.

Ogata, N., Vogel, S. M., and Narahashi, T. (1988). Lindane but not deltamethrin blocks a component of GABA-activated chloride channels, *FASEB J.,* 2, 2895–2900.

Rice, D. C. (1990). Principles and procedures in behavioral toxicology testing, In *Handbook of In Vivo Toxicity Testing* (D. L. Arnold, H. C. Grice, and D. R. Krewski, eds.), Academic Press, San Diego, CA, pp. 383–408.

Richardson, R. J. (1992). Interactions of organophosphorus compounds with neurotoxic esterase. In *Organophosphates: Chemistry, Fate, and Effects* (J. E. Chambers and P. E. Levi, eds.), Academic Press, San Diego, CA, pp. 299–323.

Richie, J. M. (1979). A pharmacological approach to the structure of sodium channels in myelinated axons, *Annu. Rev. Neurosci.,* 2, 341–362.

Schaeppi, U. and Fitzgerald, R. E. (1989). Practical procedures of testing for neurotoxicity, *J. Am. Coll. Toxicol.,* 8, 29–34.

Sivam, S. P., Norris, J. C., Lim, D. K., Hoskins, B., and Ho, I. K. (1983). Effect of acute and chronic cholinesterase inhibition with DFP on muscarinic, dopamine, and GABA receptors of the rat striatum, *J. Neurochem.,* 40, 1414–1421.

Tilson, H. A. and Mitchell, C. L. (1984). Neurobehavioral techniques to assess the effects of chemicals on the nervous system, *Annu. Rev. Pharmacol. Toxicol.,* 24, 425–450.

U. S. Congress, Office of Technology Assessment (1990). *Neurotoxicity: Identifying and Controlling Poisons of the Nervous System* (OTA-BA-436): U. S. Government Printing Office, Washington, DC.

[USEPA] U. S. Environmental Protection Agency (1991). *Neurotoxicity Testing Guidelines,* National Technical Information Service, Springfield, VA.

[USEPA] U. S. Environmental Protection Agency (1993). Draft report: Principles of neurotoxicity risk assessment, *Fed. Reg.,* 58, 41556–41599.

Weiss, B. L., Forster, G., and Kupfer, D. J. (1976). Cholinergic involvement in neuropsychiatric syndromes. In *Biology of Cholinergic Function* (A. M. Goldberg and I. Hanin, eds.), Raven Press, New York, pp. 609–617.

Wu, C. H. and Narahashi, T. (1988). Mechanism of action of novel marine neurotoxins on ion channels, *Annu. Rev. Pharmacol. Toxicol.,* 28, 141–161.

Zigmond, M. J. and Stricker, E. M. (1989). Animal models of parkinsonism using selective neurotoxins: Clinical and basic implications, *Int. Rev. Neurobiol.,* 31, 2–60.

# 13
# Immunotoxicity Testing

**Kathleen Rodgers**
*University of Southern California*
*Los Angeles, California*

## I. BACKGROUND

### A. Function of the Immune System

Immunotoxicology is a subdiscipline in toxicology that examines the effects of xenobiotics on the immune system (NRC, 1992; Smialowicz and Holsapple, in press). As reviewed in Chapter 6, this system confers resistance of the host to infection by bacteria, viruses, and parasites; functions in the rejection of allografts; and may eliminate spontaneously occurring tumors (Mims, 1982). Proper function of the immune system is exquisitely sensitive to disruptions in physiological homeostasis (Folch and Waksman, 1974; Heiss and Palmer, 1978; Jose and Good, 1973; Monjan and Collector, 1977; Purtilo et al., 1972). The immune response is highly regulated; however, there is a great deal of duplication in the immune system, in that different mechanisms may be used to eliminate a foreign antigen. Therefore, a toxicant may affect one facet of the host defense against an infective agent without altering the ability of the host to survive challenge by another such agent.

### B. Overview of Immunotoxicology

Several recent reviews have surveyed the effects of various xenobiotics on the immune system (Smialowicz and Holsapple, in press; Dean et al., in press). The classes and types of chemicals found to be immunotoxic are too extensive to be reviewed in this chapter. However, pesticides are one class of compound that is immunotoxic. A summary of the pesticides that have an effect on the immune system can be found in Table 1 (reviewed in Rodgers, in press). The strength of evidence for the ability of these chemicals to affect the immune system is widely varied, from one study showing a small change after in vitro exposure, to well-characterized effects on an immune response with an attempt to define the mechanism of action of the chemical. Each study and the body of evidence for the immunotoxic potential for a compound should be analyzed

**Table 1**   Pesticides That Affect the
Immune System

Organochlorine pesticides
    Chlordane
    Dichlorodiphenyltrichloroethane (DDT)
    Dieldrin
    Heptachlor
    Lindane
    Mirex
    Toxaphene
Organophosphate pesticides
    Carbophenothion
    Crufomate
    Demeton-*o*-methyl
    Dichlorovos
    Diisopropylethyl phosphate
    Dimethoate
    Malathion
    Methyl parathion
    Monocrotophos
    *O,O,O*-Trimethyl phosphorothioate
    *O,O,S*-Trimethyl phosphorothioate
    *O,S,S,*-Trimethyl phosphorodithioate
    Parathion
    Soman
    Tetra-*o*-cresyl piperazinyldiphosphoramidate
    Triphenyl phosphate
    Triphenyl phosphine oxide
    Tris(2,3-dichloropropyl)phospate
Carbamate
    Aldicarb
    Aminocarb
    Carbaryl
    Carbofuran
    Ethyl carbamate
    Methyl carbamate
Pyrethroid
    Allethrin
    Cypermethrin
    Deltamethrin
    Fenpropathrin
    Permethrin
Herbicides
    Atrazin
    Diuron
    Mecoprop
    Propanil

*Source:* Reviewed by and originally referenced in Rodgers
(Immunotoxicology of Pesticides).

before extrapolation of the data to effects on human health. Factors that should be considered in such an analysis include the relevance of the dose administered to human exposures, the route of administration, the site of action of the chemical, and the level of immune alteration noted (Table 2). Only with such a detailed and careful analysis of the information can the relevance of animal studies to effects on human health be determined.

## C. Generation of an Immune Response

The generation of an immune response results in the formation of effector cells, either cytotoxic T lymphocytes (CTL) or antibody-secreting plasma cells. The humoral response, which protects against bacterial and viral infections, is mediated by the collaboration of the macrophage, the regulatory T lymphocyte, and the B lymphocyte. Protein factors, called lymphokines, cytokines, or interleukins, are released from all three cell types and provide signals for lymphocyte and macrophage differentiation and interaction (Oppenheim and Cohen, 1983). The plasma cell generated by this response is a terminally differentiated B lymphocyte that secretes an antibody monospecific for the antigen that stimulated the immune response. These antibodies mediate the clearance of antigen by several mechanisms. The cell-mediated immune response eliminates cells that do not express the normal self-antigens (virally infected cells, neoplastic cells, or tissue allografts). This response results from the interaction between macrophages, regulatory T lymphocytes, and precursors of CTL. The CTL eliminates the antigen through direct cell–cell contact and subsequent lysis of the cell bearing the antigen.

## D. Nonspecific Immunity

Many defenses against incoming antigens do not require a time lag or previous exposure to the antigen to be effective (Werb and Goldstein, 1987). Mononuclear phagocytes, polymorphonuclear neutrophils (PMN), and natural killer cells are effector cells in the mediation of nonspecific immunity. Natural killer cells, through a mechanism similar to, but not identical with, lysis by CTL, lyse tumor cells that express proteins which render them sensitive to natural

**Table 2** Considerations for Immunotoxicity Testing

Examination of nontoxic dose
    To eliminate complications of other toxic effects
    To reduce the influence of stress
Selection of species
    Metabolism
    Manipulation of the system
    Comparability with human immune response
Ability to be included in standard toxicity screen
    Usually examine basal immunity
    Typically least sensitive to modulation
Considerations for use of in vitro exposure
    Influence of metabolism
    Pharmacokinetics
    Indirect effects on immune system
    Relevance of concentration to in vivo exposure

killer cells. The PMNs are effective in the elimination of invading bacteria through the release of cytocidal factors. Macrophages are important in protecting the host against tumors and intracellular parasites. The function of the macrophage and PMN is multifaceted, in that they can remove particulate matter through phagocytosis, generate oxygen radicals through a respiratory burst, and secrete many inflammatory mediators and proteases. The macrophage is also key in the generation of a specific immune response and is involved in several other systems, including inflammatory response, coagulation, and wound healing.

Other aspects of nonspecific immunity include the barrier between the body and the outside world that is provided by the skin and gut. These initial defenses are very important in the maintenance of physiological well-being, and many possible antigens are eliminated before the generation of a specific immune response by these systems.

## II. CONSEQUENCES OF IMMUNE MODULATION

### A. Immune Enhancement

Normally, the protection of the host against infection and neoplastic disease is accomplished in the absence of extensive destruction of the surrounding tissues, owing to tolerance of self-antigens through mechanisms not currently understood. However, a number of diseases involve hypersensitivity of the immune system to either foreign (e.g., allergy) or self (auto-immunity) antigens. Allergic responses occur in response to numerous environmental antigens, including ragweed and domesticated animals (Terr, 1987). Allergy is the result of the formation of allergen-specific IgE antibodies, which bind to mast cells or basophils and lead to degranulation of these cells on subsequent exposure to antigen, and allergen-specific T-cell activation. Autoimmune diseases include juvenile diabetes (which may result from a viral infection of the pancreatic islet cells and their subsequent destruction), penicillin-induced hemolytic anemia, and myasthenia gravis (which is the result of the formation of antibodies to receptors for acetyl-choline) (Theofilopoulos, 1987). The etiology of autoimmune disease is complex, multifaceted, and not yet well understood.

### B. Immune Suppression

The study of human immunodeficiency disease syndromes reveals a clear association between the suppression or absence of an immunological function and an increased incidence of infectious or neoplastic diseases (Ammann, 1987). Immunosuppressive agents are used in treating autoimmune disease and as adjunctive therapy in organ transplantation procedures to prevent rejection of the donor tissue. Studies in this area provide information on the clinical effects of chronic, low-level immunosuppression. These types of therapies have resulted in an increase in the incidence of parasitic, viral, fungal, and bacterial infections. There is a well-established association between the therapeutic use of chemical immunosuppressive agents and an increased incidence of infections and neoplastic diseases in humans (Penn, 1985).

The acquired immunodeficiency syndrome (AIDS) provides another example of the consequences of immunosuppression, in which the loss of immune responsiveness is associated with an increased incidence of disease, most notably from *Pneumocystis carinii* and other opportunistic pathogens, and the development of Kaposi's sarcoma, a rare form of cancer.

## III. CONSIDERATIONS IN SCREENING FOR IMMUNOTOXICITY

As stated, the immune system is designed to respond to influences from the external environment and to defend the host from the invading antigens. As a result, the function of the immune system is very susceptible to alterations in the physiology of the host. For example, stress and pregnancy will substantially alter the ability of an animal to generate an immune response to antigen (Monjan and Collector, 1977; Purtilo et al., 1972). Therefore, care should be taken to design experiments that will minimize alterations in the physiological homeostasis of the laboratory animal (see Table 2). This distinguishes the direct immunotoxic effects (i.e., the immune system is the most sensitive target for the compound) from alterations in immune function owing to toxicity. This does not mean, however, that alterations in immune function as a result of indirect effects are not important to acknowledge and determine.

## A. Examination of Nontoxic Doses

To reduce the contribution of stress, or the release of corticosteroids in response to tissue damage by the compound, when examining the effects of an agent on the immune system, initial studies should be conducted at nontoxic doses, as measured by the most sensitive parameter to assess toxicity. For example, inhibition of red blood cell acetylcholinesterase is currently thought to be a sensitive indicator of organophosphate toxicity. Therefore, studies of the immunotoxicity of organophosphate compounds should be conducted at doses that do not inhibit the activity of the blood enzyme (i.e., noncholinergic doses) (Rodgers and Ellefson, 1992).

## B. Selection of Species

The mouse is the species most often used in the assessment of the immunotoxic effects of a chemical. However, the effects of a chemical on the immune system may vary from species to species. The differences among species may be due to differences in the pharmacokinetics of the compound or to those within the immune system. These differences should be acknowledged and compensated. For example, if possible, studies should be conducted on an animal species for which the metabolic capability is similar to humans. In addition, if the immune response under consideration differs from species to species, the site of action should be determined. For example, the number of mast cells or basophils in a given organ varies from animal to animal. This identification of the site of action allows a further understanding of the effects a compound may have on the human immune system and indicates potential differences between animals and humans. That is, if the site of action of a compound can be determined and the importance of the analogous site to the function of the human immune system can be established, then the ability of the animal model to predict the risk to human health by exposure to a given chemical can be more fully evaluated.

Recent studies on the immune system of fish and other nonmammalian species of interest in ecotoxicological studies indicate that similar types of immune responses can be examined in these species (Zelikoff, in press).

## C. Inclusion in Standard Toxicology Screen

Pathological evaluation can be a useful immunotoxicological assessment because it can be incorporated into the standard toxicological assessment of new chemicals (Vos, 1980). Therefore, it would not be necessary to use more animals than those required in the standard toxicological bioassay. Immunopathological evaluation includes assessment of hematological values, as well as weight, histopathology, and the cellularity of lymphoid organs (Kuper et al., in press).

However, as will later be discussed further, immunopathological analysis is not a sensitive parameter and does not measure an immune function. Additional models are being generated to minimize the number of animals that would be added to a toxicological study to assess the effects of a compound on immune function. Exon and others (1986) have developed a system in the rat that allows the assessment of several immune parameters simultaneously after in vivo immunization. Alternatively, the animals could be treated with the compound in vivo, to allow consideration of the pharmacodynamics of the compound in immunotoxicological testing, followed by in vitro stimulation of the immune response, thereby allowing assessment of several parameters simultaneously (Rodgers et al., 1986). However, in vitro stimulation of the immune response may not allow the detection of the immunotoxic potential of compounds that act at a site present only in the activated macrophage or lymphocyte or through an indirect mechanism.

## D.  Considerations for In Vitro Testing

Although assessment of immune function after in vivo administration of a compound is optimal for several reasons, in vitro exposure to a chemical is often used in immunotoxicology. Several factors should be considered when in vitro exposure is used. These factors include the influence (1) of metabolism on the immunotoxicological potential of the compound; (2) of crossing physiological barriers on the concentration of the compound at the target site; (3) of the endocrine or nervous system on the immune system; and (4) of culture conditions (i.e., concentration of a stimulant, serum type, concentration of the compound, and so on) on the immunotoxic potential of the compound. For example, it is possible to achieve very high concentrations of the chemical in the culture and, thereby, produce immunotoxic effects that would not be observed after in vivo administration. This route of exposure is very useful in that it would measure a direct effect of the chemical on the immunocyte. In addition, the number of animals and subsequently the cost of the experiments is reduced because multiple chemicals can be examined using the cells from a single animal.

## IV.  GENERAL TESTS OF IMMUNE STATUS: BASAL

In the following two sections, several techniques to study immune function are mentioned. The specific methodology for most of these immune function parameters can be found in a recent book entitled *Modern Methods in Immunotoxicology,* edited by Drs. G. R. Burleson, J. H. Dean, and A. E. Munson.

The status of the basal, unstimulated immune system is the easiest to assess during standard toxicological analysis (NRC, 1992). This includes examination of the structure and cellularity of lymphoid organs, the basal levels of immunoglobulins circulating in the peripheral blood, and analysis of the numbers and types of specific immunocyte populations in lymphoid organs by flow cytometric analysis (Kuper et al., in press; Cornacoff et al., in press). However, these measures of immunity are quite insensitive to modulation by environmental toxicants, because the cells and immunoglobulins have long half-lives, and it may require overt cytotoxicity or alterations in the patterns of immunocyte homing to cause a measurable effect. The level of immunoglobulins and the number of cells of a given subpopulation would be a more sensitive measure of immunotoxicity, if these parameters were assessed after administration of an antigen or immunostimulant. However, this would preclude the incorporation of these studies into toxicological examinations as they are currently designed.

As discussed earlier, immunopathological examination of the immune system includes the assessment of hematological parameters and histopathological examination of lymphoid organs. The hematological parameters that would indicate alterations in the immune system include the lymphocytes, PMNs, basophils, eosinophils, and monocytes. The lymphoid organs that should be examined are the thymus, spleen, lymph nodes, bone marrow, and peripheral blood.

Flow cytometric analysis of the subpopulations of cells of the immune system involves the use of reagents called monoclonal antibodies (labeled with fluorescein to allow detection), which recognize proteins specific for certain populations (e.g., CD4, a protein expressed by T cells and macrophages; CD3, a protein associated with the T-cell receptor and expressed on T cells, and others), in various combinations to allow the identification of these populations (Cornacoff et al., in press). By using sophisticated equipment that is readily available in many clinical laboratories—the flow cytometer—the number of cells expressing these markers can be quantitated. The usefulness of this parameter to detect immunotoxicity may increase if it is assessed following stimulation of the immune system. After stimulation of the immune system, new cells infiltrate into the organ in question, and the cells present before stimulation may change the proteins expressed on the cell surface. Interference with this process by a chemical would be immunotoxicity and should be more sensitive to modulation than at basal levels.

## V. SPECIFIC TESTS OF IMMUNE ENHANCEMENT

Hypersensitivity reactions are the most common type of immunotoxicity associated with chemical exposure (Trizio et al., 1988). Hypersensitivity responses and susceptibility to autoimmune disease are strongly influenced by genetics and variations in the neurological–hormonal balance. Animal models are under development to detect and elucidate the mechanisms of hypersensitivity reactions mediated by chemicals (Kimber, in press; Stern, in press; Karol, in press; Sarlo and Clark, in press). However, significant differences in the immunological and inflammatory responses between various laboratory animals have made it difficult to interpret data obtained. The guinea pig is commonly used to evaluate asthmatic and contact sensitivity responses to chemicals (Buehler, in press). The techniques using this species have been refined and validated as sensitive indicators of pulmonary and dermal hypersensitivity, and they show promise as predictors of these disorders in humans (Karol, in press; Buehler, in press). Hypersensitivity reactions are divided into several categories that differ in the kinetics of expression, the cells involved in the generation, and the adverse effects that occur as a result of the response.

### A. Immunoglobulin E- and Immunoglobulin G-Mediated Immediate Reactions

One category of hypersensitivity is immediate hypersensitivity. An immediate hypersensitivity response usually can be identified in routine toxicological studies. Daily exposure of animals to a chemical provides an opportunity to induce an immune response and allows adverse effects to be identified. The guinea pig is considered a sensitive animal for hypersensitivity reactions, as evidenced by erythema, edema, urticaria, pulmonary distress, and other clinical signs of anaphylactic shock that are indicators of the hypersensitivity reaction.

### B. Contact Hypersensitivity

The contact hypersensitivity response, another category of hypersensitivity reaction, is mediated by T cells (i.e., is cell-mediated and transferable with T cells) and is classically demonstrated 24–48 hr after challenge. The response decreases after 48 hr. Many skin sensitization procedures are available and are commonly used to detect this reaction. The following assays (many using the guinea pig) are used to measure this reaction: Buehler test, open epicutaneous test, guinea pig maximization test, Draize test, optimization test, Freund's complete adjuvant test, split adjuvant technique, and mouse ear swelling test (Buehler, in press; Gad, in press). The reactions are complex and require the interaction of many cell types and cytokines during both the sensitization and elicitation phases. These tests differ in the ability of the chemical to penetrate into the skin and in the use of various adjuvants to amplify the immunological response that occurs. A number of parameters are tested in these models from gross examination of the area of treatment, to assessment of cell and protein infiltration using radiolabeled reagents.

## C.  Autoimmunity

Autoimmune disease occurs when the tolerance of the immune system to the host is broken. This breakdown of immune tolerance results in destruction of the person's own tissues. Autoimmune disease has been associated with exposure to xenobiotics (NRC, 1992). The symptoms of autoimmunity manifest after exposure to the chemical and go into remission after removal from exposure. However, there are very few models of autoimmunity currently used in the assessment of the immunotoxicological potential of a chemical (Rose and Bhatia, in press). Since the etiology of the diseases is complex, genetic predisposition or concurrent exposure to self-antigens may interact with the chemical to produce autoimmune disease. There are strains of animals that are genetically predisposed to develop various autoimmune diseases, such as autoimmune diabetes and systemic lupus erythematosus. Autoimmunity can also be induced by injection of autoantigens and an appropriate adjuvant into these animals. However, chemically induced autoimmunity is also possible. Some of the xenobiotics that were shown to cause autoimmune disease in humans were studied in animals with variable results. These studies, for the most part, were conducted in animals not prone to autoimmune disease. Parameters that were examined in these animals include the generation of glomerulonephritis, antinuclear antibodies, anti-DNA antibodies, and glucose and protein in urine.

## VI.  SPECIFIC TESTS OF IMMUNE SUPPRESSION

## A.  Humoral Immunity

The humoral immune response results in the production of antibodies by differentiated B cells. Although the studies of basal immunity, discussed earlier, would be of use in the assessment of the status of the humoral immunity, a determination of immune function should also be conducted. Because of the complexity of this response (see foregoing), the ability of immuno-cytes to generate a primary immune response is a sensitive indicator of immune dysfunction caused by immunotoxicants.

A humoral immune response can be generated after either in vivo or in vitro immunization. Several types of antigens can be used to generate a humoral immune response, with varying degrees of regulatory T-lymphocyte involvement. After in vivo immunization, the response can be measured either by quantitation of the serum antibody titer to the antigen (measured by immunoassay or hemagglutination), or by counting the cells that produce antigen-specific antibodies (through determining the number of plaque-forming cells) (Holsapple, in press; Exon and Talcott, in press). The humoral immune response can also be assessed by the ability of immunocytes to proliferate in response to a mitogen, such as lipopolysaccharide.

## B.  Cellular Immunity

A cellular immune response results in the generation of effector cells that phagocytose or lyse invading antigens. Two assay systems are used to measure the effect of environmental toxi-cants on the in vivo generation of a cell-mediated immune response. One is the generation of a delayed-type hypersensitivity response to antigens, such as keyhole limpet hemocyanin. This response is measured by the area of induration formed, the ability of radiolabeled mono-cytes to migrate and become macrophages, or the amount of radiolabeled albumin that infiltrates the area, all as a result of antigen challenge. The second parameter that can be measured after either in vivo or in vitro exposure to antigen is the generation of CTL to alloantigen (House and Thomas, in press). The level of response is assessed by the ability of immunized cells to lyse target cells that have the same major histocompatibility locus as that of the immunizing antigen. Both of these assay systems involve complex interactions of many cell types and cytokines (House, in press).

The mixed leukocyte response (MLR) is also a measure of the cellular arm of the immune system (Smialowicz, in press). It assesses the ability of the lymphocytes to proliferate in response to alloantigen. Although MLR does not measure the ability of the effector cells to eliminate antigen, it is sensitive to perturbation by chemicals known to affect cellular immunity and is generally more sensitive to changes than the proliferative response to mitogens, which cause polyclonal activation of lymphocytes. The mitogens used to stimulate the proliferation of T cells are the plant lectins phytohemagglutinin and concanavalin A.

## C. Nonspecific Immunity

The immune system is able to eliminate antigen before the generation of specific immune responses through nonspecific mechanisms. Natural killer cells can lyse tumor cells that are sensitive to them at the time of initial exposure (i.e., time to generate a specific immune response is unnecessary; Djeu, in press).

Macrophages and PMNs also participate in the first-line of defense against foreign invaders. Standard assays for nonspecific leukocyte function include quantitation of peritoneal macrophage and PMN number (basal and in response to in vivo stimuli) and quantitation of macrophage phagocytosis (basal and stimulated; Becker, in press; Neldon et al., in press). Currently, standardized assays to measure the function of PMN are lacking, but some are under development, such as phagocytosis and bactericidal activity. Additional estimates of macrophage function that can be measured and are sensitive to modulation by environmental toxicants include quantitation of ectoenzymes, bactericidal activity, tumoricidal activity, modulation of cell surface markers, the respiratory burst activity, nitric oxide formation, the secretion of inflammatory mediators and cytokines, and the presentation of antigen to immunc T cells (Lewis, in press; Rodgers, in press, b; Dietert et al., in press; Qureshi and Dietert, in press). These assays are useful in determining the site of action of various environmental toxicants on the macrophage and the generation of immune responses.

## D. Bone Marrow

The reservoir of stem cells that replenish erythroid, myeloid, and lymphoid cells is found in the bone marrow. This replenishment is necessary following systemic depletion of lymphocytes, granulocytes, macrophages, or red blood cells by chemical destruction or natural attrition. In addition, the bone marrow can supply additional immunocytes, as needed, to fight infection. Because this organ contains many highly proliferating cells, it is sensitive to toxic agents that modulate cellular proliferation. Therefore, a change in the cellularity of the bone marrow could be a useful indicator of a general toxicity, or may lead to immunotoxic effects in circumstances for which it is necessary to call on the reserve of the bone marrow. Two assays currently used to assess the effects of toxicants on the bone marrow are (1) determination of the number of cells that form colonies in the spleen after intravenous injection (colony-forming units; CFU-S) and (2) determination of the number of cells that form granulocyte–monocyte colonies in vitro in response to necessary nutrients (CFU-GM) (Deldar et al., in press).

## VII. HOST RESISTANCE

There are many models of host resistance currently used to assess the integrity of the immune system after exposure to toxicants (Bradley, in press). These assays are expensive to conduct, require special housing to isolate infected animals, and require special facilities to grow the pathogens. Most contract laboratories that conduct immunotoxicity testing have such tests available, but these models are not generally feasible for individual investigators to undertake. Because of the expense and the insensitive (but definitely clinically relevant) endpoint currently used in these assays, these models should not be used to screen the immunotoxic potential of a chemical. However, once an alteration in one area of immune function is noted, the appropriate model (as discussed later) could be used to determine the effect of the toxicant on the integrated immune system to respond to an invader (Luster et al., 1988).

The ability of the body to resist infection by some pathogens is mediated by the humoral immune response. A decrease in the resistance of mice to influenza virus is associated with suppression of the number of plaque-forming cells (measure of humoral immunity) and in the mitogenic responses of B cells. The production of antibodies that opsonize (coat bacteria with antibodies to allow more efficient ingestion by phagocytes) and fix complement and the levels of complement are involved in the elimination of streptococcal infection. In addition, a decrease in humoral immune responses results in increased parasitemia after infection with *Plasmodium yoelli* (the parasite that causes malaria in mice).

Alterations in cell-mediated immunity have also been associated with increased susceptibility to disease. A change in the ability of the host to resist influenza virus, herpes simplex virus, *Listeria monocytogenes* (an obligate intracellular microbe), and *Plasmodium yoelli* infections, and to eliminate the tumor PYB6 was correlated with alterations in MLR. Changes in T-cell responses to mitogen and cell-mediated responses are correlated with the ability of the mouse to eliminate *Listeria monocytogenes,* herpes simplex virus, PYB6 tumor, and *Plasmodium yoelli.*

## VIII. HUMAN IMMUNOTOXICOLOGY

Methods for testing the immune function in human populations have been adopted from clinical immunology (NRC, 1992). In this setting, an unusual susceptibility to infections is characteristic of a defect in immunity, whether primary or secondary. In addition, as reviewed in Chapter 6, immune hypersensitivity or autoimmune disease can result from overactivity of the immune system. A systemic approach to the evaluation of immunocompetence is based on simple screening procedures, followed by appropriate specialized tests of immune function. Currently, the tests are not sensitive enough to detect modest immunodeficiency caused by toxic agents. This is because a wide range of responses in normal individuals resulting from day-to-day and person-to-person variability in these responses. The testing methods to assess immune function parameters in human populations are reviewed in Reese and Betts (1991), Aloisi (1988), and the NRC publication of *Biologic Markers in Immunotoxicology* (1992). The tier-testing regimen outlined in the NRC publication involves a series of currently recommended assays. The first tier presents a series of simple tests that can be done on all individuals to screen for immunodeficiency. The fraction of the population that is found to be outside the normal range in the first tier would undergo the testing outlined in tiers 2 and 3 in this scheme. Currently available tests examine the ability of the immune system to respond to secondary recall antigens (antigens previously exposed to during childhood vaccinations or normal illnesses). Because this secondary recall response is less sensitive to modulation than a primary immune response, it is recommended that antigens be developed that could be given to test a primary immune response (i.e., the human population has not been previously exposed to the antigen) and to which it would be safe to expose the general population. Currently, keyhole limpet hemocyanin (KLH) is one such antigen under consideration. However, it is necessary to develop additional primary antigens for evaluation of the immune system in longitudinal studies.

## IX. IMMUNOTOXICITY TESTING IN RISK ASSESSMENT

The place of immunotoxicity testing in the assessment of the risk of an adverse effect in response to a chemical is currently under development. Many agencies are establishing guidelines for the use of immunotoxicity testing in the regulation of chemicals. In some instances, the effects of a chemical on the immune system is relatively well-defined and the immune system is the organ most sensitive to the effects of the chemical. In a few instances, the U. S. Environmental Protection Agency (USEPA) has chosen to use these data obtained from immunotoxicity testing to establish regulatory guidelines.

Attempts have been made in the scientific community to determine (1) which tests of immune function can detect chemicals that have immunotoxic potential with the greatest reliability, and (2) what level of immune suppression is correlated with an increase in the sensitivity to disease (Luster et al., 1992; Luster et al., in press). The generation of a primary humoral immune response to an antigen that requires the interaction of the B cell with regulatory T lymphocytes was the most sensitive parameter to modulation by a chemical (i.e., the testing of this characteristic identified 78% of the immunotoxic chemicals). Various immune measurements, in conjunction with the generation of a primary immune response, were able to detect greater than 90% of the remaining immunosuppressive chemicals. These studies suggest that two or three tests of immune function, used together, could detect most immunosuppressive chemicals, regardless of the mechanism of action.

Additional studies showed that, contrary to what was thought previously, a slight suppression of immune function could result in an increase in the susceptibility to disease if the population being examined was large enough. These studies indicate that immunotoxicity testing of a chemical is important and could be accomplished using relatively few assays.

As always, however, the drawback to animal testing is the extrapolation of the data obtained from administration of high doses of a single chemical in laboratory animals to the assessment of the risk of the same effect occurring in humans after exposure to a low dose of the chemical in a complex environment. Studies in research laboratories that establish the mechanism by which a chemical acts to modulate an immune response are useful in the risk assessment process. Once a site of action is determined, the contribution of this site to the resistance of the host against disease or in the generation of a hypersensitivity reaction in the human and animal species can be assessed, and a more reasonable determination of the risk can be reached.

In summary, although the contribution of the field of immunotoxicity to risk assessment is still being established, inroads have been made into the definition of such a contribution.

## REFERENCES

Aloisi, R. M. (1988). *Principles of Immunology and Immunodiagnostics,* Lea & Febiger, Philadelphia.

Ammann, A. J. (1987). Immunodeficiency diseases. In *Basic and Clinical Immunology* (D. P. Stites, J. D. Stobo, J. V. Wells, eds.), Appleton & Lange, Norwalk, CT, pp. 317–355.

Becker, S. E. (in press). Fc-mediated macrophage phagocytosis. In *Modern Methods in Immunotoxicology* (G. R. Burleson, J. H. Dean, and A. E. Munson, eds.), John WIley & Sons, New York.

Bradley, S. G. (in press). Host resistance: Introduction. In *Modern Methods in Immunotoxicology* (G. R. Burleson, J. H. Dean, and A. E. Munson, eds.), John Wiley & Sons, New York.

Buehler, E. V. (in press). Prospective testing for delayed contact hypersensitivity in guinea pigs: The Buehler method. In *Modern Methods in Immunotoxicology* (G. R. Burleson, J. H. Dean, and A. E. Munson, eds.), John Wiley & Sons, New York.

Cornacoff, J. B., Graham, C. S. and LaBrie, T. K. (in press). Phenotypic identification of peripheral blood mononuclear leukocytes by flow cytometry as an adjunct to immunotoxicity evaluation. In *Modern Methods in Immunotoxicology* (G. R. Burleson, J. H. Dean, and A. E. Munson, eds.), John Wiley & Sons, New York.

Deldar, A., House, R. B., Wierda, D. (in press). Bone marrow colony forming assays. In *Modern Methods in Immunotoxicology* (G. R. Burleson, J. H. Dean, and A. E. Munson, eds.), John Wiley & Sons, New York.

Dietert, R. R., Hotchkiss, J. H, Austic, R. E. and Sung, Y. J. (in press). Production of reactive nitrogen intermediates by macrophages. In *Modern Methods in Immunotoxicology* (G. R. Burleson, J. H. Dean, and A. E. Munson, eds.), John Wiley & Sons, New York.

Djeu, J. Y. (in press). Natural killer activity. In *Modern Methods in Immunotoxicology* (G. R. Burleson, J. H. Dean, and A. E. Munson, eds.), John Wiley & Sons, New York.

Exon, J. H., Koller, L. D., Talcott, P. A., O'Reilly, C. A., and Henningsen, G. M. (1986). Immunotoxicity testing: An economical approach multiple-assay approach, *Fundam. Appl. Toxicol.,* 7, 387–397.

Exon, J. H. and Talcott, P. (in press). Enzyme-Linked immunosorbent assay (ELISA) for detection of specific IgG antibody in rats. In *Modern Methods in Immunotoxicology* (G. R. Burleson, J. H. Dean, and A. E. Munson, eds.), John Wiley & Sons, New York.

Folch, H. and Waksman, B. H. (1974). The splenic suppressor cell. I. Activity of thymus dependent adherent cells: Changes with age and stress, *J. Immunol.,* 113, 127–139.

Gad, S. C. (in press). The mouse ear swelling test. In *Modern Methods in Immunotoxicology* (G. R. Burleson, J. H. Dean, and A. E. Munson, eds.), John Wiley & Sons, New York.

Heiss, L. I. and Palmer, D. L. (1978). Anergy in patients with leukocytosis, *Am. J. Med.,* 56, 323–333.

Holsapple, M. P. (in press). The plaque forming cell (PFC) response in immunotoxicology: An approach to monitoring the primary effector function of B-lymphocytes. In *Modern Methods in Immunotoxicology* (G. R. Burleson, J. H. Dean, and A. E. Munson, eds.), John Wiley & Sons, New York.

House, R. V. (in press). Cytokine bioassays and assessment of immunomodulation. In *Modern Methods in Immunotoxicology* (G. R. Burleson, J. H. Dean, and A. E. Munson, eds.), John Wiley & Sons, New York.

House, R. V. and Thomas, P. T. (in press). In vitro induction of cytotoxic T-lymphocytes. In *Modern Methods in Immunotoxicology* (G. R. Burleson, J. H. Dean, and A. E. Munson, eds.), John Wiley & Sons, New York.

Jose, D. J. and Good, R. A. (1973). Quantitative effects of nutritional essential amino acid deficiency upon immune responses to tumors in mice, *J. Exp. Med.,* 137, 1–9.

Karol, M. H. (in press). Assays to evaluate pulmonary hypersensitivity. In *Modern Methods in Immunotoxicology* (G. R. Burleson, J. H. Dean, and A. E. Munson, eds.), John Wiley & Sons, New York.

Kimber, I. (in press). The local lymph node assay. In *Modern Methods in Immunotoxicology* (G. R. Burleson, J. H. Dean, and A. E. Munson, eds.), John Wiley & Sons, New York.

Kuper, C. E., Schuurman, H.-J., and Vos, J. G. (in press). Pathology in immunotoxicology. In *Modern Methods in Immunotoxicology* (G. R. Burleson, J. H. Dean, and A. E. Munson, eds.), John Wiley & Sons, New York.

Lewis, J. G. (in press). State of macrophage activation: Tumor cell cytolysis. In *Modern Methods in Immunotoxicology* (G. R. Burleson, J. H. Dean, and A. E. Munson, eds.), John Wiley & Sons, New York.

Luster, M. I., Munson, A. E., Thomas, P. T., Holsapple, M. P., Fenters, J. D. White, K. L., Jr., Lauer, L. D., Germolec, D. R., Rosenthal, G. J., and Dean, J. H. (1988). Methods evaluation: Development of a testing battery to assess chemical-induced immunotoxicity: National Toxicology Program's guidelines for immunotoxicity evaluation in mice, *Fundam. Appl. Toxicol.,* 10, 2–19.

Luster, M. I., Portier, C., Pait, D. G., White, K. L., Jr., Gennings, C., Munson, A. E., and Rosenthal, G. J. (1992). Risk assessment in immunotoxicology I. Sensitivity and predictability of immune tests, *Fundam. Appl. Toxicol.,* 18, 200–210.

Luster, M. I., Portier, C., Pait, D. G., Rosenthal, G. J., and Germolec, D. R. (in press). Immunotoxicology and risk assessment. In *Modern Methods in Immunotoxicology* (G. R. Burleson, J. H. Dean, and A. E. Munson, eds.), John Wiley & Sons, New York.

Mims, C. A. (1982). *The Pathogenesis of Infectious Diseases,* Academic Press, San Diego, CA.

Monjan, A. A. and Collector, M. I. (1977). Stress induced modulation of the immune response, *Science,* 196, 307–308.

Neldon, D. L., Lange, R. W., Rosenthal, G. J., Comment, C. E., and Burleson, G. R. Macrophage nonspecific phagocytosis assays. In *Modern Methods in Immunotoxicology* (G. R. Burleson, J. H. Dean, and A. E. Munson, eds.), John Wiley & Sons, New York.

[NRC] National Research Council, Subcommittee on Immunotoxicology, Committee on Biologic Markers (1992). *Biologic Markers in Immunotoxicology,* National Academy Press.

Oppenheim, J. J. and Cohen, S. (1983). *Interleukins, Lymphokines and Cytokines,* Academic Press, San Diego, CA.

Penn, I. (1985). Neoplastic consequences of immunosuppression. In *Immunotoxicology and Immunopharmacology* (J. H. Dean, M. I. Luster, and A. E. Munson, eds.), Raven Press, New York, pp. 79–89.

Purtilo, D. T., Halgrew, M., and Yunis, E. J. (1972). Depressed maternal lymphocyte responses to phytohemagglutin in human pregnancy, *Lancet,* 1, 769–771.

Qureshi, M. A. and Dietert, R. R. Bacterial uptake and killing by macrophages. In *Modern Methods in Immunotoxicology* (G. R. Burleson, J. H. Dean, and A. E. Munson, eds.), John Wiley & Sons, New York.

Reese, R. E. and Betts, R. F., eds. (1991). *A Practical Approach to Infectious Diseases,* 3rd ed., Little, Brown & Co., Boston.

Rodgers, K. E. and Ellefson, D. D. (1992). Mechanism of the modulation of murine peritoneal cell function and mast cell degranulation by low doses of malathion, *Agents Actions,* 35, 57–63.

Rodgers, K. E., Imamura, T., and Devens, B. H. (1986). Organophosphate pesticide immunotoxicity: Effects of *O,O,S*-trimethyl phosphorothioate on cellular and humoral immune response systems, *Immunopharmacology,* 12, 193–202.

Rodgers, K. E. (in press). Immunotoxicology of pesticides. In *Immunotoxicology* (R. J. Smialowicz and M. I. Luster, eds.), CRC Press, Boca Raton, FL.

Rodgers, K. E. (in press). Measurement of the respiratory burst of leukocytes for immunotoxicological analysis. In *Modern Methods in Immunotoxicology* (G. R. Burleson, J. H. Dean, and A. E. Munson, eds.), John Wiley & Sons, New York.

Rose, N. R. and Bhatia, S. (in press). Autoimmunity: Animal models of human autoimmune disease. In *Modern Methods in Immunotoxicology* (G. R. Burleson, J. H. Dean, and A. E. Munson, eds.), John Wiley & Sons, New York.

Smialowicz, R. J. (in press). In vitro lymphocyte proliferation assays: The mitogen stimulated response and the mixed lymphocyte reaction in immunotoxicity testing. In *Modern Methods in Immunotoxicology* (G. R. Burleson, J. H. Dean, and A. E. Munson, eds.), John Wiley & Sons, New York.

Smialowicz, R. and Holsapple, M., eds. (in press). Immunotoxicology, CRC Press, Boca Raton, FL.

Stern, M. L. (in press). A radioisotopic method to assess allergic contact hypersensitivity. In *Modern Methods in Immunotoxicology* (G. R. Burleson, J. H. Dean, and A. E. Munson, eds.), John Wiley & Sons, New York.

Terr, A. I. (1987). Allergic disease. In *Basic and Clinical Immunology* (D. P. Stites, J. D. Stobo, J. V. Wells, eds.), Appleton–Lange, Norwalk, CT, pp. 435–456.

Theofilopoulos, A. N. (1987). Autoimmunity. In *Basic and Clinical Immunology* (D. P. Stites, J. D. Stobo, J. V. Wells, eds.), Appleton–Lange, Norwalk, CT, pp. 128–158.

Trizio, D., Basketter, D. A., Botham, P. A., Graepel, P. H., Lambre, C. I., Magda, S. J., Pal, T. M., Riley, A. J., Ronneberger, H., Van Sittert, N. J., and Bontinck, W. J. (1988). Identification of immunotoxic effects of chemicals and assessment of their relevance to man, *Food Chem. Toxicol.,* 26, 527–539.

Vos, J. G. (1980). Immunotoxicity assessment: Screening and function studies, *Arch. Toxicol.,* 4 (Suppl.), 95–108.

Werb, Z. and Goldstein, I. M. (1987). Phagocytic cells: Chemotaxis and effector functions of macrophages and granulocytes. In *Basic and Clinical Immunology* (D. P. Stites, J. D. Stobo, and J. V. Wells, eds.), Appleton–Lange, Norwalk, CT, pp. 96–113.

Zelikoff, J. T. (in press). Fish immunotoxicology. In *Immunotoxicology and Immunopharmacology* (J. Dean, M. Luster, A. Munson, and I. Kimber, eds.), Raven Press, New York.

# PART III
## BASIC ELEMENTS AND APPROACHES IN RISK ASSESSMENT

**Charles O. Abernathy**
*United States Environmental Protection Agency*
*Washington, D.C.*

*Risk* is the probability of an adverse effect occurring after exposure to an agent, whereas *risk assessment* is the process used to quantify that risk. According to the National Academy of Sciences paradigm, risk assessment is a stepwise process consisting of a hazard identification, dose–response evaluation, and exposure assessment, all of which are then integrated into a final risk characterization. Risk assessment can be either qualitative or quantitative, depending on the database used to develop it. Currently, for human health risk assessments, emphasis is put on using existing data to quantitatively extrapolate to individual or population risk.

The underlying principles for risk assessment are covered in this section. Although these can be applied to assessing the risk of almost any activity (e.g., driving automobiles or accidents in the home), this section will concentrate on environmental chemical risk assessments. Accordingly, the focus will primarily be on environmental agents and their relevant routes of human exposure (i.e., dermal, oral, and inhalation).

In environmental toxicology, chemicals have been commonly separated into two classes; those with carcinogenic effects and those producing other types of health effects. Accordingly, risk assessment of environmental chemicals has been generally dichotomous. For assessing noncarcinogenic effects of chemicals that occur after oral exposure, the U. S. Environmental Protection Agency (USEPA) uses a Reference Dose (RfD) methodology (the RfD concept is similar to that of the Acceptable Daily Intake in both theory and practice). The RfD procedure is based on a "threshold" theory that assumes that a "range of exposures from zero to some finite amount can be tolerated by the organism with essentially no chance of expression of the toxic effect."

Recently, the "zero" part of the threshold assumption has been modified to accommodate the essential trace elements (ETEs). With any ETE, a zero exposure can lead to deleterious effects (since an element essential to the well-being of the organism would be lacking) as well as an excessive exposure (which can lead to toxicity). However, the lower end within the range of essentiality does not obviate the presence of a finite upper bound threshold for the lack of toxic effects. In addition, the relative risks to specific subpopulations and new methods for dose–response modeling are being examined by the USEPA. These aspects are covered in the chapter on noncancer risk assessment.

For carcinogens, cancer slope factors are developed to express the carcinogenic potency of the chemicals. In general, agents that can cause cancer, either in experimental animals or humans, have been considered as though there is no threshold for cancer induction. In other words, it is assumed that there is no level of chemical exposure that is "safe," and any exposure poses some risk to the organism, unless there are data that demonstrate otherwise. The chapter on cancer risk assessment covers this subject from its historical aspects to current perspectives. In addition, it discusses many issues that are currently being debated during the revision of USEPA's cancer guidelines. Until the revision is finalized, however, the 1986 guidelines are still in effect.

Calculation of a RfD, or a cancer slope factor, is only one of the first steps in the risk assessment process. This information must then be used in conjunction with various exposure scenarios that are encountered in the environment. Depending on the types of exposure occurring to humans (e.g., exposure to a chemical by ingestion of soil by children, or by ingesting of food or drinking water by a specific population), "real-life" risk assessments are performed. Such aspects are considered in the chapter on medium-specific and multimedium risk assessments.

The final part of the risk assessment paradigm is risk characterization. This step describes the strengths and weaknesses of the database, integrates all the information considered, and gives a carefully weighed discussion of the conclusions presented in the preceding hazard identification, dose–response evaluation and exposure assessment. At times, little emphasis has been placed on this facet, and it has been neglected by some as playing an important role in risk assessment. However, this discussion is of paramount importance. Risk characterization summarizes and integrates the database on a chemical to provide an understanding of the overall quality of the risk assessment. This overall characterization is discussed in the chapters on cancer and noncancer risk assessment.

# 14

# Cancer Risk Assessment: Historical Perspectives, Current Issues, and Future Directions*

**Susan F. Velazquez**
*Toxicology Excellence for Risk Assessment*
*Cincinnati, Ohio*

**Rita Schoeny and Glenn E. Rice**
*United States Environmental Protection Agency*
*Cincinnati, Ohio*

**Vincent J. Cogliano**
*United States Environmental Protection Agency*
*Washington, D.C.*

## I. INTRODUCTION

### A. Historical Perspectives

In the simplest terms, *cancer* may be defined as a disease of unregulated growth. Although it is common to refer to cancer as a distinct entity, in actuality, cancer encompasses a multitude of different diseases having different etiologies, varying manifestations, and different prognoses for treatment and cure.

Cancer has been associated with the natural process of aging, but causal associations have also been inferred between the development of various cancers and diverse types of exposures, including the following: radiation, biological agents (e.g., cytomegalovirus, schistosomial parasites), naturally occurring plant products (e.g., aflatoxins, cycasin), solid-state materials (e.g., asbestos), inorganics (e.g., nickel refinery dust), and organic materials (e.g., vinyl chloride). Many lifestyle and natural factors appear to modify the carcinogenic process, either providing protection from, or increasing the likelihood of, a neoplastic response. These include genetic predisposition or resistance, dietary influences, immunocompetency, age, and endogenous hormonal factors. The scope of this chapter will focus on the risk assessment of chemical carcinogens, but will briefly consider numerous other factors that influence carcinogenesis.

Chemical carcinogenesis was first reported in 1775 by Dr. Percival Pott, the English surgeon who linked the occurrence of human scrotal cancer with exposures to the mixture of materials found in chimney soot (Pott, 1775). Nearly 150 years later this observation was extended to other

---

*The opinions in this manuscript are those of the authors and do not necessarily reflect the opinion or policies of the U.S. Environmental Protection Agency.

mammals. Yamagiwa and Ichikawa (1915, 1918) described the elicitation of a neoplastic response on the ears of rabbits and later on mouse skin following the dermal application of coal tar. Subsequent work by Kennaway (1924a,b) dealt with fractionation of coal tars into less complex mixtures; treatment of animals with specific chemical compounds, rather than mixtures, soon followed (reviewed in Pitot, 1981).

This pattern of initial identification of carcinogenicity in humans followed by experimental demonstration was also seen for another important class of chemical carcinogens: namely, the aromatic amines. Rehn, a German physician, reported on a cluster of bladder cancers observed among dye workers in Germany in the early 1800s (Rehn, 1895). One of the constituents of their exposure, β-naphthylamine (2-aminonaphthalene), was shown to be carcinogenic in dogs in 1937 (Williams and Weisburger, 1991). Vinyl chloride and cigarette smoke are other agents determined to be carcinogenic, first in humans and, subsequently, in animal models. From the standpoint of human health, this is not the preferred sequence of events. The goal of the risk assessment process is the identification of the type and extent of potential human hazards so that avoidance or remediation can be implemented to prevent negative impacts on human health.

## B. Mechanisms of Carcinogenesis

Chemical carcinogens have been grouped as being either genotoxic (those that cause a permanent change in DNA) or nongenotoxic. Mechanisms of nongenotoxic chemicals are diverse, and may be specific for the species, strain, sex, or organ involved. A discussion of nongenotoxic carcinogenesis is found in Section III.B.

For those compounds interacting with DNA, some are direct acting (e.g., *N*-nitroso-*N*-methylurea), but the majority require metabolism to reactive electrophilic species, as demonstrated by the pioneering work by Miller and Miller (1981). Once formed, electrophilic metabolites bind covalently to nucleophilic sites found on proteins, DNA bases, and other cellular macromolecules. Because of the many types and high concentrations of metabolizing enzymes present in the liver, this organ has the largest capacity for the biotransformation of carcinogens. Several other organs, including skin, kidney, and lung, also have the ability to metabolize chemicals to active species.

The metabolic activation of carcinogens represents one major rate-limiting step for subsequent chemical–DNA interactions (e.g., the formation of DNA adducts), which may be linked to the development of cancer. Route of exposure, exposure regimens, and species, sex, and age differences have roles in defining the metabolic fate of a chemical.

Once nuclear DNA has been damaged, several repair mechanisms may come into play. Most repair processes result in error-free restoration of the original DNA sequence. Some unrepaired altered base sequences are themselves mutagenic (e.g., $O^6$-methylguanine adducts, which cause mispairing). It appears, however, that the majority of permanent, heritable changes in DNA structure are the consequences of errors made during some DNA repair processes. These types of repair may be called into play when DNA replication occurs before repair of damaged sequences or when damage to the genome is extreme or at multiple sites. Mutations can take many forms, including single-base changes; small additions or deletions, resulting in a shift of the message-reading frame; large deletions; translocations, inversion of sequences, and amplification of sequences.

Carcinogenesis has been recognized for some time as a process that results after multiple events have occurred on the cellular level. Studies that have been conducted to discern whether distinct stages of the carcinogenic process could be defined led to the adoption of operational terms such as initiation, promotion, and progression. *Initiation* has traditionally been defined as an irreversible first step involving DNA mutations that have become permanently integrated into the cell's genetic information and are passed on to all subsequent generations of cells.

Likely targets for initiation are oncogenes and tumor suppressor genes. These genes are normal constituents of the genome, and generally code for proteins that play a role in physiological processes involved in various aspects of cell division and growth regulation. Specific mutations to these oncogenes, or the loss or inactivation of tumor suppressor genes, can result in genetic changes, leading to altered protein products that are defective in performing their normal roles in growth regulation. Alternatively, the normal proteins may be over- or under-expressed. Many oncogenes and tumor suppressor genes, either through activating mutations or altered expression, have been shown to play a role in many cancers, both in humans and in experimental animal models (reviewed in Bos and van Kreijl, 1992; Harris, 1992).

In the classic initiation–promotion theory of carcinogenesis, an initiated cell can remain quiescent or undergo limited proliferation. Various stimuli can then cause the initiated cell(s) to begin a clonal expansion. It is this stage, during which the cells no longer respond appropriately to normal growth control signals, that has been referred to as promotion or progression. This process can be facilitated by chemical-promoting agents (e.g., phorbol esters), physiological factors (e.g., hormonal influence), or physical stresses (e.g., wounding) that lead to a proliferative response.

The terms initiation, promotion, and progression were coined from experiments demonstrating that different agents can elicit a carcinogenic response when administered in a specific order (i.e., a single dose of an initiator followed by repeated administration of a promoter). Although it appears that some temporal requirements exist for different stages in the carcinogenic pathway, it is clear that many of these stages may occur simultaneously, or they may be reversed with an equal carcinogenic outcome. A good example of this is colon cancer, for which multiple genetic changes must occur, the order and specificity of which are not rigidly defined (Fearon and Vogelstein, 1990).

Chemical carcinogens are generally identified from animal bioassays or epidemiological observations, in which the incidence of tumors at various sites is measured. Generally these studies give very little indication about how the chemical acted in increasing the incidence of tumors. The most commonly available "mechanistic" information has to do with the ability of the agent to produce DNA damage or mutation. Initiation–promotion assays, primarily in skin or liver, can tell whether the chemical fits some functional definition: *initiator* (something that needs to be given only once or a few times to produce neoplasia when followed by a promoter); or *promoter* (something that is generally given repeatedly and after an initiator to produce tumors). This terminology, however, is overly restrictive in that chemical carcinogens do not generally fit into narrowly defined mechanistic categories. A central goal in modern cancer risk assessment is to develop and employ mechanistic information, resulting in a more detailed and more complete characterization of the circumstances leading to carcinogenicity.

## II. OVERVIEW OF CANCER RISK ASSESSMENT BY THE U.S. ENVIRONMENTAL PROTECTION AGENCY

In 1986, the U.S. Environmental Protection Agency (USEPA) published general guidelines to be used by agency scientists in developing and evaluating risk assessments for carcinogens (USEPA, 1986). Although a general framework is presented that describes the process to be used for cancer risk assessments, it is stated at the outset that "the guidelines emphasize that risk assessments will be conducted on a case-by-case basis, giving full consideration to all relevant scientific information." To promote consistency in scientific decisions, particularly in areas of uncertainty or controversy, the guidelines offer science policy guidance or a preferred agency approach. The USEPA's guidelines follow the risk assessment paradigm described by the National Research Council in 1983 (NRC, 1983), which defines four components of risk assessment: hazard identification, dose–response assessment, exposure assessment, and risk characterization. It is also consistent with the underlying scientific and policy basis of other federal agencies (e.g., Office of Science and Technology Policy; see OSTP, 1985).

## A.  Hazard Identification of Carcinogens

Hazard identification refers to the process of determining if a compound has the potential to elicit a carcinogenic response in humans. Many types of information may be used to determine the overall weight-of-evidence of carcinogenicity: epidemiological information, chronic animal bioassays, mutagenicity tests, other short-term tests, structure–activity relationships, metabolic and pharmacokinetic properties, toxicological effects, and physical and chemical properties (USEPA, 1986).

The current guidelines specify that information be categorized into one of three types: human data, animal data, and supporting data. All information contributes to the assignment of the agent into a category based on the weight of evidence that the material is a carcinogen for humans. The process is done in two steps. In the first step, the animal and human data are evaluated for adequacy and are described in the following terms: sufficient, limited, inadequate, no data, and no evidence of carcinogenicity. The guidelines define some requirements for each of these judgments. For example, *sufficient human data* may consist of "evidence of carcinogenicity, which indicates that there is a causal relationship between the agent and human cancer"; the guidelines indicate that life-threatening benign neoplasms in humans are included in the evaluation. The guidelines for animal bioassay data deal with such topics as the relevance of specific tumor types to human cancer; the use of benign neoplasms (generally included); the number of observations required for sufficient data (generally two independent studies); use of tumors with high background incidence; and the use of information from studies conducted at the maximum tolerated dose (MTD). The human and animal data on the agent (including nonpositive studies) are then used to make a preliminary judgment on the likelihood that it may produce tumors in humans. This judgment is expressed in terms of the following categories:

Group A: Carcinogenic to humans
Group B*: Probably carcinogenic to humans
Group C: Possibly carcinogenic to humans
Group D: Not classifiable for human carcinogenicity
Group E: Evidence of noncarcinogenicity for humans

The second step is to evaluate the supporting data (e.g., genotoxicity, mechanistic data, and pharmacokinetic information). The level of concern indicated by evaluation of the supporting data is used to elevate or downgrade the classification. For a description of the amount and type of data required for a chemical to be assigned to any one of these groups, the reader is referred to the guidelines (USEPA, 1986).

The principal issues for hazard identification are twofold: (1) whether the bioassay demonstrates an association between the amount of agent administered and an increase in carcinogenic outcome; and (2) if so, what the implications are for human carcinogenicity. Statistical tests can

---

*Group B includes the categories B1 and B2. Limited human evidence of carcinogenicity is necessary for placement of a chemical in Group B1. Group B2 includes chemicals with sufficient animal evidence, but inadequate human evidence for carcinogenicity.

help answer the first of these questions, as described in the following. The implications for human carcinogenicity are discussed in Section III.

### 1. Trend Tests Versus Pairwise Comparison Tests

The primary unit of analysis is an experiment involving all dose groups for one sex and strain of animal. The typical National Toxicology Program (NTP) protocol, for example, provides four experiments: male rats, female rats, male mice, and female mice. Each tumor type is considered separately. Benign lesions are generally counted together with malignant tumors if they are of the same histological origin and can progress to malignancy. This practice also recognizes that cancer bioassays are typically terminated while most animals are expected to be alive, so that a benign lesion at the end of the study can represent a malignancy that would have developed had the animal lived out its total life span. The USEPA follows the guidance provided by the National Toxicology Program (McConnell et al., 1986) for determining which benign and malignant lesions are appropriate to combine.

Any set of tumor incidences from a cancer bioassay involves some uncertainty because of sampling error: If the experiment were repeated, some difference in the observed incidences would be expected, based on chance alone. To determine whether chance is a plausible explanation for an apparent increase in carcinogenic activity, statistical tests are used. They estimate, given the number of animals tested and the size of the increase in incidence, the probability that the observed results could have been due to chance alone. If chance is an unlikely explanation, then confidence is increased in the existence of a biological explanation for the observed results. Two kinds of statistical tests—trend tests and pairwise comparison tests—have been used to answer the question of whether the tumor incidences for one sex and strain of animal show an increase in carcinogenic activity.

*Trend Tests.* Trend tests focus on whether the results in all dose groups, considered together, as a whole, increase in accordance with the level of dose. One commonly used trend test is the Cochran–Armitage trend test (Snedecor and Cochran, 1980). This test fits a straight-line regression of the tumor incidences across all dose groups as a function of dose level. The result is a $p$ value that estimates the probability that the slope of the regression line could be zero, which would be true if the tumor incidences showed no overall upward or downward trends with dose. If this probability is small (typically below 5%), indicating that the trend is not likely to be due to chance, then the dose–incidence trend is said to be statistically significant. The Cochran–Armitage trend test also provides a test for nonlinearity, estimating a $p$ value that can be used to determine whether the dose–incidence data differ significantly from a linear relationship.

*Pairwise Comparison Tests.* These tests focus on whether the incidence in one particular dose group, considered separately from the others, is increased over the control group incidence. The most commonly used pairwise comparison test is the Fisher exact test (Fisher, 1932). It provides a $p$ value representing the probability that differences as large as those observed between the dose group and the control group would happen by chance. If this probability is small (typically below 5%), indicating that the difference is not likely to be due to chance, then the tumor incidence in the dose group is said to be statistically significantly increased over the control.

These two kinds of statistical tests have different strengths and limitations, and they can sometimes give conflicting results. Significance in a pairwise comparison test is highly dependent on the numbers of animals in the dose and control groups. If the numbers of animals are small, a pairwise comparison test may report statistical significance for only large increased incidences; this can make it unlikely to report statistical significance for carcinogens of low to medium potency. This limitation can be overcome by using a trend test. Because a trend test considers all dose groups together, the sample sizes across all dose groups are effectively pooled, providing greater power to identify a small, but real, increase in incidence as statistically significant.

On the other hand, significance in a trend test depends on the presence of an overall trend across all dose groups. If tumor incidences for the highest doses are sharply reduced because of competing mortality, no overall trend may be apparent. This limitation can be overcome by adjusting for competing risks or by dropping animals from the group if they are not considered to be at risk for tumors.

There are other cases for which an overall trend may not be apparent. Suppose a chemical is carcinogenic through metabolic activation, and metabolism becomes saturated below the doses tested in the bioassay. Then all dose groups (except controls) would receive approximately equal doses of the carcinogenic metabolite. If there were several dose groups, the dose–response curve would appear to be mostly flat, no trend would be apparent, and a trend test would be unlikely to report statistical significance.

The USEPA generally considers statistical significance in a trend test as signifying a positive experiment. The examples described illustrate why further analysis and judgment are usually necessary to determine whether the experimental protocol or the chemical's activity would affect the behavior or appropriateness of any statistical test in a particular set of circumstances. Multiple statistical tests can sometimes provide greater insight. It is not, however, an appropriate use of multiple statistical tests to require confirmation of a significant trend test with significance in a pairwise comparison or other test.

### 2. Historical Versus Concurrent Controls

Whenever possible, concurrent controls are used to analyze the results of an experiment. Concurrent controls usually share much in common with the other animals in an experiment: source and age of animals; dates, location, room conditions, protocol, personnel, and other experimental conditions; as well as slide preparation, evaluation criteria, personnel, and pathological evaluation. There are, however, some circumstances when additional perspective may be gained by using historical controls in an analysis.

Which animals are appropriate to include as historical controls can be a complex matter requiring careful judgment. Many animal strains have exhibited a *genetic drift,* in which the control tumor incidence is not stable, but has changed over time. Criteria governing pathological evaluations have changed over time for some tumors. The experiments may have been conducted in different laboratories, and the slides may have been evaluated by different pathologists. The experiments may have been conducted under somewhat different protocols; age and health of the animals, for example, may be particularly important. It is important to select only those historical controls that are representative of the background incidence of the animals in the experiment in question. A reasonable rule of thumb is to consider only historical control data from the concurrent control-testing laboratory, and within a 3- to 5-year period of the assay.

With rare tumors, historical control data are essential to understanding the rarity of the tumor type. Experience with 50 concurrent controls does not provide the proper perspective that comes from a thorough knowledge of the experience of a particular strain at a particular laboratory. For example, a concurrent control incidence of 0:50 does not take on the same importance as an overall historical control incidence of 0:2000, or even 1:2000. This is an important consideration in determining which statistical tests are appropriate in an analysis. Pairwise comparison tests, which are highly dependent on the number of animals, can give misleading results when only concurrent controls are used in a comparison for a rare tumor.

Sometimes it is desirable to look to historical control information to determine whether the experience of a concurrent control group is an aberration. For example, if the tumor incidence in the concurrent control group is uncharacteristically low, an experiment may give a false-positive indication. Conversely, if the tumor incidence in the concurrent control group is uncharacteristically high, an experiment may give a false-negative indication.

Historical control information, by its nature, cannot satisfactorily resolve this question. Although historical control information can add valuable insight into whether the experience of the animals in a particular bioassay is unusual, it cannot be used to conclude that only the concurrent control group is unusual, whereas the dosed groups are not. That is, differences between concurrent controls and historical controls are not an explanation for differences observed between concurrent controls and dosed animals—it is just as reasonable to conclude that the background tumor rate for all animals in an experiment happened to be somewhat higher or lower than usual. In view of the presumption that concurrent controls are generally the most representative of the animals in an experiment, careful judgment must be applied before the interpretation of results using concurrent controls is altered by the use of historical controls.

## B. Dose–Response Assessment for Carcinogens

Dose–response evaluation is considered appropriate for those materials judged to be group A, human carcinogens, and group B, probable human carcinogens. Dose–response evaluation is done on a case-by-case basis for those agents categorized as group C, possible human carcinogen. This assessment is distinct from the weight-of-evidence approach used to determine the probability that a chemical possesses a carcinogenic potential for humans. As emphasized in the guidelines, the "calculation of quantitative estimates of cancer risk does not require that an agent be carcinogenic in humans."

Ideally, the estimation of the carcinogenic potency of a chemical would be based on human data. Epidemiological data, however, are not generally available or suitable for use in quantitative dose–response assessments, requiring that animal models be used a surrogates. The guidelines suggest that "data from a species that responds most like humans should be used, if information to this effect exists." In practice, information is usually not available to suggest that, for a given chemical, one species is definitely better able to serve as a model for carcinogenesis in humans than another. Since humans may be as susceptible as the most sensitive animal species, the data set demonstrating the greatest tumor response (and thus leading to the most conservative risk estimate) has traditionally been used. There are certain types of tumors, however, that have been demonstrated to have no relevance to human cancer, and these are now considered as being inappropriate as a basis for hazard identification or dose–response assessment. These are discussed in more detail later in this chapter.

The initial step is to identify the data set(s) to be used for the dose–response evaluation. Although relevance to humans is a consideration, the quantitative estimate does not attempt to predict a tumor type or tumor site to be found in humans. Tumor types not found in humans, or tumors in animal organs not present in humans, may indicate carcinogenic potential and thus can be used to estimate potency. Other considerations in the choice of data sets include study quality, route of exposure (i.e., relevance to environmental exposures), and statistically significant increases in incidence. Generally, benign tumors are included in the total incidence to be modeled, unless there is scientific evidence to indicate that these tumors would not progress to malignancy.

After identifying the study that is most appropriate for developing a quantitative risk estimate, the next step is to transform the doses to which the animals were exposed into human-equivalent doses. In concert with other federal agencies, the USEPA (1992) has recently proposed the use of a cross-species scaling factor of (body weight)$^{3/4}$, which is based on a body surface area adjustment. This scaling factor, representing a consensus opinion of several federal agencies, was chosen over other options, such as the previously used scaling factor of (body weight)$^{2/3}$ (also based on surface area) or scaling on the basis of a straight body weight conversion. Analysis of the variation of key physiological parameters as a function of body size was performed across several mammalian species, and supported the cross-species scaling factor of (body weight).$^{3/4}$ After having transformed the administered doses to human equivalent doses, the next step is to model the dose–response information to determine the carcinogenic potency of the chemical at low doses. This is accomplished with the use of statistical models, described in the following.

Cancer bioassays are generally performed in laboratory animals at very high doses relative to levels at which humans are actually exposed. These high doses are necessary to produce a statistically measurable effect, given the relatively small number of animals used. Dose–response assessment, however, is concerned with estimating quantitative carcinogenic risk associated with environmental exposures. Alternatively, risk managers may be interested in setting standards for exposures by various media (e.g., air or drinking water) based on a carcinogenic risk level that is considered to be de minimis (e.g., 1:1 million risk). Data from a cancer bioassay can generally provide information only about the dose associated with a statistically significant tumor incidence, from 5 to 100% (Clayson, 1978). To determine experimentally the shape of the dose–response curve down to a low tumor incidence (e.g., 1%), thousands of animals would be required. For example, the "ED$_{01}$" study, by the National Center for Toxicological Research (NCTR), used 24,192 rodents at considerable expense (Cairns, 1979). Since the use of thousands of animals is not feasible for routine testing, the question becomes how best to estimate the shape of the dose–response curve at very low levels of cancer risk (i.e., below those that can be determined experimentally).

In the absence of mechanistic data to support a threshold mechanism, it has been assumed by the USEPA and most regulatory agencies that any dose of a carcinogen is associated with some increased risk. The results of the ED$_{01}$ study are consistent with this idea for a genotoxic agent. This study involved exposing over 24,000 female BALB/c mice to low doses of 2-acetylaminofluorene (2-AAF) for up to 33 months (Gaylor, 1979). Carcinogenic responses attributed to 2-AAF were observed in the liver and bladder. For liver tumors, a linear relationship was apparent over the range of experimental doses, supporting a nonthreshold mechanism of tumor induction. The incidence of bladder tumors was not linear, but decreased dramatically at the lower end of the dose range. As time was extended, however, the incidence of bladder tumors increased at the lower doses, so that no threshold could be determined. It was concluded by Gaylor (1979) that the ED$_{01}$ study "demonstrates the impossibility of establishing time–dose thresholds, even with large numbers of animals."

The nature of the curve at levels of exposure below the lowest experimental dose is unknown. Several models have been developed to estimate cancer risk in this region. Some stochastic models are based on biological theory of distinct events (e.g., DNA damage) that are responsible for the carcinogenic response elicited by a chemical. These include the one-hit (Hoel et al., 1975), multihit (Rai and Van Ryzin, 1981), multistage (Crump, 1979; Crump et al., 1976), and two-stage models (Moolgavkar and Knudson, 1981; Thorslund et al., 1987). Although these models are based on assumptions of biological events leading to carcino-genesis, they are, in reality, arbitrary because relatively little is actually known about these events (Munro and Krewski, 1981). Other models are more purely statistical. These include, for example, the logit (Doll, 1971; Cornfield et al., 1978), probit (Mantel and Bryan, 1961), and Weibull (Carlborg, 1981) models. These models assume that each animal exposed to a carcinogen has its own level of tolerance. Although thresholds may exist for individuals, the variance for these individuals precludes the demonstration of a population threshold (see Munro and Krewski, 1981 for review).

Another type of modeling takes into account changes in the latency period, or time-to-tumor, induced by a carcinogen. This type of model is based on the idea that treatment with a carcinogen may affect the length of time before a tumor develops, and this process may be dose–dependent (WHO, 1978). It was demonstrated in the $ED_{01}$ study that the time-to-tumor of bladder tumors became progressively longer as the dose decreased, leading to speculation that, whereas a threshold may appear to be present for a certain tumor type, an alternative explanation is that a decreased dose results in an increased latency period that eventually exceeds the length of the observation period (Gaylor, 1979).

Still other modelers have attempted to incorporate knowledge of the kinetics of a carcinogen into shaping the low region of the dose–response curve. The model proposed by Cornfield (1977) refers to a dose–response relationship in the shape of a hockey stick, resulting from a fairly low increase in tumor incidence until one reaches a dose level at which one or more physiological processes (e.g., deactivating metabolism) are saturated. After this point, there is a significant rise in tumor incidence with increasing dose.

Application of different mathematical models to a cancer data set can result in broad differences in the estimates of risk at low doses. The model used most often by the USEPA is adapted from the multistage model, originally proposed by Armitage and Doll (1954, 1961), which assumes that cancer is the result of a sequence of changes in a cell or organ and that exposure to a carcinogen can increase the transition rate between these stages, leading to malignancy. To simplify the mathematical computations, a more flexible model, with fewer constraints than the Armitage–Doll model, was proposed by Crump et al. (1976). However, that the Crump formulation could sometimes produce numerically unstable low-dose risk estimates, when changing the results of only one or two animals could affect low-dose risk estimates by several orders of magnitude. Accordingly, the 95% upper confidence limit of the linear component of this model is generally used as an upper-bound estimate of cancer potency (formerly referred to as the $q_i^*$ by the USEPA), because it is numerically more stable than a central estimate and also is in keeping with the low-dose linear approach adopted for cancer risk assessments (USEPA, 1986). The 1986 guidelines provide the latitude for other models that can be validated to be used in low-dose extrapolations for the estimation of cancer potencies (USEPA, 1986). There are generally no data to demonstrate that one model is superior to another. The linearized multistage model (LMS) has traditionally been the model of choice because it provides a plausible and stable upper-bound estimate that is not likely to underestimate the cancer risk, but recognizes that, at very low doses, the response could be zero. This model is consistent with the theory of the multistage, nonthreshold nature of cancer. It is also recognized that exposure to carcinogenic agents, particularly those acting by nongenotoxic mechanisms, may elicit effects that add to background processes (e.g., increased mitogenesis) and, as such, may also be represented by low-dose linear extrapolation. As more mechanistic data become available and statistical models are further refined, cancer risk assessment will become oriented toward developing chemical-specific low-dose extrapolation models.

## III.  BIOLOGICAL ISSUES IN CANCER RISK ASSESSMENT

In the absence of adequate epidemiological studies, the process of hazard identification and dose–response assessment is often highly dependent on controlled experiments on laboratory animals. The assumption is that, unless there is evidence to the contrary, chemicals or other agents shown to elicit a carcinogenic response in other species may be considered to have a similar tumorigenic potential in humans. Although risk assessors adopt this as a default position, it is also widely recognized that this underlying assumption may not be valid in some circumstances.

For some chemicals, tumorigenic potential across species may be quite comparable. Perhaps the best known example of a carcinogen with similar activity in several species is that of vinyl chloride, which causes liver cancer in every mammalian species tested, including humans, by several modes of administration. For other chemicals, the target organ(s) is species-specific. Following exposure to β-naphthylamine, dogs, hamsters, monkeys, and humans develop bladder cancer; mice develop hepatomas; however, cats, rabbits, and rats do not develop cancer (Clayson, 1975; Shubik and Clayson, 1976).

To fully understand the potential a chemical has for inducing cancer in humans, it is necessary to understand the mechanism by which it is causing cancer. The potential for the same or a related mechanism to be operative in humans would then provide the basis for extrapolation from other animal species to estimate the risk of cancer to humans. The following is a description of some mechanisms, specific tumor types, and specific chemicals for which there are indications that methods other than the traditional low-dose extrapolation may be more appropriate.

## A.  Use of Data from Animals Tested at the Maximum Tolerated Dose

Many of the carcinogen risk assessments developed by the USEPA are based on repeated, daily administration of an agent to animals (generally rodents) at an array of dose intervals. In these bioassays, the animals in the highest-dose group are administered what is considered to be the MTD. A National Cancer Institute (NCI) report defined the *MTD* as "the highest dose of a test agent during the chronic study that can be predicted not to alter the animals' longevity from effects other than carcinogenicity" (Sontag et al., 1976). The MTD is generally derived from a shorter-term (e.g., 90 days) study employing a broad dose range of the same compound and test species from which one dose level, found to be slightly toxic, is selected as the highest dose to be administered in the lifetime bioassay. The objective of testing at the MTD is to elicit a measurable toxic response in a group of exposed animals, without causing excessive lethality or toxicity (Chhabra et al., 1990).

The validity of conclusions based on carcinogenicity testing at the MTD continues to be the subject of debate, an in-depth review of which can be found in NRC (1993). Testing at the MTD has been defended by some as being a necessary component of the hazard identification process. Proponents of this dosing strategy have justified its use by citing the importance of considering uncertainties associated with extrapolation of a carcinogenic response and dose–response from test species (usually rodents) to humans (Kociba, 1987). If no carcinogenic response, but also no toxic response, is demonstrated in a chronic study, then one may argue that the doses tested were not sufficient to elicit any measurable response. Consequently, a study that fails to achieve an MTD and also fails to elicit a neoplastic response, does not definitively answer the question of the potential for this chemical to be a carcinogen. Carr and Kolbye (1991) state that the original intent of the MTD was to minimize the possibility of not detecting a carcinogen by providing the greatest opportunity to exhibit carcinogenicity. In other words, maximizing the exposure minimizes the possibility of nondetection (false-negative result).

Opponents of this testing regimen argue that administration of certain types of compounds (e.g., nongenotoxic chemicals having no specific cellular receptor) at the MTD leads to a proliferative response. This response could result from repeated cell damage followed by reparative hyperplasia that ultimately evolves into uncontrolled cell growth. Mechanisms that elicit a carcinogenic response at the MTD, therefore, may not be relevant at the relatively low environmental levels of carcinogenic agents to which humans are generally exposed (Ames and Gold, 1990). Alternatively, proponents of the MTD argue that all events leading up to clinical cancer diagnosis are not known; toxicity and increased proliferation can certainly be two important contributing factors, but are probably not the only critical events (Weinstein, 1992). In fact, for different types of cancers, a wide array of different cellular or organ events may be critical.

Two multichemical analyses of chronic (2-year) NTP bioassays showed that chemically induced cell proliferation and organ toxicity did not always correlate with cancer in rodents. Tennat et al. (1991) examined the relation between mutagenicity, toxicity, and carcinogenicity for 31 compounds, which NTP had tested between 1987 and 1989 in the same rodent species and strains. Chemically induced toxicity and hyperplasia did not always result in a neoplastic response for either mutagenic or nonmutagenic compounds. It was concluded that other elements (e.g., tumor suppressor genes, immune factors, chromosomal perturbations) may effectively limit the expression of carcinogenicity in these nonpositive bioassays (Weinstein, 1992). The results of Tennant et al. support the earlier work of Hoel et al. (1988) in which similar test animal endpoints were evaluated for 99 NTP compounds.

Opponents of the MTD-based testing regimen state that the problem of the MTD starts with its imprecise definition. Further arguments are based on three points: (1) high doses lead to toxicity, mitogenicity, and ultimately cancer; (2) abnormal physiological processes that result from chronic high-dose testing may be responsible for the carcinogenic response; and (3) empirically, many compounds that seemingly have no effect in humans test positively in animals at the MTD.

Cell division is an important element in the multifactorial process of cancer. Cellular progression from a normal to a transformed state can be "locked in" (i.e., permanently integrated into the DNA) only during replication (Cohen and Ellwein, 1991). Long-term high dosing has the capacity to cause repeated cell insult and death, leading to compensatory hyperplasia. Because replicating cells have an elevated mutation risk by chance alone, the MTD-related mitogenesis may, in part, be responsible for increased mutagenesis and carcinogenesis. This has contributed to a belief that mechanistic studies of carcinogenesis may be more valuable when determining human risk than bioassays involving exposure to the MTD (Ames and Gold, 1990).

Second, animals and humans are not normally subjected over a long period to the high levels of compounds used in cancer bioassays. Long-term exposure to high doses may upset physiological or homeostatic mechanisms leading to, for example, hormonal imbalance, immune dysfunction, and diminished DNA repair capabilities (Carr and Kolbye, 1991). Increased cancer incidence has also been linked to advancing age; the MTD testing regimen may cause physiological changes, similar to aging, to occur earlier in life. The elevated metabolic rate of rodents may exacerbate this artificial aging.

The USEPA (1986) guidelines for cancer risk assessment support the use of bioassays that expose animals to the MTD. This subject has been evaluated recently by the National Academy of Sciences Committee on Risk Assessment Methology (CRAM) (NRC, 1993). A number of criticisms of the MTD testing regimen were cited:

1. The mechanism by which some agents induce cancer at high doses (e.g., induction of cell proliferation) may not be operative at lower doses; therefore, they may not be relevant to human exposures.
2. Even when effects are present at low doses, tumor incidence data generated at the MTD may provide little insight into the nature of the dose–response relationship at lower doses.
3. Strong correlations have been shown between toxicity and carcinogenicity, leading some to suggest that the two are inherently related. It was noted, however, that this is not true for all chemicals.

The majority of this committee recommended that the MTD should continue to be used as the highest tested dose in carcinogenicity bioassays, but that to facilitate interpretation, the rationale for dose selection should be clearly explained. The CRAM report states that "the MTD bioassay as currently conducted in rodents is most useful as a qualitative screen to determine whether a chemical has the potential to induce cancer. It does not provide (nor was intended to provide) all the information useful for low-dose human risk assessment" (NRC, 1993). For chemicals that induce cancer at the MTD, it was suggested that additional data are necessary to determine the relevance of the response to human health risk assessment. In particular, data should be obtained on the chemical-specific mechanisms of carcinogenicity. No conclusions were given, however, on how this information may be used in consort with data from an MTD-bioassay to establish a quantitative cancer potency estimate.

The minority view point, also outlined in the CRAM report, maintains that dose selection should not be based on the MTD, but should be selected only after analysis of preliminary studies is completed to gain information about the mechanisms of toxicity and the dose–response relationship for toxic effects. The highest dose chosen for a cancer bioassay, then should be such that it is "expected to yield results relevant to humans, not the highest dose that can be administered to animals without causing early mortality from causes other than cancer" (NRC, 1993).

## B. Nongenotoxic Carcinogens

Clayson (1989) has described *nongenotoxic carcinogens* as "agents that fail either directly or indirectly to interact in a biologically significant manner with cellular DNA." The question of whether an agent induces cancer by genotoxic mechanisms is significant because of the assumptions that are made in low-dose extrapolations using statistical models. These models generally assume that carcinogens operate without a threshold and that some degree of risk is associated with any exposure. This assumption may not be valid for some nongenotoxic carcinogens, which may demonstrate a threshold below which they pose no carcinogenic risk.

It has been suggested that separate approaches to the risk assessment of carcinogens be adopted for genotoxic and nongenotoxic compounds (Clayson and Clegg, 1991). A decision tree approach has been described by Butterworth and Eldridge (1992) to help a risk assessor decide whether chemical-specific data support the use of the linearized low-dose extrapolation, or whether a quantitative risk estimate could be better determined by other methods (e.g., the NOAEL/uncertainty factor approach).

Nongenotoxic carcinogens may elicit their effects in a number of ways, involving such mechanisms as diverse as cytotoxicity or chronic tissue damage, leading to reparative proliferation, hormonal imbalances, immunological deficits, and impaired DNA repair mechanisms (reviewed in Butterworth and Eldridge, 1992). Because the mechanisms of nongenotoxic carcinogens are diverse, and often not well characterized, they are also difficult to define. The one factor that appears to be operative for most nongenotoxic carcinogens is their ability to stimulate cell proliferation (Ramel, 1992).

In a review of 139 chemicals determined to be carcinogenic by the NTP, Ashby and Tennant (1988) reported that 57 (42%) were not mutagenic in the salmonella mutation assay, commonly referred to as the Ames test (Ames et al., 1973a,b). Although this in vitro assay has been acknowledged as only one measure of genotoxicity, and other assays may reveal additional types of gene mutation, the salmonella assay is a sensitive first-level screening tool for identifying genotoxic compounds. Although it is difficult to develop screening tools to detect nongenotoxic carcinogens, Ramel (1992) suggested that the most appropriate endpoint of choice would be an ability to induce cell proliferation.

The types of tumors that are found to result from the administration of nonmutagenic chemicals to animals tend to be limited to a more narrow range of target tissues than those of genotoxic carcinogens (Ashby and Tennant, 1988). The best-studied systems demonstrating tumorigenesis after exposure to nongenotoxic carcinogens include the liver of the B6C3F1 mouse, male rat kidney, rat thyroid, and rat bladder and urinary tract. These are discussed in more detail later.

## C. Peroxisome Proliferators

One mechanism by which a diverse group of chemicals has been hypothesized to induce liver cancer in rodents involves peroxisomal proliferation. Peroxisomes are organelles (found preponderantly in the liver) that contain a variety of enzymes, including those that are responsible for the β-oxidation of fatty acids. Under normal conditions, metabolism by peroxisomal enzymes is secondary to other cellular metabolic routes (Stott, 1988).

Some chemicals that induce liver tumors in rodents also cause proliferation of peroxisomes (Stott, 1988). Agents suggested to induce cancer by a mechanism involving peroxisomal proliferation are diverse, and include commercial plasticizers, such as di(2-ethylhexyl)phthalate (DEHP); chlorophenoxy acid herbicides; some polychlorinated biphenyl isomers; the fibrate hypolipidemic drugs (e.g., clofibrate, ciprofibrate); and even high-fat diets (see Gibson, 1993 for review). Although the morphological characteristics of liver tumors induced by peroxisome proliferators are similar to those induced by genotoxic carcinogens, some notable differences have been observed; namely, lack of expression of γ-glutamyltranspeptidase, alpha + fetoprotein, or glutathione *S*-transferase-P (reviewed in Reddy and Rao, 1991).

Although the mechanisms of peroxisomal proliferation and of the subsequent carcinogenic response are not fully known, it appears that a receptor-mediated process, possibly related to the nuclear steroid receptor superfamily, is involved (Issemann and Green, 1990). The requirement for an interaction with a cellular receptor helps explain the cell-specific effects observed for peroxisomal proliferators, which induce the proliferation of these organelles only in the liver, despite their presence in virtually all cell types (Reddy and Rao, 1992).

Peroxisome proliferators are nongenotoxic both in vivo and in vitro (Butterworth et al., 1987; Cattley et al., 1988). The induction of cancer by peroxisome proliferators has been postulated to involve at least three possible mechanisms involving oxidative stress, cell proliferation, and promotion of spontaneously initiated cells. The oxidative stress attributed to peroxisome proliferators is believed to result from receptor-mediated activation of specific genes, such that hydrogen peroxide-generating enzymes are produced at levels that far outweigh the minimal increases in peroxide-degrading enzymes (e.g., catalase) (Reddy and Rao, 1992). By using a hydroxylated base (i.e., 8-hydroxydeoxyguanosine) as a measure of oxidative DNA damage, Takagi et al. (1990) have shown that, indeed, peroxisome proliferators are capable of inducing DNA damage that is consistent with the hypothesis of oxidative stress.

Marsmen et al. (1988) suggested that the extent of cellular proliferation, perhaps resulting from oxidative damage, is more closely associated with the development of liver tumors than is the degree of actual peroxisomal proliferation. This observation supported a theory that the operative mechanism for peroxisome proliferators involved cellular proliferation. Because increased cellular proliferation increases the chance for spontaneous mutations, any agent inducing cellular division may ultimately be responsible for an increased incidence of neoplasia (Stott, 1988). The role of cellular proliferation in peroxisome proliferator-induced carcinogenesis has been minimized, however, by investigators who have shown that the induction of a mitogenic response is highest during the initial week of exposure to peroxisome proliferators, with the response decreasing over time, despite continued exposure (Rao and Reddy, 1989). Although the induction of cellular proliferation is losing favor as a mechanism by which peroxisome proliferators induce cancer, it may still play an important role, insofar as it may be involved in the stages of tumor progression (Cattley et al., 1991; Rao and Reddy, 1992).

The relevance of peroxisomal proliferation as a mechanism for human carcinogenesis has been questioned by some. Peroxisomal proliferation appears to be greater in smaller species, particularly rodents, but is less active in larger species, including primates (Cohen and Grasso, 1981). Epidemiological studies of hyperlipidemic patients treated with peroxisome proliferators have not shown increases in cancer, and biopsies have failed to demonstrate the proliferation of peroxisomes (Cattley et al., 1992). The degree of peroxisomal proliferation that is induced may not be the endpoint of concern, however. More recent findings demonstrating the interaction of peroxisome proliferators with a cytosolic receptor suggest that this may be the key to subsequent biological effects. As with other receptor-mediated events, it is possible that no threshold can be demonstrated for the effects of peroxisome proliferators. The role that these agents may play in human carcinogenesis, and the mechanisms by which they may elicit their effects are not yet known. It is clear, however, that the potential for receptor-mediated effects that are relevant to human carcinogenesis, possibly involving effects on other nuclear genes, cannot be ruled out.

## D. Liver Tumors in the Male B6C3F1 Mouse

The liver of the male B6C3F1 mouse is the most common target organ observed in animal carcinogenesis testing by the National Toxicology Program (NTP) (Maronpot et al., 1987). Of the chemicals tested by the NTP that were found to have carcinogenic activity in mice, rats, or both (141 chemicals out of 278 tested through 1984), about 50% (71/141) caused liver tumors in mice (Haseman et al., 1985). For 26 of these 71 chemicals, mouse liver was the *only* organ demonstrating a neoplastic response. Because of the frequency with which chemicals induce mouse liver cancer in 2-year bioassays, a great deal of attention has been focused on the import of murine hepatocarcinogenesis. The European Society of Toxicology devoted a symposium to this topic, the proceedings of which provide a good review of the issues (Maronpot et al., 1987).

The relevance of mouse liver cancer to human health has been challenged on several bases. Whereas liver cancer is observed at very high frequencies in certain strains of mice, it is a rare cancer in humans in most parts of the world (although it is more common in developing countries). In relation to the prevalence of other types of cancer, liver ranks 14th in developed countries, but 7th in developing countries (WHO, 1990). The geographic distribution shows a good correlation between higher incidence areas (e.g., sub-Saharan Africa, East and South-East Asia) and the prevalence of hepatitis B and also aflatoxin contamination of foodstuffs (WHO, 1990).

The relevance of liver cancer in the male B6C3F1 mouse has been questioned because many widely divergent chemicals (e.g., pesticides, phenobarbital, butylated hydroxyanisole [BHA], chlorinated hydrocarbons) are able to induce a dose-related increase in mouse liver tumors, but not in rat liver or in any other organ system. Most of the chemicals shown to be uniquely carcinogenic to murine liver do not appear to be genotoxic, supporting an argument by many that the etiology of these tumors may not be operative in other organs or in other species.

Genetic differences among inbred mouse strains have resulted in variable, and often high, levels of spontaneous liver tumor formation. For example, C57BL and BALB/c mice exhibit relatively low frequencies of spontaneous liver cancer (1–4%), whereas C3H mice and B6C3F1 mice (used in the NTP bioassay) are much more susceptible (20–80%) (Buchmann et al., 1991). These substantial strain differences have raised questions about the validity of using mouse liver tumors in susceptible strains in both the hazard identification and dose–response assessment of carcinogens.

Apart from strain variations, male mice are more susceptible than females to liver cancer. Analyzing the tumor incidence data from control (untreated) B6C3F1 mice in 59 studies, Haseman et al. (1985) reported an average liver tumor (adenoma or carcinoma) incidence of 30 ± 8% for males, but only 8 ± 4% for females. In males, the incidence of carcinomas was about twice that of adenomas, whereas incidences were similar for females. A hormonal basis for this difference between male and female mice has been postulated.

Strain differences in susceptibility to hepatocarcinogenesis have been attributed, to a large extent, to a genetic predisposition termed *hcs* (hepatocarcinogen-sensitivity locus) that is involved in the regulation of cell division (Hanigan et al., 1990). Genetic linkage analysis has recently demonstrated that there are at least three separate genes that are involved in determining murine susceptibility to liver cancer (Gariboldi et al., 1993). *Hcs-1* is located on chromosome 7, in the same region as the H-*ras* oncogene (Hillyard et al., 1992). The H-*ras* oncogene is activated (e.g., acquire transforming properties) by point mutations in hot spots of the gene (i.e., codons 12 and 61). The H-*ras* oncogene is activated, to a large extent, in both spontaneous and chemically induced tumors of sensitive strains (e.g., B6C3F1), but rarely in insensitive strains (e.g., C57BL, BALB/c; Buchmann et al., 1991). Activation of *ras* oncogenes is also quite rare in rat liver tumors (Stowers et al., 1988).

A small percentage of human liver cancers have been attributed to genetic factors (reviewed in Dragani et al., 1992), but these do not appear to be related in any way to the genetic predispositions seen in certain strains of mice. The most striking difference between liver cancer in humans and mice is that cirrhosis is a major risk factor in the development of liver cancer in humans, but develops very rarely in mice. Likewise, whereas *ras* activation is highly prevalent in susceptible mouse strains, it is rarely found in human hepatocellular carcinoma (Tada et al., 1990). This suggests that the mechanisms involved in human liver cancer may not be the same as those in B6C3F1 mouse liver. It is possible, however, that mechanisms similar to those operative in mouse liver (such as activation of the *ras* oncogene) may be relevant for human organs other than liver. This possibility is supported by reports that *ras* oncogenes are activated in a wide variety of human tumors (reviewed in Bos, 1989).

Species-specific metabolic differences have also been purported to contribute to the high frequency of mouse liver tumors. Chemical carcinogenesis often involves the metabolic oxygenation of the parent compound to reactive intermediates (e.g., epoxides, quinones). The formation of reactive oxygen radicals (e.g., superoxy anion or hydroxy radical) may also result from metabolic activities. Oxidative metabolism, which takes place primarily in the liver by mixed-function oxidases, varies inversely with body size. The mouse may be particularly susceptible to DNA damage resulting from its high rate of oxidative metabolism. For many xenobiotics, this rate is about 50 times greater than that of humans (Davidson et al., 1986).

For the forgoing reasons, the relevance of mouse liver tumors to human cancer risk has been questioned. The B6C3F1 mouse continues to be used in bioassays conducted by the National Toxicology Program, largely because of the large amount of historical information on this strain, and also because of the moderately low incidence of liver tumors in female B6C3F1 mice. Until more conclusive evidence disallows the use of this strain (in particular, data on liver tumors), it cannot be assumed that the operative mechanisms leading to liver cancer are not also possible in humans. The USEPA (1986) guidelines provide the latitude and guidance for less weight to be given to male mouse liver tumors in the hazard identification of carcinogens, and for dose–response on murine liver cancers to be considered less appropriate than data from other target organs for use in the determination of a quantitative cancer risk estimate. The quantitative assessment verified by USEPA's Carcinogen Risk Assessment Verification Endeavor (CRAVE) Work Group for pentachlorophenol (PCP), a group B2 carcinogen, is an example (USEPA, 1993). Multiple tumor types were induced in B6C3F1 mice, including liver tumors, pheochromocytomas, and hemangiosarcomas in female mice, and liver tumors and pheochromocytomas in male mice. The most conservative risk estimate (0.5 per (mg/kg)/day) would have resulted from the use of liver tumors and pheochromocytomas in male mice. However, based on the greater biological significance of the hemangiosarcomas in female mice, this was considered to be "the tumor of greatest concern," and the verified slope factor for PCP (0.12 per (mg/kg)/day)) was ultimately based on the combined incidences of hemangiosarcomas, hepatocellular tumors, and pheochromocytomas in female mice.

Determination of the genetic and metabolic similarities and differences between humans and rodents used in carcinogenicity testing, and the relation between genetic makeup and the development of cancer, will contribute greatly to the development of more meaningful risk assessments. Until a greater understanding is reached on the operative mechanisms of carcinogenesis in humans and rodents, however, the induction of liver tumors in the male B6C3F1 mouse should continue to be included in the weight-of-evidence assessment to determine the carcinogenic classification of a chemical.

## E. Male Rat Kidney Tumors

"Classic" renal carcinogens such as nitrosamines, lead acetate, and aflatoxin $B_1$ (Hard, 1990) generally induce cancer in both male and female rats, as well as in other sites and in other species of animals. These compounds are generally genotoxic and are capable of inducing renal tubule cancer in well over half, and sometimes approaching 100% of the exposed animals (USEPA, 1991). Several chemicals, however, induce a significant tumorigenic response exclusively in the kidney of male rats. These tumors are morphologically indistinguishable from either spontaneous kidney tumors or those induced by classic renal carcinogens. Their development, however, proceeds by a specific process involving the accumulation of the male rat-specific protein, $\alpha_{2\mu}$-globulin.

In male rats, normal physiological concentrations of low molecular weight plasma proteins (e.g., $\alpha_{2\mu}$-globulin) are maintained by renal filtration. Removal of these proteins from the plasma is followed by either excretion into the urine or reabsorption and catabolism in the proximal tubules of the kidney. The reabsorbed proteins that accumulate in the renal tubule cells are catabolized in hyaline droplets, which are formed by the fusion of lysosomes with protein-containing endocytic vacuoles. Hyaline droplets in the tubules of male rats contain $\alpha_{2\mu}$-globulin, which, because it is not broken down easily, results in the formation of crystalline structures in the tubule cells (Alden, 1986).

The following events are thought to be involved: accumulation of $\alpha_{2\mu}$-globulin appears to play a causative role in the formation of kidney tumors resulting from certain chemical exposures. These chemicals form complexes with $\alpha_{2\mu}$-globulin that are more resistant to degradation than is uncomplexed $\alpha_{2\mu}$-globulin. Chemicals that form such complexes include unleaded gasoline, pentachloroethane, $d$-limonene, methyl isobutyl ketone, decalin, isophorone, and certain jet fuels (USEPA, 1991).

The consequential accumulation of the chemical–$\alpha_{2\mu}$-globulin complex in the renal tubule leads to an overload of lysosomal protein, and eventually cell death (Swenberg et al., 1989). This, in turn, leads to regenerative proliferation (which is sustained as long as the chemical exposure continues), the formation of foci of hyperplasia and, ultimately, renal tubule tumors. Several investigators have concluded that this series of renal effects that are seen in male rats is not likely to occur in the absence of $\alpha_{2\mu}$-globulin (Flamm and Lehman-McKeeman, 1991; Green et al., 1990).

Although many low molecular weight proteins appear to be common to both males and females and to play similar roles in different species, the $\alpha_{2\mu}$-globulin appears to be species- and sex-specific. It was first characterized in the urine of male rats (Roy and Neuhaus, 1967) and has since been found to be present in most strains of male rats, including F344, Sprague–Dawley, Buffalo, and Brown Norway rats (Ridder et al., 1990). The one exception is the NCI Black–Reiter (NBR) rat (Chatterjee et al., 1989). The accumulation of $\alpha_{2\mu}$-globulin-containing hyaline droplets has not been demonstrated in female rats or in any other species, including mice, hamsters, guinea pigs, dogs, and monkeys (USEPA, 1991). Likewise, $\alpha_{2\mu}$-globulin does not appear to play a role in humans; only about 1% of the concentration of $\alpha_{2\mu}$-globulin in rat urine is found in human urine (Olson et al., 1990).

The Risk Assessment Forum (RAF) of the USEPA has evaluated this unique tumor type and has published its conclusions in a report providing extensive scientific background and policy discussion (USEPA, 1991). The RAF has formulated the following science policy statement:

> Male rat renal tubule tumors arising as a result of a process involving $\alpha_{2\mu}$-globulin accumulation do not contribute to the qualitative weight-of-evidence that a chemical poses a human carcinogenic hazard. Such tumors are not included in dose–response extrapolations for the estimation of human carcinogenic risk.

The RAF also takes this policy statement one step farther to conclude that male rat nephropathy associated with $\alpha_{2\mu}$-globulin accumulation is likewise not suited as an endpoint for determining noncarcinogenic hazard. To apply this policy, enough scientific data must be available to show that, in exposed male rats, the administered chemical was responsible for an increased number and size of hyaline droplets in the renal proximal tubule cells, that the protein accumulating in the hyaline droplets was identified as $\alpha_{2\mu}$-globulin, and that the specific histopathological sequence of lesions caused by $\alpha_{2\mu}$-globulin is present (USEPA, 1991). This sequence starts with the demonstration of an excessive accumulation of hyaline droplets containing $\alpha_{2\mu}$-globulin in renal proximal tubules, followed by cytotoxicity, single-cell necrosis, and regenerative tubule cell proliferation. Subsequently, intralumenal granular casts and papillary mineralization develop, followed by the formation of foci of tubule hyperplasia, and finally renal tubule tumors (USEPA, 1991).

It is important to recognize that not all kidney tumors of male rats involve an accumulation of $\alpha_{2\mu}$-globulin. The use of this tumor type is considered to be appropriate for use in human cancer risk assessments *unless* sufficient evidence exists to implicate $\alpha_{2\mu}$-globulin as playing a causative role.

## F.  Thyroid Follicular Cell Tumors

Another tumor type that presents a unique situation to cancer risk assessors is that of the thyroid follicular cell. In this case, it is not suggested that humans cannot develop thyroid cancer with an etiology similar to that operative in experimental animals. Rather, the question is whether a threshold model should be used for dose–response modeling, and whether there is sufficient evidence to conclude that humans are less sensitive than experimental animal models.

The cause of most thyroid follicular cell tumors (TFCTs) involves a disturbance of the intricate feedback mechanism between the hypothalamus, the anterior pituitary of the brain, and the thyroid gland. Thyroid hormones (THs, also known as triiodothyronine [T3] and thyroxine [T4]) are produced by the thyroid in response to stimulus by the pituitary in the form of thyrotropin (thyroid-stimulating hormone; TSH). The TSH, in turn, is controlled by the amount of thyrotropin-releasing hormone (TRH), secreted by the hypothalamus, and also by the amount of circulating $T_3$ and $T_4$. Thyroid hormones, essentially combinations of iodinated tyrosyl residues, are involved in numerous roles associated with the regulation of metabolism, growth, and maintenance of an animal. Control over the level of THs in the circulation is achieved homeostatically by a negative-feedback system in which a sufficient amount of circulating THs suppresses the release of TSH. Conversely, low levels of $T_3$ and $T_4$ stimulate the pituitary to secret more TSH, in an effort to produce more of the thyroid hormones.

In laboratory animals, many agents that cause a disturbance in the thyroid–pituitary relationship can elicit a tumorigenic response in the thyroid. These include partial thyroidectomy (Dent et al., 1956), iodine deficiency (Schaller and Stevenson, 1966), ionizing radiation (NAS, 1980), and goitrogenic compounds found in foodstuffs (e.g., cabbage; reviewed in Van Etten, 1969). In addition, many synthetic compounds have demonstrated the potential for inducing TFCTs, including several thionamides, aromatic amines, and polyhydric phenols (see Paynter et al., 1986 for review). The mechanisms by which these agents induce cancer are different, but the common denominator is a disturbance of the feedback mechanism between the thyroid and the pituitary. If exposure to an agent causes circulating levels of TH to decrease, the pituitary responds by secreting increased levels of TSH, thereby stimulating a hypertrophic and, eventually, hyperplastic response in the thyroid. After prolonged stimulation, neoplasia may develop. If exposure to the causative agent is terminated and normal homeostatic regulation of thyroid hormones can be resumed, this process is considered to be reversible.

A technical panel of the USEPA's RAF was convened to investigate more fully the mechanisms by which thyroid follicular cell tumors develop and to provide guidance on the use of this tumor type in the risk assessment process. Although no final guidance has been issued by the USEPA, the conclusions of this group have been published by Hill et al. (1989). As suggested by numerous investigators, the technical panel supported the notion that TFCTs may develop as a result of chronic imbalances in the thyroid–pituitary feedback mechanism and that this mechanism may be considered to have a threshold below which neoplasia will not develop. The panel also concluded that, although humans do respond to goitrogens in a manner similar to that observed in experimental animals, the development of TFCTs in humans is relatively rare; ionizing radiation is the only known human thyroid carcinogen (NCRP, 1985).

## G. Bladder Tumors

There has been a great deal of controversy over some well-known rodent bladder carcinogens, which are particularly visible because of their use as artificial sweeteners. Perhaps the best studied of these is saccharin. In contrast with the classic genotoxic bladder carcinogen 2-acetylaminofluorene, saccharin is not genotoxic, appears to operate only at high doses, and induces bladder cancer in rats, but not in mice, hamsters, or monkeys (reviewed in Ellwein and Cohen, 1990). It has also been demonstrated that susceptibility is higher for male rats than females, higher for the F344 strain than Sprague–Dawley rats, and is highly dependent on the type of diet consumed (Garland et al., 1989).

In addition to the species, strain, and sex-specific susceptibilities to saccharin-induced bladder cancer, urinary pH also appears to be a determining factor. The dietary effect may be attributed to differences in the urinary pH that result from the administration of different feeds; rats given the semisynthetic AIN-76A diet have little tumorigenic response to saccharin, apparently because of the low urinary pH associated with this diet (Okamura et al., 1991). Other urinary factors, such as sodium concentration and volume, also play a role in bladder carcinogenesis in the rat (reviewed in Chappel, 1992).

The mechanism for saccharin-induced bladder cancer has been hypothesized to involve the binding of saccharin to urinary proteins, initiating the subsequent formation of silicate-containing precipitate and crystals (Cohen et al., 1991). These urinary crystals act as an abrasive to the bladder epithelium, causing cytotoxicity with resultant regenerative hyperplasia. Cohen et al., (1991) have further hypothesized that the sex-, species-, dose- and diet-specific effects of saccharin may be related to the formation of these crystals.

Numerous epidemiological studies have not demonstrated any clear relationship between bladder cancer in humans and sodium saccharin consumption (reviewed in Elcock and Morgan, 1993). Furthermore, it may be relevant that although bladder stones have been tumorigenic in rodents (Jull, 1979), they have not been related to cancer in humans (Dodson, 1970), raising the question of whether nongenotoxic chemicals that cause only bladder stone-related bladder cancer in rodents are relevant to human carcinogenesis. The issues, then, for determining the relevance of nongenotoxic rat bladder carcinogens to human health are twofold: first, whether the mechanism operative in rats is also operative in humans; and second, whether this mechanism operates with a true threshold, and if so, how can that threshold be determined for humans? These questions have been the subject of active debate and research, the answers to which will provide more meaningful risk assessments of nongenotoxic bladder carcinogens.

## IV. FUTURE DIRECTIONS: REVISIONS TO THE USEPA GUIDELINES

In August of 1988, USEPA initiated a review of the existing guidelines, with several goals in mind. One goal was to update the guidelines to include new information in areas on mechanisms of carcinogenesis (e.g., those described for the association of renal cancer in male rats with the species- and sex-specific $\alpha_{2\mu}$-globulin protein). Such mechanistic information may substantially impinge on the determination of whether a chemical poses a real concern for issues of human cancer. Also, several areas of scientific controversy remained for which no current policy had been established (e.g., how to deal with tumor promoters).

The USEPA convened two workshops to address these issues (USEPA, 1989). The first, in January 1989, convened experts in various areas of science germane to cancer risk assessment. Work groups met to discuss the following topics: use of animal data; weight-of-evidence schemes; and dose–response assessment. A second workshop (June 1989) was held on use of human data in cancer risk assessment. Subsequent to these meetings working groups of USEPA scientists were assembled under the aegis of the RAF to turn the ideas generated in the workshops into a draft of revised Guidelines for Risk Assessment of Carcinogens. In 1992, case studies were run by three groups of USEPA risk assessors to test the application of draft guidance on hazard identification and dose response assessment. At the end of 1992, a working draft of revised guidelines was shared with scientists at a colloquium sponsored by the Society for Risk Analysis. As of this writing, the working draft is being revised, but does not constitute agency policy. Until formal announcement by USEPA is made in the *Federal Register,* the policies set forth in the 1986 carcinogen guidelines remain in effect.

The working draft reflects some major changes of emphasis and procedure for both qualitative and quantitative assessment. The working draft stipulates that a narrative statement be used to express the weight-of-evidence for human carcinogenicity. It has not yet been decided whether to use an alphanumeric-rating system, such as is currently the practice. The working draft specifies that data on carcinogenicity be characterized as either human observational data or experimental data. The latter category includes not only evidence from long-term animal bioassays, but also those types of data considered "supporting data" in the 1986 guidelines (e.g., data on genotoxicity, pharmacokinetics, or structure–activity relationships). Emphasis is on the use and interpretation of mechanistic data in the determination of an agent's potential for human carcinogenicity. The working draft indicates that certain types of animal data judged by the scientific community to be irrelevant to human carcinogenicity be excluded from consideration in the weight of evidence. The example cited in the draft is increased incidence of male rat kidney tumors attributable to $\alpha_{2\mu}$-globulin. The narrative classification can include qualifying statements on likelihood of human carcinogenicity specific to exposures conditions; for example, agent X is not likely to be a human carcinogen under conditions of environmental exposure (dealing with effects secondary to toxicity seen only at a high dose); or agent Y is likely to be a carcinogen by inhalation, but there are not data to indicate a carcinogenic effect by ingestion (route-dependent carcinogenicity).

The working draft indicates that there should be a closer link between the qualitative and quantitative judgments; the mechanism of action of the agent should be an essential consideration in both judgments. The narrative statement can indicate whether and what type of low-dose extrapolation is appropriate.

The dose–response assessment would be done in two steps. The first step would be to fit a model to data in the observed range. The second step, if needed, would be to use an extrapolation procedure to estimate risk in the range of human exposure. In both steps, the preferred approach is to use a biologically based model if there are sufficient data. The draft indicates that data other than tumor incidence (e.g., information on DNA adducts) can be used in the extension of the dose–response below the observable range. A change of emphasis in this document involves the use of a linear procedure as a default in low-dose extrapolation. In the revision, the process would be to provide justification for the use of the LMS (or any other model) instead of justifying a departure from the default. Moreover, the draft contemplates use of a margin of exposure analysis in lieu of a model when a threshold is likely to exist in the dose–response relationship. The draft recommends using all appropriate data in the analysis, in contrast with the selection of a single data set for modeling. Options for presenting results include use of a single data set (if justified), combining data sets for modeling, combining all animals with tumors in a single study, and presenting ranges of estimates and combinations of these options. The goal is to present the results in the way that best represents the biological data.

## V. CONCLUSIONS

Humans are exposed to a multitude of chemicals that pose varying health risks. A mandate for regulatory agencies, such as the USEPA, is to identify those agents that occur, or have the potential to be released into the environment at levels that warrant concern. This chapter has attempted to outline various topics that must be addressed when characterizing the carcinogenic risk posed by a chemical. Biological and statistical issues come into play for assessments of both hazard identification (i.e., the likelihood of a chemical being a human carcinogen) and dose–response (i.e., the dose of a chemical likely to result in a carcinogenic response of a certain magnitude). In addition to hazard identification and dose–response assessments, the actual characterization of carcinogenic risk posed by a chemical also entails a determination of the extent of human exposure, a topic beyond the scope of discussion for this chapter. These assessments each involve the use of many assumptions and estimations, the magnitude of which may be decreased by the incorporation of more information (e.g., mechanistic studies, pharmacokinetic data, improved low-dose extrapolation models). To acquire these data and to establish guidelines for incorporating them into the risk characterization process remain goals; the process of cancer risk assessment will become more sophisticated as we attain a greater understanding of the disease and its causes.

## REFERENCES

Alden, C. L. (1986). A review of unique male rat hydrocarbon nephropathy, *Toxicol. Pathol.*, 14, 109–111.

Ames, B. N. and L. S. Gold (1990). Chemical carcinogens: Too many rodent carcinogens, *Proc. Natl. Acad. Sci. USA*, 87, 7772–7776.

Ames, B. N., F. Lee, and W. Durston, (1973a). An improved bacterial test system for the detection and classification of mutagens and carcinogens, *Proc. Natl. Acad. Sci. USA*, 70, 782–786.

Ames, B. N., W. Durston, E. Yamasaki, and F. Lee (1973b). Carcinogens are mutagens: A simple test system combining liver homogenates for activation and bacteria for detection, *Proc. Natl. Acad. Sci. USA*, 70, 2281–2285.

Armitage, P., and R. Doll (1954). The age distribution of cancer and a multistage theory of carcinogenesis, *Br. J. Cancer,* 8, 1–12.

Armitage, P., and R. Doll (1961). Stochastic models for carcinogenesis. In *Proceedings of the Fourth Berkeley Symposium on Mathematical Statistics and Probability,* University of California Press, Berkeley, 4, 19–38.

Ashby, J., and R. W. Tennant (1988). Chemical structure, *Salmonella* mutagenicity and extent of carcinogenicity as indicators of genotoxic carcinogenesis among 222 chemicals tested in rodents by the U.S. NCI/NTP, *Mutat. Res.,* 204, 17–115.

Bos, J. L., and C. F. van Kreijl (1992). Genes and gene products that regulate proliferation and differentiation: Critical targets in carcinogenesis. In *Mechanisms of Carcinogenesis in Risk Identification* (H. Vainio, P. N. Magee, D. B. McGregor, and A. J. McMichael, eds.), International Agency for Research on Cancer, Lyon, pp. 57–66.

Buchmann, A., R. Bauer-Hofmann, J. Mahr, N. R. Drinkwater, A. Luz, and M. Schwarz (1991). Mutational activation of the c-Ha-*ras* gene in liver tumors of different rodent strains: Correlation with susceptibility to hepatocarcinogenesis, *Proc. Natl. Acad. Sci. USA,* 88, 911–915.

Butterworth, B. E., and S. R. Eldridge (1992). A decision tree approach for carcinogen risk assessment: Application to 1,4-dichlorobenzene, *CIIT Activities,* Vol. 12 (11–12), Nov.–Dec., 11 pp.

Butterworth, B. E., D. J. Loury, T. Smith-Oliver, and R. C. Cattley (1987). The potential role of chemically induced hyperplasia in the carcinogenic activity of hypolipidemic carcinogens, *Toxicol. Ind. Health,* 3, 129–149.

Cairns, T. (1970). The $ED_{01}$ study: Introduction, objectives and experimental design, *J. Environ. Pathol. Toxicol.,* 3, 1–7.

Carlborg, F. W. (1981). Dose–response functions in carcinogenesis and the Weibull model, *Food Cosmet. Toxicol.,* 19, 255–263.

Carr, C. J., and A. C. Kolbye (1991). A critique of the use of the maximum tolerated dose in bioassays to assess cancer risks from chemicals, *Regul. Toxicol. Pharmacol.,* 14, 78–87.

Cattley, R. C., T. Smith-Oliver, B. E. Butterworth, and J. A. Popp (1988). Failure of the peroxisome proliferator WY-14,643 to induce unscheduled DNA synthesis in rat hepatocytes following in vivo treatment, *Carcinogenesis,* 9, 1179–1183.

Cattley, R. C., D. S. Marsman, and J. A. Popp (1991). Age-related susceptibility to the carcinogenic effect of the peroxisome proliferator WY-14,643 in rat liver, *Carcinogenesis,* 12, 469–473.

Cattley, R. C., D. S. Marsman, R. B. Conolly, and J. A. Popp (1992). Cell proliferation and promotion in peroxisome proliferator-induced rodent hepatocarcinogenicity, *CIIT Activities,* Chemical Industry Institute of Toxicology, Research Triangle Park, NC, 12(3), 1–4.

Chappel, C. I. (1992). A review and biological risk assessment of sodium saccharin, *Regul. Toxicol. Pharmacol.,* 15, 253–270.

Chatterjee, B., W. F. Demyan, C. S. Song, B. D. Garg, and A. K. Roy (1989). Loss of androgenic induction of $\alpha_{2\mu}$-globulin gene family in the liver of NIH black rats, *Endocrinology,* 125, 1385–1388.

Chhabra, R. S., J. E. Huff, B. S. Schwetz, and J. Selkirk (1990). An overview of prechronic and chronic toxicity/carcinogenicity experimental study designs and criteria used by the National Toxicology Program, *Environ. Health Perspect.,* 86, 313–321.

Clayson, D. B. (1975). The chemical induction of cancer. In *Biology of Cancer,* 2nd ed. (E. J. Ambrose and F. J. C. Roe, eds.), Ellis Horwood, Chichester, pp. 163–179.

Clayson, D. B. (1978). Overview, fact, myth and speculation, *J. Environ. Pathol. Toxicol.,* 2, 1–8.

Clayson, D. B. (1989). Can a mechanistic rationale be provided for nongenotoxic carcinogens identified in rodent bioassays? *Mutat. Res.,* 221, 53–67.

Clayson, D. B., and D. J. Clegg (1991). Classification of carcinogens: Polemics, pedantics, or progress? *Regul. Toxicol. Pharmacol.,* 14, 147–166.

Cohen, A. J., and P. Grasso (1981). Review of the hepatic response to hypolipemic drugs in rodents and assessment of its significance to man, *Food Cosmet. Toxicol.,* 19, 585–605.

Cohen, S. M., and L. B. Ellwein (1991). Genetic errors, cell proliferation, and carcinogenesis, *Cancer Res.,* 51, 6493–6505.

Cohen, S. M., M. Cano, R. A. Earl, S. D. Carson, and E. M. Garland (1991). A proposed role for silicates and protein in the proliferative effects of saccharin on the male rat urothelium, *Carcinogensis, 12,* 1551–1555.

Cornfield, J. (1977). Carcinogenic risk assessment, *Science,* 198, 693–699.

Cornfield, J., F. W. Carlborg, and J. Van Ryzin (1978). Setting tolerance on the basis of mathematical treatment of dose–response data extrapolated to low doses. In *Proceedings of First International Congress on Toxicology: Toxicology as a Predictive Science* (G. L. Plaa and W. A. M. Duncan, eds.), Academic Press, New York, pp. 143–164.

Crump, K. S. (1979). Dose response problems in carcinogenesis, *Biometrics,* 35, 157–167.

Crump, K. S., D. G. Hoel, C. Langley, and R. Peto (1976). Fundamental carcinogenic processes and their implications for low dose risk assessment, *Cancer Res.,* 36, 2973–2979.

Davidson, I. W. F., J. C. Parker, and R. P. Beliles (1986). Biological basis for extrapolation across mammalian species, *Regul. Toxicol. Pharmacol.,* 6, 211–237.

Dent, J. N., E. L. Godsden, and J. Furth (1956). Further studies on induction and growth of thyrotropic pituitary tumors in mice, *Cancer Res.,* 16, 171–174.

Dodson, A. T. (1970). *Urological Surgery,* 4th ed., C. V. Mosby, St. Louis, 350 pp.

Doll, R. (1971). Age distribution of cancer, *J. R. Stat. Soc. Ser. A,* 134, 133–166.

Dragani, T. A., G. Manenti, M. Gariboldi, F. S. Falvella, M. A. Pierotti, and G. Della Porta (1992). Genetics of hepatocarcinogenesis in mouse and man. In *Oncogenes and Transgenic Correlates of Cancer Risk Assessment. NATO ASI Series A, Life Sciences* (C. Zervos, ed.), Plenum Publishing, New York, 232, 71–90.

Elcock, M., and R. W. Morgan (1993). Update on artificial sweeteners and bladder cancer, *Regul. Toxicol. Pharmacol.,* 17, 35–43.

Ellwein, L. B., and S. M. Cohen (1990). The health risks of saccharin revisited, *Crit. Rev. Toxicol.,* 20, 311–326.

Fearon, E. R., and B. Vogelstein (1990). A genetic model for colorectal tumorigenesis, *Cell,* 61, 759–767.

Fisher, R. A. (1932). *Statistical Methods for Research Workers,* 4th ed., Oliver & Boyd, London.

Flamm, W. G., and L. D. Lehman-McKeeman (1991). The human relevance of the renal tumor-inducing potential of *d*-limonene in male rats: Implications for risk assessment, *Regul. Toxicol. Pharmacol.,* 13, 70–86.

Gariboldi, M., G. Manenti, F. Canzian, F. S. Falvella, M. A. Pierotti, G. D. Porta, G. Binelli, and T. A. Dragani (1993). Chromosome mapping of murine susceptibility loci to liver carcinogenesis, *Cancer Res.,* 53, 209–211.

Garland, E. M., T. Sakata, M. J. Fisher, T. Masui, and S. M. Cohen (1989). Influences of diet and strain on the proliferative effect on the rat urinary bladder induced by sodium saccharin, *Cancer Res.,* 49, 3789–3794.

Gaylor, D. W. (1979). The $ED_{01}$ study: Summary and conclusions. In *Innovations in Cancer Risk Assessment ($ED_{01}$ Study)* (J. A. Staffa, and M. A. Mehlman, eds.), International Toxicology Books, Kingston, NJ, pp. 179–186.

Gibson, G. G. (1993). Peroxisome proliferators: Paradigms and prospects, *Toxicol. Lett.,* 68, 193–201.

Green, T., J. Odum, J. A. Nash, and J. R. Foster (1990). Perchloroethylene-induced rat kidney tumors: An investigation of the mechanisms involved and their relevance to humans, *Toxicol. Appl. Pharmacol.,* 102, 77–89.

Hanigan, M. H., M. C. Winkler, and N. R. Drinkwater (1990). Partial hepatectomy is a promoter of hepatocarcinogenesis in C57BL/6J male mice but not in C3H/HeJ male mice, *Carcinogenesis,* 11, 589–594.

Hard, G. C. (1990). Tumors of the kidney, renal pelvis and ureter. In *Pathology of Tumors in Laboratory Animals.* Vol. 1: *Tumors of the Rat,* 2nd ed. (V. S. Turuscov and U. Mohr, eds.), International Agency for Research on Cancer, Lyon, IARC Scientific Publication No. 99.

Harris, C. C. (1992). Tumour suppressor genes, multistage carcinogenesis and molecular epidemiology. In *Mechanisms of Carcinogenesis in Risk Identification* (H. Vainio, P. N. Magee, D. B. McGregor, and A. J. McMichael, eds.), International Agency for Research on Cancer, Lyon, pp. 67–86.

Haseman, J. K., J. E. Huff, G. N. Rao, J. E. Arnold, G. A. Boorman, and E. E. McConnell (1985).

Neoplasms observed in untreated and corn oil gavage control groups of F344/N rats and (C57BL/6N x C3H/HeN)F1 (B6C3F1) mice, *JNCI* 75, 975–984.

Hill, R. N., L. S. Erdreich, O. E. Paynter, P. A. Roberts, S. L. Rosenthal, and C. F. Wilkinson (1989). Review: Thyroid follicular cell carcinogenesis, *Fundam. App. Toxicol.,* 12, 629–697.

Hillyard, A. L., D. P. Doolittle, M. T. Davisson, and T. H. Roderick (1992). Locus map of mouse with comparative map points of human on mouse, The Jackson Laboratory, Bar Harbor, ME.

Hoel, D. G., D. Gaylor, R. Kirschstein, U. Saffiotti, and M. Schneiderman (1975). Estimation of risks of irreversible delayed toxicity, *J. Toxicol. Environ. Health,* 1, 133–151.

Hoel, D. G., J. K. Haseman, M. D. Hogan, J. Huff, and E. E. McConnel (1988). The impact of toxicity on carcinogenicity: Implications for risk assessment, *Carcinogenesis,* 9, 2045–2052.

Issemann, I., and S. Green (1990). Activation of a member of the steroid hormone receptor superfamily by peroxisome proliferators, *Nature,* 347, 645–650.

Jull, J. W. (1979). The effect of time on the incidence of carcinomas obtained by the implantation of paraffin wax pellets in the mouse bladder, *Cancer Lett.,* 6, 21–25.

Kennaway, E. L. (1924a). On cancer-producing tars and tar fractions, *J. Ind. Hyg.,* 5, 462–488.

Kennaway, E. L. (1924b). On the cancer-producing factor in tar, *Br. Med. J.,* 1, 564–567.

Kociba, R. J. (1987). Issues in biochemical applications to risk assessment: How should the MTD be selected? *Environ. Health Perspect.,* 76, 169–174.

Mantel, N., and W. R. Bryan (1961). Safety testing of carcinogenic agents, *JNCI,* 27, 455–470.

Maronpot, R. R., J. K. Haseman, G. A. Boomran, S. E. Eustis, G. N. Rao, and J. E. Huff (1987). Liver lesions in B6C3F1 mice: The National Toxicology Program, experience and position. In *Mouse Liver Tumors: Proceedings of the European Society of Toxicology,* (P. L. Chambers, D. Henschler, F. Oesch, eds.), *Arch. Toxicol. Suppl.* 10. Springer-Verlag, New York, pp. 10–28.

Marsman, D. S., R. C. Cattley, and R. A. Popp (1988). Contrasting effects of di(2-ethylhexyl)phthalate and Wyeth 14,643 on hepatocyte proliferation and carcinogenicity in male F344 rats [abstract], *Proc. Am. Assoc. Cancer Res.,* 29, 87.

McConnell, E. E., H. A. Solleveld, J. A. Swenberg, and G. A. Boorman (1986). Guidelines for combining neoplasms for evaluation of rodent carcinogenesis studies, *JNCI,* 76, 283–289.

Miller, E. C., and J. A. Miller (1981). Searches for ultimate chemical carcinogens and their reactions with cellular macromolecules, *Cancer,* 47, 2327–2345.

Moolgavkar, S., and A. Knudson (1981). Mutation and cancer: A model for human carcinogenesis, *JNCI,* 66, 1037–1052.

Munro, I. C., and D. R. Krewski (1981). Risk assessment and regulatory decision making, *Food Cosmet. Toxicol.,* 19, 549–560.

[NAS] National Academy of Sciences (1980). The effects of populations of exposure to low levels of ionizing radiation, National Research Council, National Academy of Sciences, Washington, DC.

[NCRP] National Council on Radiation Protection (1985). Induction of thyroid cancer by ionizing radiation, NCRP Report 80, National Council on Radiation Protection and Measurement, Bethesda, MD.

[NRC] U.S. National Research Council, Commission on Life Sciences, Committee on the Institutional Means for Assessment of Risks to Public Health (1983). *Risk Assessment in the Federal Government: Managing the Process,* National Academy Press, Washington, DC.

[NRC] U.S. National Research Council, Commission on Life Sciences, Committee on Risk Assessment Methodology (1993). Use of the maximum tolerated dose in animal bioassays for carcinogenicity. In *Issues in Risk Assessment,* National Academy Press, Washington, DC. pp. 14–77.

Okamura, T., E. M. Garland, T. Masui, T. Sakata, M. St. John, and S. M. Cohen (1991). Lack of bladder tumor promoting activity in rats fed sodium saccharin in AIN-76A diet, *Cancer Res.,* 51, 1778–1782.

Olson, M. J., J. T. Johnson, and C. A. Reidy (1990). A comparison of male rat and human urinary proteins: Implications for human resistance to hyaline droplet nephropathy, *Toxicol. Appl. Pharmacol.,* 102, 524–536.

[OSTP] Office of Science and Technology Policy (1985). Chemical carcinogens: Notice of review of the science and its associated principles, *Fed. Reg.,* 50, 10372–10442.

Paynter, O. E., G. J. Burin, R. B. Jaeger, and C. A. Gregario (1986). Neoplasia induced by inhibition of thyroid gland function (guidance for analysis and evaluation), Hazard Evaluation Division. U.S. Environmental Protection Agency, Washington, DC.

Pitot, H. C. (1981). *Fundamentals of Oncology,* 2nd ed., revised and expanded. Marcel Dekker, New York, Chaps. 1 and 3.

Pott, P. (1775) Chirurgical observations relative to the cancer of the scrotum, London. [Reprinted (orig. 1775) in *NCI Monogr.* 10, 7–13].

Rai, K., and J. Van Ryzin (1981). A generalized multi-hit dose-response model for low-dose extrapolation, *Biometrics,* 37, 341–352.

Ramel, C. (1992). Genotoxic and nongenotoxic carcinogens: Mechanisms of action and testing strategies. In *Mechanisms of Carcinogenesis in Risk Identification* (H. Vainio, P. N. Magee, D. B. McGregor, and A. J. Michael, eds.), International Agency for Research on Cancer, Lyon, pp. 195–209.

Rao, M. S., and J. K. Reddy (1989). The relevance of peroxisome proliferation and cell proliferation in peroxisome proliferator-induced hepatocarcinogenesis, *Drug Metab. Rev.,* 21, 103–110.

Rao, M. S., and J. K. Reddy (1991). An overview of peroxisome proliferator-induced hepatocarcinogenesis, *Environ. Health Perspect.,* 93, 205–209.

Reddy, J. K., and M. S. Rao (1992). Peroxisome proliferation and hepatocarcinogenesis. In *Mechanisms of Carcinogenesis in Risk Identification* (H. Vainio, P. N. Magee, D. B. McGregor, and A. J. Michael, eds.), International Agency for Research on Cancer, Lyon, pp. 225–235.

Rehn, L. (1895) Blasengeschwülste bei Fuchsin-Arbeitern, *Arch. Klin. Chir.,* 50, 588–600.

Ridder, G. N., E. C. Von Bargen, C. L. Alden, and R. D. Parker (1990). Increased hyaline droplet formation in male rats exposed to decalin is dependent on the presence of $\alpha_{2\mu}$-globulin, *Fundam. Appl. Toxicol.,* 15, 732–743.

Roy, A. K., and O. W. Neuhaus (1967). Androgenic control of a sex-dependent protein in the rat, *Nature,* 214, 618–620.

Schaller, R. T., and J. K. Stevenson (1966). Development of carcinoma of the thyroid in iodine deficient mice, *Cancer,* 19, 1063–1080.

Shubik, P., and D. B. Clayson (1976). Application of the results of carcinogen bioassays to man. In *Environmental Pollution and Carcinogenic Risks* (C. Rosenfeld, W. Davis, eds.), International Agency for Research on Cancer, Scientific Publications, Paris, 13, 241–252.

Snedecor, G. W., and W. G. Cochran (1980). *Statistical Methods,* Iowa State University Press, Ames, IA.

Stott, W. T. (1988). Chemically induced proliferation of peroxisomes: Implications for risk assessment, *Regul. Toxicol. Pharmacol.,* 8, 125–159.

Stowers, S. J., R. W. Wiseman, J. M. Ward, E. C. Miller, J. A. Miller, M. W. Anderson, and A. Eva (1988). Detection of activated proto-oncogenes in *N*-nitrosodiethylamine-induced liver tumors: A comparison between B6C3F$_1$ mice and Fischer 344 rats, *Carcinogenesis,* 9, 271–276.

Swenberg, J. A., B. Short, S. Borghoff, J. Strasser, and M. Charbonneau (1989). The comparative pathobiology of $\alpha_{2\mu}$-globulin nephropathy, *Toxicol. Appl. Pharmacol.,* 97, 35–46.

Tada, M., M. Omata, and M. Ohto (1990). Analysis of *ras* gene mutations in human hepatic malignant tumors by polymerase chain reaction and direct sequencing, *Cancer Res.,* 50, 1121–1124.

Tennant, R. W., M. R. Elwell, J. W. Spalding, and R. A. Griesmer (1991). Evidence that toxic injury is not always associated with induction of chemical carcinogenesis, *Mol. Carcinog.,* 4, 420–440.

Thorslund, T. W., C. C. Brown, and G. Charnley (1987). Biologically motivated cancer risk models, *Risk Anal.,* 7, 109–119.

[USEPA] U.S. Environmental Protection Agency (1986). Guidelines for carcinogen risk assessment, *Fed. Reg.* 51 (33992), 1–17.

[USEPA] U.S. Environmental Protection Agency (1989). Workshop Report on EPA Guidelines for Carcinogen Risk Assessment, Risk Assessment Forum, Technical Panel on Carcinogen Guidelines, Washington, DC. EPA/625/3-89/015, March.

[USEPA] U.S. Environmental Protection Agency (1991). alpha$_{2\mu}$-globulin: Association with chemically induced renal toxicity and neoplasia in the male rat, Prepared for the Risk Assessment Forum, Washington, DC. EPA/625/3-91/019F, September.

[USEPA] U.S. Environmental Protection Agency (1992). Draft report: A cross-species scaling factor for carcinogen risk assessment based on equivalence of mg/kg$^{3/4}$/day; Notice. 57, *Fed. Reg.*, 109, 24252–24173.

[USEPA] U.S. Environmental Protection Agency (1993). Integrated Risk Information System (IRIS) [Online], Office of Health and Environmental Assessment, Environmental Criteria and Assessment Office, Cincinnati, OH.

van Etten, C. H. (1969). Goitrogens. In *Toxic Constituents of Plant Foodstuffs* (I. E. Liener, ed.), Academic Press, New York, pp. 103–142.

Weinstein, B. (1992). Toxicity, cell proliferation, and carcinogenesis. *Mol. Carcinog.*, 5, 2–3.

[WHO] World Health Organization (1978). *Environmental Health Criteria, No. 6: Principles and Methods for Evaluating the Toxicity of Chemicals,* World Health Organization, Geneva, 1, 25–61.

[WHO] World Health Organization (1990). *Cancer: Causes, Occurrence and Control* (L. Tomatis, ed.), IARC Scientific Publications, No. 100, Oxford University Press, New York, p. 59.

Williams, G. M., and J. H. Weisburger (1991). Chemical carcinogenesis. In *Toxicology* (M. O. Amdur, J. Doull, and C. D. Klaassen, eds.), Pergamon Press, New York, pp. 127–200.

Yamagiwa, K., and K. Ichikawa (1915). Experimentelle Studie über die Pathogenese der Epithelialgeschwülste, *Mitt. Med. Fak. Univ. Tokio,* 15, 295–344.

Yamagiwa, K., and K. Ichikawa (1918). Experimental study of the pathogenesis of carcinoma, *J. Cancer Res.,* 3, 1–29.

Yamasaki, H., K. Enomoto, D. J. Fitzgerald, M. Mesnil, F. Katoh, M. Hollstein (1988). Role of intercellular communication in the control of critical gene expression during multistage carcinogenesis. In *Cell Differentiation, Genes and Cancer* (T. Kakunaga, T. Sugimura, L. Tomatis, and H. Yamasaki, eds.), IARC Scientific Publication 92, International Agency for Research on Cancer, Lyon, 57–75.

# 15

# Risk Assessment: Principles and Methodologies

**Welford C. Roberts***
*United States Army Materiel Command*
*Alexandria, Virginia*

**Charles O. Abernathy**
*United States Environmental Protection Agency*
*Washington, D.C.*

## I. INTRODUCTION

Various federal, state, and other local governmental agencies have statutory requirements to regulate contaminants to protect human health and the environment. For each chemical, biological, or physical agent, it is necessary to identify whether it causes a harmful effect, to determine the potency of the agent, and to estimate the potential risk imposed by exposure to that contaminant. The process of estimating and characterizing potential risks from various agents is called *risk assessment*. Translation of the risk assessment into a regulation involves *risk management*. The public is informed of risk assessment and risk management actions through *risk communication*. This chapter will focus on risk assessment and will consider only briefly risk management and communication.

## A. What Is Risk?

Webster's unabridged dictionary (1970) defines *risk* as

1. The chance of injury, damage, or loss; a dangerous chance; a hazard.
2. In insurance (a) the chance of loss; (b) the degree of probability of loss; (c) the amount of possible loss to the insuring company: in full, *amount at risk;* (d) a person or thing with reference to the risk involved in insuring him or it; (e) the type of loss that a policy covers, as life, fire, etc. *to run (or take) a risk;* to expose oneself to the chance of injury or loss; to endanger oneself; to take a chance

For this discussion, risk is considered the possibility of an injury, disease, or death, resulting from an exposure to an environmental agent. Risk assessment is the estimate of the risk

---

*Current affiliation:* Uniformed Services University of the Health Sciences, Bethesda, Maryland

associated with a specific set of conditions (Abernathy and Roberts, 1994). By this definition "risk" has two principal components:

1. The existence of a hazard
2. The likelihood of being exposed to a hazard

## B.  Why Worry About Risk?

There are two reasons to be concerned with risk. Exposure to an agent poses a real probability of an adverse health effect. Second, the public perceives risk from a potential exposure to an agent.

"Risk perception" is a relative concept that is influenced by a variety of social and psychological factors. The degree of risk that a person or society is willing to accept depends on the level of tolerance that exists for undesirable consequences when the possible, and usually perceived as the more probable, outcome of a situation will be favorable. Even though this presentation of the topic addresses primarily health effects, the concept of risk assessment is broader and encompasses many experiences. For example, risk can be applied to economic outcomes. When one selects an investment vehicle, such as a stock option, the decision process requires a consideration of the possibility that there will be no income generated from the transaction, and there could be a financial loss. People who encounter such situations, and make decisions about the pursuit of a course of action, go through a risk assessment process to identify and determine the probability of a successful versus an unsuccessful outcome.

Even though risk and risk assessment can be defined for a variety of situations, this chapter will focus on definitions and dynamics associated with health. Thus, the major concerns are the identification, assessment, and subsequent prevention or diminution of adverse health effects.

In terms of health effects, people may accept certain levels of risk to derive benefits that provide "a better way of life." There are many examples of common practices and events that have some risk associated with them; however, these activities provide comforts and services to society and the risks, then, are accepted. Table 1 lists some events that exemplify this concept. It shows that a variety of acceptable and even expected activities (e.g., working, driving, smoking, drinking coffee and alcoholic beverages, and recreational activities [swimming, bicycling]) can shorten life. This table illustrates that this is not a risk-free society and suggests that some "acceptable" risks shorten life span more than environmental risks. For a detailed review and quantitative assessment of loss of life expectancy for a large variety of risks, the reader is referred to an article by Cohen (1991).

We make choices of lifestyle, diet, and occupation that have associated risks; the choices reflect the level of tolerated risk. This tolerance/acceptance is influenced by a variety of factors, which include individual and group needs, societal needs and practices, level of technology, economics, and geography. These factors may be beneficial (economic growth, employment, increased standard of living and quality of life, revenues generated) or detrimental (decreased quality of life, emotional difficulties, health effects, lawsuits, loss of environmental resources, loss of work, medical payments) (Klaassen, 1986). Tolerance is also influenced by the way risk is perceived. Risk perception may be influenced by the visibility of the risk, fear associated with it, and by the degree of control that one believes he or she may have, or believes to have, on the risk factor (Zeckhouse and Viscusi, 1990). Santos (1990) implies that the public may view risks differently from regulatory and other public agencies, and that there are a number of factors that can influence the perception. Table 2 contains some of the factors that she identifies that were originally characterized by Sandman (Sandman, 1993; Chess et al., 1988), who described them as "outrage factors" (i.e., "everything about a risk except how likely it is to cause harm").

**Table 1**  Loss of Life Expectancy from Various Societal Activities and Phenomena

| Risk factor | Loss of life expectancy (days) |
|---|---|
| Cancer risks associated with environmental pollutants | |
| Indoor radon | 30 |
| Worker chemical exposure | 30 |
| Pesticide residues in food | 12 |
| Indoor air pollution | 10 |
| Consumer products use | 10 |
| Stratospheric ozone depletion | 22 |
| Inactive hazardous waste sites | 2.5 |
| Carcinogens in air pollution | 4 |
| Drinking water contaminants | 1.3 |
| Noncancer risks associated with environmental pollutants | |
| Lead | 20 |
| Carbon monoxide | 20 |
| Sulfur dioxide | 20 |
| Radon | 0.2 |
| Air pollutants (e.g., benzene, carbon tetrachloride, chlorine, etc.) | 0.2 |
| Drinking water materials (e.g., lead, pathogens, nitrates, chlorine disinfectants, etc.) | 0.2 |
| Industrial discharge into surface water | Few minutes |
| Sewage treatment plan sludge | Few minutes |
| Mining wastes | Few minutes |
| Lifestyle/demographic status | |
| Being an unmarried male | 3500 |
| Smoking cigarettes and being male | 2250 |
| Being an unmarried female | 1600 |
| Being 30% overweight | 1300 |
| Being 20% overweight | 900 |
| Having less than an 8th-grade education | 850 |
| Smoking cigarettes and being female | 800 |
| Being poor | 700 |
| Smoking cigars | 330 |
| Having a dangerous job | 300 |
| Driving a motor vehicle | 207 |
| Alcohol | 130 |
| Accidents in the home | 95 |
| Suicide | 95 |
| Being murdered | 90 |
| Misusing legal drugs | 90 |

*Source:* Adapted from Cohen and Lee (1979) and Cohen (1991).

## C.  Historical Perspective

The concept of assessing risk probably has existed as long as people have been on this planet and capable of making decisions. A report to the Secretary, Health and Human Services provides a historical perspective of risk acceptability by indicating how temporal changes in technology, socioeconomic factors, and lifestyle affect the types and nature of the risks that are of concern (DHHS, 1985). It states that

**Table 2**  Risk Perception Factors

| |
| --- |
| Voluntary or involuntary |
| Controlled by the system or controlled by the individual |
| Fair or unfair |
| Having trustworthy or untrustworthy sources |
| Morally relevant or morally neutral |
| Natural or artificial |
| Exotic or familiar |
| Memorable or not memorable |
| Certainty or uncertainty |
| Undetectable or detectable |
| Dreaded or not dreaded |

*Source:* Adapted from Chess et al., (1988), Santos (1990), and Sandman (1993).

What was acceptable in the past may not be acceptable today. As exposures alter, as mores change, as prevention and control techniques improve, as the laws evolve, as needs arise, as information on health hazards increase, as alternatives become available, acceptability changes.

In the United States, our ancestors had to contend with health risks from infectious diseases, caused by poor sanitation, spoiled food, and poor water. However, because of advances in epidemiological and microbiological techniques, improvements in sanitation, water purification, and the development of vaccines, these risks have decreased. With increased technological advances and environmental awareness, the tolerance for accepting risks in this country is ever decreasing. This may be different in other less-developed nations of the world, where disease and poor sanitation still are major causes of decreased life expectancy. In such areas where there also may be depressed economies, few jobs, low wages, and hunger, the risks that people are willing to tolerate to acquire basic needs (food, water, shelter) may be greater than those acceptable in a well-developed nation. In well-developed nations there is a greater chance that such needs are met and risks are compared with factors of comfort and general well-being, rather than basic survival.

However, even within well-developed nations, there are depressed areas where basic needs are difficult to obtain and where people are willing to accept greater risks to acquire basic resources than the general population. There are current concerns about whether such areas incur greater environmental and health impact because potentially hazardous operations and facilities were preferentially located in neighborhoods and towns that may be less concerned about long-term risk and more concerned about immediate needs. The U. S. Environmental Protection Agency (EPA) has proposed specific ways of addressing environmental equity issues in the risk assessment and risk management process (USEPA 1992a,b; *EPA Journal,* 1992). Such measures include elucidating the ethnic and cultural diversity of exposed populations to determine if there are groups that have some likelihood of being affected differently from the rest of the population.

## D.  United States Laws That Require or Imply Risk Assessments

Many decisions concerning the welfare of people and society require the review of alternative courses of actions that have varying degrees of adverse consequences and risk. There are a variety of existing environmental health and safety statutes (discussed in more detail elsewhere in this book) that require or imply the conduct of risk assessments (Federal Focus, 1991). For

**Table 3** United States Safety, Health, and Environmental Statutes That Imply Risk Assessments

| Act | Statute | Agency[a] |
|---|---|---|
| Atomic Energy Act | 42 U.S.C. 2011 | NRC, EPA |
| Comprehensive Environmental Response Compensation and Liability Act | 42 U.S.C. 9601 | EPA |
| Clean Air Act | 42 U.S.C. 7401 | EPA |
| Clean Water Act | 33 U.S.C. 1251 | EPA |
| Consumer Product Safety Act | 15 U.S.C. 2051 | CPSC |
| Eggs Products Inspection Act | 21 U.S.C. 1031 | DOA |
| Federal Food, Drug, and Cosmetics Act | 21 U.S.C. 301 | HHS, EPA |
| Federal Hazardous Substances Act | 15 U.S.C. 1261 | CPSC |
| Federal Insecticide, Fungicide, and Rodenticide Act | 7 U.S.C. 136 | EPA |
| Federal Meat Inspection Act | 21 U.S.C. 601 | DOA |
| Federal Mine Safety and Health Act | 30 U.S.C. 801 | DOL |
| Hazardous Liquid Pipeline Safety Act | 49 U.S.C. 1671 | DOT |
| Hazardous Materials Transportation Act | 49 U.S.C. 1801 | DOT |
| Lead-Based Paint Poisoning Act | 42 U.S.C. 4801 | HUD, HHS, CPSC |
| Lead Contamination Control Act of 1988 | 42 U.S.C. 300j-21 | EPA, CPSC |
| Marine Protection, Research, and Sanctuaries Act | 16 U.S.C. 1431 | EPA, DA |
| Motor Carrier Safety Act | 49 U.S.C. 2501 | DOT |
| National Traffic and Motor Vehicle Safety Act | 15 U.S.C. 1381 | DOT |
| Natural Gas Pipeline Safety Act | 49 U.S.C. 2001 | DOT |
| Nuclear Waste Policy Act | 42 U.S.C. 10101 | EPA |
| Occupational Safety and Health Act | 29 U.S.C. 651 | DOL |
| Poison Prevention Packaging Act | 15 U.S.C. 1471 | CPSC |
| Poultry Products Inspection Act | 21 U.S.C. 451 | DOA |
| Resource Conservation and Recovery Act | 42 U.S.C. 6901 | EPA |
| Safe Drinking Water Act | 42 U.S.C. 300f | EPA |
| Toxic Substances Control Act | 7 U.S.C. 136 | EPA |

[a]Abbreviations: NRC, Nuclear Regulatory Commission; EPA, Environmental Protection Agency; CPSC, Consumer Safety Product Commission; DOA, Department of Agriculture; HHS, Health and Human Services; DOL, Department of Labor; DOT, Department of Transportation; HUD, Housing and Urban Development; DA, Department of the Army.
*Source:* Adapted from Federal Focus (1991).

example, the EPA routinely conducts risk assessments to regulate contaminants under the provisions of the Clean Air Act and the Safe Drinking Water Act, and the Department of Labor does so under the Occupational Safety and Health Act. Other examples of risk assessment statutes are shown in Table 3.

## II. RISK ASSESSMENT: DEFINITION

There are various definitions for risk assessment; all, however, have a common theme. A definition offered by the U. S. Department of Health and Human Services (DHHS, 1985) is that risk assessment is "the use of available information to evaluate and estimate exposure to a substance(s) and its consequent adverse health effects." The EPA (USEPA, 1990a,b,c; 1991a,b,c) notes that risk assessment involves analyzing past exposures, determining the types and amounts of adverse effects, and predicting the outcome from subsequent exposure. In addition to the predictive aspect of risk assessment, Brown (1985) indicates that there also can be retrospective uses for risk assessment and offers cancer and radiation as an example. He exemplifies this concept by asking the question "What is the likelihood that a person's cancer is related to a previous exposure to a hazard?" All of these definitions focus on potential adverse health as the outcome of exposure to a contaminant.

In 1983 the National Academy of Sciences (NAS) published a report that evaluated risk assessment practices by federal agencies (NAS, 1983). In the report risk assessment was defined as

> ... the characterization of the potential adverse health effects of human exposure to environmental hazards. Risk assessments include several elements: description of the potential adverse health effects based on the evaluation of the results of epidemiological, clinical, toxicologic, and environmental research; extrapolation from those results to predict the type and estimate the extent of health effects in humans under given conditions of exposure; judgments as to the number and characteristics of persons exposed at various intensities and durations; and summary judgments on the existence and overall magnitude of the public health problem.

From this definition, NAS identifies four components of the risk assessment process:

1. Hazard identification
2. Dose–response assessment
3. Exposure assessment
4. Risk characterization

This definition, which includes processes that may be qualitative or quantitative, is used by the EPA and many other agencies for most current risk assessments. This is the definition and approach that is used in this chapter.

The relation between the components of the risk assessment process are illustrated in Fig. 1. Hazard identification precedes the dose–response assessment. When these are combined with an exposure assessment, a risk characterization can be developed. In a report that discusses

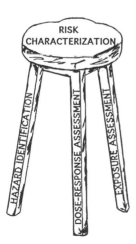

**Figure 1**   The relationship between the components of the risk assessment paradigm is only as stable as any "leg" (i.e., hazard identification, dose-response assessment, or exposure assessment) that supports the overall risk characterization. If any component is weak or missing, then the overall characterization is unstable.

methods for assessing risk from combustion sources, the EPA suggests that risk assessments proceed from the source to the receptor (USEPA, 1990b). According to this process, the source is characterized first, and contaminant movement away from the source is then modeled to estimate the exposure to the receptor. Health effects are then predicted based on the estimated exposure.

## III. RISK MANAGEMENT AND RISK COMMUNICATION

There are two activities that are related to and sometimes confused with the risk assessment. These are risk management and risk communication. Both are important in addressing and regulating risk, but are concepts that are separate from risk assessment. Risk management and risk communication are dependent on a risk assessment. A risk assessment usually is not dependent on or based on risk management or risk communication parameters or needs. However, risk management can frame the risk assessment. For example, if technological constraints limit contaminant removal from air, water, or soil, a risk assessment may characterize the residual risk that remains after remediation. The risk assessment is based on the best scientific data and independently precedes the other two risk activities.

Risk management is the process of weighing policy alternatives and selecting the most appropriate regulatory action, integrating the results of risk assessment with engineering data and with social, economic, and political concerns, to reach a decision (NAS, 1983). It is the process of forming and implementing a strategy for accepting or abating risks (Brown, 1985). *Risk management* may be defined simply as "the process of deciding what to do about a problem," which requires the integration of a broader spectrum of scientific and nonscientific disciplines. It combines risk assessment with regulatory directives, and with social, economic, technical, political, and other considerations (USEPA, 1986). There is an overlap between the risk assessment process and risk management as shown in Fig. 2. Risk characterization, the last step in risk assessment, can be considered the first step in risk management. Figure 2 depicts the

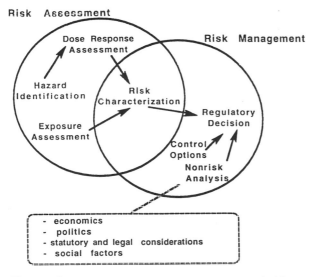

**Figure 2** Relation between risk assessment and risk management with examples of nonrisk analysis factors.

**Table 4**  Key Principles of Risk Communication

| |
|---|
| Accept and involve the public as a legitimate partner. |
| Plan carefully and evaluate your efforts. |
| Listen to the public's specific concerns. |
| Be honest, frank, and open. |
| Coordinate and collaborate with other credible sources. |
| Meet the needs of the media. |
| Speak clearly and with compassion. |

*Source:* Chess et al., (1988), Santos (1990), and Sandman (1993).

relation between risk assessment and risk management and provides examples of some of the parameters that may be considered in managing a risk.

Although risk assessment may be one component of risk management, it also can be totally left out of the management process, and control strategies can be based solely on nonrisk parameters. For example, the decision to control an environmental contaminant can be based on a perceived hazard, rather than one defined by a risk assessment. Another example is regulating environmental contaminants at zero concentration levels when adverse health effects do not occur below higher (e.g., threshold) levels.

*Risk communication* is a method for informing the public about the risks associated with hazards and the control strategies that are being considered to mitigate them. Several definitions are discussed by Santos (1990), who summarizes them in basic communication theory that recognizes that the process must be "two-way" requiring both a "source" and a "receiver." She also explains that risk communication helps explain technical information to the general public. In this effort, both the risk assessment and risk management processes may be presented. Concepts often associated with risk communication include informing the public early and involving them in the decision-making process, use of the media, and presentation of truthful and frank information (USEPA, 1990b, 1989a). Some key rules of effective risk communication are shown in Table 4.

Although both risk management and risk communication are vitally important, they are not the focus of this chapter and are presented only to eliminate any confusion with risk assessment. For additional information, the reader may consult an annotated bibliography of risk assessment, management, and communication sources published by the EPA (USEPA, 1991b).

## IV.  COMPONENTS OF THE RISK ASSESSMENT PARADIGM

## A.  Hazard Identification

*1.  Definition*

*Hazard identification,* the first step in the risk assessment, is defined by NAS as the "process of determining whether an agent can cause an increase in the incidence of a health condition (cancer, birth defect, etc.)" (NAS, 1983). Usually there are few human data available. Thus, experimental laboratory animal tests, as well as with *in vitro* tests, and chemical structure–activity relationships are generally used to estimate hazard to exposed persons. Most of the available toxicity database is the result of animal studies. When using animal data, it is assumed that the deleterious effects observed in animals will occur, or are expected to occur, in humans (Abernathy and Roberts, 1994).

This initial step requires a review of the biological properties of the agent of interest and elucidation of the toxic effects that are statistically or biologically significant. Adverse systemic effects may include organ system dysfunction, gross organ pathology, histopathology, metabolic and physiological impairment, and clinical and blood chemistry abnormalities. Cancer and gene mutation also are considered in the hazard identification process.

Hazards can be physical, chemical, or biological, and can result in injury, disease, or death when there is sufficient exposure (i.e., adequate quantity of agent and exposure duration) to a susceptible receptor (e.g., people, animals, or an ecosystem).

Physical hazards generally involve an energetic interaction between physical agents and a receptor. Categories of physical hazards (Key et al., 1977) are

*Radiation:* Ionizing radiation (e.g., x-ray, gamma-ray, alpha-particle, beta-particle, proton, and neutron) and nonionizing radiation (e.g., ultraviolet, infrared, visible, microwave, radio-frequency, and laser)
*Atmospheric variations:* heat, cold, air pressure
*Oscillatory vibrations (acoustic energy):* noise, vibration

Examples of physical agent effects are discussed in a National Institute of Occupation Safety and Health (NIOSH) manual, which addresses occupational exposures to chemical, biological, and physical insults (Key et al., 1977). Effects from ionizing radiation include somatic and genetic damage, exemplified by exposures to radiation workers (e.g., effects from nuclear accidents and exposures to radium dial painters). Such effects include radiodermititis, epilation, acute radiation syndrome, cancer, leukemia, cataracts, sterility, and life span shortening. Nonionizing radiation affects the skin and eyes primarily through heat generation and may cause cataracts. Heat and cold ambient temperature extremes can cause conditions that range from reversible incapacitation, through irreversible tissue damage, to death. Excess air pressure causes barotrauma, which is tissue damage that results from expansion or contraction of gas spaces found within or adjacent to the body, and can occur either during compression or decompression. Pressure changes also affect the partial pressure of nitrogen, oxygen, and carbon dioxide, which can cause these gases to become toxic (Key et al., 1977).

Auditory and nonauditory effects occur from exposure to acoustic energy. Excessive increases in local atmospheric pressures may traumatically affect the ear and cause hearing loss or blast overpressure effects (e.g., internal organ hemorrhages). Vibration phenomena include whole body vibration, segmental vibration, acceleration, and resonance (Key et al., 1977). Vibration effects may include increases in oxygen and pulmonary ventilation (whole-body vibration), difficulty in maintaining posture (whole-body vibration), and Reynaud's phenomenon (segmental vibration).

For detailed examples of risk assessments associated with physical phenomena (as well as chemical and biological agents), the reader may wish to consult the U. S. Army Health Hazard Assessment Program, which was created to identify, assess, and eliminate or control health hazards associated with the life cycle management of weapons systems, munitions, equipment, clothing, training devices, and materiel/information systems (Gross and Broadwater, 1994).

Chemical hazards are associated with effects from exposure to substances during various durations of time. Chemicals can be classified according to their effect either as systemic toxicants or as carcinogens. Some chemicals have systemic effects when exposure duration is acute, subchronic, or chronic, and are carcinogenic when there is chronic exposure. Animal toxicity data may be acute (usually one exposure), subacute (14 days), subchronic (90 days), or chronic (2 years), for general toxicity studies. Other toxicity tests, such as reproductive, developmental, and mutagenic assays use protocols specifically designed to examine these endpoints (USEPA, 1990a).

A chemical effect can vary with the exposure (e.g., route and duration) or type. For example, short exposures to high concentrations of a variety of organic solvents can affect nerve cells, probably from physical alteration of the cell membranes (Andrews and Snyder, 1986), and produce central nervous system effects that range from dizziness, euphoria, and disorientation, to death from respiratory depression or cardiac arrest. Longer-term exposures to low solvent concentrations (e.g., in an occupational setting) may also cause neurotoxicity, as well as cancer, reproductive, hematological, dermatological, cardiovascular, respiratory, gastrointestinal, and renal effects (Roberts, 1990).

Data on the effects of chemicals on humans are scant. Most of the human data come from case reports, correlation assessments, and occupational or epidemiological cohort studies. The most desirable and informative are the epidemiological cohort studies. They examine populations that have been exposed to an agent and compare them with a matched control population. This type of study is the most valuable, since it provides information on humans exposed to environmental concentrations (USEPA, 1990a).

Biological hazards are associated with the diseases that may occur when one is exposed to microorganisms, including bacteria, viruses, rickettsia, chlamydia, and fungi. Some parasites (protozoa, helminths, or arthropods) also cause biological hazards (Key et al., 1977). Examples are shown in Table 5.

### 2. Deficit Versus Excess Toxicity

One intuitively associates a hazard with the presence of an undesirable agent; however, adverse health effects also can develop from the absence of essential nutrients (e.g., amino acids, vitamins, and trace elements). This dichotomy in hazard definition is exemplified by the focus of the sciences of toxicology and nutrition. Toxicologists generally evaluate health outcomes associated with exposures to excess amounts of agents (e.g., neurotoxicity from excess carbon disulfide exposure or carcinogenicity from exposure to excess amounts of benzene).

Nutritionists, on the other hand, assess health effects of both excesses and deficiencies in the diet. Some essential nutrients have adverse health conditions associated with both dietary excesses and deficiencies and, therefore, have an optimal dose range that must be maintained for proper physiological functioning. For example, nutritional iron deficiency may result in anemia, whereas an excess may cause hemosiderosis. Another example is copper deficiency, which may cause microcytic and normochromic anemia; excessive tissue deposition of copper is seen in persons with Wilson's disease, with hepatolenticular degeneration (White et al., 1973; Latham et al., 1972).

## B.  Dose–Response Assessment

### 1. Definition

An important tenet of toxicology is that "the dose makes the poison." This concept is discussed by Doull and Bruce (1986) who offer a quote from Paracelsus (16th century):

> All substances are poisons; there is none that is not a poison. The right dose differentiates a poison and a remedy.

This quote is germane to the dose–response section of the risk assessment process.

The NAS (1983) defines *dose–response assessment* as "the process of characterizing the relationship between the dose of an agent administered or received and the incidence of an adverse health effect in exposed populations and estimating the incidence of the effect as a function of human exposure to the agent." This definition has two implications:

**Table 5**  Examples of Biological Hazards

| Diseases | Agent |
|---|---|
| Viruses | |
| Rabies | Rhabdovirus |
| Milker's nodules | Paravaccinia virus |
| Newcastle disease | Newcastle virus (paramyxovirus) |
| Viral hepatitis | Hepatitis types A and B viruses |
| Rickettsia and Chlamydia | |
| Rocky Mountain spotted fever | *Rickettsia rickettsii* |
| Q-fever | *Coxiella burnetti* |
| Ornithosis | *Chlamydia psittaci* |
| Bacteria | |
| Tetanus | *Clostridium tetani* |
| Anthrax | *Bacillus anthracis* |
| Brucellosis | *Brucella* spp. |
| Leptospirosis | *Leptospira* spp. |
| Plague | *Pasturella pestis* |
| Food poisoning | *Clostridium perfringens* |
| | *Staphylococcus aureus* |
| Tuberculosis | *Mycobacterium tuberculosis* |
| Erysipeloid | *Erysipelothrix* spp. |
| Tularemia | *Francisella tularensis* |
| | (*Pasturella tularens*) |
| Fungi | |
| Candidiasis | *Candida albicans* |
| Aspergillosis | *Aspergillis* spp. |
| Coccidioidomycosis | *Coccidioides immitis* |
| Histoplasmosis | *Histoplasma capsulatum* |
| Mycetoma | *Monosporum apiospermum* |
| | *Allescheria boydii* |
| Sporotrichosis | *Sporothrix schenkii* |
| Chromoblastomycoses | *Fonsecaea* (*Cladosporium*) spp. |
| Dermatophytosis | *Phialphora verrucosa* |
| | Tinea groups |
| Parasites | |
| Swimmer's itch | *Schistosoma* spp. |
| Creeping eruption | Hookworm (filariform stage) |
| Hookworm disease | Hookworm |
| Ascariasis | Nematode |

*Source:* Klainer and Geis (1973), Davis et al., (1973), Key et al. (1977), and Jawetz et al., (1974).

1. Assessing the quantitative relation between an agent and health outcome from a given set of data
2. Given this data, predicting an effect

The need to predict alludes to the fact that most of the definitive health effects data are based on animal studies, usually at doses higher than those expected in human exposures from environmental exposures. Therefore, extrapolations (e.g., animal-to-human and high-to-low dose) are required to define potential human responses. When reliable data from humans are available, the quantitation of adverse effects is generally considered more reliable and more easily made (Abernathy and Roberts, 1994). Data from animal studies must be examined critically, since most toxic effects are observed after relatively high doses. In addition, animals may have susceptibilities different from those of humans, and strains of experimental animals are less genetically diverse than the populations of humans. On the positive side, it is possible to carefully control experimental variables for animal studies; a situation not possible in human epidemiological studies.

It is common to identify levels (doses and exposures) that are associated with biological effects, adverse effects, frank effects, and absence of effects. Markers of such effects [e.g., no-observed-adverse-effect level (NOAEL), lowest-observed-adverse-effect level (LOAEL), reference dose (RfD), reference concentration (RfC), benchmark dose, and such] are discussed in Chapter 16. Sometimes dose–response curves may be constructed to assess the severity of effects or, such as in estimating cancer risks, to derive potency factors (unit risk factors), and determine the change in the severity of effect per unit of contaminant (i.e., dose or exposure). The steepness (slope) of the dose–response curve (i.e., those that are linear or have a linear component in the area of interest) may be directly related to the severity of effect (Fig. 3). However, steep curves for minor effects are not as severe as shallow curves for more severe endpoints. Curve slopes also may be related to population heterogeneity.

A variety of mathematical models are used to estimate the risk of developing cancer subsequent to exposure to a carcinogen. These models extrapolate experimental data to estimate effects at lower exposure levels and consist of several types to include distribution models (log-probit, Mantel–Bryan, logit, and Weibull), mechanistic models (one-hit, gamma-multihit, multistage, and linearized multistage), pharmacokinetic, and time-to-tumor (Klaassen, 1986). These models vary in their assumptions about how cancer develops or who is susceptible and, therefore, can produce risk estimates that vary by orders of magnitude.

### 2. Selected Toxicological Principles

*Dose.* Basic toxicological principles, especially those associated with exposure and pharmacokinetic or toxicokinetic dynamics, must be addressed when assessing the dose–response component of the risk assessment paradigm. These principles are presented earlier in this text,

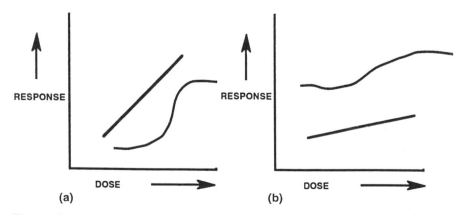

**Figure 3** Relation between dose–response and severity of effect. The slopes of the curves in panel a are greater than those of panel b. Thus, the effects represented in panel a are greater (more severe) than those of panel b.

and the reader should be familiar with them to fully appreciate the significance and limitations inherent in the dose–response assessment. A few of these principles will be reiterated in the following paragraphs.

When dose–response relationships are evaluated, it is important to consider how the agent was delivered to the body. The route of delivery sometimes affects the type of response that is elicited. Some chemicals produce the same effect regardless of the route of entry. For example, the polycyclic aromatic hydrocarbons (PAHs)—dibenz[*a,h*]anthracene and benzo[*a*]pyrene—produce cancer in animals when administered orally or to the skin (ATSDR, 1990). Inhalation of benzo[*a*]pyrene by animals produced cancer, and persons exposed by inhalation to emissions that contain PAH mixtures (coke oven emissions, roofing tar emissions, and cigarette smoke) also developed cancer (ATSDR, 1990). Therefore, it appears that some PAHs may be carcinogenic by all exposure routes. In contrast, some chemicals have vastly different effects that vary according to the exposure route. Oral exposures introduce agents directly to the gastrointestinal system, with subsequent entry to the hepatic–portal system, where the liver can metabolically alter (detoxify or increase toxicity) the substance's activity. The liver is the primary site for chemical metabolism. However, inhalation and dermal exposures can allow substances to be absorbed either unchanged directly into the circulatory system or can modify them with local skin or lung enzymes in an extrahepatic metabolic process. Antimony is an example of a compound that has exposure route differences. When administered by inhalation, antimony induced lung neoplasms in rats; however, there was no evidence of carcinogenicity in two lifetime studies in which rats and mice were given antimony in drinking water (USEPA, 1993). Other examples of chemical exposures for which inhalation and oral exposure routes result in different cancer risk assessments are asbestos and cadmium (Ohanian, 1992).

Sometimes one route of exposure can be used to estimate dose by another exposure route (i.e., "route-to-route extrapolation"); however, specific physiological and metabolic conditions must exist (USEPA, 1989c).

Another concern of dose–response relationships is relating exposures (e.g., contaminant concentrations in air, food, or water) to the actual dose that is delivered to the body and, finally, to the target organ. Factors such as absorption, distribution, and metabolism can qualitatively and quantitatively modify the chemical that actually reaches and affects the target. Advances in physiological and biological-based pharmacokinetic modeling have resulted in a tool that can be used by the risk assessor to estimate target doses (USAF, 1990).

*Response.*   The response that is considered in the risk assessment step is a biologically, and usually statistically, significant change (increase or decrease) in a health outcome that is related to an agent. The types of responses can be general (e.g., effects on body weight or food and water intake); they can be more specific (e.g., organ weight, physiological, enzyme, and histological changes); or, most frequently, a combination of the two.

It should be emphasized that the presence of biological significance is more important than statistical significance. This is partly due to the nature of statistical science, which recognizes that most methods have some inherent degree of error. 1,4-Dithiane is an example for which biological significance outweighs statistical significance (Deardorff et al., 1994). Results of oral dosing studies showed that female rat brain weights were significantly lighter in the high- and low-dose groups. However, brain weights of the middose group were not significantly lighter and the differences in weights of the treated and control groups were within that expected from removing and handling the brains. Thus, even though there was statistical significance, biological significance was not demonstrated. Another endpoint (nasal lesions) was identified as the critical health effect.

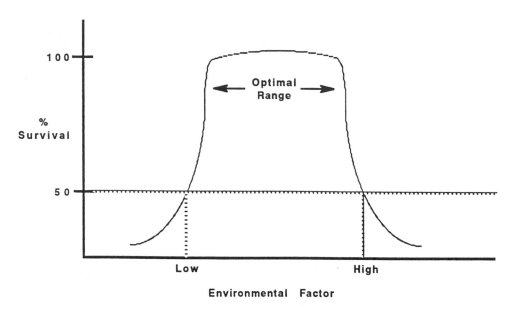

**Figure 4**  The "law of limiting factors" defines an optimal range of tolerance (also called the essential range) to an environmental factor for the survival of organisms. At environmental factor levels above or below the optimal range, organism survival will decline.

*Law of the Minimum; Limits of Tolerance.*  In the previous section (Sec. IV.A), there is a discussion concerning toxic effects either because of the presence of excess contaminants or the absence of essential nutrients. This obviously is a dose phenomenon that should be recognized in the risk assessment process. There are several essential trace elements (ETE), such as zinc, molybdenum, and selenium, with health-based criteria that consider both excess and deficit amounts in the daily diet (Abernathy et al., 1993; Donohue et al., 1994; USEPA, 1988). This concept is not new and was recognized in the 19th and early 20th centuries by a German biochemist, Justus Liebig, and an American ecologist, Victor Shelford (Nadakavukaren, 1986). Liebig studied problems of fertility in agricultural soils and observed that crop yields were affected by the absence of nutrients (c.g., copper) that were needed in minute amounts. Based on such observations, he developed the *law of the minimum* stating that "the growth of a plant is dependent on the amount of foodstuff which is presented to it in a minimum quantity." Victor Shelford demonstrated that too much of a limiting factor can be as harmful as not enough. For such substances, organisms have an ecological maximum and minimum, and the range in between the two extremes are the organism's *limit of tolerance* (Fig. 4).

## V.  EXPOSURE ASSESSMENT

### A.  Definition

*Exposure assessment,* the third step in the risk assessment paradigm, is the process of measuring or estimating the intensity, frequency, and duration of the human exposure to an agent currently present in the environment, or of estimating the hypothetical exposure that might arise from the release of new chemicals into the environment (NAS, 1983). It involves physical contact with the agent, and a variety of factors should be considered when assessing the potential risk that an environmental contaminant poses. These include exposure route and duration, elucidation of the size and composition of the exposure population, and determination of the magnitude and frequency of exposure.

## B. Exposure Route and Duration

Exposure (and dose) routes were discussed previously relative to hazard identification (this chapter) and toxicological impact (see Part I). The exposure route also is important in determining the significance of an exposure to a contaminant. The exposure routes include dermal (skin, cutaneous), oral (ingestion of food and water), inhalation (air), and parenteral (skin injection, intraperitoneal). The *total absorbed dose* is a summation of the dose absorbed by each route.

Exposure sites may have differences in absorption and metabolism that can affect the significance of an exposure. For example, 2,4,6-trinitrotoluene (TNT), 1,2-dichloroethane, 1,2-dichloroethylene, and *p*-dioxane are reported to cause significant adverse health effects when humans or experimental laboratory animals are exposed by either inhalation, dermal absorption, or oral ingestion (Nadakavukaren, 1986; Roberts and Hartley, 1992). An exposure assessment of these chemicals, thus, should consider media such as air, water, and food as exposure routes in a risk assessment. By contrast, gases, such as carbon monoxide, ozone, and sulfur chloride, pose health effects only from inhalation; therefore, only air should be considered as an exposure route (Key et al., 1977).

As discussed earlier in this book, short-term (acute and subacute) exposures from a particular chemical may result in effects that differ from longer-term (subchronic, chronic, and lifetime) exposure to the same chemical, thus indicating the relation of exposure duration to toxicity. Table 6 shows examples of chemicals that were evaluated for drinking water toxicity for which the critical effect, which was the basis for the recommended exposure limits, varies with the exposure duration.

## C. Contact Probability Versus Number Exposed

The final area of concern for exposure assessment is the potential for people to be exposed. There are two components:

1. The *probability* that people will contact the agent
2. The *number* of people that can actually or potentially come in contact with the agent

Regardless of an agent's toxicity or its degree of hazard, there simply is no risk if no exposure occurs. Therefore, as the probability that persons can come into contact with a hazardous agent increases, then the risk increases. Figure 5 illustrates how both exposure potential and the number of exposed persons relate in the determination of risk to an agent that has an adverse health effect. When both contact potential and number of exposed persons are low, then the risk of adverse health effects also is low. Conversely, high-exposure potential and large numbers of exposed persons result in high risk. When one parameter is high and the other is low, the risk may be considered to be medium (the relative importance of this type of classification may be more appropriately determined in a risk management process). The figure illustrates extreme possibilities for contact potential and number of exposed persons, but in reality, there are infinite categories. Because of inherent uncertainties in risk assessment and exposure assessment, it is usually difficult to fit a characterization into a neat box. Scientific experience and judgment thus become important factors in this process.

The relation between risk and the number of exposed persons is exemplified by the production of munitions chemicals. Munitions, such as hexahydro-1,3,5-trinitro-1,3,5-triazine (RDX), nitroguanidine, and octahydro-1,3,5,7-tetranitro-1,3,5,7-tetrazocine (HMX), have demonstrated mammalian toxicity. However, because of their limited use, production and en-

**Table 6** Examples of Adverse Health Effects That Vary by Exposure Duration

| Chemical | Critical effect by duration[a] | | | | Ref. |
|---|---|---|---|---|---|
| | 1 day | 10 day | Longer term[b] | Lifetime[c] | |
| Aciflouren | | Developmental toxicity | Liver weight | NA (carcinogen) | USEPA, 1989a |
| Ametryn | | Body weight gain, histopathology | Fatty liver, histopathology | Fatty liver, histopathology | USEPA, 1989a |
| Bromocil | | Hepatoxicity | No observed adverse effect at highest dose | Body weight gain, thyroid hyperplasia | USEPA, 1989a |
| Butylate | | Teratogenesis | Reproductive toxicity | Body weight gain | USEPA, 1989a |
| 2, 4, 6-Trichlorophenoxyacetic acid | | Developmental toxicity | Reproductive toxicity | Biochemical parameters, histopathological and gross pathology | USEPA, 1989a |
| Propazine | | Teratogenesis | Body weight gain | Body weight gain, hematology, urinalysis | USEPA, 1989a |
| White phosphorus | Lethality | Lethality | Lethality | Reproductive toxicity | Roberts and Hartley, 1992 Ware, 1988 |
| 1, 1-Dichloromethylene | Serum chemistry, liver histopathology | | Decreased kidney weight | Hepatotoxicity | |
| Dichlorodifluoromethane | Based on 10-day | Organ weights, histopathology | Body weight gain, serum chemistry, hematology, histopathology | Survival, histopathology | USEPA, 1991c |

[a]Discussion of the basis and assumptions associated with exposure durations can be found in any of the references noted above.
[b]Approximately a 7-year exposure duration.
[c]Approximately a 70-year exposure.

| CONTACT POTENTIAL | NUMBER OF EXPOSED PEOPLE | | |
|---|---|---|---|
| | NONE | LOW | HIGH |
| NONE | NO RISK | NO RISK | NO RISK |
| LOW | NO RISK | LOW RISK | MEDIUM RISK* |
| HIGH | NO RISK | MEDIUM RISK* | HIGH RISK |

**Figure 5** Relation between risk and two elements of exposure assessment. *The relevance and actual classification of risk based on these conditions may be defined differently in the risk management process.

vironmental occurrence of these chemicals are limited both geographically and quantitatively (Nadakavukaren, 1986). Therefore, when one considers the entire United States population, there is little potential for exposure, and the human risk from such munitions is minimal to nonexistent. An example of the opposite condition is carbon monoxide (CO), which is a significant urban air pollutant primarily because of automotive emissions, but also from industrial and power plant emissions. (Nadakavukaren, 1986; Salvato, 1982). It also is a common indoor air pollutant that originates from sources, such as cigarette smoke; emissions from gas, wood, or kerosene stoves; appliances; and vehicle exhaust. Given the wide use of vehicles in the United States, CO is present in large quantities, which between 1968 and 1975 were estimated to be between 94.6 and 100.1 million tons (Ware, 1988). Coupled with the large number of people who live in urban areas, both the exposure potential and the number of exposed persons are high for this chemical.

## VI. RISK CHARACTERIZATION

## A. Definition

The final step in the risk assessment process is the *risk characterization*. The NAS (1983) definition for this step is "the process of estimating the incidence of a health effect under the various conditions of human exposure described in exposure assessment. It is performed by combining the exposure and the dose–response assessments. The summary effects of the uncertainties in the preceding steps are described in this step." The reader is referred to Fig. 1 for the integration of the hazard identification, dose–response assessment, and exposure assessment. Risk characterization is the product of the risk assessment process that can be used by a risk manager to develop control and remediation strategies, and it can be used by a risk communicator to inform the public about the type, magnitude, and potential for persons to develop adverse health effects. In addition to summarizing the other three risk assessment processes, the risk characterization should discuss major assumptions, scientific judgments, and the uncertainties of the process (USEPA, 1986). It is only as reliable as the information generated by each phase in the evolution of the risk characterization. Its adequacy is determined by enumeration of both the strengths and weaknesses of each part of the qualitative and quantitative assessment (USEPA, 1986).

## B. Qualitative Versus Quantitative Risk Characterization

*1. Systemic Effects: Threshold Effect*

A risk characterization may be qualitative or quantitative. Most frequently it is both qualitative and quantitative. A *qualitative risk characterization* is a narrative that describes the elements of the risk assessment paradigm for a particular hazard and may express hazard, exposure, and risk potential in semiquantitative terms, such as "negligible," "minimal," "moderate," or "severe." Comparisons with common, perhaps acceptable, hazards and risks may be made and comparative terms, such as "less than," "equal to," or "greater than," may be used to define the nature of the risk.

A *quantitative risk characterization* expressed hazard and risk in numerical terms. It can indicate a finite amount of hazard per unit dose or exposure of an agent (e.g., percentage change in response for each milligram of agent per kilogram of animal body weight). The factors that are derived for quantitative assessments are discussed in detail in Chapter 16.

Examples of quantitative risk characterizations used by the EPA for chemicals that have health effects other than cancer and gene mutations are discussed by Barnes and Dourson (1988) and include the *estimated exposure dose* (EED) and the *margin of exposure* (MOE). The EED, which can be measured or calculated and should include all sources and routes of exposure, is compared with the RfD or RfC* for a particular agent. When the EED is less than the RfD or RfC, the need for regulatory action should be small. The MOE is the ratio between a NOAEL and EED:

$$MOE = \frac{NOAEL \text{ (experimental dose)}}{EED \text{ (human dose)}} \qquad (1)$$

When the MOE is greater than or equal to the product of the UF and MF the need for regulatory action is small.

For noncancer effects, a threshold mechanism is assumed. As stated by Barnes and Dourson (1988), this assumption is based on the theory that a "range of exposures from zero to some finite value can be tolerated by the organism with essentially no chance of expression of the toxic effect." Although this statement appears valid for most chemicals, it does not apply to one specific group of chemicals. For essential trace elements (ETEs), zero exposure would result in deleterious effects (Abernathy et al., 1993). However, for ETEs, the concept of a finite upper-bound threshold for nontoxicity is also supported by experimental data (NRC, 1989). Therefore, the essentiality requirement does not prevent risk assessment of an ETE, it only means that the essential nature of the chemical must be considered during evaluation (Abernathy et al., 1993).

For noncancer effects, a RfD is derived. The RfD is defined as "an estimate (with an uncertainty spanning perhaps an order of magnitude) of a daily exposure to the human population (including sensitive subgroups) that is likely to be without appreciable risk of deleterious effects during a lifetime" (USEPA, 1988). The RfD concept is similar to the acceptable daily intake (ADI) used by some regulatory and risk assessment groups. The EPA has introduced the term RfD to obviate the use of such prejudicial words as "acceptable" and "safety" (Barnes and Dourson, 1988). In the RfD process, a no-observed-adverse-effect level (NOAEL) or a lowest-

---

*The RfC is a relatively recent development by the U. S. EPA that is descriptive of substances that have an inhalation exposure and is similar in concept to the RfD, which is based on substances that have oral exposures. The RfCs were not discussed in the paper by Barnes and Dourson (1988). The reader is referred to Jarabek et al. (1990) for a discussion of RfCs.

observed-adverse-effect level (LOAEL) is determined by evaluating the toxicity database of a chemical. The appropriate NOAELs or LOAELs are selected, primarily, from animal studies or from human studies. Many factors such as toxicity endpoint, appropriateness of the species studied, methodology, route and length of exposure are critically reviewed. For example, in studies of similar quality, a human study would be selected over an animal study. In addition, for drinking water regulations, data from oral exposures are preferable. The most relevant study is selected and the endpoint of toxicity is considered to be the "critical" effect. The NOAEL (or LOAEL) is divided by uncertainty factors (UFs) and, sometimes, a modifying factor (MF; Table 7) to obtain an RfD:

$$RfD = \frac{NOAEL \ (or \ LOAEL)}{UFs \times MF} \tag{2}$$

The units for the RfD are in milligrams of the chemical per kilogram of body weight per day (mg/kg day$^{-1}$). The EPA derives RfC values for airborne chemicals; the reader is referred to Jarabek et al. (1990) for a discussion of this process.

## 2. Carcinogenicity: Nonthreshold Effects

Those agents that cause cancer in humans or in animals are considered to have no-threshold (i.e., there is no "safe" exposure level unless there are data to the contrary). With these chemicals, any exposure has some risk and, as exposure increases, the probability of a carcinogenic response increases (USEPA, 1986).

The EPA evaluates potential carcinogenicity from both a qualitative and a quantitative

**Table 7** General Description of Standard Uncertainty and Modifying Factors Used in Deriving Reference Doses[a]

| Basis for UF[a] | General comments |
|---|---|
| Human (intraspecies) | A tenfold factor normally is utilized to account for variability of responses in human populations. |
| Animal (interspecies) | A tenfold factor generally is used to account for differences in responses between animal species and humans. |
| Subchronic to chronic | A tenfold factor may be used when chronic data are unavailable and a 90-day study is used for RfD[b] derivation. |
| LOAEL to NOAEL[b] | A tenfold factor may be used when a LOAEL instead of a NOAEL is used to derive the Rfd. For "minimal" LOAELs, an intermediate UF of 3 may be used. |
| Data gaps | A factor, usually three- to tenfold is applied for "Incomplete" data bases (i.e., missing studies). It is meant to account for the inability of any study to consider all toxic endpoints. The intermediate factor of 3 (½ log unit) is often used when there is a single data gap exclusive of chronic data. |
| Modifying factor | Usually applied for differences in absorption rates, tolerance to a chemical, lack of sensitive endpoint, or other toxicokinetic/dynamic parameters. The default value is 1. |

[a]Professional scientific judgment is used to determine the appropriateness of each UF. Values ranging from 1 to 10 (usually 1, 3, or 10) may be used for each UF. The tenfold value is the most commonly used.
[b]Abbreviations: UF, uncertainty factor; LOAEL, lowest-observed-adverse-effect level; NOAEL, no-observed-adverse-effect level; RfD, Reference dose.
*Source:* Barnes and Dourson (1988), Abernathy et al., (1993), IRIS (1993), and Jarabek et al., (1990).

standpoint. In the qualitative evaluation, EPA uses a "weight-of-evidence" approach to determine the potential carcinogenicity of a chemical. Factors include

Occurrence (or lack of) cancers in various species
Dose–response data, number(s) of tumor sites
Decreases in time-to-tumor
Effects on different sexes
Mutagenicity
Human case reports and epidemiology studies

Each chemical is then placed in a category (Table 8).

Quantification of carcinogenic responses is accomplished by using mathematical models. Although there are several models, EPA generally uses the linearized multistage model (LMS). It is a conservative model, and the value obtained from the LMS risk model gives a plausible upper-bound estimate of the cancer risk. A chemical's carcinogenic potency after oral administration is given by a slope factor ($q_1$*; Fig. 6). Use of such models are generally necessary, since relatively high doses are given to experimental animals, and the EPA needs to estimate risk at the relatively low doses that may be encountered in environmental situations. When there is appropriate pharmacokinetic, metabolic, or other mechanistic data, a model other than the LMS may be applied to develop the risk estimate (USEPA, 1986).

Carcinogenic risk can be expressed as the product of the actual human dose and risk per unit dose developed from dose response modeling (USEPA, 1990b). The EPA *Risk Assessment Guidelines for Carcinogens* (USEPA, 1986) presents three ways of expressing estimates of cancer risks:

1. *Unit Risk:* Assuming low-dose linearity, this is the excess risk from continuous constant lifetime exposure of 1 unit (e.g., ppm or ppb in food and water (mg/kg day$^{-1}$) by ingestion, or ppb or $\mu g/m^3$ in air) of carcinogen concentration.
2. *Dose corresponding to a given level of risk:* Use when nonlinear extrapolation models estimate different unit risks at different dose levels.
3. *Individual and population risks:* Use when risk may be characterized either in terms of individual lifetime risks, the excess number of cancers produced per year in the exposed population, or both.

**Table 8**  EPA Cancer Classification Categories[a]

| Category | Description |
|---|---|
| A | Human carcinogen |
| B | Probable human carcinogen |
|   |     B1: Limited human data |
|   |     B2: Sufficient animal data and inadequate human data |
| C | Possible human carcinogen |
| D | Not classifiable |
| E | Evidence of noncarcinogenicity |

[a]The EPA is presently revising the cancer guidelines and this classification system will be modified.
*Source:* EPA Risk Assessment Guidelines of 1986 (USEPA, 1987).

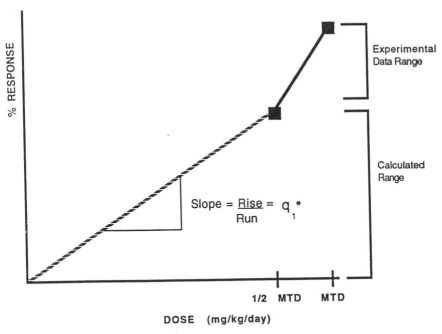

**Figure 6** Schematic presentation of calculation of a slope factor ($q_1^*$) for a chemical that is carcinogenic after oral administration. The solid line represents actual dose levels, whereas the dotted line represents area of extrapolation. The upper-bound estimate of the risk response is calculated by multiplying the ($q_1^*$) times the daily dose. MTD, maximum tolerated dose.

Since the various mathematical models that estimate the risk can vary by orders of magnitude, a risk characterization for cancer risk may contain a range of risk estimates (Ohanian, 1992).

## C. What Should Be Included in a Risk Characterization: EPA Risk Assessment

Methods of characterizing risks and presenting the characterization may vary with the nature of the hazard (e.g., carcinogen vs. noncarcinogen), the exposure source, and characteristics of the exposed population. Because of the complexities in toxicology, risk assessment methodology, and assumptions and uncertainties inherent in the process, there are various ways that federal, state, and local agencies perform and express risk assessments (USEPA, 1990c).

### 1. Risk Assessment: Threshold Versus Nonthreshold

When chemicals exert systemic effects, they are considered to have a threshold mechanism, and a RfD approach is used to assess their risk. Carcinogenic chemicals are assumed to have nonthreshold effects (USEPA, 1990a; Fig. 7). Cancer potential is determined by a weight-of-evidence approach, and the linearized multistage mathematical model is used to estimate potency.

### 2. Risk Management

Under the Safe Drinking Water Act (SDWA) of 1974, as amended in 1986 (USC, 1974; Public Law 99-339, 1986), the EPA is required to establish maximum contaminant level goals (MCLGs)

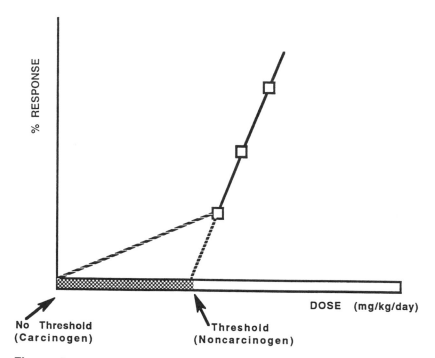

**Figure 7** Diagrammatic representation of threshold and nonthreshold concepts. A dose up to the threshold intercept can be tolerated by an organism without expression of adverse health effects (see text).

and maximum contaminant levels (MCLs) or treatment techniques. The risk assessment process gives a scientific estimate of the magnitude of the health risk of a chemical, and this information is used to set an MCLG. The MCLG reflects risk assessment (RfD or cancer classification) and is health based; it is not enforceable.

The MCL is a risk management decision. To promulgate an MCL under the SDWA, risk managers start with the risk characterization and then factor in such considerations as economic impact, analytical and treatment techniques, political, legal and social aspects, to arrive at an MCL (see Fig. 2). The resulting MCL is legally enforceable (USC, 1974; Public Law 99-339, 1986). For a more complete discussion on MCLG and MCL see references (USEPA, 1989b, 1991b).

## 3. Risk Communication

Risk communication is the process by which the public participates in and is aware of drinking water standards. Before, during, and after promulgating a standard, the EPA shares risk assessment and risk management information with the public by publishing notices of impending actions in the *Federal Register.*

The EPA also has another mechanism for sharing chemical information with the public. It maintains an electronic database, called the Integrated Risk Information System (IRIS). All of the available data used by EPA in its risk assessments for each chemical (Table 9) is listed on this system. To obtain additional information on this system, contact IRIS User Support in Cincinnati, OH at (513) 569-7254.

**Table 9** General File Structure for Chemicals Listed on the Integrated Risk Information System[a]

| |
|---|
| Substance identification and CAS number[b] |
| Chemical and physical properties |
| RfD/RfC: oral and inhalation reference doses for chronic noncarcinogenic health effects |
| CRAVE: oral and inhalation slope factors and unit risks for chronic exposures to carcinogens |
| Drinking water health advisories: recommended estimates of concentrations of contaminants in drinking water that people could be exposed to for 1-day, 10-days, longer-term (7 years), or a lifetime without causing any anticipated adverse noncancer effects |
| Aquatic toxicity data |
| Exposure standards: a summary of EPA regulatory actions |
| References |

[a]Certain data sets (i.e., RfC) may be missing if an RfC has not been verified for that chemical.
[b]Abbreviations: CAS number, Chemical Abstract Services registry number; RfD, reference dose; RfC, reference concentration; CRAVE, carcinogen risk assessment verification endeavor (cancer assessments).

## VII. SUMMARY

Risk assessment is a dynamic science that continually evolves as a result of both scientific advancements and increased public interest. It requires a multidisciplinary approach that integrates many scientific disciplines (e.g., toxicology, biochemistry, pathology, pharmacology, biostatistics, and so on). Currently risk assessment has inherent uncertainties that reduce accuracy in estimating and predicting human health effects. Some of these uncertainties include

Extrapolating effects observed in animals to predict effects to humans
Relating exposure to body burden and target organ dose; and
Extrapolating high, tissue-damaging dosing studies in animals to low-dose, non–tissue-damaging exposures that persons experience (Kimbrough, 1991)

As biological and health sciences continue to improve, so will risk assessment methodology. Scientists strive to improve the methods that they employ to estimate and predict chemical, biological, and physical agent effects on persons to enhance the risk management decisions that regulators must make. Ohanian (1992) identifies some research that should be pursued to improve risk assessment methodology:

1. Use of data on mechanisms of action in cancer classification scheme
2. Application of maximum tolerated dose and its implication in risk assessment
3. Risk assessment of complex mixtures using a toxicity equivalency factor (TEF) approach
4. Role of essentiality versus toxicity in risk assessment of trace elements
5. Application of benchmark dose approach in the derivation of reference dose
6. Consideration of mechanism of carcinogenicity in the selection of risk assessment model (i.e., two-stage, receptor-mediated and such)
7. Incorporation of data on active metabolites in assessing cancer risk
8. Estimation of human exposure parameters using physiologically based tissue dosimetry and response models
9. Development and validation of human exposure models designed to generate realistic prediction of exposure to chemicals

These and other research efforts will reduce the uncertainties that are inherent in the risk assessment process. They will improve risk assessment accuracy for estimating and predicting adverse health effects and better protect the public's health and improve the quality of life.

## REFERENCES

Abernathy, C. O., and W. C. Roberts (1994). Risk assessment in the Environmental Protection Agency, *J. Hazard Subst.*, 39, 135–142.

Abernathy, C. O., R. Cantilli, J. T. Du, and O. A. Levander (1993). Essentiality versus toxicity: Some considerations in the risk assessment of essential trace elements, *Hazard Assess. Chem.*, 8, 81–113.

Andrews, L. S., and R. Snyder (1986). Toxic effects of solvents and vapors. In *Casarett and Doull's Toxicology,* 3rd ed. (C. D. Klaassen, M. O. Amdur, and J. Doull, eds.), Macmillan Publishing, New York, pp. 636–638.

[ATSDR] Agency for Toxic Substances and Disease Registry (1990). Toxicological profile for polycyclic aromatic hydrocarbons, U. S. Department of Health and Human Services, Public Health Service, Atlanta, GA, (ATSDR/TP-90-20)

Barnes, D. G., and M. Dourson (1988). Reference dose (RfD): Description and use in health risk assessments, *Regul. Toxicol. Pharmacol.*, 8, 471–486.

Brown, S. L. (1985). Quantitative risk assessment of environmental hazards, *Annu. Rev. Public Health,* 6, 247–267.

Chess, C., B. J. Hance, and P. Sandman (1988). *Improving Dialog With Communities: A Risk Communication Manual for Government,* Environmental Communication Research Program, Rutgers University, New Brunswick, NY.

Cohen, B. L. (1991). Catalog of risks extended and updated, *Health Phys.,* 61, 317–335.

Cohen, B. L., and I-S. Lee (1979). A catalog of risks. *Health Phys.,* 36, 707–722.

Davis, B. D., R. Dulbecco, H. N. Eisen, H. S. Ginsberg, W. B. Wood, and M. McCarty (1973). *Microbiology,* Harper & Row, Hagerstown, MD.

[DHHS] Department of Health and Human Services (1985). Risk assessment and risk management of toxic substances: A report to the Secretary, Department of Health and Human Services from the Executive Committee, DHHS Committee to Coordinate Environmental and Related Programs (CCERP), DHHS.

Deardorff, M. B., B. R. Das, and W. C. Roberts (1994). 1,4-Dithiane. In *Drinking Water Health Advisory: Munitions 2* (W. R. Hartley, W. C. Roberts, and B. J. Commons, eds.), P.A.S., Ann Arbor, MI.

Donohue, J. M., L. Gordon, C. Kirman, W. C. Roberts, and C. O. Abernathy (1994). Zinc chloride and other zinc compounds. In *Drinking Water Health Advisory: Munitions* 2 (W. R. Hartley, W. C. Roberts, and B. J. Commons, eds.), P.A.S., Ann Arbor, MI.

Doull, J., and M. C. Bruce (1986). Origin and scope of toxicology. In *Casarett and Doull's Toxicology: The Basic Science of Poisons,* (C. D. Klaassen, M. O. Amdur, J. Doull, eds.) Macmillan Publishing, New York, pp. 3–10.

*EPA Journal* (1992). Washington, DC: U. S. Environmental Protection Agency. 18(1), 6–61.

Federal Focus, Inc. (1991). Towards common measures: Recommendations for a presidential executive order on environmental risk assessment and risk management policy. Federal Focus, Inc. and The Institute for Regulatory Policy, Washington, DC.

Gross, R. A., and W. T. Broadwater (1994). Health hazard assessments. In *Textbook of Military Medicine,* Vol. 2, *Occupational Health: The Soldier and the Industrial Base,* Part 3: *Disease and the Environment,* Department of the Army, Office of the Surgeon General, The Bordon Institute, Washington, DC, pp. 165–205.

Jarabek, A. M., M. G. Menach, J. H. Overton, M. L. Dourson, and F. J. Miller (1990). The U. S. Environmental Protection Agency's inhalation RfD methodology: Risk assessment for air toxics, *Toxicol. Ind. Health,* 6, 279–301.

Jawetz, E., J. L. Melnick, and E. A. Adelberg (1974). *Review of Medical Microbiology,* Lange Medical Publications, Los Altos, CA.

Key, M. M., A. F. Henschel, J. Butler, R. N. Ligo, I. R. Tabershaw, and L. Ede, eds. (1977). *Occupational*

*Diseases: A Guide to Their Recognition.* U. S. Government Printing Office, Washington, DC, [DHEW (NIOSH) publication 77-181].

Kimbrough, R. D. (1991). Uncertainties in risk assessment, Appl. Occup. Environ. Hyg., 6, 759–763.

Klaassen, C. D. (1986). Principles of toxicology. In *Casarett and Doull's Toxicology: The Basic Science of Poisons.* (C. D. Klaassen, M. O. Amdur, J. Doull, eds.), Macmillan Publishing, New York, pp. 11–32.

Klainer, A. S., and I. Geis (1973). *Agents of Bacterial Disease,* Harper & Row, Hagerstown, MD.

Latham, M. C., R. B. McGandy, and F. J. Stare (1972). *Scope Manual On Nutrition,* The Upjohn Company, Kalamazoo, MI.

McKechnie, J. L., ed. (1970). *Webster's New World Dictionary of the English Language,* Unabridged, 2nd ed. The Publisher's Guild, New York.

Nadakavukaren, A. (1986). *Man and Environment: A Health Perspective,* Waveland Press, Prospects Heights, IL, pp. 17–19.

[NAS] National Academy of Science (1983). Risk assessment in the federal government: Managing the process, NAS, Washington, DC.

[NRC] National Research Council (1989). *Recommended Dietary Allowances,* 10th ed., National Academy Press, Washington, DC.

Ohanian, E. V. (1992). New approaches in setting drinking water standards, *J. Am. Coll. Toxicol.,* 11, 321–324.

Public Law 99-339. The Safe Drinking Water Act Amendments of 1986.

Roberts, W. C. (1990). Vestibular function after solvent exposure, dissertation, University of South Carolina, School of Public Health.

Roberts, W. C., and W. R. Hartley, eds. (1992). *Drinking Water Health Advisory: Munitions,* Lewis Publishers, Boca Raton, FL.

Salvato, J. A. (1982). *Environmental Engineering and Sanitation.* John Wiley & Sons, New York.

Sandman, P. (1993). *Responding to Community Outrage: Strategies for Effective Risk Communication,* American Industrial Hygiene Association, Fairfax, VA.

Santos, S. L. (1990). Developing a risk communication strategy, *J. AWWA,* (Nov.), 45–49.

[USAF] U. S. Air Force (1990). *Development and Validation of Methods for Applying Pharmacokinetic Data in Risk Assessment,* Vol. 1–7, Harry G. Armstrong Aerospace Medical Research Laboratory, Wright-Patterson AFB, OH, (AAMRL-TR-90-072). Available from the National Technical Information Service, Springfield, VA. NTIS order Nos. AD-A237-365 through 371.

USC 4. (1974). The Safe Drinking Water Act. seq. 3e.

[USEPA] U. S. Environmental Protection Agency (1993). *Office of Water Health Advisories, Health Advisories for Drinking Water Contaminants,* Lewis Publishers, Chelsea, MI.

[USEPA] U. S. Environmental Protection Agency (1992a). *Environmental Equity: Reducing Risk for All Communities,* Vol. 2. *Supporting Documentation,* Washington, DC (EPA230-R-92-008A).

[USEPA] U. S. Environmental Protection Agency (1992b). *Environmental Equity: Reducing Risk for All Communities,* Vol. 1, *Supporting Documentation,* Washington, DC (EPA230-R-92-008A).

[USEPA] U. S. Environmental Protection Agency (1991a). General quantitative risk assessment guideline for noncancer health effects, Washington, DC (draft).

[USEPA] U. S. Environmental Protection Agency (1991b). Risk assessment, management, communication: A guide to selected sources, Washington, DC (EPA/560/7-91-008).

[USEPA] U. S. Environmental Protection Agency (1991c). *Office of Drinking Water Health Advisories. Drinking Water Health Advisory: Volatile Organic Compounds,* Lewis Publishers, Chelsea, MI.

[USEPA] U. S. Environmental Protection Agency (1990a). Seminar publication: Risk assessment, management and communication of drinking water contamination, U. S. Environmental Protection Agency, Washington, DC (EPA/625/4-89/024).

[USEPA] U. S. Environmental Protection Agency (1990b). Methodology for assessing health risks associated with indirect exposure to combustor emissions, Washington, DC (EPA/600/6-90/003).

[USEPA] U. S. Environmental Protection Agency (1990c). Risk assessment methodologies: Comparing EPA and state approaches, Washington, DC (EPA570/9-90-012).

[USEPA] U. S. Environmental Protection Agency (1989a). *Office of Drinking Water Health Advisories. Drinking Water Health Advisory: Pesticides,* Lewis Publishers, Chelsea, MI.

[USEPA] U. S. Environmental Protection Agency (1989b). Guidelines for authors of EPA Office of Water Health Advisories, Washington, DC.

[USEPA] U. S. Environmental Protection Agency (1989c). Interim methods for development of inhalation reference doses, Washington, DC (EPA/600/8-88/066F).

[USEPA] U. S. Environmental Protection Agency (1988). Reference dose (RfD): Description and use in health risk assessments, Integrated Risk Information System (IRIS). Online: Intra-Agency Reference Dose Workgroup, Office of Health and Environmental Assessment, Environmental Criteria and Assessment Office, Cincinnati, OH.

[USEPA] U. S. Environmental Protection Agency (1987). The risk assessment guidelines of 1986, Washington, DC (EPA/600/8-87/045).

[USEPA] U. S. Environmental Protection Agency (1986). Guidelines for carcinogen risk assessment, *Fed. Reg.,* 51(33992), 1–17.

Ware, G. W., ed. (1988). *Reviews of Environmental Contamination and Toxicology,* Vol. 106, U. S. Environmental Protection Agency Office of Drinking Water Health Advisories. Springer-Verlag, New York.

White, A., P. Handler, and E. L. Smith (1973). *Principles of Biochemistry,* 5th ed., McGraw-Hill, New York, pp. 1149.

Zeckhouse, R.J., and W. K. Viscusi. (1990). Risk within reason, *Science,* 248, 559–564.

# 16
# Medium-Specific and Multimedium Risk Assessment

**Brian K. Davis and A. K. Klein**
*California Department of Toxic Substances Control*
*Sacramento, California*

## I. INTRODUCTION

Risk assessment is a method used to determine potential health risks to humans or to ecological receptors resulting from exposure to contaminants. The primary message of this chapter is that the risk assessor must consider the totality of exposure and risk from all contamination sources and all exposure pathways. The chapter describes how to evaluate and sum the risk components from different media (surface water, groundwater, air, soil, food) to estimate a total risk. In addition to summing risk over different media, consideration is also given to the need to sum over time, over different chemicals, and over different sources.

It is sometimes valid to evaluate exposure to various chemicals from only one medium, but in general, all media should be considered. Summation of exposure levels should be done by exposure route (ingestion, inhalation, dermal contact), since the toxicity of a contaminant is often dependent on the exposure route. Therefore, exposure levels are not totaled for a specific medium, because exposure to that medium may occur through more than one exposure route. For example, a human receptor may be exposed to the medium of soil by incidentally ingesting soil, inhaling dust, and having direct skin contact with soil. The appropriate summation is for each route of exposure from all media.

Alternatively, summation can be deferred until the risk characterization step. Risk is characterized by comparing exposure levels of the contaminants to health-based criteria values for noncarcinogens, and by determining an upper bound estimate on risk based on exposure levels and the cancer slope factor for carcinogens (see Chapters 14 and 17 for criteria description). The total risk or hazard is determined by totaling over different media for carcinogens and noncarcinogens.

Although logic and prudence dictate that all media should be considered, unless evidence to the contrary is available, single-medium risk assessments are often performed in response to legal mandates. The law may require that only one medium be addressed and may not give authority to regulators to consider other media. This is discussed in Section V.A.

## II.  MEDIUM-SPECIFIC EXPOSURE ASSESSMENT

## A.  Overview

### 1.  The Role of Exposure Assessment

Exposure assessment is one of four components of risk assessment (see Chapter 15). The first of the components is hazard identification, in which the sources of contamination, such as toxic waste sites or smoke stack emissions, are considered and contaminants of concern are identified. The second component is dose–response, in which the toxicity of the contaminants is described in quantitative terms and used to derive health-based criteria. The third component is exposure assessment in which the exposure of the receptor to the contaminants is assessed, considering each individual medium and the routes of ingestion, inhalation, and dermal contact. Exposure assessment evaluates fate and transport of contaminants in air, water, and soil, and derives estimates of the doses over time to the various receptors. The fourth component is risk characterization in which the nature and magnitude of the health hazard or risk is described by relating the estimated doses to the health-based criteria for the contaminants being evaluated.

### 2.  Routes of Exposure

The routes of exposure are inhalation, ingestion, and dermal contact. The primary route by which organisms are exposed to contaminants varies for different media; ingestion for food and water and inhalation for air. Secondary routes of exposure may also be important. Inhalation of chemicals volatilizing from water and dermal contact with contaminants in water may result in significant exposure. Ingestion and dermal contact are the most important routes of exposure for soil, but inhalation of volatilized contaminants and contaminated dust also contribute to exposure.

   The route of exposure is a critical factor for risk assessment because the harmful effects of a chemical are often route-dependent. Since dermal absorption is usually less than absorption from either the gastrointestinal tract or the lungs, dermal exposure often leads to less toxicity than similar levels of exposure by ingestion or inhalation. Even for exceptional compounds, such as carbon tetrachloride and benzene, which are readily absorbed across the skin, each route and each medium must be considered separately.

### 3.  Chemical Changes or Transformation

Chemicals are not immutable in the contaminated medium. Fate and transport of contaminants is a description of chemical changes and movement of contaminants from one medium to another. Chemical changes may result from physical or biological activity and may lead to either decreased or increased toxicity. Examples of the effect of physical aspects of the environment are the photooxidation of chemicals in air by sunlight, and the hydrolysis of chemicals in water. Parathion, a common insecticide, can be photooxidized in air to paraoxon, a more toxic chemical. This photooxidation is dependent both on sunlight and the presence of atmospheric pollutants (Woodrow et al., 1978). Parathion and paraoxon are eventually hydrolyzed in the environment to *p*-nitrophenol, a less toxic chemical (Woodrow et al., 1977) and, ultimately, degraded completely. As an example of environmental transformation resulting from biological activity, mercury ores are primarily mercuric sulfide (cinnabar), a compound with low toxicity, but microbes in soil, sediment, and the gut can transform mercuric sulfide into much more toxic organic forms of mercury such as methylmercury (Wade et al., 1993).

### 4.  Transport among Media

Chemicals can move from one medium into other media. This may be unidirectional, as in the transfer of a chemical from contaminated soil into groundwater, surface water, or air followed by its movement away from the source of contamination. Alternatively, an equilibrium may develop, with a chemical cycling from one medium to another and back. The principal force behind the transfer of a chemical from one medium to others is fugacity, the tendency of the chemical to escape from gas, solid, or liquid phases, eventually leading to the partitioning of the chemical among the environmental media of soil, air, biota, sediment, and water. An equilibrium develops when the escaping tendencies of a chemical present in two media are equal. At equilibrium, the concentration of the chemical in one medium will always be proportional to its concentration in the other medium. This is described by a partition coefficient $K$, which represents the partitioning between any two media, such as soil and water, water and air, or air and biota. For example, to predict whether there is a potential for exposure to a surface water contaminant by the inhalation route, the relevant partition coefficient is Henry's constant, $K_H$. In simple terms, $K_H$ is the ratio of the concentration of the chemical in air to the concentration of the chemical in water. The concentration of the chemical in air is dependent on its vapor pressure, the tendency of the chemical to escape to a gaseous compartment, and the concentration of the chemical in water is dependent on its solubility in water. A chemical with a high Henry's constant would have a greater tendency to volatilize and move into air than to remain in water. Such a chemical is expected to be found as a vapor in air, even if it had originally been released into water.

During the establishment of a distributional equilibrium among media, chemical changes may also occur. For example, when mercuric sulfide is transformed into volatile forms, such as elemental mercury or methylmercury, it moves into the air. It can later be redeposited in soil or water. Thus, as mercury cycles through air, water, and sediments, a variety of chemical species are involved (Wade et al., 1993). A metal such as mercury achieves equilibria among its chemical species as well as among various media.

## B.  Rationale for Single-Medium Risk Assessments

There are several circumstances in which it may be appropriate to consider only a single medium in a risk assessment. In some instances, the contaminating chemical is released to a single medium and is not readily transferred to other media. Some examples are the release of a volatile chemical into the air from a smokestack, the release of a soluble chemical with low volatility into a lake, or the release of a chemical that becomes tightly bound to soil particles in soil.

A second circumstance in which a single-medium risk assessment is appropriate is when receptors are exposed to only one medium. For example, a chemical contaminant in soil may move into groundwater and into air, but if conditions prevent exposure to soil (such as restricted access) or groundwater (such as no current use), then exposure assessment may be restricted to the airborne contaminant.

Finally, there may be circumstances for which exposure is from several media, but is only significant from one medium. It is important to notice that the key word, *significant,* refers to significance relative to some health-based standard or criterion and not relative to exposure to the same contaminant in other media. If an air contaminant poses an unacceptable health risk, it is still unacceptable, even when it pales by comparison with the health risk from the same contaminant in a different medium, such as water.

This discussion has cited three conditions in which the logic for evaluating only one medium is based on physical, chemical, and biological considerations. Single-medium risk assessments are also done in response to legal mandates. A government agency may be mandated to address risks and hazards from contaminants only in one medium. The discussion of statutory authorities (see Sec. V of this chapter) illustrates this point with examples of statutes and the responsible regulatory agencies that carry them out.

Consideration of the combined effects of different media is included in the risk characterization step of risk assessment. This is discussed at length later (see Sec. III.D.2).

## C. Water

### 1. Surface Water

Surface water in streams, rivers, and lakes has been a convenient place to dispose of wastes, not only from boats, but also from industry, agriculture, and residences. In addition to deliberate dumping, wastes are washed into lakes, rivers, and streams by rainwater. Eventually, surface waters deposit a portion of the contaminants in the oceans. Along the way chemicals may change form, may be lost to the air through volatilization, or may settle and be trapped in sediment. The concentrations also diminish through dilution as transport occurs.

### 2. Groundwater

Although protected from the immediate effects of surface activities by a layer of earth, groundwater can be contaminated with a variety of chemicals. Since aquifers are replenished by rainwater, one would expect that other liquids as well as chemicals dissolved in water could also move into them. This expectation is borne out by the frequency of contaminated wells. In a survey of 466 randomly selected drinking water systems using groundwater, Westrick et al. (1984) found that 30 (6.4%) had trichloroethylene at levels ranging from 0.2 to 78 µg/L (compared with a drinking water standard of 50 µg/L). The United States Environmental Protection Agency (USEPA) (1984) has independently estimated that 3.6% of the nation's ground water supplies for drinking water are contaminated with trichloroethylene. It is well-established that certain chemicals can move through the soil from sources of contamination to groundwater. Sabel and Clark (1984) showed that trichloroethylene leached to groundwater from a Minnesota municipal solid waste landfill. They measured trichloroethylene at 0.7–125 parts per billion (ppb) in leachate samples. The rate of movement depends on both soil characteristics and the nature of the chemical contaminants. The concentrations change within the soil, as discussed later, and within the groundwater. Similar to surface water, concentrations in groundwater diminish by dilution, if for no other reason.

### 3. Routes of Exposure

Humans can be directly exposed to contaminants in surface water. Direct exposure while swimming is primarily dermal, with some incidental ingestion and some inhalation of volatile chemicals. Surface water and groundwater are both sources of water for agricultural and residential use.

Ingestion of contaminants can result directly from drinking the water, or indirectly, from eating food that has become contaminated through one or more intermediate steps. Contaminants can be transferred from water to plants in irrigating commercial fields and home gardens. This contamination may be on the external plant surfaces or in internal plant structures. Contaminated plants may be eaten by humans or fed to livestock, introducing another step before consumption by humans. The final concentrations and forms of the chemicals reaching the receptor depend on many variables, including the types of water treatment for residences, the kinds of foods, and methods of food preparation.

A complete exposure assessment should consider ingestion pathways for food, which may include fruits, vegetables, and grains irrigated with contaminated water; milk, meat, and eggs from animals consuming water or feed contaminated by the transfer of chemicals from irrigation water; and fish and other seafood taken from contaminated water. Another food-related pathway is the use of tap water in cooking.

In addition to exposure pathways involving the ingestion route, exposure to water contaminants by the inhalation route can be important. Significant inhalation exposure to chemicals volatilized from water can result from use of residential water in showering, washing dishes and clothes, and flushing toilets (McKone, 1987). McKone and Knezovich (1991) have shown that, in households using tap water contaminated with trichloroethylene, a volatile organic chemical, the inhalation exposure while taking a shower could exceed ingestion exposure.

This discussion demonstrates the importance of considering fully the fate of contaminants in a specific medium. It is not sufficient to think only of the obvious, direct route of exposure, which in this instance, would be ingestion of drinking water. Contaminants in water can readily move to air and food, and exposure can be through the skin (dermal contact) and the lungs (inhalation). The exposure from these pathways may individually or collectively exceed that from the direct drinking water pathway.

## D. Air

The medium of air may be considered as two separate, but connected compartments: outdoor and indoor air. Sources of contamination of outdoor air include discharges from industries and refineries, pesticide applications, automobile exhausts, and hazardous waste sites. Sources of indoor air contamination include radon in belowground rooms; tap water containing volatile chemicals that are released during showering, bathing, washing dishes and clothing, and flushing toilets; tobacco smoking; and various consumer products, such as cleaning agents, paints, and adhesives. Although environmental regulations have focused on identifying and controlling contaminants in outdoor air, recent studies have shown that an average person in the United States spends more than 94% of their time indoors, resulting in a substantial risk from the indoor air pollution generated by various consumer products (Ott, 1990).

The two-compartment model for outdoor and indoor air is an oversimplification. First, it assumes homogeneity of contaminants within each compartment. Like other media, the air within each compartment is, in fact, heterogeneous; contaminant concentrations vary according to the location of the source and the extent of air movement.

It may also assume that the two compartments are independent, ignoring the exchange between outdoor air and indoor air. Under constant conditions, the concentration of a contaminant from an outdoor source will eventually reach the same level in indoor air as in the ambient outdoor air. The structure of the building impedes air exchange, but eventually the concentrations must equilibrate. The converse is also relevant. That is, air exchange through the building moves contaminants from indoor sources into outdoor air. However, the contribution of nonindustrial indoor sources to outdoor pollution is usually insignificant because of the large volume of outdoor air. The important consequence of movement of indoor air to outdoor air is to reduce the concentration of indoor contaminants. Energy conservation measures that reduce the flow between indoor and outdoor air also contain serious indoor pollutants such as radon.

Air contaminants are present either as vapors of volatile chemicals or bound to dusts or particles. For example, benzene from gasoline is present as a vapor in air near gas stations and freeways, whereas lead may be present in house dust from lead-based paint and other sources.

### 1. Effects of Weather Conditions on Potential Exposure

Weather plays a central role in the dispersion and migration of contaminants in outdoor air. Dry, stable weather and temperature inversions may keep airborne contaminants at elevated levels for longer periods, whereas winds and precipitation both tend to rapidly decrease air contaminant levels. Prevailing airflow patterns may dictate exposure patterns. For example, prevailing winds carrying airborne contaminants from the northeast can result in greater exposure of receptors southwest of the source. Because outdoor air is an exceedingly large compartment, concentrations of outdoor air contaminants decrease rapidly by dilution.

Weather conditions influence indoor air levels only to the extent that they affect the ventilation of indoor airspaces. Levels of contaminants in indoor air can remain stable for longer periods relative to outdoor air and, thus, may pose a greater long-term exposure hazard to human receptors.

### 2. Chemical-Specific Characteristics

The vapor pressure of a chemical is the most important chemical characteristic to consider when deciding whether the medium of air should be considered in an exposure assessment. Chemicals with high vapor pressure are more stable in the gaseous phase and are important air contaminants. Chemicals with high vapor pressure and relatively low water solubility or high vapor pressure and poor adsorption to soil particles move readily from water or soil into the air. Some examples of chemicals with high vapor pressures that are important indoor air contaminants are those in dry-cleaned goods, paints, new fabrics, household cleaners, and adhesives. Chemicals adsorbed onto soil particles can be resuspended into the air on dust particles and subsequently inhaled. On the other hand, adsorption onto atmospheric dust particles with eventual removal from air by rain and deposition to surfaces can act to remove chemicals from air.

Chemicals with high water solubility may dissolve in fog droplets and be transported in air for some distance before being deposited onto soil or plants (Glotfelty et al., 1987). These airborne chemicals, once deposited, may then be ultimately ingested.

### 3. Routes of Exposure

Humans can be directly exposed to contaminants in indoor and outdoor air by the inhalation of vapors or respirable particles. Respirable particles are those with a diameter of 10 μm or less (Casarett, 1972) that can penetrate past the terminal bronchioles of the lung. Because humans inhale through the mouth as well as by nose, quite large (greater than 100 μm) particles can be inspired. These larger particles enter the lungs, but are excluded from the bronchioles. Along with a proportion of smaller particles, they are captured by the mucus and the ciliated cells in the upper respiratory tract, returned to the pharyngeal area, and ingested.

Like chemical contaminants in water, air contaminants can also be transferred to surfaces and internal structures of plants. Humans can then be exposed by eating contaminated plants or livestock, as was discussed for chemicals in water. A complete exposure assessment of contaminants in air should consider ingestion as well as inhalation.

## E. Soil

Soil is usually the primary source of contamination at hazardous waste sites. Soil contaminants can be rinsed from surface soil by rainwater, can migrate through soil to groundwater, or can volatilize and move to outdoor air or through cracks in foundations to indoor air. Soil consisting of fine particles, such as clays and silts, can also become suspended in air as a result of wind erosion or can be tracked indoors to add to the indoor dust level.

### 1. Soil Layers

The greatest exposure to soil by humans is to surface soil. For risk assessment purposes, surface soil is usually defined to include the soil at shallow depths (1–2 ft; 30–60 cm) below surface as well as the actual surface. For sites where construction could occur or where soil may be excavated and redeposited on the surface, soil concentrations of chemicals down to 10–12 ft (3–3.6 m) below the surface may have to be considered in an assessment of exposure. Humans can be directly exposed to surface soil by dermal contact, incidental ingestion, and inhalation of dust. The level of exposure is affected by the type of soil, moisture content of the soil, and soil cover (vegetation, asphalt, concrete, or other "caps").

Subsurface soil refers to root-zone soil, extending from just below surface to about 39 in. (99 cm) in depth. Direct contact with this soil layer can occur with construction, agricultural, or gardening activities. Plant roots can transfer contaminants from subsurface soil into plant structures and to surface soil. The broad definition of surface soil in the previous paragraph overlaps with subsurface soil, as defined here. These are operational definitions that account for the potential of direct contact with surface soil and contamination of plants through the roots in subsurface soil.

The primary concern about deep soil contamination is the possibility of that mass of contamination acting as a reservoir for leaching into groundwater. The rate of leaching depends on soil characteristics, as described in the following section.

## 2. Kinds and Properties of Soil

Soil characteristics are too varied and complex to be presented here. This section contains a brief discussion of organic carbon content and soil particle size, two soil properties that are important for the transfer of contaminants through soil and from soil to skin.

Organic carbon content is a major factor in the ability of many nonionic organic chemicals to adsorb to soil particles. Soils with little organic carbon adsorb chemicals poorly and, consequently, transfer contaminants more readily into aquifers. Similarly, contaminants in soils with low organic carbon content can be transferred more easily to skin (soil to skin partitioning) following direct soil contact.

Particle size is another important characteristic. Water and other fluids move more easily through sand and gravel, which consist of large particles, than through clay, which is made up of small particles. Particle size also influences the rate of exposure to contaminants in soil from direct dermal contact. The poorer adherence to skin of soils with a high content of sand or gravel limits the time of contact with the soil and its contaminants. Clay soils adhere better to skin, providing more time for the transfer of contaminants from soil to skin.

The movement of water and contaminants through clays is usually much slower than through sand and gravel soils. This is because clay soils generally have a high organic carbon content and small particle size, whereas sand and gravel soils generally have lower organic carbon content and larger particle size. However, soils with high clay content may form deep cracks during dry weather that can act as conduits to deep soil and aquifers.

## 3. Chemical-Specific Characteristics

Chemicals bind to soil particles because of their affinity for organic components of soil or dust. This affinity is primarily influenced by two chemical-specific characteristics. First, larger molecular weight compounds tend to be less water-soluble and have more electrons with more opportunities for interactions with the organic fraction of soil. In other words, large molecules are more likely to adsorb to soil particles. Second, the *pK* value of the chemical, that is, the relative strength of the chemical to function as a weak acid or base, influences the tendency of the chemical to adsorb to soil.

## 4. Routes of Exposure

Humans are directly exposed to contaminants in soil by the inhalation, ingestion, and dermal contact routes. Activities responsible for soil contamination include industrial and manufacturing processes; transport, storage, and disposal of hazardous wastes; application of pesticides to gardens and lawns; surface water runoff; and fallout from municipal incinerators and smelters.

Contaminated soil is suspended as dust in outdoor air, particularly in construction and agricultural work. Soils can also be a component of indoor dust, either from exchange with outside air or following tracking of soil into a building.

Inadvertent ingestion of contaminated soil by adults occurs by eating foods contaminated by soil from the hands, or by other hand-to-mouth activities, such as smoking. Ingestion of contaminants can also occur through indirect pathways, such as eating foods that have been contaminated by the transfer of chemicals from surface or root-zone soil, or by drinking water contaminated by the transfer of chemicals from soil or sediment.

Children ingest larger amounts of soil than adults because of their increased mouthing behavior and because of play activities in dirt (Clausing et al., 1987; Calabrese et al., 1989). Some children exhibit a "pica" behavior, craving and ingesting large amounts of dirt. Thus, exposures to contaminants in soil per unit of body weight are higher for children and may be considerable in pica children.

Dermal exposure to contaminants in soil can occur during gardening, landscaping, construction, trenching, recreation, and agricultural activities.

## F.  Problems with Medium-Specific Focus

The sections on water, air, and soil discussed the importance of transport of contaminants among these media. As mentioned in Section II.B., there are conditions in which it is logical or legally mandated to evaluate only one medium in a risk assessment. However, it is usually necessary to evaluate the potential exposure from all media and routes to reach the conclusion that consideration of a single medium in isolation from other media is appropriate.

## III.  MULTIMEDIUM RISK CHARACTERIZATION

## A.  Environmental Fate and Transport

The preceding discussions of single media have argued that concentrations, chemical species, and environmental locations of chemical contaminants are not constant. These changes in contaminants are collectively referred to as environmental fate and transport. The chemical and physical characteristics of the contaminant and the characteristics of the medium determine the nature and rates of the changes.

The importance of fate and transport is illustrated by the distinction between a source medium and a contact medium. A source medium is the medium that is initially contaminated, whereas a contact medium is the medium from which the receptor contacts the chemical contaminants. Contaminants can move from the source medium to the contact medium directly or indirectly through an intermediate or transport medium. Movement from medium to medium is called *transport*. As discussed in Section II.A.4, the direction of transfer among media is primarily from the source medium. A contaminant can be subjected to numerous reactions, such as, photooxidation in air, hydrolysis in water, and biodegradation in soil, which will change its nature and concentration. Changes in chemical composition are called "fate."

Although the distinction between source and contact media might appear to be obvious, confusion does arise. This is illustrated by the field of hazardous waste site regulation for which there is strong pressure to specify generic soil remediation levels for common chemical contaminants. Some states (New Jersey, Washington) are considering adoption of this approach. The application of generic soil remediation levels for all cases makes no allowance for site-specific conditions of fate and transport that can drastically alter contaminant concentrations in the contact media.

A hypothetical, but not unrealistic example, follows. Suppose facility A releases a high concentration of a contaminant into the soil at the site (the source medium), but because of sunny, hot conditions, the contaminant rapidly volatilizes and is degraded in the air. Furthermore, the small level of remaining contaminant is blown away from the area of concern (area A) by prevailing winds. Suppose facility B releases a moderate concentration of the same contaminant onto the soil at its site, but there is little degradation under the conditions of this area. The contaminant moves rapidly through the soil into an aquifer that is used for residential water by the area of concern (area B). The concentration in the air over the area A (the contact medium) may be insignificant, whereas the concentration in the residential water, the contact medium for area B may be of concern. Application of the same generic soil remediation level to these two sites could lead to inappropriate actions for both. The soil remediation goal might require costly and unnecessary activity at facility A, but insufficient remediation at facility B.

The usefulness of generic, chemical-specific soil remediation values has been argued by analogy to maximum contaminant levels (MCLs) for drinking water, which is a contact medium. The MCLs are generic, chemical-specific drinking water standards that apply to all drinking water (see Secs. V.A.1. and V.A.2. following). The MCLs are based on considerations of technical feasibility, economic and societal effects, as well as health. The source of the chemicals and the pathway they took to reach the drinking water is irrelevant. The MCL compliance is usually at the point where water enters the distribution system of a public water system.

The analogy of MCLs to soil remediation levels fails, because the contaminated soil at a facility or site is the source medium and may or may not be a contact medium. Contaminated soil is not equivalent to the contact medium of residential drinking water. Site-specific soil remediation levels should be based on a fate and transport analysis to determine contaminant concentrations and potential exposure from the contact medium.

Indeed, it is inappropriate to use MCLs as criteria to evaluate a source medium, such as groundwater at the origin of the contamination, although this is sometimes done. On the one hand, it may be wasteful and unnecessary to purify groundwater, the source medium, based on an MCL that has been set for drinking water, the contact medium. On the other hand, the collective health effects of several chemical contaminants might exceed acceptable levels when added. For example, if two contaminants in an aquifer are both carcinogens and each is removed (or "remediated") to the target level of risk based on MCLs, the total excess cancer risk is the sum of the two risk levels or twice the target level. Finally, since MCLs are based on other considerations, in addition to health, reliance on them for remediation goals may be under-protective in some instances and overprotective in others. These problems are avoided by performing a risk assessment that takes into account the specific conditions at hand, rather than applying generic numbers to the source medium in all situations.

The problems with generic chemical-specific remediation levels are similar in soil. Health-based levels that are set for the contact medium are inappropriate for the source medium. Environmental fate and transport should be considered in assessing the risks and hazards from exposure to contact media that are based on existing conditions. Acceptable levels of contaminants in the source medium can then be based on health protective levels in the contact media. The procedures for setting site-specific remediation goals based on risk assessment are described in Section III.E.

## B. Determining the Outcome of Fate and Transport

It may seem obvious that the best way to determine the outcome of environmental fate and transport is the empirical approach of simply measuring contaminant levels in the contact medium of interest. In many instances, this is true: however, the complexity of the fate and transport systems can make adequate sampling of the contact medium extremely difficult. This is often true for transfer of chemicals from contaminated soil to breathing-zone air. Movement of the air depends on factors such as surface topography, wind speed and direction, and temperature. These factors can vary considerably over space and over time, both daily and seasonally. Sample data means are reflective of the true contact medium means only insofar as the samples are representative. The variability may make this impossible to achieve.

Furthermore, it may be important to relate the contamination in the source medium to that in the contact medium. If several sources are contributing to a contaminated contact medium, the relative contributions of each source may be important for establishing liability.

The alternative to sampling the contact medium is to model the dispersion of contaminants in the medium of interest. There are several models currently in use for modeling the dispersion of contaminants in air. Obviously, the models also suffer from the difficulty in addressing the complexities described earlier. They attempt to predict contaminant concentrations only at an average location under average conditions.

Similarly, the transfer of contaminants from soil to groundwater and the movement within the groundwater can be modeled or measured. Sampling of groundwater also presents difficulties, but not as many as sampling air.

## C.  Intake Equations

Up to this point we have considered the movement of contaminants among environmental media and the ways in which receptors may be exposed. Intake equations apply this information to calculate the amount of contaminant that a receptor will actually take into the body.

*1.  Generic Intake Equations*

The Risk Assessment Guidance for Superfund (USEPA, 1989) gives the following general intake equation:

$$I = \frac{C \times CR \times EFD}{BW \times AT} \tag{1}$$

where

$I$ = intake or the amount of chemical at the exchange boundary (skin or membrane) in units of milligrams of chemical per kilogram of body weight per day [mg/(kg × day)].

$C$ = chemical concentration in the contact medium or the average concentration contacted over the exposure period in units of milligrams of chemical per liter (mg/L) for water, milligrams of chemical per cubic meter (mg/m$^3$) for air, and milligrams of chemical per kilogram (mg/kg) for soil.

$CR$ = contact rate or amount of contaminated medium contacted per unit of time or event in units of liters per day for water, cubic meters per day for air, and kilograms per day for soil.

$EFD$ = exposure frequency and duration describing how long and how often exposure occurs in units of days.

$BW$ = body weight in kilograms.

$AT$ = averaging time, or the period over which exposure is averaged in days.

This generic intake equation is applicable to any length of exposure time (e.g., subchronic, chronic) and, with modifications, to any route of exposure. The *EFD* term may be divided into exposure frequency (*EF*), the number of days of exposure per year, and exposure duration (*ED*), the number of years of exposure.

Notice that the intake is defined as administered dose or the amount of chemical at the exchange boundary (i.e., absorption is not taken into account). The exception to this is the consideration of dermal exposure to chemicals. The intake equations for dermal exposure given in the Risk Assessment Guidance for Superfund (USEPA 1989) calculate absorbed dose or uptake of the chemical by the skin, rather than calculating simple contact with the skin. The equation for dermal contact with chemicals in water is

$$I = \frac{C \times SA \times PC \times ET \times EF \times ED \times CF}{BW \times AT} \tag{2}$$

where

$I$ = dermal uptake (absorbed dose) in units of milligrams of chemical per kilogram of body weight per day [mg/(kg × day)].

$C$ = chemical concentration in the contact medium or the average concentration contacted over the exposure period in units of milligrams of chemical per liter of water (mg/L).

$SA$ = skin surface area available for contact in units of square centimeters ($cm^2$).

$PC$ = dermal permeability constant in units of centimeters per hour.

$ET$ = exposure time in hours per day.

$EF$ = exposure frequency in days per year.

$ED$ = exposure duration in years.

$CF$ = conversion factor used to convert units in the equation.

$BW$ = body weight in kilograms.

$AT$ = averaging time, or the period over which exposure is averaged in days.

An analogous equation estimates dermal uptake from contact with chemicals in soil.

The intake rates predicted by Eqs. (1) and (2) are compared with health-based criteria, either a health-protective dose level, called a reference dose (RfD) for noncarcinogenic endpoints (see Chapter 17) or multiplied by a slope factor for carcinogenicity (see Chapter 14). Most, although not all, reference doses and slope factors for oral and inhalation exposure are determined from administered dose levels in epidemiology studies or toxicology studies with animals. They must be compared with estimated intakes that are also administered dose levels.

For inhalation exposures, reference concentrations (RfCs) have been established that are compared with the chemical concentration in breathing-zone air (the contact medium), rather than the calculated intake.

Occasionally, health-based criteria must be adjusted for absorption. One example is when the absorption rates are known to be different for humans and the experimental animal on which the reference dose or slope factor is based, and they have not been taken into account in determining that criterion. A second example is the use of a health-based criterion for a related compound because no criterion is available for the compound being evaluated. If absorption rates for the two compounds are established, an adjustment is appropriate. A third example is the use of a criterion for a different route because no criterion is available for the route being evaluated. This is most common with dermal exposures, for which experimental data are usually lacking, and few health-based criteria values exist. Adaptation of an oral or inhalation criterion involves correcting for differences in absorption so that the adjusted criterion is compared with dermal uptake derived from Eq. (2), which is calculated as an absorbed dose.

## 2. Assumptions

Several major assumptions apply to intake [see Eqs. (1) and (2)]. First, the chemical concentration $C$ is the concentration in the contact medium, the medium from which the receptor is exposed to the chemical, as discussed in Section III.A. It is not appropriate to use the chemical concentration in the source medium or transport medium as the $C$ value. If there are no sample data, the concentration of the chemical in the contact medium can be estimated from concentrations in the source medium based on fate and transport. Second, the exposure parameter estimates used in these equations may be quite variable and uncertain; indeed, some parameters can never be accurately described by single values. For example, it is not realistic to use a single value for the contact rate for incidental soil ingestion by a child over an exposure duration of years. The effect of the variability and uncertainty inherent in each of the parameters on the calculated intake or uptake values needs to be considered in any risk assessment.

## D. Risk Estimation

Risk estimation is performed by calculating the intake of a chemical and then comparing the result with health-based criteria for that chemical. Health-based criteria are reference doses or reference concentrations for noncarcinogenic toxicity and cancer slope factors.

### 1. Eliminating Exposure Pathways

Before calculating intakes, exposure pathways that are not applicable should be eliminated. If the chemical under consideration has not or cannot contaminate a particular medium because that medium is not present (such as a site where groundwater cannot be contaminated because there is no underlying aquifer), the chemical has little or no affinity for the medium, or there is a barrier preventing movement of the chemical to the medium, then that medium and all exposure pathways involving that medium are eliminated from consideration. If it can be shown that there is no possibility that persons will ingest foods, water, or soil contaminated by the chemical originating from the site, will have dermal contact with contaminated water or soil, or will inhale contaminated particles or vapors coming from the source or site, then these exposure pathways may be excluded from further consideration for human health risk assessment. It is necessary to do a similar evaluation for ecological receptors.

After calculating intakes, insignificant exposure pathways may also be eliminated. These are pathways that occur, but do not add significantly to total exposure. However, the availability of computer spreadsheets to complete the calculations obviates the incentive to eliminate minor pathways. Instead, intakes from all pathways for an exposure route can be added to get the overall inhalation and ingestion intakes and dermal uptake for each chemical.

If circumstances dictate the elimination of insignificant exposure pathways, the approach begins by identifying the most significant pathway for each exposure route. Then intakes of all the other pathways for that exposure route are compared with the intake of the major pathway. Any pathway with an intake that is an insignificant fraction of the major pathway can be eliminated, unless the magnitude of exposure from that pathway is so great that it remains of concern.

Alternatively, the risks and hazards for each chemical can be calculated for each exposure pathway, as described in the next section, and summation can be done in the risk characterization step.

### 2. Converting Intakes to Risks and Hazards

Carcinogenic effects are expressed as the incremental probability or risk of an individual developing cancer over a lifetime as a result of exposure to a potential carcinogen. The equation (USEPA 1989) is

$$\text{Risk} = \text{chronic daily intake} \times \text{slope factor} \tag{3}$$

Risk = the probability that an individual will develop cancer (unitless).

Chronic daily intake = the intake averaged over an averaging time (AT) of 70 years in units of $[\text{mg}/(\text{kg} \times \text{day})]$.

Slope factor = a constant that relates intake averaged over a lifetime and incremental risk of cancer; units are $[\text{mg}/(\text{kg} \times \text{day})]^{-1}$.

Chronic daily intake is the intake calculated in Eqs. (1) and (2) with 70 years (an average lifetime) as the averaging time. This distinguishes intake for carcinogens from shorter times, such as subchronic exposure.

A carcinogen or cancer-causing chemical may have a different slope factor for each exposure route. If intakes for all the pathways for each exposure route for a chemical have been added, then the summed value for each exposure route is used with the corresponding slope factor to get the cancer risk for that exposure route. Risks are then added for all exposure routes to get the total risk for that chemical. Alternatively, the risk for each pathway can be calculated separately for all chemicals being considered. Then the risks may be totaled to get the pathway-specific risk and summed again to get the total cancer risk from exposure to multiple chemicals. Either procedure will yield the same excess cancer risk estimate.

Several points should be kept in mind about this estimate of total cancer risk. First, it is not always appropriate to add risks from different chemicals, for reasons given later in Section IV.B. Second, this is an estimate of excess cancer risk, the risk from the exposure under consideration, which is additional to the background cancer risk all individuals face. Finally, the cancer slope factors are upper-bound estimates and, therefore, the cancer risk is also an upper-bound estimate. The true excess cancer risk from the exposure might be far less.

Noncarcinogenic hazards are not measured by risk, but rather, by a direct comparison of the exposure intake with a chemical-specific reference dose. When the intake value is for a specific chemical in a specific exposure pathway, the ratio is called a hazard quotient and is expressed as follows:

$$\text{Hazard quotient} = \frac{\text{intake}}{\text{reference dose}} \tag{4}$$

where

Hazard quotient = the ratio of the exposure intake to a reference dose (unitless).
Intake = the intake over a specific exposure duration in units of $[mg/(kg \times day)]$.
Reference dose = a level of exposure below which no adverse health effects are expected $[mg/(kg \times day)]$.

In this ratio, the intake and reference dose values must have the same units, reflect the same route of exposure, represent the same exposure duration (chronic, subchronic, short-term), and both be administered doses, or both be absorbed doses. As was described for the estimation of carcinogenic risks, the hazards may be either calculated and added by chemical, or calculated for each pathway for each chemical, added by pathway, and summed to get the total hazard from all chemicals under consideration.

A sum of hazard quotients is called a *hazard index*. This hazard index must have the same value, regardless of the summation sequence. Hazard quotients and hazard indices are not probabilities like cancer risks. If the hazard index is less than 1, no harm is expected, because the exposure is below the threshold for an adverse effect. If the hazard index is greater than 1, the threshold has been exceeded and toxicity may occur.

## E. Reverse Risk Assessment

Instructions are provided in the Risk Assessment Guidance for Superfund (USEPA, 1989) for calculating risk-based preliminary remediation goals. Although risk assessment estimates health risks and hazards based on existing contaminant concentrations, reverse risk assessment does the opposite. It solves for target contaminant concentrations based on acceptable risks and hazards.

For carcinogenicity, the total risk for a chemical in a specific environmental medium is calculated by adding the risks from all pathways that involve that environmental medium (such as the ingestion of groundwater and the inhalation of vapors from groundwater). As shown in Eq. (3), risk equals the cancer slope factor multiplied by the intake. In reverse risk assessment, the risk equation is expanded to include the intake equation, which, in turn, includes the concentration of the chemical and the exposure parameters. This is done by substituting the right side of intake from Eq. (1) or Eq. (2) in Eq. (3). Since the total risk is a sum of risks for individual pathways and routes, there must be a substitution for each intake value. That is,

$$\text{Total risk} = (\text{intake}_{\text{oral}} \times \text{slope factor}_{\text{oral}})$$
$$+ (\text{intake}_{\text{inhalation}} \times \text{slope factor}_{\text{inhalation}})$$
$$+ (\text{intake}_{\text{dermal}} \times \text{slope factor}_{\text{dermal}})$$

Each of the three intake values can be replaced with the right side of the appropriate intake equation. Each term in the substituted equation includes the contaminant concentration in the medium of interest [$C$ in Eqs. (1) and (2)]. The equation can then be rearranged to solve for the concentration corresponding to any assigned target risk level.

A similar technique applies to noncarcinogenic effects. The hazard index for a chemical in a specific environmental medium is the total of the hazard quotients for that chemical for all exposure pathways involving the environmental medium. The right side of the appropriate intake equation is substituted for the intake in the numerator of each term (hazard quotient) in the hazard identification. The hazard index equation can then be rearranged to solve for a target concentration of chemical in the environmental compartment by setting the hazard index equal to 1. By using the appropriate exposure parameter values, these total risk and hazard index equations calculate the risk-based remediation goals for soil, groundwater, and surface water for the land use scenarios of interest (residential, industrial, commercial, or other).

A simpler method is to apply the following ratio:

$$\frac{\text{Target medium level}}{\text{Current medium level}} = \frac{\text{target risk}}{\text{current risk}} \tag{5}$$

and, therefore,

$$\text{Target medium level} = \frac{\text{target risk}}{\text{current risk}} \times \text{current medium level} \tag{6}$$

where

Target medium level = the remediation level for the chemical in the medium in units of milligrams per kilogram (mg/kg) soil, milligrams per cubic meter (mg/m$^3$) air, or milligrams per liter (mg/L) water.

Current medium level = the measured or modeled concentration of the chemical in the medium in units of mg/kg soil, mg/m$^3$ air, or mg/L water.

Target risk = the risk determined to be protective of health (unitless).

Current risk = the risk associated with the present concentration of the chemical in the medium (unitless).

For noncarcinogenic effects, the corresponding equations are

$$\frac{\text{Target medium level}}{\text{Current medium level}} = \frac{\text{target HI}}{\text{current HI}} \tag{7}$$

and, therefore,

$$\text{Target medium level} = \frac{\text{target HI}}{\text{current HI}} \times \text{current medium level} \tag{8}$$

where

Target medium level = the remediation level of the chemical in the medium in units of mg/kg soil, mg/m$^3$ air, or mg/L water.

Current medium level = the measured or modeled concentration of chemical in the medium in units of mg/kg soil, mg/m$^3$ air, or mg/L water.

Target HI = the hazard index determined to be protective of health, a value of 1 (unitless).

Current HI = the hazard index associated with the current concentration of the chemical in the medium (unitless).

## IV. SUMMING RISKS OR HAZARDS: BEYOND MULTIMEDIUM RISK ASSESSMENT

### A. Overview

The goal of risk assessment is to evaluate the likelihood of humans or ecological receptors being harmed by exposure to chemical contaminants. In discussing the conversion of intake estimates to risk and hazard estimates (see Sec. III.D.2), it was pointed out that summation must be done to assess the total potential for problems. This can be achieved at the intake level by adding all pathways for each route of exposure and then totaling risks from all routes and hazard quotients from all routes. Alternatively, risks and hazard quotients can be determined for each pathway and then added.

This section deals with other important considerations in evaluating total risks and hazards. These include exposure to more than one chemical, exposures over time, and exposures from different sources.

### B. Exposure to More Than One Chemical

Everyone is exposed to a multitude of chemicals, both synthetic and natural, in work and home environments. Nonetheless, risk assessment often focuses on a single chemical. Risk assessment for a pesticide is based on exposures to that single chemical, in most cases ignoring the plethora of other exposures. Similarly, risk assessment for an abandoned mercury mine is based on exposures only to those mercury compounds.

Some facilities work with hundreds of chemicals and a risk assessment may consider all of them. Even in this situation, exposure to chemicals from other sources is not considered.

Toxicity of two chemicals may be synergistic, antagonistic, or additive. Although there are examples of interactions, such as the insecticide synergism of piperonyl butoxide with pyrethrins and rotenone, and the possible potentiation of the neurotoxicity of *n*-hexane by methyl ethyl ketone (Abdel-Rahman et al., 1976; Couri et al., 1978), in most instances, little information is available. In the absence of specific studies, it is assumed that chemicals that produce the same toxic endpoint do so additively.

If we assume additivity, hazard quotients can be added for each target organ or system and, similarly, cancer risk estimates can be summed. For example, all hazard quotients based on toxicity to the immune system can be added to provide a cumulative estimate of possible health hazard.

This procedure can be refined if information about mechanisms of toxicity is available. For example, several metals are potent nephrotoxins. Since the toxicity to the kidneys (necrotic proximal tubules with proteinaceous debris in the lumens) appears to be similar, it seems reasonable to add the hazard quotients. In contrast, the drugs atropine and quinacrine are both toxic to the eyes, but the former causes glaucoma, whereas the latter causes corneal edema. There is no basis for thinking that these two chemicals would have additive toxicity. Adding the hazard quotients for atropine and quinacrine would likely exaggerate the hazard. These examples are at the descriptive level. Knowledge of the underlying biochemical mechanisms can provide a firm rationale for making decisions about the additivity of chemical toxicities.

Just as there are many mechanisms of noncarcinogenic toxicity, carcinogenesis proceeds through a variety of pathways. It is sometimes appropriate to add the excess cancer risks from different chemicals and sometimes inappropriate, depending on the availability of information for making such a judgment. Because an understanding of the underlying mechanisms of carcinogenesis is only now being elucidated, regulatory agencies currently add risks from all carcinogens.

## C.  Exposure Over Time

Exposure to a chemical has two components: concentration of the chemical in the contact medium and time. Risk assessment methods consider the fraction of a lifetime and the fraction of time during that lifetime that an individual is exposed. For example, an average worker may be assumed to work for 25 years at the location of interest and to work for 8 h/day, 5 days/week, and 50 weeks/year.

The implication of this procedure is that when the individual leaves the workplace, he or she enters a pristine environment. From the point of view of assigning responsibility, this is a reasonable approach, but from the health standpoint, it may disregard considerable exposure. The individual continues to be exposed to chemical contaminants in his life away from the job. Exposure may be to the same chemicals, or to other chemicals with the same target organs. The individual's health would be best protected by considering total exposure to chemicals at all times.

## D.  Exposure from All Sources

Consideration of all sources of chemical contaminants is also important. An evaluation of the potential effects of release of a chemical often considers a single facility. For a common air pollutant, such as benzene, the risk assessment may conclude that the facility is not creating a health hazard, even though the concentration of benzene from all sources is hazardous. This is also reasonable for purposes of assigning responsibility, but unreasonable from the health perspective. There needs to be an assessment of health concerns considering air quality and water quality as a whole.

The contamination released by a facility adds to the background levels. Background contamination may be naturally occurring, as with metals, or may be contamination from other human sources, such as pesticides. The organochlorine pesticide DDT [1,1,1-trichloro-2,2-bis-(p-chlorophenyl)ethane] was widely used around the world and is quite persistent. Its ubiquitous spread to the most isolated areas and to the adipose tissues of essentially the entire population of the world have been well documented (ATSDR, 1993). Although registration for almost all uses of DDT was cancelled in the United States on January 1, 1973, it and its metabolites (DDE and DDD) are still found in surprisingly high concentrations.

Background concentrations from any source may be treated differently for threshold and nonthreshold toxicity. For nonthreshold toxicity (some mechanisms of carcinogenicity and mutagenicity) the level of exposure from a specific source generates an excess risk that is independent of background exposure. Therefore, an argument can be made for subtracting the background level of concentration in performing a risk assessment. In contrast, for threshold toxicity (noncarcinogenicity), whether exposure reaches the threshold depends on contaminant contributions from all sources. It is inappropriate to subtract background levels.

## V. STATUTORY AUTHORITIES

Environmental statutes that require human health risk assessments are summarized in this section. Several of these statutes are quite comprehensive, covering multiple aspects of the environmental issue addressed, such as the Safe Drinking Water Act, in which treatment techniques and legal remedies, as well as treatment standards are specified. Chapter 35 gives a more detailed discussion of these laws. The following summaries pertain only to those requirements in the statutes that are applicable to the performance or content of human health risk assessments.

Environmental statutes provide regulatory authority to specific agencies or departments within government over specific environmental issues. In turn, these agencies provide guidance or promulgate regulations to carry out and enforce such laws. In the area of health assessments, these laws, guidance, regulations, and the policies behind them have often mandated a medium-specific focus. More importantly, these laws have created medium-specific regulatory programs. Thus, government may unintentionally promote a medium-specific approach. Examples of medium-specific and multimedium assessments performed under federal and California statutes will be given.

These laws and regulations have shaped and will continue to define the performance of human health risk assessments. This is because many health risk assessment reports are either done by scientists in the regulatory agencies or are submitted by outside contractors to those scientists for their review. In either event, the reports must conform to statutory and regulatory requirements.

### A. Statutes Focusing on One Medium

#### 1. Federal

*The Clean Air Act.* The Clean Air Act sets primary ambient air standards for air pollutants, based on the protection of public health. This act calls for environmental health assessments for specific hazardous air pollutants identified in the statute. The statute also specifies what must be included in the assessment. Each assessment must contain a comprehensive review of the toxicological and epidemiological information for the chemical relative to its acute, subacute, and chronic adverse health effects, and levels of exposure that pose a significant threat to human health. The assessment must identify gaps in information relating to health effects and exposure levels as well as the experiments necessary to fill those gaps. This act also requires that the methods used to determine carcinogenic risks and hazards of other effects, such as birth defects and reproductive dysfunctions associated with hazardous air pollutant exposure, be reviewed by the National Academy of Sciences.

This act gives authority to the National Institute of Environmental Health Sciences (NIEHS) to provide funds for "basic research to identify, characterize, and quantify risks to human health from air pollutants." The cumulative effect of this act relative to assessing health risks is that it requires specific components to be contained within a human health risk assessment and federal guidelines for conducting a risk assessment to be subjected to critical scientific review. In addition, through its grant-funding authority, the act can influence the direction of health risk research toward the study of air pollutants.

*The Safe Drinking Water Act.* The Safe Drinking Water Act mandates the setting of drinking water quality standards, called maximum contaminant level goals (MCLG) and maximum contaminant levels (MCL), for specific chemicals known or anticipated to occur in public water systems. The MCLG for a chemical is the estimate of a concentration in drinking water at which no adverse health effects would occur. The MCLG must have an adequate margin of safety for the protection of public health. The MCLG is a nonenforceable goal and is strictly health-based, determined by a risk assessment. The maximum contaminant level or MCL is the enforceable concentration of a chemical in drinking water and is a level deemed to be feasible, given technology and cost considerations. The MCL must be set as close to the MCLG as possible, but may be higher because it includes considerations other than the risk assessment results.

The effect of this act is to create a regulatory program for a single medium that has the potential to underestimate health risk as discussed earlier. The derivation of the MCL and MCLG includes a "relative source contribution" assumption that a certain fraction of the total intake of a chemical is from contaminated drinking water. This accounts for exposure to a chemical from different sources. The process does not account for cumulative risk from multiple chemicals in drinking water.

## 2. California

*The Toxic Air Contaminant Act.*  The Toxic Air Contaminant Act (AB 1807) requires the evaluation of chemicals, including pesticides, for possible identification as toxic air contaminants. This evaluation takes the form of a human health risk assessment of each candidate chemical. If the risk assessment shows that a chemical may cause or contribute to adverse health effects from exposure in air, that chemical is listed in regulation as a toxic air contaminant, and appropriate measures to control the levels found in air may be instituted.

This statute requires for each chemical a review of the scientific literature relating to physical and chemical properties, environmental fate, and human health effects. The statute also provides funding for measuring ambient concentrations of the chemical in air. From the review and the measurements taken, an estimate is made of the range of risk to humans resulting from current or anticipated exposure to the chemical in the air.

Because the toxic air contaminant statute is concerned with a single medium, risk assessment performed under this authority emphasize air, even if partitioning of dose among other exposure media is done. This emphasis is reflected by the fact that the chemicals considered under this act are chemicals that would be expected to be in air because of their volatility, such as ethylene oxide and perchloroethylene, or because they can be inhaled as dusts or fibers, such as some metals and asbestos.

*The Safe Drinking Water Act.*  The Safe Drinking Water Act of 1989 (AB 21) requires the review of maximum contaminant levels (MCLs) every 5 years and the development of recommended public health levels (RPHLs). Similar to federal MCLGs and MCLs, California RPHLs are strictly health-based and California MCLs include consideration of economic impact and technical feasibility. The statute requires risk assessment methods in the development of both MCLs and RPHLs.

*The Air Toxics "Hot Spots" Information and Assessment Act.*  The Air Toxics "Hot Spots" Information and Assessment Act (AB 2588) mandates human health risk assessments for specific sources of air pollution that are close to locations of sensitive populations, such as hospitals, residences, day care centers, and schools. This statute does not specify components to be included in the risk assessment, but requires conformity to guidelines provided by the state. Such guidelines have been published. Risk assessments performed following these guidelines consider other media as transfer conduits. For example, the deposition of contaminants on soil from air is considered with the subsequent assessment of soil and plant contact.

Since this statute addresses only air emissions from facilities, the resulting health assessments are necessarily blind to possible primary contamination of soil or water by hazardous substances released from those facilities.

*The Pesticide Contamination Prevention Act.*  The Pesticide Contamination Prevention Act (AB 2021) requires that adverse health effects be identified for pesticides and their degradation products that have the potential to reach groundwater. Under certain circumstances, a risk assessment must identify the adverse health effects as carcinogenic, mutagenic, teratogenic, or neurotoxic. A level must be identified that does not cause any adverse health effects and has an adequate margin of safety.

This statute establishes procedures to identify and track potential and actual groundwater contaminants, to evaluate chemicals detected in groundwater or in soil as a result of agricultural use, and to modify or cancel the use of these chemicals.

## B.  Statutory Authorities Covering All Media

*1. Federal*

*The Federal Insecticide, Fungicide, and Rodenticide Act.*  The Federal Insecticide, Fungicide, and Rodenticide Act (FIFRA) mandates that specific data be submitted before pesticides are permitted to be registered and sold. These data include acute, subchronic, and chronic toxicological studies. The risk assessment process is not explicitly mandated in this statute, but is used in carrying it out.

*The Comprehensive Environmental Response, Compensation, and Liability Act.*  The Comprehensive Environmental Response, Compensation, and Liability Act (CERCLA or Superfund) and *Superfund Amendments and Reauthorization Act* (SARA) mandate human health risk assessments for hazardous wastes at abandoned or inactive sites. These risk assessments are used to establish baseline risks, as well as to help evaluate alternative cleanup options and to justify the cleanup option chosen.

The guidelines published by the USEPA under this statute provide specific instructions for performing a site-specific multimedium human health risk assessment (USEPA, 1989). These guidelines describe environmental media in terms of their roles in the fate and transport of the chemical in question, such as exposure medium, release medium, transport or retention medium, and receiving medium. In the exposure model for hazardous substances release sites recently developed by McKone and Daniels (1991), two types of media are described (see also foregoing Sec. III.A). The exposure medium is the medium that humans contact (personal air, tap water, food, household dust, soil). Environmental media are ambient air, surface soil, root-zone soil, surface water, and groundwater. It is essential to consider all exposure and environmental media in risk assessments performed under this statutory authority.

The CERCLA also established the Agency for Toxic Substances and Disease Registry (ATSDR), mandated to perform health risk assessments for every site on the Superfund (National Priorities) List. The content of these health risk assessments is specified in the statute and includes the consideration of potential pathways of exposure, such as ground- or surface water contamination, air emissions, and food chain contamination.

Much of the codification of the risk assessment process used by regulatory agencies has taken place in the regulations and guidance associated with CERCLA.

*The Resource Conservation and Recovery Act.*  Under certain circumstances, the Resource Conservation and Recovery Act (RCRA) mandates a human health assessment before a permit to operate a hazardous waste facility will be issued. This statute states that the assessment must include an estimation of the potential normal and accidental releases of hazardous substances from the facility, the potential exposure pathways, and the magnitude of human exposure to those exposure pathways.

### 2. California

*The Hazardous Waste Account and the Hazardous Substances Control Account.* The Hazardous Waste Account and the Hazardous Substances Control Account provide California with a state superfund program equivalent to the federal CERCLA and a program of permitting and overseeing facilities that transport, treat, dispose of, and/or store hazardous waste, similar to the federal RCRA. Under this act the California Environmental Protection Agency (CalEPA) reviews human health risk assessments of sites and facilities where hazardous substances have been or are being released to the environment. Like the USEPA, CalEPA requires multimedium human health risk assessments for these sites or facilities and recommends that CERCLA guidance (USEPA, 1989) be followed (CDTSC, 1992).

*The Safe Drinking Water and Toxic Enforcement Act.* The Safe Drinking Water and Toxic Enforcement Act (Proposition 65) requires that chemicals known to the state of California to cause cancer or reproductive effects be listed in regulation and that safe levels of the chemicals be established. Health risk assessments of listed chemicals are carried out under this statutory authority to estimate those environmental concentrations considered to pose "no significant risk." For a chemical that causes cancer, the no-significant-risk level is specified as that level that may result in 1 excess case of cancer in 100,000 persons exposed over their lifetime (excess risk = $1 \times 10^{-5}$).

*The Birth Defects Prevention Act.* The Birth Defects Prevention Act of 1986 (SB950) identifies health effects data for pesticides that must be submitted to the state of California before registration and sale. Pesticides are ranked, based on the nature of the adverse health effects and the magnitude of occupational and environmental exposures. Like the Federal Insecticide, Fungicide, and Rodenticide Act the California Birth Defects Prevention Act does not specifically call for risk assessment. State toxicologists perform risk assessments to determine how significant the adverse effects are and whether they can be mitigated by protective measures.

## REFERENCES

Abdel-Rahman, M. S., L. B. Hetland, and D. Couri (1976). Toxicity and metabolism of methyl *n*-butyl ketone, *Am. Ind. Hyg. Assoc. J.*, 37, 95–102.

[ATSDR] Agency for Toxic Substances and Disease Registry, U. S. Department of Health and Human Services (1993). Toxicological profile for DDT, DDE, and DDD.

Calabrese, E. J., R. Barnes, E. J. Stanek, H. Pastides, C. E. Gilbert, P. Veneman, X. Wang, A. Lasztity, and P. T. Kostecki (1989). How much soil do young children ingest: An epidemiologic study, *Regul. Toxicol. Pharmacol.*, 10, 123–137.

California Air Resources Board (1992). *California Air Pollution Control Laws.*

Casarett, L. J. (1972). The vital sacs: Alveolar clearance mechanisms in inhalation toxicology. In *Essays in Toxicology,* Vol. 3. (W. J. Hayes, Jr., ed.), Academic Press, New York.

[CDTSC] California Department of Toxic Substances Control (1992). Supplemental guidance for human health multi-media risk assessments of hazardous waste sites and permitted facilities, Office of the Science Advisor.

Clausing, P., B. Brunekreef, and J. H. Van Wijnen (1987). A method for estimating soil ingestion by children, *Int. Arch. Occup. Environ. Health,* 59, 73–82.

Couri, D., M. S. Abdel-Rahman, and L. B. Hetland (1978). Biotransformation of *n*-hexane and methyl *n*-butyl ketone in guinea pigs and mice, *Am. Ind. Hyg. Assoc. J.,* 39, 295–300.

Federal Environmental Laws (1992). West Publishing, St. Paul, MN.

Glotfelty, D. E., J. N. Seiber, and L. A. Liljedahl (1987). Pesticides in fog, *Nature,* 325, 602–605.

McKone, T. E. (1987). Human exposure to volatile organic compounds in household tap water: The indoor inhalation pathway, *Environ. Sci. Technol.*, 21, 1194–1201.

McKone, T. E., and J. P. Knezovich (1991). The transfer of trichloroethylene (TCE) from a shower to indoor air: Experimental measurements and their implications, *J. Air Waste Manage. Assoc.*, 41, 832–837.

McKone, T E., and J. I. Daniels (1991). Estimating human exposure through multiple pathways from air, water, and soil, *Regul. Toxicol. Pharmacol.*, 13, 36–61.

Ott, W. R. (1990). Total human exposure: Basic concepts, EPA field studies, and future research needs, *J. Air Waste Manage. Assoc.*, 40, 966–975.

National Research Council (1991). *Environmental Epidemiology,* Vol. 1: *Public Health and Hazardous Wastes,* National Academy Press, Washington, DC.

Sabel, G. V., and T. P. Clark (1984). Volatile organic compounds as indicators of municipal solid waste leachate contamination, *Waste Manage. Res.*, 2, 119–130.

[USEPA] U. S. Environmental Protection Agency (1984). National primary drinking water regulations; Proposed rulemaking, *Fed. Reg.* 49(114), 24329.

[USEPA] U. S. Environmental Protection Agency (1989). *Risk Assessment Guidance for Superfund,* Vol. 1, *Human Health Evaluation Manual,* Part A, EPA/540/1-89/002.

Wade, M. J., B. K. Davis, J. S. Carlisle, A. K. Klein, and L. M. Valoppi (1993). Environmental transformation of toxic metals. In *Occupational Medicine: State of the Art Reviews. De Novo Toxicants: Combustion Toxicology, Mixing Incompatibilities, and Environmental Activation of Toxic Agents,* Vol. 8, No. 3 (D. J. Shusterman and J. E. Peterson, eds.), Hanley & Belfus, Philadelphia, pp. 575–601.

Westrick, J. J., J. W. Mello, and R. F. Thomas (1984). The groundwater supply survey, *J. Am. Water Works Assoc.*, 76, 52–59.

Woodrow, J. E., D. G. Crosby, T. Must, K. W. Molianen, and J. N. Seiber (1978). Rates of transformation of trifluralin and parathion vapors in air, *J. Agric. Food Chem.*, 26, 1312–1316.

Woodrow, J. E., J. N. Seiber, D. G. Crosby, K. W. Molianen, C. J. Soderquist, and C. Mourer (1977). Airborne and surface residues of parathion and its conversion products in a treated plum orchard environment, *Arch. Environ. Contam. Toxicol.*, 6, 175–191.

# 17

# Noncancer Risk Assessment: Present and Emerging Issues

**John L. Cicmanec**
*United States Environmental Protection Agency*
*Cincinnati, Ohio*

**Michael L. Dourson**
*Toxicology Excellence for Risk Assessment*
*Cincinnati, Ohio*

**Richard C. Hertzberg**
*United States Environmental Protection Agency*
*Atlanta, Georgia*

## I. INTRODUCTION

One of the primary goals of this chapter is to provide the risk assessor with principles and guidelines to assist in the interpretation and integration of available scientific information for noncancer risk assessment of chemicals. It is recognized that, although this information is essential, the difficult task concerns the use of this knowledge by the risk assessors and the judgments they will make. Not all guidelines apply at all times. For experts, these guidelines should serve to aid in organizing factual information and scientific interpretations. In some situations, these guidelines will provide a framework to use in preparing or reviewing dose–response assessment and in defining the critical issues to be discussed with colleagues. The purpose of this section is to define high-quality, state-of-the-art risk assessment approaches. This material should also aid in formulating judgments concerning the nature and magnitude of a hazard. Ideally, this discussion will reflect sufficient flexibility to accommodate new knowledge and innovative methods. Also it will present scientifically supportable risk assessment procedures.

## II. HAZARD IDENTIFICATION

Hazard identification is the first step in the risk assessment of a chemical. The process is initially based on evaluating scientific reports of human or animal exposure to a potentially toxic substance. Specifically, this process focuses on the adverse effects associated with exposure to that chemical. The hazard assessment process involves characterizing the adverse effects on the subject and the overall physiological significance of these effects, defining the magnitude of effects and selecting which effects are most crucial or represent the most serious compromise to normal function. Ultimately, the evaluation of animal studies hinges on determining the significance to human health of the key adverse effects described in the study. This process depends on experience in evaluating scientific reports and the use of professional judgment. A chemical may cause many toxic effects in animals and one of the key decisions is to determine the biological significance of the effect and distinguishing between reversible and irreversible endpoints. The *critical effect* is defined as the adverse effect, or its known precursor, that first appears as dose levels are increased and becomes more severe as the dose is increased.

The critical effect serves as the basis for dose–response assessment, a topic that will be discussed more fully later. The critical effects caused by the same chemical may change among toxicity studies of different durations, they may be influenced by responses in other organs, and they may differ depending on the availability of data and on the pattern of the response.

## A.  Principal and Supporting Studies

Human studies provide the most direct evidence that observed adverse effects will have significance in humans. Although epidemiological reports often provide extensive documentation of many clinical and pathological effects, the quantitative aspects of the risk assessment process must be often done indirectly, as only approximate doses can be determined in many cases. In most instances for which human exposures have served as the basis for risk assessment, the exposures were accidental and involved large populations living in remote areas. Two examples are the methylmercury exposure in Iraq (Clarkson et al., 1975; Bakir, 1978) and hexachlorobenzene exposure in Turkey (Peters et al., 1982). In some rare instances, widespread human exposure to compounds, such as fluoride in drinking water, can serve as the basis for risk assessment (Hodge, 1950). In these cases, the database and quantitative aspects are ideal. Even for instances in which the human studies or reports do not provide sufficient information to do a quantitative risk assessment, they are still of benefit because the human reports provide a basis to determine whether the animal studies will accurately predict the response in humans. When reviewing the summaries of animal studies, it is important to verify that the observed effects in animals include the specific type of adverse effect noted in humans, even if the data for humans is taken from case reports.

The more common circumstance involves using animal studies as the basis for risk assessment. For many environmental pollutants, a database of animal studies, involving two or three common laboratory species, is available for review. The usual database also contains animal studies of varying length of exposure and varying detail of study design and endpoints assessed. A basic responsibility for the risk assessor is to select the most appropriate study to predict the corresponding adverse effect to be observed in humans. In many instances, one animal study will not provide a definitive answer for quantitative risk assessment. In these cases, other studies provide important supportive data, even though they are not the critical study. When reviewing the database, it is important to determine that collectively the studies have examined a broad range of possible adverse effects, including reproductive and developmental endpoints. This is necessary so that the endpoint selected as the critical adverse effect truly reflects the most sensitive endpoint for that particular compound. Critical effects may change among toxicity studies of different durations, and these effects may be influenced by toxicity in other organs; however, it is the task of the risk assessor to single out that endpoint which is most indicative of the circumstance with which he or she is working. It should be recognized that, for many compounds, there may be a very limited database; hence, a compromise judgment is employed in making the risk assessment.

## B.  Quality of Study

Certain basic features of study design relate directly to the quality of the study. This includes adequate characterization of the test compound and possible contaminants, animal group size, inclusion of both sexes for testing, selection of animals of suitable age, selection of a wide range of dosages that are likely to define the no-observed adverse effect level (NOAEL) and lowest-observed adverse effect level (LOAEL), and proper characterization of the animal subjects chosen for the study. It is also essential to carefully describe the types of observations and methods of laboratory analysis. It is important that appropriate statistical analysis of the data has been performed. The study report should also provide sufficient background description of the toxicological response being investigated, a description of the study rationales, and the reasons why that particular study might aid in predicting the critical response in humans.

Animal and human studies that are judged to be inadequate for quantitative risk assessment may, nevertheless, provide important supporting evidence. The most apparent example is of human case reports that indicate a toxicity endpoint similar to the one observed in animal studies, even though the human report cannot provide quantitative information. Many animal studies can contribute to the supporting database, even though they are inadequate for quantitative risk assessment because of improper study duration, inadequate number of doses, or too few test subjects. Such studies may demonstrate a pattern of response similar to the critical study and provide additional points on the dose–response curve not contained in the critical study. The combining data from studies that are not of identical design must be done with caution. Often the key study, although very thorough, may not examine all critical endpoints; hence, the supporting studies take on greater significance. Data obtained from in vitro studies often provide insights of results and information useful for comparative purposes, although not directly providing definitive conclusions for risk assessment. One useful example of in vitro data would be the toxicity equivalency factors for various dioxin congeners. For practical reasons, it is unlikely that animal testing of each of the congeners will ever be completed, yet the in vitro tests provide a measure of comparative data for use by the risk assessor.

The criteria for evaluating epidemiological studies are well defined. They include factors such as proper selection and characterization of confounding factors and a description of how they were considered; and an attempt to establish doses or level of exposure when possible. It is important that the description of an epidemiological study reflect the ability of the study to detect specific adverse effects, and the statistical power of the methods employed should be included in the assessment. As with determining the adequacy of studies, expert judgment is necessary to determine the weight of evidence for or against a specific effect. This judgment is primarily based on experience in dealing with a variety of risk assessment challenges and from interaction with other risk assessors.

## C. Route, Source, and Duration of Exposure

Human exposure to a chemical pollutant may be by more than one route of entry. In addition, the bioavailability of a chemical ingested from one source (food) may differ from that from another source (water), even though the route of entry is the same. Usually, the toxicity database for a compound does not provide data on all available routes and sources of administration. In the absence of data on a specific route of exposure, the risk assessor should consider the potential for toxicity from reports by another particular route. However, for quantitative comparison, the exact formulas for extrapolation are not often available, which increases the need for scientific judgment. Consideration must be also given for potential differences in absorption or metabolism resulting from different routes of exposure.

Toxic effects may vary with magnitude, frequency, and duration of exposure. Animal studies differ in exposure duration (acute, less than 90 days; subchronic, 90 days to 2 years; and chronic, 2 years up to lifetime), in dosing schedules (single, intermittent, or continuous), and by route. Among the possible routes of administration, oral, inhalation, and dermal exposure are the most common avenues employed. For oral exposure, the compound may be added to the food or drinking water, or it may be administered by gavage, particularly when the compound is distasteful or irritating. In some instances, the investigator may choose oral gavage to be sure that a very specific dose is administered for each day of dosing. Inhalation exposure often varies by the duration of exposure (i.e., 6 h/day, 5 days/week) and, depending on properties of the compound, the exposure may be nose-only or entire body. Dermal exposure is usually performed on a shaved portion of the animal that is inaccessible by mouth and cannot be scratched. The duration of dermal exposure may be for a prescribed period for certain irritating substances. However, in most instances, the compound is simply left in place until the next day when a new dose is applied. The risk assessor must consider each factor when evaluating studies.

## D.  Assessing Toxicological Significances

Adverse toxicological effects are either manifest as a clinical sign, a biochemical change, a functional impairment, or a pathological lesion. Furthermore, an adverse effect impairs performance and reduces the ability of the organism to respond to additional challenge and to carry on normal physiological functions. The presence of change alone is not necessarily indicative of an adverse effect. The results of animal studies are often reported in terms of which changes show statistical significance. In other instances, values for the test and control groups are stated, and a range of normal values is listed. Statistical and biological significance of an observed effect must not be equated, and are often considered as sequential. The determination of adversity should involve careful toxicological evaluation, for which statistics are only a tool used for clarifying the implications of the data. The actual decision of whether an effect is adverse should be based primarily on a biological basis. Any animal that is clearly in a state of physiological compromise should be judged as exhibiting an adverse effect.

Apparent differences can arise when effects that are toxicologically insignificant show statistical significance when the data are analyzed. For example, a 5% decrease in body weight in an experimental group that is statistically significant when compared with a control group in a chronic study is often judged not biologically significant if both groups were fed ad lib, since a decrease in body weight is often associated with increased longevity. In most of these cases, the problem is determining the biological relevance of a change that is statistically significant. Ultimately, these decisions are based on use of professional judgment and experience.

## III.  DOSE–RESPONSE ASSESSMENT

A basic tenet of toxicology is that as the dosage of a chemical is increased, the toxic response increases (Doull et al., 1980). This increase can occur for both the severity of the response and the proportion of the population that is affected as the dosage increases. Dose–response assessment involves the quantitative evaluation of toxicity data to determine the likelihood of similar associated effects in humans.

Data available for dose–response assessment range from well-conducted and well-controlled epidemiological studies of human exposures, in addition to many well-characterized exposures and supportive studies in several animal species, to a complete lack of human and animal toxicity data, with only structure–activity relationships to guide the evaluation. Nevertheless, the risk assessor must develop a criteria for the minimal amount of information of sufficient quality to perform a dose–response assessment for a compound.

## A. Structure–Activity Relationship

The Food and Drug Administration (FDA), the Environmental Protection Agency (EPA), and the pharmaceutical industry independently have developed an approach for risk assessment of chemicals for which little or no test data exist. This approach depends on evaluating data from studies of structurally related compounds; hence, the name structure–activity relationship.

The first step involves the evaluation and interpretation of descriptive information for the compound, such as physicochemical characteristics for the compound and structurally similar compounds. The second step involves the evaluation of toxicological and pharmacological data for analogous substances and potential metabolites. Analogues are selected on the basis of two factors: (1) structural, functional, and mechanistic similarities that control the biological activity of the substances, and an attempt is made to identify analogues with similar overall structural similarities that would have biological activity comparable with the chemical under study; and (2) the availability of pertinent toxicological data for the analogues that would be useful in the assessment. Potential analogues are identified either directly by expert pharmacokinetists, or by using guidance from computerized substructure searchable databases, such as the Structure and Nomenclature Search System (SANSS). In addition, key potential metabolites of the chemical under study are identified through the application of principles of metabolism, or less frequently, on the basis of actual test data for that particular chemical. Emphasis is given to potential metabolic pathways that lead to activation or inactivation. The third component involves the use of mathematical expressions for biological activity or "quantitative structural–activity relationships" (QSARs). The QSARs are generated to estimate physical and chemical properties such as water solubility, partition coefficient, and vapor pressure, that provide useful information in the selection of analogues. Estimation of the log $p$ and water solubility of a chemical assists greatly in determining its potential for absorption through the skin, lungs, and gastrointestinal tract.

Once this information is gathered, the judgment of the risk assessor, used in concert with biochemists and pharmacologists, estimates a range and pattern of toxicological response for that chemical. In performing the evaluation, this group of scientists must consider a variety of parameters as they apply directly to the chemical under study and in comparison with its analogues. These parameters include potential for dermal, pulmonary, and gastrointestinal absorption; biotransformation pathways; and distribution and excretion.

If the analogues are reasonably close to the subject chemical and the toxicity data are reliable, then a risk estimate can be calculated. As the analogues become more remote and the database is less complete, meaningful risk analyses are less likely to be achieved.

## B. Chronic Reference Dose

The chronic reference dose (RfD) is an estimate (with uncertainty spanning an order of magnitude) of a daily exposure to the human population (including sensitive subgroups) that is likely to be without appreciable risk of deleterious effects during a lifetime (IRIS, 1993). The RfD is determined by use of the following equation.

$$\text{RfD} = \frac{\text{NOAEL or LOAEL}}{\text{UF} \times \text{MF}}$$

where

NOAEL is the exposure level at which there are no statistically or biologically significant increases in the frequency or severity of adverse effects between the exposed population and its appropriate control; some effects may be produced at this level, but they are not considered as adverse, nor precursor to specific adverse effects. In an experiment with several NOAELs, the regulator should focus primarily on the NOAEL seen at the highest dose. This leads to the common usage of the term NOAEL to mean the highest exposure without adverse effect.

LOAEL = the lowest exposure level at which there are statistically or biologically significant increases in frequency or severity of adverse effects between the exposed population and its appropriate control group.

Uncertainty factor (UF) = one of several, generally tenfold, factors used in operationally deriving the RfD from experimental data.

Modifying factor (MF) = an uncertainty factor that is greater than zero and less than or equal to 10; the default value for the MF is 1.

The RfD is useful as a reference point for gauging the potential effects of other doses. Doses at or below the RfD are not likely to be associated with health risks. In contrast, as the amount of the chemical that an individual is exposed to increases above the RfD, the probability that an adverse effect will be seen also increases. Unfortunately, the conclusion that all doses below the RfD are acceptable and that all doses above the RfD are unacceptable cannot be categorically stated. The precision of the RfD depends on the overall magnitude of the composite uncertainty and modifying factors used in its calculation. The precision is usually one significant figure and more likely is in the range of one order of magnitude.

The determination of an RfD requires scientific judgment on the appropriate NOAEL and associated UF and MF. The reasoning behind these judgments and the underlying assumptions and their limitations are discussed later.

## 1. Selection of Toxicity Data

Once a hazard identification has been conducted and the critical effect(s) are identified, the risk assessor must select the experimental dose from the study that represent the highest level tested at which no critical effect(s) was demonstrated. This value (i.e., the NOAEL) is the key datum gleaned from the toxicologist's review of the entire database for that chemical, and it is the first component in the estimation of an RfD. Use of this NOAEL assumes that the critical effect does not occur at a lower dose and, thus, prevents all other "threshold" toxic effects caused by that chemical. When quantitative human toxicity data are available for use in the estimation of an RfD, it will be used in the selection of a NOAEL. Clearly, use of this data has the advantage of avoiding the uncertainty inherent with interspecies extrapolation.

In the absence of appropriate human data, the animal database becomes the primary focus of concern. The primary advantages in using data from animal studies are that the chemical dose is carefully controlled and is free of contaminants, heterogeneity of the exposed populations is controlled, and other environmental conditions are standardized. In reviewing animal study data, the risk assessor should identify the specific animal species and strain that is most similar in response to humans. This decision is based on a biological rationale and makes use of available comparative pharmacokinetic information. In the absence of a clearly most relevant species, the risk assessor should choose the critical study and species that shows an adverse effect at the lowest administered dose unless he or she has specific metabolic data indicating that species is more sensitive than humans.

## 2. Confidence in the Reference Dose

The highest degree of confidence will be obtained when the test circumstances most closely resemble the "real-world" application; that is, human exposure in a semicontrolled situation. Since this type of information is available only in rare instances, the risk assessor should attempt to construct a complete database, including many animal species and a variety of exposure scenarios, from which to determine the RfD. Ideally, the database should include

1. Two adequate mammalian chronic toxicity studies in which dosing was administered by the appropriate route in two separate species.
2. One adequate mammalian multigeneration reproductive toxicity study in which the chemical was administered by the appropriate route
3. Two adequate mammalian developmental toxicity studies in separate species in which the chemical was administered by the appropriate route.

If there is a complete database, it is unlikely that further toxicological testing would determine an NOAEL much different from the one determined from this collection of studies. Consequently, the risk assessor can have high confidence that the RfD will not change. However, some chemicals pose only an acute health hazard, and general toxicity studies may indicate the need for special studies to assess neurotoxic or immunotoxic effects. In such cases, the database will not be complete without these special studies.

The risk assessor can consider a single, well-conducted subchronic mammalian bioassay by the appropriate route as the minimum database for estimating an RfD. As can be seen, in these instances, the likelihood that the RfD will change following additional toxicity testing is higher; therefore, the confidence in the RfD derived from the minimum database is low.

Developmental toxicity data, if they constitute the sole source of information, are not considered an adequate basis for estimation of a chronic RfD. This is because such data are often generated from acute and short-term chemical exposures and have limited relevance in predicting the threshold for adverse effects from chronic exposure. However, if a developmental toxicity endpoint has been established as the critical adverse effect from a complete database, then the chronic RfD may be derived from the developmental data.

### 3. Selection of Uncertainty Factors

The choice of the appropriate UF and MF reflects case-by-case judgment by experienced risk assessors (Table 1). This process should account for each of the applicable areas of uncertainty and any nuances in the available data that might change the magnitude of any factor. The primary reason for using UFs is to account for several areas of scientific uncertainty that are inherent in toxicity databases. Application of UFs reduces the dose rate working from the NOAEL: Interhuman variability (designated as $UF_H$) is intended to account for the variation in sensitivity among members of the human population. The susceptibility of human infants to nitrate poisoning, usually through oral exposure in drinking water, and that of developing fetuses to certain neurotoxicants are examples of sensitive subpopulations among humans (Walton, 1951).

Experimental animal-to-human variability (designated as $UF_A$) is intended to account for the uncertainty in extrapolating animal data to circumstances of human exposure for a specific chemical. This is primarily due to differences in toxicokinetics and toxicodynamics between species. Subchronic to chronic variability (designated as $UF_S$) is intended to account for the uncertainty in extrapolating from less than chronic NOAELs (or LOAELs) to chronic exposures. (Note that determination of RfDs for exposure for less than chronic conditions, such as developmental toxicity, obviate the need for this particular uncertainty factor). The LOAEL-to-NOAEL variability (designated as $UF_L$) is intended to account for the uncertainty in extrapolating from LOAELs to NOAELs. Database completeness (designated as $UF_D$) is intended to account for the inability of any single study to adequately address all possible adverse outcomes. This may also be used to account for a very limited number of studies that do not examine all significant endpoints.

Each of these areas is generally addressed by the risk assessor with an order of magnitude

**Table 1** Description of Uncertainty and Modifying Factors for Deriving Chronic Reference
Doses (RfDs)

| Standard uncertainty factors | General guidance |
| --- | --- |
| H (interhuman) | Use of a tenfold factor when extrapolating from experimental or occupational human exposure. This factor is intended to account for variation in sensitivity among humans. |
| A (experimental animals to man) | Use a tenfold factor when extrapolating from results of a long-term animal study when results of long-term human exposure are not available or are inadequate. The purpose of this factor is to account for the uncertainty in extrapolating from animals to humans. |
| S (subchronic to chronic) | Use of a tenfold factor when adjusting from less than chronic results to true chronic exposure in experimental animals or humans. |
| L (LOAEL to NOAEL) | Use of a tenfold factor when deriving an RfD from a LOAEL instead of a NOAEL. |
| D (incomplete database to complete) | Use a tenfold factor when a database does not contain results from at least chronic studies in two species and when reproductive and developmental results are missing. Some adjustments are made when part of these requirements are met. |

factor (i.e., 10). In practice, the magnitude of any composite UF is dependent on professional
judgment for the total uncertainty in all areas. If uncertainties in all areas have been resolved the
risk assessor can use a onefold UF to estimate the RfD. When uncertainties exist in one, two, or
three areas it is a standard practice to use a 10-, 100-, or 1000-fold UF, respectively. When
uncertainties exist in four areas it is standard practice to use a 3000-fold UF. When a single
subchronic animal study does not define the NOAEL, and it is the only toxicity data available
for that substance, then uncertainty exists in all five areas, and an uncertainty factor of 10,000
is used. If a toxicity database is weaker than a single, animal subchronic bioassay that does not
define a NOAEL, then that database is considered inadequate for quantitative risk assessment.

Risk assessors occasionally use a factor less than 10 or even a factor of 1, if the existing
data reduce or obviate the need to account for a particular area of uncertainty. For example, the
use of a 1-year rat study as the basis of an RfD may reduce the need for a tenfold factor for the
area of subchronic to chronic extrapolation to threefold. It has been empirically demonstrated
that 1-year rat NOAELs are closer in magnitude to chronic values than are 3-month NOAELs.
A rather recent publication investigates more fully this concept of variable UF through an
analysis of expected values (Lewis, 1990).

Uncertainty factor reduction follows the general guideline for composite UFs and is
done in a fashion that reflects the imprecision of uncertainty factors. It may not be appropriate to employ an UF of 270 (i.e., $10 \times 3 \times 3 \times 3$) based on $UF_H \times UF_A \times UF_S \times UF_L$ when
the uncertainties in A, S, and L are partial, since 270 indicates more preciseness than uncertainty factors are designed to reflect. The appropriate choice is a UF of 300 (i.e., 10 $UF_H \times 30$
$UF_A \times UF_S \times UF_L$). The intermediate factor of 3 is used since 3 is the approximate logarithmic
mean of 1 and 10.

### 4. Selection of Modifying Factors

In addition to the use of uncertainty factors, modifying factors may also be applied in the
calculation of some RfDs. The reason for the use of modifying factors is that the areas of

scientific uncertainty of H, A, S, L, or D, do not represent all of the uncertainties involved in the estimation of an RfD. For example, when too few animals are used in a dosing group, the NOAEL may be set too low, since an adequate number of subjects were not included in the trial. Consideration of this type of database would argue for modifying the standard use of 10-fold factors—a 100-fold UF might be raised to 250 if only a limited number of animals were used in a chronic study. Although scientifically reasonable, it introduces the perception that selection of the UFs is arbitrary, and a number such as 250 indicates more precision than is actually present when placing numeric values on uncertainty. Through the use of MFs some of these problems are avoided while, at the same time, maintaining the consistency of the standard use of uncertainty factors.

*Assumptions and Limitations.* A basic assumption in the development of an RfD is that a threshold exists in the dose rate for each compound, above which an adverse effect will be induced in the animal. This concept is supported by the known methods of toxicity that show that a physiological reserve must be depleted and the repair capacity of the organism must be overcome before toxicity occurs (Doull et al., 1980).

Another assumption is that the RfD represents an estimate of a population threshold dose rate; that is, it adequately protects sensitive humans within the larger group. As described previously, one of the UFs accounts for the variability of individual thresholds. For certain compounds there is sufficient evidence of hypersusceptibility or chemical idiosyncrasy to warrant concern whether or not the adjustment through the use of a factor of 10 is always sufficient to fully account for threshold for the entire population. In truth, many of the chemical idiosyncrasies for certain individuals may be so far below the standard population that no adjustment to the RfD will be protective for this subgroup. An example is the dermal hypersensitivity of some persons to nickel (Kaaber et al., 1978).

The third assumption in the development of an RfD relates to the definition of critical effect. Risk assessors assume that, if the critical effect is prevented, then other adverse threshold effects that occur at higher doses will also be prevented. However, since the RfD procedure generally ignores the dose–response slope, then if other adverse effects have less abrupt slopes, estimating the RfD on the basis of the critical effect may not be sufficiently protective. For this reason, information on slopes of dose–response curves may be used to determine the critical effect in the benchmark dose approach. Other assumptions are used as well.

## C. Dose–Response Modeling

Another risk assessment goal is to estimate, through the use of a theoretical dose–response model, the likely human response to a variety of exposure levels to a selected contaminant. However, it is necessary to have sufficient data before a dose–response model can be employed. By way of definition, *dose–response* refers to the relationship between dose (or inhalation exposure) and toxic responses. In some instances, response might equate to prevalence of a sign or symptom for an exposed population. The toxicity data that might be used in a dose–response model can be derived from laboratory or clinical studies, or from epidemiological data.

The initial step for using a mathematical model for dose–response analysis is to describe the risk assessment goal. The next step is to evaluate the quality of the toxicity data and to consider its suitability for meeting the stated goal. Once this has been accomplished, the risk assessor must select the appropriate mathematical model and its parameters. The final step involves evaluating the overall quality of the model in describing the toxicity data and clearly stating the key assumptions and uncertainties involved in using the model. There is a wide variety in the content and quality of toxicity data that might be used; therefore, it is necessary that professional judgment and experience be used in application of dose–response models to risk assessment.

Certain models require that exposure values be stated in a specific form, such as daily intake rate. In these instances, assumptions may be required to convert the reported units of exposure into the required form. Referring to standard biological conversion tables may assist with this part of the exercise; in other cases, broader assumptions and interpretation may be needed. Quite often the goal is to be able to state an internal dose, such as steady-state concentration or blood level, for a particular pollutant. If these values can be derived, then no additional dose adjustment is needed. If information suggests other factors that influence toxic response, then additional scaling factors or dose adjustment may be calculated, but such modifications must be justified in each case.

When chemical-specific factors for dosimetry are not available, then conventional conversion steps should be used for estimating daily intake for oral exposures (stated in units of mg/kg-day) or average daily air concentration for inhalation exposures (state in units of $mg/M^3$). Interspecies scaling of dose so that experimental animal data can be applied to humans may involve use of a default tenfold reduction.

Duration is scaled according to fraction of lifespan for exposures greater than 90 days. Procedures for scaling duration with shorter-term data, such as using actual time exposed and duration by using the multiplied product (Haber's principle), should be justified in each case.

For exposure–response data, models that have been used for response rates are the probit–logit class, the multistage–multihit class, and the Weibull. The Weibull model is most commonly used when modeling systemic toxicity from animal data (Crump, 1984). When low-dose behavior is the goal (i.e., exposure estimates for negligible risk), then major critical effects should be modeled, and the lowest dose corresponding to the target level of negligible risk will be used. The choice of using the central tendency estimate or confidence limit will always be made separately. Parameters will be estimated by maximum likelihood, and mode acceptability will be judged by the $X^2$-statistic.

Exposure–intensity models describe the dependence of a measured biological parameter on exposure level. The application of such a model must compare the modeled value for the measured parameter with healthy individuals. For these comparisons, the recommended model is the exponential–polynomial class of mathematical functions. In these cases the literature source for the parameter range for normal values needs to be referenced.

### 1. Exposure–Severity Data

Toxicological responses will be placed into four progressive categories of no-effect, nonadverse effects, mild-to-moderate adverse effects, and severe or lethal effects. By design these categories resemble the dose categories used in determining an RfD; namely, no-observed effect level (NOEL), NOAEL, LOAEL, and frank effect level (FEL). Since all of the data are used in the regression, there is no need to specify a LOAEL. Instead, the term adverse effect level (AEL), is used, since one is dealing with the lowest dose showing mild-to-moderate adverse effects. Logistic regression on ordered categories (Harrell, 1986; Hertzberg, 1989) will be used to determine model parameters. Parameters will be estimated by maximum likelihood. Model acceptability by the risk assessor will be judged by several factors, including the model $X^2$-statistic. Additional fitting statistics to consider are correspondence statistics, correlation coefficients, and model parameter significance levels. Visual judgment of the graphs and tables generated by these techniques is also necessary. A recommended technique is the use of graph of dose versus duration, with each point represented by a different symbol to denote categories with model results represented by a curve showing the exposure levels that predict 10% and 1% of risks for an AEL or FEL.

## D.  Benchmark Dose

The Benchmark approach has been the subject of numerous publications (Gaylor, 1983; Dourson et al., 1985; Kimmel and Gaylor, 1988; Kimmel, 1990, Brown and Erdreich, 1989). The primary advantage of this approach is that it provides a fuller explication of the dose–response curve, which the RfD approach does not. Also, the reference dose approach does not take into account the variability of the data. The NOAEL from a small study will likely be higher than the NOAEL from a larger study in the same species, whereas the opposite may be true when variability is considered. Additionally, the NOAEL must be one of the experimental doses, and the number and spacing of doses in a study will influence the dose that is chosen for the NOAEL. Since the NOAEL is defined as a dose that does not produce an observable change in adverse responses from control levels, and is dependent on the power of the study, then theoretically the risk associated with that dose may fall anywhere between zero and an incidence just below that detectable from control levels. This value is usually in the range of from 7 to 10% for quantal data. Crump (1984) and Gaylor (1989) have estimated the upper confidence limit for developmental risk at the NOAEL for several data sets to vary between 2 and 6%.

The benchmark dose is based on a model-derived estimate of a particular incidence level, such as 1 or 10%. More specifically, the benchmark dose is the lower confidence limit for the effective dose that produces a certain increase in the incidence above control levels. The benchmark dose is derived by modeling the data in the observed range, calculating the upper confidence limit on the dose–response curve, and selecting the point on the upper confidence curve corresponding to a 10% increase in incidence of an effect. The dose corresponding to the model estimate for a 10% increase in incidence is the *effect dose* for 10% of the population ($ED_{10}$), whereas the benchmark dose is that dose corresponding to the upper confidence limit of the 10% incidence is the *lowest effective dose* for 10% ($LED_{10}$). With the benchmark approach, an $LED_{10}$ will be calculated for each agent for which there is an adequate database. In some cases the data may be adequate to also estimate the $ED_{01}$ or $ED_{05}$, incidence levels that may be closer to a true no-effect dose. A level between the $ED_{01}$ and $ED_{10}$ is usually the lowest level or risk that can be estimated adequately for binomial endpoints from standard developmental toxicity studies.

### 1.  Assessing Risk for Less-Than-Lifetime Exposures

In contrast with the risks associated with lifetime exposure, there is also a need for risk assessment for short-term exposures. The hazard identification process is used similarly for acute, intermittent, or other less-than-lifetime exposures as it is for chronic, low-level exposures. For less-than-lifetime exposures, the risk assessor selects the appropriate toxicity data, identifies adverse effects, and considers the significance of these effects on public health. Once the data are analyzed, the risk assessor draws conclusions from this information and presents the weight-of-evidence needed for the assessment of hazard. Ideally, human toxicity data will be available for short-term exposures and can then be used in conjunction with animal data. In these cases, the process is more straightforward and often involves direct application of the human data to a specific exposure scenario. When animal data are the sole basis of the dose–response assessment, then uncertainty factors are applied to the NOAEL or LOAEL, in a process similar to chronic exposure. Less research data may be available for intermittent or less-than-lifetime exposures than for chronic exposures, and often, greater uncertainty is associated with use of the research data.

A common risk assessment problem is concerned with episodic releases, similar to intermittent use of a chemical product or periodic releases for a site where a toxicant is used or made. Most often the exposure patterns from such releases frequently do not match those of animal studies in either dose or duration. Judgment is required in determining the relevance of available experimental data to the analysis of effects for the exposure pattern of concern. Scientific judgment is also required in considering other factors such as the potential for recovery between exposures, data on pharmacokinetics and pharmacodynamics of the compound, and the potential for bioaccumulation. These factors greatly influence conclusions on the likelihood and extent of toxicity for particular exposures. Some of the issues that should be considered are as follows.

### 2.  Selection of Studies and Identification of Effects

Studies that can assist in the identification of effects include studies of acute, high-dose exposures relative to tests of subchronic duration at a dose level closer to the potential range of human exposure. In some instances, the test of low-dose, chronic exposure may be of value. The effects observed at high doses for short duration are often more severe than chronic, low-dose exposure, and they may involve entirely different organ systems and clinical effects. Acute and short-term toxicity studies do not always assess the more subtle toxic effects, nor the effects requiring a latent period before manifestation. The risk assessor should constantly review study reports with these considerations in mind. Some chemicals, such as carbamates and organophosphorus compounds, show acute and chronic toxicity that are very similar, since they are rapidly metabolized and excreted. In contrast with this, other substances accumulate and result in chronic toxicity at doses much lower than those for acute exposure. As might be expected, results from chronic, low-dose exposure are often not at all applicable to high-dose, acute exposures.

### 3.  Quantifying Risk

Selection of a study as the basis for quantitative risk estimation should be governed by attaining the closest possible association between dose rate and duration relative to the human exposure of concern. Quantifying the toxicity from short-term, high exposure will be defined not only by all of the processes that determine tissue dose, but also by the potential for recovery after the exposure ceases or between repeated exposures. Some chemicals cause delayed toxicity after a single dose. In addition, short-term, high exposure may cause a pronounced vulnerability to the effect of other toxicants present in food or medication, or by other environmental exposure or resident microorganisms.

## IV.  RISK CHARACTERIZATION

Risk characterization is the crucial link between a risk assessment and its application in risk management. Good risk characterization provides a solid framework for communicating the technical basis of a risk assessment to risk managers and the public. It is important that the risk assessors communicate their confidence in, and the potential limitations for, each risk assessment. Without an appropriate analysis of key assumptions and uncertainties, misinterpretation and misunderstanding of risk estimates are likely. It should be clear that very few risk assessments are based on a fully satisfactory database; therefore, the strengths and limitations of the assessment should be provided, in addition to the quantitative value that is routinely provided. This step is necessary to ensure objectivity and balance in the characterization of risk.

Formal integration of the strengths and weaknesses from the first three steps of a risk assessment greatly clarifies the estimated risks, the uncertainties in these estimates, and the critical assumptions are organized to summarize their impact on risk estimates. Multiple risk descriptors should be provided as well as the range of possible exposures, definition of the high end of individual risk, and the particular population that may be at risk. It is also necessary to define important subgroups within the population. The desired result is that the risk managers will have a comprehensive overview allowing them to prioritize control options and to effectively communicate risk management decisions to the public.

Risk characterization flows directly from the first three steps of the assessment. It should represent both a summary and integration of the previous key findings and conclusions, discuss the quality of the risk characterization, and briefly state ongoing or potential research that could support the risk assessment. In addition, appropriate caveats to the description and interpretation of risk should be included, to minimize overconfidence in point estimates. Many of these concepts were recently summarized in a memorandum prepared by Mr. F. Henry Habicht, then Deputy Administrator of EPA (Habicht, 1992).

## A. An Integrated View of the Evidence

In developing the hazard characterization, dose–response and exposure sections of the risk assessment, the assessor makes judgments concerning the relevance and appropriateness of the data and methodology. These judgments are summarized with the hazard characterization, dose–response, and exposure characterization sections. As a guide, the summaries may include the following:

1. Hazard identification: the qualitative, weight-of-evidence conclusions concerning the potential that a chemical may pose a specific hazard to human health; the nature and incidence of observed effects, and a description of the route by which these effects are expected to occur.
2. Dose–response characterization: a discussion of the dose–response behavior of the critical effects; dose levels and ranges of the various studies; exposure duration relative to the test animal's lifespan; choice of an NOAEL or LOAEL, benchmark dose; the magnitude of the uncertainty and modifying factors; information defining the shape and slope of the dose–response curves, mechanism of toxic action, and a description of how this information was used for dose–response assessment.
3. Exposure characterization: the estimates of range of exposure; the route, duration, and pattern of exposure; relevant pharmacokinetics; and a description of the population exposed.

In the process of integrating these summaries, the risk assessor should determine if all segments of the assessment are compatible; that is, are the cancer and noncancer endpoints placed in the correct perspective and are the constraints of the available data properly addressed. It is also important to present data for all endpoints for which assessments are available for each compound.

## B. Key Assumptions and Uncertainties

Within risk characterization, the key assumptions and defined uncertainties concerning the analysis and interpretation of data are explained, and the risk manager should be given a clear understanding of the degree of scientific consensus that exists about risk assessment. Whenever more than one interpretation of the dose–response assessment is supported by the data and choosing between them is difficult, all views should be presented. The rationale for the selected approach should be given and all approaches should be discussed.

If quantitative uncertainty analysis of the data is appropriate, it is summarized in the risk characterization; in virtually all cases qualitative discussion of important uncertainties should be included. If other organizations such as the EPA or FDA also published risk assessments, they should also be summarized and included.

## C.  Descriptors of Risk

Risk may be described in a variety of qualitative and quantitative ways. For quantitative assessment, the risk qualifiers are often presented in more than one fashion so that the risk manager is presented with a complete picture.

The range of confidence placed in a particular risk assessment can vary considerably. The most accurate way to describe risk will depend on the database. If data on actual incidence of disease in humans are available, then projections about disease incidence in a human population exposed to similar doses may be possible. For example, by knowing that a certain percentage of patients with angina experience chest pain on exertion at a known experimental concentration of carbon monoxide, it may be possible to estimate the percentage of similar patients expected to experience symptoms when exposed to similar concentrations.

It is essential that the risk assessor communicate to the risk manager that projections between dissimilar populations is much more tentative, and the final decisions will rely more heavily on professional judgment. For example, there is as yet no completely reliable method to estimate the percentage of persons exposed to 2 mg of toluene per kilogram per day through drinking water who will develop hepatic or renal toxicity. A risk assessor can state that an exposure of 0.2 mg/kg per day (the oral RfD) is likely to be without appreciable risk for exposed populations. This value was derived following application of appropriate UFs to the NOAEL taken from an animal subchronic study, but the currently used methods of risk assessment do not provide a substantiated method for calculating risk above the RfD.

### 1.  *Estimation of Incidence of Effect Within a Population*

Presentation of population risk in terms of incidence (i.e., cases per thousand individuals in a population) or in actual numbers of expected cases for the population of interest is another way of expressing the hazard associated with exposure to a pollutant. For cancer risks, this is usually presented in terms such as "for the 4 million people in this city, we project no more than 1 additional cancer per year." The usefulness of risk information depends on how well the risk is understood and the degree of confidence that can be placed in it. With each risk assessment, the risk manager should be given information on (1) the biological nature of the risk, (2) the information used to determine if the exposure will have consequences for humans, and (3) the degree of confidence that the risk assessor places in the database and numerical descriptors of risk.

Risk managers often have the responsibility to communicate the results of a risk assessment to the public; therefore, some examples of practical conclusions about the risk should be part of the information associated with those risk assessments.

In unusual cases sufficient data exist for human exposure to estimate a similar effect for noncancer endpoints. Techniques do not yet exist to give a quantitatively precise extrapolation procedure for noncancer effects from experimental animals to humans. It is also impossible at this time to accurately predict incidence for noncancer toxicological endpoints. Determining the critical effect for the most sensitive experimental animal species and dividing by a $UF_S$ is a straightforward procedure, but of limited precision and accuracy. Other procedures, such as establishing a benchmark dose, hold promise of improving this segment of the risk assessment process, but they also have deficiencies.

At best, without a more complete understanding of the mechanisms of toxicity, existing animal toxicity data provide only a general trend in the staging of chemical-induced disease for humans at doses higher than the reference dose. Presently risk assessment methodology is being rapidly expanded and mechanism-based, dose–response models will likely improve the methods by which this descriptor will be determined.

## 2. Estimation of the Number of Individuals Higher Than a Specified Risk

Another common way to present risks is to specify a "cutoff point," such as an RfD, and then estimate the percentage of persons exceeding this dose. There are several variations of this descriptor. For example, the RfD is described as a dose that is likely to be without appreciable risk for deleterious effect during a lifetime. Presentation of a population in terms of the number at or below the RfD ("probably not at risk") and above the RfD ("may be at risk") may be useful information for risk managers. For some hazardous health effects, the existence of a toxicity "threshold" is presumed. This presumption aids in resolving the potential risk management decision of dividing the population into "probably at risk" and "probably not at risk" segments. For clarity, the RfD should not be considered as an estimate of a threshold dose for humans, but rather, as a subthreshold dose.

This method is particularly useful to a risk manager considering possible actions to ameliorate risk for a population. If the number of persons in the "at risk" category can be estimated in the baseline (before contemplated action) case and also after a contemplated action is taken, the number of persons removed from the "at-risk" category can be used as an indication of the efficacy of the contemplated action.

## 3. Specific Risk Estimated for Highly Exposed Individuals

The purpose of this procedure is to estimate the magnitude of exposure at the upper end of the exposure distribution to be used as an indicator of the risk for those individuals falling into the high-risk category. Calculation of this special area of risk allows risk managers to determine if certain individuals are at an unacceptably high degree of risk.

Even in the absence of a complete database, it is often possible to estimate the specific risk to a portion of the population that is at high risk. This circumstance is more likely to happen, since animal testing is initially done at higher doses, which matches more closely with high-dose human exposure. Whenever possible it is important to express the number of individuals in the selected high-exposure group and to also show the range in the estimate of health risk. If population data are not available, it may be possible to describe a scenario representing high-dose exposures using upper percentile or judgment-based values for exposure variables. In these instances, caution should be used in applying assumptions that may raise the variables so that an "unreasonable" exposure estimate results.

## 4. Estimating Risk for Highly Sensitive or Susceptible Individuals

Any risk assessment exercise should attempt to identify sensitive or susceptible populations to the toxic effect of concern. Sensitive or susceptible individuals are those within the exposed population at increased risk of experiencing the critical adverse effect. Some examples that are readily apparent are pregnant women, infants, or asthmatics. However, for many toxic substances, it is often impossible to predict before exposures occur what segment of the population may be most sensitive. Unfortunately, for most substances, a wide range of individuals are usually exposed before a meaningful decision can be made about which subgroups are particularly more sensitive. This lack of predictability is primarily due to lack of knowledge of the mechanism of toxicity for most toxic substances. Consideration of factors, such as age, genetic subgroups, and preexisting disease, can aid in predicting highly sensitive groups.

## 5. Other Risk Descriptors

Working from the existing database, the actual quantitative risks frequently cannot be estimated for most toxic substances. In these instances, risk assessors can use indicators, such as "margin of error," to compare the available information for the hazard identification and dose–response assessment with the estimated human dose determined from a possible exposure scenario. The *margin of exposure* indicates the magnitude by which the NOAEL exceeds the estimated human dose when expressed as milligrams per kilogram per day or milligrams per cubic meter.

$$\text{Margin of exposure} = \frac{\text{NOAEL (experimental dose)}}{\text{estimated human dose}}$$

If the margin of exposure (MOE) is equal to or more than the total uncertainty used as a basis for determining the RfD for that substance, then the need for regulatory concern is small. Margins of exposure can also be calculated for occasions for which the RfD has not been estimated. In these cases, the use of MOE is more uncertain, and additional guidance by risk assessors is needed. Since MOEs do not estimate risks per se, they do permit the risk manager to sense how close certain exposures or doses from different exposure scenarios are to the range at which there may be concern.

Calculating theoretical upper-bound risks, or very conservative worst-case risks, may lead to the conclusion that the risk is quite small; even in the worst case. This information is useful for risk managers and, like the MOE, provides a perspective of which areas of the assessment are unimportant from a risk management viewpoint. The preferred way of expressing these risks is to use "less-than" terms such as "less than $10^{-7}$," which clearly shows the range of risk, while at the same time, that additional effort to quantify the risk more accurately was not necessary owing to the very low level of risk involved in this segment of the assessment.

## D. Communicating Results: Providing a Perspective

Once the risk characterization is complete the results must be communicated to the risk manager. The risk manager will then use the results of the risk characterization, together with social and economic considerations, as well as the important technological factors in reaching a regulatory decision. Nevertheless, because of the way these risk management factors may impact different cases, consistent risk management judgments must be made on a case-by-case basis. It is possible that a chemical with a specific risk characterization may be regulated differently under different statutes and media. The technical information provided in this chapter does not provide guidance for consideration of the nonscientific aspects of risk management decisions.

## REFERENCES

Brown, K. G., and L. S. Erderich (1989). Statistical uncertainty in the no-observed-effect-level, *Fundam. Appl. Toxicol.,* 13, 235–244.

Clarkson, T. W., L. Amin-Zaki, and S. K. Al-Tiikiti (1975). An outbreak of methylmercury poisoning due to consumption of contaminated grain, *Fed. Proc.,* 35, 2395–2399.

Crump, K. S (1984). A new method for determining allowable daily intakes, *Fundam. Appl. Toxicol.,* 4, 854–871.

Doull, J., C. Klaasen, and M. Auder (1980). *Casarett and Doull's Toxicology,* 2nd ed., MacMillan, New York, p. 718.

Dourson, M. L., R. C. Hertzberg, R. Hartung, and K. Blackburn (1985). Novel approaches for the estimation of acceptable daily intake, *Toxicol. Ind. Heatlh,* 1, 23–41.

Gaylor, D. W. (1983). The use of safety factors for controlling risk, *J. Toxicol. Environ. Health,* 11, 329–336.

Habicht, F. H. (1992). Memorandum to Assistant Administrators and Regional Administrators of the U. S. Environmental Protection Agency regarding "Guidance on Risk Characterization for Risk Managers and Risk Assessors."

Harrell, F. (1986). *The Logist Procedure,* SUGI Supplemental Library Users Guide, Ver. 5th ed. SAS Institute, Cary, NC.

Hertzberg, R. C. (1989). Fitting a model to categorical response data with application to species extrapolation of toxicity, *Health Phys.,* 57, 405–409.

Hodge, H. C. (1950). The concentration of fluorides in drinking water to give the minimum caries with maximum safety, *J. Am. Dent. Assoc.,* 48, 436–439.

Kaaber, K., N. K. Veien, and J. C. Tjell (1978). Low nickel diet in the treatment of patients with chronic nickel dermatitis, *Br. J. Dermatol.,* 98, 197–201.

Kimmel, C. A., and D. W. Gaylor (1988). Issues in qualitative and quantitative risk analysis for developmental toxicity, *Risk Anal.,* 8, 15–20.

Kimmel, C. W. (1990). Qualitative approaches to human risk assessment for noncancer health effects, *Neurotoxicology,* 11, 189–198.

Lewis, S. C., J. R. Lynch, and A. I. Nikiforov (1990). A new approach to deriving community exposure guidelines from no-observed-adverse-effect levels, *Regul. Toxicol. Pharmacol.,* 11, 314–330.

Peters, H. A., D. J. Gocmen, D. J. Cripps, C. T. Bryan, and J. Dobramiacis (1982). Epidemiology of hexachlorobenzene-induced porphyria in Turkey. Clinical and laboratory follow-up after 25 years, *Arch. Neurol.,* 39, 744–749.

[USEPA] United States Environmental Protection Agency (1989). Interim procedures for estimating risks associated with exposure to mixtures of chlorinated dibenzo-*p*-dioxins and -dibenzofurans (CDDs and CDFs), 1989 update. EPA/625/3-89/016. USEPA, Washington, DC.

Walton, G. (1951). Survey of literature relating to infant methemoglobinemia due to nitrate-contaminated water, *Am. J. Public Health,* 41, 986–996.

# PART IV
## RISK ASSESSMENT OF CHEMICAL MIXTURES AND CHEMICAL INTERACTIONS

**Edward J. Calabrese**
*University of Massachusetts*
*Amherst, Massachusetts*

The evaluation of chemical interactions within the context of risk assessment is an extremely important issue, since exposure to multiple agents and complex mixtures is, in fact, the norm. The following section will provide the reader with the theoretical foundations of how modern toxicology and epidemiology approach the study, evaluation, interpretation, and application of the knowledge of chemical interaction within a public health and risk assessment framework. The information provided within this section is also directly relevant to the rapidly emerging area of ecological risk assessment.

Despite the extensive amount of toxicological research effort in the area of chemical interactions and the documenting of factors that affect such interactions, it is important that the reader appreciate the limitations in current knowledge on the mechanistic explanation of how agents interact and how difficult it can be to finally achieve such toxicological clarity. For example, in 1978 Mehendale and colleagues first reported that a 15-day prior dietary dosage of kepone (10 ppm) enhanced the lethality of $CCl_4$ by 67-fold in male Sprague-Dawley rats. Nearly 20 years later, there remains considerable mechanistic uncertainty concerning how the prior exposure to kepone enhances the initial and profound toxicity of $CCl_4$, despite an impressive series of follow-up studies by the same investigators as well as other research groups.

This example serves to illustrate not only how challenging the unraveling of interaction mechanisms can be, but also the potential risk that humans and other organisms experience in the face of exposure to agents that, given current understandings and predictive methods, would not be expected to produce such an enhancement of toxicity.

The recognition of the markedly enhanced toxicity of $CCl_4$ by prior exposure to low dosages of kepone was not only important because of the enhanced toxicity (e.g., organ damage), but more importantly, because the interaction prevented tissue repair and recovery, with profound lethality being the result. These types of enhancements of toxicity and their effect on survival have lead to the more recent emphasis on defining the outer boundaries of interaction responses.

As a result of such recent progress in assessing toxicological interactions the concept of "superinteractions" and how they may be predicted has emerged. Although the kepone $CCl_4$ interaction is profound, with enhanced toxicity approaching two orders of magnitude, lead has been shown to enhance the toxicity of endotoxin by up to 100,000-fold, depending on the temporal aspects of the joint exposure. That two commonly encountered agents have the potential to affect superinteractions, resulting in a profound enhancement of lethality, should make all realize that understanding how environmental toxins interact is not only a toxicological problem, but one of potentially great public health concern. The following chapters will strive to place this important area of toxicological research in proper public health perspective.

# 18
# Predicting the Toxicological Consequences of Multiple Chemical Interactions

**Edward J. Calabrese**
*University of Massachusetts*
*Amherst, Massachusetts*

## I.  INTERACTION: A CONCEPTUAL FRAMEWORK

Over the past two decades considerable debate has occurred within the biostatistical–epidemiological, pharmacological, and toxicological communities over the concept of interaction (Calabrese, 1991). This debate, which was spearheaded by a 1974 report by Rothman, led to a successful attempt by Rothman et al. (1980) to develop a conceptual framework within which to consider the term *interaction*. Before addressing their conceptual framework, a brief recapitulation of the debate is instructive, since it illustrates pitfalls and interdisciplinary communication challenges in dealing with the concept of interaction.

In his initial report, Rothman (1974) argued that synergy or antagonism between two or more causes of disease should be evaluated by a specific criterion that equated *independence of the causes* with the situation in which the *joint effect was equal to the sum of the separate effects*, with *effect* defined as "excess risk." In addition, he noted strongly the distinction between biological and statistical interaction, stating that biological interaction, in contrast with statistical interaction, could not be defined with arbitrariness in the choice of scale of measurement.

This initial articulation by Rothman (1974) brought forth an intense debate in which Walter and Holford (1978) argued that the selection of statistical models of independence is contingent on the specification of the causal models under consideration, which varied according to different etiologic situations. Furthermore, selection of a statistical model of independence may at times reflect statistically convenient properties of the model. Kupper and Hogan (1978) also argued persuasively that the existence of interaction is model-dependent. A subsequent report by Blot and Day (1979) noted the distinction between synergy and interaction and claimed that public health objectives need to be considered separately from, and given priority over, statistical objectives in assessing whether two agents are synergistic.

From this debate Rothman et al. (1980) distilled four broad contexts in which the concept of interaction should be discussed. One must be aware of the context in which one is working to effectively and clearly communicate in the area of interaction. These four broad contexts are *statistical, biological, public health,* and *individual decision-making.* Each of these contexts, according to Rothman et al. (1980), have different implications for the evaluation of interaction. It was argued by these authors that past disagreements, concerning the methodological principles needed to assess interaction derived from a failure to separate these four contexts.

*Statistical interaction* denotes the interdependence between the effects of two or more factors within the limits of a given model of risk. The assessment of the interaction depends on the model chosen. If the choice of model is entirely based on a desire for statistical convenience without consideration of biological mechanism, no scientific inference about biological interaction can be made (Walter and Holford, 1978; Kupper and Hogan, 1978). Clearly, the closer the mathematical model corresponds to the biological process, the more accurate the prediction.

*Biological interaction* is defined as "the interdependent operation of two or more causes to produce disease." Rothman et al. (1980) argued that if the biological model of interaction is explicit and its implications can be deduced, the issue of whether the causes act synergistically or independently is moot. Specification of the biological model replaces the purely abstract and vague concept of interdependence of effects with a specific form of interdependence that is testable. Furthermore, they state that little information about the biological process can be gathered from classifying the proposed biological mechanism as synergistic or independent. They provide the simple, yet relevant, example of the initiation–promotion model of carcinogenesis. In this example, assume that agent A increases the number of cells susceptible to carcinogen B, which can transform a susceptible cell into malignant cells. Thus, although both A and B contribute to the development of cancer, some may say they interact synergistically, whereas others may say they act independently. The key, as noted earlier, is better specification of the model. Two areas of considerable general interest are those in which etiologic factors act interchangeably in the same step of a multistep process or, alternatively, act at different steps in the process. These two broad categories are believed to correspond to mathematical models in which the effects of factors are additive or multiplicative, respectively.

*Public health interaction* is concerned with the number of cases of disease within a population and the proportional contribution of each risk factor to the case burden. For public health purposes, Rothman et al. (1980) indicate that interaction between risk factors is equivalent to a departure from additivity of incidence rate differences ("attributable risks"). Consider their example of the risk of lung cancer from two risk factors (i.e., smoking and asbestos). Assume that the risk of lung cancer is a defined period of time is 1:100 persons for those not exposed to either risk factor:

> Suppose that the risk for smokers who are not exposed to asbestos is 10 per thousand in the same time period. For those with asbestos exposure, the risks are three and 30 per thousand for nonsmokers and smokers, respectively. The risk ratio is identical for smoking (and for asbestos) at each level of the other risk factor. To some data analysts, this might indicate statistical or biologic independence, but for public-health applications it is not appropriate to consider the effects of smoking and asbestos as independent. The number of cases of lung cancer caused by cigarette smoking depends on how many of the smokers are also exposed to asbestos (or symmetrically, the number caused by asbestos depends on how many of those exposed to it are also smokers). Consequently, the public-health implications of the effects of smoking and asbestos depends on the proportion of the population in [whom] these factors occur jointly. No alternative exists to an additive criterion for evaluating independ-

ence of effects for the public-health viewpoint, as long as the public-health burden is directly proportional to the number of cases. (Rothman et al., 1980)

*Interaction in individual decision making* is considered to parallel that in public health decision making. Thus, departure from additivity of risk differences is the focus, regardless of the underlying biological mechanisms.

In summary, Rothman et al. (1980) concluded:

> In statistical contexts, independence and interaction may well be defined in an arbitrary manner. In biologic contexts addressing specific causal mechanisms, defining interaction or synergy between factors is unnecessary, since these terms do not enhance the intelligibility of a mechanism which is already specified in detail . . . . in public-health contexts synergy and antagonism should ordinarily be interpreted as departures from additivity of incidence rate differences, and analogously, in the context of individual decision-making, synergy and antagonism should ordinarily be interpreted as departures from additivity of risk differences.

## II. PHARMACOKINETIC AND PHARMACODYNAMIC FOUNDATIONS OF INTERACTIONS: A CONCEPTUAL OVERVIEW

### A. Temporal Factors and Toxic Endpoints

In testing of possible interactions, one must deal with several important considerations. These include temporal (time) factors and response–endpoint considerations (Murphy, 1980, 1983; NAS [National Academy of Sciences], 1980).

#### 1. The Time Factor

Although most screening tests for interactions employ simultaneous exposure, this type of exposure approach has the chance of reducing the likelihood of detecting some potential interactions, as, for example, when the two agents in question affect the same cellular mechanism to cause a toxic effect, but have markedly different times of onset. If a critical threshold of reversible cellular injury is required for the adverse effect, tests of acute toxicity of combinations given simultaneously may show antagonism, whereas an additive action may be seen if the dosing is spaced to cause the maximum effect. A specific example of this temporal influence relative to interaction is seen between initiators and promoters of chemical carcinogenesis. More specifically, dermal exposure to an initiating agent, such as benzo[*a*]pyrene must take place before the exposure to the promoter (e.g., croton oil) for the interaction to occur.

#### 2. The Toxic Effect

Since most toxic substances have multiple toxic effects, the nature of any chemical interaction may vary, depending on the response that one measures. For example, since chlorinated insecticides and halogenated solvents produce liver injury independently, they may be reasonably expected to act in an additive or synergistic manner when combined (Table 1). However, the insecticide is likely to be a central nervous system stimulant, whereas the solvent may be a central nervous system depressant. Thus, in this case, their joint action may result in an antagonistic response (Murphy, 1980, 1983).

### B. Chemical Interactions

There are numerous instances under which direct chemical-to-chemical interaction alters toxicological activity in both the medical–pharmaceutical (Griffin et al., 1988; Smith and Dodd,

**Table 1** Chemical and Biological Bases of Toxicant Interactions

| | Examples | |
|---|---|---|
| Basis of interaction | Synergism or potentiation | Antagonism |
| Chemical | Formation of nitrosamines from nitrites and amines | Dimethyl hydrazine reacts *in vivo* with pyridoxal phosphate (vitamin $B_6$) to form a hydrazone, thus rapidly depleting tissue stores of this enzymatic cofactor (Cornish, 1969) |
| Biological absorption | Neurotoxicity of EPN (o-ethyl o-p-nitropheny phenylphosphorothioate) enhanced by aliphatic hexacarbons due in part to increased skin absorption (Abou-Donia et al., 1985) | Dietary zinc inhibits lead toxicity in part by decreasing the percent dietary lead absorbed (Cerklewski and Forbes, 1976) |
| Distribution | Increased lead levels in brain after treatment with dithiocarbamate/thiuram derivatives (Oskarsson and Lind, 1985) | The mechanisms by which selenium protects against cadmium toxicity include decreasing the concentration of cadmium in liver and kidney and the redistribution of cadmium in the testes from the low-to-high molecular weight Cd-binding proteins (Chen et al., 1975) |
| Excretion | Decreased renal excretion of penicillin when co-administered with probenecid | Arsenic antagonizes the effects of selenium in part by enhancing the biliary excretion of selenium (Levander and Argrett, 1969) |
| Metabolism | Organophosphorous compounds (profenfos, sulprofos, DEF) potentiate the toxicity of fenvalerate and malathion by inhibiting esterase which detoxifies many pyrethroid insectides (Gaughan et al., 1980) | Selenium inhibits 2-acetylaminofluorene-induced hepatic damage and liver tumor incidence in part by shifting metabolism toward detoxification (ring hydroxylation) relative to metabolic activation (N-hydroxylation) Marshall et al., 1979) |
| Interaction at receptor sites (receptor antagonism) | No information available | Blocking of acetyl-receptor sites by atropine after poisoning with organophosphates |
| Interaction among receptor sites (functional antagonism) | No information available | Interaction of histamine and norepinephrine on vasodilation and blood pressure (antagonism) |
| Interaction at DNA | No information available | Induction of DNA repair by exposure to alkylating agents |

*Source:* EPA (1988).

1982; Smith, 1985) and environmental health (EPA, 1988) areas. On the environmental side, perhaps the interaction that has received the most attention is the formation of nitrosamines from nitrites and amines at low pH values in the stomach (Calabrese, 1980). The Environmental Protection Agency (EPA, 1988) reported the formation of arsine and stibine from ores containing arsenic and antimony, respectively, when they contact the strong acids of the stomach. Although these limited examples represent an enhancement of toxicity, the types of responses vary across the entire spectrum of response possibilities.

Chemical–chemical interactions have been extensively documented in the medical–pharmaceutical areas and include in vivo interactions, such as the use of chelating agents to complex with metal ions, the inactivation of heparin by binding to protamine, and the oral antidotal use of ammonia, which converts ingested formaldehyde to hexamethylenetetramine (Goldstein et al., 1974; EPA, 1988). Much concern has also been directed to the occurrences of in vitro drug interactions. According to Griffin et al. (1988), such interactions may be of considerable medical importance and may take place during the formulation of drugs to existing formulations (e.g., additives to intravenous fluids), or during storage of a formulation in its container (i.e., with container materials such as plastics). These authors indicate that, although the in vivo chemical interaction of drugs may be expected to result in either drug toxicity or drug inefficiency, the in vitro interaction almost always results in a diminished bioavailability (that is, reduced drug efficiency) during dosage. In their review, Griffin et al. (1988) provided information on types of in vitro drug interaction. These included (1) excipients in drug formulations; (2) additives to intravenous fluids; (3) drug–container interactions, especially those involving drug–plastics interactions; and (4) drug–contact lens interactions.

Excipients are additional ingredients, the function of which is to enhance the formulation of the active drug substance into a stable and uniform preparation with the necessary bioavailability and release characteristics. A wide range of pharmaceutical excipients exist and may compose the bulk of an oral dosage form. The spectrum of excipients includes aerosol propellants, antioxidants, binders, colors, disintegrants, fillers, flavors, lubricants, preservatives, solubilizers, solvents, surfactants, suspending agents, sweeteners, thickeners, and so on (Griffin et al., 1988). Even though these agents have generally been considered inert, numerous emerging examples have illustrated that modern synthetic excipients should not be considered inactive (Smith and Dodd, 1982; Smith, 1985). Examples in these papers indicted cases for which the excipient was toxic itself or modified the bioavailability of the active drug. There is the classic example given by Tyrer et al. (1970) that attributed the outbreak of phenytoin intoxication in Australia to a change in capsule fillers from calcium sulfate to lactate. This resulted in an increased dissolution rate, and increased bioavailability and toxicity.

Of particular current interest are emerging research concerns associated with toxic side effects of proprietary versus generic formulations. For example, Sanderson and Lewis (1986) have observed significantly more side effects (34.6 vs. 24.8%) in patients receiving a generic formulation (i.e., propranolol) as compared with those patients receiving the proprietary drug (Inderal). These authors suggested that the way in which the tablets were formulated may have been responsible for the difference in the incidence of side effects.

## C. Pharmacokinetic Interactions

### 1. Interactions Affecting Gastrointestinal Absorption

Numerous factors—such as acid–base balance in the gastrointestinal lumen, gut motility, and blood flow to the intestines—may affect absorption of xenobiotics (Prescott, 1969a,b, 1974; Griffin, 1981). From a practical perspective, it is important to differentiate between interactions that (1) enhance or diminish the *rate* of absorption and (2) enhance or decrease the *amount* of xenobiotic absorbed. According to Kristensen (1976), the rate of absorption is often not important for drugs exhibiting a long plasma half-life that are administered in multiple doses to achieve a steady-state concentration (e.g., warfarin, psychotherapeutics, and most antihypertensive drugs). However, a diminished rate of absorption may be important in a clinical situation when a quick onset of drug effect is desired.

*Acid–Base Balance and Drug Interaction.*   The passive absorption of drugs across the gastro-intestinal epithelium may be contingent on the hydrogen ion concentration (pH). For example, salicylic acid is absorbed, in experimental conditions, at a fivefold greater rate at pH 1 compared with pH 8 (Brodie, 1964). At pH 1 the salicylic acid is in a readily diffusible, nonionized, and lipid-soluble state. In contrast, acetylsalicylic acid is absorbed more rapidly in physiological situations from buffered alkaline solutions than from unbuffered solutions of pH 2.8 (Cooke and Hunt, 1970). This is most likely due to a greater dissolution rate of and aqueous solubility of acetylsalicylic acid in alkaline solution and in an increase in gastric-emptying rate at higher pH values (Kristensen, 1976).

Griffin et al. (1988) have noted that antacids and adsorbents that are frequently employed in drug pharmaceutical preparations may interact with a wide range of primary drugs affecting their absorption. Of potential clinical significance are interactions involving ferrous sulfate and antacid, isoniazid and antacid, and tetracyclines and antacid. These three interactions have been classified as ones having good evidence of actual or potential importance in patients or in relevant studies on normal subjects (D'Arcy, 1987).

The drug cimetidine, which is a $H_2$-receptor blocker, causes a rise in the gastric pH. This has resulted in its affecting the gastrointestinal absorption of several agents, including aspirin (Khoury et al., 1979) and tetracycline (Cole et al., 1980; Rogers et al., 1980).

*Gastric Emptying and Drug Interaction.*   Various drugs markedly alter the rate of gastric emptying. For example, Nimmo et al. (1973) reported that propantheline and metoclopramide delay and accelerate gastric emptying, respectively. Propantheline markedly diminishes the rate of acetaminophen (paracetamol) absorption, whereas, in contrast, metoclopramide enhances the rate of acetaminophen absorption. However, the total amounts of acetaminophen absorbed in both instances were similar. The anticholinergic drugs (e.g., atropine, hyoscine, tricyclic anti-depressants) and the opiates (e.g., morphine, codeine, pethidine) slow down gastric emptying and diminish the absorption of other ingested drugs.

*Binding and Chelating Mechanisms and Drug Interaction.*   Prescott (1969a,b) demonstrated that the salts of divalent or trivalent metals ($Ca^{2+}$, $Fe^{2+}$, $Mg^{2+}$, $Al^{3+}$) may interact with drugs in the intestine to produce insoluble and nonabsorbable complexes. Of particularly widespread interest is the example of the interaction between $Ca^{2+}$ and tetracyclines. The calcium phosphate filler markedly reduces the absorption of tetracycline. These interactions, of potential clinical significance, are avoidable if the drugs are given in properly spaced time intervals (Neuvonen and Turakka, 1974; Neuvonen, 1976). An interesting interaction has been described by Griffin et al. (1988), who noted that the gastrointestinal absorption of an oral dose of minocycline on tetracycline is particularly inhibited by food and milk. However, the absorption of minocycline was significantly less affected than tetracycline, indicating a possible explanation for why minocycline seems more effective than tetracycline in treating acne in teenagers who ingest large amounts of milk.

The anion-exchange resin cholestyramine binds acidic drugs, such as warfarin, and dimin-ishes the amount of warfarin absorbed (O'Reilly, 1974; Robinson et al., 1971). Again, temporal factors are important, since this interaction may also be avoided by giving warfarin an hour or more before the cholestyramine. Another chelating resin, colestipol, reduces the absorption of chlorothiazide (Kauffman and Azarnoff, 1973) and digitalis glycoside (Phillips et al., 1976).

An area of considerable interest is the influence of food on xenobiotic bioavailability and toxicity. For comprehensive reviews see D'Arcy and Merkus (1980), Toothmaker and Welling (1980), Welling (1980), and Welling and Tse (1982). A variety of factors may be simultaneously operational, including levels of divalent cations, protein, dietary fats, gastric emptying, bile flow, or other, that may alter normal absorption efficiencies.

## 2. Plasma Protein and Tissue Binding

Numerous drugs are extensively bound to plasma proteins, and it is the free (i.e., nonprotein-bound) drug fraction that displays pharmacological activity. An extensive literature now exists that indicates the displacement of a drug from its binding site on albumin by other drugs. The extent to which such interactions affecting plasma protein binding occur and have clinical relevance are discussed in detail elsewhere (Calabrese, 1991).

## 3. Metabolism

*Introduction.* Numerous agents, including commonly ingested drugs and ubiquitous environmental contaminants, stimulate the capacity of various metabolically active organs, especially the liver, to metabolize a wide range of chemical agents. Other compounds may inhibit the capability of the liver to metabolize pharmaceutical agents and environmental contaminants. The implications of being able to modify how the liver or other tissues metabolize potentially toxic agents are believed to be profound. In fact, it is now recognized that the insecticide synergists (i.e., agents that, when administered along with insecticides, markedly enhance the insecticide's ability to kill insects) act by blocking the enzymes normally effecting insecticide detoxification. For example, the toxicity of the insecticide carbaryl against susceptible female houseflies has been enhanced greater than 200-fold by certain chemical synergists. Here, therefore, is an example for which researchers are learning to predict the occurrence of chemical interactions based on an understanding of how insecticides are detoxified by the insect. In this example, they are using this knowledge to develop more effective formulations for exposing insects that may have developed resistance to the original insecticide, and they are also trying to find ways of using less insecticide, while still obtaining a highly effective insecticidal performance.

In the foregoing example, the investigators were attempting to use the concept of synergism to develop more efficient insecticidal formulations. However, the problem for public health agencies is different, in that they try to avoid human exposures to potentially dangerous mixtures. For example, in 1957, Frawley et al. reported the first synergistic interaction of two organophosphate insecticides (i.e., malathion and EPN), and this led to the development by the Food and Drug Administration (FDA) of regulations requiring that every newly registered organophosphate insecticide would have to be evaluated for possible synergisms with all registered organophosphate insecticides. As more organophosphate insecticides were developed, this regulatory requirement became an extreme testing burden. However, with the unfolding of the biochemical mechanism for this interaction, it became possible to assess possible interactions of organophosphate insecticides by biochemical means. This thereby circumvented the laborious and impractical toxicological testing of such possible interactions in whole animals without sacrifice to the protection of the public's health. Thus, in both examples—making a more efficient insecticidal preparation and predicting adverse public health effects from multiple agent exposures—predictions can be markedly enhanced with a clear understanding of the mechanisms of toxicity.

*Cytochrome P-450 Enzymes.* Since many, if not most, environmental toxins require bioactivation to highly reactive intermediate forms capable of causing a wide array of toxic cellular and molecular lesions, the importance of cytochrome P-450 enzymes in the development of environmentally induced diseases is theoretically profound. The cytochrome P-450 enzymes are involved in the oxidative metabolism of not only an enormous range of endogenous molecules, such as steroids, prostaglandins, and biogenic amines, among others, but also of innumerable drugs, chemical carcinogens, mutagens, and environmental contaminants. Given this critical role of cytochrome P-450 enzymes in the operation of phase I metabolism of xenobiotics of environmental concern, it is not surprising that genetic variations in P-450 enzyme activities and their relative capacities for induction are likely to markedly affect susceptibility to an enormous array of environmental contaminants. Consequently, the cytochrome P-450 enzymes are given a special distinction in this analysis of interaction factors affecting susceptibility to environmental agents. The field of P-450 molecular biology, according to Nebert and Gonzales (1987), has "literally exploded" in the current decade, with advances occurring in the multiple facets that surround P-450 research, such as chemicals that induce P-450 activities (Nebert, et al., 1981; Waterman and Estabrook, 1983), association of P-450 to cancer (Pelkonen and Nebert, 1982; Conney, 1982; Wolf, 1986; Conzalez et al., 1987), genetic differences in P-450 expression (Nebert et al., 1982), and others.

Since the 1980s, considerable progress has been made concerning the family of P-450 enzymes. In brief, the field of P-450 molecular biology has shown enormous expansion. For example, the first two P-450$_3$ cDNA probes were reported in 1980, and the first P-450 full-length cDNA sequence appeared in 1983. By 1986, there were 67 complete P-450 cDNA or protein sequences in eight eukaryotic species and one prokaryote. It is now known that there are ten P-450 gene families, eight of these existing in mammals. From the cDNA nucleotide sequencing, coherent theories of P-450 gene evolution have emerged (Nebert and Gonzales, 1987). In 1987, Nebert and Gonzales proposed a standardized P-450 gene nomenclature involving the use of Roman numerals and capital letters that facilitates the matching of previously characterized P-450 proteins with the newly defined gene families and subfamilies. The mammalian P-450 families are given as from I to VIII. For example, the P-450 I family in rats, rabbits, mice, and humans has two genes ($P_1$ and $P_3$) that rare inducible by polycyclic aromatic hydrocarbons (PAHs) and tetrachlorodibenzo-$p$-dioxin (TCDD). In essence, the human $P_1$ enzyme is what has been called aryl hydrocarbon hydroxylase (AHH) and is associated with the increased risk to cigarette smoking-induced bronchogenic carcinoma. In contrast with $P_1$, $P_3$ is highly correlated with cancer induced by 2-acetylaminofluorene and aminobiphenyls in animal models (Kamataki et al., 1983). The P-450 II gene family was initially referred to as the phenobarbital-inducible family. This gene family is now organized to comprise five subfamilies (A through E) with subfamily IID represented by debrisoquine 4-hydroxylase (P-450IID1). Within the IIE subfamily are at least two P-450 proteins that are induced by ethanol, imidazole, acetone, trichloroethylene, and pyrazole. According to Nebert and Gonzales (1987), the P-450 activity showing the highest induction rates includes the oxidation of aniline, alcohols, and nitrosamines. These authors anticipate the initiation of clinical studies attempting to correlate restriction fragment length polymorphism (RFLPs) patterns of these genes with individual risk of cancer. Relative to the P-450 III gene family, macrolide antibiotics, such as triacetyloleandromycin and griseofulvin, induce at least one gene of this family. Nebert and Gonzales (1987) suggest that clinical studies of the human orthologues of these P-450 III genes are likely to yield important insights for predicting macrolide antibiotic response or toxicity caused by these agents. The hypolipidemic peroxisomal proliferators (e.g., clofibrate) are found within the P-450 IV gene family. They induce a protein (P450LA$w$) that displays a total lack of immunocross-reactivity with P-450s induced by polycyclic hydrocarbons or phenobarbital.

The principal point here is that, within the unfolding of our understanding of the P-450 system, lies a major foundation for predicting toxic chemical interactions. The major advances, as just summarized, are providing a coherent framework for understanding the biochemical responses of the individual to complex arrays of chemical exposures. Often the literature reports are simply descriptive; that is, compound A induces a form of cytochrome P-450 that enhances the metabolism of compound B. More recently, the data are beginning to link such induction with a specific family of cytochrome P-450. With this type of specificity, it is possible to begin developing theoretical constructs for the prediction of interactions.

## 4. *Interactions at Receptor Sites and Critical Cellular Targets*

According to Griffin et al. (1988), xenobiotic agents may interact by antagonizing each other at the same receptor site (competitive antagonism) or at separate, but physiologically related, sites (physiological antagonism). There are also instances in which a drug interacts with its own metabolite at a common receptor. Although previous mechanisms of interactions affecting absorption, distribution, excretion, and metabolism that principally affect the amount of toxicant reaching the primary receptor have yielded both antagonistic and synergistic responses, interaction at the receptor site is generally believed to yield antagonistic interactions (e.g., histamines and antihistamines, including $H_2$-blockers, atropine and cholinergic drugs, morphine and nalorphine). As stated over 30 years ago by Veldstra (1956):

> ... we may say that the effect of a combined action of two compounds at the same site of primary action will not result in a synergism, but will, generally, even be unfavorable. The competition for the receptor will usually decrease the frequency of the best interactions, and with decreasing intrinsic activity of one of the components the combined action will more and more take the form of a competitive antagonism.

## 5. *Excretion*

Several general mechanisms exist by which xenobiotic interactions are affected by renal excretory processes. The two mechanisms of greatest importance involve passive reabsorption and active secretion. Under normal circumstances, a non–protein-bound xenobiotic often undergoes glomerular filtration and becomes progressively concentrated as water is reabsorbed along its passage through the nephron. A concentration gradient is thus created and, if the xenobiotic is lipid-soluble and capable of permeating the tubular epithelium, the agent will be passively reabsorbed back into systemic circulation.

One of the key features in the study of drugs is that many are weak electrolytes, with the degree of ionization of the drug being determined by the pH of the renal environment. It is now well established that weak bases are excreted more rapidly when the urine has a low pH, and more slowly at high urinary pH, whereas the reverse is true for weak acids. Griffin et al. (1988) indicated that the effects of pH in the renal environment on the excretion of weak electrolytes is of clinical importance if the $pK_a$ value of the drug is in the range of about 7.5–10.5 for bases and 3.0–7.5 for acids, and if a significant proportion of the drug is normally excreted unchanged in the urine.

The link to chemical interactions is that one agent may affect the excretion pattern of another by affecting the pH of the renal environment. The classic example of such a pH-mediated interaction concerns administration of sodium bicarbonate during amphetamine treatment. The sodium bicarbonate treatment increases the pH, and this will delay the excretion of the amphetamine, a weak base. More specifically, approximately 30–40% of a dose of amphetamine is excreted in the urine as unchanged drug over 48 h under normal circumstances of fluctuating urinary pH. If the urine is made more acidic (pH 5) for the same 48-h period, the proportion of unchanged drug excreted is increased to 60–70%.

The second major excretory mechanism involved in renal excretory interactions involves active secretion in the proximal tubule. Numerous drugs are secreted by the proximal convoluted tubule. Offerhaus (1981) indicated that drug interactions can be expected if drugs that are principally secreted by the proximal convoluted tubule are given simultaneously. Griffin et al. (1988) noted that the plasma half-life of penicillin may be increased by a variety of drugs, including probenecid, which is a well-known interaction, and also by aspirin, phenylbutazone, sulfonamides, indomethacin, thiazide diuretics, furosemide, and ethacrynic acid.

## III.  CARCINOGENESIS

## A.  Introduction

That the process of carcinogenesis can be modified significantly by other chemical agents has long been known. The ways in which such modulation occurs are extremely diversified and numerous. Over the past decade, concepts such as cocarcinogenesis and promotion have become significantly clarified as a result of advances in our understandings of the carcinogenic process, but also more complex as the intricacies of highly diversified processes are revealed. This section will provide an introduction to the concepts of carcinogenesis, promotion, and syncarcinogenesis, including terminology and definitions, as well as operational characteristics and mechanistic differences.

## B.  Cocarcinogenesis

The term *cocarcinogenesis* was initially defined as the enhancement of neoplasm induction brought about by noncarcinogenic factors that act in conjunction with an initiating carcinogen (Berenblum, 1974; Sivak, 1979). Cocarcinogenesis thereby encompassed several kinds of enhancements, including promotion, during which the enhancing agent facilitates tumorigenesis following completion of initiation. Despite this broad conceptual framework, cocarcinogenesis has been operationally differentiated from promotion as the enhancement of carcinogenicity resulting from the administration of a modifying agent either just before or together with a carcinogen, with *promotion* referring to enhancement caused by an agent administered after a carcinogen. Such a conceptual distinction is of considerable usefulness, since it provides differentiation between the enhancement of the process of neoplastic conversion by cocarcinogenesis and the enhancement of neoplastic development by promotion. At the level of mechanism, cocarcinogenesis may be viewed as "the enhancement of carcinogenesis resulting from effects produced either immediately before or during carcinogen exposure or at a time after carcinogen exposure when chemical damage is still persistent" (Williams, 1984).

Differentiating the action of a cocarcinogen from a promoter can, at times, be difficult. For instance, promoters, like cocarcinogens, can enhance cancer development when administered along with a carcinogen. Under such conditions of exposure, it is hard to discern whether the enhancement of carcinogenesis is caused by the cocarcinogenic or the promotional activity. Williams (1984) believes that such agents should be considered promoters unless it can be shown that the process of neoplastic conversion is enhanced.

A variety of possible nongenotoxic mechanisms have been proposed through which cocarcinogens may operate (Williams, 1984). These could include (1) increased uptake of the carcinogen, (2) increased proportion of carcinogen activated, (3) depletion of competing nucleophiles, (4) inhibition of the rate or fidelity of DNA repair, and (5) enhancing conversion of DNA lesions to permanent alterations. Specific examples of cocarcinogens exist, including the carcinogenic capacity of ferric oxide to enhance the occurrence of benzo[*a*]pyrene-induced lung neoplasms in hamsters (Saffiotti et al., 1968). In this instance, it is believed that the mechanism of ferric oxide cocarcinogenesis involves the facilitated uptake of the carcinogen by bronchial epithelial cells (Kennedy and Little, 1974) and pulmonary alveolar macrophages (Autrup et al., 1979). However, the mechanism of cocarcinogenesis may vary according to the specific circumstances. For example, ferric oxide is believed to enhance the carcinogenesis of diethylnitrosamine (DEN; Montesano et al., 1970; Feron et al., 1972) by enhancing the effects of the interaction of the DEN with cellular constituents (Williams, 1984).

Other important ways by which chemical cocarcinogens act are through the inhibition of detoxification, or by enhancing the activation of genotoxic carcinogens. Berry et al. (1977) have provided an example of the first mechanism. Here, the carcinogenicity of polycyclic aromatic hydrocarbons is enhanced by trichloropropane oxide. This agent inhibits the enzyme epoxide hydrolase that inactivates the reactive epoxide of the carcinogens. Relative to the activation mechanism is the action of enzyme inducers; for example, ethanol enhances the hepatocarcinogenesis of vinyl chloride (Radiki et al., 1977) and *n*-nitrosopyrrolidine (McCoy et al., 1981).

It has been suggested that cocarcinogens may also cause their effects by the inhibition of DNA repair. However, Williams (1984) indicated that most agents that inhibit repair do so in a nonspecific manner that also diminishes replicative synthesis. Consequently, there is a longer overall interval available for repair before replication; therefore, the reduced repair has not usually been associated with an increased yield of permanent alterations in DNA. However, agents that act specifically on DNA repair processes (e.g., 3-aminobenzamide) have increased the effect of hepatocarcinogenic agents (Takahashi et al., 1982).

## C. Syncarcinogenic Effects

The additive or synergistic effects of two or more carcinogens in neoplasm production has been defined as *syncarcinogenesis* (Nakahara, 1970; Schmahl, 1970). Syncarcinogenesis may occur when two carcinogens are given either in a sequential form (Odashima, 1959), or concurrently (MacDonald et al., 1952). Williams (1984) has emphasized that these two forms of syncarcinogenesis may have different mechanisms and may be distinguished from initiation–promotion concepts of carcinogenesis. Promotion and carcinogenesis have been distinguished from syncarcinogenesis on the basis that the cocarcinogen or promoter is theoretically considered noncarcinogenic. From a mechanistic perspective, the principal difference is that cocarcinogens and promoters are not genotoxic. Furthermore, in sequential syncarcinogenesis, the order of treatment can be reversed and the effect still occurs (Williams and Furuya, 1984). This is not the situation with either cocarcinogenesis or promotion unless the agent has properties of both types of processes, and the exposure to the chemical is close to that of the carcinogen to be able to produce cocarcinogenesis.

The phenomenon of syncarcinogenesis has been reported in various organs, including the skin (Steiner, 1955); liver (MacDonald et al., 1952); and bladder (Deichmann et al., 1965a,b). The syncarcinogenic effect occurs when both agents have the same target organ (Schmahl, 1980).

## D. Tumor Promotion

### 1. Introduction

The concept of tumor promotion was first brought forward by John Hill in 1761 in the publication *Cautions Against the Immediate Use of Snuff* (Boutwell, 1974). Hill notes that "whether or not [cancers], which attend Snufftakers are absolutely caused by that custom, or whether the principles of the disorder [nose cancer] were there before, and Snuff only initiated the parts, and hastened the mischief, I shall not pretend to determine; but even supposing the latter only to be the case, the damage is certainly more than the indulgence is worth; for who is to say, that the Snuff is not the absolute cause, or that he has not the seeds of such a disorder which Snuff will bring into action." Thus, Hill was not only the first to propose a cause for cancer that remains with us today, but also he proposed the possibility of more than one causative agent, with snuff acting as what modern toxicology calls a promoter to "bring into action . . . the seeds of the disorder."

The first major experimental advance occurred in 1915, when Yamagiwa and Ichikawa demonstrated that a similar lesion could be produced by the repeated treatment of coal tar condensate to the ears of rabbits (Yamagiwa and Ichikawa, 1915). Three years later Tsutsui

(1918) reported that mice were also responsive, developing skin cancer after repeated exposure to coal tar. Since the coal tar treatment produced inflammation and wounds, it was considered that continuous or repetitive irritation may cause cancer. Subsequent studies by Rous and Kidd (1941) and Friedwald and Rous (1944) further clarified the role of irritation, wounding, and the resulting stimulation of rapid cell division in the process of tumor formation. In fact, they employed a two-stage technique for the development of skin tumors in rabbits. They reported that agents and procedures that cause hyperplasia (e.g., turpentine, chloroform, and wounding) often enhanced the occurrence of tumors caused by a prior treatment with methylcholanthrene or tar. In their reports, Rous and colleagues (1941) emphasized the tumor initiation to describe action of the carcinogen to create "latent tumor cells" that would then be later revealed by subsequent administration of the same skin with a nonspecific tumor-enhancing factor. These authors referred to this process as *tumor promotion*. Subsequent research by Berenblum (1941) ushered in the modern era by his discovery that croton oil promoted the development of 3,4-benzpyrene-induced skin cancer in mice, and Mottram (1944), who noted that benzpyrene needed to be applied only once in a small subcarcinogen dose to have tumors elicited by the promotional action of croton oil.

The concept of tumor promotion, therefore, has had a long history, but was principally derived from the early experimental research of Rous, Berenblum, and Mottram. In these studies it was found that a single application of coal tar or a polycyclic hydrocarbon to the skin of rabbits or mice in subcarcinogen amounts would initiate the process of skin carcinogenesis if it were followed by a promotional event.

From the historical and voluminous subsequent research, operational criteria have been defined to describe the characteristics of a promoter in the mouse skin model (McGee, 1987). These criteria are

1. That it should not be carcinogenic per se
2. That it should not increase tumor yield if administered before the initiating carcinogen
3. That when applied after an initiating, subcarcinogenic dose of the carcinogen, it should accelerate the rate of development of tumors and, thus, increase the total, time-related tumor incidence
4. That the total yield of tumors produced should be dose-related to the initiator, not to the promoter, providing the promoter is used in excess of the minimum amount required to promote all initiated cells
5. That, unlike initiation, which can take place rapidly during a single exposure to the initiator and which is a permanent event, promotion requires long exposure to the promoter before the changes induced become irreversible

These criteria, as noted by McGee (1987), have been the guideline for the application of the concept of promotion to tumor induction in other organs, including the liver, bladder, and colon.

Given the foregoing description of the historical foundations of promotion action and the operational criteria, it is possible to define the term tumor promotion. Tumor promotion may be operationally defined as: the process by which an agent brings about the selective expansion of initiated cells that increase the probability of malignant transformation. From a mechanistic perspective, this expansion of initiated cells is the result of altered gene expression induced by the presence of a promoting agent.

## 2. Mechanism

The promotional agent for which biochemical effects have been best characterized is the phorbol ester 12-*O*-tetradecanoylphorbol-13-acetate (TPA). When normal fibroblasts are exposed in culture to TPA, there occurs a "mimicry of transformation." In other words, when normal cells are exposed to TPA, they display many properties of cells stably transformed by oncogenic viruses or chemical carcinogens. More specifically, the cells look morphologically transformed, cell-to-cell orientation is lost, saturation density increases, serum requirements decrease, protease plasminogen activator is increased, ornithine decarboxylase and polyamine syntheses are increased, and transport of deoxyglucose and certain ions is enhanced, along with decreased calcium requirements. In addition, tumor promoters, such as TPA, inhibit terminal differentiation. Given that tumors characteristically display aberrant differentiation, this represents a particularly significant property of tumor promoters. From these collective observations, Weinstein (1980) proposed a coherent hypothetical scheme for how a promoter, such as TPA, may act. He maintained that the cell surface represents a signaling mechanism that enables the cell to respond to extracellular environments. Hormones or agents like TPA lock onto very specific receptors that then modify the flow of signals from the cell surface to the cytoplasm and nucleus. Although initiating agents act at the level of DNA, such alterations are often insufficient to produce malignant transformation. According to Weinstein (1980), it is necessary to reprogram the cell's previous pattern of gene expression to produce a cancer cell. As for TPA, it is believed that its reprogramming function acts through modifications at the cell surface. The reprogramming would likely result in altered differentiation, such that terminal differentiation is blocked and cells are set forth into a type of exponential division. Such a process leads to the promotion of a clone of initiated cells subsequent to a benign tumor, thereby setting the stage for variant cell progression to a malignant tumor.

## ACKNOWLEDGMENT

This paper was based on material published in the book *Multiple Chemical Interactions,* Calabrese, E. J., 1991, Lewis Publishers, Chelsea, MI.

## REFERENCES

Autrup, H., C. C. Harris, P. W. Schafer, B. F. Trump, G. D. Stonner, and I. Hsu (1979). Uptake of benzo[*a*]pyrene–ferric oxide particulates by human pulmonary macrophages and release of benzo[*a*]pyrene and its metabolites, *Proc. Soc. Exp. Biol. Med.,* 161, 280–284.

Berenblum, I. (1941). The cocarcinogenic action of croton resin, *Cancer Res.,* 1, 44.

Berenblum, I. (1974). *Carcinogensis as a Biological Problem* (A. Neuberger and E. L. Tatum, eds.), American Elsevier, New York.

Berry, D. L., T. J. Slaga, A. Viaje, N. M. Wilson, J. DiGiovanni, M. R. Juchau, and J. K. Selkirk (1977). Effect of trichloropropene oxide on the ability of polyaromatic hydrocarbons and their "K-region" oxides to initiate skin tumors in mice and to bind to DNA in vitro, *JNCI,* 58, 1051–1055.

Blot, W. J., and N. E. Day (1979). Synergism and interaction: Are they equivalent? [letter], *Am. J. Epidemiol.,* 110, 99–100.

Boutwell, R. K. (1974). The function and mechanism of promoters of carcinogenesis. *Crit. Rev. Toxicol.,* 2, 419–433.

Brodie, B. B. (1964). Physico-chemical factors in drug absorption. In *Absorption and Distribution of Drugs,* (Binns, ed.), Livingston, Edinburg, pp. 46–48.

Calabrese, E. J. (1980). *Nutritional and Environmental Health,* Vol. 1, *The Vitamins,* John Wiley & Sons, New York.

Calabrese, E. J. (1991). *Multiple Chemical Interactions,* Lewis Publishers, Chelsea, MI, pp. 704.

Cole, J. J., B. G. Charles, and P. J. Ravenscroft (1980). Interaction of cimetidine with tetracycline absorption, *Lancet* 2, 536.

Conney, A. H. (1982). Induction of microsomal enzymes by foreign chemicals and carcinogenesis by polycyclic aromatic hydrocarbons: G. H. A. Clowes Memorial Lecture, *Cancer Res.,* 42, 4875–4917.

Cooke, A. R., and J. N. Hunt (1970). Absorption of acetylsalicyclic acid from unbuffered and buffered gastric contents, *Am. J. Dig. Dis.*, 15, 90–102.

D'Arcy, P. F. (1987). Drug interactions and reactions update. Drug–antacid interactions: Assessment of clinical importance. *Drug Intell. Clin. Pharm.* 21 (cited in Griffin et al., 1988).

D'Arcy P. F., and F. W. H. M. Merkus (1980). Food and drug interactions: Influence of food on drug bioavailability and toxicity, *Pharm. Int.*, 1, 238–244.

Deichmann, W. B., J. Radomski, E. Glass, W. A. D. Anderson, M. Coplan, and F. Woods (1965a). Synergism among oral carcinogens. III. Simultaneous feeding of four bladder carcinogens to dogs, *Ind. Med. Surg.*, 34, 640–649.

Deichmann, W. B., T. Scotti, J. Radomski, E. Bernal, M. Coplan, and F. Woods (1965b). Synergism among oral carcinogens. II. Results of the simultaneous feeding of bladder carcinogens to dogs, *Toxicol. Appl. Pharmacol.*, 7, 657–659.

[EPA] Environmental Protection Agency (1988). Technical support document on risk assessment of chemical mixtures. U. S. EPA Environ. Criteria and Assessment Office. Office of Health and Environmental Assessment, U. S. EPA, Cincinnati, OH.

Feron, V. J., P. Emmelot, and T. Vossenaar (1972). Lower respiratory tract tumours in Syrian golden hamsters after intratracheal instillations of diethylnitrosamine alone and with ferric oxide, *Eur. J. Cancer*, 8, 445–449.

Frawley, J. P., H. Fuyat, E. Hagan, J. Blake, and O. Fitzhugh (1957). Marked potential in mammalian toxicity from simultaneous administration of two anti-cholinesterase compounds, *J. Pharmacol. Exp. Ther.*, 121, 96–106.

Friedwald, W. F., and P. Rous (1944). The initiating and promoting elements in tumor production, *J. Exp. Med.*, 80, 101–125.

Goldstein, A., L. Aronow, and S. M. Kalman (1974). *Principles of Drug Action: The Basis of Pharmacology*, 2nd ed., John Wiley & Sons, New York.

Gonzalez, F. J., A. K. Jaiswal, and D. W. Nebert (1987). P-450 genes: Evolution, regulation, and relationship to human cancer and pharmacogenetics, *Cold Spring Harbor Symp. Quant. Biol.*, 51, 879–890.

Griffin, J. P. (1981). Drug interactions occurring during absorption from the gastrointestinal tract, *Pharmacol. Ther.*, 15, 79–88.

Griffin, J. P., P. F. D'Arcy, and C. J. Speirs (1988). *A Manual of Adverse Drug Interactions*, 4th ed., John Wright & Sons.

Kamataki, R., K. Maeda, Y. Yamazoe, N. Matsuda, K. Ishii, and R. Kato (1983). A high-spin form of cytochrome P-450 highly purified from polychlorinated biphenyl-treated rats, *Mol. Pharmacol.*, 24, 146–155.

Kauffman, R. E., and D. L. Azarnoff (1973). Effects of colestipol on gastrointestinal absorption of chlorothiazide in man, *Clin., Pharmacol. Ther.*, 14, 886–890.

Kennedy, A. R., and J. B. Little (1974). The transport and localization of benzo[*a*]pyrene–hematite and hematite–po in the hamster lung following intratracheal instillation, *Cancer Res.*, 34, 1344–1352.

Khoury, W., K. Geraci, and A. Askari (1979). The effect of cimetidine on aspirin absorption, *Gastroenterology*, 76, 1169.

Kristensen, M. B. (1976). Drug interactions and clinical pharmacokinetics, *Clin. Pharmacokinet.*, 1, 351–372.

Kupper, L. L., and M. D. Hogan (1978). Interaction in epidemiologic studies, *Am. J. Epidemiol.*, 108, 447–453.

Macdonald, J. C., E. C. Miller, J. A. Miller, and H. P. Rusch (1952). The synergistic action of mixtures of certain hepatic carcinogens, *Cancer Res.*, 12, 50–54.

McCoy, G. D., S. S. Hecht, S. Katayama, and E. L. Wynder (1981). Differential effect of chronic ethanol consumption on the carcinogenicity of *N*-nitrosopyrrolidine and *N*-nitrosonorcinotine in male Syrian golden hamster, *Cancer Res.*, 41, 2849–2854.

McGee, P. N. (1987). Comments for the EPA workshop on risk assessment methodologies for tumor promotion, U. S. EPA, Washington, DC, pp. C35–C40.

Montesano, R., U. Safiotti, and P. Shubik (1970). The role of topical and systemic factors in experimental respiratory carcinogenesis. In *Inhalation Carcinogenesis* (M. G. Hanna, P. Nettesheim, and J. R. Gilbert, eds.), Proc. Biol. Div., Oak Ridge National Laboratory, Oak Ridge, TN, p. 353.

Mottram, J. C. (1944). A developing factor in experimental blastogenesis. *J. Pathol. Bacteriol.,* 56, 181.

Murphy, S. D. (1980). Assessment of the potential for toxic interactions among environmental pollutants. In *Principles and Methods in Modern Toxicology* (C. L. Galli, et al., eds.), Elsevier/North Holland-Biomedical Press, Amsterdam, pp. 277–294.

Murphy, S. D. (1983). General principles in the assessment of toxicity of chemical mixtures, *Environ. Res.,* 48, 141–144.

Nakahara, W. (1970). Mode of origin and characterization of cancer. In *Chemical Tumor Problems* (W. Nakahara, ed.), Japanese Society for the Promotion of Science, Tokyo, pp. 287–330.

National Academy of Sciences (NAS). (1980). Predicting effects from chemical mixtures. National Academy Press, Washington, DC.

Nebert, D. W., H. J. Eisen, M. Negishi, M. A. Lang, and L. M. Hjeimeland (1981). Genetic mechanisms controlling the induction of polysubstrate monoxygenase (P-450) activities, *Annu. Rev. Pharmacol. Toxicol.,* 21, 431–462.

Nebert, D. W., and F. J. Gonzales (1987). P-450 genes: Structure, evolution, and regulation, *Annu. Rev. Biochem.,* 56, 945–993.

Nebert, D. W., M. Negishi, M. A. Lang, L. M. Hjeimeland, and H. J. Eisen (1982). The *Ah* locus, a multigene family necessary for survival in a chemically adverse environment: Comparison with the immune system, *Adv. Genet.,* 21, 1–52.

Neuvonen, P. J. (1976). Interactions with the absorption of tetracyclines, *Drugs,* 11, 45–54.

Neuvonen, P. J., and H. Turakka (1974). Inhibitory effect of various iron salts on the absorption of tetracycline in man, *Eur. J. Clin. Pharm.,* 7, 357–360.

Nimmo, J., R. C. Heading, P. Tothill, and L. F. Prescott (1973). Pharmacological modification of gastric emptying: Effects of propantheline and metoclopromide on paracetamol absorption, *Br. Med. J.,* 1, 587–589.

Odashima, S. (1959). Development of liver cancers in the rat by 20-methylcholanthrene painting following initial 4-dimethylaminoazobenzene feeding, *Gann,* 50, 321–345.

Offerhaus, L. (1981). Drug interactions at excretory mechanisms, *Pharmacol. Ther.,* 15, 45–68.

O'Reilly, R. A. (1974). Drug interactions involving oral anticoagulants, *Cardiovasc. Clin.,* 6(2), 23–41.

Pelkonen, O., and D. W. Nebert (1982). Metabolism of polycyclic aromatic hydrocarbons: Etiologic role in carcinogenesis, *Pharmacol. Rev.,* 34, 189–222.

Phillips, W. A., J. M. Ratchford, and J. R. Schultz (1976). Effects of colestipol hydrochloride on drug absorption in the rat, *J. Pharm. Sci.,* 65, 1285–1291.

Prescott, L. F. (1969a). Pharmacokinetic drug interactions, *Lancet,* 2, 1239–1243.

Prescott, L. F. (1969b). Drug absorption interactions—gastric emptying. In *Drug Interactions* (Morselli, Garattini, and Cohen, eds.), Raven Press, New York, pp. 11–20.

Prescott, L. F. (1974). Drug adsorption interactions—gastric emptying. In *Drug Interactions,* (Morselli, Garattini, and Cohen, eds.), Raven Press, New York, pp. 11–20.

Radiki, M. S., K. L. Stemmer, P. G. Brown, E. Larson, and E. Bingham (1977). Effect of ethanol and vinyl chloride on the induction of liver tumours: Preliminary report, *Environ. Health Perspect.,* 21, 153–155.

Robinson, D. S., D. M. Benjamin, and J. J. McCormack (1971). Interaction of warfarin and nonsystemic gastrointestinal drugs, *Clin. Pharmacol. Ther.,* 12, 491–495.

Rogers, H. J., F. R. House, P. J. Morrison, and I. D. Bradbook (1980). Interaction of cimetidine with tetracycline absorption, *Lancet,* 2, 694.

Rothman, K. J. (1974). Synergy and antagonism in cause–effect relationships, *Am. J. Epidemiol.,* 99, 385–388.

Rothman, K. J. (1976). Synergy and antagonism in cause–effect relationships, *Am. J. Epidemiol.,* 103, 506–511.

Rothman, K. J., S. Greenland, and A. M. Walker (1980). Concepts of interaction, *Am. J. Epidemiol.,* 112, 467–470.

Rous, P., and J. G. Kidd (1941). Conditional neoplasms and subthreshold neoplastic states: A study of tar tumors of rabbits, *J. Exp. Med.,* 73, 365–390.

Saffiotti, U., F. Cefis, and L. H. Kolb (1968). A method for the experimental induction of bronchogenic carcinoma, *Cancer Res.,* 28, 104–124.

Sanderson, J. H., and J. A. Lewis (1986). Differences in side-effect incidence in patients on proprietary and generic propranolol, *Lancet,* 1, 967, 968.

Schmahl, D. (1970). Syncarcinogenesis: Experimental investigations. In *Chemical Tumor Problems* (W. Nakahara, ed.), Japanese Society for the Promotion of Science, Tokyo, p. 1018.

Schmahl, D. (1980). Combination effects in chemical carcinogenesis, *Arch. Toxicol. Suppl.,* 4, 29–40.

Sivak, A. (1979). Cocarcinogenesis, *Biochim. Biophys. Acta,* 560, 67–89.

Smith, J. M. (1985). Appendix 2, Adverse reactions attributed to pharmaceutical excipients. In *Textbook of Adverse Drug Reactions,* 3rd ed. (D. M. Davies, ed.), Oxford University Press, Oxford, pp. 726–742.

Smith, J. M. and T. R. P. Dodd (1982). Adverse reactions to pharmaceutical excipients, *Adverse Drug React. Acute Poisoning Rev.,* 1, 93–142.

Steiner, P. E. (1955). Carcinogenicity of multiple chemicals simultaneously administered, *Cancer Res.,* 15, 632–635.

Takahashi, S., T. Ohnishi, A. Denda, and T. Y. Konishi (1982). Enhancing effect of 3-aminobenzamide on induction of $\gamma$-glutamyl transpeptidase positive foci in rat liver, *Chem. Biol. Interact.,* 39, 363–368.

Toothmaker, R. D., and P. G. Welling (1980). The effect of food on drug bioavailability, *Annu. Rev. Pharmacol. Toxicol.,* 20, 173–199.

Tsutsui, H. (1918). Uber das kunstlich erzcugte cancroid bei der maus, *Gann,* 12(2), 17.

Tyrer, J. H., M. J. Eadie, J. M. Sutherland, and W. D. Hooper (197)). Outbreak of anticonvulsant intoxication in an Australian city, *Br. Med. J.,* 2, 271–273.

Veldstra, H. (1956). Synergism and potentiation, *Pharmacol. Rev.,* 6, 339–367.

Walter, S. D., and T. R. Holford (1978). Additive, multiplicative, and other models for disease risks, *Am. J. Epidemiol.,* 108, 341–346.

Waterman, M. R., and R. W. Estabrook (1983). *Mol. Cell. Biochem.,* 53/54, 267–278.

Weinstein, B. (1980). Evaluating substances for promotion, cofactor and synergy in the carcinogenic process, *J. Environ. Pathol. Toxicol.,* 3, 89–101.

Welling, P. G. (1980). Effect of food on bioavailability of drugs, *Pharm. Int.,* 1, 14–18.

Welling, P. G., and F. L. S. Tse (1982). The influence of food on the adsorption of antimicrobial agents, *J. Antimicrob. Chemother.,* 9, 7–27.

Williams, G. M. (1984). Modulation of chemical carcinogenesis by xenobiotics, *Fundam. Appl. Toxicol.,* 4, 325–344.

Williams, G. M., and K. Furuya (1984). Distinction between liver neoplasm promoting and syncarcinogenic effects demonstrated by reversing the order of administering phenobarbital and diethylnitrosamine either before or after *N*-2-fluorenylacetamide, *Carcinogenesis,* 5, 171–174.

Wolf, C. R. (1986). Cytochrome P-450s: Polymorphic multigene families involved in carcinogen, *Trends Genet.,* 2, 209–214.

Yamagiwa, K., and K. Ichikawa (1915). Experimental study of the pathogenesis of carcinoma, *J. Cancer Res.,* 3, 1.

# 19

# Interaction: An Epidemiological Perspective for Risk Assessment

**Kenneth A. Mundt**
*University of Massachusetts*
*Amherst, Massachusetts*

**Carl M. Shy**
*University of North Carolina*
*Chapel Hill, North Carolina*

## I. INTRODUCTION

Interaction in epidemiological research theoretically occurs if two or more causal factors in a population act together in some way to produce an event, usually disease or death, at a rate greater or less than would be expected if the effects of each of these risk factors were summed. In other words, interaction results if the causes of a disease do not operate independently of each other.

Despite the apparent straightforwardness of this concept, and the numerous scientific fields (such as toxicology, pharmacology, genetics, and others) already accommodating this and closely related phenomena, epidemiologists have not yet resolved many of the controversies pertaining to interaction, which were briskly debated in the late 1970s and early 1980s. Until epidemiologists reach general consensus on the concept of interaction and more broadly subscribe to standard approaches to the assessment and interpretation of interaction, other health professionals reading and interpreting the epidemiological literature face a great challenge. At the heart of this challenge lie several major issues, some of which remain unclear to many epidemiologists. These include the following:

1. Lack of a standard terminology describing and differentiating among subtle conceptual variations related to interaction in epidemiology
2. Inadequate appreciation of the many forms of interaction that operate within epidemiological research, their causes, implications for study validity, and interpretational consequences
3. Failure to plan for assessment of interaction at the design phase of epidemiological studies, often limiting the capability to adequately address interaction after the study is completed
4. Disagreement on the proper analytical methods to apply in the assessment of interaction
5. Limited guidance available on how to interpret either the presence or absence of interaction in a given study

The purpose of this chapter is to acquaint the reader with the various epidemiological perspectives on interaction and to provide the necessary background to allow a reasonable evaluation of interaction in an epidemiological study.

For risk assessment, the identification of risk factors participating in an interaction should be of great interest and utility. In the chapter entitled "Evaluation of Epidemiologic Information" in the text, *Epidemiology and Health Risk Assessment,* Szklo acknowledges that interaction has only recently become one of the concerns of epidemiologists. Szklo notes that this recent interest is in contrast with the extensive attention given the notion of susceptible subgroups in toxicology, citing Dahl's classic studies of genetic susceptibility or resistance to salt-induced hypersensitivity in rats (Dahl et al., 1960). Szklo suggests that discrepancies between epidemiological studies might be due to undetected interactions, and that interaction should be an integral part of study hypotheses (Szklo, 1988). Furthermore, identification of interaction may be of practical interest, as the effect attributable to a given factor may be considerably larger (or smaller) in the presence of one or more additional risk factors. In other words, failure to account for the interaction will result in an underestimation (or overestimation, in the case of an antagonism) of risk. Conversely, intervention of risk factors that operate interdependently with other factors should lead to preventive benefits greater (or less) than would be gained if the factors acted independently (Bulterys et al., 1990; Wacholder and Weinberg, 1986).

Unfortunately, several issues remain to be resolved before epidemiologists or risk assessors may fully benefit from even a modest grasp of the concepts and methods. At present, many obstacles severely limit the valid interpretation of interaction within epidemiological research to elucidate mechanisms involved in the pathological process.

## II. OPERATING ASSUMPTIONS

Epidemiology is subject to numerous methodological and interpretive challenges and pitfalls (such as study design options, various selection and information biases, confounding, random and systematic measurement error, and so on), the discussion of which is beyond the scope of this chapter. Therefore, most of the discussion on interaction to follow assumes that the epidemiological studies described in terms of their interaction, are free from any serious or "fatal" flaws, and that the study results are otherwise valid. It is further assumed that the reader is reasonably familiar with the principles of basic epidemiology, including, as a minimum, the following: study designs, such as cohort and case–control (and their relative strengths, weaknesses, and range of applications); measures of disease occurrence, including estimates of absolute and relative risk; identification and prevention of selection bias and information bias; the role of random error, or chance; the identification, control, and interpretation of confounding data. Readers not familiar with these might wish to consult one of several available introductory epidemiology texts (Hennekens et al., 1987; Kelsey et al., 1986).

## III. TERMINOLOGY AND DEFINITIONS

In this chapter, the term *interaction* is used generically to indicate all forms and perspectives of both observed nonindependence and theorized interdependence of causal factors. However, numerous terms have been and continue to be used throughout the field. Some of these will be defined in the next section, not to suggest a standard usage, but rather, to expose the reader to the range of terms and perspectives likely to be encountered in the epidemiological literature.

Some confusion arising out of the epidemiological literature on interaction no doubt stems from the lack of standardized terms and definitions for various aspects of interaction, or "nonindependence" among two or more risk factors for a disease outcome. There are several possible reasons for the current lack of consensus among epidemiologists. One main reason is that methodological epidemiology has enjoyed only a relatively short history of about three decades, with most of the quantitative advancements formalized only in the latter half of this period. This relative youth of quantitative epidemiological concepts and methods results in general inexperience with them, and subsequently the "preferred" terminology for various phenomena have not been finally decided. Because other scientific fields had addressed interaction-related issues previously, epidemiology has imported some of this terminology. With borrowed terms, however, come borrowed concepts and definitions, some of which may not be entirely compatible with their new application. For example, "synergism" has historically been used to describe the joint effect of two or more factors when neither factor alone produces an effect. In common epidemiological usage, *synergism* is synonymous with any positive interaction.

Another explanation for the apparent confusion is related to the inherent dualism of interaction in epidemiology, eloquently differentiated by Miettinen as "*ontological* and *epistimological*" aspects. Although this specific point will be discussed throughout the chapter, its relevance to the present topic of terminology will be described briefly here. Ontologically, interaction in epidemiology refers to and reflects the true nature, or "cooperation" of two or more factors or agents that act together physically, chemically, or biologically. Although the specific mechanism of this interaction may not be known, it is believed to cause the outcome (disease) of interest beyond that caused by either or both factors individually, and includes effects entirely caused by the joint action. However, this true nature may not be inferred from epidemiological research (Miettinen, 1982). Epidemiological terminology most closely related to this perspective of interaction includes effect modification, synergism, and antagonism, although terms such as biological interaction, causal interdependence, and preventive interdependence have been used.

Epistemologically, interaction in epidemiology has to do with the ways in which joint effects are detected, measured, and interpreted from observational data. These aspects are distinct from joint actions among true causes mentioned in the foregoing paragraph in that the methods for assessing interaction in epidemiology are limited to the manipulation and analysis of observational data, representing an entire range of possibilities from "true" interaction effects, to spurious effects caused by possible biases (including confounding bias, selection bias, information bias) and measurement error. Perhaps one of the most important influences distancing epidemiological assessment of interaction from elucidating true causal interdependencies is the widespread reliance on surrogate and indicator measures for underlying or unknown causal parameters. Many of these variables may be intercorrelated in complex and indirect ways and, when considered in the context of a multivariate analysis, may behave nonindependently. To interpret this interedependence as interaction among causal factors (i.e., ontologically), would be mistaken. The most common term reflecting this category of interaction is *statistical interaction*.

Many epidemiologists do not differentiate between these two realms of interaction in epidemiology, or identify the specific context in which a particular term is used, and terms are often used interchangeably. Much of the confusion and controversy surrounding interaction in epidemiology stems from, and is reflected by, this indiscriminate use of terminology. For this reason, qualifiers or modifiers will clarify how terms used in this chapter are being used. For example, the term *interaction* may be modified to specify "interaction among true causes" or "observed interaction among risk indicators."

## A. Definitions

Several common definitions for terms used in epidemiology to describe interaction are presented in the following from *A Dictionary of Epidemiology,* 2nd ed., edited by John Last (1988). The dictionary compiled the definitions and views of nearly 140 contributing and corresponding editors, among them many of the leading names in epidemiology. Although various definitions are available in textbooks and published articles, this single source should most closely represent a consensus among epidemiologists. Nevertheless, several ambiguities remain, as will be discussed further.

As a starting point, it seems useful to describe interaction's complement, or what in general interaction *is not,* i.e., independence.

> *independence:* two events are said to be independent if the occurrence of one is in no way predictable from the occurrence of the other. Two variables are said to be independent if the distribution of values of one is the same for all values of the other. Independence is the antonym of association. (Last, p. 64)

Note that this definition chooses to address the issue of independence in two contexts: the relationship between *events* and between *variables.* Both reflect an applied epidemiological perspective in that they are based entirely on observed qualities or behaviors. No inference is made, however, as to how, or if, the true underlying causes of the events or the measured variables (which are mathematical representations of attributes) act entirely separately to produce the observed effects, or if some other explanation (such as measurement error) produced the appearance of independence. Furthermore, the distinction between independent distribution (i.e., a factor is distributed in the population without consideration of the distribution of the other factors) and independent action (two or more factors act identically in either the presence or absence of the other factors) should be highlighted.

We have chosen interaction as the most generic term to describe phenomena—biological and statistical—but caution the reader to consider the range of ways in which this term continues to be used. The three different view points expressed in the dictionary definition below reflect this generic quality:

> *interaction:*
> 1. The interdependent operation of two or more causes to produce or prevent an effect. *Biological interaction* means the interdependent operation of two or more causes to produce, prevent or control disease
> 2. Differences in the effects of one or more factors according to the level of the remaining factor(s)
> 3. In statistics, the necessity for a product term in a linear model (Last, p. 68).

The first part of the definition focuses specifically on causes producing or preventing a nonspecified event, or in the case of biological interaction, producing, preventing, or controlling a disease. In contrast with the definition provided for independence, this definition does not necessarily address what can be observed in an epidemiological study. Kleinbaum et al. (1982) argued that "biologic interaction can be characterized only in terms of experimentally verifiable biologic models describing modes of action of substances at the cellular level." They further chose to avoid using the term interaction to describe the mechanisms of causes.

The second part describes what epidemiologists commonly call "effect modification." For convenience in discussion, and because of the overlapping meanings of effect modification and the second definition of interaction, the definition for effect modification is presented here:

*effect modifier/modification:* A factor that modifies the effect of a putative causal factor under study. Effect modification is detected by varying the selected effect measure for the factor under study across levels of another factor (Last, p. 41).

Both the definition of effect modifier and description number two of interaction accommodate an epidemiological perspective in that it describes what has been observed without any inference about the biological or chemical interdependence of causes. However, the definitions avoid (rather than clarify) an area of confusion in the epidemiological literature by not identifying the specific context—either the population base or simply in the study database—in which the interaction operates (Miettinen, 1974). Specific terms for these distinct phenomena include "population interaction" (Kleinbaum et al., 1982) for the population-based effect, and "statistical interaction" (Checkoway, et al. 1989) for the data-based effect. Interestingly, in their respective epidemiology textbooks, Kleinbaum et al. chose to use the term interaction for both effects, whereas Checkoway et al. selected effect modification for both, noting that both effect modification and statistical interaction are merely statistical concepts (in contrast with biological or causal) that depend upon the statistical methods used to evaluate them (Checkoway et al., 1989).

To illustrate the continuing confusion, and lack of consensus within epidemiology for these specific terms and their interpretation, consider two recent publications. First, in the introductory chapter of *Introduction to Occupational Epidemiology,* Hernberg views the importance of identifying effect modifiers as a matter of study validity: "in order to give a more complete picture of the nature of the occurrence relation" (Hernberg, 1992). However, effect modification is mentioned only once subsequently, and that in the context of an example illustrating possible effect modification by smoking of an association between carbon disulfide exposure and coronary heart disease. Hernberg states, "Scrutinizing such possible effect modification could help shed more light on the mechanism whereby carbon disulfide contributes to the causation of CHD" (Hernberg, 1992). Although this example also illustrates complications in the interpretation of observed effect modification, this aspect will be discussed later.

A second example, directly related to risk assessment, comes from a chapter called "Biomarkers" by Nauman et al. in a new text, *Environmental Epidemiology and Risk Assessment.* In this chapter, biomarkers of susceptibility are described as "indicators of an inherent or acquired limitation of an organism's ability to respond to the challenge of exposure to a specific xenobiotic substance" (Nauman et al., 1993). Subsequently, these susceptibility markers—which clearly address biological or physiological qualities and are not simply statistical concepts—are equated with effect modifiers (Naumann et al., 1993; Hulka, 1990).

The third part of the foregoing interaction definition describes one statistical context, that of a linear regression. Because interaction may be assessed statistically on any mathematical scale—not just linear—this definition is incomplete and potentially misleading. Narrowly speaking, if effect modification were to be statistically evaluated in the context of a linear regression, then an interaction term, defined as the product of two (or more) of the model's independent terms, may improve the fit of the model to the data, depending on the nature of the interdependence, and on how the terms are measured and coded.

An additional pair of terms—synergism and antagonism—has been used variously to describe the directionality of specific examples of both biological and statistical interaction. Although there is usually little confusion over the direction of the effect of interaction described by these terms, the context is unclear, as epidemiologists use the terms to describe biological and chemical mechanisms (Kleinbaum et al., 1982) as well as statistical relationships (Rothman, 1974, 1976a,b, 1986; Hertz-Picciotto et al., 1992).

After acknowledging that the definition of synergism has been controversial in epidemiology, the following are offered in the dictionary:

*synergism:*

1.   A situation in which the combined effect of two or more factors is greater than the sum of their solitary effects.
2.   In bioassay, two factors act synergistically if there are persons who will get the disease when exposed to both factors but not when exposed to either alone (Last, p. 127).

*antagonism:*

1.   The situation in which the combined effect of two or more factors is smaller than the solitary effect of any one of the factors.
2.   In bioassay, the situation in which a specified response is produced by exposure to either of the two factors but not by exposure to both together (Last, p. 6).

Note that the first definitions for each of these terms are not specific relative to the context (biological or statistical), whereas the second addresses biological interactions. The first definitions are also not entirely congruous in that the reference point for synergism is the sum of the solitary effects, whereas the reference point for antagonism is any one of the factors. Thus, the definition for antagonism does not allow for partial antagonism, where the combined effect of two or more factors is greater than any solitary effect, but less than their combined effects. This latter definition appears to be common in epidemiological applications (Rothman, 1976a,b).

Finally, there occasionally exists an oddity in epidemiological assessment of interaction in which an observed effect (between one factor and the outcome, such as an occupational exposure and the incidence of bladder cancer) appears positive, or harmful, for one level of the second factor (such as for males), but for the other level (females) the factor is *protective* of bladder cancer. This situation has been called a crossover effect, or qualitative interaction (Thompson, 1991).

An alternative way to refer to the evaluation of interaction in an epidemiological study is an assessment of joint effects. This term is attractive in that it does not assume any biological or statistical relationship, and includes all possibilities such as positive and negative effect modification (or synergism or antagonism), as well as independence. In evaluating and describing joint effects in statistical terms, however, modifiers clearly identifying the mathematical scale are required. One disadvantage of the term joint effects (which is not defined in the dictionary) is that it connotes and in some ways denotes the simultaneous consideration of exactly two terms, whereas the assessment of interaction may involve any number of factors.

Because only a modest proportion of all epidemiological studies take into consideration some aspect of interaction, and these attempts often use terminology and methods differently, and interpret results inconsistently, the resulting impression may be that interaction is either unimportant or incompletely understood. Since this lack of solidity in the field is reflected in the main textbooks as well as the published scientific literature, students of epidemiology do not acquire a firm grasp of the concepts and terminology; therefore, the application of methods and interpretation of results also vary. One first step toward improving our understanding of interaction, and enhancing our appreciation of its importance, would be to establish a standard terminology, and clearly differentiate between specific concepts and terms as they apply to epidemiology. With a more concerted effort toward a standard terminology, and more widespread application, a greater range of experience with various aspects of interaction will be generated. This experiential base will allow epidemiological methodologists to determine the true practical usefulness of assessing interaction in epidemiological data, in terms of improving study validity and elucidating disease processes and mechanisms, a notion that currently remains largely theoretical.

## IV. CONCEPTS OF INTERACTION IN EPIDEMIOLOGY

Although interaction and related phenomena have been recognized in various medical and health-related sciences, such as toxicology and pharmacology, the conceptual and methodological basis for interaction in epidemiology remained undeveloped until the 1970s. At that time, much discussion and debate over epidemiological theories of causality inevitably led to the consideration of the causal action of more than one etiological factor. Schools of thought in epidemiology diverged at this time, possibly as epidemiology evolved between, and somewhat out of, two often discordant realms: medicine, with a focus on the individual and on specific biological and pathological processes; and population mathematics, which addresses phenomena—biological or statistical—on groups of individuals. Modern epidemiology owes much to each perspective, and it is not difficult to see how two or more contentious views on interaction each might have gained reasonable support. The tension between observational methods and biological mechanisms was illustrated in the description and definition of interaction-related terminology in the foregoing.

Another aspect of the evolution of epidemiological methods that has contributed to the distancing of the biological mechanisms from the epidemiological methods comes from the proliferation of high-powered and complicated analytical techniques. These tools, such as logistic, poisson, and other nonlinear multivariable regression techniques, have been made possible only through the rapid advances made in computer technology. Now, every epidemiologist, whether adequately prepared to use such tools appropriately or not, has access to advanced analytical procedures on microcomputers that previously were available only on costly mainframe computer systems. With the advent of these procedures in epidemiology, and appropriate recognition of their tremendous positive potential, came an infatuation with them, and often an abandonment of the usual cautious and deliberate analytical approach. In these situations, the desire to apply an available analytical method might win over the need to employ a model that best describes the biological or other relationships among various measures or parameters of interest.

Throughout the early development of epidemiological concepts of interaction it is not clear to what extent the relationships observed in epidemiological research mimicked the underlying disease mechanisms. Although it is now known that concordance may be disappointingly poor, epidemiologists have been, and continue to be, optimistic that their study measures, including those of exposures and potential confounding variables, validly represent the phenomena of interest. Perhaps the first key to concordance between the epidemiological representation of population-based associations and the relevant underlying biological mechanisms is the degree to which the epidemiologist has directly and validly measured the appropriate causal factor. The second key, that of selecting the appropriate mathematical model to represent the relationship, will be discussed later.

In his classic paper entitled "Causes," Rothman established a simple conceptual model for multicausality of disease that has survived as a paradigm in epidemiology (Rothman, 1976a). Rothman's model, which used causal pies to represent sufficient causes, or specific combinations of component causes (pie slices) that, in an individual, are sufficient to lead to inception of disease. It is possible that, more than any other single reason, this conceptual model provided a basis for all epidemiologists to consider the range of roles individual risk factors might play in the etiology of disease, ultimately leading to divergent perspectives on and controversy over the proper assessment and interpretation of interaction.

Throughout the presentation, illustration and discussion of Rothman's causal model, all component causes are referred to as true-risk factors for a specific outcome and, therefore, the model, though highly useful for improving our understanding of the possible variety of relationships among multiple causal factors, remains theoretical. In practice, epidemiologists usually measure what is convenient or easy to measure, as surrogate measures for the "true" risk factors. This is especially common if the true risk factors are unknown. Furthermore, for most disease processes, the full range of component causes for any sufficient cause are likely to be unknown, and assessment of the relationship among risk indicators is limited to those recognized and measured. The result is that the theoretical model can rarely be determined through observational studies. Nevertheless, epidemiologists continue to describe the relationships among their measured variables as if they were directly measured causal factors, and the observed relationships (depending on how closely they indicate the true causal factors) may have little bearing on the biological relationship among the true component causes.

From these causal pies, Rothman proposed a set of definitions for various possible interrelationships among risk factors for disease (component causes), including independence, complete synergy, combinations of synergy and independent action, as well as antagonism. Specifically, *independence* was described as the scenario in which two causes are components of two different sufficient causes, but are not comembers of any other sufficient causes for the same disease. Thus, these component causes act (in conjunction with other component causes of the respective sufficient causes) independently of each other. Synergy is described by two component causes within the same sufficient cause, neither having any effect without the other present. If neither component cause serves as a component cause within other sufficient causes, the entire effect can be described as *complete synergy:* that is, neither has an independent role in determining risk. Technically, by definition, all component causes for a specific sufficient cause act synergistically; that is, no effect results unless all component causes are present. On the other hand, what is most often observed is something *less than complete synergy,* which can be described in this model as the combination of synergism and independent action, stemming from one or both of the component causes participating both in the synergy and acting as a component cause in one or more other sufficient causes. *Antagonism,* according to this model, would be represented by a pie in which one of the component causes might consist of one or the other of two factors, but not both of the two factors (in which case the component cause and, therefore, the sufficient cause, would not be satisfied, and the disease would not occur).

This conceptual model is attractive because of its simplicity, but also because of its ability to be extended to describe highly complex situations. At a very basic level, outcome or disease risks associated with various sufficient causes may be contrasted and compared. If such contrasts are carefully selected, it is at least theoretically possible to isolate and quantify the risk of the disease attributable to a specific causal factor. Although the concept of attributable risk generally oversimplifies the true interrelationships probably operating among component causes of a disease, it does provide a baseline, or default, value of expectation under the assumption that a given factor operates independently of other causes.

This baseline value can then be compared with the observed level of risk as an indicator of interaction. For example, suppose the risk of some cancer in an occupational population exposed to factor A, as measured by the cumulative incidence in this population, is 4:100,000 per year. We can assume that this observed risk estimate reflects the combination of risk from all sufficient causes among the population (background risk), plus at least one sufficient cause in which A participates. If we examine the incidence of this same cancer in a population not exposed to A, we can assume that this rate (say 1:100,000 per year) represents the combination of risk from all causes, except that of A. Often, such comparison rates are obtained from the general U. S. population, when it is reasonable to assume that the exposure of interest is rare in the general population. To obtain the amount of risk attributable to A among those exposed to A, the background risk from the general population referent is subtracted from the risk observed among those exposed to A, leaving a quantity known as attributable risk, or absolute risk (in this example, 3:100,000 per year). A clear assumption of this measure is that A operates independently of all other background causal factors present. Unfortunately, there is no practical way that this assumption can be verified, especially if no specific causes of the disease are known.

After extending this approach to a second occupational risk factor or exposure of interest (factor B), the default independent relationship may be quantified in terms of absolute or attributable risk. If the incidence of disease within a population exposed to B (and for simplicity, not to A; likewise, that those who were exposed to A were not also exposed to B) is 2.5:100,000 per year, then the absolute or attributable risk due to B may be estimated as 1.5:100,000 per year by subtracting the background risk of 1:100,000 per year. If we then assume that A and B act completely independently of each other to cause the cancer, then the best estimate of the risk expected among a subpopulation exposed to both A and B would be 5.5:100,000 per year, estimated as the sum of the background (1:100,000 per year) and the absolute risk from A (3:100,000 per year) and the absolute risk from B (1.5:100,000 per year). If the risk of disease among persons exposed to both A and B is observed to be different from that expected, this would detract from the null hypothesis of independence.

## V.  EVOLUTION OF METHODS FOR ASSESSING INTERACTION

In 1976, Rothman popularized the direct assessment of interaction between two factors by developing and publishing an intuitive method for estimating the degree of interaction present between two (or more) factors in an epidemiological study (Rothman, 1976a). This approach, first introduced in 1974, differed from the then prevailing method of eliminating interactions "by adept transformations of scale" in that it dealt with, rather than avoided, the possible interaction (Rothman, 1976a). The need to characterize and measure interaction was justified, according to Rothman, for purposes of completeness in describing causal relationships, which "warrants evaluation of synergy or antagonism as part of the general description leading to full elaboration, in principle, of the determinants of a given effect" (Rothman, 1976a). He further postulated that as more risk factors for disease were identified, epidemiologists would increasingly turn to the question of interaction.

The measure proposed by Rothman, was an index ($S$) derived from the ratio of the joint effect (of factors A and B) observed in a study to the joint effect hypothesized under the hypothesis of no interaction, or independence, as follows:

$$S = \frac{R_{11} - R_{00}}{R_{10} + R_{01} - 2R_{00}}$$

where

$R_{11}$ represents the risk (incidence) among individuals with both factors A and B.

$R_{00}$ represents the risk among individuals with neither factor.

$R_{10}$ represents the risk among individuals with factor A, but not factor B.

$R_{01}$ represents the risk among individuals with factor B but not factor A.

For relative risk estimators, including the odds ratio obtained from a case–control study, a variation of this formulation can be derived (by dividing both sides of the equation by the background risk, $R_{00}$):

$$S = \frac{RR_{11} - 1}{RR_{10} + RR_{01} - 2}$$

where

$RR_{11}$ represents the risk among individuals with both factors A and B, relative to those with neither factor.

$RR_{10}$ represents the risk among individuals with factor A only, relative to those with neither factor.

$RR_{01}$ represents the risk among individuals with factor B only, relative to those with neither factor.

Values of $S$ substantially exceeding unity indicate synergism, values substantially less than unity indicate antagonism, and for values at or near unity, no interaction is present. Note that the default relationship between A and B, indicating no interaction, is additive.

Shortly after this method was published, several other authors elaborated on the concepts, and extended the methodologies with new statistics. Increasing attention was paid to the assessment of interaction among variables measured on continuous scales as well as categorically, but other than the typical (0,1) coding. Concurrently, issues pertaining to the mathematical scale on which variables were evaluated (such as additive or multiplicative), and the implications on interaction assessment moved to the forefront.

For example, Koopman criticized Rothman's conceptualization and model for interaction as being incomplete, and offered examples of additional sources which might produce interaction in epidemiological studies (Koopman, 1977). In 1981, Koopman published a paper on interaction between discrete causes, in which he supported the choice of a model of additive risks as the most reasonable. By using the interaction contrast of disease rates (ICDR) proposed by Hogan et al. for detecting interaction in the additive model, Koopman demonstrated that values for this measure (ICDR) are always zero (or slightly negative) when the assumption of no interaction in Rothman's sufficient-component discrete causes model holds (Koopman, 1981; Rothman, 1976a). Thus, Koopman advocated the use of the ICDR as a screening tool for interaction, suggesting that more specific models to describe and elucidate the relationship between discrete causes be sought when values for ICDR differ from zero. Furthermore, he cautioned against using multiplicative models, despite their "statistical convenience" of producing relative measures of association, in screening for interaction. Specifically, Koopman noted that, although positive interaction on a multiplicative scale always indicates positive interaction on an additive scale, the situation of obtaining an indicator for negative interaction on a multiplicative scale might be interpreted on an additive scale in various cases as negative interaction, no interaction, or possible even weak positive interaction (Koopman, 1981).

In the same year, Walker (1981) broadened the perspective in which the assessment of interaction might prove to be useful as a basis for making decisions about personal risk or public health interventions. Noting that decisions for risk are subject to interactions present, Walker proposed an approach, based on the additivity of attributable risk, that would indicate the extent to which information on one factor (for example, B) must be taken into account concomitantly when making a decision involving the risk associated with A. The suggested measure, called the index of interaction, takes a value of zero if information on B is irrelevant (i.e., B is independent) and a value of 1 if no rational decision could be made *without* information on B. Walker's method, however, does not address the relevance of the interaction model to identify plausible mechanisms of disease production, but does reflect the additivity inherent to decision-making criteria, such as net expected value or attributable risk (Walker, 1981).

Concurrently, Siemiatycki and Thomas (1981) addressed the issue of which biological relationship might be inferred from epidemiological studies demonstrating interaction. Specifically, they cited three examples published in the epidemiological literature in which the relation between the individual relative risks for two risk factors and their joint effects was multiplicative: cigarette smoking and alcohol consumption as risks for esophageal cancer, as well as cigarette smoking and ionizing radiation, and cigarette smoking and asbestos as risk factors for lung cancer. The authors argue that although it is tempting to use these examples to support certain multistage models of carcinogenesis, the use of such epidemiological evidence could arise from a variety of scenarios. By using a simple representation of the multistage theory of carcinogenesis, they demonstrate, with a simulation approach, that two carcinogens, each having no effect on the other's mode of action (i.e., independent actions), might nevertheless lead to additive, multiplicative, or other statistical relationship (Siemiatycki and Thomas 1981).

Despite this fairly early recognition of the severe limitations in the interpretation of, and the biological inference that can be drawn from, interactions detected in epidemiological data, many epidemiologists and biostatisticians continued to attempt to refine the quantitative methods for the assessment of interaction. Many of the papers published during the 1980s fell into one of the following topical categories, each reflecting a major area of debate and controversy: selection of multiplicative versus additive scale; power and efficiency of interaction assessment; coding and types of variables involved; regression techniques and alternatives; and biological inference. Some of these issues are discussed further in the following.

In several papers, Greenland (1983, 1985, 1993; Greenland and Poole, 1988; Greenland and Morgenstern, 1989; Greenland and Robins, 1986; Thomas and Greenland, 1985) addressed statistical aspects of interaction assessment, focusing mainly on power and efficiency in the context of two binary risk factors. Greenland reviewed a number of tests, both additive and multiplicative, used to evaluate interaction in epidemiological studies. In general, he concluded that the power of the tests, under commonly encountered situations, was very low, and that several of the statistics performed poorly, rendering many of them useless (Greenland, 1983). He did reiterate that the power of tests for interaction were much improved if instead of two binary variables, risk factors were measured on a continuous scale; however, additional difficulties arose. Specifically, with continuous factors, assessment of joint effects must also specify the shape of the dose–response relationship. In a later paper, Greenland (1985) presented and illustrated some general methods for determining power, sample size, and smaller detectable effects for epidemiological studies addressing multiple risk factors simultaneously, under assumptions of both additive and multiplicative models. Thomas and Greenland (1985) examined the more specific scenario of assessing interaction in case–control studies matching on one of the factors involved in the possible interaction. Interestingly, they found that in nearly all situations, efficiency was lost by matching. Other disadvantages of matching, relative to interaction assessment, included loss of ability to estimate the main effect of the matching variable, inability to fit nonmultiplicative models, and (as in any closely matched case–control study) increased restrictiveness in selecting controls.

The late 1980s also produced numerous epidemiological publications on a diversity of quantitative approaches to assessing interaction in epidemiological studies. Many of these papers explored various criteria for determining the "best" mathematical model for the evaluation of interaction. Breslow and Storer (1985) proposed a family of parametric relative risk functions that covered a range from subadditive to supramultiplicative, by varying the exponent in a power transformation for the log relative risk. In an example showing interaction between cigarette smoking and alcohol consumption and the development of esophageal cancer based on three different relative risk models (additive, intermediate, and multiplicative), they demonstrate that the choice of model greatly influences the results. For example, under the additive model, heavy alcohol consumption is associated with an extremely high risk of cancer, regardless of smoking category (which implies independence). However, the interaction between these two factors appears to be quite striking under the multiplicative model. Ironically, the additive, multiplicative, and a range of intermediate models appeared to fit the data about equally well. The authors noted that the observed quantitative differences have profound implications for the mechanistic interpretation of these results and for any public health intervention or recommendation. More recently, Coughlin et al., (1991) compared additive and multiplicative attributable risk models and presented improved additive-model methods for use when an additive approach is determined to be appropriate based on goodness-of-fit evaluation. In a very recent paper, Greenland (1993) revisited the context of matched case–control studies, and demonstrated that, in stratified studies, additive relative risk models do not assure the absence of causal interaction, or departure from additivity.

Moolgavkar and Venzon (1987) reviewed several different parametric families of general relative risk functions, and noted that results were often based on the way in which even binary covariates were coded. Greenland and Poole (1988) further demonstrated that the effects of interdependent factors can vary with the choice of the referent category, but that "reference-invariant properties of joint effects" exist that may be studied, even if the appropriate referent category is not obvious.

Thus, it is evident that development of epidemiological methods for assessing interaction will continue, as will the debate and controversy. Despite the sophistication of biostatistical techniques available to epidemiologists for the detection and evaluation of interaction in epidemiological research, there has not been a parallel development in the understanding of the concepts underlying joint effects observed. The next section will look at several of the ways in which interactions in epidemiological studies might arise and the subsequent difficulties in drawing biological inference from these occurrences.

## VI. SOURCES OF INTERACTION IN EPIDEMIOLOGY

The need to describe (preferably quantitatively) what has been observed in an epidemiological study represents an epidemiological approach somewhat different from clinical and toxicological research, which examines the action of a treatment randomly assigned to groups of participants. These groups, because of the randomization, are intended to be identical except for the treatment. The action of the treatment is often understood in terms of biochemistry or other mechanism, and the experiment is conducted to conform or fail to confirm the anticipated action. At a minimum, the treatment is clearly identified as the main factor in the experiment, and reasonably valid measures of dose may be available. In contrast, much of epidemiological research sets out to describe what is observed among human populations, often not driven by an understanding of the mechanisms of action, and sometimes without knowing which, if any, of the study measures are the main risk factors. From this fairly statistical perspective, description of a relation among indicators of risk (which is usually all we have) may or may not reflect a similar relation among underlying causal factors. In fact, it is possible, if not likely, that no such true relation exists, and that what was observed represents an artifact of the methodology. Proper interpretation of these situations is difficult, partly because of difficulties differentiating between true and artifactual effects, among all observed effects.

The debates that took place over the concepts and methods of assessing interaction in epidemiological research largely reflect these two diverse epidemiological approaches: the clinical–toxicological and the statistical–descriptive. As discussed earlier, some of the confusion surrounding interaction may be attributed to the blurring of these perspectives. Even in Rothman's pioneering descriptions of interaction among causes (using component and sufficient causes), discussion was limited to true causes, and did not elaborate on the nearly inevitable use of risk indicators and surrogate measures in epidemiological studies. In differentiating between confounding and effect modification (the form of interaction addressed), Rothman described confounding as occurring only in the context of a particular study, and specifically not representing an inherent relation among variables. In contrast, he described effect modification as the inherent characteristic of the relation between two causes of an effect, and a possibly useful way to describe nature (Rothman, 1976a,b)

In his recent commentary, Thompson (1991) reiterates this state of affairs, and concludes that "definitive conclusions regarding synergistic and antagonistic effects are generally beyond our grasp." Nevertheless, in this review, Thompson does attempt to identify a core conceptual and interpretive issue in the interest of unifying the field with respect to interaction assessment, and urges epidemiologists to (1) recognize the limitations of our methods, (2) give careful consideration to possible mechanisms when evaluating individual factors, and (3) to exercise "extreme caution" when considering interactions.

Possible sources of interaction in epidemiological studies may be divided into two broad theoretical categories: those reflecting true interactions operating among causal factors in the mechanisms of the disease process; and those arising out of the way in which the factors involved in the interaction were selected, measured, evaluated, or interpreted. In practice, however, it is usually impossible to differentiate between these sources. One exception may be when a specific mechanism of interaction is known, and the factors involved are correctly identified, measured, and analyzed in the epidemiological study, in which case, the interaction assessment may reflect the underlying biological or causal interaction.

## A. Biological–Causal Mechanisms

The following theoretical models are used to illustrate how various forms of causal interaction may be expressed in an epidemiological study if parameter measures are correctly identified and validly measured. These examples assume that the epidemiological study had adequate power to detect the interaction and are free from other methodological and analytical problems such as bias caused by selection of study participants, differential quality of information collected, or failure to control for confounding.

### 1. Sufficient-Component Cause Model

Rothman's causal model, discussed previously, states that when all component causes (pie slices) of a sufficient cause (causal pie) are present, the outcome inevitably results. Under this model, two risk factors, or component causes, participating in different sufficient causes, will have independent (additive) effects. For interaction to occur, two component causes must be part of the same sufficient cause, each factor having no individual effect without the presence of the other factor (Rothman, 1974, 1976a,b). Illustrating this model with examples of component causes makes it clear that the model is highly accommodating of various causal mechanisms. For example, sufficient causes for a given outcome (disease) might include host factors (such as genetic susceptibility, immunity, nutritional status, or other), environmental factors (such as environmental exposures, pollutants or agents, physical attributes of the environment, such as heat, humidity, noise, radiation, and so on), or events along a pathogenic process. Essentially any aspects contributing to the disease process may be considered component causes of a disease, and the number of potential component causes is limitless (Koopman, 1981). However, this generic model does not specify *how* or *when* each component cause might act, and the application of this model to epidemiological data becomes problematic. For example, if the component causes of a sufficient cause have a necessary temporal sequence, then two individuals with the same factors or exposures, but in a different order, will have different disease experiences.

Koopman further pointed out that under the sufficient-component cause model, two component causes may not always appear to interact in an epidemiological investigation. They will appear to interact when all other component causes are present except for the two (or more) risk factors under study. When both factors are present, the outcome will occur, but not when either one alone is present. On the other hand, in the situation for which one of the study risk factors participates in one or more other sufficient causes, no interaction may be seen in the presence of both, as only one of the two factors completes that sufficient cause. Finally, if both component causes are present, but some other component cause is missing, no disease will result, and consequently no interaction between causes will be detected (Koopman, 1981).

## 2. Toxicological–Chemical Interaction

Perhaps the most straightforward scenario in which interaction occurs is when two or more chemical agents combine, or their effects combine, resulting in a joint effect much greater than, or different from, that expected if each acts independently (Weinberg, 1986). For example, numerous dramatic drug interactions are known in which each pharmaceutical agent has a beneficial action on health individually, but in combination result in a serious side effect, possibly including death (Calabrese, 1991).

Perhaps the classic example of chemical interaction most often used to illustrate interaction in epidemiological research is the joint effect of asbestos and cigarette smoking on the incidence of lung cancer. Relative to nonsmokers with no exposure to asbestos, individuals with asbestos exposure alone experience roughly a fivefold increase in risk of lung cancer; individuals with smoking exposure alone have a tenfold increase; and among those with both exposures simultaneously, risk is elevated about 50-fold—far exceeding the expected increase of about 14 times if these two operated independently (i.e., if the excess risks were additive). Other examples of interaction among hazardous agents and cigarette smoking leading to greater-than-expected rates of lung cancer include alpha and gamma radiation (Checkoway et al., 1988) and arsenic (Hertz-Picciotto, 1992; Cohn, 1992; Hertz-Picciotto et al., 1992). Note, however, that although these examples all involve lung cancer and cigarette smoking, it is not possible to determine whether more than one constituent is participating in the perceived interaction, nor if any other chemical interactions are operating among the hundreds of potentially hazardous substances present in cigarette smoke (Steenland and Thun, 1986; Thomas and Whittermore, 1988).

## 3. Susceptible Subgroups

The effect on health of an agent or risk factor is believed to vary in a population because of biological variability among individuals. This variability, in an epidemiological study, is believed to result in small deviations about an average "effect," and appear similar to (and indistinguishable from) random measurement error. Theoretically, in this situation, whatever determines the variability of response could be considered an unmeasured effect modifier. If this factor were validly and precisely measured, then the difference in risk related to the factor could be quantified.

The appearance of such effect modification may reflect the presence of a determinant or risk factor for the outcome related to specific individuals in a population that makes them a subgroup more susceptible to the action of some risk factor. Frequently, age—especially very young or very old—functions as an indicator of a subgroup of the population at greater risk of a disease outcome relative to the rest of the population. For example, very young age might serve as an indicator of vulnerability of the rapidly developing nervous system to environmental neurotoxins; or advanced age might serve as a surrogate for the loss of a chromosomal repair function increasing the risk of certain cancers. More specific identification and measurement of the potential effect modifier defining a susceptible subgroup (such as a genetic trait) will lead to an increase in the relative effect (or relative risk) associated with the joint effect with the exposure or agent (Schulte, 1987). For example, if increasing age were correlated with a loss in the ability to excise dimers (or correct other chromosomal damage) in the dermal layer caused by solar radiation, then age might appear in an epidemiological study of skin cancers to be an effect modifier (i.e., an interaction with age would result). If, however, some test for dimer repair function (a more direct measure of susceptibility) were applied, the magnitude of the observed interaction would substantially increase. Note that the mathematical relationship between the interaction terms (susceptibility measure and solar radiation) is a function of the directness and quality of the epidemiological measure used to represent each.

## 4. No-Hit Model

Several mechanisms for disease induction have been proposed, and the roles of independence and interaction examined. One such model, proposed by Walter and Holford (1978), has been called the no-hit model. Under this model, disease results if one or more beneficial events fail to occur. If two factors act independently in increasing the rate at which the beneficial event occurs, then the observed relative risk for both factors combined will be the product of the risks associated with each factor alone. Thus, the expected relationship reflecting independence is multiplicative, and interaction between factors would be expressed as a departure from multiplicativity. Note that an additive relationship between risks would be interpreted as negative interaction, or antagonism, according to this model.

## 5. Single-Hit Model

Walter and Holford (1978) also described a mechanistic model in which a single adverse event is sufficient for disease inception. Under this model, two risk factors acting independently to increase the rate at which the adverse event occurs would appear to have additive risks, and departures from additivity would indicate interaction.

## 6. Multistage Models

Perhaps the most popular disease models, especially those describing carcinogenesis, have been multistage models (Armitage and Doll, 1954; Moolgavkar and Venzon, 1987). Among the simplest of these, as well as the one most familiar to epidemiologists, is the two-stage, initiator–promotor model. Under this model, a precursory cellular transformation (initiation) results from exposure to one risk factor or agent, followed by a second transformation (promotion) by another factor, leading to disease; here, a malignant tumor.

The relation between the two risk factors involved in initiation and promotion, respectively, may take a variety of forms under this simple model. Siemiatycki and Thomas (1981) have demonstrated that if each factor acts exclusively at either the first or the second stage, then the incidence rate observed for the joint effects will be approximated by the product of the incidence rates observed among those with only one of the risk factors. However, a number of additional interpretations are possible. Consider an example in which the initiator must be present for the first transformation to occur, and the promotor must follow, otherwise the cancer does not occur. In this case, individuals with only one of the factors, or with neither, should experience the same background rate of incident tumors, and whether the product of these rates describes the rate experienced by individuals with both the initiator and promotor is a matter of circumstance. Theoretically, if there is no other causal mechanism than that involving these two risk factors, then the background rate will be zero, and the rate among those with both factors, in relative terms, will be enormous.

Among individuals with both the initiator and promotor risk factors present, some variability of risk will result from the specific timing of these events. If initiation and promotion can be accomplished nearly simultaneously, or at least within a very narrow period, then the presence of both risk factors concurrently should not interfere with tumor inception. However, if initiation must precede promotion by some substantial period, then the timing of exposure becomes critical. For instance, among employees exposed over a work history within a plant to both an initiator and a promotor, no increase in risk is expected among those exposed only to the promotor first, a large increase is expected among those exposed to the initiator and the promotor in the ideal time sequence, and possibly some intermediate level of increase among those with other combinations over time. This highlights the importance of the quality of risk factor measurements made for epidemiological studies, relative to the time and nature of exposures, especially if the study results are to be used in elucidating the disease process and mechanisms.

## B. Epidemiological–Statistical

### 1. Multiple (Correlated) Surrogate Measures

Parameters used as risk factors in epidemiology tend to be those attributes or agents that are most conducive to being measured, and may not necessarily be direct measures of the true risk factor. For example, measures of cigarette consumption in pack-years serves reasonably well as a risk indicator for lung cancer, even though the carcinogen(s) responsible are not directly identified or measured in terms of dose. The degree to which epidemiological measures are surrogates or indicators of a true causal factor probably varies from nearly direct measurement, such as isolating a pathogenic organism in the tissue of an infected individual, to greatly removed surrogates, such as male gender as a measure of an occupational exposure more likely sustained by males.

In principle, the more highly correlated a measured variable is with the underlying causal factor, the closer it will reflect the true level of risk, or the strength of association with the outcome of interest. Conversely, the weaker the association between the measured variable and the causal factor, the weaker the measure of association will be as well. Therefore, suppose that two imperfect surrogates, such as gender and occupation, are measured jointly, and each appears to be a weak to moderate risk factor for a specific outcome, such as bladder cancer. In this example, males might be at increased risk because they traditionally have been more likely to work in the dye manufacturing industry. Likewise, those with a specific job title (such as chemical operator) might have been more likely to have been exposed to the carcinogenic agent. In a given epidemiological study, however, those with both of these risk factors (male gender and chemical operator) might appear to have a level of risk far greater than the sum of risks indicated by the separate effects, an interpretation consistent with an interaction. The apparent interaction has resulted from the creation of a better risk indicator of exposure to carcinogens (the joint measure) than either measure taken alone. This effect is quite likely to occur, as epidemiologists almost always rely on indirect measures of risk factors.

## 2. *Unmeasured Intervening Variables*

Thompson (1991) described a related source of interaction stemming from the inevitable inclusion of measures in epidemiology that are related to, but imperfect measures of the phenomena that participate in the causal mechanism. He postulated that in most epidemiological settings there will be one or more unmeasured intervening variables between those risk factors measured and the outcome of interest. In epidemiology, intervening variables are measures along a sequence of events leading to a disease endpoint. For example, suppose exposure to a toxicant in the environment leads to a certain tissue dose which, in turn, results in metabolic production of a carcinogenic metabolite, and when a clearance mechanism is saturated, the metabolite accumulates, leading to a carcinogenic mutation and a malignancy. Although the exposure, which is measured in ambient air, is the risk factor, and cancer is the outcome, the sequence of events between these measures can greatly influence the occurrence of the outcome. One example related to this illustration might be some nutritional factor that regulates the rate of metabolite clearance. In this example, two factors might exert their influence on the incidence of disease through a common intervening variable, resulting in an interrelationship exceeding that of additivity of rates and, therefore, resembling an interaction. Thompson further elaborates on this basic model to demonstrate that two or more factors need not act directly on the common intervening variable, but may act indirectly through one or more other factors along a causal chain of events.

## 3. *Chance–Multiple Comparisons*

Epidemiological analyses employ numerical representations, or coding, of various phenomena such as risk factors as well as disease outcomes. Because of random measurement error, however, study results may be entirely due to this measurement error. If the error truly is random, that is, no systematic bias is present, the average association observed over many repeated studies will represent the true effect. Although the distribution of all possible study outcomes will be a bell-shaped normal distribution curve centered on the true value, a small proportion of the time the result will be substantially different from this value. From basic biostatistics, recall that with an alpha (predetermined probability level at which the null hypothesis is rejected) set at the traditional 0.05 level, 5% of all null hypotheses still will be rejected, even if there is no such association or effect, simply because of measurement error.

Similarly, detection of an interaction, in the absence of all other biases, may result entirely because of the random error associated with the two or more factors involved in the interaction. Despite that a particular statistical test may suggest that a result is statistically significant at a specified alpha level, there is always a chance (directly proportional to the selected alpha level) that the test represents a false-positive owing to random error. If a statistically significant interaction is observed in a single study, but not in additional similar investigations, one explanation may be that the result was observed because of measurement error. Because the probability of actually obtaining a false-positive test for interaction is related to the number of tests performed, epidemiologists attempting to evaluate every possible joint effect among all study risk measures will be more likely to encounter an interaction that, despite being statistically significant, is spurious.

### 4. *Databased Interaction*

Another interpretation of interaction which has not yet been described well in the literature is databased interaction. Similar to random measurement error described earlier, databased interaction results from the peculiar distribution of two or more factors within a study database. In the real world, these two factors might be distributed completely independent of each other, yet in the epidemiological study, because of the way in which study participants were selected, information collected, and such, may be interrelated. This description may be an extension of what occurs with databased confounding, in which a measure of association is influenced by the differential distribution in the study database of a second risk factor for the disease outcome of interest (Axelson, 1989). In the presence of a databased interaction, it may be advisable to "control" for it in a statistical model, as it may behave like a confounder and spuriously influence the coefficient of the main risk factors of interest. Unfortunately, there is very little experience with this available in the published literature.

### 5. *Scale–Coding Issues*

The choice of mathematical scales on which to evaluate interaction has been a topic of debate for many years (Walter and Holford, 1978; Kupper and Hogan, 1978). As can be seen in the conceptual models presented above, interaction may be defined as an observed departure from the expected or hypothesized relationship. Thus, if under the sufficient–component cause model, two risk factors act independently, then the risks should be additive. If, however, we observe that the joint effect is best represented by the product of the individual risks, there is a departure from additivity and, therefore, an interaction. On the other hand, under a different disease model, the expected relation might be multiplicative, and the finding of an additive relationship would represent an interaction (specifically, antagonism).

Note that in any situation that interaction is assessed, it necessarily will be found when the "inappropriate" disease model is invoked. In most epidemiological scenarios in which no disease mechanism is known, selection of the mathematical scale on which to evaluate interaction may be arbitrary, and detection or failure to detect an interaction a matter of chance selection of scale. In epidemiological studies evaluating the joint effects of two risk factors when no specific disease model is known or postulated, it is best to simply describe the relationship present in the data, whether it be additive or multiplicative, or some exponential function. Then, if it is determined later that the disease mechanism should produce a multiplicative relationship, the previous results may be evaluated in this light. Given the numerous ways in which risk factors may appear to act jointly in some manner other than expected, extreme caution is urged in interpreting any example of interaction occurring in an epidemiological study.

## VII.  REASONS INTERACTION IS NOT ASSESSED

In most epidemiological studies, interaction is not routinely assessed. There may be several reasons for this, most of which are not scientific. For example, as mentioned throughout this chapter, the topic of interaction in epidemiology has been surrounded with a degree of confusion and controversy, largely unresolved to date. Epidemiologists then must face the dilemma of whether to engage in the methodological uncertainties of interaction assessment and risk the interpretational ambiguities that might arise. Yet, if interaction assessment is not attempted in individual studies, qualitative metanalyses, such as that recently published on synergism between arsenic and cigarette smoking may not be possible (Hertz-Picciotto et al., 1992).

Specific justifications for not attempting to evaluate the joint effects of risk factors in an epidemiological study include the following:

1. *Lack of power:* Statistical power to detect interactions is drastically lower than for the main effects (Greenland, 1983, 1985). Epidemiologists rarely take this into account before starting a study, possibly because study sizes are frequently limited by logistical or budgetary constraints.
2. *Interest in only main effects:* If one or more main effects are actually involved in an interaction, the results of an epidemiological study ignoring these effects may be quite different, and possibly invalid. The degree of this bias may be quite small or be substantial, and is not predictable.
3. *Confusion over proper assessment methods:* This is probably quite common at the present, but should diminish as more of a consensus is reached, and more direction is available to the epidemiologist unfamiliar with the concepts of interaction.
4. *A priori knowledge of independence, or lack of biologically plausible rationale for interaction:* Depending on the objective of the epidemiological analysis, these may be good reasons for not evaluating interaction. As discussed earlier, however, interaction may be present in a database, possibly influencing the validity of the study results. Also, interaction frequently may occur between variables that have no direct biological interrelationship, but by virtue of their direct or indirect relation with a common underlying causal factor, or an unmeasured intervening variable, do interact.
5. *Fear of finding interaction:* Because of the analytical and interpretational challenges associated with assessing interaction and accounting for it in subsequent analyses, many investigators either do not investigate the possibility of an interaction in their studies, or do not know how to address those which are discovered, in which case, the interaction may not be fully explored and reported. Again, as more guidance becomes available and agreed on, this problem should subside.

In many epidemiological studies, several of these issues may be relevant, making the analytical decisions more difficult. Combined with the limited ability of detected interactions to elucidate the biological and pathological processes operating to cause disease, it is no wonder that many epidemiologists currently prefer to avoid interaction assessment. For this reason, one should not assume that the absence of mention of interaction in a published epidemiological study means that no interaction was present. On the other hand, given the numerous factors that may influence the presence or absence of interaction, interpretation of studies seeking and finding or failing to uncover interactions may not be straightforward. The net result is that despite the intuitive and conceptual usefulness of interaction in epidemiology, in practice, biological inference from observed (or not observed) interaction may not be valid, except in rare cases. Unfortunately, these cases cannot be detected without some toxicological or biological confirmation (Thompson, 1991).

## VIII.  RECOMMENDATIONS FOR RISK ASSESSORS

Risk assessors, as well as other health scientists, frequently turn to the results of epidemiological studies in pursuit of insights on human health that cannot be obtained from any other discipline (Smith, 1988). In many cases, this is appropriate, and the public health rewards may be recognized in terms of identifying interventions and establishing regulations that prevent disease and protect health. Much of the ability to implement appropriate interventions depends on identifying risk factors on which one might intervene, such as identifying respiratory health risks in the environment that may be reduced by tighter air pollution regulations. Another important aspect, in the interest of economy of limited resources and reaching those most in need of an intervention, lies in the ability to identify subgroups of human populations who are at greatest risk of death or disease caused by an etiologic agent.

Both of these central public health goals can be approached through epidemiology. Furthermore, the ability to achieve both of these goals is theoretically enhanced through the identification of interactions among risk factors for disease. First, successful identification of risk factors acting together to produce disease at a greater-than-expected rate necessarily means that intervention on any of these should result in prevention of a relatively greater proportion of disease than would be accomplished through intervention on a single factor acting independently to cause disease. Secondly, identification of risk factors that may be personal characteristics and that participate in a causal interaction might also be factors that identify susceptible subgroups of human populations. This information is valuable, both to the clinical scientists attempting to understand the pathological process and disease mechanism, and to the public health scientist and risk assessor attempting to protect the health of these more susceptible individuals.

Although these interests in interaction in epidemiology are compelling, the state of the art in epidemiology may not be ready to assume these noble challenges. For numerous reasons discussed throughout this chapter, epidemiologists have not been able to resolve some basic issues concerning the assessment of interaction, including use of the appropriate mathematical scale, a default choice of disease model or mechanism, sources of "spurious" interaction, limited statistical power, and so on. Nevertheless, discussion of interaction in epidemiology has not ceased, and great strides have been achieved over the short history of this topic, a trend that is expected to continue as creative minds are engaged on the subject and more practical experience accrues. In the meantime, unfortunately, interaction in epidemiological research will be of limited value to the risk assessor.

In conclusion, the following recommendations are made for risk assessors and other health scientists interested in interactions in epidemiological studies. First, keep in mind that interaction is a relatively new topic of discussion, largely stimulated by rapid advances made recently in computing science. Highly complex relationships among many risk factors may be modeled mathematically by nearly any epidemiologist or biostatistician with access to a microcomputer. However, much of the conceptual basis for interpreting and using these results have yet to be refined and better understood. Second, because of the nature of the measures used by epidemiologists to represent observed phenomena, interactions may occur for reasons other than causal interdependence of the factors, or coparticipation in a single disease process. In practical terms this suggests that observed interactions should not be assumed to reflect a basic biological or chemical mechanism underlying the measures. Third, lack of any observed interaction cannot definitively be interpreted as independence in action (if any) between two risk indicators. This may be due to a simple lack of statistical power to detect an interaction, improper choice of mathematical or mechanistic model, or most likely, selection of imperfect surrogate or indicator variables to represent the true risk factors for an outcome.

The limited situations in which interactions demonstrated in epidemiological studies might provide useful insights on the disease process are those in which some consistency is found over several studies, for which the variables participating in the interaction are highly specific (unlike gender or race—both of which are surrogates for many health-related phenomena), or for which the biological or toxicological mechanism is at least partly understood. Epidemiological studies concluding that an interaction is present should identify the assumed underlying biological and mathematical models used to determine the presence of the interaction. In situations for which no mechanism is known, analytical techniques should be used that assume no specific underlying relation and the actual relationship present should be described.

# REFERENCES

Armitage, P., and R. Doll (1954). The age distribution of cancer and a multi-stage theory of carcinogenesis, *Br. J. Cancer,* 8, 1–12.

Axelson, O. (1989). Confounding from smoking in occupational epidemiology, *Br. J. Ind. Med.,* 46, 505–507.

Breslow, N. E. and B. E. Storer (1985). General relative risk functions for case–control studies, *Am. J. Epidemiol.,* 122, 149–162.

Bulterys, M. G., S. Greenland, and J. F. Kraus (1990). Chronic fetal hypoxia and sudden infant death syndrome: Interaction between maternal smoking and low hematocrit during pregnancy, *Pediatrics,* 86, 535–540.

Calabrese, E. J. (1991). *Multiple Chemical Interaction.* Lewis Publishers, Inc., Chelsea, Michigan.

Checkoway, H., N. E. Pearce, D.J. Crawford-Brown and D. Cragle (1988). Radiation doses and cause-specific mortality among workers at a nuclear materials fabrication plant, *Am. J. Epidemiol.,* 127, 255–266.

Checkoway, H., N. Pearce and D. J. Crawford-Brown (1989). *Research Methods in Occupational Epidemiology.* Oxford University Press, New York.

Cohn, S. E. (1992). Synergism between occupational arsenic exposure and smoking in the induction of lung cancer [letters], *Epidemiology,* 3, 471.

Coughlin, S. S., C. C. Nass, L. W. Pickle, B. Trock, and G. Bunin (1991). Regression methods for estimating attributable risk in population-based case–control studies: A comparison of additive and multiplicative models, *Am. J. Epidemiol.,* 133, 305–313.

Dahl, L. K., M. Heine, and I. Tassinari (1960). High salt content of Western infant's diet: possible relationship to hypertension in the adult, *Nature* 198, 1204–1205.

Greenland, S. (1983). Tests for interaction in epidemiologic studies: A review and a study of power, *Stat. Med.,* 2, 243–251.

Greenland, S. (1985). Power, sample size and smallest detectable effect determination for multivariate studies, *Stat. Med.,* 4, 117–127.

Greenland, S. (1993). Additive risk versus additive relative risk models, *Epidemiology,* 4, 32–36.

Greenland, S. and H. Morgenstern (1989). Ecological bias, confounding, and effect modification, *Int. J. Epidemiol.,* 18, 269–274.

Greenland, S. and C. Poole (1988). Invariants and noninvariants in the concept of interdependent effects, *Scand. J. Work Environ. Health,* 14, 125–129.

Greenland S. and J. M. Robins (1986). Identifiability, exchangeability, and epidemiological confounding, *Int. J. Epidemiol.,* 15, 413–419.

Hennekens, C. H., J. E. Buring, and S. L. Mayrent (1987). *Epidemiology in Medicine*. Little, Brown and Company, Boston, Massachusetts.

Hemberg, S. (1992). *Introduction to Occupational Epidemiology*. Lewis Publishers, Inc., Chelsea, Michigan.

Hertz-Picciotto, I. (1992). Synergism between occupational arsenic exposure and smoking in the induction of lung cancer [Letter, authors reply], *Epidemiology*, 3, 471–472.

Hertz-Picciotto, I., A. H. Smith, D. Holtzman, M. Lipsett, and G. Alexeeff (1992). Synergism between occupational arsenic exposure and smoking in the induction of lung cancer, *Epidemiology*, 3, 23–31.

Hulka, B. S., T. C. Wilcosky, and J. D. Griffith (1990). *Biological Markers in Epidemiology*. Oxford University Press, New York.

Kelsey, J. L., W. D. Thompson and A. S. Evans (1986). *Methods in Observational Epidemiology*. Oxford University Press, New York.

Kleinbaum, D. G., L. L. Kupper and H. Morgenstern (1982). *Epidemiologic Research*. Lifetime Learning Publications, Belmont, California.

Koopman, J. S. (1977). Causal models and sources of interaction, *Am. J. of Epidemiol.*, 106(6):439–444.

Koopman, J. S. (1981). Interaction between discrete causes, *Am. J. of Epidemiol.*, 113(6):716–724.

Kupper, L. L. and M. D. Hogan (1978). Interaction in epidemiologic studies, *Am. J. of Epidemiol.*, 108(6):447–453.

Last, J. M. (1988). *A Dictionary of Epidemiology*. Oxford University Press, New York.

Miettinen, O. S. (1974). Confounding and effect-modification, *Am. J. Epidemiol.*, 100, 350–353.

Miettinen, O. S. (1982). Causal and preventive interdependence, *Scan. J. Work Environ. Health*, 8, 159–168.

Moolgavkar, S. H. and D. J. Venzon (1987). General relative risk regression models for epidemiologic studies, *Am. J. of Epidemiol.*, 126(5):949–961.

Nauman, C. H., J. Griffith, J. N. Blancato and T. E. Aldrich (1993). Biomarkers in environmental epidemiology, in *Environmental Epidemiology and Risk Assessment*, (Aldrich and Griffith, eds.), Van Nostrand Reinhold, New York.

Rothman, K. J. (1974). Synergy and antagonism in cause-effect relationships, *Am. J. of Epidemiol.*, 99(6):385–388.

Rothman, K. J. (1976a). Causes, *Am. J. of Epidemiol.*, 104, 587–592.

Rothman, K. J. (1976b). The estimation of synergy or antagonism, *Am. J. of Epidemiol.*, 103, 506–511.

Rothman, K. J. (1986). Interactions between causes. In *Modern Epidemiology*, Little, Brown & Company, Boston.

Schulte, P. A. (1987). Simultaneous assessment of genetic and occupational risk factors, *J. Occup. Med.*, 29, 884–891.

Siemiatycki, J., and D. C. Thomas (1981). Biological models and statistical interactions: An example from multistage carcinogenesis, *Int. J. Epidemiol.*, 10, 383–387.

Smith, A. H. (1988). Epidemiologic input to environmental risk assessment, *Arch. Environ. Health*, 43, 124–127.

Steenland, K., and M. Thun (1986). Interaction between tobacco smoking and occupational exposures in the causation of lung cancer, *J. Occup. Med.*, 28, 110–118.

Szklo, M. (1988). Evaluation of Epidemiologic Information in *Epidemiology and Health Risk Assessment*, (L. Gardis, ed.), Oxford University Press, New York.

Thomas, D., and S. Greenland (1985). The efficiency of matching in case–control studies of risk-factor interactions, *J. Chron. Dis.*, 38, 569–574.

Thomas, D. C., and A. S. Whittemore (1988). Methods for testing interactions, with applications to occupational exposures, smoking, and lung cancer, *Am. J. Ind. Med.*, 13, 131–147.

Thompson, W. D. (1991). Effect modification and the limits of biological inference from epidemiologic data, *J. Clin. Epidemiol.*, 44, 221–232.

Wacholder, S., and C. R. Weinberg (1986). Selecting subpopulations for invervention, *J. Chron. Dis.*, 39, 513–519.

Walker, A. (1981). Proportion of disease attributable to the combined effect of two factors, *Int. J. Epidemiol.*, 10, 81–85.

Walter, S. D., and T. R. Holford (1978). Additive, multiplicative and other models for disease risks, *Am. J. of Epidemiol.*, 108(5):341–346.

Weinberg, C. R. (1986). Applicability of the simple independent action model to epidemiologic studies involving two factors and a dichotomous outcome, *Am. J. Epidemiol.*, 123, 162–173.

# 20

# The Median Effect Equation: A Useful Mathematical Model for Assessing Interaction of Carcinogens and Low-Dose Cancer Quantitative Risk Assessment

**James Stewart**
*Harvard University
Cambridge, Massachusetts*

**Edward J. Calabrese**
*University of Massachusetts
Amherst, Massachusetts*

## I. INTRODUCTION

Developing a clear understanding of the biochemical complexity of dose–response relationships for even single agents represents a major toxicological achievement. Such apparent understandings have rarely been achieved, even after concerted and multidimensional research efforts. However, despite the complexity of biochemical interactions in each affected system, a fundamental rule to which the typically unknown biochemical details of each system's responses conforms is the law of mass action. Thus, even though different enzymes catalyze different reactions, with various numbers of substrates and products, and with various sequences (e.g., ordered, Ping-Pong, or randomly), and with different rate constants, the basic rates and chemical reaction behavior can be generalized by either the Michaelis–Menten equation (1913) or the Hill equation (1913). These equations are governed by the mass action law. From this perspective, it follows that dose–response relationships can be evaluated by the application of the law of mass action. Although one may certainly want to develop a detailed understanding of the mechanisms of specific biochemical interactions with a large number of rate constants, even simple enzyme reactions often contain numerous rate constants for multidirectional reactions. Even when this complexity has been apparently effectively described in biochemical terms, it still has been sufficiently incomplete to offer only modest practical usefulness. Although the approach of delineating detailed mechanisms is theoretically sound, and efforts will continuously be made in that direction, progress will be limited by lack of resources and technological advances. Given these limitations, and in the interest of developing sound predictions of dose–response relationships, Chou and Talalay (1981, 1984, 1987) have advocated the development of a generalized equation that can be employed in a clear and straightforward manner for evaluating dose–responses of cellular and in vivo systems. The issue, then, was how to take this concept and apply the principle of mass action with the Michaelis–Menten and Hill equations to a mathematical form that would be practical. To accomplish this task, Chou and Talalay (1981) derived what they referred to as the median effect equation. This equation, in essence, *normalizes all types of dose–response results* by a uniform method that, according to Chou and Talalay (1984), is "based on sound fundamental considerations (i.e., mass action law) that have physiochemical and biological validity in simpler systems."

The median effect equation operationalizes this concept by describing the equality of two dimensionless ratios, with dose on the right side of the equation versus effect or response on the left of the equation. The dose is normalized relative to the median effect dose ($ED_{50}$), and this value is raised to the power of the slope, with the effect being normalized to the control values.

## II. MEDIAN EFFECT ANALYSIS

The median effect equation, as derived by Chou (1976), relates dose and response in a way much different and less complicated than the models discussed previously. The assumptions underlying the median effect equation are that the mass action law applies to the system, and that the system operates at steady state. The assumption of applicability of the mass action law and the steady-state assumption are common in biochemistry, chemistry, physical chemistry and pharmacokinetic modeling, receptor-binding theory, and others (Michaelis and Menten, 1913; Mortimer, 1971; Laitinen and Harris, 1975; Hoel, 1985; Cornfield, 1977; Hoel et al., 1975; Scatchard, 1949). In fact, in Hoel et al. (1975, 1985), the model of metabolic fate of carcinogens assumes that activation, detoxification, DNA repair, and binding of the activated carcinogen to DNA, all obey the mass action law and steady-state conditions are present. Cell growth kinetics have been modeled using the law of mass action (Weiss and Kavanau, 1957). Weiss and Kavanau assumed that cell mass growth was dependent on cell births, cell deaths, and cell transformations. They also assumed steady-state conditions and applied the mass action law to develop the equations to model cell mass growth. Assumptions on cell births, deaths, and transformations are also part of the two-stage of Moolgavkar and Knudson (1981) discussed earlier.

Specific examples of equations incorporating the median effect concept are the: Michaelis–Menten equation (Michaelis and Menten, 1913), Hill equation (Hill, 1913), Scatchard equation (Scatchard, 1949), and the pH ionization equation of Henderson and Hasselbach.

The median effect equation, as derived in Chou (1976) is given by

$$\frac{F_a}{F_u} = \left(\frac{d}{d_m}\right)^m \tag{1}$$

where $F_a$ = fraction affected, $F_u$ = fraction unaffected at dose $d$, $d$ = the dose, $d_m$ = the median effect dose (i.e., the dose required for 50% effect), and $m$ = Hill-type coefficient. Equation 1 describes a relatively simple relationship between dose and response. The Hill-type coefficient ($m$) determines the sigmoidicity of the dose–response curve (Chou, 1976; Totter and Finamore, 1978) and is an estimate of the stoichiometric ratio/kinetic order of the interaction between carcinogen and target.

The median effect equation can be fit to a variety of shapes of dose–response curves, depending on the magnitude $m$ and the $d_m$. In some cases $m$, which theoretically should be an integer, may take on noninteger values (Chou, 1976). If $m$ is not an integer, it is taken to not represent the actual stoichiometric ratio, but rather, the next lowest integer value is the *minimum* estimated stoichiometric ratio. For example, in the Hill and Scatchard equations, $m$ represents an estimate of the number of binding sites on a protein molecule or enzyme (e.g., four oxygen molecules bind to one hemoglobin molecule). The number of binding sites or binding events is a concept similar to the stage concept of the multistage model or hit theory of the multihit and one-hit models.

## A. Biological Plausibility of the Median Effect Equation

In this most general form, the median effect equation can be thought of as describing a reaction between a B and a chemical dose D. In the context of cancer quantitative risk assessment, B = target and D = carcinogen.

$$D + B \Leftrightarrow DB \Leftrightarrow cancer \tag{2}$$

Under constant chronic dosing of carcinogen the animal system may respond to the chemical insult by acting on the chemical enzymatically; having cellular targets interact with the chemical; repairing the targets; stimulating cells to divide, and so on. Since the dosing is constant over time, it is hypothesized that the system will adjust to the presence of the chemical, and a new state will be achieved in which enzyme levels may be different. DNA adducts may be formed, DNA adducts may be repaired, the chemical may bind to cellular receptors, the chemical may separate from cellular receptors. The system, although dynamic in its detail, will reach a "steady state." Once steady state is achieved DB will not change. It is not important that the identity of DB be known. Therefore, DB can be an intermediate, a receptor–agonist complex, DNA adduct, or whatever. What is important is the assumption that the system will achieve a steady state.

If cancer is the measured effect and $K_{50}$ (i.e., the median effect dose) the dose required to produce a 50% effect, then $F_a$, the fraction of B affected by dose D, can be calculated from Eq. (3). Equation 3 is valid when the stoichiometry of the reaction of D and B is one and the interaction is steady state.

$$F_a = \frac{1}{1 + (K_{50}/D)} \tag{3}$$

Equation (3) is equivalent to the Michaelis–Menten equation when $F_a = v/V_{max}$; $F_u = 1 - (v/V_{max})$; $D = S$ and $K_{50} = K_m$.

If the stoichmetry of the reaction of D and B is not equal to 1, then the equation becomes

$$F_a = \frac{1}{1 + (K_{50}/D)^m} \tag{4}$$

where the largest integer value of $m$ is an estimate of the minimum number of molecules of D that bind to a molecule of B to produce the observed effect (Hill, 1913; Chou, 1976). In Eq. (4), $F_a$ is the fraction affected by the dose; the $K_{50}$ is the dose necessary to produce the effect in 50% of the targets; and D is the dose. Equation (4) is also a form of the median effect equation of Chou (1976) where $d_m = K_{50}$. Equation (4) also describes the relationship between the carcinogen dose and fraction affected for the target–carcinogen system described in Eq. (2).

An important assumption of the median effect equation is reversibility of the reaction to produce DB. The concept of reversibility is not consistent with either the two-stage model of Moolgavkar and Knudson (1981) or the multistage model of Crump et al. (1976). Both of these models assume that the stages are irreversible (Moolgavkar et al., 1988; Crump et al., 1976). A recent example of steady-state reaction between a carcinogen and a target is DNA adduct formation and destruction (Buss et al., 1990). In this study, which supported the median effect equation, the concentration of DNA adducts took approximately 4 weeks to reach steady state. Another supportive example includes the relationship between cell growth, death, and differentiation. Weiss and Kavanau (1957) modeled cell mass growth under the assumption of steady state; in biochemistry enzymes appear to bind and release substrates under steady-state conditions (Rawn, 1983); in pharmacokinetic modeling, compartments are assumed to operate under steady-state conditions (Hoel et al., 1983; Cornfield, 1977; Gehring and Blau, 1977; Hoel, 1985); in addition, in the Hartley–Seilken time-to-tumor model of carcinogenesis, the compartments are assumed to operate a steady state and to follow first-order kinetics (i.e., $m = 1$ in the median effect equation; Hartley and Seilken, 1977). Steady-state reactions, by definition, adhere to the mass action law and are a necessary condition for the Michaelis–Menten equation (Michaelis and Menten, 1913); the Scatchard equation (Scatchard, 1949); the Hill equation (Hill, 1913); the Henderson–Hasselbach equation; the adsorption isotherm of Langimuir (Lanimuir, 1918); and the median effect equation (Chou, 1976). No matter how many steps or what type of biochemical mechanism is used to produce cancer, if the system operates at steady state, then the median effect equation can theoretically model the system (Chou, 1976; 1980).

The assumption that the mass action law is obeyed and that steady-state conditions are maintained, appears to be biologically plausible. No assumptions need be made concerning the hypothesized number of stages, hits, receptors, and such. The median effect equation requires only the two assumptions and Eq. (2). This equation and assumptions establish the biological plausibility of the median effect equation as a mathematical model for the cancer process.

## B.   Median Effect Equation and the Two-Stage Model of Carcinogenesis

To provide a framework for discussing the median effect equation, the two-stage model of carcinogenesis will be used (Knudson, 1979; Moolgavkar and Knudson, 1981; Moolgavkar et al., 1988). A graphic depiction of the two-stage model is given in Fig. 1. The two-stage process

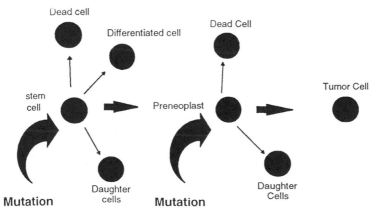

**Figure 1**   Two-stage model of carcinogenesis. (From Moolgavkar and Knudson, 1980.)

of carcinogenesis begins with a stem cell undergoing mutation. This mutation can occur in a variety of ways, most of which are not definitively known (EPA, 1986). One way it may occur is the direct interaction of a xenobiotic with DNA (Marks and Furstenburger, 1987; EPA, 1986) to form a DNA adduct. Once the DNA adduct is formed, it may result in frameshift mutations, deletions, point mutations or other (Schaaper et al., 1990). From the most basic levels of chemistry and biochemistry the direct interaction of one molecule with another is assumed to adhere to the mass action law (Mortimer, 1971; Rawn, 1983). If the interaction adheres to the mass action law and occurs at steady state, the reaction, by definition, must be reversible. The assumption of reversibility allows the DNA–adduct to revert back to normal DNA. If a mutation occurs in a critical site, the product (under the two-stage model) is a preneoplastic cell (Moolgavkar et al., 1988). The preneoplastic cell is not a cancer cell, but rather, a cell that has undergone a heritable genomic event. It is also assumed that this genomic event is essential to the cancer process.

One important feature of the two-stage model is its incorporation of the concept of clonal expansion. By increasing the growth of preneoplastic cells, an expanded pool of target cells is available for the second stage. Clonal expansion has been described as an altering of the balance between dying and newly produced cells (Farber and Sarma, 1987). In liver cancer, during the clonal expansion phase, the cell growth factor increases from 4%, with no clonal expansion, to 8%, with clonal expansion. The cell death fraction increases from 3%, with no clonal expansion, to 7%, with clonal expansion (Farber and Sarma, 1987). Thus, modeling cell growth has used the assumption of a steady-state condition (i.e., a controlled relationship between cell growth and cell death; Weiss and Kavanau, 1957). The two-stage model of Moolgavkar and Knudson (1981) also incorporates rates of cell births, cell deaths, and cell conversion. Since the median effect equation assumes that the system adheres to the mass action law and the system is at steady state, it implicitly incorporates the same concepts. The median effect equation also provides the option of the preneoplastic cell reverting back to a normal stem cell, as is seen in skin papilloma regression after removal of promoting agent (Reddy and Failkow, 1990). The multistage and two-stage models assume that the conversion is permanent and irreversible (Crump et al., 1976; Moolgavkar et al., 1988). Reversion phenomena would be expected under the mass action law and median effect analysis, but not under the two-stage model of Moolgavkar and Knudson (1981) or the multistage model of Crump et al. (1976).

Under the two-stage model, once the preneoplastic cells are formed and clonal expansion occurs, another mutation is necessary to transform the preneoplastic cell into a cancer cell. The second stage of the two-stage model requires that the second stage be a mutation. Again, with the possible exception of retinoblastoma, exactly how the second mutation occurs is unknown. Once the mutation occurs the cell is transformed into a cancer cell.

Potential mechanisms of cancer causation may involve activation of oncogenes and inactivation of tumor suppressor genes (Bishop, 1991). Oncogenes are thought to act through several different mechanisms (Bishop, 1991; Goustin et al., 1986; Cross and Dexter, 1991). To activate a protooncogene, it is considered necessary that the protooncogene undergo a mutation (Varmus, 1989; Bishop, 1991). Tumor suppressor genes have been identified as having a role in a number of cancers (e.g., Wilms' tumor, colon carcinoma, lung carcinoma, neuroblastoma, and kidney carcinoma; Dowdy et al., 1991; Bishop, 1991). In fact, it was hypothesized by Dowdy et al., that there may be three genetic loci involved in Wilms' tumor. Under the steady-state assumption, the rates of activation and deactivation would reach a steady state; therefore, the effects–concentrations of the products produced as a result of activated oncogenes or deactivated tumor suppressor genes would also reach a steady state. To further illustrate the broad applicability of the median effect equation, consider the current controversy concerning the mechanism of action of TCDD (dioxin; Gallo et al., 1991; Roberts, 1991; Holloway, 1990). It has been argued that dioxin must first bind to a cell surface receptor, then (for cancer to occur) the receptor–dioxin complex must travel to the nucleus and interact with DNA. This assumed mechanisms has been used to reestimate safe levels of exposure. In the context of the median effect equation, it does not matter what the underlying mechanism is (i.e., direct interaction with DNA, interaction with the receptor, or interaction with a number of cellular targets); it only matters that the system, as a whole, operates at steady state and adheres to the mass action law. In an analysis of dioxin data conducted in Stewart et al. (1992a) dioxin has an $m = 2.2$, indicating a sublinear dose response. Whether dioxin binds to a receptor, to DNA, or to some other cellular target, does not affect the biological basis for applying the median effect equation.

## III.  COMPARISON OF EQUATIONS FOR THE EFFECTS OF MULTIPLE AGENTS BASED ON THE MEDIAN EFFECT PRINCIPLE (Chou and Talalay, 1984; Calabrese, 1992)

The biological plausibility of the median effect equation can be extended to include the effects of multiple agents (Chou and Talalay, 1987). The following series of equations reflect the application of the median effect equation in a variety of scenarios, ranging from similar modes of action (*additivity*) to independent modes of action (*synergism* or *antagonism*). The equations are described further in Chou and Talalay (1987) and Greco et al. (1988).

### A.  First-Order Conditions

1.  For two mutually exclusive drugs that obey first-order ($m = 1$) conditions:

$$\frac{(F_a)_{1,2}}{(F_u)_{1,2}} = \frac{(F_a)_1}{(F_u)_1} + \frac{(F_a)_2}{(F_u)_2} = \frac{(D)_1}{(ED_{50})_1} + \frac{(D)_2}{(ED_{50})_2} \tag{5}$$

where $ED_{50}$ is the concentration of the drug that is required to produce a 50% effect.

2.  For two mutually nonexclusive drugs that obey first-order ($m = 1$) conditions (note the extra term):

$$\frac{(F_a)_{1,2}}{(F_u)_{1,2}} = \frac{(F_a)_1}{(F_u)_1} + \frac{(F_a)_2}{(F_u)_2} + \frac{(F_a)_1(F_a)_2}{(F_u)_1(F_u)_2} \tag{6}$$

### B.  Higher-Order Conditions

1.  For two mutually exclusive drugs that obey higher-order conditions (this means that each drug has a sigmoidal dose–response curve):

$$\left(\frac{(F_a)_{1,2}}{(F_u)_{1,2}}\right)^{1/m} = \left(\frac{(F_a)_1}{(F_u)_1}\right)^{1/m} + \left(\frac{(F_a)_2}{(F_u)_2}\right)^{1/m} = \frac{(D)_1}{(ED_{50})_1} + \frac{(D)_2}{(ED_{50})_2} \tag{7}$$

2.  For two mutually nonexclusive drugs that obey higher-order conditions:

$$\left(\frac{(F_a)_{1,2}}{(F_u)_{1,2}}\right)^{1/m} = \left(\frac{(F_a)_1}{(F_u)_1}\right)^{1/m} + \left(\frac{(F_a)_2}{(F_u)_2}\right)^{1/m} + \left(\frac{(F_a)_1(F_a)_2}{(F_u)_1(F_u)_2}\right)^{1/m} \tag{8}$$

Greco et al. (1988) derived additional equations representing other situations, specifically when additivity is assumed and also for synergism or antagonism. The equation representing additivity (no interaction) when $m_1 = m_2 = m$ is given by:

$$u = \frac{\left[(D_1/D_{m1}) + (D_2/D_{m2})\right]^m}{1 + \left[(D_1/D_{m1}) + (D_2/D_{m2})\right]^m} \tag{9}$$

For synergism–antagonism with $m_1 = m_2 = m$ the equation becomes:

$$u = \frac{\left[(D_1/D_{m1}) + (D_2/D_{m2}) + (\alpha D_1 D_2/D_{m1}D_{m2})\right]^m}{1 + \left[(D_1/D_{m1}) + (D_2/D_{m2}) + (\alpha D_1 D_2/D_{m1}D_{m2})\right]^m} \tag{10}$$

where $\alpha = 1$ if the toxins are nonmutually exclusive and zero if they are mutually exclusive (Chou and Talalay, 1987). From Greco et al. (1988) for additivity when $m_1 \neq m_2$, the equation becomes:

$$1 = \frac{D_1 + D_2}{\left(D_{m1}[u/1-u]^{1/m_1}\right) + \left(D_{m2}[u/1-u]^{1/m_2}\right)} \tag{11}$$

whereas for synergism–antagonism the equation becomes:

$$1 = \frac{D_1 + D_2 + \alpha D_1 D_2}{\left(D_{m1}[u/1-u]^{1/m_1}\right) + \left(D_{m2}[u/1-u]^{1/m_2}\right) + \left(D_{m1}D_{m2}[u/1-u]^{1/m_2}\right)\left([u/1-u]^{1/m_2}\right)} \tag{12}$$

where $u$ = fraction affected.

## C.  Previous Applications of the Median Effect Equation

A useful form of the median effect equation can be obtained by taking the logarithm of both sides of Eq. (1) yielding a linear equation given by

$$\ln\left(\frac{F_a}{F_u}\right) = m\ln(d) - m\ln(d_{0.5}) \tag{13}$$

Thus the quantity $\ln(F_a/F_u)$ is linear in $\ln(d)$ with slope $m$ and intercept $-m \ln(d_m)$. Note that estimates of $F_a$, $F_u$, and $\ln(d)$ can be calculated readily from experimental carcinogenesis bioassay data. Crude estimates of $m$ and $d_m$ are obtained from the plot of Eq. (5). Once the median effect dose is determined and the slope $m$ is known, the effect at any dose $d$ can be estimated from Eq. (6).

$$F_a = \frac{1}{1 + (d_m/d)^m} \tag{14}$$

The median effect equation has been applied to a limited number of dose–response studies of carcinogens. Chou (1980, 1981, 1987) used the data from Bryan and Shimkin (1943) and Peto et al. (1975) to show that the data from both acute administration (i.e., single injection) of a carcinogen and chronic administration were explainable by the median effect equation. Also investigated in Chou (1987) was the data of Peto et al. (1975). These data involve chronic skin exposure of mice to benzo[*a*]pyrene twice a week for 100 weeks. The total accumulated dose (in micrograms per mouse) was then analyzed using the median effect equation. The slope was much steeper ($m = 4.569$ vs. 1.388) in the chronic exposure study versus the acute exposure study. The resulting $d_m$'s also varied substantially, 98.86 µg/mouse (point estimate) in the acute study versus 1579 µg/mouse in the chronic study. Thus, it seems from these data that for a given total dose of carcinogen, a single injection (acute exposure) is much more hazardous than chronic exposure. To illustrate this, the dose necessary to produce a risk of 1:1 million was calculated for each type of exposure. For acute exposure $4.70 \times 10^{-3}$ µg/mouse is necessary, whereas for chronic exposure the dose necessary is 76.77 µg/mouse, a factor of 16,760 greater. Interestingly, 76.77 µg/mouse equates to $3.94 \times 10^{-1}$ µg/application, again indicating that for this data, chronic exposure appears less hazardous than acute exposure. This interpretation must be tempered by the fact that the routes of exposure were different, which could well account for some or all of the difference.

Chou (1980) conducted another analysis of the data of Peto (1975) and Bryan and Shimkin (1943) to compare the results of median effect analysis and analysis by the power law:

$$F_a = bd^k \tag{15}$$

where $d$ = dose, $k$ and $b$ are constants, and $F_a$ is the fraction affected. In the analysis of the Peto data, instead of micrograms per mouse as the measure per dose, Chou used weeks of application of carcinogen as a surrogate measurement of dose. He then fit the median effect equation and the power law equation to both the Peto data and the Bryan and Shimkin data and found that the chronic exposure data fit the median effect equation better in the high-dose range and that the two equations produced similar results in the low-dose range. The low dose, for Chou (1980), was $F_a < 0.05$, not the $10^{-5}$ or $10^{-6}$ range usually discussed in quantitative risk assessment.

The most extensive application of the median effect equation was made by Totter and Finamore (1978). They analyzed 38 datasets representing direct-acting carcinogens, indirect-acting carcinogens, transplacental chemical carcinogens, and radiation. The systems tested included cell cultures, mice, rats, hamsters, chicks, fungi, drosophila, and barley seeds. The 38 datasets were taken from the literature and included exposure by different routes. Totter and Finamore found that the 38 datasets, although different in many ways, were explainable by median effect analysis. The $m$ values ranged from 0.33 to 3.13. Totter and Finamore excluded those data points that occurred after the maxima or minima of the dose–response curve. This trimming of data should be partially responsible for the good fit obtained. Totter and Finamore also did not account for background incidence.

## IV. ILLUSTRATION OF THE APPLICATION OF THE MEDIAN EFFECT EQUATION TO MULTIPLE CHEMICAL INTERACTIONS

One of the limitations of median effect analysis and, for that matter, other types of analysis of multiple chemical interactions, is the need for large amounts of data. Since it has been demonstrated that chemicals may interact synergistically at one dose, additively at another, and even antagonistically at yet another dose, testing chemicals at one concentration or one mixture is not sufficient (NRC, 1988; Chou and Talalay, 1987). Therefore, any testing protocol must involve different mixtures and different doses if the analysis is to be meaningful. These extensive

**Table 1** Parameter Estimates Obtained from Greco et al., (1988) after Fitting Eq. (11) to Data for Le Pelley and Sullivan (1936)

| Chemical | $d_m$ | $m$ |
|---|---|---|
| Rotenone | $0.151 \pm 0.0019$ | $2.64 \pm 0.081$ |
| Pyrethrins | $0.884 \pm 0.011$ | $2.49 \pm 0.073$ |

data requirements are not practical for long-term studies (NRC, 1988); however, they may be feasible for short-term studies. Mathematical modeling, if based on the biology, may provide some useful insights for long-term exposure scenarios.

Le Palley and Sullivan (1936) applied rotenone and pyrethrins to houseflys and measured the fraction killed at each dose. In this study, rotenone and pyrethrins were given separately and jointly, thereby allowing measurement for interaction. Greco (1988) fit Eqs. (11) and (12) to these data and obtained estimates of the median effect doses ($d_m$) for rotenone and pyrethrins.

In Table 1, the 95% confidence intervals for $m$ overlap, indicating that the dose–response curves are parallel. Since the $m_1 = m_2 = m$ application of Eq. (10) is appropriate, to obtain parameter estimates for Eq. (10) the statisical software package BMDP-PC90, 1990 was used. The nonlinear regression program, with maximum likelihood parameter estimation, was selected and Eq. (10) fit to the Le Pelley and Sullivan data. The parameter estimates obtained are displayed in Table 2.

As with the multistage model and the two-stage model, the median effect model implies that at low dose the effects will be additive, since the interaction term approaches zero faster than either of the individual dose terms [see Eq. (10)]. To demonstrate this, Eq. (10) was applied to a theoretical dataset where $d_{m1} = 10$, $d_{m2} = 10$, $m = 3$, and $\alpha = 0$ or 1. From this data, two curves were obtained and graphed simultaneously. The results of this graph are displayed in Fig. 2. The curves for $\alpha = 1$ and $\alpha = 0$ are indistinguishable at a low dose, and the interaction occurs only at a high dose. (Low dose in this context is 0.001 that of the $d_m$.) A question that needs to be answered in the general sense is: "How low is low dose?" Work is underway to investigate this question. If there is a relation between $d_m$ (i.e., the TD$_{50}$; Stewart et al. 1993) and low-dose additivity, then the importance of interaction can be assessed by the relation of the exposure to the TD$_{50}$.

**Table 2** Parameter Estimates Obtained from Fitting Eq. (10) to Data for Le Pelley and Sullivan (1936). Equation Fit Using BMDP-PC90 Nonlinear Regression Program 3R Using Maximum Likelihood ($m_1 = m_2 = m$)

| Chemical | $d_m$ | $m$ |
|---|---|---|
| Rotenone | $0.147 \pm 0.0018$ | $2.57 \pm 0.047$ |
| Pyrethrins | $0.895 \pm 0.011$ | |

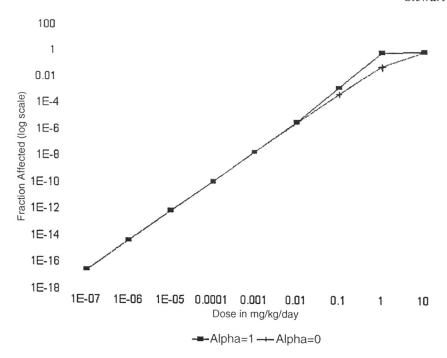

**Figure 2** Effect of interaction term on Eq. (11) at low and high dose. (Data from Le Pelley and Sullivan, 1936.)

## REFERENCES

Ackland, S. P., R. I. Schilsky, M. A. Beckett, and R. R. Weichselbaum (1988). Synergistic cytotoxicity and DNA strand break formation by bromodeoxyuridine and bleomycin in human tumor cells, *Cancer Res.,* 48, 4244–4249.

Anderson, E. L. (1983). Quantitative approaches in use to assess cancer risk, *Risk Anal.,* 3, 277–295.

Armitage, P., and R. Doll (1954). The age distribution of cancer and a multistage theory of carcinogenesis, *Br. J. Cancer,* 8, 1–12.

Armitage, P., and R. Doll (1961). *Stochastic Models for Carcinogenesis From the Berkeley Symposium on Mathematical Statistics and Probability,* University of California Press, Berkeley, CA, pp. 19–38.

Berkson, J. (1944). Application of the logistic function to bioassay, *J. Am. Stat. Assoc.,* 39, 357–365.

BMDP (1988). BMDP Statistical Software, BMDP Statistical Software, Los Angeles, CA.

Bishop, J. M. (1991). Molecular themes in oncogenesis, *Cell,* 64, 235–248.

Bregman, M. D., and F. L. Meyskens (1986). Difluoromethylornithine enhances inhibition of melanoma cell growth in soft agar by dexamethasone, clone a interferon and retinoic acid, *Int. J. Cancer,* 37, 101–107.

Bryan, W. R., and M. B. Shimkin (1943). Quantitative analysis of dose response data obtained with three carcinogenic hydrocarbons in strain C3H male mice, *JNCI,* 3, 503–531.

Burns, F. J., M. Vanderlaan, A. Sivaki, and R. E. Albert (1976). Regression kinetics of mouse skin papillomas, *Cancer Res.,* 36, 1422–1427.

Buss, P., M. Caviezel, and W. K. Lutz (1990). Linear dose–response relationships for DNA adducts in rat liver from chronic exposure to aflatoxin $B_1$, *Carcinogenesis,* 11, 2133–2135.

Chou, T. C. (1976). Derivation and properties of Michaelis–Menton type and Hill type equations for reference ligands, *J. Theor. Biol.,* 59, 253–276.

Chou, T. C. (1980). Comparison of dose–effect relationships of carcinogens following low-dose chronic exposure and high-dose single injection: An analysis by the median effect principle, *Carcinogenesis,* 1, 203–213.

Chou, T. C. (1981). Carcinogenic risk assessment by the mass-action law principle: Application to large scale chronic feeding experiment with 2-acetylaminofluorene (2-AAF), *Proc. Am. Assoc. Cancer Res.,* 22, 141.

Chou, T. C., and P. Talalay (1977). A simple generalized equation for the analysis of multiple inhibitions of Michaelis–Menton kinetic systems, *J. Biol. Chem.,* 252, 6438–6442.

Chou, T. C., and P. Talalay (1987). Application of the median effect principle for the assessment of low dose risk of carcinogens and for the quantitation of synergism and antagonism of chemotherapeutic agents. In *New Avenues in Developmental Cancer Chemotherapy,* Academic Press, New York, 37–64.

Cohen and Ellwein (1990). Cell proliferation in carcinogenesis, *Science,* 249, 1007–1011.

Cornfield, J. (1977). Carcinogenic risk assessment, *Science,* 198, 693–698.

Cornfield, J., K. Rai, and J. Van Ryzin (1980). Procedures for assessing risk at low levels of exposure, *Arch. Toxicol.,* Suppl. 3, 295–303.

Cross, M., and M. Dexter (1991). Growth factors in development, transformation and tumorigenesis, *Cell,* 64, 271–280.

Crump, K. S., D. Hoel, C. Langley, and R. Peto (1976). Fundamental carcinogenic processes and their implications for low dose risk assessment, *Cancer Res.,* 36, 2973–2979.

Day, N. E., and C. C. Brown (1980). Multistage models and the primary prevention of cancer, *JNCI,* 64, 977–989.

Dowdy, S. F., C. L. Fasching, D. Araujo, L. Kin-Man, E. Livanos, B. F. Weissman, and E. J. Stanbridge (1991). Suppression of tumorigenicity in Wilms' tumor by the p15.5-p14 region of chromosome 11, *Science,* 254, 293–295.

Durand, R. E., and P. L. Olive (1987). Enhancement of toxicity from $N'$-(chloroethyl)-$N'$-cyclohexyl-$N$-nitrosourea in V79 spheroids by a nitrofuran. *Cancer Res.,* 47, 5303–5309.

[EPA] Environmental Protection Agency (1986). *The Risk Assessment Guidelines of 1986,* EPA/6008-87/045, USEPA, Washington, DC.

Farber, E., and D. S. R. Sarma (1987). Chemical carcinogenesis: The liver as a model, In *Concepts and Theories in Carcinogenesis* (Maskens et al., eds.), Elsevier Science Publishers, Amsterdam.

Food Safety Council (1980). Quantitative risk assessment, *Food Cosmet. Toxicol.,* 18, 711–714.

Gehring, P. I., and G. E. Blau (1977). Mechanisms of carcinogenesis: Dose response, *J. Environ. Pathol. Toxicol.,* 1, 163–167.

Goustin, A. S., E. B. Leof, G. D. Shipley, and H. L. Moses (1986). Growth factors and cancer, *Cancer Res.,* 46, 1015–1029.

Hartley, H. O., and R. L. Sielken (1977). Estimation of safe doses in carcinogenic experiments, *Biometrics,* 33, 1–7.

Hill, A. V. (1913). The combination of hemoglobin with oxygen and with carbon monoxide, *J. Biochem.,* 7, 471–480.

Hoel, D. G., D. W. Gaylor, R. L. Kirschstein, U. Saffiotti, and M. A. Schneiderman (1975). Estimation of risks of irreversible, delayed toxicity, *J. Toxicol. Environ. Health,* 1, 133–140.

Hoel, D. G., N. L. Kaplan, and M. W. Anderson (1983). The implication of nonlinear kinetics on risk estimation in carcinogenesis, *Science,* 219, 1032–1034.

Holloway, M. (1990). "A great poison" dioxin helps elucidate the function of genes, *Sci. Am.,* Nov.

Illmensee, K., and B. Mintz (1976). Totipotency and normal differentiation of single teratocarcinoma cells cloned by injection into blastocysts, *Proc. Nat. Acad. Sci.,* 73, 549–553.

Iverson, S., and N. Arley (1950). On the mechanism of experimental carcinogenesis, *Acta Pathol. Microbiol. Scand.,* 27, 773–803.

Kano, Y., T. Ohnuma, T. Okano, and J. F. Holland (1988). Effects of vincristine in combination with methotrexate and other antitumor agents in human acute lymphoblastic leukemia cells in culture, *Cancer Res.,* 48, 351–356.

Kong, X. B., M. Andreeff, M. P. Fanucchi, J. J. Fox, K. A. Watanabe, P. Vidal, and T. C. Chou (1987). Cell differentiation effects of 2'-fluoro-1-β-D-arabinofuranosyl pyrimidines in HL-60 cells, *Leukemia Res.,* 11, 1031–1039.

Knudson, A. G. (1971). Mutation and cancer: Statistical study of retinoblastoma, *Proc. Nat. Acad. Sci.,* USA 68, 820–823.

Krewski, D., and J. Van Ryzin (1981). Dose response models for quantal response toxicity data. In *Statistics and Other Topics* (J. Sxorgo, D. Dawson, J. N. K. Rao, E. Saleh, eds.), North Holland, New York, pp. 201–231.

Laitinen, H. A., and W. E. Harris (1975). *Chemical Analysis,* 2nd ed., *McGraw-Hill Series in Advanced Chemistry,* NY, pp. 5–6.

Langmuir, I. (1918). The adsorption of gases on plane surfaces of glass, mica and platinum, *J. Am. Chem. Soc.,* 40, 1361–1403.

Mantel, N., and W. Bryan (1961). "Safety" testing of carcinogenic agents, *JNCI,* 27, 455–470.

Marks, F., and G. Furstenburger (1990). The conversion stage of skin carcinogenesis, *Carcinogenesis,* 11, 2085–2092.

Michaelis, L., and M. L. Menton (1913). Die Kinetik der Invertinwirkung, *Biochem. Z.,* 49, 333–369.

Mintz, B., and K. Illmensee (1975). Normally genetically mosaic mice produced from malignant teratocarcinoma cells, *Proc. Nat. Acad. Sci.,* USA 72, 3585–3589.

Moolgavkar, S. H. (1986). Hormones and multistage carcinogenesis, *Cancer Surv.,* 5, 635–648.

Moolgavkar, S. H., and A. G. Knudson (1981). Mutation and cancer: A model for human carcinogenesis, *JNCI,* 66, 1037–1052.

Moolgavkar, S. H., and D. J. Venzon (1979). Two event models for carcinogenesis: Incidence curves for childhood and adult tumors, *Math. Biosci.,* 47, 55–77.

Moolgavkar, S. H., A. Dewanji, and D. J. Venzon (1988). A stochastic two stage model for cancer risk assessment. I. The hazard function and the probability of tumor, *Risk Anal.,* 8, 383–392.

Mortimer, C. E. (1971). *Chemistry: A Conceptual Approach,* 2nd ed., Van Nostrand Reinhold, New York, 484–512.

Naomoto, Y., and N. Tanaka (1987). In vitro synergistic effects of natural tumor necrosis factor and natural interferon-α, *Jpn. J. Cancer Res.,* 78, 87–92.

[OSTP] Office of Science and Technology Policy (1985). Chemical carcinogens: A review of the science and its associated principles, *Fed. Reg.,* 50, 10372–10442.

Peto, R., F. J. C. Roe, L. Levy, and J. Clark (1975). Cancer and aging in mice and men, *Br. J. Cancer,* 32, 411–426.

Rai, K., and J. Van Ryzin (1981). A generalized multihit dose response model for low dose extrapolation, *Biometrics,* 37, 341–352.

Rawn, J. D. (1983). *Biochemistry,* Harper & Row, New York.

Reddy, A. L., and P. J. Failkow (1990). Evidence that weak promotion of carcinogen-initiated cells prevents their progression to malignancy, *Carcinogenesis,* 11, 2123–2126.

Reed, L. J., and J. Berkson (1929). Application of the logistic function to experimental data, *J. Phys. Chem.,* 33, 760–779.

Roberts, L. (1991). Dioxin risks revisited, *Science,* 251, 624–626.

Scatchard, G. (1949). The attractions of proteins for small molecules and ions. *Ann. N. Y. Acad. Sci.,* 51, 660–672.

Schaaper, R. M., N. Koffel-Schwartz, and R. P. P. Fuchs (1990). *N*-Acetoxy-*N*-acetyl-aminofluorene-induced mutagenesis in the *lacI* gene of *Escherichia coli, Carcinogenesis,* 11, 1087–1095.

Stewart, J. H., D. W. Hosmer, and E. J. Calabrese (1995a). Part 2: Development of the median effect equation for use as a model in cancer quantitative risk assessment, *Human and Ecological Risk* (submitted for publication).

Stewart, J. H., D. W. Hosmer, and E. J. Calabrese (1995b). Part 3: Preliminary application and testing of the median effect equation as a model in quantitative risk assessment, *Human and Ecological Risk* (submitted for publication).

Totter, J. R., and F. J. Finamore (1978). Dose response to cancerogenic and mutagenic treatments, *Environ. Int.,* 1, 233–244.

Trosko, J. A., and C. C. Chang (1985). Role of tumor promotion in affecting the multihit nature of carcinogenesis, *Basic Life Sci.,* 33, 261–284.

Van Ryzin, J. (1980). Quantitative risk assessment, *J. Occup. Med.,* 22, 321–326.

Varmus, H. (1989). An historical overview of oncogenes. In *Oncogenes and the Molecular Origins of Life* (R. A. Weinberg, ed.), Cold Spring Harbor Press, New York.

Weiss, P., and J. L. Kavanau (1957). A model of growth and growth control in mathematical terms. *J. Gen. Physiol.,* 41, 1–47.

Ziese, L., R. Wilson, and E. A. C. Crouch (1987). Dose response relationships for carcinogens: A review, *Environ. Health Perspect.,* 73, 259–308.

# 21

# Genetic Toxicology and Risk Assessment of Complex Environmental Mixtures*

**Virginia Stewart Houk and Michael D. Waters**
*United States Environmental Protection Agency*
*Research Triangle Park, North Carolina*

## I. INTRODUCTION

In 1983, a U. S. National Academy of Sciences (USNAS, 1983) publication described what is now commonly referred to as the risk assessment paradigm. The assessment of risk is divided into four stages: hazard identification, dose–response assessment, exposure assessment, and risk characterization. *Hazard identification* and *dose–response assessment* characterize the relationship between exposure, dose, and an adverse health effect. *Exposure assessment* measures (or models) the magnitude of human contact with a substance and explains the pathways by which materials gain access to the body. *Risk characterization,* the product of the risk assessment process, combines dose–response and exposure data to estimate the risks to public health (Fig. 1).

With few exceptions, humans are exposed to complex mixtures of chemicals, rather than to single chemicals. *Mixtures* have been defined as "any combination of two or more chemical substances regardless of source or of spatial or temporal proximity" (USEPA, 1986a). Many are anthropogenic in origin; however, a variety are generated by natural processes, such as the photooxidation of atmospheric hydrocarbons. Cigarette smoke, automobile exhaust, and drinking water are examples of complex environmental mixtures encountered in everyday life.

The assumptions and uncertainties associated with risk assessments of single chemicals also apply to mixtures of chemicals. However, the complexity and diversity of chemical mixtures make them intrinsically difficult to characterize, compromising an already controvertible assess-

---

*This document has been reviewed by the Health Effects Research Laboratory, U. S. Environmental Protection Agency, and approved for publication. Approval does not signify that the contents reflect the views of the agency, nor does mention of trade names or commercial products constitute endorsement or recommendation for use.

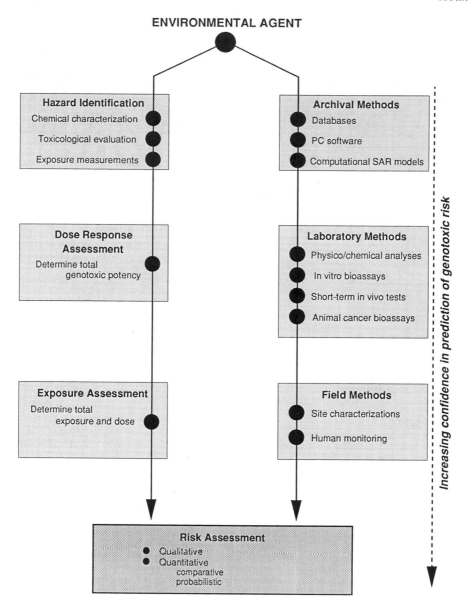

**Figure 1** The elements of risk assessment and the methods that provide supportive genotoxicity data. (Adapted from Lewtas et al., 1994a.)

ment process. Data available on mixtures vary considerably in both quality and quantity. A complex mixture may contain hundreds or thousands of chemicals, many of which cannot be identified or quantified by current analytical capabilities. As the number of compounds in the mixture increases, the uncertainties of assessment increase. Toxicological data on identified constituents may be scant or nonexistent. Dose–response models, which often are based on biological mechanisms of single compounds, may not apply to a heterogeneous mixture of chemicals. Exposure assessments of complex mixtures are especially problematic because of their highly variable temporal exposure patterns and the potential for effects at multiple endpoints. Insufficient empirical data at any of these stages confounds the characterization of risk.

Because of the unique problems that exist with risk assessments of complex mixtures, several approaches have been proposed that supplement the NAS risk assessment paradigm. These schemes are designed to overcome uncertainty and to provide a degree of flexibility when discussing potential outcome. One such example is the *Guidelines for the Health Risk Assessment of Chemical Mixtures* (USEPA, 1986a), which provides guidance for several approaches, rather than recommending a single procedure. Selection of an option relies on the availability and quality of information gathered from three possible sources: the mixture of concern, a mixture similar to the one in question (a surrogate), or the mixture's constituents. The best risk assessments are those conducted on the mixture of concern or a reasonably similar mixture. When data are available for only select components of the mixture, the additivity model is typically invoked, and the toxicities associated with individual constituents are summed to predict the overall toxicity of the whole mixture.

Risk characterization is both a qualitative and quantitative exercise, and it relies on three levels of information: archived data, laboratory data, and field data (see Fig. 1). Archived data include databases and the application of computational methods. Laboratory-derived data includes analyses of physicochemical properties, in vitro and other short-term test results, and findings from long-term animal bioassays. Field data include site characterizations (in which environmental samples, plants, and feral animal species are monitored) and epidemiological investigations (in which human populations are studied). Risk methods attempt to integrate these diverse data sets to provide a cohesive characterization of risk. A weight-of-evidence scheme, which determines the relevancy and strength of the available data, is often applied to the overall analysis. In general, field data are held in higher regard, but laboratory data, especially results from animal bioassays, provide valuable supplemental evidence.

When data are limited in quality or quantity, or when only a crude characterization of risk is sought, a qualitative risk assessment is made. Qualitative assessments alert the investigator to potential problem areas and also help guide research efforts. Quantitative risk assessments, on the other hand, are made when there is sufficient evidence of relevance to humans or when there are appropriate data to support quantitative analysis.

Quantitative assessments may be probabilistic or comparative, depending on the strength of available data. When extensive dose–response and exposure data are available for the mixture of concern, or for specific components of that mixture, it may be possible to estimate the probability of a health effect outcome. Such probabilistic assessments yield unit risk estimates (e.g., lifetime risk per microgram of particulate matter per cubic meter of air). However, the application of risk estimates to whole mixtures is often problematic, because the evaluation favors data-sparse and model-intensive techniques (Owen and Jones, 1990). As a result, inferential methods, such as toxicity equivalency factors (TEF) or comparative potency, are gaining acceptance (Schoeny and Margosches, 1989). These comparative approaches to risk assessment rely on relative decision making in which estimates of risk are based on rankings of hazard or toxicity. Such assessments are useful when data are available for surrogate mixture(s) or when a mixture comprises chemical cogeners or homologues, the toxicity of which can be related to an isomer possessing an extensive health effects database.

The following discussion will attempt to identify and resolve some of the unique concerns that have evolved from risk assessments of complex mixtures, especially relative to the field of genetic toxicology. *Genetic toxicity* is any toxic effect associated with the hereditary material (DNA). Deleterious health effects resulting from genetic damage include cancer, birth defects, cardiovascular disease, and aging. The characterization and management of genetic risks not only helps protect human health, but also helps ensure species vigor and diversity by protecting the gene pool. The elements of risk assessment—as they relate to genotoxicity—are outlined in Fig. 1. The data used to support this process fall along a continuum in which confidence in the probability of human response increases as one develops increasingly more relevant (and complex) datasets.

Generally speaking, the risk assessment process is driven by formulaic guidelines provided by federal agencies and statutes. Prescribed methods for each stage of the process are discussed in Section II. For various reasons, actual risk assessments of complex environmental mixtures often diverge from this somewhat doctrinaire approach. Therefore, subsequent sections of this chapter will present issues relevant specifically to risk assessments of complex mixtures. Included are approaches for assessing a mixture for potential hazard (Sec. III), methodologies that provide information in support of the risk assessment process (Sec. IV), and examples of real-world risk assessments of complex mixtures, ranging from qualitative to quantitative (Sec. V).

## II. ELEMENTS OF RISK ASSESSMENT

### A. Hazard Identification

Simply put, hazard identification is a qualitative articulation of whether an agent is causally linked to an adverse effect. Data supporting causality may be qualitative or quantitative and may be obtained from sources as diverse as computer databases and epidemiology studies. Hazard identification is the initial step in determining whether sufficient evidence exists for the subsequent assessment of dose–response and exposure.

Because of the universality of DNA as the genetic material across species, data from phylogenetically different test systems—from microorganisms to humans—may be incorporated into the hazard identification process. Data provided by genetic bioassays are interpreted by risk assessors according to the category of the test and the endpoint detected by the test. All relevant information contributes to the weight-of-evidence scheme, and consistent results across different test systems or species strengthen the evaluation.

The EPA's Office of Prevention, Pesticides, and Toxic Substances has released guidelines proposing the use of a battery of genetic bioassays (Fig. 2) to detect potential carcinogens and germ cell mutagens (Dearfield et al., 1991). The initial three-test battery provides qualitative criteria for hazard identification. In addition, a hierarchical weight-of-evidence scheme for mutagenicity hazard identification has been formulated by EPA based on target tissue and target species (Fig. 3). For carcinogens, evidence from human and animal studies are heavily favored, with data from short-term and in vitro tests providing supplemental information on the specific nature of the genetic response and potential mechanism of action.

Complex chemical mixtures present a difficult challenge for hazard identification, in that most are poorly defined and vary in composition. The most comprehensive characterizations involve the merger of chemical and toxicological data. Various computational, labora-

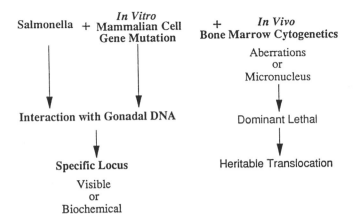

**Figure 2** The current mutagenicity testing scheme of the U. S. EPA Office of Prevention, Pesticides, and Toxic Substances. Note: Not all tests are necessarily required following completion of the base set of three tests. (From Dearfield et al., 1991.)

tory, and field methods (discussed in detail in Sec. IV) may be applied to help define the hazards of the mixture.

## B.  Dose–Response Assessment

This component of the risk assessment process defines the relation between the dose of an agent and the magnitude of response. That relation may be expressed quantitatively as the potency of the agent. For mutagens, two fundamental expressions of potency are typically used: (1) the calculated slope of the dose–response curve, and (2) the dose at which a specific response is observed [such as the dose at which a 50% response is obtained ($ED_{50}$), or the lowest effective dose (LED)]. Both estimates of potency can be used in probabilistic or comparative assessments of risk (Fig. 4). For carcinogens, similar forms of quantitation are available. Slopes may be calculated from dose–response curves obtained from animal cancer bioassays, and these potency estimates converted to "unit risk" estimates for humans (CAG, 1980). Because the goal is to estimate human cancer risk at low doses, potency is derived from the slope of the curve at its low-dose end. The multistage model, widely used in federal carcinogen regulation and discussed in greater detail later (see Sec. II.D), relies on this kind of analysis to establish an upper confidence limit on suspected cancer risk. Alternatively, a $TD_{50}$ may be calculated, in which potency is expressed as the chronic dose rate that halves the probability of animals remaining tumor-free throughout the standard life span of the species (Gold et al., 1984). This measure of potency has an extensive database (Gold et al., 1993), and its usefulness has been demonstrated in a variety of studies, including carcinogen potency ranking (Nesnow, 1991).

| *In Vivo* | > | *In Vitro* |
|---|---|---|
| Germ Cell | > | Somatic Cell |
| Mammalian | > | Submammalian |
| Eukaryotes | > | Prokaryotes |

**Figure 3** Hierarchical weight-of-evidence scheme for mutagenicity hazard identification used by the U. S. EPA. (Adapted from Jarabek and Farland, 1990.)

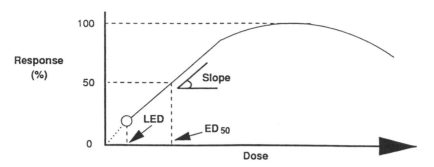

**Figure 4**   The use of slope, lowest effective dose (LED), and effective dose causing 50% response ($ED_{50}$) in determining mutagenic potency.

Critical uncertainties must be addressed when modeling dose response, including high-to-low dose and interspecies extrapolations. Low-dose extrapolations introduce uncertainty, partly because of questions surrounding the shape of the dose–response curve in the low-dose region. Although the field of pharmacokinetics is adding to our understanding of low-dose extrapolation through physiologically and biologically based models, such models are problematic for mixture assessments owing to difficulties, for example, with mass–balance equations (Krewski and Thomas, 1992).

For complex mixtures, consideration also must be given to the combined effects of the components constituting the mixture. In the absence of empirical evidence on interactions within the mixture, component additivity is assumed. Response additivity asserts that the components act on different receptor systems and that the toxicity of the mixture can be approximated by summing the known toxicities of the components. Dose additivity assumes that the components in the mixture have the same mode of action and that the overall toxic response can be predicted by summing the individual doses (USEPA, 1986a). Although evidence favors the additivity of risks at low doses, there are inherent problems with this approach, including the lack of complete data on chemical composition, the improbability that mixture components elicit similar effects or have similar modes of action, and the likelihood of interactions among chemicals. Many in vitro studies of genotoxicity do not support the additivity assumption for highly complex mixtures (Houk, 1992). For carcinogenicity studies, additive relative risk has been demonstrated for joint exposure to two carcinogens affecting the same stage of carcinogenesis, but exposures affecting different stages led to supra-additive or supramultiplicative relative risks (Brown and Chu, 1989; Kodell et al., 1991). Moreover, at high-exposure levels, synergistic effects have been demonstrated in both toxicological and epidemiological studies of carcinogens (Krewski and Thomas, 1992).

## C.  Exposure Assessment

Exposure assessment generally consists of three steps: (1) characterization of the exposure setting (i.e., the physical environment and potentially exposed populations), (2) identification of exposure pathways, and (3) quantification of exposure by estimates of concentration and intake. Although exposure customarily refers to interactions at exchange boundaries (e.g., skin or lung) before uptake, efforts to measure internal exposure at the cellular and molecular level are increasingly common. Methods for quantifying exposure include direct chemical measurements (such as personal monitoring devices or human blood levels) and indirect measurements (such as ambient concentrations or results from fate and transport models).

Direct measurements are growing in acceptance owing to the preference for microenvironmental data and body-burden estimates.

Exposure data are integrated to develop a qualitative or quantitative estimate of the magnitude of human contact with the agent(s) of concern. To assess total human exposure, environmental- and human-monitoring studies are often conducted. In environmental-monitoring studies, contaminants are identified and quantified in a microenvironment, and their distribution and movement through various media are described. In biomonitoring, personal exposure devices are used to collect external data, which are then combined with information from biological markers of internal dose and response (using body fluids, cells, or tissues).

Genotoxicity assays have been used for many years in environmental-monitoring studies to detect causative agents, to monitor their fate, to apportion sources of toxicity, and to demonstrate—through the use of sentinel organisms—direct associations between exposures and genotoxic response (see Sec. IV.C). Because results do not rely on prior identification of specific chemicals, these techniques are particularly suited to studies of complex mixtures. Genetic bioassays also have been used in human studies to detect genetic damage in tissues or body fluids. Recently developed biomarkers, such as DNA adducts, are especially useful because they can facilitate construction of the relations between external dose, internal exposure, and response. It also is now possible to couple genetic bioassays with personal exposure-monitoring methods (J. Lewtas, personal communication). The development of these new sampling, chemical, and bioassay procedures has led to remarkable progress in this field and, when combined with available molecular dosimetry data, should result in better understanding of human exposures to genotoxic agents.

## D. Risk Characterization and Assessment

Risk characterization integrates the information produced by the other three components of the risk assessment process to estimate the overall likelihood of a health effect given specific conditions of exposure. The nature and magnitude of human risk are described in both qualitative and quantitative terms. The various strengths and weaknesses associated with the estimate of risk are summarized, and biological and statistical assumptions and uncertainties are explained.

For genotoxic substances, risk characterizations are made in two areas: carcinogenicity and heritable genetic risk. The EPA has developed guidelines for risk assessment in both of these areas (USEPA, 1986b,c). Each of these guidelines rely on a weight-of-evidence approach to classify chemicals or mixtures into categories, incorporating estimates of exposure into the final risk analysis. The EPA also has developed guidelines for risk assessments of chemical mixtures (USEPA, 1986a). Criteria to evaluate the quality of data for mixtures are provided in three categories: information on exposure, health effects, and interactions. Figure 5 is a decision tree illustrating the way in which decisions on risk assessment approaches may be made, depending on the availability and adequacy of these data elements.

Risk assessments generally fall into two categories: qualitative and quantitative (comparative or probabilistic). The specific assessment strategy chosen will depend on the strength of available data, as well as on risk management objectives. Human data, although preferred to animal data, are often unavailable or inadequate to perform risk assessments. Consequently, results from long-term animal bioassays are typically used to estimate human cancer risk.

To predict human risk from animal tumorigenicity studies requires extrapolation modeling. Mathematical models of dose–response, which combine both biological and statistical premises, are pivotal to quantitative cancer risk assessment. Tolerance–distribution models (probit, logit, and Weibull) and stochastic models (one-hit and multistage) form the core of quantitative cancer risk assessment (Morris, 1990). Tolerance–distribution models assume that each individual has

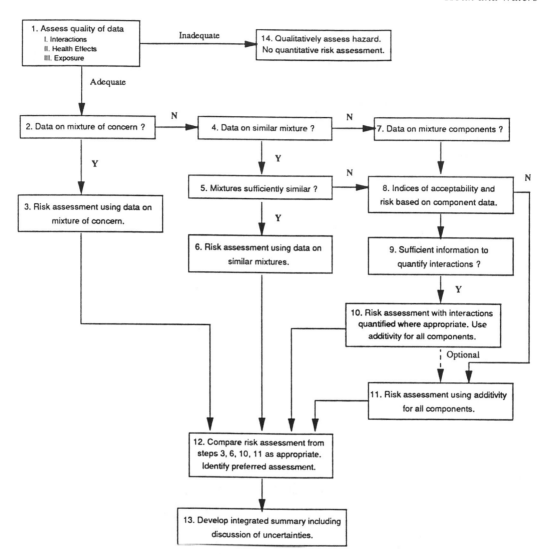

**Figure 5** Decision tree of the risk assessment approach recommended by the U. S. EPA for chemical mixtures. (From USEPA, 1986a.)

a tolerance level to a carcinogen. Stochastic models assume that everyone is equally susceptible to cancer, and that cancer is initiated by one or several independent, random events.

Of these models, the multistage model most effectively expresses the current biological thinking about cancer (i.e., that cancer is a disease requiring multiple events in the progression of a normal cell to a malignant one; Fig. 6). The multistage model was first proposed in the 1950s (Armitage and Doll, 1954), and a variation of this model (Guess and Crump, 1976, 1978; Crump et al., 1976, 1977) has provided the framework for regulatory cancer risk assessment at the federal level. However, recent advances in the theory of cancer induction have uncovered important deficiencies in multistage models, such as their disregard for separate mechanisms known to be involved in tumor initiation and promotion. Consequently, biologically based models of cancer risk assessment are receiving considerable attention. Moolgavkar and Knudson

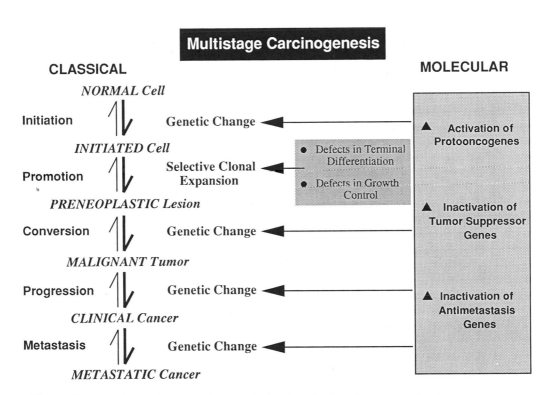

**Figure 6**  Steps in multistage carcinogenesis showing classic and molecular details.

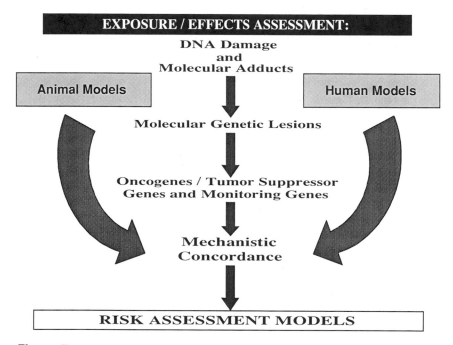

**Figure 7**  The use of animal and human models to provide evidence of mechanistic concordance for biologically based cancer risk assessment models.

(1981), for example, have developed a popular two-stage model of cancer risk, based on evidence linking mutation induction with tumor formation. Their model assumes that the first event in the formation of a tumor is the induction of a mutation that transforms a normal cell to a preneoplastic ("initiated") cell. The second transition is from initiated cell to malignant cancer cell. This two-stage cancer model has gained widespread acceptance because it is interpretable in biological terms and explains many of the phenomena observed with human cancers (Thorslund et al., 1987). It is evident, however, from more recent research (specifically, the colorectal cancer model based on the work of Vogelstein et al., 1988, 1989) that a two-stage model cannot accurately explain the multiple biological processes involved in tumor development. As our understanding of the molecular mechanisms of carcinogenesis advances, the development of more realistic, biologically based cancer risk models will follow (Harris, 1991). Ideally, biologically based cancer risk assessment models will be based on evidence of mechanistic concordance between animal and human model systems, as illustrated in Fig. 7.

## III. SPECIAL CONSIDERATIONS INVOLVING COMPLEX MIXTURES

### A. Integrating Chemical and Toxicological Data

Critical to any assessment of complex mixtures is the integration of chemical and biological information. Chemical analyses are indispensable for identifying and quantitating the hazardous constituents of the mixture; toxicological assessments determine which compounds or mixtures pose the greatest risk. Combining data from both disciplines provides a more thorough and conclusive evaluation of potential hazard than either in isolation.

Matrix evaluation, which involves the manipulation of selected variables to define a mixture, can be used to map or plot the chemical or biological characteristics of the mixture. The goal of matrix sampling for chemical analysis and biotesting is to define the boundary conditions that permit the positioning of effects of a given mixture within a matrix of related mixtures (NRC, 1988). If mixtures can be mapped onto a broad representation of critical physicochemical variables, many of the uncertainties concerning interpretation of toxicological tests on chemical mixtures may be resolved (Fig. 8). Conversely, as indicated in the same figure, a matrix or profile of biological data can be used to direct the application of analytical chemical techniques (see also discussion on GAPs, Sec. IV.A, and Table 2).

### B. Characterization of Complex Mixtures

The composition of a complex environmental mixture (urban air, industrial effluent, river water, or other) will vary from one locale to another and from one collection point to another. Consequently, it is important to define the mixture a priori as carefully as possible and, when testing an actual sample, to collect material that is representative of the mixture of concern. Randomized sampling techniques should be followed, and standardized sampling methodologies should be conformed to (see, e.g., USEPA, 1980).

To analyze a collected sample for potential hazard, one of two generalized test strategies may be employed: (1) the whole mixture (heterogeneous sample) may be analyzed, or (2) the mixture may be broken into constituent parts (individual compounds or classes of compounds) for analysis. Selection of the appropriate technique is dependent on the physical and chemical characteristics of the sample, the purpose for which data are intended, the tests to which a sample may be assigned, and budgetary restrictions.

If individual component chemicals are to be considered, a detailed chemical profile is required. Gas chromatography or high-performance liquid chromatography may be used to survey the compounds making up the mixture. Following such an evaluation, the toxic potential

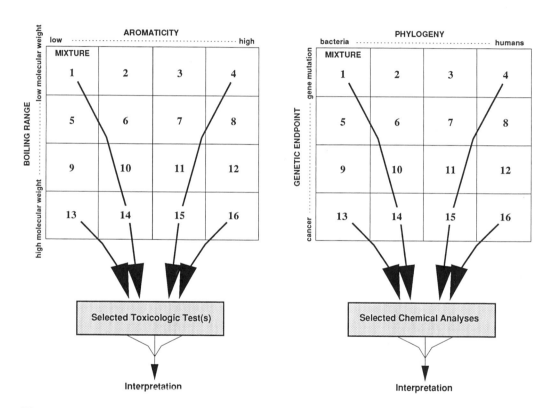

**Figure 8**   Example of matrix testing in which critical physicochemical and genotoxicological variables for a series of mixtures are identified to define boundary conditions for interpreting results of chemical and toxicological testing. (Adapted from NRC, 1988.)

of each constituent must be determined. This information can be retrieved from preexisting toxicological databases, or it can be generated by individually testing each identified compound in appropriate assays. If the identified chemicals have assigned potency values (such as mutagenicity slope values, LEDs, cancer $TD_{50}$, or unit risk numbers), a quantitative risk assessment may be performed by invoking the additivity model and summing the individual toxicities to predict the overall toxicity of the mixture (USEPA, 1986a).

The advantage of chemical-specific analysis is that particularly hazardous chemicals can be detected, whereupon control measures can be implemented. However, several factors make this approach indeterminate. Even a relatively detailed chemical analysis may fail to detect or identify toxic chemicals owing to the insensitivity of the analytical technique, the sheer number of components to be resolved, the relatively small amount of chemical present in the mixture, or the lack of appropriate standards. The evaluation of a multitude of identified chemicals is both costly and time-consuming. Searches of preexisting databases may yield limited information, or worse, no information. Finally, the additivity model ignores chemical interactions, possible physicochemical matrix effects, and transformation or degradation.

In practice, it is usually not possible to carry out complete chemical characterization of a complex environmental mixture. Accordingly, such mixtures are often partitioned into separate chemical fractions for toxicity testing. Two principal separation methods exist: liquid–liquid partitioning and chromatography (NRC, 1988). Table 1 provides a list of conventional separation techniques. One especially successful method of partitioning complex mixtures is bioassay-directed fractionation (NRC, 1988). In this approach, each fraction is bioassayed until the major class or specific chemical(s) responsible for the activity can be isolated and chemically characterized (Fig. 9). As an example, cigarette smoke condensate was fractionated and tested in mouse skin carcinogenicity bioassays, which led to the identification of fractions containing tumor-initiating activity and tumor-producing activity (Bock et al., 1969; Hoffman and Wynder, 1971). Subsequent studies using short-term mutagenicity and cellular transformation bioassays were able to identify specific chemicals in biologically active fractions that were responsible for the genotoxic activity (DeMarini, 1983).

The advantages of fractionation include the separation of active constituents from inactive or toxic components and the extrication of active chemicals present in small quantities. Disadvantages include the limited amount of sample available for testing following processing,

**Table 1** Conventional Methods for Separating Complex Mixtures into Fractions Suitable for Testing

| Type | Variations | Materials |
|---|---|---|
| Liquid–liquid partitioning | Solvent–solvent; solvent–acid/base | Organic solvents of different polarity; aqueous acid/base solutions |
| Chromatography | Column (open), thin-layer (TLC) | |
| | Adsorption | Aluminum, silica gel, polyamide, Florisil |
| | Partition | Cellulose |
| | Molecular exclusion | Porous polymers, gels |
| | Ion-exchange | Ion-exchange resins (anionic, cationic) |
| | High-performance liquid (HPLC) | |
| | Adsorption | Aluminum, silica gel, polyamide, Florisil |
| | Partition | Cellulose, bonded phases |
| | Molecular exclusion | Porous polymers, gels |
| | Ion-exchange | Ion-exchange resins (anionic, cationic) |

*Source:* NRC, 1988.

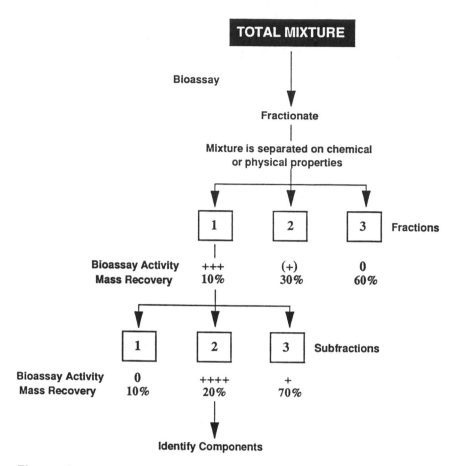

**Figure 9** Diagrammatic representation of bioassay-directed fractionation in which the mixture is sequentially separated into fractions that are subjected to bioassay. Fractions showing highest activity are pursued with additional fractionation and bioassay to identify the most active components. (From NRC, 1988.)

the likelihood of spillover of chemical classes between fractions, and the possible loss or modification of components with fractionation.

A final alternative for testing a complex environmental mixture is to treat the mixture as a single entity and analyze it in its crude state. Although uncommon, such studies can provide useful information. Houk and DeMarini (1988), DeMarini et al. (1987, 1989), and Simmons et al. (1988) administered crude industrial waste samples to several short-term biological systems, including bacterial assays for mutagenicity and DNA damage, and rodent assays to detect DNA adducts, lethality, hepatotoxicity, nephrotoxicity, and urinary mutagenicity. The usefulness of such an approach was demonstrated when a crude waste that was genotoxic in vitro also produced urinary mutagens in the rat and DNA adducts in bladder tissue.

The obvious advantages of this approach include the relevancy of the tested sample to its environmental counterpart, decreased potential for artifact formation, and the elimination of the need for modeling interactive effects. Moreover, if the mixture is representative of others in its class (e.g., diesel emissions from different sources would share certain characteristics), it may be possible to extrapolate results across samples. This method also circumvents the labor-intensive process of individually testing multiple chemicals. But sometimes a complex mixture is too cytotoxic to be tested directly in a bioassay. Furthermore, it may be incompatible with the test system because of its physical matrix. Other disadvantages include the inability to specify the constituent(s) of the mixture responsible for the toxicity, as well as potential masking effects (e.g., the masking of mutagenicity by cytotoxicity).

## IV.  IN SUPPORT OF THE RISK ASSESSMENT PROCESS

### A.  Archived Data

Computerized databases and models are valuable reservoirs of information that support the risk assessment process by augmenting hazard identification and by guiding test efforts. Moreover, dose–response information is contained in many datasets, and, by combining individual chemical component concentration and toxicity data, situational exposure assessments may be possible.

Numerous databases are available from which to extract information on the genetic toxicity or carcinogenicity of chemical constituents of a mixture, or on the mixture itself. Examples include detailed monographs on the carcinogenic hazards of individual chemicals and complex mixtures, such as those produced by the International Agency for Research on Cancer (IARC); books such as *Atmospheric Chemical Compounds: Sources, Occurrence, and Bioassay* by Graedel et al. (1986), which contains information on structures, properties, detection methodologies, and sources of chemicals; reviews such as "The genotoxicity of industrial wastes and effluents" (Houk, 1992), which is a comprehensive analysis of the genotoxicity of wastes classified according to industrial source; personal computer software such as the Genetic Activity Profile (GAP) database (Waters et al., 1990a), which provides a computer-generated graphic representation of an array of genetic bioassay data as a function of chemical dose (see later example); data listings, such as the carcinogenic potency database compiled by Gold et al. (1993), which includes calculations of carcinogenicity $TD_{50}$ values; and on-line computer databases such as EPA's Integrated Risk Information System (IRIS), which contains EPA consensus scientific positions on human health hazard, or the Registry of Toxic Effects of Chemical Substances (RTECS), which contains some toxicological data on complex mixtures.

Computerized databases can complement data from in vitro tests, animal bioassays, or epidemiology studies to assist in the evaluation of potential human health risks. For example, the information contained in genetic activity profiles (GAPs) may be combined with data from other sources to estimate the genetic activity and potential carcinogenic hazard of complex mixtures (Waters et al., 1990b). The GAPs represent graphic displays of short-term test results, either positive or negative, for individual chemicals or complex mixtures and the doses at which these results are obtained (Fig. 10). Information is collected from the open literature, and either the LED or highest ineffective dose (HID) is recorded for each agent and each bioassay system. The presentation format is a bar graph representing the tests that have been applied to a given agent. Positive results for these individual tests are displayed as LED values superimposed on bars projected upward from the origin. Negative results are displayed as HID values on bars projected downward from the origin. The dose scale on the *y*-axis is constructed such that the length of the bar in the upward direction represents the average LED for the agent—the longer the bar, the lower the average LED for the agent. The length of the bar in the downward direction represents the average HID for the agent—the longer the bar, the higher the dose applied to the test in the absence of an extreme toxic response. The GAPs are presented with tests in either a phylogenetic sequence or an endpoint sequence. Thus, GAPs permit direct visual assessment of

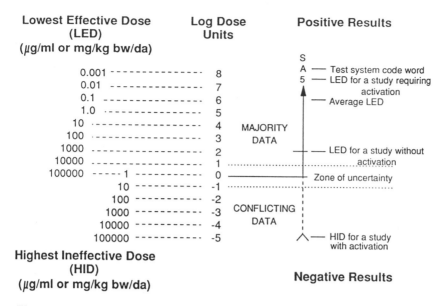

**Figure 10** Diagrammatic representation of a genetic activity profile showing graphic layout, units, and abbreviations.

the responses of an array of short-term tests to the agent and facilitate a limited comparative assessment of a test system's usefulness in evaluating the particular agent.

In approaching the evaluation of the genetic activity of a complex mixture, knowledge of chemical partitioning can indicate which chemicals are likely to be found in which chemical fractions. However, since chemical analysis is usually performed sequentially, substantial effort may be required for chemical speciation. If the chemicals likely to be present in a particular chemical fraction are known, then a search of available short-term test data, particularly as represented by GAPs, can indicate the kinds of bioassays that are most appropriate for the anticipated chemicals. Furthermore, it is possible to use computer-based GAP-matching techniques (Garrett et al., 1984, 1986) to find chemicals displaying the pattern of biological response represented by the types or classes of chemicals expected in the chemical fraction. Table 2 defines a logical sequence for the application of analytical chemical techniques, bioassay methods, genetic activity profiles, and rodent carcinogenicity data to estimate the genetic activity and potential carcinogenic hazard of a complex environmental mixture or mixture fraction.

Finally, in addition to their role in the organization, representation, and interpretation of relevant databases, computers are a valuable tool for use in the development of structure–activity relationships (SAR). The SAR modeling uses the structural features of a chemical to alert the investigator to its potential toxicity, mutagenicity, or carcinogenicity (see Richard et al., 1989). Structural classification schemes tend to be based on common organic functionalities (e.g., esters) or on chemical classes associated with toxicity (e.g., nitroaromatics). Statistically based SAR methods use existing toxicity data to infer relevant molecular features, and these "descriptors" are then used to predict the toxicity of chemicals for which there are no data. Computational SAR methods can be used to develop rational bioassay strategies and to probe underlying mechanisms of toxicity. They provide a quantitative basis for defining a chemical class and for differentiating between class members. Ideally, continuing feedback should exist between quantitative computational SAR studies, the development of bioassay data, knowledge regarding mechanisms of action, and assessment needs.

**Table 2** Use of GAPs in Estimating the Genetic Activity and Potential Carcinogenic Hazard of a Complex Environmental Mixture or Mixture Component

1. Collect a representative sample of the complex mixture.
2. Partition the sample by using chemical fractionation methods.
3. Use generalized chemical analytical methods to determine that fractionation has been successful and to provide an inventory of likely chemicals within the component fractions.
4. Refer to published inventories of chemicals detected in complex mixture sources of the type represented by the sample (e.g., Graedel et al., 1986).
5. Collect GAPs for all chemicals known or suspected to be present in the fractions derived from the complex mixture sample (cf. Waters et al., 1988).
6. Using GAPs, make a selection of bioassay systems to be applied to the fractions that should detect known or suspected component chemicals.
7. If the number of GAPs for chemicals in any fraction is large, use GAP-matching techniques to group chemicals according to the similarity of their biological activity. Select tests that are appropriate to detect the activity represented by such groups of chemicals.
8. From the LEDs indicated in GAPs, determine if chemicals at known quantity within a given fraction could be detected by the genetic bioassays to be applied to that fraction.
9. Carry out genetic bioassays on fractions of the complex mixture sample as directed by qualitative and quantitative information from GAPs.
10. Determine if chemicals having GAPs are rodent or human carcinogens and the dose range over which carcinogenicity may be detected (cf., Gold et al., 1987, 1989).
11. Determine whether these chemicals are present in the complex mixture sample at levels that could lead to cancer in animals exposed over their lifetime.
12. Determine the human exposure to the chemicals contained in the complex mixture.

## B. Laboratory Data

### 1. Physicochemical Analyses

When assessing complex mixtures, it is advantageous to identify properties that exacerbate risk. Concentration, mobility and transport capabilities, solubility, electrophilicity, persistence, reactivity, and bioavailability are important pieces of information that can be considered, together with toxicity data, to substantiate potential hazard. Information on melting points, octanol/water coefficients, $pK_a$, and other data, are readily retrievable from archived sources (e.g., Karcher and Devillers, 1990), but usually only for individual chemical compounds. For complex mixtures, archived information is typically unavailable (except on individual compounds that compose the mixture), and an accurate assessment of physicochemical properties often requires laboratory analyses. Physicochemical data may be used not only in a preliminary hazard assessment, but in exposure and pharmacokinetic modeling as well (Reitz, 1990).

### 2. In Vitro and Short-Term In Vivo Genotoxicity Studies

Short-term bioassays are screening tools for the toxicological evaluation of complex mixtures. They are rapid, inexpensive, sensitive indicators of a sample's potential to induce damage. Short-term genetic bioassays are based on the cellular and subcellular mechanisms underlying the carcinogenic process and are used to ascertain different types of genetic damage. Commonly studied endpoints include DNA damage, gene mutation, chromosomal aberrations, micronuclei, sister-chromatid exchange, aneuploidy, and cell transformation. The type of lesion is important because it conveys information about the intrinsic nature of the genetic (or related) hazard (Lewtas et al., 1994a).

More than 200 short-term tests employing bacteria, yeast, fungi, cultured cells, plants, insects, and animals have been developed to assist the identification of agents that pose a genetic hazard to humans (Waters et al., 1988). The Ames *Salmonella typhimurium* mutagenicity assay is by far the most widely used. An extensive analysis of the performance of this test on a chemical class basis (Claxton et al., 1988) has shown that the sensitivity of the assay by chemical class varies from 0.63 to 0.92. The bioassay is very efficient in detecting carcinogens that are nitro-containing organics or hydrocarbons, but not very efficient in detecting carcinogens that are halogenated or inorganic compounds. A conservative approach in the interpretation of short-term tests would be to consider any short-term or long-term bioassay that performs with as much sensitivity and specificity as a rodent bioassay to be acceptable for the screening of complex mixtures for carcinogenicity. Brusick (1983) showed that when rat and mouse bioassay data are compared, the sensitivity value ranges from 0.70 to 0.85 and specificity ranges from 0.58 to 0.75. Combining all evaluations of the performance of the *Salmonella* assay yields a sensitivity value of 0.77 and a specificity of 0.64. These values support the usefulness of the *Salmonella* assay as a primary screen for complex mixtures. Furthermore, *Salmonella* detects most of the IARC Group I human carcinogens; exceptions include benzene, diethylstilbestrol, arsenic, nickel, and asbestos (Shelby and Zeiger, 1990).

The *Salmonella* assay has been used to measure the mutagenic activity of numerous complex environmental mixtures, including cigarette smoke condensate (DeMarini, 1983), automobile exhaust (Lewtas, 1983), ambient air (Barale et al., 1990), industrial wastes (Houk, 1992), and drinking water (Meier, 1988). But the usefulness of the *Salmonella* assay (and in vitro tests in general) extends beyond the mere detection of mutagens and carcinogens in a mixture. Such tests also may be used to determine the contribution of specific environmental sources to the genotoxicity of the whole mixture (Van Hoof and Verheyden, 1981; Lewis et al., 1988); to evaluate parameters—such as sunlight—that may influence genotoxicity (Nestmann et al., 1984; Claxton et al., 1990); to monitor environmental sites (Donnelly et al., 1983; McGeorge et al., 1985; Driver et al., 1990); to compare responses in target and nontarget human cells and tissues (Lewtas et al., 1993); and to monitor human exposures (Matsushita et al., 1990).

Recent advances in the molecular analysis of mutations in *Salmonella* have suggested that the mutation spectra produced by complex mixtures is reflective of the predominance of a single (or a few) mutagenic chemical class(es) within the mixture (Fig. 11). For example, the base-pair substitution mutation spectrum produced by MX (a chlorinated hydroxyfuranone compound common to drinking water) is virtually identical with that produced by chlorinated drinking water (DeMarini et al., 1993). This finding substantiates the results of Meier (1988), who showed that MX contributes up to 60% of the mutagenicity detected in chlorinated drinking water. Molecular analyses are beginning to contribute important information to mutagenicity and carcinogenicity risk assessment, especially considering recent evidence that suggests striking similarities between the types of mutations induced in *Salmonella,* rodents, and human cancer cells exposed to the same complex mixture (D. M. DeMarini, personal communication).

Short-term in vivo tests also have been used to evaluate the genotoxicity of complex mixtures (Das and Nanda, 1986; DeMarini et al., 1989; Gallagher et al., 1990, 1993; Lewtas et al., 1993). In this type of test, an organic extract of the mixture—or sometimes the crude mixture itself—is administered to the whole animal, and, over the course of a few days, tissues or body fluids are collected and evaluated. Bioindicators of genetic damage include urinary metabolites, the formation of DNA adducts, and the detection of micronuclei.

## 3. Animal Bioassays

Results from studies of laboratory animals, particularly mammalian species, are held in high regard in the cancer risk assessment process. Because human data are generally unavailable, long-term carcinogenicity experiments in animals are often the primary source of relevant

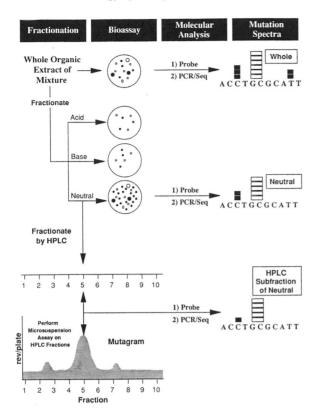

**Figure 11** Fractionation, bioassay, molecular analysis, and construction of mutation spectra for fractions of a complex mixture separated by liquid–liquid (acid–base) partitioning, followed by high-pressure liquid chromatography (HPLC) of the neutral fraction. (Note: A microsuspension *Salmonella* assay has been performed to create a mutagram.) Molecular analysis including colony probe hybridization (probe) and polymerase chain reaction (PCR) followed by DNA sequencing yields data used in the construction of mutation spectra for the whole organic extract, the neutral fraction, and an HPLC subfraction of the neutral fraction. (From Lewtas et al., 1994b.)

information for human response and are the most universally accepted means (other than epidemiological investigations) of determining carcinogenic hazard. The acceptability of animal data is based on the premise that biological effects may be extrapolated across mammalian species. Animal bioassays actually offer some advantages over human data, in that experiments can be controlled, high doses can be administered, and invasive techniques can be used (Morris, 1990).

To evaluate human carcinogenic potential, most chemicals are tested in 2-year bioassays conducted in rats and mice (Huff et al., 1991). Chemicals tested in this manner have produced responses ranging from no effects in either species, to the induction of neoplasms in multiple tissues in both species. A weight-of-evidence scheme proposed for classifying carcinogens (Ashby et al., 1990) asserts that activity in several species, and a correspondence of tumor sites across species, are important in the identification of a human cancer hazard. This observation has been reiterated by Tennant (1993), who states that transspecies, multiple site, mutagenic rodent carcinogens should be considered first priority for attention for human cancer risk. Weakest evidence is reflected in a restricted pattern of tumor induction (i.e., at a specific site in a single sex of a single species).

In addition to carcinogenicity, animal cancer models may be effectively used to study the nature and level of DNA adducts arising from exposures to complex mixtures, by use of techniques such as $^{32}$P-postlabeling. The DNA adducts derived from the polycyclic aromatic compounds emitted from tobacco smoke, coke ovens, smelters, coal-burning, diesel exhaust, and urban air pollution have been investigated using mouse skin tumor initiation models (Lewtas, et al., 1993).

## C.  Field Data

Field data are those gathered from an environmental site or from a human population. Often, data are temporal or spatial in nature, permitting the tracking, regulation, or control of the parameter being measured (Houk et al., 1993). Environmental- and human-monitoring techniques are integral to every level of the risk assessment process (Fig. 12).

### 1.  Site Characterizations

The objective of site characterization is to determine the nature and magnitude of toxic substances that may be present in the air, waste, soil, or water proximal to a site. Investigators should attempt to describe the source of the toxicity, to determine how the toxic material is released into the environment and whether the release is transient or prolonged, to assess the distribution of the toxic material throughout different environmental media, and to predict the exposure potential for each possible exposure pathway. A good example of the approaches used to characterize sites is provided by EPA's Office of Emergency and Remedial Response (USEPA, 1989). Their manual explains how data gathered at Superfund sites are applied to the risk assessment process and how such information can be used to perform human health evaluations.

The methods described earlier under Sections IV.A and IV.B can also be applied to site characterizations. Inventories may be available onsite (e.g., from an industry) describing the

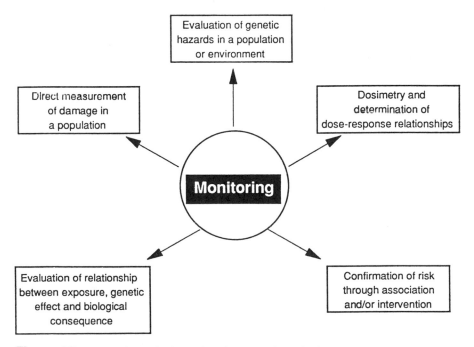

**Figure 12**  Five major objectives of environmental monitoring. (From Lewtas et al., 1994a.)

chemicals manufactured or disposed of, or the content of emissions. Alternatively, laboratory techniques (such as analytical chemistry or biological testing) can be used to monitor a site. Measurements may be made either by collecting environmental samples and analyzing them in the laboratory, or by performing in situ monitoring.

In situ monitoring employs indigenous species collected at a site or a test species introduced to a site. These species are called indicator, or sentinel, organisms. The in situ approach monitors environmental pollution by two basic methods: It measures the bioaccumulation of toxic chemicals in the tissues of the organisms, and it measures the adverse effects of the toxicants on the organism. This monitoring technique is especially important because it represents a real-world exposure scenario in which complex physical and chemical interactions in the environment affect outcome. Several reviews have been published on this subject area (Sandhu et al., 1990; McBee and Bickham, 1990).

Genetic bioassays have been used at every level of field application. They have been used to analyze and rank sources of environmental genotoxicity (Houk, 1992), to identify causative agents and to trace them to their source (Van Hoof and Verheyden, 1981; Lewis et al., 1988), to monitor the effectiveness of process modifications implemented by an industry (McGeorge et al., 1985), to monitor rural and urban airsheds (Watts et al., 1988, Barale et al., 1990), to monitor cleanup at Superfund sites (Hughes et al., 1993), and to monitor human exposures (Leonard et al., 1985; Matsushita et al., 1990). In situ applications include the introduction of sentinel organisms to detect genotoxic hazards at a petrochemical complex (Lower et al., 1983), at industrial sites (Schairer et al., 1979), and at a Superfund site (Hughes et al., 1993). In addition, feral animals, pets, and indigenous plant species have been collected from various settings and examined for evidence of genotoxic damage. Feral rodents collected at Superfund sites were used to demonstrate an association between hazardous waste exposures in both chromosomal aberrations and micronuclei (Thompson et al., 1988; Tice et al., 1987; McBee et al., 1987). Pet dogs were used in a recent study by Backer et al. (1993) to link exposure to Superfund sites with increased micronuclei frequency. Klekowski and Levin (1979) utilized a fern growing along a heavily polluted river to demonstrate the cytogenetic effects of a pulp and paper mill effluent.

## 2. Human Monitoring

Epidemiological studies provide the most compelling evidence for characterization of hazard. By definition, confirmation of a "human" carcinogen requires evidence from humans. However, the deficiencies normally associated with epidemiological studies (long latency periods, lack of sensitivity, selection of control populations, and so forth) are compounded when trying to establish a causal link between exposure to a *mixture* and an adverse health effect.

To be of use in quantitative risk assessments of mixtures, epidemiological analyses must provide quantitative dose–response functions which, in turn, rely on accurate exposure characterizations. Direct measurements of body burden may be performed to verify uptake by exposed individuals or to estimate internal dose. Because it is not possible to measure the concentration of all xenobiotics in bodily tissues or fluids, surrogate compounds (mixture component chemicals) are often used as indicators of exposure to a mixture. For example, the detection of benzo[a]pyrene (B[a]P) would suggest exposure to polyaromatic hydrocarbons (PAHs). Radio-labeled surrogate carcinogens can be used to study the low-dose response for DNA adduct formation, thereby enhancing the application of this approach (Lutz et al., 1990). Another indicator of internal dose to humans is the measurement of urinary mutagens with the *Salmonella* assay. This method has been used to detect exposure to tobacco smoke, as well as to occupational chemicals (Everson, 1986).

Methods also are available to measure early biologic response or preclinical effects

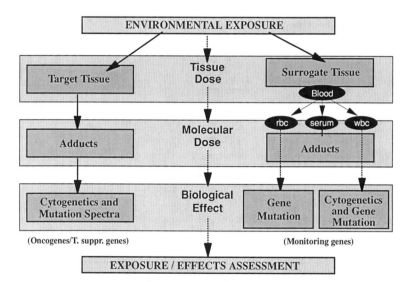

**Figure 13**  The use of DNA adduct dosimetry to enhance exposure assessment.

(the biologically effective dose). These methods, called biomarkers, reveal information about the relation between exposure, response or effect, and individual susceptibility. Because biomarkers are manifested before disease onset, they are particularly attractive to cancer epidemiology. Chromosomal aberrations, sister-chromatid exchanges, and somatic gene mutations are examples of indices of nonspecific exposure to mutagenic or carcinogenic substances. However, their observation does not necessarily result in a deleterious health outcome.

DNA adducts are another example of a biomarker of carcinogen exposure. Because of evidence indicating that carcinogens initiate the malignant process by specifically altering DNA structure by binding to DNA bases, it has been suggested that carcinogen–DNA adducts are markers of tumor initiation. The DNA adducts have been used as biomarkers of exposure in a variety of studies involving complex mixtures, including occupational exposures (Phillips et al., 1988; Perrera et al., 1988), lifestyle exposures (Mumford et al., 1993; Savela and Hemminki, 1991), industrial exposures (Lewtas et al., 1993), and ambient exposures (Hemminki et al., 1990). In the future, determination of carcinogen–DNA adduct levels in humans may be compared with the levels known to produce tumors in experimental animals (a variation of the parallelogram method) to provide relevant extrapolation from animal tests to human health risk. Figure 13 illustrates the use of DNA adduct dosimetry in potential tumor–target sites and in surrogate tissues to provide correlative information on molecular dose which, in turn, may be linked to data on biological effects, such as gene mutation (including activation of oncogenes or inactivation of tumor suppressor genes) and chromosomal aberration. The combination of data in target and surrogate tissues can provide a more rational basis for exposure–effects assessment as a major component of the risk assessment process.

## V. THE RISK ASSESSMENT STRATEGY

The selection of a risk assessment strategy depends on the strength of the data gathered at each stage of the risk assessment paradigm (see Fig. 1). The following discussion separates risk assessment into three groups: qualitative; quantitative, using comparative methods; and quantitative, using probabilistic methods. For complex mixtures, the amount of useful information significantly declines as one moves from qualitative to more quantitative levels.

## A. Qualitative Risk Assessment

The largest obstacle to generating health risk estimates for complex mixtures is the lack of relevant data. It is impossible to quantitate all of the constituent chemicals in a mixture; moreover, most toxicity testing has been conducted at high exposure levels on single chemicals, rather than on combinations of chemicals.

Nonetheless, risk can be crudely classified with limited information. Depending on response in genotoxicity tests and prevalence in the environment, simple classification schemes can be developed based on weight-of-evidence evaluations. For example, genotoxic agents can be classified as possible, probable, or demonstrated human (somatic) mutagens, depending on available data (Lewtas et al., 1994a). When combined with information on exposure, a qualitative categorization of risk from high to low may be possible. Such assessments can alert investigators to potential problem areas, or they can provide guidance in the selection of agents for additional study.

An example of this kind of analysis is provided by Houk (1992) in which complex mixtures (industrial wastes and effluents) were ranked according to mutagenic potency in the *Salmonella* assay (Table 3). Mutagenic potency data were then combined with information on industrial emission rates to calculate a daily mutagenic burden to the surrounding environment.

**Table 3**  Distribution of the Mutagenic Potencies of Industrial Wastes and Effluents Based on Activity per Unit Mass (Revertants per milligram [rev/mg][a])

| Potency (rev/mg) | Waste |
|---|---|
| $10^7$ | |
| | Plastics tar |
| Extreme | Composited organic wastes from a hazardous waste incineration facility |
| | Petrochemical waste oil (coke plant waste and waste paints), crude waste |
| $10^6$ | |
| High    $10^5$ | |
| | Chemical manufacturing (industrial organics) |
| $10^4$ | Condensate blend of wastewater from munitions production; herbicide manufacturing (acetone/water) |
| | Effluent from the manufacture of dyes and epoxy resins; chlorination stage effluent; pulp and paper mill effluent, biotreated; coke plant effluent; refinery waste (API oil–water separator sludge), basic fraction |
| | Pulp and paper waste; wastewaters from the manufacture of hair dyes and herbicides; used crankcase oil |
| Moderate    $10^3$ | Paper dyeing and manufacture; plasticizer waste; chemical (peroxides) manufacturing effluent; wood preserving waste, acid fraction; textile dyeing; pharmaceutical manufacturing; petrochemical plant waste (API oil–water separator sludge), acid fraction; combined API/slop-oil emulsions; neutral fraction; stormwater runoff, neutral fraction; foundry effluent; vinyl chloride production waste (EDC tar); resins manufacturing effluent; paper dyeing; wood-preserving bottom sediment, crude waste; petroleum refinery effluent (2 independent studies) |
| $10^2$ | Kraft pulp mill fiber waste (water-soluble compounds); acetonitrile bottom stream, basic fraction |
| Low | |
| Below detection | Pharmaceutical wastewater; electroplating effluent; resin manufacturing; surfactants manufacture; PVC wastewater |

[a]See Houk (1992) for additional explanation.

By using published data on the range of mutagenic potency for other complex environmental mixtures (e.g., automobile exhaust), the mutagenic risks posed by industrial effluents could be compared with those of other environmental sources (Table 4). This represents a simple, but effective, way to qualitatively rank hazards (based on a single endpoint) and to express relative risk. Such efforts can be used to target contaminant sources for mitigation or to set priorities for regulatory action.

## B. Quantitative Risk Assessment Using Comparative Methods

Comparative assessments of risk rely heavily on experimental data to infer human risk. The information produced by this process may be used to compare or rank risks between mixtures and to establish priorities for action, but it should not be considered a measure of absolute risk, nor can it predict the probability of an adverse effect.

One approach for characterizing the risks associated with complex mixtures is the *hazard index* (Svendsgaard and Hertzberg, 1993). This quantitative decision aid relies on the concept of response additivity. Constituents of the mixture are identified and assigned human cancer potency values (when available), and the risk values are then summed to estimate the overall risk of the mixture (USEPA, 1986a). The product of this exercise is a hazard, or toxicity, index that can assist in assigning priorities for action. The most notable deficiency of this approach is the potential for incomplete data—both chemical and toxicological—on chemicals composing the mixture.

**Table 4**  Comparison of Mutagenic Potencies of Complex Mixtures Based on Results Generated by the Salmonella Mutagenesis Assay[a]

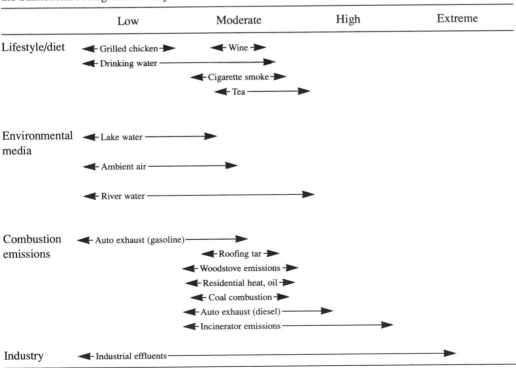

[a]For details see Houk (1992).

In certain circumstances, data on mixture components may be incomplete, but it may be conjectured that the mixture consists of chemical congeners or homologues. In such instances, the EPA recommends the toxicity equivalency factor (TEF) approach (see Schoeny and Marogosches, 1989). The carcinogenic potency (from animal bioassays) of the individual chemical congeners that make up the mixture are compared with the carcinogenic potency of a signature isomer possessing a relatively extensive health effects database. The potency of each congener relative to the signature compound is then calculated, and these relative potencies are multiplied by their concentration in the mixture and summed to estimate the total cancer risk. This approach has been proposed to estimate risks associated with mixtures of chlorinated dioxins and furans using the isomer tetrachlorodibenzo-*p*-dioxin (TCDD) as the signature compound (Bellin and Barnes, 1987). In this scheme, TCDD is assigned a value of 1, and the dioxins and furans are assigned a toxicity equivalency factor relative to TCDD. The estimated risks for each component are summed, and exposure data are incorporated to estimate the potential human hazard. Another example is provided by Thorslund (1991), who suggests that risks from mixtures containing PAHs can be estimated by using the carcinogenic potency of B[*a*]P to establish "B[*a*]P equivalents" for each PAH. This method may be useful for simple mixtures or for complex mixtures for which it can be shown that the chemical congeners account for the majority of the carcinogenicity of the whole mixture. However, as with the hazard index, this method assumes that either doses or responses are additive. It thereby ignores the potential for interactions among components and does not take into account agents that may display dissimilar modes of action.

In contrast, comparative potency methods, which relate the genotoxic potency of one mixture to another, do not exclude the potential for interactions. Moreover, comparative potency offers the advantage of evaluating the whole mixture, rather than its constituents. The comparative potency method was initially conceptualized to estimate lung cancer risks for diesel emissions (Lewtas et al., 1981; Harris, 1981). Data from short-term mutagenicity assays and animal tumorigenicity studies were combined with epidemiological cancer data for specific occupational and high-dose exposures (cigarette smoke, coke oven, and roofing tar emissions). This approach provided a comparative basis by which to estimate the lung cancer risk for a similar combustion emission (diesel) for which human data were not available. Human lung cancer unit risks for diesel emission sources were then calculated (Albert et al., 1983), illustrating the ability of comparative potency methods to yield absolute estimates of risk (Fig. 14). Since these initial studies were conducted, additional comparative potency values have been developed for gasoline vehicle emissions and coal, oil, and wood combustion (Lewtas, 1988). A high correlation was demonstrated between the mutagenic potency in the *Salmonella* assay and the tumorigenic potency in mice for diesel and gasoline emission engines. These tumorigenic and mutagenic potencies, in turn, were highly correlated with the concentration of nitrated PAHs and PAHs in the extracts of polycyclic organic matter. This evidence suggests that the chemical similarity of these automotive emissions may justify the use of short-term mutagenicity assays to estimate the comparative human risk for mixtures that are chemically similar.

## C.  Quantitative Risk Assessment Using Probabilistic Methods

Probabilistic assessments of risk involve evidence that is directly relevant to humans; that is, they rely on data obtained from studies of human populations or studies of experimental animals closely linked to humans. A numerical risk estimate, which expresses the likelihood or probability that an adverse effect will occur, is derived from the data.

For mutagenicity, this expression reflects the likelihood that a change in mutation rate will occur. This change in mutation rate may be measured by an increase of genetic disease per

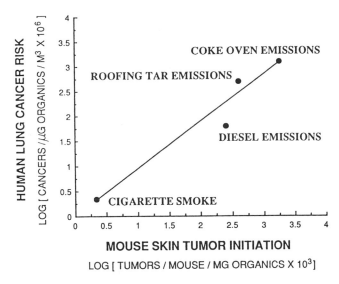

**Figure 14** Correlation between unit cancer risks from epidemiology data and mouse skin tumorigenicity data. The correlation constant is 0.95. (Adapted from Nesnow, 1990.)

generation or by the fractional increase in the assumed spontaneous human mutation rate (Jarabek and Farland, 1990). Estimation of the probability of heritable genetic disease from exposure to a genotoxic agent currently relies on in vivo mammalian germ cell mutagenicity data (USEPA, 1986b). To date, no known human heritable gene mutagen has been identified, making this endpoint of limited significance for regulatory purposes (Farland, 1992).

For carcinogens, numerical estimates are expressed as *unit-risk values,* defined as the lifetime probability of cancer death given a specified lifetime exposure. Unit risk values are derived from a combination of experimental and epidemiological findings, and are predicated on the linear nonthreshold extrapolation model to estimate human cancer risk at low doses. To illustrate, human lung cancer unit risk values were calculated for three emission sources—cigarette smoke, roofing tar, and coke ovens—using data from animal tumorigenicity studies and lung cancer epidemiology investigations (Albert et al., 1983).

An extension of this research and an example of an integrated cancer risk assessment is provided by the work of Mumford et al. (1987, 1990, 1993) in which several kinds of exposure and effects information were used to examine the etiologic link between indoor air pollution and lung cancer. These researchers conducted a study of residents of Xuan Wei, a rural county in China, with an unusually high rate of lung cancer mortality. The high-mortality rate could not be attributed to tobacco use or occupational exposures, but rather, was related to exposure to emissions in poorly ventilated homes from smoky coal, a fuel used for both heating and cooking. Studies were designed to evaluate the relation between domestic fuel and lung cancer by monitoring both the immediate environment and the affected population. Information on three different fuel types—smoky coal, smokeless coal, and wood—was gathered and analyzed. Air samples were collected at each site and analyzed for PAHs and nitrogen-containing PAHs known to cause cancer in animals. Concentrations of airborne particles and their size distribution were measured. Genotoxicity tests (including in vitro mutagenicity assays in *Salmonella* and mouse lymphoma cells, as well as cell transformation in rodent epithelial cells) were performed using extracts of the air samples. The mouse skin carcinogenicity assay was used as a two-stage cancer model to study both the initiation and promotion activity of the samples. The mouse skin tumorigenicity data was then combined with air-monitoring data (for exposure estimates) and compared with epidemiological data to investigate the etiological link between smoky coal combustion and lung cancer. Finally, tissues (placenta, cord blood, and peripheral blood) were obtained from exposed and control populations and analyzed for the presence of DNA adducts.

Results from these studies, both collectively and individually, consistently showed a strong etiologic link between indoor smoky coal and lung cancer. Each of the elements of this scientific investigation contributed pertinent information to the assessment of human health hazard and risk and extended the comparative potency database. It is when such consistent findings are demonstrated among chemical, physical, toxicological, and epidemiological findings that one obtains the accumulated evidence suggesting strong etiologic links between exposure to complex environmental mixtures and human cancer or other genetically mediated health effects.

## VI.  FUTURE DIRECTIONS

The future of risk assessment research on complex environmental mixtures, especially in the field of genetic toxicology, is indeed promising. New molecular technologies have enabled direct investigation of the effect of exposures to genetic toxicants on the structure and function of DNA. These same molecular technologies are providing information on individual susceptibilities conferred by genetic heritage. Thus, it should be possible from the scientific perspective to identify those individuals who will exhibit a greater health risk from exposure to genetic toxicants, and perhaps to encourage minimization of such exposures.

This new knowledge of the molecular genetics of cancer and genetically mediated diseases may be expected to enhance our understanding of the *interactions* between genetic susceptibilities and environmental factors. Such interactions are believed to account for the major influence of environmental exposures on cancer and genetic disease, with "purely" genetic and "purely" environmental factors individually making much smaller contributions.

Key mutational events in cancer causation (e.g., mutation in the tumor suppressor gene *p53*) are rapidly being discovered. These findings present unique aids in cancer diagnostics, useful biomarkers for cancer epidemiology, and tools for the development of new biologically based risk assessment models. Such models, now in their infancy, may be expected to guide the implementation of more appropriate and scientifically defensible risk assessment procedures.

Nothing said in the foregoing is to imply that current technologies involving the use of short-term tests and whole-animal chronic studies, analytical chemical methods, and environmental exposure monitoring will not be of future importance. These technologies have made important contributions to risk assessments for complex environmental mixtures, and the importance of this research will only increase as these technologies develop and as they are combined with the new molecular tools for toxicological research. Thus, advances in toxicological research will be paralleled by advances in analytical chemistry and monitoring technology. For example, apportionment methods, such as source dispersion modeling (the modeling of ambient dispersion of various source emissions) and receptor modeling (the modeling of source tracers through the ambient environment as they reach the receptor), will have major effects on the assessment of human exposures to complex environmental mixtures.

Critical to future risk assessments of complex mixtures will be the proper identification and pursuit of research targets of opportunity to more carefully define the linkages between exposures to complex mixtures and genetic alterations (biomarkers) in human populations. These targets of opportunity exist now in those parts of the world that have suffered severe environmental degradation. Such research to understand the long-term effects of genetic damage to human somatic and germinal tissues is essential to future environmental health protection and genetic risk assessment.

## REFERENCES

Albert, R., J. Lewtas, S. Nesnow, T. Thorslund, and E. Anderson (1983). Comparative potency method for cancer risk assessment: Application to diesel particulate emissions, *Risk Anal.*, 3, 101–117.

Armitage, P., and R. Doll (1954). The age distribution of cancer and a multistage theory of carcinogenesis, *Br. J. Cancer*, 8, 1–12.

Ashby, J. et al. (1990). A scheme for classifying carcinogens, *Regul. Toxicol. Pharmacol.*, 12, 270–295.

Backer, L. C., C. B. Grindem, and J. L. Hunter (1993). Biomarkers in pet dogs—a sentinel for human health effects from environmental pollution? Abstracts from the International Congress on the Health Effects of Hazardous Waste, U. S. Department of Health and Human Services, p. 216.

Barale, R., L. Migliore, B. Cellini, L. Franncioni, F. Giogelli, I. Barai, and N. Loprieno (1990). Genetic toxicology of airborne particulate matter using cytogenetic assays and microbial mutagenicity assays. In *Genetic Toxicology of Complex Environmental Mixtures* (M. D. Waters, F. B. Daniel, J. Lewtas, S. Nesnow, and M. Moore, eds.), Plenum Press, New York, pp. 57–71.

Bellin, J., and D. G. Barnes (1987). Interim procedures for estimating risks associated with exposures to mixtures of chlorinated dibenzo-*p*-dioxins and -dibenzofurans (CDDs and CDFs), Risk Assessment Forum, EPA 625/3-87/012, March, 1987.

Bock, F. G., A. P. Swain, and R. L. Stedman (1969). Bioassays of major fractions of cigarette smoke condensate by accelerated technic, *Cancer Res.*, 29:584–587.

Brown, C. C., and K. C. Chu (1989). Additive and multiplicative models and multistage carcinogenesis theory, *Risk Anal.*, 9, 99–105.

Brusick, D. (1983). Evaluation of chronic rodent bioassays and Ames assay tests as accurate models for predicting human carcinogens. In *Application of Biological Markers to Carcinogenicity Testing* (H. A. Millman and S. Sell, eds.), Plenum Press, New York, pp. 153–163.

Brusick, D. J., H. N. B. Gopalan, E. Heseltine, J. W. Huismans, and P. H. M. Lohman (1992). *Assessing the Risk of Genetic Damage,* United Nations Environment Programme, Nairobi, 52 pp.

[CAG] Carcinogenic Assessment Group (1980). *Method for determining the unit risk estimate for air pollutants,* Carcinogenic Assessment Group, U. S. Environmental Protection Agency, Washington, DC.

Claxton, L. D., T. E. Kleindienst, E. Perry, and L. T. Cupitt (1990). Assessment of the mutagenicity of volatile organic air pollutants before and after atmospheric transformation. In *Genetic Toxicology of Complex Environmental Mixtures* (M. D. Waters, F. B. Daniel, J. Lewtas, S. Nesnow, and M. Moore, eds.), Plenum Press, New York, pp. 103–111.

Claxton, L., A. G. Stead, and D. Walsh (1988). An analysis by chemical class of *Salmonella* mutagenicity tests as predictor of animal carcinogenicity, *Mutat. Res.*, 205, 197–225.

Crump, K. S., D. G. Hoel, C. H. Langley, and R. Peto (1976). Fundamental carcinogenic processes and their implications for low dose risk assessment, *Cancer Res.*, 36, 2973–2979.

Crump, K. S., H. A. Guess, and K. L. Deal (1977). Confidence intervals and test of hypothesis concerning dose response relationships inferred from animal carcinogenicity data, *Biometrics,* 33, 437–451.

Das, R. K., and N. K. Nanda (1986). Induction of micronuclei in peripheral erythrocytes of fish *Heteropneustes fossilis* by mitomycin C and paper mill effluent, *Mutat. Res.*, 175, 67–71.

Dearfield, K. L., A. E. Auletta, M. C. Cimino, and M. M. Moore (1991). Considerations in the U. S. Environmental Protection Agency's testing approach for mutagenicity, *Mutat. Res.*, 258, 259–283.

DeMarini, D. M. (1983). Genotoxicity of tobacco smoke and tobacco smoke condensate, *Mutat. Res.*, 114, 59–89.

DeMarini, D. M., J. P. Inmon, J. E. Simmons, E. Berman, T. C. Pasley, S. H. Warren, and R. W. Williams (1987). Mutagenicity in *Salmonella* of hazardous wastes and urine from rats fed these wastes, *Mutat. Res.*, 189, 205–216.

DeMarini, D. M., J. E. Gallagher, V. S. Houk, and J. E. Simmons (1989). Toxicological evaluation of complex industrial wastes: Implications for exposure assessment, *Toxicol. Lett.*, 49, 199–214.

DeMarini, D. M., D. A. Bell, J. G. Levine, M. L. Shelton, A. Abu-Shakra (1993). Molecular analysis of mutations induced at the *hisD3052* allele of *Salmonella* by single chemicals and complex mixtures, *Environ. Health Perspect.,* 101 (Suppl. 3), 207–212.

Donnelly, K. C., K. W. Brown, and B. R. Scott (1983). The use of short-term bioassays to monitor the environmental impact of land treatment of hazardous wastes. In *Short-term Bioassays in the Analysis of Complex Environmental Mixtures, III* (M. D. Waters, S. S. Sandhu, J. Lewtas, L. Claxton, N. Chernoff, and S. Nesnow, eds.), Plenum Press, New York, pp. 59–78.

Driver, J. H., H. W. Rogers, and L. D. Claxton (1990). Mutagenicity of combustion emissions from a biomedical waste incinerator, *Waste Manage.,* 10, 177–183.

Everson, R. B. (1986). Detection of occupational and environmental exposures by bacterial mutagenesis assays of human body fluids, *J. Occup. Med.,* 28, 647–655.

Farland, W. H. (1992). The U. S. Environmental Protection Agency's Risk Assessment Guidelines: Current status and future directions, *Toxicol. Ind. Health,* 8, 205–212.

Gallagher, J. E., M. A. Jackson, M. H. George, and J. Lewtas (1990). Dose related differences in DNA adduct levels in rodent tissues following skin application of complex mixtures from air pollution sources, *Carcinogenesis,* 11, 63–68.

Gallagher, J. E., M. George, M. Kohan, C. Thompson, T. Shank, and J. Lewtas (1993). Detection and comparison of DNA adducts after in vitro and in vivo diesel emission exposures, *Environ. Health Perspect.,* 99, 225–228.

Garrett, N. E., H. F. Stack, M. R. Gross, and M. D. Waters (1984). An analysis of the spectra of genetic activity produced by known or suspected human carcinogens, *Mutat. Res.,* 134, 89–111.

Garrett, N. E., H. F. Stack, and M. D. Waters (1986). Evaluation of the genetic activity profiles of 65 pesticides, *Mutat. Res.,* 168, 301–325.

Gold, L. S., C. B. Sawter, R. McGraw, G. M. Buckman, M. deVecidna, R. Levinson, N. K. Hooper, W. R. Havender, L. Bernstein, R. Peto, M. C. Pike, and B. N. Ames (1984). A carcinogenic potency database for the standardized results of animal bioassays, *Environ. Health Perspect.,* 58, 9–319.

Gold, L. S., M. B. Manley, T. H. Slone, G. B. Garfinkel, L. Rohrbach, and B. Ames (1993). The fifth plot of the Carcinogenic Potency Database: Results of animal bioassays published in the general literature through 1988 and by the National Toxicology Program through 1989, *Environ. Health Perspect.,* 100, 65–168.

Graedel, T. E., D. T. Hawkins, and L. D. Claxton (1986). *Atmospheric Chemical Compounds: Sources, Occurrence, and Bioassay,* Academic Press, Orlando, FL, 732 pp.

Guess, H. A., and K. S. Crump (1976). Low-dose extrapolation of data from animal carcinogenicity data, *Environ. Health Perspect.,* 22, 149–152.

Guess, H. A., and Crump, K. S. (1978). Best-estimate low-dose extrapolation of carcinogenicity data, *Environ. Health Perspect.,* 22, 149–152.

Harris, J. E. (1981). *Potential Risk of Lung Cancer from Diesel Engine Emissions,* National Academy Press, Washington, DC.

Harris, C. C. (1991). Chemical and physical carcinogenesis: Advances and perspectives for the 1990s, *Cancer Res.,* 51, 5023S–5044S.

Hemminki, K. E., E. Grzybowska, M. Chorazy, K. Twardowska-Saucha, J. W. Srocynski, K. L. Putnam, K. Randerath, D. H. Phillips, A. Hewer, R. M. Santella, T. L. Young, and F. P. Perera (1990). DNA adducts in humans environmentally exposed to aromatic compounds in an industrial area of Poland, *Carcinogenesis,* 11, 1229–1231.

Hoffman, D., and E. L. Wynder (1971). A study of tobacco carcinogenesis. XI. Tumor initiators, tumor accelerators, and tumor promoting activity of condensate fractions, *Cancer,* 27, 848–864.

Houk, V. S. (1992). The genotoxicity of industrial wastes and effluents: A review, *Mutat. Res.,* 277, 91–138.

Houk, V. S., and D. M. DeMarini (1988). Use of the microscreen phage-induction assay to assess the genotoxicity of 14 hazardous industrial wastes, *Environ. Mol. Mutagen.,* 11, 13–29.

Houk, V. S., D. M. DeMarini, R. R. Watts, and J. Lewtas (1993). Toxicological evaluations of hazardous effluents and emissions using genetic bioassays. *Effective and Safe Waste Management. Interfacing Sciences and Engineering with Monitoring and Risk Analysis* (R. L. Jolley and R. Wang, eds.), Lewis Publishers, Ann Arbor, MI, pp. 265–280.

Huff, J., J. Haseman, and D. Rall (1991). Scientific concepts, value, and significance of chemical carcinogenesis studies, *Annu. Rev. Pharmacol. Toxicol.,* 31, 621–652.

Hughes, T. J., K. C. Klein, B. S. Gill, E. Perry, T. Liles, R. Williams, L. Claxton, and B. C. Casto (1993). Biomonitoring studies at a Superfund site in North Carolina, *Environ. Mol. Mutagen.,* 21, 31.

Jarabek, A. M., and W. H. Farland (1990). The U. S. Environmental Protection Agency's risk assessment guidelines, *Toxicol. Ind. Health,* 6, 199–216.

Karcher, W., and J. Devillers (1990). *Practical Applications of Quantitative Structure–Activity Relationships (QSAR) in Environmental Chemistry and Toxicology,* Kluwer Academic Publishers, Boston, MA.

Klekowski, E., and D. E. Levin (1979). Mutagens in a river heavily polluted with paper recycling wastes: Results of field and laboratory mutagen assays, *Environ. Mutagen.,* 1, 209–219.

Kodell, R. L., D. Krewski, and J. Zielinski (1991). Additive and multiplicative relative risk in the two-stage clonal expansion model of carcinogenesis, *Risk Anal.,* 11, 483–490.

Krewski, D., and R. D. Thomas (1992). Carcinogenic mixtures, *Risk Anal.,* 12, 105–113.

Leonard, H., M. Duverger-Van Bogaert, A. Bernard, M. Lambotte-Vandepaer, and R. Lauwerys (1985). Population monitoring for genetic damage induced by environmental physical and chemical agents, *Environ. Monit. Assess.,* 5, 369–384.

Lewis, C. W., R. E. Baumgardner, L. D. Claxton, J. Lewtas, and R. K. Stevens (1988). The contribution of woodsmoke and motor vehicle emissions to ambient aerosol mutagenicity, *Environ. Sci. Technol.,* 22, 968–971.

Lewtas, J. (1983). Evaluation of the mutagenicity and carcinogenicity of motor vehicle emissions in short-term bioassays, *Environ. Health Perspect.,* 47, 141–152.

Lewtas, J. (1988). Genotoxicity of complex mixtures: Strategies for the identification and comparative assessment of airborne mutagens and carcinogens from combustion sources, *Fundam. Appl. Toxicol.,* 10, 571–589.

Lewtas, J., R. Bradow, R. Jungers, B. Harris, R. Zweidinger, K. Cushing, B. Gill, and R. Albert (1981). Mutagenic and carcinogenic potency of extracts of diesel and related environmental emissions: Study design, sample generation, collection and preparation, *Environ. Int.,* 5, 383–387.

Lewtas, J., J. Mumford, R. Everson, B. Hulka, T. Wilcosky, W. Kozumbo, C. Thompson, M. George, L. Dobias, R. Sram, X. Li, and J. Gallagher (1993). Comparison of DNA adducts from exposure to complex mixtures in various human tissues and experimental systems, *Environ. Health Perspect.,* 99, 89–97.

Lewtas, J., D. M. DeMarini, J. Favor, D. W. Layton, J. T. MacGregor, J. Ashby, P. H. M. Lohman, R. H. Haynes, and M. L. Mendelsohn (1994a). Risk characterization strategies for genotoxic environmental agents. In *Methods for Genetic Risk Assessment,* Lewis Publishers, Ann Arbor, MI, pp. 125–169.

Lewtas, J., L. C. King, and D. M. DeMarini (1994b). New approaches to bioassay- and biomarker-directed identification of genotoxic components in complex mixtures: DNA adduct identification and mutation spectra. In *Toxicology of Complex Mixtures: From Real Life Examples to Mechanisms of Toxicological Interactions* (R. S. H. Yang, ed.), Academic Press, San Diego, pp. 385–398.

Lower, W. R., V. K. Drobney, B. J. Aholt, and R. Politte (1983). Mutagenicity of the environments in the vicinity of an oil refinery and a petrochemical complex, *Teratology Carcinog. Mutagen.,* 3, 65–73.

Lutz, W. K., P. Buss, A. Baertsch, and M. Caiezel (1990). Evaluation of DNA binding in vivo for low-dose extrapolation in chemical carcinogenesis. In *Genetic Toxicology of Complex Environmental Mixtures* (M. D. Waters, F. B. Daniel, J. Lewtas, S. Nesnow, and M. Moore, eds.), Plenum Press, New York, pp. 331–342.

Matsushita, H., S. Goto, and Y. Takagi (1990). Human exposures to airborne mutagens indoors and outdoors using mutagenesis and chemical analysis methods. In *Genetic Toxicology of Complex Environmental Mixtures* (M. D. Waters, F. B. Daniel, J. Lewtas, eds.), Plenum Press, New York, pp. 33–56.

McBee, K., J. W. Bickham, K. W. Brown, and K. C. Donnelly (1987). Chromosomal aberrations in native small mammals (*Peromyscus leucopus* and *Sigmodon hispidus*) at a petrochemical waste disposal site: I. Standard karyology, *Arch. Environ. Contam. Toxicol.,* 16, 681–688.

McBee, K., and J. W. Bickham (1990). Mammals as bioindicators of environmental toxicity, In *Current Mammalogy,* Vol. 2 (H. H. Genoways, ed.), Plenum Press, New York, pp. 37–88.

McGeorge, L. J., J. B. Louis, T. B. Atherholt, and G. J. McGarrity (1985). Mutagenic analyses of industrial effluents: Results and considerations for integration into water pollution control programs. In *Short-Term Bioassays in the Analysis of Complex Environmental Mixtures IV,* (M. D. Waters, S. S. Sandhu, J. Lewtas, L. Claxton, G. Strauss, and S. Nesnow, eds.), Plenum Press, New York, pp. 247–268.

Meier, J. R. (1988). Genotoxic activity of organic chemicals in drinking water, *Mutat. Res., 196,* 211–246.

Moolgavkar, S. H., and A. G. Knudson (1981). Mutation and cancer: A model for human carcinogenesis, *JNCI, 66,* 1037–1052.

Morris, S. C. (1990). *Cancer Risk Assessment. A Quantitative Approach,* Marcel Dekker, New York, 408 pp.

Mumford, J. L., X. Z. He, R. S. Chapman, S. R. Cao, D. B. Harris, X. M. Li, Y. L. Zian, W. Z. Jiang, C. W. Xu, J. C. Chuang, W. E. Wilson, and M. Cooke (1987). Lung cancer and indoor air pollution in Xuan Wei, China, *Science, 235,* 217–220.

Mumford, J. L., C. T. Helmes, X. Lee, J. Seidenberg, and S. Nesnow (1990). Mouse skin tumorigenicity studies of indoor coal and wood combustion emissions from homes of residents in Xuan Wei, China with high lung cancer mortality, *Carcinogenesis, 11,* 397–403.

Mumford, J. L., X. Lee, J. Lewtas, T. L. Young, and R. M. Santella (1993). DNA adducts as bio-markers for assessing exposure to polycyclic aromatic hydrocarbons in tissues from Xuan Wei women with high exposure to coal combustion emissions and high lung cancer mortality, *Environ. Health Perspect., 99,* 83–87.

[NRC] National Research Council (1988). *Complex Mixtures. Methods for in vivo Toxicity Testing,* Washington, DC, National Academy Press, 227 pp.

Nesnow, S. (1990). Mouse skin tumors and human lung cancer: Relationships with complex environmental emissions, In *Complex Mixtures and Cancer Risk* (H. Vanio, M. Sorsa, and A. J. McMichael, eds.), International Agency for Research on Cancer, Lyon, pp. 44–54.

Nesnow, S. (1991). A multifactor ranking scheme for comparing the carcinogenic activity of chemicals, *Environ. Health Perspect., 96,* 17–21.

Nestmann, E. R., D. J. Kowbel, O. P. Kamra, and G. R. Douglas (1984). Reduction of mutagenicity of pulp and paper mill effluent by secondary treatment in an aerated lagoon, *Haz. Waste, 1,* 67–72.

Owen, B. A., and T. D. Jones (1990). Hazard evaluation for complex mixtures: Relative comparisons to improve regulatory consistency, *Regul. Toxicol. Pharmacol., 11,* 132–148.

Perrera, F. P., K. Hemminki, T. L. Young, D. Brenner, G. Kelly, and R. M. Santella (1988). Detection of polycyclic aromatic hydrocarbon DNA adducts in white blood cells of foundry workers, *Cancer Res., 48,* 2288–2291.

Phillips, D. H., K. Hemminki, A. Alhonen, A. Hewer, and P. L. Grover (1988). Monitoring occupational exposure to carcinogens: Detection by $^{32}$P-postlabeling of aromatic DNA adducts in white blood cells from iron foundry workers, *Mutat. Res., 204,* 531–541.

Reitz, R. H. (1990). Distribution, persistence, and elimination of toxic agents (pharmacokinetics), In *Progress in Predictive Toxicology* (D. B. Clayson, I. C. Munro, P. Shubik, and J. A. Swenberg, eds.), Elsevier, Amsterdam, pp. 79–90.

Richard, A. M., J. R. Rabinowitz, and M. D. Waters (1989). Strategies for the use of computational SAR methods in assessing genotoxicity, *Mutat. Res., 221,* 181–196.

Ruiz, E. F., V. W. E. Rabago, S. U. Lecona, A. B. Perez, and T. Ma (1992). Tradescantia-micronucleus (Trad-MCN) bioassay on clastogenicity of wastewater and in situ monitoring, *Mutat. Res., 270,* 45–51.

Sandhu, S. S., W. R. Lower, F. J. de Serres, W. A. Suk, and R. R. Tice, eds. (1990). *In Situ Evaluation of Biological Hazards of Environmental Pollutants,* Plenum Press, New York, 277 pp.

Savela, K., and K. Hemminki (1991). DNA adducts in lymphocytes and granulocytes of smokers and nonsmokers detected by the $^{32}$P-postlabeling assay, *Carcinogenesis, 12,* 503–508.

Schairer, L. A., J. Van't Hof, C. G. Hayes, R. M. Burton, and F. J. de Serres (1979). Measurement of biological activity of ambient air mixtures using a mobile laboratory for in situ exposures: Preliminary results from the *Tradescantia* plant test system. In *Application of Short-term Bioassays in the Analysis of Complex Environmental Mixtures* (M. D. Waters, S. Nesnow, J. L. Huisingh, S. Sandhu, and L. Claxton, eds.), Plenum Press, New York, pp. 421–440.

Schoeny R. S., and E. Margosches (1989). Evaluating comparative potencies: Developing approaches to risk assessment of chemical mixtures, *Toxicol. Ind. Health, 5,* 825–837.

Shelby, M., and E. Zeiger (1990). Activity of human carcinogens in the *Salmonella* and rodent bone-marrow cytogenetics tests, *Mutat. Res.*, 234, 257–261.

Simmons, J. E., D. M. DeMarini, and E. Berman (1988). Lethality and hepatotoxicity of complex waste mixtures, *Environ. Res.*, 46, 74–85.

Svendsgaard, D. J., and R. C. Hertzberg (1994). Statistical methods for the toxicological evaluation of the additivity assumption as used in EPA's Chemical Mixture Risk Assessment Guidelines, In *Toxicology of Complex Mixtures: From Real Life Examples to Mechanisms of Toxicological Interactions* (R. S. H. Yang, ed.), Academic Press, San Diego pp. 599–642.

Tennant, R. W. (1993). Stratification of rodent carcinogenicity bioassay results to reflect relative human hazard, *Mutat. Res.*, 286, 111–118.

Thompson, R. A., G. D. Schroder, and T. H. Connor (1988). Chromosomal aberrations in the cotton rat, *Sigmodon hispidus,* exposed to hazardous waste, *Environ. Mol. Mutagen.*, 11, 359–367.

Thorslund, T. W. (1991). *Development of Relative Potency Estimates for PAHs and Hydrocarbon Combustion Product Fractions Compared to Benzo(a)pyrene and Their Use in Carcinogenic Risk Assessment.* ICF/Clement International, Washington, DC.

Thorslund, T. W., C. C. Brown, and G. Charnley (1987). Biologically motivated cancer risk models, *Risk Anal.*, 7, 109–119.

Tice, R. R., B. G. Ormiston, R. Boucher, C. A. Luke, and D. E. Paquette (1987). Environmental biomonitoring with feral rodent species. In *Short-term Bioassays in the Analysis of Complex Environmental Mixtures V* (S. S. Sandhu, D. M. DeMarini, M. J. Mass, M. M. Moore, and J. L. Mumford, eds.). Plenum Press, New York, pp. 175–180.

[USEPA] U. S. Environmental Protection Agency (1980). Samplers and sampling procedures for hazardous waste streams, EPA600/2-80-18, Washington, DC. January 1980.

[USEPA] U. S. Environmental Protection Agency (1986a). Guidelines for the health risk assessment of chemical mixtures. *Fed. Reg.*, 51(185), 34014–34025.

[USEPA] U. S. Environmental Protection Agency (1986b). Guidelines for mutagenicity risk assessment. *Fed. Reg.*, 51(185), 34006–34012.

[USEPA] U. S. Environmental Protection Agency (1986c). Guidelines for carcinogen risk assessment. *Fed. Reg.*, 51(185), 33992–34003.

[USEPA] U. S. Environmental Protection Agency (1989). Risk assessment guidance for Superfund, Volume 1: Human Health Evaluation Manual (Part A), Office of Emergency and Remedial Response, Washington, DC, EPA/540/1-89/002, December 1989.

[USNAS] U. S. National Academy of Sciences (1983). *Risk Assessment in the Federal Government: Managing the Process.* Commission on Life Sciences. National Research Council. National Academy Press, Washington, DC, 191 pp.

Van Hoof, F., and J. Verheyden (1981). Mutagenic activity in the River Meuse in Belgium, *Sci. Total Environ.*, 20, 15–22.

Vogelstein, B., E. R. Fearon, S. R. Hamilton, S. E. Kern, A. C. Peresinger, M. Leppert, Y. Nakamura, R. White, A. M. M. Smits, and J. L. Bos (1988). Genetic alterations during colorectal-tumor development, *N. Engl. J. Med.*, 319, 525–532.

Vogelstein, B., E. R. Fearon, S. E. Kern, S. R. Hamilton, A. C. Peresinger, Y. Nakamura, and R. White (1989). Allelotype of colorectal carcinomas, *Science,* 244, 207–211.

Waters, M. D., H. F. Stack, A. L. Brady, P. H. M. Lohman, L. Haroun, and H. Vainio (1988). Use of computerized data listings and activity profiles of genetic and related effects in the review of 195 compounds, *Mutat. Res.*, 205, 295–312.

Waters, M. D., L. D. Claxton, H. F. Stack, A. L. Brady, and T. E. Graedel (1990a). Genetic activity profiles in the testing and evaluation of chemical mixtures, *Teratogenesis Carcinog. Mutagen.*, 10, 147–164.

Waters, M. D., L. D. Claxton, H. F. Stack, and T. E. Graedel (1990b). Genetic activity profiles—application in assessing potential carcinogenicity of complex environmental mixtures, In *Complex Mixtures and Cancer Risk* (H. Vainio, M. Sorsa, and A. J. McMichael, eds.), IARC, Lyon, pp. 75–88.

Watts, R. R., R. J. Drago, R. G. Merrill, R. W. Williams, E. Perry, and J. Lewtas (1988). Wood smoke impacted air: Mutagenicity and chemical analysis of ambient air in a residential area of Juneau, Alaska, *JAPCA,* 38, 652–660.

# 22

# The Effect of Combined Exposures of Chlorine, Copper, and Nitrite on Methemoglobin Formation in Red Blood Cells of Dorset Sheep

**Cynthia J. Langlois, James A. Garreffi,
Linda A. Baldwin, and Edward J. Calabrese**
*University of Massachusetts
Amherst, Massachusetts*

## I.  INTRODUCTION

Simultaneous exposure to agents that can oxidize the hemoglobin of the red blood cell to methemoglobin is common. Although the effects of some of these agents have been documented individually, few studies have assessed the interaction potential of such agents. Moore and Calabrese (1980), in their in vitro study with sheep red blood cells, reported an additive effect in the formation of methemoglobin induced by copper and chlorite. That study, however, was limited in that the effects of only one test level of copper and chlorite (3 m$M$) were examined.

This chapter presents two in vitro studies that extend the initial data of Moore and Calabrese (1980) by modification of study design and provide insight into the current risk assessment assumptions of mixtures. Sheep were chosen as the animal model because, unlike rodents, their methemoglobin-reducing capabilities are similar to humans (Smith and Beutler, 1966). In addition, sheep are also a model for glucose-6-phosphate dehydrogenase (G6PD) deficiency (Calabrese and Horton, 1986). Copper, chlorite, and nitrite were selected as methemoglobin-forming agents because they are ubiquitous and exposure to them is common.

## II.  STUDY 1

The first study comprised two separate experiments designed to assess various levels of oxidizing agents, concurrently, on nonpregnant, female Dorset sheep red blood cells (Calabrese et al., 1992).

The two experiments assessed joint concentrations of copper and nitrite (experiment 1) and

**Table 1** Methemoglobin Production for Part A, Copper and Nitrite Interaction, Mean Percent ± Standard Deviation

| | | Concentration of Nitrite, m$M$ | | | | | |
|---|---|---|---|---|---|---|---|
| | | 0 | 0.0625 | 0.125 | 0.25 | 0.50 | 0.75 |
| | 0 | 1.62 | 2.34 | 3.43 | 5.24 | 9.15 | 13.28 |
| | | 0.48 | 0.43 | 0.47 | 0.81 | 1.76 | 2.39 |
| | 0.0625 | 2.77 | 3.26 | 4.09 | 5.97 | 9.96 | 12.76 |
| | | 0.91 | 0.79 | 0.69 | 0.81 | 0.99 | 0.89 |
| | 0.125 | 3.28 | 4.11 | 5.10 | 7.43 | 10.98 | 13.91 |
| Concentration of Copper, m$M$ | | .97 | 1.17 | 1.74 | 1.53 | 1.38 | 1.24 |
| | 0.25 | 5.20 | 6.89 | 7.92 | 8.87 | 13.02 | 15.69 |
| | | 1.27 | 1.29 | 1.92 | 1.85 | 2.62 | 2.16 |
| | 0.50 | 10.19 | 10.53 | 10.91 | 13.70 | 17.18 | 21.18 |
| | | 4.78 | 2.94 | 2.79 | 4.87 | 6.40 | 5.50 |
| | 0.75 | 13.70 | 14.97 | 15.34 | 19.06 | 23.40 | 27.59 |
| | | 6.44 | 5.40 | 5.46 | 8.60 | 9.90 | 10.50 |

copper and chlorite (experiment 2) that produced methemoglobin levels of 1.25, 2.5, 5.0, 10.0 and 15.0% separately.

## A. Copper and Nitrite Joint Exposure (Experiment 1)

Analysis of methemoglobin values observed in Table 1 revealed that the effect of this mixture was additive across all levels of concurrent exposure. Table 2 likewise supports the additive nature of the concurrent exposure, based on the high degree of similarity between the expected and observed values throughout the entire dose range. In addition, the generally parallel nature of the dose–response curves (Fig. 1) support the lack of interaction of the copper and nitrite exposure. The statistical analyses revealed that the additive hypothesis was not rejected ($p > 0.05$), thereby further substantiating the additive relationship.

**Table 2** Methemoglobin Production for Part B Copper/Chlorite Interaction, Mean Percent ± Standard Deviation

| | | Concentration of Chlorite, m$M$ | | | | | |
|---|---|---|---|---|---|---|---|
| | | 0 | .25 | .50 | 1.0 | 2.0 | 3.0 |
| | 0 | 1.36 | 1.77 | 2.22 | 4.12 | 9.50 | 14.63 |
| | | 0.29 | 0.52 | 0.73 | 1.93 | 2.55 | 3.32 |
| | 0.0625 | 2.13 | 2.03 | 2.68 | 4.15 | 9.65 | 14.47 |
| | | 0.52 | 0.56 | 0.59 | 1.04 | 1.04 | 2.91 |
| | 0.125 | 3.03 | 3.42 | 3.64 | 5.31 | 9.65 | 15.20 |
| Concentration of Copper, m$M$ | | 0.60 | 0.56 | 0.68 | 1.16 | 2.42 | 4.40 |
| | 0.25 | 5.06 | 5.20 | 5.96 | 7.93 | 12.44 | 16.74 |
| | | 0.98 | 0.66 | 0.91 | 1.44 | 2.86 | 3.47 |
| | 0.50 | 8.61 | 9.57 | 10.00 | 10.73 | 17.35 | 25.84 |
| | | 1.85 | 1.57 | 1.09 | 2.87 | 4.04 | 7.51 |
| | 0.75 | 13.11 | 14.34 | 15.44 | 16.10 | 24.43 | 30.23 |
| | | 2.80 | 2.40 | 2.70 | 4.40 | 5.90 | 6.60 |

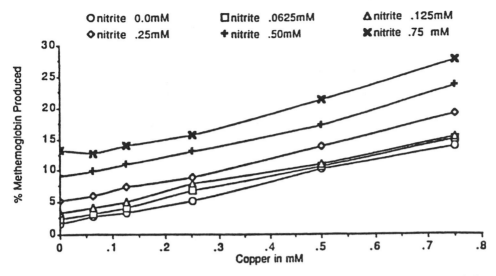

**Figure 1**   Combination copper and nitrite concentrations versus percentage methemoglobin in part A.

## B.   Copper and Chlorite Joint Exposure (Experiment 2)

As in the copper and nitrite joint exposures, the levels of methemoglobin observed in the concurrent copper and chlorite experiment suggest that effects were additive (Table 3). Table 4 supports the additive relationship of the concurrent exposure, based on the similarity between the expected and observed values throughout the entire dose range evaluated. Furthermore, the generally parallel nature of the dose–response curves (Fig. 2) confirm the lack of interaction of the combined copper and chlorite exposure. However, the statistical analysis rejected the additive hypothesis ($p < 0.05$). Although the statistical analysis did not support the additive relationship, the deviation from additivity is quite modest, given the generally parallel nature of the dose–response curves and the similarity of observed and expected values.

**Table 3**   Observed Versus Expected Values for Part A

| | | Concentration of Nitrite, m*M* | | | | | |
|---|---|---|---|---|---|---|---|
| | | 0 | 0.0625 | 0.125 | 0.25 | 0.50 | 0.75 |
| Concentration of Copper, m*M* | 0 | 1.62 | 2.34 | 3.43 | 5.24 | 9.15 | 13.28 |
| | | 1.14 | 2.09 | 3.04 | 4.94 | 8.74 | 12.54 |
| | 0.0625 | 2.77 | 3.26 | 4.09 | 5.97 | 9.96 | 12.76 |
| | | 2.24 | 3.19 | 4.14 | 6.04 | 9.84 | 13.64 |
| | 0.125 | 3.28 | 4.11 | 5.10 | 7.43 | 10.98 | 13.91 |
| | | 3.34 | 4.29 | 5.24 | 7.14 | 10.94 | 14.74 |
| | 0.25 | 5.20 | 6.89 | 7.92 | 8.87 | 13.02 | 15.69 |
| | | 5.54 | 6.49 | 7.44 | 9.34 | 13.14 | 16.94 |
| | 0.50 | 10.19 | 10.53 | 10.91 | 13.70 | 17.18 | 21.18 |
| | | 9.94 | 10.98 | 11.84 | 13.74 | 17.54 | 21.34 |
| | 0.75 | 13.70 | 14.97 | 15.34 | 19.06 | 23.40 | 27.59 |
| | | 14.34 | 15.29 | 16.24 | 18.14 | 21.92 | 25.74 |

**Table 4**   Observed Versus Expected Values for Part B

|  |  | Concentration of Chlorite, m$M$ | | | | | |
| --- | --- | --- | --- | --- | --- | --- | --- |
|  |  | 0 | 0.25 | 0.50 | 1.0 | 2.0 | 3.0 |
|  | 0 | 1.36 | 1.77 | 2.22 | 4.12 | 9.50 | 14.63 |
|  |  | 1.22 | 1.72 | 2.32 | 3.64 | 9.40 | 15.19 |
|  | 0.0625 | 2.13 | 2.03 | 2.68 | 4.15 | 9.65 | 14.47 |
|  |  | 1.51 | 2.01 | 2.61 | 3.93 | 9.79 | 15.48 |
|  | 0.125 | 3.03 | 3.42 | 3.64 | 5.31 | 9.65 | 15.20 |
|  |  | 2.23 | 2.82 | 3.42 | 4.74 | 10.60 | 16.29 |
| Concentration of Copper, m$M$ | 0.25 | 5.06 | 5.20 | 5.96 | 7.93 | 12.44 | 16.74 |
|  |  | 4.41 | 4.91 | 5.51 | 6.38 | 12.69 | 18.38 |
|  | 0.50 | 8.61 | 9.57 | 10.00 | 10.73 | 17.35 | 25.84 |
|  |  | 9.30 | 9.80 | 10.04 | 11.72 | 17.58 | 23.27 |
|  | 0.75 | 13.11 | 14.34 | 15.44 | 16.10 | 24.43 | 30.23 |
|  |  | 14.56 | 15.06 | 15.66 | 16.98 | 22.84 | 28.53 |

## III.   STUDY 2

The second study involved a series of experiments in which four levels of each chemical were tested in all possible combinations (Langlois and Calabrese, 1992). The concentrations employed were those that produced 0, 2.5, 5, and 10% methemoglobin. See Table 5 for means and standard deviations, and Table 6 for observed versus expected values.

## A.   Two-Way Interactions

The two-way interactions between cupric plus chlorite and cupric plus nitrite were strictly additive; as was expected. Figures 3 and 4 show the parallelism of the dose–response curves, which further suggests additivity. One interesting finding was that the other two-way interaction, chlorite plus nitrite, was not additive. The observed values were significantly lower than the

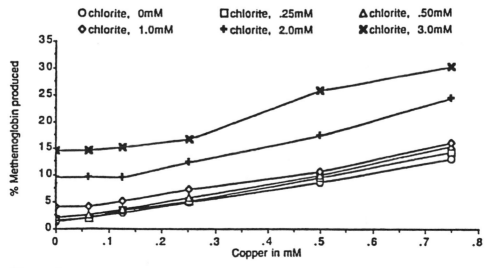

**Figure 2**   Combination copper and chlorite concentrations versus percentage methemoglobin in part B.

**Table 5** Results in Mean Percent Methemoglobin ± Standard Deviation

| Nitrite levels (mM) | 0 mM chlorite | | | | 0.5 mM chlorite | | | | 1 mM chlorite | | | | 2 mM chlorite | | | |
|---|---|---|---|---|---|---|---|---|---|---|---|---|---|---|---|---|
| | 0 | 0.125 | 0.25 | 0.5 | 0 | 0.125 | 0.25 | 0.5 | 0 | 0.125 | 0.25 | 0.5 | 0 | 0.125 | 0.25 | 0.5 |
| 0mM cupric | 1.66 ± 0.44 | 3.34 ± 0.77 | 4.95 ± 0.50 | 11.37 ± 1.03 | 2.32 ± 0.82 | 4.60 ± 1.08 | 6.43 ± 1.26 | 11.41 ± 1.04 | 3.94 ± 0.85 | 6.02 ± 1.21 | 8.15 ± 1.04 | 12.56 ± 1.33 | 7.67 ± 2.14 | 8.39 ± 2.49 | 9.19 ± 1.79 | 13.73 ± 1.33 |
| 0.125 mM cupric | 2.77 ± 0.92 | 4.68 ± 1.05 | 6.83 ± 1.40 | 12.17 ± 1.14 | 3.28 ± 0.92 | 5.27 ± 1.47 | 7.70 ± 0.98 | 12.03 ± 0.71 | 4.49 ± 1.36 | 6.31 ± 1.85 | 9.34 ± 1.29 | 12.42 ± 1.34 | 7.43 ± 2.35 | 9.36 ± 2.74 | 10.99 ± 1.49 | 14.43 ± 1.81 |
| 0.25 mM cupric | 4.02 ± 1.61 | 6.06 ± 1.18 | 7.80 ± 0.91 | 13.63 ± 2.43 | 4.72 ± 0.99 | 6.67 ± 1.87 | 9.11 ± 1.62 | 13.40 ± 1.26 | 6.45 ± 1.49 | 8.21 ± 2.82 | 8.73 ± 1.77 | 14.01 ± 2.07 | 8.80 ± 1.99 | 8.75 ± 2.38 | 10.63 ± 1.30 | 15.65 ± 3.10 |
| 0.5 mM cupric | 5.15 ± 3.02 | 7.29 ± 2.14 | 9.69 ± 1.84 | 16.24 ± 2.39 | 6.37 ± 2.72 | 8.48 ± 2.63 | 10.79 ± 1.09 | 15.56 ± 2.41 | 8.69 ± 1.86 | 10.58 ± 4.18 | 10.78 ± 1.64 | 17.05 ± 3.04 | 10.58 ± 2.72 | 12.57 ± 3.05 | 12.24 ± 2.18 | 18.93 ± 3.76 |
| 0.5 mM Na acetate | 1.35 ± 0.73 | 2.14 ± 0.71 | 5.51 ± 1.42 | 11.15 ± 1.29 | 2.82 ± 0.79 | 3.97 ± 1.33 | 7.03 ± 2.40 | 10.67 ± 0.67 | 4.49 ± 0.88 | 5.56 ± 1.42 | 8.02 ± 2.80 | 10.79 ± 2.40 | 6.56 ± 1.24 | 7.88 ± 2.16 | 10.31 ± 1.74 | 14.82 ± 3.38 |

**Table 6**  Observed (top) Versus Expected (bottom) Values in Percentage Methemoglobin

| Nitrite levels (mM) | 0 mM chlorite | | | | 0.5 mM chlorite | | | | 1 mM chlorite | | | | 2 mM chlorite | | | |
|---|---|---|---|---|---|---|---|---|---|---|---|---|---|---|---|---|
| | 0 | 0.125 | 0.25 | 0.5 | 0 | 0.125 | 0.25 | 0.5 | 0 | 0.125 | 0.25 | 0.5 | 0 | 0.125 | 0.25 | 0.5 |
| 0mM cupric | 1.66 | 3.34 | 4.95 | 11.37 | 2.32 | 4.60 | 6.43 | 11.41 | 3.94 | 6.02 | 8.15 | 12.56 | 7.67 | 8.39 | 9.19 | 13.73 |
|  |  |  |  |  |  | 4.00 | 5.61 | 12.03 |  | 5.62 | 7.23 | 13.65 |  | 9.35 | 10.96 | 17.38 |
| 0.125 mM cupric | 2.77 | 4.68 | 6.83 | 12.17 | 3.28 | 5.27 | 7.70 | 12.03 | 4.49 | 6.31 | 9.34 | 12.42 | 7.43 | 9.36 | 10.99 | 14.43 |
|  |  | 4.45 | 6.06 | 12.48 | 3.43 | 6.77 | 8.38 | 14.80 | 5.05 | 8.39 | 10.00 | 16.42 | 8.78 | 12.12 | 13.73 | 20.15 |
| 0.25 mM cupric | 4.02 | 6.06 | 7.80 | 13.63 | 4.72 | 6.67 | 9.11 | 13.40 | 6.45 | 8.21 | 8.73 | 14.01 | 8.80 | 8.75 | 10.63 | 15.65 |
|  |  | 5.70 | 7.31 | 13.73 | 4.68 | 8.02 | 9.63 | 16.05 | 6.30 | 9.24 | 11.25 | 17.67 | 10.03 | 13.37 | 14.98 | 21.40 |
| 0.5 mM cupric | 5.15 | 7.29 | 9.69 | 16.24 | 6.37 | 8.48 | 10.79 | 15.56 | 8.69 | 10.58 | 10.78 | 17.05 | 10.58 | 12.57 | 12.24 | 18.93 |
|  |  | 6.83 | 8.44 | 14.86 | 5.81 | 9.15 | 10.76 | 17.18 | 7.43 | 10.77 | 12.28 | 18.80 | 11.16 | 14.50 | 16.11 | 22.53 |
| 0.5 mM Na acetate | 1.35 | 3.49 | 5.51 | 11.15 | 2.82 | 3.97 | 7.03 | 10.67 | 4.49 | 5.56 | 8.02 | 10.79 | 6.56 | 7.88 | 10.31 | 14.82 |
|  |  | 3.03 | 4.74 | 11.06 | 2.01 | 5.35 | 6.96 | 13.38 | 3.63 | 6.97 | 8.58 | 15.00 | 7.36 | 10.70 | 12.31 | 18.73 |

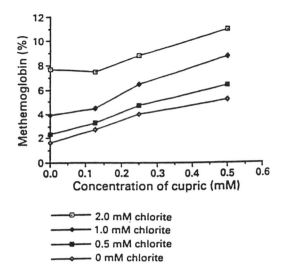

**Figure 3** Combination chlorite and cupric acetate concentrations versus percentage methemoglobin.

expected ones. Also, the dose–response curve shows a clear deviation from parallelism and additivity (Fig. 5). This antagonism was also statistically significant.

## C. Three-Way Interactions

When all three chemicals were combined, the result was slightly less than additive at some points, but this was not statistically significant. The slight deviation from additivity can be seen in Fig. 6. Overall, this response was additive.

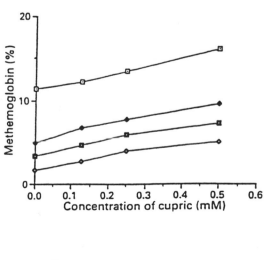

**Figure 4** Combination cupric acetate and nitrite concentrations versus percentage methemoglobin.

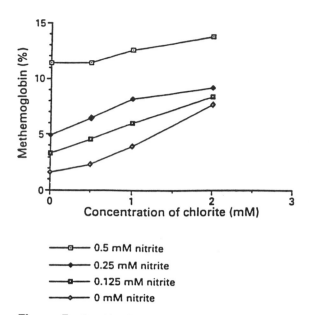

**Figure 5**  Combination chlorite and nitrite concentrations versus percentage methemoglobin.

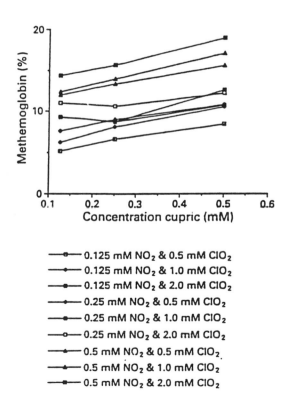

**Figure 6**  Combination chlorite, nitrite, and cupric acetate concentrations versus percentage methemoglobin.

## IV. DISCUSSION

Because many chemicals must be taken into account when studying environmental contamination, a variety of methods have been proposed for assessing the toxicity of complex mixtures.
A common feature of all approaches is that an additive response is usually assumed. For the
most part, the data support this assumption. However, to determine the type of interaction, the
biochemical mechanism of action must be taken into account. The current studies were not
designed to determine such information.

### A. Study 1

The study 1 in vitro assessment of the concurrent exposures of copper and chlorite and
copper and nitrite revealed that the responses observed from combining these methemoglobin-
producing agents, with some exception, are principally additive. Such findings, although of an
in vitro nature, provide support for the U. S. Environmental Protection Agency (USEPA)
guidance recommendations concerning assumptions for how to estimate responses from mixtures (USEPA, 1986).

In the copper plus chlorite experiment, at the lower levels (0.25 m$M$ chlorite), there is very
little difference in the methemoglobin levels produced, when compared with the zero dose for
chlorite. A possible explanation for this observation is that chlorite is considered to be primarily
a hemolytic agent and only secondarily does it cause methemoglobin formation. At the higher
levels, after the chlorite has marked lower red cell reduced glutathione levels, the levels of not
only chlorite, but of the H$_2$O$_2$ produced by the presence of chlorite, may be responsible for the
increased methemoglobin formation (Kiese, 1974; Heffernan et al., 1979).

The copper plus chlorite additive effect described earlier by Moore and Calabrese (1980) is
supported by the present study when one examines the upper levels of exposure in this
experiment (2 m$M$ chlorite and 0.5 and 0.75 m$M$ copper). That study (Moore and Calabrese,
1980) was limited in that it studied the effects that only one test level of copper and chlorite
(millimolar each) had on methemoglobin production and may be the reason for the divergence
with the work presented here (i.e., slight antagonism) at lower concentrations.

### B. Study 2

A mechanistic explanation can be proposed for the one nonadditive response of chlorite
plus nitrite. It could be related to the stability of the ions. Cupric ion and chlorite ion are
both relatively stable. Nitrite, on the other hand is not; it is readily oxidized to nitrate ion.
It is reasonable to assume that chlorite has the ability to oxidize nitrite. Chlorite has what is
known as a nonmetallic character. The more nonmetallic a species is, the greater its tendency to
gain electrons and become negatively charged (Zajicek, 1990). Metals, on the other hand, have
the tendency to maintain a positive charge. The chlorine atom is more nonmetallic than the
nitrogen atom. In light of this, chlorine is likely to remove an electron from nitrite, even though
they have the same oxidation potential. This would reduce methemoglobin formation, since
nitrate is less potent than nitrite. Chlorite is probably reduced to chloride ion or hypochlorite.
The latter agent is capable of producing methemoglobin. This could explain the observed
antagonism. The reaction between chlorite and nitrite suggests that these two chemicals would
not be found in significant amounts in the same water supply. However, since nitrite and copper
have other sources (food, air) it is possible that simultaneous exposure to all three of these
chemicals does indeed occur. When all three chemicals were considered, the antagonism seemed
to have been masked.

Although this study was designed to assess the interactive potential of the three oxidants tested, the broad response range assessed suggests that the findings may have relevance across a broad spectrum of possible exposure scenarios. However, caution needs to be exercised in extrapolation, given the in vitro nature of the study along with the use of a nonhuman model.

In conclusion, this in vitro study shows that the response of combining these methemoglobin-producing agents is additive. The combination of chlorite and nitrite alone produces a less-than-additive response. Generally, though, these preliminary results support the EPA's current assumptions about mixtures (USEPA, 1986).

## ACKNOWLEDGMENT

The findings reported in this chapter were previously published in Langlois and Calabrese, 1992; Calabrese et al., 1992.

## REFERENCES

Calabrese, E. J., and H. Horton (1986). An evaluation of animal models for G-6-PD deficiency, *Drug Metab. Rev.,* 17, 261–281.

Calabrese, E. J., J. A. Garreffi, Jr., and E. J. Stanek (1992). The effects of joint exposures to environmental oxidants on methemoglobin formation: Copper/nitrite and copper/chlorite, *J. Environ. Sci. Health,* A27, 629–642.

Heffernan, W., C. Gulon, and R. Bull (1979). Oxidative damage to the erythrocyte induced by sodium chlorite, in vivo, *J. Environ. Pathol. Toxicol.,* 2, 1487–1499.

Kiese, M. (1974). *Methemoglobinemia: A Comprehensive Treatise,* CRC Press, Cleveland.

Langlois, C. J., and E. J. Calabrese (1992). The interactive effect of chlorine, copper and nitrite on methaemoglobin formation in red blood cells of Dorset sheep, *Hum. Exp. Toxicol.,* 11, 223–228.

Moore, G., and E. Calabrese (1980). The effects of copper and chlorite on normal and G-6-PD deficient erythrocytes, *J. Environ. Pathol. Toxicol.,* 4, 271–280.

Smith, J., and E. Beutler (1966). Methemoglobin formation and reduction in man and various animal species, *Am. J. Physiol.,* 210, 347–350.

[USEPA] U. S. Environmental Protection Agency (1986). Guidelines for the health risk assessment of chemical mixtures, *Fed. Reg.,* 51(185), FRL 2984-2.

Zajicek, O. T. (1990). Professor of chemistry. University of Massachusetts, personal communication.

# PART V
# MODELS AND STATISTICAL METHODS

**D. Krewski**
*Health Canada*
*Ottawa, Ontario, Canada*

Statistical models and methods play an important role in toxicological risk assessment. Statistical tests are used to identify potential human health hazards based on the results of laboratory experiments. Once a potential hazard has been identified, estimates of the level of risk may be obtained using mathematical models to describe the dose response relationship in quantitative terms. A judicious choice of the experimental design can maximize the value of the information obtained for purposes of both hazard identification and risk estimation.

In this section, the use of statistical methods for toxicological risk assessment is discussed. Zhu and Fung describe tests for the increasing trend in fetotoxicity and teratogenicity in developmental toxicity studies, as well as models that can be used to describe dose response relationships for these critical endpoints. The analysis of developmental toxicity data is complicated by the multinomial nature of the response variate (a fetus may die before term, be born with one or more anomalies, or lead to a normal birth) and the fact that such data exhibit overdispersion relative to the multinomial distribution. A simple data transformation can be used to eliminate such overdispersion, thereby permitting the use of statistical methods for the analysis of multinomial data.

Receptor mediated processes play an important role in chemical carcinogenesis. Denes et al. review mathematical models for receptor binding, including the Hill equation used to describe binding of TCDD to the Ah receptor. Such models have important implications for the prediction of risks at low doses. Receptor binding models can be used in conjunction with other pharmacokinetic and pharmacodynamic models to develop comprehensive, biologically based models of carcinogenesis for use in toxicological risk assessment.

Genetic toxicology has evolved to a number of short-term laboratory tests for mutation. The Ames Salmonella/microsome assay and the transgenic mouse assay are widely used for evaluating the mutagenic potential of chemical substances. Piegorsch describes statistical tests for trends in heritable mutations induced in laboratory animals. As in the analysis of overdispersed developmental toxicity data discussed by Zhu and Fung, provision is made for overdispersion relative to the Poisson distribution commonly used to describe count data.

Dinse describes statistical tests for increased tumor occurrence rates in long-term animal cancer studies. Since the pioneering paper by Peto [*Br. J. Cancer, 29,* 101–105, (1974)], a number of different tests for increased tumor occurrence rates have been proposed in the literature. One of the difficulties encountered in the development of such tests is the fact that tumor onset times are not generally observable with occult tumors, thereby necessitating the use of statistical techniques for interval censored failure time data.

While risk assessment methods for discrete data are relatively well established, methods for continuous outcomes have received relatively little attention. Chen et al. discuss risk assessment methods for use with continuous indicators of toxicity, including neurotoxic effects.

Pharmacokinetic models are used to describe the uptake, distribution, metabolism, and excretion of xenobiotics once they enter the body. Such models can be used to predict the dose of reactive metabolites reaching target tissues, thereby affording an opportunity for more accurate estimates of risk. Physiologically based pharmacokinetic (PBPK) models are of particular interest because of their biological basis: The body is described in terms of a small number of physiologically relevant homogeneous organ and tissue compartments, with chemical disposition within the compartmental system characterized by a series of nonlinear partial differential equations. Chu and Ku provide a detailed discussion of their development of a PBPK model for phenanthrene.

Building on the early work of Armitage and Doll on multi-stage models of carcinogenesis, Moolgavkar and his colleagues have developed biologically based cancer models that have now been used in a number of applications for quantitative cancer risk assessment. The two-stage clonal expansion model discussed by Luebeck and Moolgavkar represents an improvement over the Armitage-Doll model in that it provides for both tissue growth and cell kinetics. Biologically based cancer models have a number of advantages over empirical models used in cancer risk assessment. In particular, biologically based models invite questions about the mechanisms of carcinogenesis, leading to a deeper understanding of the fundamental biological events involved in malignant transformation of normal cells.

# 23
# Statistical Methods in Developmental Toxicity Risk Assessment

**Yiliang Zhu**
*University of South Florida*
*Tampa, Florida*

**Karen Fung**
*University of Windsor*
*Windsor, Ontario, Canada*

## I. INTRODUCTION

Exposure to environmental agents may induce developmental aberrations in the offspring of exposed parents, particularly as a consequence of maternal exposure. Because epidemiological evidence of adverse effects on fetal development may not be available for specific chemicals encountered in the environment, laboratory experiments in small mammalian species provide an alternative source of evidence essential for identifying potential developmental toxicants. Animal studies afford a greater level of control than is possible in epidemiological studies, and they can be conducted in advance of human exposure. At present, risk assessment and regulation of developmental toxicants are largely based on data from laboratory studies. This chapter discusses statistical methods for analyzing data arising from developmental toxicity, or segment II, experiments.

## A. Developmental Toxicity Data

Developmental toxicity studies are designed to investigate the potential of the test agent to cause structural abnormalities, prenatal death, and growth alterations (EPA, 1991). Functional deficits, another major manifestation of developmental toxicity, are not presently evaluated in these studies. Test animals are selected on the basis of species, strains, age, weight and health status. Typically, groups of 20–30 mated females, usually rats, mice, or rabbits, are exposed to one of three to four doses, in addition to an unexposed control, during the period of major organogenesis. The highest dose is chosen to produce some minimal maternal toxicity, ranging from marginal body weight reduction to not more than 10% mortality (EPA, 1991). Routes of exposure are chosen relative to major human exposure conditions.

Developmental toxicity is evaluated by examining the uterine contents of pregnant animals just before term or following birth, depending on the protocol of the experiment. The number of implantation sites is counted. An implant may be resorbed at different stages during gestation, or die before birth; if it survives, growth reduction, such as weight loss, may occur; it may further exhibit variuos types of structural variation, or even one or more types of malformation. In addition to these multiple indicators on each implant or fetus, summary data, such as the incidence of prenatal death (resorption or death) and the incidence of fetal malformation among live pups within the same litter, are most frequently used as measures of developmental toxicity. A sketch of these multiple outcomes on each dam is given in Fig. 1.

Because of genetic similarity and the same treatment conditions, offspring of the same mother behave more alike than those of another mother. This has been termed *litter effect* in the literature. As a consequence, the binary and continuous responses on different fetuses within the same litter are likely to be correlated, inducing extra variation in data relative to those associated with the common binomial or multinomial distribution. As an important characteristic of developmental toxicity data, this extra variation must be taken into account in statistical analyses. Since exposure to the test agent takes place after implantation, the number of implants, a random variable, is not expected to be dose-related; hence, it is an ancillary statistic containing no information relative to the dose–response relationship. This suggests that statistical analyses be conditioned on the number of implants, and litters should be treated as experimental units.

## B.  Two Examples

Throughout this chapter, we will use data from two experimetns conducted under the U. S. National Toxicology Program (NTP) to illustrate the statistical methods to be discussed. The first

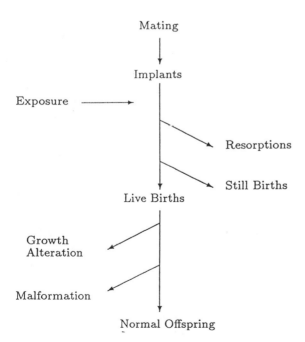

**Figure 1**  Schematic representation of the outcomes from a dam in a developmental toxicity experiment.

experiment involved 30, 26, 26, 24, and 25 pregnant mice, and the second involved 24, 23, 22, 24, and 25 pregnant rats, both exposed to diethylhexalphthalate (DEHP) at concentration levels of 0, 0.025, 0.05, 0.1, and 0.15%; and 0, 0.5, 1.0, 1.5, and 2.0% in diet, respectively (Tables 1 and 2). For present purposes, only the number of implants $m$, the number of prenatal deaths $r$, and the number of malformed fetuses $y$ among $s = m - r$ live births per litter are given. In practice, a specific type of malformation, such as cleft palate, may be of particular interest. For convenience of illustration, we consider a live fetus with any types of malformation as a malformed fetus. It can be seen for these two studies that the incidences of malformation $y/s$ and the prenatal death $r/m$ are both dose-related. In the rat data, for example, the incidence of malformations increased from about 1% in controls to about 4% in the highest-dose group; the proportion of implants resulting in either resorption or death increased from about 4% in controls to nearly 57% in the highest-dose group.

**Table 1** Trinomial Counts of Prenatal Death and Malformed Fetus from Experiment on Mice Exposed to Diethylhexalphthalate (DEHP)[a]

| Concentration (% in diet) | | | | |
|---|---|---|---|---|
| 0.00 | 0.025 | 0.05 | 0.10 | 0.15 |
| (5, 0, 8) | (1, 0, 4) | (3, 0, 6) | (1, 0, 1) | (9, 0, 9) |
| (2, 0, 9) | (3, 0, 8) | (0, 0, 8) | (2, 0, 2) | $(10, 0, 10)_2$ |
| $(1, 0, 10)_2$ | (0, 0, 9) | (2, 0, 8) | (4, 0, 4) | $(11, 0, 11)_4$ |
| (0, 0, 11) | (2, 0, 9) | (1, 2, 9) | (6, 0, 6) | (7, 4, 11) |
| (3, 0, 11) | (1, 0, 10) | (1, 0, 11) | (10, 0, 10) | $(12, 0, 12)_4$ |
| $(0, 0, 12)_2$ | (0, 0, 11) | (4, 1, 11) | (2, 1, 10) | (10, 2, 12) |
| (4, 0, 12) | (1, 0, 11) | (0, 2, 11) | (1, 1, 11) | (6, 6, 12) |
| (4, 1, 12) | $(1, 0, 12)_2$ | (1, 3, 11) | (2, 2, 11) | $(13, 0, 13)_4$ |
| (0, 2, 12) | (1, 1, 12) | (2, 4, 11) | (2, 4, 11) | (4, 4, 13) |
| $(0, 0, 13)_3$ | $(0, 0, 13)_2$ | (0, 0, 12) | (3, 6, 11) | (8, 4, 13) |
| (1, 0, 13) | $(1, 0, 13)_4$ | (0, 1, 12) | (12, 0, 12) | (4, 9, 13) |
| (4, 0, 13) | (2, 1, 13) | (2, 1, 12) | (10, 2, 12) | (14, 0, 14) |
| (1, 1, 13) | (3, 1, 13) | (0, 2, 12) | (7, 3, 12) | (9, 5, 14) |
| (0, 3, 13) | $(1, 0, 14)_2$ | (1, 0, 13) | (9, 3, 13) | (10, 6, 16) |
| (0, 0, 14) | (2, 0, 14) | (2, 2, 13) | (0, 5, 13) | (13, 4, 17) |
| (1, 0, 14) | $(1, 0, 15)_2$ | (0, 0, 14) | (2, 0, 14) | |
| (5, 0, 14) | (4, 0, 15) | $(2, 0, 14)_2$ | (2, 4, 14) | |
| (2, 1, 14) | (1, 1, 15) | (3, 1, 14) | (6, 4, 14) | |
| (0, 0, 15) | (1, 1, 16) | (3, 2, 14) | (6, 5, 14) | |
| (0, 0, 16) | | (3, 5, 14) | (5, 6, 14) | |
| (1, 0, 16) | | (3, 6, 14) | (3, 0, 15) | |
| (9, 0, 16) | | (2, 0, 15) | (9, 6, 15) | |
| (10, 0, 16) | | (1, 1, 15) | (16, 1, 18) | |
| (0, 1, 16) | | (2, 1, 15) | (19, 0, 19) | |
| (1, 0, 17) | | (2, 4, 16) | | |
| (11, 0, 18) | | | | |

[a]Data $(r, y, m)_k$ represent $r$ deaths and $y$ malformed fetuses among $m$ implants in a single litter; the subscript $k$ denotes the multiplicity of litters producing the same responses.

**Table 2** Trinomial Counts of Prenatal Death and Malformed Fetuses from Experiment on Rats Exposed to Diethylhexalphthalate (DEHP)[a]

| Concentration (% in diet) | | | | |
|---|---|---|---|---|
| 0.0 | 0.5 | 1.0 | 1.5 | 2.0 |
| $(0, 0, 6)$ | $(0, 0, 1)$ | $(0, 0, 8)$ | $(0, 0, 8)$ | $(2, 0, 5)_2$ |
| $(0, 0, 9)$ | $(1, 0, 5)$ | $(1, 0, 9)$ | $(0, 0, 9)_2$ | $(8, 0, 8)$ |
| $(1, 0, 9)$ | $(0, 0, 8)$ | $(0, 1, 9)_2$ | $(0, 1, 9)$ | $(3, 0, 9)$ |
| $(0, 0, 10)_3$ | $(1, 0, 8)$ | $(0, 0, 10)_4$ | $(1, 0, 10)_4$ | $(9, 0, 9)$ |
| $(1, 1, 10)$ | $(0, 0, 9)_2$ | $(1, 0, 10)$ | $(0, 1, 10)$ | $(1, 0, 10)$ |
| $(0, 0, 11)_5$ | $(0, 0, 10)_5$ | $(0, 0, 11)_3$ | $(0, 0, 11)_4$ | $(3, 0, 10)$ |
| $(1, 0, 11)_2$ | $(1, 0, 10)_2$ | $(1, 0, 11)_4$ | $(1, 0, 11)_2$ | $(0, 0, 10)_4$ |
| $(2, 0, 11)$ | $(0, 0, 11)_2$ | $(1, 2, 11)$ | $(2, 0, 11)_2$ | $(1, 0, 11)$ |
| $(2, 1, 11)$ | $(1, 0, 11)_3$ | $(0, 0, 12)_3$ | $(0, 1, 11)$ | $(3, 0, 11)_2$ |
| $(0, 0, 12)_3$ | $(0, 0, 12)_3$ | $(1, 0, 12)$ | $(1, 1, 11)_2$ | $(4, 0, 11)$ |
| $(1, 0, 12)$ | $(1, 0, 12)$ | $(4, 0, 12)$ | $(0, 0, 12)_2$ | $(11, 0, 11)$ |
| $(0, 1, 12)$ | $(2, 0, 13)$ | | $(0, 1, 12)$ | $(0, 1, 11)$ |
| $(0, 0, 13)$ | | | $(0, 2, 12)$ | $(2, 1, 11)$ |
| $(1, 0, 13)_2$ | | | | $(1, 0, 12)$ |
| | | | | $(2, 0, 12)$ |
| | | | | $(12, 0, 12)_2$ |
| | | | | $(13, 0, 13)_2$ |
| | | | | $(3, 2, 13)$ |

[a]Data $(r, y, m)_k$ represent $r$ deaths and $y$ malformed fetuses among $m$ implants in a single litter; the subscript $k$ denotes the multiplicity of litters producing the same responses.

## C. Hierarchical Models

Since the random variable $m$ is an ancillary statistic, statistical analyses on the incidence of prenatal death, the incidence of malformation, and fetal weight may be based on the distribution

$$\mathbf{P}(r,w,y\,|\,m) \,-\, \mathbf{P}(y\,|\,w,s,m)\mathbf{P}(w\,|\,s,m)\mathbf{P}(r\,|\,m) \tag{1}$$

conditional on the number of implants $m$, where $w$ denotes average fetal weight per litter. Given $m$ and the constraint $s + r = m$, the number of live births or litter size $s$ and the number of prenatal deaths $r$ can be used interchangeably. The model in Eq. (1) can be easily adpated for the multiple responses on individual implant/fetus in the same litter. In this case, $y$ would be a vector of 0 or 1, indicating a normal or malformed live fetus, respectively; $r$ would be a vector indicating whether or not an implant leads to a live birth; and $w$ would be the vector of individual fetal weight. Then, individual fetal weight can be modeled in conjunction with its malformation status, for example. The three models on the right-hand side of Eq. (1), $\mathbf{P}(r\,|\,m)$, $\mathbf{P}(w\,|\,r,m)$, and $\mathbf{P}(y\,|\,w,s,m)$, reflect the biological risks in a way that is mathematically convenient: an implant is at the risk of resorption or death; surviving this risk, it may be subject to growth alteration such as weight reduction; it may further become malformed with a specific type of malformation. Nevertheless, the biological connection between weight reduction and malformation is not clear (Catalano et al., 1993).

Statistical analyses of the incidence of prenatal death $r/m$ and the incidence of malformation $y/s$ may be based on the distribution

$$\int \mathbf{P}(r,w,y\,|\,m)d\mathbf{P}(w) \;=\; \mathbf{P}(r,y\,|\,m) \;=\; \mathbf{P}(y\,|\,s,m)\mathbf{P}(r\,|\,m) \tag{2}$$

(Chen et al., 1991; Ryan, 1992, Chen and Li, 1994; Zhu et al., 1994; Krewski and Zhu, 1994). Here, the conditional probabilities $\mathbf{P}(r\,|\,m)$ and $\mathbf{P}(y\,|\,s,m)$ characterize the fetal malformation rate and the prenatal death rate, respectively.

Joint analyses on the outcomes from live births, that is, fetal weight and the incidence of fetal malformation, may be conducted on the basis of

$$\mathbf{P}(y,w\,|\,s) \;=\; \mathbf{P}(y\,|\,w,s)\mathbf{P}(w\,|\,s) \tag{3}$$

as reported by Ryan et al. (1991), Catalano and Ryan (1992), and Chen (1993).

The foregoing discussion indicates that various submodels of Eq. (1) may serve as a basis for analyzing one or more developmental toxicity endpoints. For example, $\mathbf{P}(r\,|\,m)$ in Eq. (2) may be used to analyze the incidence of prenatal death alone, regardless of its correlation with other endpoints. The choice of jointly analyzing several outcomes versus separately analyzing a single outcome should be guided, among others, by the objectives of the study, and the statistical efficiency required for the analyses. The multiple outcomes of developmental toxicity are likely to be correlated. If these multiple outcomes are the results of different biological mechanisms, joint analyses allow the detection of all the important effects. If the multiple outcomes are manifestations of some common biological effects, joint analyses have the potential of greater statistical power than is possible in separate analysis of a single outcome. Therefore, our discussion will emphasize multivariate statistical methods associated with the models in Eqs. (1), (2), and (3), especially the joint analyses of the incidences of prenatal death and fetal malformation.

Traditionally, however, the analysis of developmental toxicity data has been separately conducted on individual outcome, such as the proportion of fetal malformation $y/s$ on the basis of the conditional distribution

$$\mathbf{P}(y\,|\,s) \tag{4}$$

Since $s$ is not an ancillary statistic relative to dose–response relationship, analyses based on Eq. (4) suffer certain degree of information loss.

## D. Scope and Organization

In Section II, methods for analyzing the proportion of fetal malformation $y/s$ are described, as they represent a traditional approach to the analysis of developmental toxicity data. Whereas a brief review is provided, emphasis is given to recent development of generalized score tests for trend and generalized estimating equations (GEEs) for dose–response modeling. These methods can be directly applied to the analysis of any outcome of proportion such as the incidence of prenatal death. In Section III, these moment-based methods are extended for the joint analysis of the incidences of prenatal death $r/m$ and fetal malformation $y/s$. A simple data transformation method that permits the transformed data to be approximated by the mean and covariance of multinomial distribution is also described. In Section IV, these methods are illustrated, using data from studies conducted under the U. S. National Toxicology Program. In Section V, relatively new methods for joint analyses of prenatal death rate, fetal weight, and malformation rate are outlined. In Section VI, the benchmark dose method for risk assessment is discussed. Our conclusion and discussion are given in Section VII. Additional technical details on the GEEs, the data transformation, and the generalized score tests for trend are enclosed in appendices.

## II.   ANALYSIS OF THE INCIDENCE OF FETAL MALFORMATION

Extensive work has been conducted on the analysis of the incidence of fetal malformation $y/s$ per litter. Because of the extrabinomial variation induced by the litter effects, β-binomial distribution has been widely used for the conditional model $P(y|s)$ (cf, Williams, 1975; Crowder, 1978; Kupper et al., 1986; Chen and Kodell, 1989; Kodell et al., 1991). Let $\pi_1$ be the probability that a live fetus may develop a specific or any type of fetal malformation and $\rho(0 \le \rho \le 1)$ be the intralitter correlation coefficient among the live fetuses within the same litter. The β-binomial distribution

$$P(y|s;\pi_1,\rho) = \binom{s}{y,s-y} \frac{\Gamma[(1-\rho)/\rho]}{\Gamma[s+(1-\rho)/\rho]} \frac{\Gamma[s-y+(1-\pi_1)(1-\rho)/\rho]}{\Gamma[(1-\pi_1)(1-\rho)/\rho]} \frac{\Gamma[y+\pi_1(1-\rho)/\rho]}{\Gamma[\pi_1(1-\rho)/\rho]} \quad (5)$$

can be derived by assuming that fetuses in the same litter may become malformed with varying probability which follows a β-distribution; and given this probability, the total number of malformed fetuses within the same litter follows a binomial distribution. This β-mixture of binomial distribution gives rise to a β-binomial distribution, and remains, moreover, a valid distribution for negative values of $\rho$ in the vicinity of zero provided

$$\rho \le \max\left\{-\frac{\pi_1}{s-1-\pi_1}, \ -\frac{1-\pi_1}{s-1-(1-\pi_1)}\right\}$$

(Prentice, 1986). Alternative distributions for correlated binary data exhibiting extrabinomial variation have also been proposed by Altham (1978), Kupper and Haseman (1978), and Paul (1987). Whereas these distributions provide a basis for likelihood-based inferences, likelihood ratio test, and maximum likelihood estimation, for example, statistical methods based on only the first two moments of the data are less restrained by strict distributional assumptions, often simple to implement, and yet maintain reasonably high statistical efficiency. Thus, in this section, we discuss generalized score tests for trend and GEEs for dose–response modeling of the incidence of fetal malformation $y/s$. These methods are immediately applicable to any proportion data, particularly the proportion of prenatal deaths $r/m$, and the proportion of overall toxicity $(y + r)/m$. To proceed, we begin with the characterization of the extrabinomial variation exhibited in the fetal malformation rate.

## A.   Extrabinomial Variation

Assume that the mean and variance for the number of malformed fetuses within the same litter are given by

$$E(y|s) = s\pi_1 \tag{6}$$

and

$$\text{Var}(y|s) = \mathbf{V} = sh^{-1}\pi_1(1-\pi_1) \tag{7}$$

respectively, where $h$ is a positive, real-valued function. When $h = 1$ and $h^{-1} = \sigma$, the variance function Eq. (7) corresponds to that of a binomial distribution and a generalized linear model, respectively. When $h^{-1} = 1 + (s-1)\rho$, Eq. (7) may be derived directly from the β-binomial distribution, and includes, moreover, the extended binomial distributions of Altham (1978), Kupper and Haseman (1978), and Paul (1987) as special cases under appropriate reparametrization. This implies the generality and flexibility in using this extended β-binomial variance function to characterize the extrabinomial variation in the fetal malformation rate $y/s$, as compared with using the β-binomial distribution.

Alternative to specifying a parametric variance function, the original data $(y,s)$ may be simply scaled by the design effect, as suggested by Rao and Scott (1992). Suppose that the experiment consists of $t$ dose groups, including a control with dose $d_1 = 0$, and that the $i$th $(i = 1, \ldots, t)$ dose group involves $n_i$ $(j = 1, \ldots, n_i)$ litters. The design effect

$$D_i = \mathbf{V}_i \Big/ \left\{ \sum_{j=1}^{n_i} \pi_{1i}(1 - \pi_{1i}) \right\} \tag{8}$$

for the $i$th dose group is essentially the ratio of the true variance $\sum_{j=1}^{n_i} s_{ij}\mathbf{V}_i = \sum_{j=1}^{n_i} \mathbf{V}_{ij}$ to the binomial variance $\sum_{j=1}^{n_i} s_{ij}\pi_{1i}(1 - \pi_{1i})$, where $\pi_{1i}$ is the mean response probability in the $i$th dose group. It can be shown (see Appendix B) that the transformed data

$$(\tilde{y}_{ij}, \tilde{s}_{ij}) = (y_{ij}, s_{ij})/D_i, \tag{9}$$

may be approximated, similar to the binomial data, by

$$E(\tilde{y}_{ij} \mid \tilde{s}_{ij}) = \tilde{s}_{ij}\pi_{1i}$$

and

$$\mathrm{Var}(\tilde{y}_{ij} \mid \tilde{s}_{ij}) \approx \tilde{s}_{ij}\pi_{1i}(1 - \pi_{1i}).$$

The transformation by Eq. (9) is similar in nature to a moment correction in large sample theory. Consequently, standard methods based on the mean and variance functions of the binomial distribution are applicable to the transformed data. Since both $\pi_{1i}$ and the true variances $\mathbf{V}_{ij}$ are unknown, sample estimates

$$\hat{\pi}_{1i} = \frac{\displaystyle\sum_j y_{ij}}{\displaystyle\sum_j s_{ij}}$$

and

$$\hat{V}_{i\cdot} = \sum_j (y_{ij} - s_{ij}\hat{\pi}_{1i})^2$$

may be used to estimate the design effects $D_i$. In Section III.A, this transformation is generalized to the case of multiple binary data.

## B. Generalized Score Tests for Trend

In the presence of extra binomial variation in the incidence of fetal malformation $y/s$, the Cochran–Armitage test for trend (Cochran, 1954; Armitage, 1955) and other tests associated with the binomial distribution cannot be used, as the type I error rate exceeds the nominal value (Portier and Hoel, 1984). Lefkopoulou et al. (1989) proposed a generalized score statistic based on GEEs derived from a logistic dose–response model and the variance of the generalized linear model with $h^{-1} = \sigma$ in Eq. (7). Ryan (1993) proposed a modified version of this latter statistic using the value of $\sigma$ estimated from Pearson's $\chi^2$ statistic. Rao and Scott (1992) suggested to simply apply the Cochran–Armitage statistic to the transformed data in Eq. (9).

These various statistics for testing trend can be unified within the framework of generalized score tests. In the present context, generalized score tests are constructed in analogy to

Neyman's $C(\alpha)$ tests (Neyman, 1959), on the basis of projected generalized score functions and GEEs (see also Sec. III.B and Appendix C).

Let $\eta_i = \eta(d_i;\gamma)$ be a monotone transformation of the dose $d_i (i = 1, \ldots, t)$ with unknown parameters $\gamma$. Suppose that the probability of observing a malformed fetus among $s$ live fetuses in the $ij$th litter is given by

$$\pi_1(d_i) = F(a + b\eta_i) \tag{10}$$

a monotone function in $\eta$, hence, in dose $d_i$. The composite null hypothesis of no dose effect is expressed by

$$H_0 : b = 0 \quad (i.e., \pi_{11} = \cdots = \pi_{1t} = \pi_{10})$$

with the value of the nuisance parameters $(a, \gamma)$, and additional dispersion parameters involved in the variance function, unspecified. To test $H_0$, the generalized score statistic

$$Z = \frac{\displaystyle\sum_{i=1}^{t}\sum_{j=1}^{n_i}(\eta_i - \bar{\eta})V_{ij}^{-1}s_{ij}y_{ij}}{\left[\displaystyle\sum_{i=1}^{t}\sum_{j=1}^{n_i}(\eta_i - \bar{\eta})^2 s_{ij}^2 V_{ij}^{-1}\right]^{1/2}} \tag{11}$$

may be used, where

$$\bar{\eta} = \sum_{i=1}^{t}\sum_{j=1}^{n_i} s_{ij}^2 V_{ij}^{-1}\eta(d_i;\gamma) \bigg/ \left\{\sum_{i=1}^{t}\sum_{j=1}^{n_i} s_{ij}^2 V_{ij}^{-1}\right\} \tag{12}$$

is a weighted average of the transformed dose, $V_{ij} = \text{Var}(y_{ij}|s_{ij})$ may be specified as in Eq. (7). The parameters $\gamma$ in $\eta$ may be estimated by solving the equation

$$\sum_{i=1}^{t}\sum_{j=1}^{n_i} s_{ij}\frac{\partial\eta}{\partial\gamma^T}V_{ij}^{-1}(y_{ij} - s_{ij}\hat{\pi}_{10}) = 0 \tag{13}$$

where $\hat{\pi}_{10} = y_{..}/s_{..}$ is the overall malformation rate for all dose groups. Here, a dot in place of a subscript denotes that a summation has taken place over the associated subscript. Equation (13) is simplified from the GEE for $\gamma$ (see Sec. II.C and Appendix A). Any additional parameters involved in the $V_{ij}$ can be estimated based on Pearson's squared residuals, or quadratic estimating equations to be discussed in Section II.C. Other $\sqrt{n}$-consistent $(n = n_1 + \cdots + n_t)$ estimates of the nuisance parameters may also be used. As $n_i \to \infty$ at comparable rates, the $Z$ statistic follows approximately the standard normal distribution. Large values of the $Z$ statistic lead to the rejection of the null hypothesis.

Since the statistics in Eq. (11) and their distribution under the null hypothesis depends on the transformation $\eta$ only, not the function $F(\cdot)$, the generalized score tests are robust against misspecification of $F(\cdot)$. This nonparametric property relative to $F(\cdot)$ has been noted by Cox (1958), and by Tarone and Gart (1980) for the score and $C(\alpha)$ statistics under the assumption of binomial distribution. On the other hand, the power for detecting a particular departure from the null bypothesis of no trend depends generally on both the model $F(\cdot)$ and the dose transformation $\eta$. The sensitivity of the generalized score statistics about the misspecification of the variance $\mathbf{V}_{ij}$ requires further investigation.

Special cases arise when we set $\eta(d; \gamma) \equiv d$: replacing $\mathbf{V}_{ij}$ with $s_{ij}\pi_{10}(1 - \pi_{10})$ ($h = 1$) yields the Cochran–Armitage statistic; substituting $\hat{\sigma}s_{ij}\pi_{10}(1 - \pi_{10})$ ($h^{-1} = \sigma$) for $\mathbf{V}_{ij}$ with the moment estimate $\hat{\sigma}$ gives the statistic proposed by Ryan (1993); replacing $\mathbf{V}_{ij}$ with any reasonable sample-based estimate results in an empirical statistic; the test statistic of Lefkopoulou et al. (1989) may be obtained by first assuming $V_{ij} = s_{ij}V$, and then replacing $s_{i\cdot}V$ by the sample estimate

$$\hat{V}_{i\cdot} = \sum_{j=1}^{n_i}(y_{ij} - s_{ij}\pi_{10})^2$$

In these foregoing quantities, $\pi_{10}$ can be simply replaced by $\hat{\pi}_{10} = y_{\cdot\cdot}/s_{\cdot\cdot}$. Note that the score statistic Eq. (11), and the Cochran–Armitage statistic in particular, in conjunction with the binomial variance can be directly applied to data after applying the Rao–Scott transformation.

## 1.  Related Results

Fung et al. (1994) conducted a simulation study comparing the small sample property of the Cochran–Armitage test applied to data after using the Rao-Scott transformation, the tests of Lefkopoulou et al. (1989) and Ryan (1993), and other related tests for trend. These tests yield type I error rates close to the nominal level in the presence of intralitter correlation, although the test of Lefkopoulou et al. (1989) appears somewhat conservative under certain conditions. In another simulation study, Chen (1993a) found that the type I error of Wald type tests for trend is more likely to exceed the nominal level than score tests when the intralitter correlation in the underlying $\beta$-binomial distribution increases with dose. Carr and Portier (1993) found that the Wald type tests based on quasi-likelihood estimation are often more powerful than the likelihood ratio tests based on the $\beta$-binomial distribution with increasing dose-dependent intralitter correlation. Moreover, statistical methods based on quasi-likelihood appear robust to certain degree against some departure from the $\beta$-binomial distribution

## C.  Dose–Response Modeling

### 1.  Models

Dose–response modeling has become an integrated part of the quantitative risk assessment process. The use of simple mathematical models of the form of Eq. (10) has been a common practice as biologically based dose–response models for developmental toxicity remain to be developed (Gaylor and Razzaghi, 1992). The models in Eq. (10) include the probit model $F(x) = \Phi(x)$ (Catalano et al., 1993), linear logistic model $F(x) = [1 + \exp(-x)]^{-1}$ (Allen et al., 1994b), both with a power transformation, and the extreme value model $F(x) = 1 - \exp[-\exp(x)]$. The latter model in conjunction with an independent spontaneous rate also yields the Weibull model

$$\pi_{1i} = 1 - \exp\left[-(a + bd_i^{\gamma})\right] \tag{14}$$

(Krewski and Van Ryzin, 1981). Because of the increased flexibility in the shape of the models that incorporate a power transformation of the dose, the phenomenon of a biological threshold, generally believed to exist, can be closely approximated by such models, even when a threshold dose is omitted. The estimates of benchmark dose (see Sec. VI), a relatively new method for risk assessment, are generally not affected whether or not a threshold is used in these models. In a simulation study conducted by Stiteler et al. (1993), the Weibull model, omitting the threshold dose, approximates the threshold phenomenon better than several other models primarily owing to the power transformation used. Krewski and Zhu (1994) found that the Weibull model is sufficiently flexible in describing various shapes, including that of a hockey stick, of the dose–response curves observed in a number of developmental toxicity studies conducted under the NTP. In the remainder, the Weibull model [Eq. (14)] will be used in dose–response modeling.

At $d = 0$, the Weibull model [Eq. (14)] gives $1 - \exp(-a)$, which reflects the probability of an anomaly occurring spontaneously in the absence of exposure to the test agent. The constraints $a \geq 0$ and $b \geq 0$ ensure $0 \leq \pi \leq 1$. The Weibull parameter $\gamma$ determines the shape of the dose–response curve. For $\gamma < 1$ the curve is concave; for $\gamma > 1$ the curve is convex when $d < \{(1 - \gamma^{-1})b^{-1}\}^{1/\gamma}$ and concave when $d > \{(1 - \gamma^{-1})b^{-1}\}^{1/\gamma}$. If the dose is scaled to be in the range of [0,1], the inflection point is a strictly increasing function of $\gamma$, and approaches 1 as $\gamma \to \infty$. When data to be modeled are not comparable with these properties, the Weibull model, however, may not be satisfactory.

It is worthwhile to mention the model

$$\pi_1 = \left[ 1 - \exp\{-(a + bd)\} \right] \exp\{-s\eta(d)\}$$

proposed by Rai and Van Ryzin (1985) in a pioneering effort to adapt the concept of single-hit kinetics and to use the litter size $s$ as a covariate to account for extrabinomial variation in the malformation rate. The use of litter size in the dose–response model alone, however, is not sufficient to characterize the extrabinomial variation. Faustman et al. (1989) applied this model to several datasets arising from the NTP studies. Kodell et al. (1991) proposed a Weibull model incorporating both a threshold dose and the litter size $s$ as covariates, but found that the inclusion of litter size $s$ did not significantly improve the goodness of fit of the model. On the other hand, Allen et al. (1994b) preferred the inclusion of litter size as a covariate. In a joint modeling of fetal malformation and prenatal death in a series of 11 NTP studies, Krewski and Zhu (1994) did not find the number of implants $m$ to be a significant covariate. Zhu et al. (1994), however, reported a contrary finding in a large-scale study with the herbicide 2,4,5-T (Holson et al., 1992) conducted by the U. S. National Center for Toxicology Research.

## 2. Model Fitting and GEEs

The maximum likelihood method based on the β-binomial distribution has been widely used for fitting dose–response models to malformation rates. However, the specification of a full likelihood function may be avoided by using the method of quasi-score functions or generalized estimating equations (GEEs) proposed by Liang and Zeger (1986). The quasi-likelihood method was used by Williams (1982) to fit a linear logistic model. Whereas the moment method, based on Pearson's $\chi^2$ statistics was used by Williams (1982), Ryan (1992), and Krewski and Zhu (1994), quadratic GEEs were used by Zhu et al. (1994), and Krewski and Zhu (1995) to estimate the overdispersion parameters involved in the variance functions.

The method of GEEs has several advantages. First, it is robust against misspecification of the underlying distribution, since only the first two moments are required. This is especially attractive in a multivariate situation for which the underlying distribution is difficult to specify. Under certain conditions, GEEs include quasi-likelihood and likelihood equations as special cases. Second, with the specification of a working covariance function, GEEs still yield consistent and asymptotically normal estimates under mild regularity conditions, although efficiency may decrease. The GEE estimators of parameters in the mean are nearly as efficient as the maximum likelihood estimators based on the Dirichlet-trinomial distribution, although those for the dispersion parameters are less efficient (Zhu et al., 1994). Third, GEEs are often computationally simpler to implement than maximum likelihood estimation.

In a recent simulation study, Carr and Portier (1993) considered the estimation of the slope in a complementary log or extreme value dose–response model under the β-binomial distribution. Their results confirm that quasi-likelihood estimation with moderate number of litters per dose group generally provides accurate parameter estimates. Moreover, maximum likelihood estimates based on the β-binomial distribution with equal intralitter correlation across dose groups are typically biased when the true correlation increases with dose (Kupper et al., 1986). They also showed that the variance estimates for the slope using quasi-likelihood, bootstrap, or jackknife methods are in general close to the true variance.

To illustrate the use of GEEs for dose–response modeling, consider the Weibull model [Eq. (14)] and the extended β-binomial variance function [Eq. (7)] with $h_{ij}^{-1} = 1 + (s - 1)\rho_i$. Here, the distinct value $\rho_i$ is postulated for each dose group to accommodate the intralitter correlation that is likely to increase with dose (Kupper et al., 1986; Zhu et al., 1994). Alternatively, it is possible to model the intralitter correlation as a smooth function of dose (Prentice, 1986; Moore, 1987; Williams, 1988), although the choice of a simple parametric function may not always be clear.

The GEEs for the parameters $\theta = (a,b,\gamma)^T$ in Eq. (14) are given by

$$\sum_{i=1}^{t} \sum_{j=1}^{n_i} \frac{1}{1 + (s_{ij} - 1)\rho_i} \frac{1}{\pi_{1i}(1 - \pi_{1i})} \frac{\partial \pi_{1i}}{\partial \theta} (y_{ij} - s_{ij}\pi_{1i}) = 0 \tag{15}$$

To estimate the dispersion parameters $\{\rho_i\}$, the quadratic GEEs

$$\sum_{j=1}^{n_i} \frac{s_{ij} - 1}{\{1 + (s_{ij} - 1)\rho_i\}} \left[ \frac{(y_{ij} - s_{ij}\pi_{1i})^2}{s_{ij}\{1 + (s_{ij} - 1)\rho_i\}\pi_{1i}(1 - \pi_{1i})} - 1 \right] = 0 \tag{16}$$

$(i = 1, \ldots, t)$ may be used, where the squared residuals $(y_{ij} - s_{ij}\pi_{1i})^2$ are used as responses (see Appendix A). The estimates $\hat{\theta}$ and $\{\hat{\rho}_i\}$ are obtained by solving the Eqs. (15) and (16) iteratively until convergence. Details concerning the estimation of the variance–covariance for these parameter estimates are given in Appendix A.

Alternative to the GEE approach based on the variance function [Eq. (7)], we can apply the Rao–Scott (1992) transformation described in Section II.A to the data, and then solve the GEEs [Eq. (15)] for $\theta$ in association with the transformed data $(\tilde{y}_{ij}, \tilde{s}_{ij})$ with the $\{\rho_i\}$ set to be zero. In this case, the estimates obtained by methods of GEEs are asymptotically equivalent to maximum likelihood estimates based on the binomial likelihood function.

## III. JOINT ANALYSIS OF DEATH AND MALFORMATION

The methods discussed in Section II for analyzing a single outcome of proportion can be generalized for jointly analyzing the incidences of prenatal death and fetal malformation on the basis of $P(y,r|m)$ in Eq. (2). It can be seen, moreover, that analyses of higher dimensional categorical data, the disaggregation of resorption and fetal death, for instance, can be conducted in analogy.

## A.  Overdispersion

Similar to the binomial counts of malformed fetuses in a given litter, the trinomial counts of malformed fetuses and prenatal deaths $(y,r)$, given the number of implants $m$ within a dam, are generally overdispersed relative to the standard trinomial distribution. Suitable characterization of this overdispersion is crucial for obtaining valid statistical inferences.

In general, Dirichlet-multinomial distribution (cf, Johnson and Kotz, 1969) provides a mechanism for describing multinomial data with certain types of overdispersion. A useful property of the Dirichlet-multinomial distribution is its collapsibility, inherited from the multinomial and Dirichlet distributions. Specifically, when a group of categories are collapsed, the original Dirichlet-multinomial distribution factors into a product of two lower-dimensional Dirichlet-multinomial distributions, one conditioning on the total counts of the collapsed groups, and the other marginal, with one category being the union of the collapsed categories. Any number of groups can be collapsed in this manner.

Consider, for example, the Dirichlet-trinomial distribution for the trinomial counts $(y,r)$ given $m$ (Chen, et al., 1991). In addition to the conditional probability $\pi_1$ that a live birth becomes malformed, let $\pi_2$ be the probability of a prenatal death, and $\phi$ be the intralitter correlation coefficient among implants. The Dirichlet-trinomial distribution is given by

$$\mathbf{P}(y,r\,|\,m;\pi_1,\pi_2,\phi) = \binom{m}{y,r,s-y} \frac{\Gamma[(1-\phi)/\phi]}{\Gamma[m+(1-\phi)/\phi]}$$
$$\times\;\frac{\Gamma[y+\pi_1(1-\pi_2)(1-\phi)/\phi]}{\Gamma[\pi_1(1-\pi_2)(1-\phi)/\phi]}\;\frac{\Gamma[s-y+(1-\pi_1)(1-\pi_2)(1-\phi)/\phi]}{\Gamma[(1-\pi_1)(1-\pi_2)(1-\phi)/\phi]}\;\frac{\Gamma[r+\pi_2(1-\phi)/\phi]}{\Gamma[\pi_2(1-\phi)/\phi]} \tag{17}$$

where $\Gamma(\cdot)$ is the $\gamma$-function. Denoting by $\mu_1 = \pi_1(1-\pi_2)$ the probability that an implant may lead to a malformed fetus and letting $\mu_2 = \pi_2$, Eq. (17) remains a valid probability function for negative values of $\phi$ so far as

$$\phi \geq \max\left\{ -\frac{\mu_k}{m-1-\mu_k};\quad k = 1,2,3;\quad m \geq 2\right\} \tag{18}$$

with $\mu_3 = 1 - \mu_1 - \mu_2$. This result holds in higher-dimensional cases (Zhu et al., 1994). Following the discussion on collapsibility, the Dirichlet-trinomial distribution $\mathbf{P}(y,r\,|\,m;\pi_1,\pi_2,\phi)$ can be expressed as a product of two $\beta$ binomial distributions, one being $\mathbf{P}(y\,|\,s,m;\pi_1,\rho)$, given in Eq. (5), and the other being

$$\mathbf{P}(r\,|\,m;\pi_2,\phi) = \binom{m}{r,s} \frac{\Gamma[(1-\phi]}{\Gamma[m+(1-\phi)/\phi]}\;\frac{\Gamma[s+(1-\pi_2)(1-\phi)/\phi]}{\Gamma[(1-\pi_2)(1-\phi)/\phi]}\;\frac{\Gamma[r+\pi_2(1-\phi)/\phi]}{\Gamma[\pi_2(1-\phi)/\phi]}$$

with the latter reflecting the distribution of the prenatal death rate $r/m$. The likelihood factorization in Eq. (17) indicates a connection between the joint and separate analyses of the incidences of prenatal death and fetal malformation. The Dirichlet-multinomial covariance further implies that the correlation coefficient $\rho$ among live fetuses is determined by $\rho = \phi[1 - \pi_2(1-\phi)]^{-1}$, given the correlation coefficient $\phi$ among implants. Fairly large amounts of computation are usually required to conduct likelihood-based inferences on the basis of the Dirichlet-trinomial distribution. Therefore, we extend the discussion in Section II on the moment-based statistical methods to the situation of jointly analyzing the incidences of prenatal death and fetal malformation. Again, we begin with how to characterize the extramultinomial variation by means of parametric covariance functions and transformation.

## 1. Parametric Covariance Function

By letting $z = (y, r)^T$, the mean and covariance of $z$ conditional on the number of implants $m$ may be described by

$$E(z \mid m) = m\mu = m \begin{pmatrix} \mu_1 \\ \mu_2 \end{pmatrix} = m \begin{pmatrix} \pi_1(1 - \pi_2) \\ \pi_2 \end{pmatrix} \tag{19}$$

and

$$\text{Cov}(z \mid m) = \mathbf{V} = mh^{-1}[\text{diag}(\mu) - \mu\mu^T] \tag{20}$$

respectively, where $h$ is a positive, real-valued function as in Eq. (7). When $h = 1$, for example, Eq. (20) corresponds to the multinomial covariance; when $h_{ij} = \sigma^{-1}$, Eq. (20) corresponds to the covariance

$$\phi m[\text{diag}(\mu) - \mu\mu^T]$$

of the generalized linear model; when $h_{ij} = [1 + (m_{ij} - 1)\phi_i]^{-1}$, Eq. (20) corresponds to the Dirichlet-multinomial covariance. The Dirichlet-trinomial covariance function is further extended when Eq. (18) holds. We may also permit $0 > \phi > -(m - 1)^{-1}$ to allow for moderate underdispersion. Because of the upper bound $\phi \leq 1$, however, the extended Dirichlet-trinomial covariance function may not be able to describe extreme overdispersion. Again, it is convenient to postulate distinct value $\phi_i$ for each dose group to allow for dose-dependence (Chen and Li, 1994; Zhu et al., 1994; Krewski and Zhu, 1994).

## 2. Transformation

Instead of specifying a parametric covariance function for the data, the Rao–Scott transformation for clustered binary data can be extended to account for the extramultinomial variation in the trinomial counts (Zhu and Krewski, 1995; see Appendix B). This transformation has several advantages over direct analysis of the original correlated data. First, since the transformation does not require the specification of a covariance function, it may enjoy certain degree of robustness. Second, since the first two moments of the transformed data can be approximated by those of the multinomial distribution, standard methods associated with the multinomial distribution are readily applicable. For example, $\chi^2$ statistics may be used as a measure of goodness-of-fit. Third, the analysis of transformed data is computationally simpler than that of the original data with a parametric covariance function. In an analysis of 11 experiments conducted under the U. S. National Toxicology Program, Krewski and Zhu (1995) found that dose–response models fitted to the transformed data were practically equivalent to models fitted to the original data using the Dirichlet-trinomial covariance function.

Specifically, the Rao–Scott transformation for the overdispersed trinomial data is defined as

$$\tilde{z}_{ij} = z_{ij}/\hat{D}_i, \quad (i = 1, \ldots, t) \tag{21}$$

where $\hat{D}_i$ is an estimate of the average design effect

$$D_i = \frac{1}{2} \text{trace} \, [\mathbf{V}_0^{-1}(\mu_i)\mathbf{V}_i] = \frac{1}{2}\left( \frac{v_{11i}}{\mu_{1i}} + \frac{v_{22i}}{\mu_{2i}} + \frac{v_{33i}}{\mu_{3i}} \right) \tag{22}$$

with $m_{i.}v_{kki}$ $(k = 1,2,3)$ being the variances for the components of the group total counts

$$(y_{i.}, r_{i.}, s_{i.} - y_{i.})$$

given the total number of implants $m_{i.}$ per dose group. To compute $\hat{D}_i$, $\mu_{1i}$, $\mu_{2i}$, and $\mu_{3i}$ are replaced by their sample estimates $\hat{\mu}_{1i} = y_{i.}/m_{i.}$, $\hat{\mu}_{2i} = r_{i.}/m_{i.}$, and $\hat{\mu}_{3i} = 1 - \hat{\mu}_{1i} - \hat{\mu}_{2i}$, respectively; and $v_{kki}$ $(k = 1,2,3)$ replaced by the corresponding sample variances

$$\hat{v}_{11i} = \frac{n_i}{(n_i - 1)m_{i.}} \sum_{j=1}^{n_i} (y_{ij} - m_{ij}\hat{\mu}_{1i})^2$$

$$\hat{v}_{22i} = \frac{n_i}{(n_i - 1)m_{i.}} \sum_{j=1}^{n_i} (r_{ij} - m_{ij}\hat{\mu}_{2i})^2$$

and

$$\hat{v}_{33i} = \frac{n_i}{(n_i - 1)mi_{.}} \sum_{j=1}^{n_i} (s_{ij} - y_{ij} - m_{ij}\hat{\mu}_{3i})^2$$

respectively. Other reasonable estimates of these quantities may also be used. Values of $\hat{D}_i$ less or greater than unity indicated overdispersion or underdispersion, respectively relative to multinomial variation.

With moderately large samples, the mean and covariance of the transformed data may be approximated by

$$E(\tilde{z}_{ij} | \tilde{m}_{ij}) = \tilde{m}_{ij}\mu_i + O(n_i^{-1/2})$$

and

$$\text{Var}(\tilde{z}_{ij} | \tilde{m}_{ij}) = \tilde{m}_{ij}[\text{diag}(\mu_i) - \mu_i\mu_i^T] + O(n_i^{-1/2})$$

respectively, which are similar in structure to those of the multinomial distribution. Therefore, methods based on trinomial distribution can be applied to the transformed data.

## B. Generalized Score Tests for Trend

Generalized score statistics can be derived in analogy to those for the incidence of fetal malformation (see Appendix C). Again, we assume that the response probabilities of prenatal death and fetal malformation are given by models of the form

$$\pi_k = F\left[a_k + b_k\eta(d, \gamma_k)\right]$$

$(k = 1,2)$ with the monotone transformations $\eta_k = \eta(\cdot, \gamma_k)$ for dose, and that the covariance function is of the form of Eq. (20). Partitioning the parameter vector $\theta$ into two sets $\theta = (\psi^T, \lambda^T)^T$, with $\psi = (b_1, b_2)^T$, and $\lambda = (a_1, a_2, \gamma_2, \gamma_2)^T$, the composite null hypothesis of no-dose effect can be expressed as

$$H_0 : \psi = (b_1, b_2)^T = (0, 0)^T \tag{23}$$

or equivalently

$$H_0 : \mu_{k1} = \cdots = \mu_{kt}; \quad (k = 1,2)$$

with the value of $\lambda$, and possibly the dispersion parameters involved in the covariance, unspecified.

To test the null hypothesis [Eq. (23)], we can use the generalized score statistics

$$
X_2 = \frac{\left[ \sum_{i=1}^{t} \sum_{j=1}^{n_i} h_{ij}(\eta_{1i} - \bar{\eta}_1)(y_{ij} - s_{ij}\pi_{10}) \right]^2}{\sum_{i=1}^{t} \sum_{j=1}^{n_i} h_{ij}m_{ij}(\eta_{1i} - \bar{\eta}_1)^2 \pi_{10}(1 - \pi_{10})(1 - \pi_{20})}
$$
$$
+ \frac{\left[ \sum_{i=1}^{t} \sum_{j=1}^{n_i} h_{ij}(\eta_{2i} - \bar{\eta}_2)(r_{ij} - m_{ij}\pi_{20}) \right]^2}{\sum_{i=1}^{t} \sum_{j=1}^{n_i} h_{ij}m_{ij}(\eta_{2i} - \bar{\eta}_2)^2 \pi_{20}(1 - \pi_{20})}
\tag{24}
$$

with

$$
\bar{\eta}_k = \frac{\sum_{i=1}^{t} \sum_{j=1}^{n_i} m_{ij}h_{ij}\eta_{ki}}{\sum_{i=1}^{t} \sum_{j=1}^{n_i} m_{ij}h_{ij}}
\tag{25}
$$

($k = 1,2$). All the nuisance parameters involved in the statistics are replaced by consistent estimates under the null hypothesis. For example, $\pi_{10}$ and $\pi_{20}$ are evaluated under the null hypothesis by

$$
\hat{\pi}_{10} = \frac{\sum_{i=1}^{t} \sum_{j=1}^{n_i} h_{ij}y_{ij}}{\sum_{i=1}^{t} \sum_{j=1}^{n_i} h_{ij}s_{ij}}
$$

and

$$
\hat{\pi}_{20} = \frac{\sum_{i=1}^{t} \sum_{j=1}^{n_i} h_{ij}r_{ij}}{\sum_{i=1}^{t} \sum_{j=1}^{n_i} h_{ij}m_{ij}}
$$

$\gamma_1$ and $\gamma_2$ involved in the transformations may be estimated by solving the equations

$$
\sum_{i=1}^{t} \sum_{j=1}^{n_i} h_{ij} \frac{\partial \eta_1}{\partial \gamma_1^T} (y_{ij} - s_{ij}\pi_{10}) = 0
$$

and

$$
\sum_{i=1}^{t} \sum_{j=1}^{n_i} h_{ij} \frac{\partial \eta_2}{\partial \gamma_2^T} (r_{ij} - m_{ij}\pi_{20}) = 0
$$

the dispersion parameters may be estimated by, for example, Pearson's $\chi^2$ statistics or by quadratic estimating equations (see Sec. III.C). Since the statistics [Eq. (24)] approximately follow the $\chi^2$ distribution with two degrees of freedom as $n_i \to \infty$ at comparable rates, large values of the statistics indicate a significant dose effect.

Similar to the generalized score statistics for fetal malformation, the statistics in Eq. (24) and their distribution under the null hypothesis are also free of $F(\cdot)$. The choice of $\eta_k$ generally has an impact on the power of these tests, although not on the type I error. Further research on the behavior of these statistics, especially under the alternative hypothesis, is useful. Note that the second term in Eq. (24) is exactly the square of the statistics in Eq. (11), as applied to the proportion of prenatal death. Moreover, the first term in Eq. (24) is similar to the square of Eq. (11) as applied to the proportion of fetal malformation, in that it can be obtained from Eq. (11) by substituting the expected number of live births $m_{ij}(1 - \pi_{20})$ for $s_{ij}$ in the denominator, and using $\eta_1$ as given in Eq. (25) instead of Eq. (12). This connection indicates that the score tests based on the trinomial counts of prenatal death and fetal malformation are more sensitive than tests conducted separately on death or malformation, especially when the dose effect is weak in one or both outcomes.

*1. Identity Transformation for Dose*

Under the identify transformation for dose, the statistics [Eq. (24)] reduce to

$$X_2 = \frac{1}{\sum_{i=1}^{t} \sum_{j=1}^{n_i} (d_i - \bar{d})^2 h_{ij} m_{ij}} \times \left[ \frac{\left\{ \sum_{i=1}^{t} \sum_{j=1}^{n_i} (d_i - \bar{d}) h_{ij} y_{ij} \right\}^2}{\hat{\mu}_{10}} \right.$$
$$\left. + \frac{\left\{ \sum_{i=1}^{t} \sum_{j=1}^{n_i} (d_i - \bar{d}) h_{ij} r_{ij} \right\}^2}{\hat{\mu}_{20}} + \frac{\left\{ \sum_{i=1}^{t} \sum_{j=1}^{n_i} (d_i - \bar{d}) h_{ij} (s_{ij} - y_{ij}) \right\}^2}{\hat{\mu}_{30}} \right]$$

and can be easily extended to the case of higher-dimensional categorical data. Various function can be chosen for $h$ to accommodate different types of variation. In particular, choosing $h = 1$ leads to a multinomial version of the Cochran–Armitage statistic, applicable to the transformed data after using the Rao–Scott transformation.

## C. Joint Dose–Response Modeling

Extending the discussion in Section II.C, we now describe joint dose–response modeling of the incidence of fetal malformation and prenatal death, using the Weibull models

$$\pi_k(d) = 1 - \exp\left\{ -(a_k + b_k d^{\gamma_k}) \right\}$$

($k = 1,2$). Given $\pi_1$ and $\pi_2$, overall toxicity is then measured by the probability

$$\pi_3(d) = 1 - \left\{ 1 - \pi_1(d) \right\} \left\{ 1 - \pi_2(d) \right\} \tag{26}$$

that an implant is either resorbed, dead, or led to a malformation.

*1. Model Fitting and GEEs*

Let $\theta_k = (a_k, b_k, \gamma_k)^T$ ($k = 1,2$). We set the working covariance matrix $\mathbf{W}_{1ij}$ equal to the extended Dirichlet-trinomial covariance in Eq. (20), with $h^{-1} = 1 + (m - 1)\phi$. The GEEs (see Appendix A) for estimating $\theta = (\theta_1^T, \theta_2^T)$ simplify to two separate sets of equations

$$\sum_{i=1}^{t} \sum_{j=1}^{n_i} \frac{1}{1+(m_{ij}-1)\phi_i} \frac{1}{\pi_{1i}(1-\pi_{1i})} \frac{\partial \pi_{1i}}{\partial \theta_1} (y_{ij}-s_{ij}\pi_{1i}) = 0 \qquad (27)$$

and

$$\sum_{i=1}^{t} \sum_{j=1}^{n_i} \frac{1}{1+(m_{ij}-1)\phi_i} \frac{1}{\pi_{2i}(1-\pi_{2i})} \frac{\partial \pi_{2i}}{\partial \theta_2} (r_{ij}-m_{ij}\pi_{2i}) = 0 \qquad (28)$$

involving $\theta_1$ and $\theta_2$ respectively.

To estimate the intralitter correlation coefficients $\{\phi_i\}$, we may use a set of quadratic equations

$$\sum_{j=1}^{n_i} \mathbf{D}_{2ij}^T \mathbf{W}_{2ij}^{-1}(Q_{ij}-\sigma_{ij}) = 0 \qquad (29)$$

$(i=1,\ldots,t)$, with

$$Q_{ij} = m_{ij}\{1+(m_{ij}-1)\phi_i\}\pi_{1i}(1-\pi_{1i})\pi_{2i}(1-\pi_{2i})(z_{ij}-m_{ij}\mu_i)^T \mathbf{W}_{1ij}^{-1}(z_{ij}-m_{ij}\mu_i),$$

$$\sigma_{ij} = \mathbf{E}(Q_{ij}) = 2m_{ij}\{1+(m_{ij}-1)\phi_i\}\pi_{1i}(1-\pi_{1i})\pi_{2i}(1-\pi_{2i})$$

and $D_{2ij} = \partial\sigma_{ij}/\partial\phi_i$. We also choose $\mathbf{W}_{2ij} = \sigma_{ij}^2$ for convenience, as the third and fourth moments of $z_{ij}$ are unknown. Note that the multivariate Pearson squared residuals $(z_{ij}-m_{ij}\mu_i)^T \mathbf{W}_{1ij}^{-1}$ $(z_{ij}-m_{ij}\mu_i)$ after fitting the Weibull models to data are treated as responses in the quadratic equations.

The parameter estimates $\hat{\theta}_1, \hat{\theta}_2$, and $\{\hat{\phi}_i\}$ are obtained by iteratively solving Eq. (27), (28), and (29), until convergence. At each iteration, Eqs. (27) and (28) are solved for $\theta_1$ and $\theta_2$, respectively, with $\{\phi_i\}$ fixed at $\{\hat{\phi}_i\}$; Eqs. (29) are solved for $\{\phi_i\}$, with $\theta_1$ and $\theta_2$ fixed at $\{\hat{\theta}_1\}$ and $\hat{\theta}_2$, respectively. For the transformed data $(\tilde{y}, \tilde{r})$ obtained using the Rao-Scott transformation, we simply set $\phi_i=0$ and solve just Eqs. (27) and (28) for $\theta_1$ and $\theta_2$, as the transformed data are approximated by the mean and covariance of the multinomial distribution.

To guard against misspecification of the covariance function $\mathrm{Var}(z_{ij}|m_{ij})$, appropriate sample moments may be used to obtain the *sandwich estimates* (Liang and Zeger, 1986; Moore and Tsiatis, 1991) for the variance and covariance of the parameter estimates. Namely, the variance estimates are given by

$$\mathbf{V}_{11} = \sum_{i=1}^{t} \sum_{j=1}^{n_i} m_{ij}^2 \mathbf{D}_{1i}^T \mathbf{W}_{1ij}^{-1}(z_{ij}-m_{ij}\mu_i)(z_{ij}-m_{ij}\mu_i)^T \mathbf{W}_{1ij}^{-1}\mathbf{D}_{1i}$$

and

$$\mathbf{V}_{22} = \mathrm{diag}\left( \sum_{j=1}^{n_i} \mathbf{D}_{2ij}^T \mathbf{W}_{2ij}^{-1}(Q_{ij}-\sigma_{ij})^2 \mathbf{W}_{2ij}^{-1}\mathbf{D}_{2ij}; \quad i=1,\ldots,t \right)$$

for $\hat{\theta}$ and $\{\hat{\phi}_i\}$, respectively, with the unknown parameters evaluated at $\hat{\theta}$ and $\{\hat{\phi}_i\}$.

## IV. APPLICATIONS

The generalized score tests and dose–response modeling techniques discussed in Section II and III can be illustrated by using both the mouse and rat data described in Section I.B.

## A. Trend Tests

Tests for trend in a single outcome (i.e., the incidence of prenatal death, the incidence of fetal malformation, or the incidence of overall toxicity) were considered. The observed statistics given in Table 3 were computed under three variance functions: the β-binomial variance $h_{ij}^{-1} = [1 + (s_{ij} - 1)\rho i]$ (BB); the generalized linear model variance $h_{ij}^{-1} = \sigma$ (GLM); and the binomial variance $h = 1$, after applying the Rao–Scott transformation (RS). Power transformations for the dose were used with the parameter γ either fixed at unity (the indentity transformation) or at the value obtained from fitting a Weibull model to data under the extended β-binomial variance. This is merely for the purpose of illustrating potential difference between using or not using a power transformation for the dose. Other nuisance parameters were all evaluated under the null hypothesis, and the dispersion parameters associated with the methods of BB and GLM were estimated by the quadratic equations and Pearson's $\chi^2$ statistic, respectively. It was assumed that the extent of overdispersion from one dose group to another is influenced only by the dose.

**Table 3** Generalized Score Statistics for Trend in the Binomial Proportions of Prenatal Death, Fetal Malformation, and Overall Toxicity

| Species | γ | Statistics[a,b] BB | GLM | RS |
|---|---|---|---|---|
| Fetal malformation | | | | |
| Mice | 2.97 | 7.46 | 8.26 | 5.76 |
| | 1.00 | 7.35 | 7.88 | 5.48 |
| Rats | 1.59 | 2.53 | 2.56 | 2.30 |
| | 1.00 | 2.38 | 2.41 | 2.16 |
| Prenatal death | | | | |
| Mice | 3.35 | 8.60 | 8.78 | 8.36 |
| | 1.00 | 8.48 | 8.52 | 8.10 |
| Rats | 19.67 | 8.07 | 8.02 | 7.95 |
| | 1.00 | 5.80 | 5.75 | 5.70 |
| Overall toxicity | | | | |
| Mice | 3.03 | 9.23 | 9.31 | 8.81 |
| | 1.00 | 9.52 | 9.51 | 9.00 |
| Rats | 11.55 | 8.12 | 8.08 | 7.99 |
| | 1.00 | 6.03 | 5.99 | 5.93 |

[a]All statistics follow the standard normal distribution.
[b]BB, β-binomial variance function; GLM, variance function of generalized linear model; RS, binomial variance applied to transformed data.

Therefore, the dispersion parameters would be identical for all dose groups under the null hypothesis. This led to the use of the pooled design effect (Rao and Scott, 1992).

$$\bar{D} = \frac{1}{t-1}\sum_{i=1}^{t}\left(1 - \frac{n_i}{n}\right)\frac{\hat{\pi}_i(1-\hat{\pi}_i)}{\hat{\pi}_0(1-\hat{\pi}_0)}\hat{D}_i$$

in the Rao–Scott transformation. Had the dose-specific design effects been used in the Rao–Scott transformation, the values of the score statistics would have been larger, indicating a gain in power for detecting the dose effect.

It is seen from Table 3 that for the mouse data, the observed values of the statistics under different variance functions are comparable for the incidences of prenatal death and overall toxicity, whether or not the power transformation was used. In the case of fetal malformation, however, the Rao–Scott transformation yielded statistics with values somewhat smaller than those of the other two methods.

For the incidences of prenatal death and overall toxicity in the rat data, the use of a power transformation under all three variance functions resulted in larger values of the statistics than without a transformation. This is mainly because DEHP had little effect on the incidences at lower dose levels, but markedly increased the incidences at the highest dose, resulting in a hockey stick type of dose–response relationship (Fig. 3). Therefore, incorporating a power transformation for the dose in the score statistics reflects such a dose effect, resulting in increased values of the statistics. We also note that the Z-scores indicate that the 3% increase in the fetal malformation rates from the control to the highest dose group is highly significant, implying a severe adverse effect of DEHP.

Multivariate score statistics for simultaneously testing trend in both the incidence of prenatal death and the incidence of malformation were also computed under the three covariance functions: the extended Dirichlet-trinomial (DT), the generalized linear models (GLM), and the multinomial covariance applied to the transformed data (RS). In the latter, a pooled design effect was used for all dose groups. The pooled design effect was obtained by substituting $\hat{\mu}_{k0}$ for $\hat{\mu}_{ki}$ in $\hat{D}_i$ and taking average of $\hat{D}_i$ using the weights $(1 - n_i/n.)$. It can be seen from Table 4 that for

**Table 4** Generalized Score Statistics for Trend in Trinomial Proportions of Prenatal Deaths and Fetal Malformations

| Species | $(\gamma_1, \gamma_2)$ | Statistics[a,b] | | |
|---------|------------------------|-----|-----|-----|
| | | DT | GLM | RS |
| Mice | (2.68, 3.16) | 122.97 | 125.25 | 111.32 |
| | (1.00, 1.00) | 126.61 | 126.91 | 112.80 |
| Rats | (2.92, 21.4) | 112.78 | 111.51 | 108.45 |
| | (1.00, 1.00) | 58.98 | 58.16 | 56.57 |

[a]All statistics follow a $\chi^2$-distribution with two degrees of freedom.
[b]DT, Direchlet-trinomial covariance function; GLM, covariance function of generalized linear model; RS, trinomial covariance applied to transformed data.

the rat data the statistics involving the power transformations yielded values approximately twice as large as those without the power transformations. Except for this difference, the observed statistics under the three covariance functions are comparable, suggesting comparable behavior of these statistics under the null hypothesis.

## B. Dose–Response Modeling

The Weibull dose–response models were both separately and jointly fitted to the incidences of prenatal death, fetal malformation, and overall toxicity, and the estimates of the model parameters based on GEEs are given in Table 5 and Table 6, respectively. The extended $\beta$-binomial variance function was used in separate modeling. For the rat data, the dose–response curves for the incidences of prenatal death, and overall toxicity exhibit the shape of a hockey stick, a common phenomenon seen in developmental toxicity data. Here, the estimates of the parameter $\gamma$ are usually accompanied by a large standard error. Since the rats in the second dose group had identically zero response rates in malformation, also a common phenomenon that may cause difficulties in analysis, this dose group was actually deleted to obtain convergence in model-fitting. Experience indicates that deletion of a dose group with zero response rates in malformation may be avoided by joint modeling of the incidences of death and malformation.

**Table 5** Estimates of the Parameters of the Weibull Models[a] Fitted to the Incidences of Death, Malformation, and Overall Toxicity Using GEEs with $\beta$-Binomial Variance (SE)

| Parameter | Mice | | | Rats | | |
|---|---|---|---|---|---|---|
| | Fetal malformation | Prenatal death | Overall toxicity | Fetal malformation | Prenatal death | Overall toxicity |
| $a$ | 0.014 | 0.104 | 0.126 | 0.012 | 0.046 | 0.053 |
| | (0.008) | (0.017) | (0.023) | (0.007) | (0.008) | (0.009) |
| $b$ | 2.179 | 1.933 | 3.887 | 0.029 | 0.794 | 0.818 |
| | (0.504) | (0.330) | (0.741) | (0.018) | (0.184) | (0.184) |
| $\gamma$ | 2.967 | 3.347 | 3.030 | 1.593 | 19.67 | 11.55 |
| | (0.448) | (0.518) | (0.419) | (1.975) | (19.25) | (2.245) |
| $\rho_1/\phi_1$ | 0.181 | 0.494 | 0.397 | −0.010 | −0.012 | 0.023 |
| | (0.117) | (0.174) | (0.128) | (0.010) | (0.022) | (0.041) |
| $\rho_2/\phi_2$ | −0.036 | −0.019 | −0.013 | [b] | −0.022 | −0.031 |
| | (0.009) | (0.018) | (0.016) | | (0.020) | (0.018) |
| $\rho_3/\phi_3$ | 0.240 | −0.013 | 0.106 | 0.022 | 0.063 | 0.089 |
| | (0.090) | (0.019) | (0.044) | (0.049) | (0.102) | (0.090) |
| $\rho_4/\phi_4$ | 0.275 | 0.446 | 0.417 | 0.003 | −0.013 | −0.030 |
| | (0.111) | (0.092) | (0.089) | (0.032) | (0.018) | (0.016) |
| $\rho_5/\phi_5$ | 0.299 | 0.409 | 0.277 | 0.006 | 0.603 | 0.564 |
| | (0.233) | (0.079) | (0.170) | (0.044) | (0.075) | (0.074) |

[a]Highest dose scaled to unity.
[b]Incidences of fetal malformation were all zero in the second dose group, and subsequently deleted to obtain convergence in model-fitting.

**Table 6** Estimates of the Parameters of the Trinomial Weibull Dose–Response Models Fitted to the Original (DT) and Transformed Data (RS)[a,b] (SE)

|  |  | Mice | | Rats | |
|---|---|---|---|---|---|
| Parameter |  | DT | RS | DT | RS[b] |
| Fetal malformation | $a_1$ | 0.011 (0.010) | 0.014 (0.009) | 0.002 (0.003) | 0.005 (0.003) |
|  | $b_1$ | 1.832 (0.524) | 1.868 (0.532) | 0.065 (0.037) | 0.064 (0.041) |
|  | $\gamma_1$ | 2.675 (0.421) | 2.675 (0.395) | 2.918 (1.993) | 3.119 (2.194) |
| Prenatal death | $a_2$ | 0.106 (0.017) | 0.116 (0.017) | 0.047 (0.008) | 0.046 (0.007) |
|  | $b_2$ | 1.888 (0.281) | 1.813 (0.278) | 0.794 (0.138) | 0.796 (0.149) |
|  | $\gamma_2$ | 3.162 (0.518) | 3.345 (0.572) | 21.38 (32.71) | 19.95 (20.69) |
| Intralitter correlation | $\phi_1$ | 0.368 (0.171) |  | 0.222 (0.130) |  |
|  | $\phi_2$ | −0.027 (0.011) |  | −0.055 (0.023) |  |
|  | $\phi_3$ | 0.083 (0.029) |  | 0.100 (0.068) |  |
|  | $\phi_4$ | 0.298 (0.061) |  | −0.005 (0.018) |  |
|  | $\phi_5$ | 0.283 (0.072) |  | 0.287 (0.115) |  |

[a]Highest dose scaled to unity.
[b]DT denotes estimates based on GEEs with the extended Dirichlet-trinomial covariance; RS denotes estimates based on GEEs with multinomial covariance function after applying the transformation to data.

Joint modeling of the incidences of fetal malformation and prenatal death was performed on both the original data, with an extended Dirichlet-trinomial covariance function (DT), and on the transformed data after applying the Rao–Scott transformation (RS). In the latter case, the estimated design effects, $\hat{D}_i$ ($i = 1, 2, 3, 4, 5$), are 3.29, 0.84, 1.64, 4.71, and 4.37 for the mouse data, and 0.95, 0.46, 1.49, 0.93, and 4.38 for the rat data. It is seen from Table 6 that the estimates of the parameters obtained by these two methods are comparable, as are the associated standard errors.

The fitted models are shown in Figs. 2 and 3 for the mouse and rat data, respectively. Here,

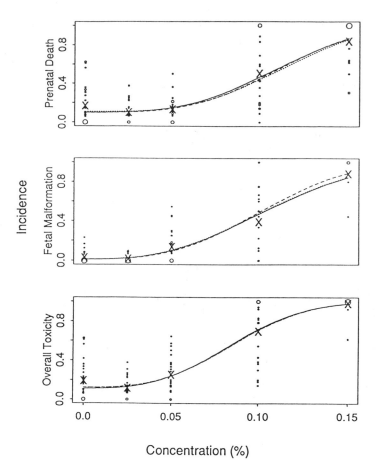

**Figure 2** Dose–response models for the incidence of prenatal death, fetal malformation, and overall toxicity in mice exposed to DEHP. Dotted lines denote models fitted to the transformed data; solid lines denote models fitted to the original data under the extended Dirichlet-multinomial covariance; dashed lines denote models fitted separately to a single outcome under the β-binomial variance. Circles denote observed response rates per litter with radii proportional to the cube-root of the number of identical observations. An "×" denotes the weighted average response rate within the same dose group.

the solid and dotted lines represent the models fitted using DT and RS methods, respectively. Models fitted separately to each of the three outcomes based on the extended β-binomial variance are represented by dashed lines. Each circle represents a number of identical proportions observed in individual litters, with the radius of the circle being proportional to the number of litters represented. An × denotes average response rate in a single dose group. The Weibull models with both the DT and RS methods appear to fit the data reasonably well. The model separately fitted to the incidence of fetal malformation in rats appears to be influenced by the removal of the second dose group.

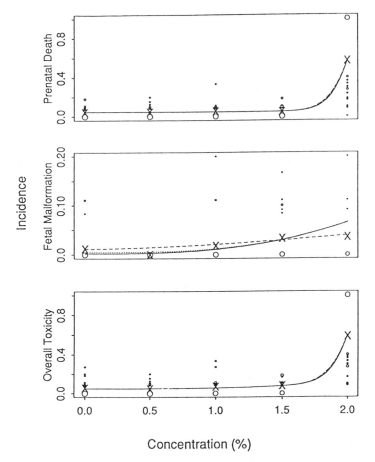

**Figure 3** Dose–response models for the incidence of prenatal death, fetal malformation, and overall toxicity in rats exposed to DEHP. Dotted lines denote models fitted to the transformed data; solid lines denote models fitted to the original data under the extended Dirichlet-multinomial covariance; dashed lines denote models fitted separately to a single outcome under the β-binomial variance. Circles denote observed response rates per litter with radii proportional to the cube-root of the number of identical observations. An "×" dnotes the weighted average response rate within the same dose group.

## V. JOINT MODELING OF DEATH, WEIGHT, AND MALFORMATION

We have discussed the joint analyses of the incidences of prenatal death and fetal malformation. Other multivariate methods have also been proposed in the literature for analyzing, for example, the data on prenatal death, fetal weight, and malformation. Lefkopoulou et al. (1989) used quasi-likelihood method in conjunction with logistic models to jointly analyze data on multiple fetal malformations. Ryan et al. (1991) explored the correlation between the outcomes of fetal weight and fetal malformation. Catalano and Ryan (1992) suggested a probit model for fetal malformation, conditional on observed fetal weight, in conjunction with a normal regression model for fetal weight. More recently, Catalano et al. (1993) proposed multistage dose–response models to include the incidence of prenatal death in the analysis of fetal weight and malformation. In this section, we briefly describe these multivariate methods.

## A.  Fetal Weight and Malformation

Although biological mechanisms inducing multiple outcomes of developmental toxicity are not well known, there has been empirical evidence showing that malformed fetuses tend to be lighter than nonmalformed fetus (Ryan et al., 1991). This correlation between the fetal weight and malformation status of an individual fetus suggests a joint analysis of these two endpoints. For this purpose, consider the model

$$\mathbf{P}(w_{ijk},y_{ijk}\,|\,s_{ij}) \;=\; \mathbf{P}(w_{ijk}\,|\,s_{ij})\mathbf{P}(y_{ijk}\,|\,w_{ijk},s_{ij}) \tag{30}$$

where $w_{ijk}$ is the weight of the $k$th fetus in the $ij$th litter ($k = 1, \ldots, s_{ij}$), and $y_{ijk} = 1$ or $0$, indicating whether or not the fetus is malformed. The conditional model $\mathbf{P}(w_{ijk}\,|\,s_{ij})$ implies that the fetal weights are correlated among littermates and may also depend on the litter size $s_{ij}$. Similarly, the model $\mathbf{P}(y_{ijk}\,|\,w_{ij},s_{ij})$ indicates that the malformation status of an individual fetus may be mathematically related to its weight and the litter size.

To use the method of GEE for dose–response modeling, the mean and variance functions are specified for the distributions $\mathbf{P}(w_{ijk}\,|\,s_{ij})$ and $\mathbf{P}(y_{ijk}\,|\,w_{ij},s_{ij})$, incorporating reasonable correlation structures between multiple responses on the same fetus, and also between littermates. The factorization in Eq. (30) suggests that a dose–response model should first be fit to the fetal weight $w_{ijk}$ using both dose and litter size as covariates, and a second model then fit to the malformation indicator variables $y_{ijk}$, conditional on the model for the fetal weight, and using dose, fetal weight, possibly litter size as covariates. A power transformation for the dose is generally useful for this purpose. An apparent advantage of the GEE approach here is that it circumvents the difficulty in specifying a joint distribution for the continuous response of fetal weight, and the dichotomous response of malformation status.

The latent variable method was used by Catalano and Ryan (1992) in which it is assumed that a fetus becomes malformed if an underlying, but unobservable, latent variable exceeds a threshold. Moreover, the latent variable and the fetal weight are assumed to follow a bivariate normal distribution. This leads to a normal regression model for the fetal weight and a probit model

$$E(y_{ijk}\,|\,w_{ijk},s_{ij}) \;=\; \Phi(\mu_{ijk})$$

for the malformation indicator $y_{ijk}$. Here, $\Phi(\cdot)$ is the standard normal cumulative distribution function, and $\mu_{ijk}$ is a linear function of the dose $d_i$, fetal weight $w_{ijk}$, and possibly also the litter size $s_{ij}$. The coefficients of this linear function turns out to depend on the underlying variance and covariance structure postulated on the bivariate normal distribution, although the parameters involved in this variance–covariance function are not all estimable. In the probit model used by Catalano and Ryan (1992), the residuals from the regression model fitted to the fetal weight was actually used as a covariate, and the interaction term of litter size and fetal weight (residual) was also included in the model. A similar approach was taken by Chen (1993b) who relied on the method of quasi-likelihood, and used a linear logistic dose–response model to describe the response probability of malformation. However, the examples used by these authors failed to provide evidences supporting a significant correlation between the incidence of fetal malformation and the litter size in the form of regression coefficient. The effectiveness of using litter size as a covariate to predict fetal malformation remains unclear here.

## B. Prenatal Death, Fetal Weight, and Malformation

The approach described in the preceding section can be extended to include the incidence of prenatal death in the analysis on the basis of the model in Eq. (1). Specifically, a dose–response model can be first fit to the proportion of prenatal death on the basis of $\mathbf{P}(r_{ij}|m_{ij})$. The fetal weight and the incidence of fetal malformation can then be analyzed as described in Section V.A. This approach was introduced by Catalano et al. (1993) to conduct risk assessment.

## VI. BENCHMARK DOSE FOR RISK ASSESSMENT

At present, human exposure guidelines for developmental toxicants are based on the no-observed adverse effect level (NOAEL) derived from laboratory studies. A *NOAEL* is defined as the highest experimental dose that fails to induce a significant increase in risk in comparison with the unexposed controls. A reference dose or reference concentration (RfD or RfC) is then obtained by dividing the NOAEL by a suitable uncertainty factor (UF) allowing for difference in susceptibility between animals and humans. The resulting RfD is then used as a guideline for human exposure. Guidelines on the magnitude of the UF to be used in specific cases were discussed by Barnes and Dourson (1988).

The NOAEL, restricted in value to one of the experimental doses, fails to properly take sample size into account (smaller and less sensitive experiments lead to higher NOAELs than larger studies), and largely ignores the shape of the dose–response curve. The risk associated with doses at or above the NOAEL is not made explicit. However, Gaylor (1992) has shown, for a series of 120 developmental toxicity experiments, that the observed risk exceeded 1% in about one-fourth of the cases. Leisenring and Ryan (1992) also found, based on the statistical properties of the NOAELs, that the NOAEL may identify a dose level associated with unacceptably high risk with a reasonably high probability. Because of the limitations associated with the use of the NOAEL (Gaylor, 1983, 1989; Kimmel and Gaylor, 1988), the EPA (1991) is considering the use of the benchmark dose (BMD) method, proposed by Crump (1984), as the basis for deriving the RfD for developmental toxicity.

The BMD is generally defined as the lower confidence limit (Crump, 1984) of the effective dose, $d_\alpha$, that induces $\alpha$-percent increase in risk (ED$_\alpha$). Although the $\alpha$-percent increase in risk may refer to the excessive risk $\pi(d_\alpha) - \pi(0) = \alpha$, or relative risk $[\pi(d_\alpha) - \pi(0)]/[1 - \pi(0)] = \alpha$, the latter takes into account the background risk in the absence of exposure, and is more sensitive to high spontaneous risk. If the background risk is $\pi(0) = 0$, then the two measures of risk are equivalent. It can be shown that the relative risk also has additional mathematical properties that facilitate computation and interpretation. The ED$_\alpha$ may be defined as the solution to the equation

$$\frac{\pi(d_\alpha) - \pi(0)}{1 - \pi(0)} = \alpha$$

where $\pi(d)$ represents an appropriate dose–response model for a particular endpoint. Crump (1984) and Chen and Kodell (1989) discussed the estimation of BMD based on dose–response model for a single endpoint. Allen et al. (1994a,b) estimated the BMDs using several dose–response models fitted to data from a large database. They found that the BMDs at 5% level are similar to NOAEL in magnitude on the average. Ryan (1992) and Krewski and Zhu (1994, 1995) used joint dose–response models to estimate the BMDs.

Under the Weibull models [Eq. (14)] for either the incidence of prenatal death or the incidence of fetal malformation, the ED$_\alpha$ is given by

$$d_\alpha = \left( \frac{-\log(1-\alpha)}{b} \right)^{1/\gamma} \tag{31}$$

where the subscript $k$ ($k = 1,2$) for the parameters $(b_k, \gamma_k)$ is suppressed for simplicity of notation. Note that the $d_\alpha$ is free of the parameter $a$ associated with the spontaneous risk. An estimate $\hat{d}_\alpha$ is obtained by evaluating Eq. (31) at $(\hat{b}, \hat{\gamma})$. The variance of $\hat{d}_\alpha$ can be approximated by

$$\text{Var}(\hat{d}_\alpha) = \gamma^{-2} d_\alpha^2 C_1^T \Omega_1 C_1 \tag{32}$$

using the $\delta$-method, with the unknown parameters involved replaced by $(\hat{b}, \hat{\gamma})$. Here, $\Omega_1$ is the covariance matrix for the estimates $(\hat{b}, \hat{\gamma})^T$ and

$$C_1 = \left( b^{-1}, \gamma^{-1} \log\{ -b^{-1} \log(1-\alpha) \} \right)^T$$

The $\text{ED}_\alpha$ for overall toxicity, based on the trinomial model $\pi_3 = 1 - (1 - \pi_1)(1 - \pi_2)$ in Eq. (26), is obtained as the solution to the equation

$$b_1 d_\alpha^{\gamma_1} + b_2 d_\alpha^{\gamma_2} = -\log(1-\alpha)$$

The variance of $\hat{d}_\alpha$ based on the $\delta$-method is given by

$$\text{Var}(\hat{d}_\alpha) = \left[ b_1 \gamma_1 d_\alpha^{\gamma_1 - 1} + b_2 \gamma_2 d_\alpha^{\gamma_2 - 1} \right]^{-2} C_2^T \Omega_2 C_2, \tag{33}$$

where $\Omega_2$ is the covariance matrix of the estimates $(\hat{b}_1, \hat{\gamma}_1, \hat{b}_2, \hat{\gamma}_2)^T$ and

$$C_2 = (d_\alpha^{\gamma_1}, b_1 d_\alpha^{\gamma_1} \log d_\alpha, d_\alpha^{\gamma_2}, b_2 d_\alpha^{\gamma_2} \log d_\alpha)^T$$

Since the variance estimates based on the $\delta$-method depend on the dose–response models and the estimates of the unknown parameters, alternative methods, such as those based on likelihood ratio (Chen and Kodell, 1989) for obtaining confidence limits of $\text{ED}_\alpha$ may be used.

The $\text{ED}_\alpha$ for overall toxicity dervied from the multivariate model $\pi_3 = 1 - (1 - \pi_1)(1 - \pi_2)$ is a more sensitive indicator of developmental toxicity than those for fetal malformation and prenatal death, in that the former is always below the minimum of the latter two (Ryan, 1992; Krewski and Zhu, 1994). In the absence of a strong dose–response relationship for one of the latter two endpoints, the $\text{ED}_\alpha$ for overall toxicity approximates their minimum. The estimates of the $\text{ED}_\alpha$ for overall toxicity-based multivariate dose–response models for the prenatal death rate $r/m$ and fetal malformation rate $y/s$ are generally expected to be more efficient than estimates based on the univariate models for the combined rate $(y + r)/m$ (Ryan, 1992). In general, risk assessment that is based on multivariate dose–response models is preferred on the ground that it can simultaneously account for each individual source of risk.

Estimates of $\text{ED}_{05}$s, along with their standard errors, for the three endpoints of interest based on three different estimation methods are given in Table 7. In these examples, the estimates, based on GEEs in conjunction with the extended Dirichlet-trinomial covariance (DT) or the Rao–Scott transformation (RS), are quite comparable. On the other hand, the estimates of $\text{ED}_{05}$ associated with the models separately fitted to an endpoint (BB) on rats are different from those associated with the methods of DT or RS. For example, the standard error of the $\text{ED}_{05}$ for overall toxicity is considerably smaller than its counterparts associated with multivariate models. But this is mainly due to the large estimate of $\gamma$ (11.55) involved in $C_1$ subsequently used to calculate the standard error. In addition, the $\text{ED}_{05}$ for the malformation rate is apparently influenced by the deletion of the second dose group, resulting in an inflated estimate.

**Table 7** Estimates of $ED_{05}$ (% in diet) of DEHP Based on the Binomial Weibull Models (BB) Separately Fitted to the Incidences of Death, Malformation, and Overall Toxicity, and Based on the Trinomial Weibull Models Fitted to the Original (DT) and Transformed (RS) Data[a]

| | Mice | | | Rats | | |
|---|---|---|---|---|---|---|
| Method[a] | Prenatal death | Fetal malformation | Overall toxicity | Prenatal death | Fetal malformation | Overall toxicity |
| BB | 0.051 | 0.042 | 0.036 | 1.740 | 2.890[b] | 1.573 |
| | (0.008) | (0.006) | (0.006) | (0.238) | (2.182) | (0.070) |
| DT | 0.048 | 0.039 | 0.034 | 1.759 | 1.842 | 1.655 |
| | (0.008) | (0.006) | (0.005) | (0.346) | (0.281) | (0.355) |
| RS | 0.052 | 0.039 | 0.035 | 1.743 | 1.867 | 1.647 |
| | (0.009) | (0.005) | (0.004) | (0.249) | (0.317) | (0.255) |

[a]BB, estimates based on GEEs with the extended β-binomial variance; DT, estimates based on GEEs with the extended Dirichlet-trinomial covariance; RS, estimates based on GEEs with multinomial covariance after transformation.
[b]Incidences were all zero in the second dose group, and subsequently deleted to obtain convergence in model-fitting.

## VII.  CONCLUSIONS

We have discussed generalized score tests for trend and dose–response modeling of multiple outcomes from developmental toxicity experiments. Conditional on the number of implants per litter, joint analyses of several outcomes are numerically more stable and statistically more efficient than separate analysis of a single outcome. The extramultinomial variation induced by the litter effects may be characterized using a parametric covariance function, such as the extended Dirichlet-multinomial covariance. Alternatively, the Rao–Scott transformation, based on the concept of generalized design effects, may be used to allow for the approximation of the multinomial mean and covariance functions to the transformed data. Simple dose–response models, the Weibull model, for example, in conjunction with a power transformation for the dose can be used to describe the dose–response relationship in developmental toxicity data.

The method of GEE has been employed for model fitting. The GEEs are not only flexible in distributional assumptions, but also computationally simpler than the maximum likelihood estimation based, for example, on the Dirichlet-multinomial distribution. The GEE estimates of the model parameter are nearly as efficient as the maximum likelihood estimates, although estimates of the dispersion parameters that are based on the quadratic estimating equations are less efficient.

Generalized score functions after local orthogonalization can be used to construct a rich class of statistics for testing increasing trends in developmental toxicity data. These generalized score functions unify many of the specific statistics previously proposed in the literature. Further investigation on the behavior of these generalized score tests under various conditions would be useful.

Joint dose–response models can be directly applied to estimate the benchmark doses in risk assessment for developmental toxicity. The BMD is currently receiving serious consideration as an alternative to the NOAEL/UF approach to establishing reference doses. The BMD, based on a multivariate dose–response model for multiple endpoints, has the advantage that it simultaneously takes into account different sources of risk. For example, the BMD for overall toxicity is a more sensitive measure of risk in that it is less than or equal to the minimum of the BMDs for fetal malformation or prenatal death.

Quantitative risk assessment is a relatively new area, and there are many open problems requiring further research. For example, biologically based dose–response models are largely unavailable. Dose–response models for continuous responses are less well developed, although some effort has been reported by Gaylor and Slikker (1990) and Slikker and Gaylor (1990) in risk assessment for neurotoxicity. The use of BMDs requires that the experimental data demonstrate clear dose–response relationships so that suitable models may be fit to the data with reasonable accuracy. This in turn requires that the current study protocol be improved so that high-quality data can be generated from a study. Therefore, it is desirable to incorporate statistical design criteria into the protocol of developmental toxicity study.

## APPENDIX A: GENERALIZED ESTIMATING EQUATIONS

By letting $E(z_{ij}|m_{ij}) = m_{ij}\mu_i$, with $\mu_i = \mu(d_i;\theta) = (\mu_{1i},\mu_{2i})^T$ specified as functions of dose and involving unknown parameters $\theta$, the GEEs for estimating $\theta$ are given by

$$\sum_{i=1}^{t} \sum_{j=1}^{n_i} m_{ij}\mathbf{D}_{1i}^T\mathbf{W}_{1ij}^{-1}(z_{ij} - m_{ij}\mu_i) = 0 \tag{34}$$

where $\mathbf{D}_{1i} = \partial\mu_i/\partial\theta^T$ and $\mathbf{W}_{1ij}$ are *working covariance* or weight matrices, preferably chosen to approximate the actual covariance matrix $\text{Var}(z_{ij}|m_{ij})$ to achieve high efficiency.

When the working covariance matrices [see Eq. (20)] involve additional dispersion parameters, these parameters need to be estimated using another set of equations. Consider, for example, the intralitter correlation coefficients $\{\phi_i\}$ in the extended Dirichlet-miltinomial covariance. By regarding the multivariate Pearson squared residuals $R_{ij} = (z_{ij} - m_{ij}\mu_{ij})^T\mathbf{W}_{1ij}^{-1}(z_{ij} - m_{ij}\mu_i)$ as responses, the GEEs for estimating the dispersion parameters are given by

$$\sum_{j=1}^{n_i} \mathbf{D}_{2ij}^T\mathbf{W}_{2ij}^{-1}(R_{ij} - 2) = 0$$

$(i = 1, \ldots, t)$, where $\mathbf{D}_{2ij} = \partial(\text{E}R_{ij})/\partial\phi_i$, and a reasonable quantity $\mathbf{W}_{2ij}$ may be taken to approximate $\text{Var}(R_{ij})$. We have chosen in Section III.C $\mathbf{W}_{2ij} = (\text{E}R_{ij})^2$ for convenience as the third and fourth moments of $z_{ij}$ are unknown. The usual Pearson moment equations are obtained by choosing appropriate $\mathbf{W}_{2ij}$. The use of the quadratic estimating equations of the form of Eq. (29) is equivalent to generalized least squares estimation when the weights $\mathbf{W}_{2ij}$ are evaluated at a fixed value of $\phi_i$. They can be viewed as a multivariate version of a class of regression equations based on absolute residuals (Davidian and Carroll, 1987, Eq. 4.1). Joint estimation of the mean and correlation parameters based on GEEs has also been discussed by Zhao and Prentice (1990) and Prentice and Zhao (1991).

Under mild regularity conditions, estimators of the unknown model parameters using the GEEs in Eqs. (27)–(29) are consistent and normally distributed as each $n_i \to \infty$ at comparable rates (cf, Zhu et al., 1994). The covariance matrix of $(\hat{\theta}^T,\hat{\phi}_1, \ldots, \hat{\phi}_t)^T$ may be estimated by

$$\begin{pmatrix} \Delta_{11} & 0 \\ \Delta_{21} & \Delta_{22} \end{pmatrix}^{-1} \begin{pmatrix} \mathbf{V}_{11} & \mathbf{V}_{12} \\ \mathbf{V}_{21} & \mathbf{V}_{22} \end{pmatrix} \begin{pmatrix} \Delta_{11} & 0 \\ \Delta_{21} & \Delta_{22} \end{pmatrix}^{-T}$$

where

$$\Delta_{11} = \sum_{i=1}^{t} \sum_{j=1}^{n_i} m_{ij}^2 \mathbf{D}_{1i}^T \mathbf{W}_{1ij}^{-1} \mathbf{D}_{1i},$$

$$\Delta_{21} = \begin{pmatrix} \sum_{j=1}^{n_i} \mathbf{D}_{21j}^T \mathbf{W}_{21j}^{-1} \delta_{1j} \\ \vdots \\ \sum_{j=1}^{n_t} \mathbf{D}_{2tj}^T \mathbf{W}_{2tj}^{-1} \delta_{tj} \end{pmatrix}$$

and

$$\Delta_{22} = \text{diag} \left( \sum_{j=1}^{n_i} \mathbf{D}_{2ij}^T \mathbf{W}_{2ij}^{-1} \mathbf{D}_{2ij}; \quad i = 1, \dots, t \right)$$

with $\delta_{ij} = -\text{E}[\partial(R_{ij} - 2)/\partial\theta^T]$. In addition to the matrices $\mathbf{V}_{11}$ and $\mathbf{V}_{22}$ given in Section III.C, we have

$$\mathbf{V}_{12} = \begin{pmatrix} \sum_{j=1}^{n_i} m_{ij} \mathbf{D}_{11}^T \mathbf{W}_{11j}^{-1} (z_{1j} - m_{1j}\mu_1)(R_{1j} - 2) \mathbf{W}_{21j}^{-1} \mathbf{D}_{21j} \\ \vdots \\ \sum_{j=1}^{n_t} m_{ij} \mathbf{D}_{1t}^T \mathbf{W}_{1tj}^{-1} (z_{tj} - m_{tj}\mu_t)(R_{tj} - 2) \mathbf{W}_{2tj}^{-1} \mathbf{D}_{2tj} \end{pmatrix}$$

Under the Dirichlet-trinomial covariance function with the observed moments in $\mathbf{V}_{11}$ replaced by their expectation, we have $\Delta_{11} = \mathbf{V}_{11}$. Therefore, the asymptotic covariance matrix for $\hat{\theta}$ reduces to $\Delta_{11}^{-1}$, which is block-diagonal with the two diagonal blocks corresponding to $\hat{\theta}_1$ and $\hat{\theta}_2$. This implies that $\hat{\theta}_1$ and $\hat{\theta}_2$ are asymptotically independent, a result also seen from the fact that the two sets of Eqs. (27) and (28) are uncorrelated. Since the dispersion parameters $\{\phi_i\}$ are involved only in the weight matrices $\mathbf{W}_{1ij}$, estimation of the $\{\phi_i\}$ affects only the efficiency of $\hat{\theta}_1$ and $\hat{\theta}_2$.

## APPENDIX B: RAO–SCOTT TRANSFORMATION

Suppose that the response probabilities $\mu_i = (\mu_{1i}, \mu_{2i})^T$ of fetuses from the $j$th litter in the $i$th dose group are constant within the dose group, and the expected number of deaths and malformed fetuses are given by

$$E(\mathbf{z}_{ij} | m_{ij}) = m_{ij}(\mu_{1i}, \mu_{2i})^T$$

For the total counts $\mathbf{z}_{i\cdot} = \sum_{j=1}^{n_i} z_{ij} = (y_{i\cdot}, r_{i\cdot})^T$ and $m_{i\cdot} = \sum_{j=1}^{n_i} m_{ij}$ within the same dose group, we write

$$\text{Var}(\mathbf{z}_{i\cdot}) = \sum_{j=1}^{n_i} m_{ij}\mathbf{V}_{ij} = m_{i\cdot}\mathbf{V}_i$$

where the dependence of $\mathbf{V}_i$ on $m_{ij}$ is suppressed for notational simplicity. In the case of the multinomial covariance function, $\mathbf{V}_i$ reduces to

$$\mathbf{V}_0(\mu_i) = \text{diag}(\mu_i) - \mu_i\mu_i^T$$

The Pearson $\chi^2$ statistic for the $i$th dose group, regardless of the true covariance function, can be written as

$$\begin{aligned}
X_i^2 &= \frac{(y_{i\cdot} - m_{i\cdot}\mu_{1i})^2}{m_{i\cdot}\mu_{1i}} + \frac{(r_{i\cdot} - m_{i\cdot}\mu_{2i})^2}{m_{i\cdot}\mu_{2i}} + \frac{(s_{i\cdot} - r_{i\cdot} - m_{i\cdot}\mu_{3i})^2}{m_{i\cdot}\mu_{3i}} \\
&= m_{i\cdot}(\hat{\mu}_i - \mu_i)^T\left[\mathbf{V}_0(\mu_i)\right]^{-1}(\hat{\mu}_i - \mu_i)
\end{aligned} \tag{35}$$

where $\mu_{3i} = 1 - \mu_{1i} - \mu_{2i}$ and $\hat{\mu}_i = \mathbf{z}_{i\cdot}/m_{i\cdot}$. Under the true value of $\mu_i$ and the true covariance matrix $m_{i\cdot}\mathbf{V}_i$, the limiting distribution of the $\chi^2$ statistic as $n_i$ tends large is

$$X_i^2 = \lambda_{i1}Z_1^2 + \lambda_{i2}Z_2^2 + O_p(n_i^{-1/2}), \tag{36}$$

a weighted sum of two independent $\chi^2$ variables $Z_k^2$ ($k = 1,2$), each having one degree of freedom, and with weights $\lambda_k > 0$ being the eigenvalues of $[\mathbf{V}_0(\mu_i)]^{-1}\mathbf{V}_i$. These eigenvalues have been called *generalized design effects* by Rao and Scott (1981), and represent a multivariate ratio of $\mathbf{V}_i$ to $\mathbf{V}_0(\mu_i)$.

After dividing $X_i^2$ by the average design effects $\overline{D}_i = (\lambda_{i1} + \lambda_{i2})/2$, we have

$$E(X_i^2/\overline{D}_i) \approx E(\chi_2^2) = 2$$

If the $\lambda_{ik}$ ($k = 1,2$) differ only slightly, we have

$$\text{Var}(X_i^2/\overline{D}_i) \approx 4(1 + \rho^2) \approx \text{Var}(\chi_2^2),$$

where $\rho = (\lambda_{i1} - \lambda_{i2})/(\lambda_{i1} + \lambda_{i2})$ is the coefficient of variation for the $\lambda_{ik}$. If the $\lambda_{ik}$ are identical in limit as $n_i \to \infty$, as when $\text{Var}(z_{ij}) = m_{ij}h_{ij}^{-1}\mathbf{V}_0(\mu_i)$ with $h_{ij}$ being a positive, real-valued function, we have

$$X_i^2/\overline{D}_i = \chi_2^2 + O_p(n_i^{-1/2}) \tag{37}$$

Since scaling $X_i^2$ by $\overline{D}_i$ is equivalent to scaling $z_{ij}$ and $m_{ij}$, Eq. (37) implies the mean and covariance functions of the transformed data can be approximated by those of the multinomial distribution.

## APPENDIX C: GENERALIZED SCORE TESTS

The generalized score statistics discussed here may be viewed as a sort of combination of the quasi-score functions, generalized estimating equations, and the $C(\alpha)$ tests. Related idea was discussed by Basawa (1991). The $C(\alpha)$ tests, based on the binomial distribution with the class of dose–response models $F(a + bd)$, was discussed by Tarone and Gart (1980).

Assuming $E(\mathbf{z}_{ij}|m_{ij}) = m_{ij}\mu_i(\theta)$ and $\mathbf{Cov}(z_{ij}|m_{ij}) = \mathbf{V}_{ij}$ with $\theta = (\psi^T, \lambda^T)^T$, the generalized score functions (GSFs) for the parameters $\psi$ and $\lambda$ are given by

$$\mathbf{g}_\psi = \sum_{i=1}^{t} \sum_{j=1}^{n_i} m_{ij} \mathbf{D}_{i\psi}^T \mathbf{V}_{ij}^{-1} (\mathbf{z}_{ij} - m_{ij}\mu_i) \tag{38}$$

and

$$\mathbf{g}_\lambda = \sum_{i=1}^{t} \sum_{j=1}^{n_i} m_{ij} \mathbf{D}_{i\lambda}^T \mathbf{V}_{ij}^{-1} (z_{ij} - m_{ij}\mu_i) \tag{39}$$

respectively, where $\mathbf{D}_{\psi i} = \partial\mu_i/\partial\psi^T$ and $\mathbf{D}_{\lambda i} = \partial\mu_i/\partial\lambda^T$. Since $\mathbf{g}_\psi$ and $\mathbf{g}_\lambda$ are correlated and may involve the entire parameter vector $\theta$, $\mathbf{g}_\psi$ may be locally orthogonalized with respect to $\mathbf{g}_\lambda$ in the sense of Cox and Reid (1987). Specifically, the locally orthogonalized GSFs for $\psi$ are given by

$$\mathbf{g}_{\psi\cdot\lambda} = \mathbf{g}_\psi - \Sigma_{\psi\lambda}\Sigma_{\lambda\lambda}^{-1}\mathbf{g}_\lambda = \sum_{i=1}^{t} \sum_{j=1}^{n_i} m_{ij}\mathbf{D}_{\psi\cdot\lambda i}^T \mathbf{W}_{ij}^{-1}(z_{ij} - m_{ij}\mu_i) \tag{40}$$

where $\Sigma_{\psi\lambda} = \text{Cov}(\mathbf{g}_\psi, \mathbf{g}_\lambda)$, $\Sigma_{\lambda\lambda} = \text{Cov}(\mathbf{g}_\lambda, \mathbf{g}_\lambda)$ and

$$\mathbf{D}_{\psi\cdot\lambda i}^T = \mathbf{D}_{\psi i}^T - \Sigma_{\psi\lambda}\Sigma_{\lambda\lambda}^{-1}\mathbf{D}_{\lambda i}^T$$

Notice that $\mathbf{D}_{\psi\cdot\lambda i}$ is effectively the residual design matrix after projecting $\mathbf{D}_{\psi i}$ onto the linear space spanned by the row vectors of $\mathbf{D}_{\lambda i}$.

The generalized score statistic is then given by

$$T_p = \mathbf{g}_{\psi\cdot\lambda}^T \Sigma_{\psi\cdot\lambda}^{-1} \mathbf{g}_{\psi\cdot\lambda} \tag{41}$$

evaluated under $H_0$, where

$$\Sigma_{\psi\cdot\lambda} = \text{Cov}(\mathbf{g}_{\psi\cdot\lambda}, \mathbf{g}_{\psi\cdot\lambda}) = \Sigma_{\psi\psi} - \Sigma_{\psi\lambda}\Sigma_{\lambda\lambda}^{-1}\Sigma_{\lambda\psi}$$

The unspecified value of $\lambda$ may be replaced by any $\sqrt{n}$-consistent estimate $\hat{\lambda}$, the GEE estimates for example. Under the null hypothesis $H_0$,

$$T_p = \chi_p^2 + O_p(n^{-1/2})$$

$(n = n_1 + \cdots + n_t)$, where $\chi_p^2$ is a chi-squared variate with degrees of freedom $p = \dim(\psi)$. Large values of $T$ lead to the rejection of the null hypothesis.

## REFERENCES

Allen, B., R. Kavlock, C. Kimmel, and E. Faustman (1994a). Dose response assessments for developmental toxicity: II. Comparison of generic benchmark dose estimates with NOAELs, *Fund. Appl. Toxicol.*, 23, 487–495.

Allen, B., R. Kavlock, C. Kimmel, and E. Faustman (1994b). Dose response assessments for developmental toxicity: III. Statistical models, *Fund. Appl. Toxicol.*, 23, 496–509.

Altham, P. M. E. (1978). Two generalizations of the binomial distribution, *Appl. Stat.*, 27, 162–167.

Armitage, P. (1955). Tests for linear trends in proportions and frequencies, *Biometrics*, 11, 375–386.

Barnes, D. G. and M. Dourson (1988). Reference dose (RfD): description and use in health risk assessment. *Reg. Tox. and Pharm.*, 8, 471–487.

Basawa, I. V. (1991). Generalized score tests for composite hypotheses. In *Estimating Functions* (V. P. Godambe, ed.), Oxford University Press, Oxford, pp. 121–132.

Carr, G., and C. Portier (1993). An evaluation of some methods for fitting dose–response models to quantal-response developmental toxicology data, *Biometrics, 49,* 779–791.

Catalano, P. J., and L. Ryan (1992). Bivariate latent variable models for clustered discrete and continuous outcomes, *J. Am. Stat. Assoc., 87,* 651–658.

Catalano, P. J., D. O. Scharfstein, L. Ryan, C. Kimmel, and G. Kimmel (1993). Statistical model for fetal death, fetal weight, and malformation in developmental toxicity studies, *Teratology, 47,* 281–290.

Chen, J. J. (1993a). Trend test for overdispersed proportions, *Biometrical J., 35,* 949–958.

Chen, J. J. (1993b). A malformation incidence dose–response model incorporating fetal weight and/or litter size as covariates, *Risk Anal., 13,* 559–564.

Chen, J. J., and R. L. Kodell (1989). Quantitative risk assessment for teratological effects. *J. Am. Stat. Assoc., 84,* 966–971.

Chen, J. J., and L. A. Li (1994). Dose–response modeling of trinomial responses from developmental experiments. *Stat. Sin., 4,* pp. 265–274.

Chen, J. J., R. L. Kodell, R. B. Howe, and D. W. Gaylor (1991). Analysis of trinomial responses from reproductive and developmental toxicity experiments, *Biometrics, 47,* 1049–1058.

Cochran, W. G. (1954). Some methods for strengthening the common $\chi^2$ tests, *Biometrics, 10,* 417–451.

Cox, D. R. (1958). The regression analysis of binary sequences (with discussion), *J. R. Stat. Soc. B., 20,* 215–242.

Cox, D. R., and N. Reid (1987). Parameter orthogonality and approximate conditional inference (with discussion), *J. R. Stat. Soc. B., 49,* 1–39.

Crowder, M. J. (1978). beta-Binomial ANOVA for proportion, *Appl. Stat., 27,* 34–37.

Crump, K. S. (1984). A new method for determining allowable daily intakes, *Fundam. Appl. Toxicol., 4,* 854–871.

Davidian, M., and R. J. Carroll (1987). Variance function estimation, *J. Am. Stat. Assoc., 82,* 1079–1091.

[EPA] Environmental Protection Agency (1991). Guidelines for developmental toxicity risk assessment, *Fed. Regist., 56,* 63797–63826.

Faustman, E. M., D. G. Wellington, W. P. Smith, and C. A. Kimmel (1989). Characterization of a developmental toxicity dose–response model, *Environ. Health Perspect., 79,* 229–241.

Fung, K. Y., D. Krewski, J. N. K. Rao, and A. J. Scott (1994). Tests for trend in developmental toxicity experiments with correlated binary data, *Risk Anal., 14,* 621–630.

Gaylor, D. W. (1983). The use of safety factors in controlling risk, *J. Toxicol. Environ. Health, 11,* 329–336.

Gaylor, D. W. (1989). Quantitative risk analysis for quantal reproductive and developmental effects, *Environ. Health Perspect., 79,* 243–246.

Gaylor, D. W. (1992). Incidence of developmental defects at the no observed adverse effect level (NOAEL), *Regul. Toxicol. Pharmacol., 15,* 151–160.

Gaylor, D. W., and M. Razzaghi (1992). Process of building biologically based dose–response models for developmental defects, *Teratology, 46,* 573–581.

Gaylor, D. W., and W. Slikker, Jr. (1990). Risk assessment for neurotoxic effects, *NeuroToxicology, 11,* 211–218.

Holson, J. F., T. B. Gaines, C. J. Nelson, J. B. LaBorde, D. W. Gaylor, D. M. Sheehan, and J. F. Young (1992). Developmental toxicology of 2,4,5-tricholorphenoxyacetic acid (2,4,5-T). I: Multireplicated dose–response studies in four inbred strains and one outbred stock of mice, *Fundam. Appl. Toxicol., 19,* 286–297.

Johnson, N. L., and S. Kotz (1969). *Discrete Distributions,* John Wiley & Sons, New York.

International Life Sciences Institute (1989). Interpretation and extrapolation of reproductive data to establish human safety standards. In *Current Issues in Toxicology,* Springer-Verlag, New York, pp. 1–133.

Kimmel, C. A., and D. W. Gaylor (1988). Issues in qualitative and quantitative risk analysis for developmental toxicology, *Risk Anal., 8,* 15–20.

Kodell, R. L., R. B. Howe, J. J. Chen, and D. W. Gaylor (1991). Mathematical modeling of reproductive and developmental toxic effects for quantitative risk assessment, *Risk Anal.*, 11, 583–590.

Krewski, D., and J. Van Ryzin (1981). Dose response models for quantal response toxicity data. In *Statistics and Related Topics* (M. Csorgo, D. A. Dowson, J. N. K. Rao, and E. Saleh, eds.), North Holland, Amsterdam, pp. 201–231.

Krewski, D., and Y. Zhu (1994). Applications of multinomial dose–response models in developmental toxicity risk assessment, *Risk Anal.*, 14, 595–609.

Krewski, D., and Y. Zhu (1995). A simple data transformation for estimating benchmark dose in developmental toxicity experiments, *Risk Anal.*, 15, 29–39.

Kupper, L. L., and J. K. Haseman (1978). The use of a correlated binomial model for the analysis of certain toxicological experiments, *Biometrics*, 34, 69–76.

Kupper, L. L., C. Portier, M. D. Hogan, and E. Yamamoto (1986). The impact of litter effects on dose–response modeling in teratology, *Biometrics*, 42, 85–98.

Lefkopoulou, M., D. Moore, and L. Ryan (1989). The analysis of multiple correlated binary outcomes: Application to rodent teratology experiments, *J. Am. Stat. Assoc.*, 84, 810–815.

Leisenring, W., and L. Ryan (1992). Statistical properties of the NOAEL, *Regul. Toxicol. Pharmacol.*, 15, 161–171.

Liang, K.-Y., and S. Zeger (1986). Longitudinal data analysis using generalized linear models, *Biometrika*, 73, 13–22.

Moore, D. F. (1987). Modelling the extraneous variation in the presence of extra-binomial variation, *Appl. Stat.*, 36, 8–14.

Moore, D. F., and A. Tsiatis (1991). Robust estimation of the variance in moment methods for extra-binomial and extra-Poisson variation, *Biometrics*, 47, 383–401.

Neyman, J. (1959). Optimal asymptotic tests of composite hypotheses. In *Probability and Statistics* (U. Grenander, ed.), John Wiley & Sons, New York, pp. 213–234.

Paul, S. R. (1987). On the beta-correlated binomial (bcb). Distribution—a three parameter generalization of the binomial distribution, *Commun. Stat. Theory Methods*, 16, 1473–1478.

Portier, C., and D. Hoel (1984). Type I error of trend tests in proportions and the design of cancer screens, *Commun. Stat. Theory Methods*, 13, 1–14.

Prentice, R. L. (1986). Binary regression using an extended beta-binomial distribution, with discussion of correlation induced by covariate measurement errors, *J. Am. Stat. Assoc.*, 81, 321–327.

Prentice, R. L., and L. P. Zhao (1991). Estimating equations for parameters in means and covariances of multivariate discrete and continuous responses, *Biometrics*, 47, 825–839.

Rai, K., and J. Van Ryzin (1985). A dose–response model for teratological experiments involving quantal responses, *Biometrics*, 41, 1–9.

Rao, J. N. K., and A. Scott (1981). The analysis of categorical data from complex sample surveys: chi-Squared tests for goodness of fit and independence in two-way tables, *J. Am. Stat. Assoc.*, 76, 221–229.

Rao, J. N. K., and A. Scott (1992). A simple method for analysis of clustered binary data, *Biometrics*, 48, 577–585.

Ryan, L. (1992). Quantitative risk assessment for developmental toxicity, *Biometrics*, 48, 163–174.

Ryan, L. (1993). Using historical controls in the analysis of developmental toxicity data, *Biometrics*, 49, 1126–1135.

Ryan, L., P. Catalano, C. A. Kimmel, and G. L. Kimmel (1991). Relationship between fetal weight and malformation in developmental toxicity studies, *Teratology*, 44, 215–223.

Slickker, W., Jr., and D. W. Gaylor (1990). Biologically-based dose–response model for neurotoxicity risk assessment, *Korean J. Toxicol.*, 6, 205–213.

Stiteler, W. M., D. A. Joly, and H. A. T. Printup (1993). Monte Carlo investigation of issues relating to the benchmark dose method. Task No. 2-30, Environmental Criteria and Assessment Office. U. S. Environmental Protection Agency, Cincinnati, OH.

Tarone, R. E., and J. J. Gart (1980). On the robustness of combined tests for trends in proportions, *J. Am. Stat. Assoc.*, 75, 110–116.

Williams, D. A. (1975). The analysis of binary responses from toxicological experiments involving reproduction and teratogenicity, *Biometrics,* 31, 949–952.

Williams, D. A. (1982). Extra-binomial variation in logistic linear models, *Appl. Stat.,* 31, 144–148.

Williams, D. A. (1987). Dose–response models for teratological experiments, *Biometrics,* 43, 1013–1016.

Williams, D. A. (1988). Estimation bias using the beta-binomial distribution in teratology, *Biometrics,* 44, 305–309.

Zhao, L. P., and R. L. Prentice (1990). Correlated binary regression using a quadratic exponential model, *Biometrika,* 77, 642–648.

Zhu, Y., D. Krewski and W. H. Ross (1994). Multinomial dose–response models for correlated multinomial data from developmental toxicity studies, *Appl. Stat.,* 43, 583–598.

# 24
# Applications of Receptor-Binding Models in Toxicology

**J. Denes, D. Blakey, D. Krewski, and J. R. Withey**
*Health Canada*
*Ottawa, Ontario, Canada*

The mechanism by which toxic substances exert their effects is an important consideration in assessing potential health risks from exposure to such agents. A number of toxic substances appear to act by binding to cellular receptors. In this chapter, we examine receptor-binding models for toxic chemicals, based on classic theories of ligand–receptor interactions. General mathematical relationships such as the Hill and Michaelis–Menten equations, used to describe the formation of ligand–receptor complexes, are examined in detail. The application of receptor-binding models in toxicological risk assessment is illustrated by a case study of the mechanism of dioxin carcinogenesis.

## I. INTRODUCTION

Toxic substances may exert their effects by a variety of mechanisms. Biologically based approaches to toxicological risk assessment require an understanding of the critical steps involved in the toxic pathways leading to the induction of adverse health effects. (Goddard and Krewski, 1995). Biologically based risk assessment models can be of great value in extrapolating toxicological data between different dose levels, different exposure patterns, and different species.

In this chapter, we focus on receptor-mediated toxic effects (Lucier, 1992). Much of the existing literature on receptor binding relates to pharmaceutical agents. The molecular theory of drug action is based on the assumption that all biological manifestations, regardless of how complex, are the consequences of physio-chemical reactions, and that a living organism is a material system subject to the same laws of nature as an inanimate system.

Ordinary chemistry is concerned with molecules made of relatively few atoms. In contrast, those that make up living cells comprise several individual molecules, each with a molecular mass of 60,000–100,000 with atoms in untold conformations. These systems may still be far removed from observable biological events.

*447*

Molecular pharmacology originated at about the turn of the century, when Langley and Erlich (1905) and others introduced the concept of receptor binding. They assumed that drugs and antibodies act by interacting with specific "receptive substances" or "receptors." Later investigations of Clarke (1933) and Ariens (1964) provided a quantitative description of receptor–drug interactions.

What are the receptors with which drugs and other agents interact? As recently as 1964, Ariens wrote in the introduction in his book *Molecular Pharmacology:*

> The terminology used—receptor, active site etc.—does not mean that we know what we are talking about. On the contrary they underline our ignorance. We need these terms about order to be able to talk on drug action on a molecular level.

Subsequently, many specific receptors have been identified, including active sites of enzymes, surface receptors, and proteins. Drug–receptor interactions may result in changes in the drug molecule, so that it becomes chemically active. There may also be changes in the receptor, such that the receptor induces changes in the surrounding molecules that initiate the sequences of physicochemical events that lead to the desired biological effect.

In Section II, we review the basic principles underlying chemical reaction rates and the law of mass action. A detailed discussion of receptor-binding models is provided in Section III. The use of receptor-binding models in toxicological risk assessment is illustrated in Section IV by means of a case study of tetrachlorobenzo-*p*-dioxin (TCDD). Our conclusions are presented in Section V.

## II. CHEMICAL REACTION RATES AND THE LAW OF MASS ACTION

In a chemical reaction certain substances A, B, . . . , called reactants, change chemically into other substances F,G, . . . , called products (Frost and Pearson, 1953). This can be expressed by the stoichiometric equation

$$A + B + \cdots \rightarrow F + G + \cdots \tag{1}$$

For example, hydrogen $H_2$ and oxygen $O_2$ react to form water:

$$2H_2 + O_2 \rightarrow 2H_2O \tag{2}$$

and hydrogen and iodine react to become hydrogen iodide:

$$H_2 + I_2 \rightarrow 2HI \tag{3}$$

The *reaction rate* is defined as the rate of change of the substances involved in the reaction, with a minus or plus sign indicating whether the substance is a reactant or a product.

At a fixed temperature, the reaction rate is a function of the concentration of the reactants. More precisely, it is proportional to the product of the concentration of the reactants. Thus, in Eq. (1), we have

$$\frac{d[F]}{dt} = k[A][B] \cdots \tag{4}$$

where the square brackets [ ] denote the concentration of a reactant or product. The rate at which water is formed by the reaction in Eq. (2) is thus

$$\frac{d[H_2O]}{dt} = k[H_2]^2[O_2] \tag{5}$$

and the rate at which iodine becomes hydrogen iodide in Eq. (3) is

$$\frac{d[\text{HI}]}{dt} = k[\text{H}_2][\text{I}_2] \tag{6}$$

In most organic reactions, the products formed also react with each other to yield the original reactants. For example, ethyl alcohol and acetic acid react with each other and yield ethyl acetate and water:

$$\text{C}_2\text{H}_5\text{OH} + \text{CH}_3\text{COOH} \rightarrow \text{CH}_3\text{COOC}_2\text{H}_5 + \text{H}_2\text{O} \tag{7}$$

Ethyl acetate and water also react to yield acetic acid and alcohol. Hence, the foregoing reaction can be written more accurately as

$$\text{C}_2\text{H}_5\text{OH} + \text{CH}_3\text{COOH} \rightleftharpoons \text{CH}_3\text{COOC}_2\text{H}_5 + \text{H}_2\text{O} \tag{8}$$

Reactions of this type are called reversible reactions. The general form of reversible reactions with two reactants and two products is given by

$$\text{A} + \text{B} \rightleftharpoons \text{C} + \text{D} \tag{9}$$

The reaction $\text{A} + \text{B} \rightarrow \text{C} + \text{D}$ has a rate $k_1[\text{A}][\text{B}]$ proportional to the product of the concentrations of A and B. Similarly, the rate of the reverse reaction $\text{C} + \text{D} \rightarrow \text{A} + \text{B}$ is $k_2[\text{C}][\text{D}]$. At equilibrium the rates of the two reactions must be equal; that is:

$$k_1[\text{A}][\text{B}] = k_2[\text{C}][\text{D}] \tag{10}$$

Hence,

$$\frac{[\text{A}][\text{B}]}{[\text{C}][\text{D}]} = \frac{k_2}{k_1} = K_{eq} \tag{11}$$

where $K_{eq}$ is the equilibrium constant.

This expression is called the *law of mass action*. This chemical law states that the product of the concentrations of the reactants of a reversible chemical reaction divided by the product of the produced substances is constant for a given temperature.

## III. RECEPTOR-BINDING MODELS

### A. Basic Ligand–Receptor Interaction: The Theory of Occupancy

The term *ligand* is used to refer to drugs, toxic materials, antibodies, and other agents that act on living cells. The active site of the cell acted on by the ligand L is the receptor R. Ligand–receptor interactions are presumed to satisfy the following assumptions (Boeynaems and Dumont, 1980):

1. The interaction between ligand and receptor is reversible.
2. The ligand can exist in two states: free or receptor-bound.
3. The biological response is measured when the interaction between ligand and the receptor has reached a state of equilibrium.
4. The biological response is proportional to the number of occupied receptors.

The interaction of the ligand and its receptor is described by the stoichiometric equation

$$L + R \underset{k_{-1}}{\overset{k_1}{\rightleftharpoons}} RL \tag{12}$$

where RL denotes the receptor–ligand complex. The biological response is proportional to [RL]. By the law of mass action, we have

$$\frac{[L][R]}{[RL]} = \frac{k_{-1}}{k_1} = K_D \tag{13}$$

at equilibrium, where $K_D$ is the constant of dissociation. Since a receptor may be either occupied or unoccupied, we have

$$[R] + [RL] = [R_T] = r \tag{14}$$

where $R_T$ is the total number of receptors.
Hence

$$\frac{[L]([R_T] - [RL])}{[RL]} = K \tag{15}$$

and

$$[RL] = r\frac{[L]}{[L] + K} \tag{16}$$

or

$$[RL] = \frac{r}{1 + \dfrac{K}{[L]}} \tag{17}$$

Let $f$ denote the fraction of receptors occupied

$$f = \frac{[RL]}{[R_T]} = \frac{[L]}{[L] + K} \tag{18}$$

The ligand concentration corresponding to a given fractional occupancy $f$ can be expressed as

$$[L]_f = \frac{Kf}{1 - f} \tag{19}$$

Hence, the ligand concentration $[L_{0.5}]$, at which half the receptors are occupied, is the dissociation constant. The range of ligand concentrations in which saturation increases from a minimal level ($f = 0.1$) to a maximal level ($f = 0.9$) is $[L_{0.9}]/[L_{0.1}] = 81$ or about two orders of magnitude.

## B.  Langmuir's Adsorption Isotherm and Ligand–Receptor Interactions

Langmuir (1918) considered the adsorption of a gas or vapor on a surface as a unimolecular layer in terms of the equilibrium between the molecules striking the surface of the adsorbent and those that evaporate after a time (cf. Weiser, 1949, pp. 51–54). Let $\mu$ be the number of molecules striking the surface per second and let $\alpha$ be the constant proportion that adheres to the surface per second. If $\vartheta$ is the fraction of the total available surface that is covered with gas molecules, then $1 - \vartheta$ is the fraction that is bare. Hence, $(1 - \vartheta)\alpha\mu$ is actual rate of adsorption of molecules per unit area of the surface. The rate at which molecules escape from the surface is proportional to the area covered, say $\vartheta v$. At adsorption equilibrium, both rates are the same; hence,

$$(1 - \vartheta)\alpha\mu = \nu\vartheta \tag{20}$$

or

$$\vartheta = \frac{\alpha\mu}{\nu + \alpha\mu} \tag{21}$$

Since Eq. (21) has the same form as Eq. (16), ligand–receptor interactions can also be explained in terms of the Langmuir isotherm.

## C. Graphic Representations of Ligand–Receptor Interactions

For brevity, let $B = [RL]$ denote the concentration of bound ligand, and let $F = [L]$ denote the concentration of free ligand. Writing $R_T$ for $[R]_T$, Eq. (16) may be reexpressed as

$$B = R_T\left(\frac{F}{F + K}\right) \tag{22}$$

Several different coordinates may be used to represent Eq. (22) graphically.

Consider first the direct plot of $B$ versus $F$ as shown in Fig. 1. This graphic representation of Eq. (22) is an equilateral hyperbola, with a horizontal asymptote at $B = R_T$ and vertical asymptote at $F = -K$. The derivative at the origin is given by

$$\left.\frac{dB}{dF}\right|_{F=0} = \frac{R_T}{K^2} \tag{23}$$

whereas the derivative at the midpoint is

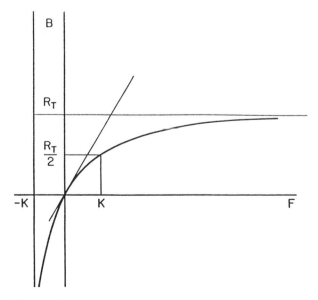

**Figure 1** A direct plot of Eq. (22) showing the concentration of bound ligand (B) as a function of the concentration of free ligand (F).

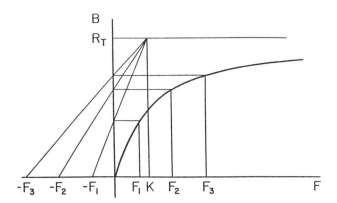

**Figure 2**  Eisenthal–Cornish–Bowden plot of Eq. (22).

$$\frac{dB}{dF}\bigg|_{F=K} = \frac{1}{4}\frac{R_T}{K^2} \tag{24}$$

The Eisenthal–Cornish-Bowden plot of Eq. (22) is shown in Fig. 2 (Eisenthal and Cornish-Bowden, 1974). This is obtained by drawing straight lines through the reflection of $F$ on the abscissa and $B$ on the ordinate. All of these straight lines will intersect at one point $(K, R_T)$.

Finally, consider the Dixon plot in Fig. 3 (Dixon, 1972). Straight lines parallel to the abscissa are drawn through the points $R_T/2$, $2R_T/3$, $3R_T/4$, ... ; straight lines are then drawn through the origin and the points where the parallel lines cut the hyperbole. They all intersect the asymptote at equidistant points. These graphic representations can be used to determine the constants $K$ and $R_T$.

## D.  The Kinetics of Ligand–Receptor Interactions

We now consider ligand–receptor interactions before they reach equilibrium. According to Eqs. (4) and (12), this is described by the differential equation

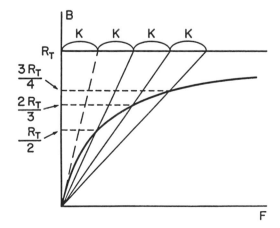

**Figure 3**  Dixon plot of Eq. (22).

$$\frac{d[RL]}{dt} = k_1[R][L] - k_{-1}[RL] \tag{25}$$

Eliminating [R], this can be written as

$$\frac{d[RL]}{dt} = [L]k_1 r - ([L]k_1 + k_{-1})[RL] \tag{26}$$

where $r = [R] + [RL]$. Assuming $[RL] = 0$ at time $t = 0$, we have

$$[RL] = \frac{k_1 r[L]}{[L]k_1 + k_{-1}} \left(1 - e^{-([L]k_1 + k_{-1})t}\right) \tag{27}$$

When equilibrium is reached at time $t = \infty$, this reduces to

$$[RL]_\infty = \frac{k_1 r[L]}{k_1[L] + k_{-1}} = r\frac{[L]}{[L] + K} \tag{28}$$

corresponding to Eq. (16).

## E.  The Combination of Hemoglobin and Gases: The Hill Equation

The uptake of oxygen and carbon dioxide by red blood cells provides a simple example of fixation of an agent by a cell. The uptake of oxygen by hemoglobin when the latter is dissolved in water in the absence of salts may be accurately described by a right-angled hyperbola of the type expressed by Eq. (16); namely,

$$[RL] = r\frac{[L]}{K + [L]} \tag{29}$$

or

$$B = R_T\frac{F}{K + F} \tag{30}$$

The oxygen present in excess and the combination formed is freely reversible.

When hemoglobin is dissolved in a salt solution, the uptake of oxygen is described by

$$[RL] = r\frac{[L]^n}{K + [L]^n} \tag{31}$$

or

$$B = R_T\frac{F^n}{K + F^n} \tag{32}$$

Hill (1910) explained this behavior under the assumption that, in the presence of salt, hemoglobin molecules are aggregated into clusters averaging $n$ molecules per cluster. The actual value of $n$ in this example is about 2.5. To arrive at Eq. (31), the stoichiometric equation

$$R + nL \rightleftharpoons RL \tag{33}$$

has to be used, rather than the simpler stoichiometric Eq. (12).

The Hill saturation function [see Eq. (31)] is best displayed by using Hill's plot, in which $\log[B/(R_T - B)]$ is plotted against $\log F$ (Fig. 4). This gives a straight line with slope $n$ that intersects the vertical axis at $-\log K$.

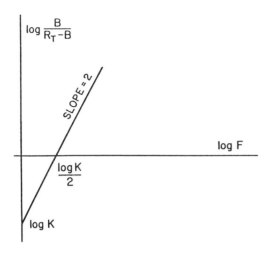

**Figure 4**  Hill plot of Eq. (32) for $n = 2$.

## F.  The Adair Saturation Function

Reactions such as the uptake of oxygen by hemoglobin can be characterized by considering hemoglobin as a receptor with $n$ equivalent binding sites (Adair, 1925). Here, the following set of reactions take place:

$$
\begin{aligned}
\text{R} + \text{L} &\overset{K_1}{\rightleftharpoons} \text{RL}_1 \\
\text{RL}_1 + \text{L} &\overset{K_2}{\rightleftharpoons} \text{RL}_2 \\
\text{RL}_2 + \text{L} &\overset{K_3}{\rightleftharpoons} \text{RL}_3 \\
&\quad \vdots \\
\text{RL}_{n-1} + \text{L} &\overset{K_n}{\rightleftharpoons} \text{RL}_n
\end{aligned}
\tag{34}
$$

The coefficients $K_s$ ($s = 1, \ldots, n$) are called the stepwise dissociation constants, characterizing each addition of a ligand to a receptor. Here, $[\text{R}] + [\text{RL}_1] + \cdots + [\text{RL}_n] = r$ is the concentration of all receptors, whether bound or free. According to the law of mass action,

$$
\begin{aligned}
\frac{[\text{R}][\text{L}]}{[\text{RL}_1]} &= K_1 \\
\frac{[\text{RL}_1][\text{L}]}{[\text{RL}_2]} &= K_2 \\
&\quad \vdots \\
\frac{[\text{RL}_{n-1}][\text{L}]}{[\text{RL}_n]} &= K_n
\end{aligned}
\tag{35}
$$

It follows that

$$[RL_1] = \frac{[R][L]}{K_1}$$

$$[RL_2] = \frac{[R][L]^2}{K_1 K_2}$$

$$\cdot$$
$$\cdot$$
$$\cdot$$

$$[RL_n] = \frac{[R][L]^n}{K_1 K_2 \cdots K_n}$$

(36)

so that

$$[R] = \frac{r}{1 + ([L]/K_1) + ([L]^2/K_1 K_2) + \cdots + ([L]^n/K_1 K_2 \cdots K_n)}$$

(37)

The fractional occupancy

$$f = \frac{([L]/K_1) + (2[L]^2/K_1 K_2) + \cdots + (n[L]^n/K_1 K_2 \cdots K_n)}{1 + ([L]/K_1) + \cdots + ([L]^n/K_1 K_2 \cdots K_n)}$$

(38)

is called Adair's formula. When $n = 1$, Eq. (38) reduces to Eq. (16). If $K_1, \ldots, K_{n-1}$ are all large, Eq. (38) approximates the Hill equation [Eq. (31)].

## G. Describing Ligand Kinetics

The rate of action of ligands, such as drugs, can be measured two ways. First, by measuring the rate at which a particular concentration produces a series of actions varying from 0 to 100% of the maximum effect, a time–action curve can be constructed. Second, by measuring the times taken by a series of concentrations to produce a particular effect, a concentration–action curve is obtained.

Equation (27) is a typical time–action curve, provided the action of the drug on the cell is proportional to the concentration of the drug–receptor complex [RL]. Here, the measured time does not necessarily indicate the time taken by the chemical reaction. (In some cases, measured time reflects the time of diffusion, or the lag time, for a particular biological response.)

Concentration–action curves are constructed by observing the time taken to produce a definite action at a series of concentrations. Frequently, the product of the concentration $C$ and time $t$ appears to be constant: $Ct =$ constant. More generally, most time–concentration curves can be represented by the following formula:

$$(C - C_m)^n t = \text{constant}$$

(39)

where $C_m$ is the concentration that just fails to produce an effect after an infinite time.

## H. Concentration–Action Curves of Disinfection

It has long been known that bacteria killed by almost any cause die in an orderly way (Clark, 1933). The number of survivors $b$ of an initial population $a$ after the passage of time $t$ satisfies the following expression:

$$\frac{\log a - \log b}{t} = k \tag{40}$$

or

$$b = ae^{-kt} \tag{41}$$

for some constant $k$, which is the form of a first-order rate process.

This formula is called the "logarithmic order of death." Initially, it was thought that this result could be explained on the basis of individual variation within the population of interest. However, it was later found that a uniform population, such as bacterial spores, also obeys the same rule.

In this paradigm, the effect of interest (death) is irreversible. However, an irreversible effect can be the result of a reversible action, provided it is the result of a chance occurrence of one or more events. For example, consider a drug that causes the coagulation of protein, which is a reversible process. Assume further that death is caused by one or more protein molecules coagulating. If a drug causes say 20% of the proteins to coagulate in every bacteria, only that fraction of the bacteria that have their vital protein molecules coagulated will die.

It follows that the number of deaths in a fixed time period will be proportional to the concentration of the $RL$ complex, so that

$$\frac{dr}{dt} = -\alpha[RL] \tag{42}$$

where $r$ is the concentration of all receptors, both bound and free. Since

$$[RL] = \frac{r[L]^n}{K + [L]^n} \tag{43}$$

if Hill's law holds, we have

$$\frac{dr}{dt} = -kr \tag{44}$$

where

$$k = \frac{\alpha[L]^n}{K + [L]^n} \tag{45}$$

Thus,

$$r = r_0 e^{-kt} \tag{46}$$

Since the number of bacteria is proportional to the number of receptors, the time–action curve is given by

$$b = ae^{-kt} \tag{47}$$

The time–concentration curve specifies the time needed to reach a given ratio; that is

$$kt = \log\frac{a}{b} = \text{constant} \tag{48}$$

or

$$\frac{\alpha[L]^n}{K + [L]^n}t = \text{constant} \tag{49}$$

If the drug concentration $[L]$ is very small in comparison with the dissociation constant $K$, the last expression can be written as

$$\frac{\alpha[L]^n t}{K} = \text{constant} \tag{50}$$

or

$$[L]^n t = \text{constant} \tag{51}$$

corresponding to Eq. (39).

## I. Enzyme Systems: The Michaelis–Menten Equation

Enzymes are proteins that act as catalysts in chemical reaction (Hayashi and Sakamoto, 1986). For example, the enzyme of the yeast that catalyzes alcoholic fermentation converts sugar into alcohol:

$$C_6H_{12}O_6 \rightarrow 2C_2H_5OH + 2CO_2 \tag{52}$$

The enzyme first forms an enzyme–substrate complex with the substrate (e.g., sugar in case of fermentation). This is a reversible process:

$$L + R \underset{k_{-1}}{\overset{k_1}{\rightleftharpoons}} RL$$

The next step, however, is irreversible:

$$RL \overset{k_2}{\rightarrow} R + P \tag{54}$$

where P is the final product. Thus, in case of fermentation of alcohol: sugar + enzyme $\rightleftharpoons$ (sugar–enzyme complex), and sugar – enzyme complex $\rightarrow$ enzyme + alcohol (+ carbon dioxide).

In general, the production of P can be expressed in terms of the following system of differential equations:

$$\frac{d[R]}{dt} = k_2[RL] - k_1[L][R] + k_{-1}[RL], \tag{55}$$

$$\frac{d[L]}{dt} = -k_1[L][R] + k_{-1}[RL], \tag{56}$$

$$\frac{d[RL]}{dt} = k_1[L][R] - k_2[RL] - k_{-1}[RL], \tag{57}$$

and

$$\frac{d[P]}{dt} = k_2[RL] \tag{58}$$

This system of differential equations can only be solved numerically. Michaelis and Menten (1913) developed an approximate solution by assuming that the concentration of the enzyme–substrate complex was constant for most of the reaction time. Under this condition,

$$0 = \frac{d[RL]}{dt} = k_1[L][R] - (k_2 + k_{-1})[RL] \tag{59}$$

so that

$$[RL] = \frac{k_1[R][L]}{k_2 + k_{-1}} \tag{60}$$

Since $[R] + [RL] = r$, we have

$$[RL] = \frac{k_1(r - [RL])[L]}{k_2 + k_{-1}}$$

$$= \frac{k_1 r[L]}{k_1[L] + k_2 + k_{-1}} \tag{61}$$

The rate of production of the final product P is

$$\frac{d[P]}{dt} = k_2[RL] \tag{62}$$

so that $V$, the reaction velocity, is given by

$$V = \frac{k_1 k_2 r[L]}{k_1[L] + k_2 + k_{-1}} \tag{63}$$

or

$$V = \frac{V_\infty k_1[L]}{k_2 + k_{-1} + k_1 L} = \frac{V_\infty}{1 + \{(k_2 + k_{-1})/k_1[L]\}} \tag{64}$$

where $V_\infty = k_2 r$. This can be reexpressed as

$$V = \frac{V_\infty}{1 + (K/[L])} \tag{65}$$

which is the usual form of the Michaelis–Menten equation.

## J.  Steady-State Expressions for More Complex Systems

Let us consider the enzymatic reaction with two enzyme-substrate complexes:

$$L + R \underset{k_2}{\overset{k_1}{\rightleftharpoons}} RL_1 \underset{k_4}{\overset{k_3}{\rightleftharpoons}} RL_2 \overset{k_5}{\rightarrow} R + P \tag{66}$$

The differential equations for this system are

$$\frac{d[R]}{dt} = k_2[RL_1] - k_1[R][L] + k_5[RL_2] \tag{67}$$

$$\frac{d[RL_1]}{dt} = k_1[R][L] - k_2[RL_1] - k_3[RL_1] + k_4[RL_2] \tag{68}$$

$$\frac{d[RL_2]}{dt} = k_3[RL_1] - k_4[RL_2] - k_5[RL_2] \tag{69}$$

and

$$\frac{d[\mathrm{P}]}{dt} = k_5[\mathrm{RL}_2] \tag{70}$$

Assuming steady-state conditions for the $\mathrm{RL}_1$ and $\mathrm{RL}_2$ complexes gives

$$k_1[\mathrm{R}][\mathrm{L}] - (k_2 + k_3)[\mathrm{RL}_1] + k_4[\mathrm{RL}_2] = 0 \tag{71}$$

and

$$k_3[\mathrm{RL}_1] - (k_4 + k_5)[\mathrm{RL}_2] = 0 \tag{72}$$

Noting that $[\mathrm{R}] + [\mathrm{RL}_1] + [\mathrm{RL}_2] = r$, Eqs. (71) and (72) can be solved for $[\mathrm{RL}_2]$, the solution being

$$[\mathrm{RL}_2] = \frac{k_1 k_3 r[\mathrm{L}]}{k_2 k_4 + k_2 k_5 + k_3 k_5 + k_1(k_3 + k_4 + k_5)[L]} \tag{73}$$

The rate of production of the final product P is

$$V = \frac{d\mathrm{P}}{dt} = k_5[\mathrm{RL}_2] \tag{74}$$

The maximum velocity when $[L] = \infty$ is given by

$$V_{\max} = \frac{k_1 k_3 k_5 r}{k_1(k_3 + k_4 + k_5)} \tag{75}$$

Thus, the velocity $V$ is given by the Michaelis–Menten formula

$$V = \frac{V_{\max}}{1 + (K_{\mathrm{m}}/[\mathrm{L}])} \tag{76}$$

where

$$K_{\mathrm{m}} = \frac{k_2 k_4 + k_2 k_5 + k_3 k_5}{k_1(k_3 + k_4 + k_5)} \tag{77}$$

## K.  The Rapid Equilibrium Method

Suppose that there exists a rapid equilibrium step, so that the formation of the ligand–receptor complex instantly reaches an equilibrium state. For example, consider the process

$$\mathrm{R} + \mathrm{L} \underset{k_{-1}}{\overset{k_1}{\rightleftharpoons}} \mathrm{RL} \overset{k_2}{\rightarrow} \mathrm{R} + \mathrm{P} \tag{78}$$

where

$$\frac{d\mathrm{P}}{dt} = k_2[\mathrm{RL}] \tag{79}$$

It follows from the law of mass action that

$$\frac{[\mathrm{R}][\mathrm{L}]}{[\mathrm{RL}]} = \frac{k_{-1}}{k_1} = K \tag{80}$$

or

$$[RL] = \frac{r[L]}{K + L} \tag{81}$$

Thus,

$$V = \frac{dP}{dt} = \frac{k_2 r[L]}{K + [L]} \tag{82}$$

This leads to the Michaelis–Menten type formula

$$V = \frac{V_{max}}{1 + (K_m/[L])} \tag{83}$$

where $V_{max} = k_2 r$ is the maximum reaction rate as $[L] \to \infty$.

## L.  The Competitive Inhibition, Affinity, and Intrinsic Activity of Drugs

The purpose of cellular receptors is to react with natural substrates or essential metabolites. The specific biological action of many drugs can be explained by supposing that the drug competes with the natural substrate for active receptor sites, thus either inhibiting or enhancing its effects. This is the principle of competitive inhibition expounded first by Ariens (1954).

This theory was an improvement over the elementary theory of drug action, but there arose phenomena that could be explained only by the competitive inhibition. Several substances were discovered that had dual effects, acting as inhibitors as well as metabolites.

As discussed previously, a drug A acts on the living cell by forming a drug–receptor complex RA with the receptor R. The action of the drug is proportional to the concentration of RA. It was shown that the concentration of RA can be expressed as

$$[RA] = \frac{r[A]}{K_A + [A]} \tag{84}$$

where $K_A$ is the dissociation constant. It follows that concentration of the receptor-bound drug at a given receptor concentration depends on the free drug concentration and the dissociation constant $K_A$. In fact, the larger the reciprocal of $K_A$ is, the more drug is bound to the receptor. Therefore, $K_A^{-1}$ is called the *affinity* of the drug relative to the receptor. Affinity is thus a constant, determining how much of the drug–receptor complex will be formed under given conditions.

The effect $E_A$ of drug A is proportional to [RA]:

$$E_A = \alpha[RA] = \frac{\alpha r}{1 + (K_A/[A])} \tag{85}$$

The proportionality constant $\alpha$ is called the *intrinsic activity* of the drug. Intrinsic activity, thus, is a substance-specific constant relating biological effects to the concentration of the receptor–drug complex. The maximum value of $E_{A(max)} = \alpha r$ is reached when [A] is large.

Let us now consider the interaction with two substances A and B with different intrinsic activities $\alpha$ and $\beta$ and with different affinities $K_A$ and $K_B$ within one receptor system. At equilibrium this interaction is represented by

$$R + A \rightleftharpoons RA \tag{86}$$

and

$$R + B \rightleftharpoons RB \tag{87}$$

Hence,

$$\frac{[R][A]}{[RA]} = K_A \tag{88}$$

and

$$\frac{[R][B]}{[RB]} = K_B \tag{89}$$

The total amount of receptor is

$$[R] + [RA] + [RB] = r \tag{90}$$

Thus, we have

$$[R] = \frac{r}{1 + ([A]/K_A) + ([B]/K_B)} \tag{91}$$

$$[RA] = \frac{rK_B[A]}{K_AK_B + K_B[A] + K_A[B]} \tag{92}$$

and

$$[RB] = \frac{rK_A[B]}{K_AK_B + K_B[A] + K_A[B]} \tag{93}$$

The combined effect of A and B is

$$E_{AB} = r\frac{\alpha K_B[A] + \beta K_A[B]}{K_AK_B + K_B[A] + K_A[B]} \tag{94}$$

When the intrinsic activity of B is near zero,

$$E_{AB} = \frac{\alpha r}{(K_A/K_B)([B]/[A]) + 1 + (K_A/[A])} \tag{95}$$

For large [A] the effect of B depends on the ratio [B]/[A], rather than the concentrations [B] and [A] themselves.

Consider now the case in which the affinity of B is greater than that of A ($K_A > K_B$) and the intrinsic activity of B is less than that of A ($\beta < \alpha$). Let us compare the effect of A alone with that of A and B together. In this case

$$E_A = r\frac{\alpha K_B[A]}{K_AK_B + K_B[A]} < r\frac{\alpha K_B[A] + \beta K_A[B]}{K_AK_B + K_B[A] + K_A[B]} = E_{AB} \tag{96}$$

It follows that

$$\frac{[A]}{K_A + [A]} < \frac{\beta}{\alpha} \tag{97}$$

If [A] is sufficiently small, then $E_A < E_{AB}$; thus, B is a metabolite of A. If [A] is sufficiently large, it is easily seen that B is an inhibitor of A.

## IV. APPLICATION TO DIOXIN RISK ASSESSMENT

### A. Toxicity of 2,3,7,8-Tetrachlorodibenzo-*p*-dioxin

2,3,7,8-Tetrachlorodibenzo-*p*-dioxin (TCDD) is a persistent environmental contaminant that induces a broad spectrum of toxicological effects, including thymic atrophy, birth defects, and immunological effects (Silbergeld and Gasiewicz, 1989). It is also considered to be the most potent carcinogen among the halogenated aromatic hydrocarbons (HAHs). Chronic treatment with as little as 10 μg/kg is sufficient to induce liver tumors in female rats (Kociba et al., 1978; NTP, 1982). One of the most remarkable properties of TCDD is the degree to which its toxicity varies among species, strains, and tissues. For example, the median lethal dose ($LD_{50}$) of TCDD ranges from 1 μg/kg in guinea pigs to 5000 μg/kg in hamsters, with mice and rats in the 50–200 μg/kg range (McConnell et al., 1978). The toxic effects of TCDD can also be gender-specific. In rats, TCDD induces liver tumors in female, but not male, animals (Kociba et al., 1978; NTP, 1982). These variable responses make it difficult to understand its mechanisms of action and, even more so, to predict human risk on the basis of results from animal experiments.

To estimate the human carcinogenic risk of TCDD, it is important to understand its mechanism of action. The multistage theory of carcinogenesis involves initiation, promotion, and an indeterminate number of steps generally referred to as tumor progression (Barett, 1992). During initiation, mutations are induced in genes that control normal cell division and differentiation. Carcinogens capable of inducing these changes are genotoxic. The induction of mutations is a stochastic process, with some possibility of mutation occurring even at low doses. Tumor promotion is a less clearly defined process that generally involves the clonal expansion of initiated cells through the stimulation of cell proliferation. Cell division may be induced in normally static cell populations by changes in the cellular environment by generation of intracellular signals. Unlike genotoxic carcinogens, tumor promoters and other nongenotoxic carcinogens induce tumors without interacting directly with the DNA of the affected cells. It is often assumed that there is a low-dose threshold for nongenotoxic components of the carcinogenic process. However, this is likely dependent on the mechanism by which these compounds lead to tumor formation.

Tetrachlorodibenzo-*p*-dioxin is a potent, nongenotoxic tumor promoter (Pitot and Campbell, 1987; Kociba, 1984). In cells treated with TCDD, no DNA adducts could be detected, even using sensitive methods capable of detecting one adduct in $10^{11}$ nucleotides (Turtletaub et al., 1991). Furthermore, TCDD is negative in the assays used to measure genotoxic activity (Wassom et al., 1977).

Clues to the mechanism of TCDD toxicity arise from its strain specificity. The induction of aryl hydrocarbon hydroxylase (AHH) activity is often used to measure responsiveness to HAHs such as TCDD. It was noted that 3-methylcholanthrene induced AHH activity in inbred mouse strain C57BL/6J, but not in the inbred mouse strain DBA/2J (Nebert et al., 1972; Thomas et al., 1972). Cross-breeding experiments between responsive and nonresponsive mice demonstrated that responsiveness to HAHs segregated as a dominant trait under the control of a single autosomal gene. The alleles were designated $Ah^b$ for responsive mice and $Ah^d$ for nonresponsive mice. Other toxic effects, including thymic involution, cleft palate, and hepatic porphyria, segregated in a manner identical with the AHH inducibility (Poland and Knutson, 1982). These studies led to the conclusion that many, perhaps most, of the biological responses to HAHs are under the control of the *Ah* locus.

The identity of the *Ah* gene product was unknown until Poland et al. (1976) reported an intracellular hepatic protein that bound [³H]TCDD saturably with high affinity in responsive, but not in nonresponsive, mice. Later, a low-affinity receptor was also identified in the nonresponsive DBA/2 mice (Okey et al., 1989). The high-affinity form of the protein in C57BL/6 mice binds to TCDD with an equilibrium binding constant of approximately $10^{-12}$–$10^{-10}$ *M*, and a binding capacity of 10–100 fmol/mg cytosol protein (Poland and Knutson, 1982; Safe, 1986; Bradfield et al., 1988; Bradfield and Poland, 1988). The low-affinity protein in DBA/2 mice has an equilibrium binding constant about tenfold lower (Okey et al., 1989). The Ah receptor also binds other aromatic hydrocarbons, but with lower affinities. Quantitative structure–activity relationship analysis revealed that the ligand-binding site on the Ah receptor is hydrophobic and that the more hydrophobic the ligand, the stronger the binding affinity (Whitlock, 1990). The most potent ligands, such as TCDD, are planar and contain halogen atoms at at least three of the four lateral positions. However, the properties required for ligand binding differ from those required for AHH induction. Therefore, it is likely that other phenomena are required for AHH induction in addition to ligand binding (Safe, 1986).

The Ah receptor is also present in human cells. As in the mouse, the human hepatic Ah receptor has an equilibrium binding constant of 0.1–1.0 n$M$ (Cook and Greenlee, 1989). There is also a human Ah receptor phenotype analogous to the nonresponsive DBA/2 mice, in which AHH induction is reduced by approximately tenfold (Manchester et al., 1987; Harper et al., 1988). It would appear, therefore, that there is a genetically determined variation in susceptibility to Ah receptor-mediated effects of TCDD in human populations.

The binding of TCDD to the Ah receptor represents only the first step in enzyme induction and other biological responses to TCDD. After the TCDD–receptor complex is formed, it undergoes conformational changes that increase the affinity of the complex for specific sites in the DNA. This process, referred to as transformation, is believed to involve other receptor-bound molecules, including the 90-kDa heat-shock protein (Perdew, 1988; Denis et al., 1988). There is some debate over whether the location of the receptor is cytosolic (Poland et al., 1976; Okey et al., 1980; Denison et al., 1986) or nuclear (Whitlock and Galeazzi, 1984), and whether binding of the ligand to the receptor occurs before or after translocation from the cytoplasm to the nucleus. Ultimately, the ligand–receptor binds to TCDD-responsive elements in the DNA, leading to increased gene expression. These binding sequences are typical of enhancers, in that they are located at relatively long distances from the target gene, and they increase the rate of gene transcription (Jones et al., 1986; Neuhold et al., 1986; Fujisawa-Sehara, 1987; Fisher et al., 1989; Hirst et al., 1989). In each TCDD–Ah receptor-binding domain in the DNA, there is a common core recognition motif that contains a copy of the sequence (Denison et al., 1988):

5′   T–GCGTG   3′
3′   A–CGCAC   5′

Unlike other receptor–DNA interactions, the ligand–Ah receptor binds preferentially to double-stranded DNA (Denison et al., 1989). The binding site is in the major groove where the receptor comes into contact with the four guanine residues of the recognition motif (Neuhold et al., 1989; Shen and Whitlock, 1989). It also differs in that the receptor is bound as a monomer, rather than a dimer (Denison et al., 1989). Differences in methylation of CpG dinucleotides within the recognition sequence can inhibit receptor–enhancer interactions (Shen and Whitlock, 1989). This may account for some of the tissue-specific effects observed in response to TCDD treatment.

The Ah receptor has at least three functional domains (Whitlock, 1990). The ligand-binding domain interacts with TCDD to convert the protein to a DNA-binding species. The DNA-binding domain recognizes a specific nucleotide sequence and positions the activated ligand receptor complex at regulatory sites in the genome. The protein-binding domain interacts with other transcriptional factors to induce expression of the target gene. Much of what is known about the Ah receptor mechanism was derived from studies that examined the activation of the *CYP1A1* gene by TCDD. CYP1A1 is a specific isozyme of cytochrome P-450 that is responsible for the activation and deactivation of many environmental contaminants, including polycyclic aromatic hydrocarbons (PAHs). The amount of CYP1A1 protein correlates well with other enzymes that also participate in the metabolic activation of carcinogens, including aryl hydrocarbon hydroxylase (AHH) and ethoxyresorufin-*O*-deethylase (EROD). As a result, the induction of CYP1A1, AHH, and EROD are used as sensitive indicators of exposure to chemicals that bind the Ah receptor. CYP1A2 is a closely related P-450 enzyme that is also induced by transcriptional activation through the Ah receptor-mediated pathway (Thomas et al., 1933; Graham et al., 1988). Although CYP1A1 can be found throughout the body, CYP1A2 is induced only in the liver (Tuteja et al., 1985).

CYP1A2 has been reported to bind TCDD, although with a somewhat lower affinity than the Ah receptor. This causes TCDD to accumulate in the liver (Leung et al., 1990a). There is also evidence that CYP1A2 can metabolize estrogen to catechol estrogen (Graham et al., 1988), reducing estradiol levels and providing a substrate for the production of free radicals that can cause mutations and cell death (Metzler, 1984).

The response of the cell to TCDD can be affected in many ways. Several of the factors that can influence Ah receptor-mediated effects were studied using variant hepatocyte cells. For a detailed review, see Whitlock (1990). For example, in one cell type, mutations at the *Ah* locus reduced the ligand-binding affinity of the receptor. In another cell type with high-binding affinity, the bound receptor never reached the nucleus, and there was no induction of AHH, even though TCDD was bound to the receptor. Assuming that a genetic locus other than the *Ah* locus controls the accumulation of the receptor in the nucleus, mutations at at least two loci can affect Ah receptor function. In a third type of variant, there are defects in both the receptor and its ability to accumulate in the nucleus. Finally, there is a fourth variant in which a dominant factor, possibly a repressor protein, inhibits normal Ah receptor function (A32). These studies indicate that there may be at least four genetic loci controlling Ah receptor function. One locus for the receptor protein itself, one for a factor that directs the cellular accumulation of the receptor, one that affects both properties, and one that inhibits Ah receptor function. This genetic diversity in Ah receptor activity may also occur in human populations.

All of the studies discussed up to this point have focused on the induction of P-450 enzymes in response to TCDD and the formation of the TCDD–Ah-receptor complex. However, the relation between Ah receptor occupancy, enzyme induction, and carcinogenesis is unclear. The C57BL/6 mice, the Ah receptor is in the 1–10 p$M$ range (Bradfield et al., 1988; Bradfield and Poland, 1988). Thus, doses of less than 1 part per trillion (ppt) TCDD should be capable of causing biological effects. However, the accumulation of TCDD to the ppt level (pg/g) does not always lead to a biological response (CDC Veterans Health Studies, 1988; CDC, 1989). This may be because dioxins partition into the lipophilic compartments of the cell (e.g., the membranes) where they cannot interact freely with the Ah receptor (Whitlock, 1990).

The agent TCDD causes a number of effects in addition to the induction of enzymes involved in the metabolism of xenobiotic agents. Effects on the endocrine system may play an even more important role in the carcinogenicity of TCDD. For example, TCDD can induce changes in steroid-metabolizing enzyme activities. This can cause alterations in hormonal levels (Goldstein and Safe, 1989; Mebus et al., 1987; Graham et al., 1988), leading to proliferative stimuli and carcinogenic activity in hormone-dependent tissues (Kociba et al., 1978). Ah receptor-dependent reductions are also induced by TCDD in epidermal growth factor receptors (Madhukar et al., 1984), estrogen receptors (Romkes et al., 1987), glucocorticoid receptors (Sunahara et al., 1989), tumor necrosis factor (Clark et al., 1991), c-*erbA* (Bombick et al., 1988), and gastrin (Mably et al., 1990). These effects can interact to stimulate cell proliferation and affect cell differentation. The interaction of TCDD, the Ah receptor, and hormones can be seen in the induction of liver tumors in rats. In normal rats, TCDD is an effective promoter of liver tumors in females, but not in males. However, in ovariectomized females, the induction of liver tumors by TCDD is reduced (Kociba et al., 1978). These studies suggest an interaction of estrogen in the carcinogenicity of TCDD. The diversity of effects of TCDD between species, strains, sexes, and tissues is a function of endocrine and metabolic status.

## B. Mathematical Models for Tetrachlorodibenzo-*p*-dioxin

Kohn and Portier (1993) developed a model for describing the action of TCDD and other halogenated aromatic hydrocarbons. Under this model it is assumed that the action of the xenobiotic is through the excess production of a particular protein, such as cytochrome P-450. This protein is produced through the presence of a natural ligand with which the xenobiotic interacts competitively. It is also produced continually, regardless of the presence of the xenobiotic or the natural ligand.

The ligand first binds to a receptor with multiple-binding sites, and the ligand–receptor complex binds to a DNA site, inducing the protein. The xenobiotic now competes with the ligand for receptor sites, and the xenobiotic–receptor complex competes with the ligand–receptor complex for DNA-binding sites. For both substances, receptor binding is expressed by the equations

$$lN + R \rightleftharpoons RN \tag{98}$$

and

$$lX + R \rightleftharpoons RX \tag{99}$$

Here, $N$ stands for the natural ligand, X for the xenobiotic, and $l$ denotes the number of binding sites on the receptor. According to Eqs. (16) and (31),

$$[RX] = \frac{r - [RN]}{1 + (K_x/[X]^l)} \tag{100}$$

and

$$[RN] = \frac{r - [RX]}{1 + (K_n/[N]^l)} \tag{101}$$

where $l$ is the Hill exponent.

Both the RN and RX complexes then bind competitively to DNA, producing the complexes DNA $\cdot$ RN and DNA $\cdot$ RX:

$$DNA + nRN \underset{k_{-1}}{\overset{k_1}{\rightleftharpoons}} DNA \cdot RN \tag{102}$$

and

$$DNA + nRX \underset{l_{-1}}{\overset{l_1}{\rightleftharpoons}} DNA \cdot RX \tag{103}$$

where $n$ is the number of DNA binding sites.

Next, the protein P is produced and the complexes RN and RX are liberated through the irreversible processes

$$DNA \cdot RN \overset{k_2}{\rightarrow} P + DNA + RN \tag{104}$$

and

$$\text{DNA} \cdot \text{RX} \xrightarrow{l_2} \text{P} + \text{DNA} + \text{RX} \tag{105}$$

It follows that

$$\frac{d}{dt} [\text{DNA} \cdot \text{RN}] = k_1 [\text{RN}]^n [\text{DNA}] - k_{-1} [\text{DNA} \cdot \text{RN}] - k_2 [\text{DNA} \cdot \text{RN}] \tag{106}$$

and

$$\frac{d}{dt} [\text{DNA} \cdot \text{RX}] = l_1 [\text{RX}]^n [\text{DNA}] - l_{-1} [\text{DNA} \cdot \text{RX}] - l_2 [\text{DNA} \cdot \text{RX}] \tag{107}$$

Assuming that the formation of the DNA–ligand complexes is the rate-limiting step, as in Eq. (59), we have

$$k_1 [\text{RN}]^n [\text{DNA}] - k_{-1} [\text{DNA} \cdot \text{RN}] - k_2 [\text{DNA} \cdot \text{RN}] = 0 \tag{108}$$

and

$$l_1 [\text{RX}]^n [\text{DNA}] - l_{-1} [\text{DNA} \cdot \text{RX}] - k_2 [\text{DNA} \cdot \text{RX}] = 0. \tag{109}$$

Solving these for the concentrations of the DNA $\cdot$ RN and DNA $\cdot$ RX complexes yields the rate of protein induction:

$$V_{\text{induct}} = \frac{V_{\text{RNmax}}}{1 + \dfrac{K_{\text{RN}}}{[\text{RN}]^n} \left( 1 + \dfrac{[\text{RX}]^n}{K_{\text{RX}}} \right)} + \frac{V_{\text{RXmax}}}{1 + \dfrac{K_{\text{RX}}}{[\text{RX}]^n} \left( 1 + \dfrac{[\text{RN}]^n}{K_{\text{RN}}} \right)}, \tag{110}$$

where $V_{\text{RNmax}} = k_2 d$, $V_{\text{RXmax}} = l_2 d$ and $d$ is the total DNA. Here, $K_{\text{RN}}$ and $K_{\text{RX}}$ are the Michaelis–Menten constants for the protein production of the RN and RX complexes.

The degradation of the protein is accomplished in the usual way through the action of some enzyme E with $p$ binding sites:

$$\text{E} + p\text{P} \rightleftharpoons \text{EP} \tag{111}$$

with

$$\text{E}_p \rightarrow \text{E} + \text{peptides} \tag{112}$$

The rate of proteolysis (prot) is assumed to follow of Michaelis–Menten kinetics

$$V_{\text{prot}} = \frac{V_{\text{prot max}}}{1 + (K_p/[\text{P}]^p)} \tag{113}$$

The xenobiotic itself is metabolized through some enzyme M:

$$\text{M} + m\text{X} \rightleftharpoons \text{MX} \tag{114}$$

$$\text{MX} \rightarrow \text{M} + \text{some product of metabolism (metab)} \tag{115}$$

and

$$V_{\text{metab}} = \frac{V_{\text{metab max}}}{1 + (K_M/[\text{X}]^m)} \tag{116}$$

Finally, the differential equations describing the temporal response of the model are given by

$$\frac{d[X]}{dt} = -V_{metab} + l_{-1}[RX] \tag{117}$$

and

$$\frac{d[P]}{dt} = V_{const} + V_{induct} - V_{prot} \tag{118}$$

where $V_{const}$ is the constant rate of production of P by a mechanism not involving the receptor R.

Kohn and Portier (1993) used this model to conduct a theoretical study on the shape of the dose–response curves of TCDD and related xenobiotics. In the absence of evidence to the contrary, the dose–response curve for chemical carcinogenesis is generally assumed to be linear in the low-dose region (EPA, 1986).

Changing the value of the constitutive (const) rate had no effect on linearity at low doses. At higher doses, however, the curve is sigmoidal. Increasing the rate $V_{constmax}$ leads to a shift in inflection point of the sigmoidal curve to lower doses.

Values for the Hill exponent of less than 1 imply supralinearity at lower doses, and shift the inflection point of the overall sigmoidal curve to lower doses. Positive cooperability, characterized by hill exponents of greater than 1, is associated with sublinearity in the low-dose region and a shift of the inflection point of the sigmoid curve to higher doses.

Further results are provided by Tritscher et al. (1992), Portier et al. (1993), and Kehn et al. (1993).

## C. Physiologically Based Pharmacokinetics for Dioxins

The pharmacokinetic behavior of dioxins has also been investigated in detail. The longitudinal pattern of tissue distribution for TCDD has been studied in the rat (Leung et al., 1990a) and the mouse (Leung et al., 1988). The physiologically based model used in these studies was very similar to that used for polychlorinated biphenyl and kepone (Bungay et al., 1979) and 2,3,7,8-tetrachlorodibenzofuran (King et al., 1983). The flow-limited model consisted of compartments assigned to the blood, liver (considered to be the only site of metabolism), fat, skin, and muscle.

The model also incorporated excretion of metabolites through the urine, bile, gut lumen, and feces. The binding of TCDD to blood components was described by a first-order linear process and two types of liver protein receptors, one having a high-affinity and low-capacity (Poland et al., 1976), and the other involving an inducible low-affinity, high-capacity microsomal protein (Voorman and Aust, 1987). Since TCDD was also known to be a potent inducer of hepatic microsomal enzymes (McConnell et al., 1984; Rose et al., 1976; Kociba et al., 1976, 1978), data from single- and multiple-dose studies were used to assess disposition and enzyme induction following oral dosing.

In a subsequent study, Leung et al., (1990b) investigated the effect of a preadministered inducing dose of TCDD, administered intraperitoneally 3 days before an intraperitoneal dose of 2-[$^{125}$I]iodo-3,7,8-trichlorodibenzo-*p*-dioxin (ITCDD), on the tissue distribution and pharmacokinetic behavior of the TCDD analogue in mice. Control animals were dosed with ITCDD alone, and these had the highest concentration in the fat. The pretreated animals had the highest concentration of ITCDD in their livers. In both control and pretreated mice, the whole-body elimination of ITCDD followed first-order kinetics, but the rate of excretion for the pretreated mice, ($t_{1/2} = 8.0$ days), was almost twice as fast as that for the control animals, ($t_{1/2} = 14.2$ days).

Microsomal ITCDD-binding protein in the liver was increased by about 12-fold in the pretreated mice, and the overall metabolism rate was increased threefold in these animals. It was clear that the principal factor that influenced the liver/fat concentration ratio was the affinity and capacity of the microsomal ITCDD-binding proteins. The principal organ concentrations, enzyme activity, and induction, as well as the interpretation of tissue concentration data for single and repeated doses, was considered to be accommodated very well by the physiological model.

A suitable physiologically based fugacity model has been used (Kissell and Robarge, 1988) to predict successfully the uptake and elimination of TCDD in humans. The data were obtained from previous reports of studies with Ranch Hand veterans who were known to have adipose tissue levels of at least 10 ppt (Wolfe et al., 1988) and from a study in which an individual ingested 105 ng of tritiated TCDD (Poiger and Schlatter, 1986). Excretion half-lives ranged from 20 to 4.4 years for veterans who had adipose levels ranging from 10 to 100 ppt and 6.7 years for the single dose in the human who had an adipose tissue concentration of 9.0 ppt. Unfortunately, these publications did not report on metabolism or binding in the liver.

In more recent studies, tissue distribution and elimination, as well as receptor interactions, have been studied (Weber et al., 1993; McKinley et al., 1993; Kedderis, 1993; McLachlan, 1993).

## V. SUMMARY AND CONCLUSIONS

The mechanism by which toxic substances exert their effects is an important consideration in toxicological risk assessment. In this chapter, we have focused on mathematical models for receptor binding mechanisms that may be involved in chemical toxicity. Of particular interest are the Hill and Michaelis–Menten equations, which have found application in a study of several toxic substances. Although the Michaelis–Menten equations are linear at low doses, the Hill equation can be linear ($n = 1$), sublinear ($n < 1$) or supralinear ($n > 1$), depending on the value of the Hill exponent $n$.

Receptor binding appears to play an important role in the induction of toxic effects of TCDD. Considerable work has been done on the development of biologically based models for both receptor binding and pharmacokinetics of TCDD. Pharmacodynamic models for tumor induction are also available (Thorslund and Charnley 1988; Tritscher et al., 1992; Luebeck et al., 1991). Ultimately, these results can be combined to obtain an integrated biologically based model of TCDD carcinogenesis (Andersen et al., 1993; Kohn et al., 1994). The receptor-binding models detailed in this paper will play an important role in the development of a comprehensive biologically based model for TCDD carcinogenesis.

## REFERENCES

Adair, G. S. (1925). The hemoglobin system vs. the oxygen dissociation curve of hemoglobin. *J. Biol. Chem.,* 63, 529.

Andersen, M. E., J. J. Mills, M. L. Gargas, L. Kedderis, L. S. Birnbaum, D. Neubert, and W. F. Greenlee (1993). Modeling receptor mediated processes with dioxin: implications for pharmacokinetics and risk assessment. *Risk Analysis,* 13, 25–36.

Ariens, E. J. (1954). Affinity and intrinsic activity in the theory of competitive inhibition, *Arch. Int. Pharmacodyn.,* 99, 32–50.

Ariens, E. J. (1964). *Molecular Pharmacology,* Academic Press, New York.

Barett, J. C. (1992). Mechanisms of action of known human carcinogens. In: *Mechanisms of Carcinogenesis in Risk Identification,* (H. Vainio, P. Magee, D. McGregor and A. J. McMichael, eds.), IARC Scientific Publications No. 116, Lyon, pp. 115–134.

Boeynaens, J. M., and J. E. Dumont (1980). *Outlines of Receptor Theory,* Elsevier/North-Holland, New York.

Bombick, D. W., J. Jankun, K. Tullis, and F. Matsumura (1988). 2,3,7,8-Tetrachlorodibenzo-*p*-dioxin causes increases in expression of c-*erb-A* and levels of protein–tyrosine kinases in selected tissues of responsive mouse strains, *Proc. Natl. Acad. Sci. USA,* 85, 4128–4132.

Bradfield, C. A., A. S. Kende, and A. Poland (1988). Kinetic and equilibrium studies of Ah receptor–ligand binding: Use of [$^{125}$I]2-iodo-7,8-dibromodibenzo-*p*-dioxin, *Mol. Pharmacol.,* 34, 229–237.

Bradfield, C. A., and A. Poland (1988). A competitive binding assay for 2,3,7,8-Tetrachlorodibenzo-*p*-dioxin and related ligands of the Ah receptor, *Mol. Pharmacol.,* 34, 682–688.

Bungay, P. M., R. L. Dedrick, and H. B. Matthews (1979). Pharmacokinetics of halogenated hydrocarbons, *Ann. N.Y. Acad. Sci.,* 7, 257–270.

[CDC] Centers for Disease Control and Prevention (1989). Preliminary report: 2,3,7,8-Tetrachlorodibenzo-*p*-dioxin exposure to humans—Seveso, Italy. *JAMA,* 261, 831–832.

[CDC] Centers for Disease Control Veterans Health Studies (1988). Serum 2,3,7,8-tetrachlorodibenzo-*p*-dioxin levels in US Army Vietnam-era veterans. *JAMA,* 260, 1249–1254.

Clark, A. J. (1933). *The Mode of Action of Drugs on Cells.* E. Arnold & Co., London.

Clark, G. C., M. J. Taylor, A. M. Tritscher, and G. W. Lucier (1991). Tumor necrosis factor involvement in 2,3,7,8-tetrachlorodibenzo-*p*-dioxin (TCDD) mediated endotoxin hypersensitivity in C57B1/6J mice congenic at the *Ah* locus, *Toxicol. Appl. Pharmacol.,* 000–000.

Cook, J. C., and W. F. Greenlee (1989). Characterization of a specific binding protein for 2,3,7,8-tetrachlorodibenzo-*p*-dioxin in human thymic epithelial cells, *Mol. Pharmacol.,* 35, 713–719.

Denis, M., S. Cuthill, A.-C. Wikstrom, L. Poellinger, and J.-A. Gustafsson (1988). Association of the dioxin receptor with the $M_r$ 90,000 heat-shock protein, *Biochem. Biophys. Res. Commun.,* 155, 801–807.

Denison, M. S., P. A. Harper, and A. B. Okey (1986). Ah receptor for 2,3,7,8-tetrachlorodibenzo-*p*-dioxin. Codistribution of unoccupied receptor with cytosolic marker enzymes during fractionation of mouse liver, rat liver and cultured Hepalc1c7 cells, *Eur. J. Biochem.,* 155, 223–229.

Denison, M. S., J. M. Fisher, and J. O. P. Whitlock, Jr. (1988). The DNA recognition site for the dioxin–Ah receptor complex: Nucleotide sequence and functional analysis, *Biochem. Biophys. Res.,* 263, 17221–17224.

Denison, M. S., J. M. Fisher, and J. P. Whitlock, Jr. (1989). Protein–DNA interactions at recognition sites for the dioxin–Ah receptor complex, *J. Biol. Chem.,* 264, 16478–16482.

Dixon, M. (1972). The graphical determination of $K_m$ and $K_i$, *Biochem. J.,* 129, 197–202.

Eisenthal, R., and A. Cornish-Bowden (1974). The direct linear plot, *Biochem. J.,* 139, 715–720.

[EPA] Environmental Protection Agency (1986). Guidelines for carcinogen risk assessment. *Federal Register,* 51, 33993–34014.

Fisher, J. M., K. W. Jones, and J. P. Whitlock, Jr. (1989). Activation of transcription as a general mechanism of 2,3,7,8-tetrachlorodibenzo-*p*-dioxin action, *Mol. Carcinog.,* 1, 216–221.

Fujisawa-Sehara, A., K. Sogawa, M. Yamane, and Y. Fujii-Kuriyama (1987). Characterization of xenobiotic responsive elements upstream from the drug-metabolizing cytochrome P-450c gene: A similarity to glucocorticoid regulatory elements, *Nucleic Acids Res.,* 15, 4179–4191.

Goddard, M. J., and Krewski, D. (1995). The future of mechanistic research in risk assessment: Where are we going and can we get there from here, *Toxicology* (in press).

Goldstcin, J. A., and S. Safe (1989). Mechanism of action and structure–activity relationships for the chlorinated dibenzo-*p*-dioxins and related compounds. In *Halogenated Biphenyls, Terphenyls, Naphthalenes, Dibenzodioxins, and Related Products* (R. D. Kimbrough and A. A. Jensen, eds.), Elsevier, New York, pp. 239–293.

Graham, F. J., G. W. Lucier, P. Linko, R. R. Maronpot, and J. A. Goldstein (1988). Increases in cytochrome P-450 mediated β-estradiol 2-hydroxylase activity in rat liver microsomes after both acute administration and subchronic administration of 2,3,7,8-tetrachlorodibenzo-*p*-dioxin in a two-stage hepatocarcinogenesis model, *Carcinogenesis,* 9, 1935–1941.

Harper, P. A., C. L. Golas, and A. B. Okey (1988). Characterization of the Ah receptor and aryl hydrocarbon hydroxylase induction by 2,3,7,8-tetrachlorodibenzo-*p*-dioxin and benzo[*a*]pyrene in the human A431 squamous cell carcinoma line, *Cancer Res.,* 48, 2388–2395.

Hill, A. V. (1910). The possible effects of the aggregation of the molecules of haemoglobin on its dissociation curves. *J. Physiol.,* 40, 4–7.

Hirst, M. A., K. W. Jones, and J. P. Whitlock, Jr. (1989). Activation of cytochrome P450IA1 gene expression buy 2,3,7,8-tetrachlorodibenzo-*p*-dioxin in wild-type and high-activity variant mouse hepatoma cells, *Mol. Carcinog.*, 2, 40–46.

Jones, P. B. C., L. K. Durrin, D. R. Galeazzi, and J. P. Whitlock, Jr. (1986). Control of cytochrome P1-450 gene expression: Analysis of dioxin-responsive enhancer system, *Proc. Natl. Acad. Sci. USA*, 83, 2802–2806.

Kedderis, L. B., M. E. Andersen, and L. S. Birnbaum (1993). Effect of dose, time and pretreatment on the biliary excretion and tissue distribution of 2,3,7,8-tetrachlorodibenzo-*p*-dioxin in the rat, *Fundam. Appl. Toxicol.*, 21, 405–411.

King, F. G., R. L. Dedrick, J. M. Collins, H. B. Matthews, and L. S. Birnbaum (1983). Physiological model for the pharmacokinetics of 2,3,7,8-tetrachlorodibenzofuran in several species, *Toxiol. Appl. Pharmacol.*, 67, 390–400.

Kissel, J. C., and G. M. Robarge (1988). Assessing the elimination of 2,3,7,8-TCDD from humans with a physiologically based pharmacokinetic model, *Chemosphere*, 17, 2017–2027.

Kociba, R. J., P. A. Keeler, C. N. Park, and P. J. Gehring (1976). 2,3,7,8-Tetrachlorodibenzo-*p*-dioxin (TCDD): Results of a 13-week oral toxicity study in rats, *Toxicol. Appl. Pharmacol.*, 35, 553.

Kociba, R. (1984). Evaluation of the carcinogenic and mutagenic potential of 2,3,7,8-TCDD and other chlorinated dioxins. In *Biological Mechanisms of Dioxin Action,* (A. Poland and R. D. Kimbrough, eds.), Cold Spring Harbor Laboratory, Cold Spring Harbor, NY, pp. 73–84.

Kociba, R. J., D. G. Keyes, J. E. Beyer, R. M. Carreon, C. E. Wade, D. A. Dittenber, R. P. Kainins, L. E. Frauson, C. N. Park, S. D. Bernard, R. A. Hummel, and C. G. Humiston (1978). Results of a two-year chronic toxicity and oncogenicity study of 2,3,7,8-tetrachlorodibenzo-*p*-dioxin in rats, *Toxicol. Appl. Pharmacol.*, 46, 279–303.

Kohn, M. C., and C. J. Portier (1993). A model of effects of TCDD on expression of rat liver proteins, *Risk Analy.*, 13, 565–572.

Kohn, M. C., G. W. Lucier, G. C. Clark, C. Sewall, A. M. Tritscher, and C. J. Portier (1993). A mechanistic model of the effects of dioxin on gene expression in the rat liver. *Toxicol. Appl. Pharmacol.*, 120, 138–154.

Langley, J. N. (1905). On the reaction of cells and nerve-endings to certain poisons, chiefly as regards to the reaction of striated muscle to nicotine and to curari. *J. Physiol.*, 33, 374–413.

Langmuir, L. (1918). The adsorption of gases on plane surfaces of glass, mica and platinum. *J. Am. Chem. Soc.*, 40, 1361–1403.

Leung, H., A. Poland, D. J. Paustenbach, F. J. Murray, and M. E. Andersen (1990b). Pharmacokinetics of [125I]-2-iodo-3,7,8-trichlorodibenzo-*p*-dioxin in mice: Analysis with a physiological modelling approach, *Toxicol. Appl. Pharmacol.*, 103, 411–419.

Leung, H., D. J. Paustenbach, F. J. Murray, and M. E. Andersen (1988). A physiologically based pharmacokinetic model for 2,3,7,8-tetrachlorodibenzo-*p*-dioxin in C57BL/2J mice, *Toxicol. Lett.*, 42, 15–28.

Leung, H. W., D. J. Paustenbach, F. J. Murray, and M. E. Andersen (1990a). A physiological pharmacokinetic description of the tissue distribution and enzyme-inducing properties of 2,3,7,8-tetrachlorodibenzo-*p*-dioxin in the rat, *Toxicol. Appl. Pharmacol.*, 103, 399–410.

Lucier, G. W. (1992). Receptor mediated carcinogenesis. In *Mechanisms of Carcinogenesis in Risk Identification* (H. Vainio, P. N. Magee, D. B. McGregor, and A. J. McMichael, eds.), IARC Scientific Publication No. 116, International Agency for Research on Cancer, Lyon, pp. 87–112.

Luebeck, E. G., S. H. Moolgavkar, A. Buchmann, and M. Schwartz (1991). Effects of polychlorinated biphenyls in rat liver: Quantitative analysis of enzyme altered foci, *Toxicol. Appl. Pharmacol.*, 111, 469–484.

Mably, T. A., H. M. Theobals, G. B. Ingall, and R. E. Peterson (1990). Hypergastrinemia is associated with decreased gastric acid secretion in 2,3,7,8-tetrachlorodibenzo-*p*-dioxin-treated rats, *Toxicol. Appl. Pharmacol.*, 106, 219–250.

Madhukar, B. V., D. W. Brewster, and F. Matsumura (1984). Effects of in vivo administered 2,3,7,8-tetrachlorodibenzo-*p*-dioxin on receptor binding of epidermal growth factor in the hepatic plasma membrane of rat, guinea pig, mouse and hamster, *Proc. Natl. Acad. Sci. USA*, 81, 7407–7411.

Manchester, D. K., S. K. Gordon, C. L. Golas, E. A. Roberts, and A. B Okey (1987). Ah receptor in human placenta: Stabilization by molybdate and characterization of binding of 2,3,7,8-tetrachlorodibenzo-*p*-dioxin, 3-methylcholanthrene, and benzo[*a*]pyrene, *Cancer Res.,* 47, 4861–4868.

McConnell, E. E., J. A. Moore, J. K. Haseman, and M. W. Harris (1978). The comparative toxicity of chlorinated dibenzo-*p*-dioxin in mice and guinea pigs, *Toxicol. Appl. Pharmacol.,* 44, 335–356.

McConnell, E. E., G. W. Lucier, R. C. Rumbaugh, P. W. Albro, D. J. Harvan, J. R. Hass, and M. W. Harris (1984). Dioxin in soil: Bioavailability after ingestion by rats and guinea pigs, *Science,* 223, 1077–1079.

McKinley, M. K., L. B. Kedderis, and L. S. Birnbaum (1993). The effect of pretreatment on the biliary excretion of 2,3,7,8-tetrachlorodibenzo-*p*-dioxin, 2,3,7,8-tetrachlorodibenzofuran, and 3,3′,4,4′-tetrachlorobiphenyl in the rat, *Fundam. Appl. Toxicol.,* 21, 425–432.

McLachlan, M. S. (1993). Digestive tract absorption of polychlorinated dibenzo-*p*-dioxins, dibenzofurans and biphenyls in a nursing infant, *Toxicol. Appl. Pharmacol.,* 123, 68–72.

Mebus, C. A., V. R. Reddy, and W. M. Piper (1987). Depression of rat testicular 1-hydroxylase and 17,20-lyase after administration of 2,3,7,8-tetrachlorodibenzo-*p*-dioxin, *Biochem. Pharmacol.,* 36, 727–731.

Metzler, M. (1984). Metabolism of stilbene estrogen and steroidal estrogens in relation to carcinogenicity, *Arch. Toxicol.,* 22, 104–109.

Michaelis, L., and M. L. Menten (1913). Die kinetik der invertinwirkung, *Biochem. Z.,* 49, 333–369.

[NTP] National Toxicology Program (1982). Bioassay of 2,3,7,8-tetrachlorodibenzo-*p*-dioxin for possible carcinogenicity (gavage study), Technical Report Series No. 102, National Toxicology Program, Research Triangle Park, NC.

Nebert, D. W., F. M. Goujan, and J. E. Gielen (1972). Aryl hydrocarbon hydroxylase induction by polycyclic hydrocarbons: Simple autosomal dominant trait in the mouse, *Nature New Biol.,* 2236, 107–110.

Neuhold, L. A., F. J. Gonzales, A. K. Jaiswal, and D. W. Nebert (1986). Dioxin-inducible enhancer region upstream from the mouse P1-450 gene and interaction with heterologous SV40 promoter, *DNA,* 5, 403–411.

Neuhold, L. A., Y. Shirayoshi, K. Ozato, J. E. Jones, and D. W. Nebert (1989). Regulation of mouse *CYP1A1* gene expression by dioxin: Requirement of two *cis*-acting elements during induction, *Mol. Cell. Biol.,* 9, 2378–2386.

Okey, A. B., L. M. Vella, and P. A. Harper (1989). Detection and characterization of a "low-affinity" form of the cytosolic Ah receptor in livers of mice "nonresponsive" to induction of cytochrome P1-450 by 3-methylcholanthrene, *Mol. Pharmacol.,* 35, 823–830.

Okey, A. B., G. P. Bondy, M. E. Mason, D. W. Nebert, et al. (1980). Temperature-dependent cytosol-to-nucleus translocation of the Ah receptor for 2,3,7,8-tetrachlorodibenzo-*p*-dioxin in continuous cell culture lines, *J. Biol. Chem.,* 255, 11415–11422.

Perdew, G. H. (1988). Association of the Ah receptor with the 90-kDa heat shock protein, *J. Biol. Chem.,* 263, 13802–13805.

Pitot, H. C., and H. A. Campbell (1987). An approach to the relative potencies of chemical agents during the stages of initiation and promotion in multistage hepatocarcinogenesis in the rat, *Environ. Health Perspect.,* 76, 49–56.

Poiger, H., and C. Schlatter (1986). Pharmacokinetics of 2,3,7,8-TCDD in man, *Chemosphere,* 15, 1489–1494.

Poland, A., and J. C. Knutson (1982). 2,3,7,8-tetrachlorodibenzo-*p*-dioxin and related halogenated aromatic hydrocarbons: Examination of the mechanism of toxicity, *Annu. Rev. Pharmacol. Toxicol.,* 22, 517–554.

Poland, A., E. Glover, and A. S. Kende (1976). Stereospecific, high affinity binding of 2,3,7,8-tetrachlorodibenzo-*p*-dioxin by hepatic cytosol, *J. Biol. Chem.,* 251, 4936–4946.

Portier, C., A. Tritscher, M. Kohn, C. Sewall, G. Clark, L. Edley, D. G. Huel, and G. Lucier (1993). Ligand/receptor binding for 2,3,7,8-TCDD: Implications for risk assessment. *Fundam. Appl. Toxicol.,* 20, 48–56.

Romkes, M., J. Piskorska-Pliszczynska, and S. Safe (1987). Effects of 2,3,7,8-tetrachlorodibenzo-*p*-dioxin on hepatic and uterine estrogen receptor levels in rats, *Toxicol. Appl. Pharmacol.,* 87, 306–314.

Rose, J. Q., J. C. Ramsey, T. H. Wentzler, R. A. Hummel, and P. J. Gehring (1976). The fate of 2,3,7,8-tetrachlorodibenzo-*p*-dioxin following single and repeated oral doses to the rat, *Toxicol. Appl. Pharmacol.,* 36, 209–226.

Safe, S. H. (1986). Comparative toxicology and mechanism of action of polychlorinated dibenzo-*p*-dioxins and dibenzofurans, *Ann. Rev. Pharmacol. Toxicol.,* 26, 371–399.

Shen, E. S., and J. P. Whitlock, Jr. (1989). The potential role of DNA methylation in the response to 2,3,7,8-tetrachlorodibenzo-*p*-dioxin, *J. Biol. Chem.,* 264, 17754–17758.

Silbergeld, E. K., and T. A. Gasiewicz (1989). Dioxins and the Ah receptor, *Am. J. Ind. Med.,* 16, 455–474.

Sunahara, G. I., G. W. Lucier, Z. McCoy, E. M. Bresnick, E. R. Sanchez, and K. G. Nelson (1989). Characterization of 2,3,7,8-tetrachlorodibenzo-*p*-dioxin-mediated decreases in dexamethasone binding to rat hepatic cytosolic glucocorticoid receptor, *Mol. Pharmacol.,* 36, 239–247.

Thomas, P. E., L. M. Reik, D. E. Ryan, and W. Levin (1983). Induction of two immunochemically related rat liver cytochrome P-450 isozymes, P-450c and P-450d, by structurally diverse xenobiotics, *J. Biol. Chem.,* 258, 4590–4598.

Thomas, P. E., R. E. Kouri, and J. J. Hutton (1972). The genetics of arylhydrocarbon hydroxylase induction in mice: A single gene difference between C57BL/6J and DBA/2J, *Biochem. Genet.,* 6, 157–168.

Thorslund, T., and G. Charnley (1988). Quantitative dose–response models for tumour promoting agents. In *Carcinogen Risk Assessment: New Directions in Qualitative and Quantitative Aspects,* (R. W. Hart and F. D. Hoerger, eds.). Barbury Report 31, Cold Spring Harbor Laboratory, Cold Spring Harbor, pp. 245–256.

Tritscher, A. M., J. A. Goldstein, C. J. Portier, Z. McCoy, G. C. Clark and G. W. Lucier (1992). Dose-response relationships for chronic exposure to 2,3,7,8-tetrachlorodibenzo-*p*-dioxin in a rat tumor promotion model: Quantification and immunolocalization of CYP1A1 and CYP1A2 in the liver, *Cancer Res.,* 52: 3436–3442.

Turtletaub, K. W., J. S. Felton, J. S. Vogel, E. G. Snyderwine, S. S. Thorgeirsson, R. H. Adamson, B. L. Gledhill, and J. C. David (1991). Low-dose DNA adduct dosimetry by accelerator mass spectrometry (AMS), *Toxicology,* 11, 131.

Tuteja, N., F. J. Gonzalez, and D. W. Nebert (1985). Developmental and tissue-specific differential regulation of the mouse dioxin-inducible P1-450 and P3-450 genes, *Dev. Biol.,* 112, 177–184.

Voorman, R., and S. D. Aust (1987). Specific binding of polyhalogenated aromatic hydrocarbon inducers of cytochrome P-450d to the cytochrome and inhibition of its estradiol 2-hydroxylase activity, *Toxicol. Appl. Pharmacol.,* 90, 69–78.

Wassom, J. S., J. E. Huff, and N. Loprieno (1977). A review of the genetic toxicology of chlorinated dibenzo-*p*-dioxins, *Mutat. Res.,* 47, 141–160.

Weber, L. W., S. W. Ernst, B. U. Stahl, and K. Rozman (1993). Tissue distribution and toxicokinetics of 2,3,7,8-tetrachlorodibenzo-*p*-dioxin in rats after intravenous injection, *Fundam. Appl. Toxicol.,* 21, 523–534.

Whitlock, J. P., Jr., and D. R. Galeazzi (1984). 2,3,7,8-Tetrachlorodibenzo-*p*-dioxin receptors in wild-type and variant mouse hepatoma cells, *J. Biol. Chem.,* 259, 980–985.

Whitlock, J. P. (1990). Genetic and molecular aspects of 2,3,7,8-tetrachlorodibenzo-*p*-dioxin action, *Annu. Rev. Pharmacol. Toxicol.,* 30, 251–277.

Wolfe, W., J. Miner, and M. Paterson (1988). Serum 2,3,7,8-tetrachlorodibenzo-*p*-dioxin levels in Air Force health study participants—preliminary report, *J. Am. Med. Assoc.,* 259, 3533–3535.

# 25
# Statistical Analysis of Heritable Mutagenesis Data

**Walter W. Piegorsch**
*University of South Carolina*
*Columbia, South Carolina*

## I. INTRODUCTION

The objective of heritable mutagenesis studies is to evaluate some toxic chemical's potential to induce genetic damage that leads to disorders in *offspring* of test subjects (i.e., transmissible genetic damage induced in the subjects' germ cells; Maxwell and Newell, 1973; Russell and Kelly, 1982; Shelby, 1988; Shelby et al., 1993). Typically, laboratory animals are employed as test subjects. For example, in a common design, male (or female) rodents are administered the agent of interest, mated with untreated partners, and their offspring are examined to determine whether or not chemically related heritable genetic effects are observed. Several different assays are available for studying such heritable damage, each of which centers its attention on a different type of genetic toxicity (Russell and Shelby, 1985). These assays include the dominant lethal test (Generoso, 1973; Generoso and Piegorsch, 1993; Green and Springer, 1973), the heritable translocation test (Bishop and Kodell, 1980; Léonard, 1975), and the specific locus test (Selby and Olson, 1981). In these assays, data are obtained on various stages of germ cell production. The data may involve embryonic or zygotic damage (Generoso et al., 1991), effects on conceptual implantation, or fetal mortality. Conceptual damage is always associated with some mutagenic event in the germ cells of the exposed parent (Shelby et al., 1993). [This contrasts with the issue of in utero developmental damage and its associated statistical concerns, as seen, e.g., in developmental teratogenicity studies (Piegorsch and Haseman, 1991; Ryan, 1992).]

There are several important statistical issues associated with the analysis of heritable mutagenesis data. These include determination of the appropriate experimental unit, the selection of appropriate methodology for data analysis, and sample size and power considerations. Each of these issues will be discussed briefly in this chapter, using as a common paradigm the male dominant lethal assay in mice (Generoso and Piegorsch, 1993). For purposes of risk assessment, this assay is often conduced as an identifying screen and, then, usually at only two treatment levels: a control and a single dose of the mutagenic stimulus. Thus, the discussion herein will center on two-group statistical comparisons for heritable mutagenesis data.

## II.  IDENTIFICATION OF THE EXPERIMENTAL UNIT

The experimental unit in any toxicity study or bioassay is the sampling unit to which the treatment is applied. Proper identification of this unit is important, since statistical analyses of the data require its precise definition. For a standard heritable mutagenesis study, the experimental unit is the exposed parent. (Technically, individual conceptuses are not exposed directly to the chemical agent under test.) For this example, data recorded on individual conceptuses from the same female's litter represent multiple observations on a single experimental unit, and it is likely that the individual conceptual responses will be correlated (Piegorsch and Haseman, 1991). If this correlation is not taken into account, any calculated test statistics or confidence intervals could be adversely affected. In particular, tests that are being performed ostensibly at the $\alpha = 0.05$ significance level may actually be operating at some higher, unknown level. Numerous investigators [e.g., Haseman and Soares (1975) and Lockhart et al. (1992)] have carried out calculations that illustrate the exaggerated significance a "per-conceptus" test can engender when applied to heritable mutagenesis data, producing misleading results. To avoid this serious form of analytic error, the experimental unit for statistical evaluation, and the level at which this evaluation and analysis occurs, should not be the conceptus. Commonly, therefore, the *litter* is taken as the experimental unit in most developmental assays.

On occasion, such as in male mouse dominant lethal testing, the male is the experimental unit, since it is technically the sampling unit that receives the exposure. It has been noted, however, that little if any additional "male effect" in these studies is observed beyond the effect caused by per-conceptus correlations within a litter (Aeschbacher et al., 1977; Epstein et al., 1972; Lockhart et al., 1992; Smith and James, 1984). Hence, the litter can serve as the unit of analysis here as well, although this lack of a male effect should be corroborated when any new data or assays are brought under study [cf, e.g., Lockhart et al. (1992)]. The statistical methods discussed in the following all consider the litter, rather than the conceptus, as the basic experimental unit.

## III.  NOTATION

Assume that there are two experimental (control plus treated) groups in a given study. If some ordered score variable, such as dose, is recorded at the treated level, we denote it by $x_1$, whereas $x_0 = 0$ is the control "dose." Within each experimental group, assume that there are $J_i$ litters ($i = 0,1$) and within each litter there are $N_{ij}$ conceptuses ($i = 0,1$; $j = 1,2, \ldots J_i$). We denote by $Y_{ijk}$ the response of the $k$th conceptus within the $j$th litter of the $i$th treatment group. This can be considered the per conceptus response. The corresponding per litter response will be the sum of these individual indicators, denoted by $Y_{ij} = \sum_{j=1}^{J_i} Y_{ijk}$.

To illustrate the notation, if the endpoint of interest is conceptual resorption, then $Y_{ijk} = 0$ if the $k$th implant in the $j$th litter of the $i$th treatment group is viable, and $Y_{ijk} = 1$ if it is a resorption. $Y_{ij}$ is then the total number of resorbed conceptuses in the $j$th litter of the $i$th treatment group.

## IV.  STATISTICAL ANALYSIS FOR DISCRETE RESPONSE VARIABLES

The primary focus of this chapter is on the analysis of discrete variables, and a variety of statistical procedures have been proposed for this purpose. The two most common approaches are (1) nonparametric (rank-based) methods, and (2) procedures based on underlying distributional assumptions and data modeling. Before discussing the various methods, however, an important preliminary issue must be addressed.

## A. Number Versus Proportion Affected

Let $Y_{ij}$ denote the total number of resorptions in the $j$th litter of the $i$th experimental group. Since the ranges of values of $Y_{ij}$ is limited by the litter size $N_{ij}$, it is logical to base statistical analyses on the proportion of affected conceptuses (i.e., $R_{ij} = Y_{ij}/N_{ij}$). Indeed, statistical analyses based on $R_{ij}$, rather than $Y_{ij}$, are recommended, since there are many problems with use of $Y_{ij}$ that can disturb or confound the statistical analysis. For instance, Haseman and Soares (1976) have shown that, for three large populations of mice, the proportion of affected conceptuses is less dependent on litter size than is the number of affected conceptuses. One simple way to avoid these problems is to correct $Y_{ij}$ by dividing it by the number at risk (i.e., take $R_{ij} = Y_{ij}/N_{ij}$).

## B. Nonparametric Methods

When interest centers on the proportion of affected conceptuses, $R_{ij} = Y_{ij}/N_{ij}$, analyses are often based on the basic sampling model for proportions: the binomial distribution. Unfortunately, this simple model does not fit well under per litter sampling (Haseman and Kupper, 1979; Haseman and Soares, 1976; Lockhart et al., 1992), and simple statistical distributions, such as the binomial, may be inappropriate to describe the sampling distribution of $Y_{ij}$ or $R_{ij}$. Thus, any analyses based on estimating parameters from the binomial model (i.e., "parametric" binomial methods) may lead to suspect or erroneous inferences about the heritable mutagenesis of the chemical or other stimulus under study.

Distribution-free (nonparametric) methods are an alternative to parametric models for the $R_{ij}$. These assume no specific parametric form for the sampling distribution of $R_{ij}$, although they do concede the existence of a parameter, $p_i$, which is the probability of resorption at treatment level $i$. Thus, the basic null hypothesis of no treatment effect translates to no difference in the underlying proportions: $H_0 : p_0 = p_1$. The alternative hypothesis is a one-sided increase due to chemical treatment: $H_a : p_0 < p_1$.

Basic forms of distribution-free tests for $H_0$ involve computations that substitute the observations with their ranks. Analyses based on ranks are well known, such as the Mann–Whitney–Wilcoxon test for two-sample comparisons (Lehmann, 1975). This method is fairly straightforward, and can be useful for per litter analyses (Piegorsch and Haseman, 1991).

These rank-based methods carry with them an implicit assumption that the variances (or, more generally, the *shapes* of the probability distributions) of the observed proportions $R_{ij}$, must be equivalent. This assumption may not always hold; it is most often invalidated when large disparities exist among the $N_{ij}$. (When large disparities are evidenced, the applicability of the Mann–Whitney–Wilcoxon test would be brought into question.) In addition, corrections are recommended if there are tied observations, especially at a single rank value (Haseman and Hoel, 1974; Lin and Haseman, 1976), since calculation of the test statistic may be ambiguous or impossible when many (tied) observations carry the same risk. The basic form of such a correction simply replaces the ranks of tied values with their midranks (i.e., for two or more tied observations, calculate the average rank among the tied values, and employ this average "midrank" for each tied observation in the test statistic). Lehmann (1975) provides further details for this approach.

For data in the form of proportions, an additional distribution-free method exists that may be applied to nonbinomial proportions (Piegorsch et al., 1994). Instead of manipulating the ranks of the observations, the method employs other statistical aspects of the data to arrive at inferences concerning treatment versus control effects. The distribution-free test statistic is based on so-called permutation methodology (Crump et al., 1991; Mantel, 1963), a paradigm that calls for rearrangement of the observations into all possible combinations under $H_0$: $p_0 = p_1$. Each rearrangement is compared with the magnitude of the actual difference, $p_1 - p_0$, observed in the data. $H_0$ is rejected if the observed difference is seen to be associated with one of the more unlikely or extreme rearrangements. No parametric statistical assumptions, such as binomial distribution sampling, are required.

In moderate to large samples—say, when $J_i \geq 10$ in both groups—calculation of the test statistic may be simplified. The test statistic is a ratio that is constructed in two stages: first, the numerator is calculated, based on a simple pairwise comparison between the two groups' *pooled* proportion of resorptions, $\bar{p}_{0+} - \bar{p}_{1+}$, where $\bar{p}_{i+} = \sum_{j=1}^{J_i} Y_{ij} / \sum_{j=1}^{J_i} N_{ij}$ ($i = 0,1$). The second stage employs an empirical estimate of variation in the denominator to gauge the strength of the difference in pooled proportions. Hence, the ratio may be termed an *empirical* test statistic:

$$Z_e = \frac{\bar{p}_{1+} - \bar{p}_{0+}}{s \left/ \sqrt{J_0 J_1 / (J_0 + J_1)}\right.}$$

where $s$ is the empirical standard deviation. The simplest choice for this estimate is based on the pooled sample variance of the $R_{ij}$'s under $H_0$; that is, calculate

$$s^2 = \frac{\sum_{i=0}^{1} \sum_{j=1}^{J_i} R_{ij}^2 - \frac{1}{J_0 + J_1} \left( \sum_{i=0}^{1} \sum_{j=1}^{J_i} R_{ij} \right)^2}{J_0 + J_1 - 1},$$

then, use $s = \sqrt{s^2}$. The one-sided test rejects when $Z_e$ is greater than an upper-$\alpha$ critical point from a standard normal reference distribution. (For example, at $\alpha = 0.05$, the upper-$\alpha$ critical point is 1.645.) Lockhart et al. (1992) showed that this empirical text exhibited very stable properties when applied to heritable mutagenesis data. They recommended it for use in settings where no distributional and parametric assumptions can be made for analyzing results from a dominant lethal experiment.

## C. Procedures Based on Assumed Parametric or Semiparametric Models

In some instances, it may be possible to accept selected assumptions on the distribution of the $R_{ij}$, or on the actual (parametric) form of the dose–response from a heritable mutagenesis experiment. If so, then parametric methods might be considered for the data analysis. (Use of any parametric model involves sacrifice of the wide applicability associated with distribution-free methods. This is in exchange for increased efficiency when the postulated model is, in fact, correct.)

One well-studied form of parametric analysis for heritable mutagenesis data is an important generalization of the basic binomial sampling model. It is known as the $\beta$-binomial sampling model, and it extends the binomial model to account for extra variability induced by the per litter sampling effect (Aeschbacher et al., 1977; Chen and Kodell, 1989; Kodell et al., 1991; Vuataz and Sotek, 1978). This extension includes an intralitter correlation parameter $0 \leq \rho_i < 1$, that measures the excess variability at each treatment level. The probability function assumed under this model is given by

$$\Pr\left[Y_{ij} = y \mid p_i, \rho_i\right] \propto \frac{\Gamma\left(y + p_i \frac{\rho_i}{1 - \rho_i}\right)\Gamma\left(N_{ij} - y + \{1 - p_i\}\frac{\rho_i}{1 - \rho_i}\right)\Gamma\left(\frac{1 - \rho_i}{\rho_i}\right)}{\Gamma\left(p_i \frac{\rho_i}{1 - \rho_i}\right)\Gamma\left(\{1 - p_i\}\frac{\rho_i}{1 - \rho_i}\right)\Gamma\left(\frac{1 - \rho_i}{\rho_i} + N_{ij}\right)}$$

$(i = 0,1; j = 1, \ldots, J_i)$, where $\Gamma(\cdot)$ is the gamma function. When $\rho_0 = \rho_1 = 0$ there is no extra-binomial variability. If this is indicated, simple binomial analyses, such as those described by Haseman and Kupper (1979), would be appropriate. However, this is typically not so with dominant lethal data, and more complex methods are often required for the statistical analysis.

Estimation under the β-binomial model proceeds by maximum likelihood (ML); that is, maximize the likelihood function

$$\mathcal{L} = \prod_{j=1}^{J_0} \Pr\left[y_{0j} \mid p_0, \rho_0\right] \times \prod_{j=1}^{J_1} \Pr\left[y_{1j} \mid p_1, \rho_1\right]$$

relative to the $p_i$ and the $\rho_i$ under the $H_0$-constraint that $p_0 = p_1$. Denote this constrained maximum as $\mathcal{L}_0$. Also calculate the unconstrained maximum likelihood $\mathcal{L}_{max}$, and then take twice the logarithm of their ratio as the test statistic (Pack, 1986): $G^2 = -2\log\{\mathcal{L}_0/\mathcal{L}_{max}\}$. The one-sided test rejects $H_0$ when the signed square root of this value,

$$Z_l = \frac{p_1 - p_0}{|p_1 - p_0|}\sqrt{G^2}$$

is greater than an upper-$\alpha$ critical point from a standard normal reference distribution. As might be expected, these calculations require a computer for their implementation (Brooks, 1984; Smith, 1983). Typically, the $p_i$ are unknown and we replace them in $Z_l$ with their estimates $\overline{P}_{it}$.

Some simplification of these likelihood-based computations is available under the β-binomial model when it may be assumed that the two correlation parameters, $\rho_0$ and $\rho_1$, are equal (i.e., when $\rho_0 = \rho_1 = \rho$; say). Here, a closed-form trend statistic may be constructed instead (Risko and Margolin, 1988). Assuming without loss of generality that we can take $x_0 = 0$ and $x_1 = 1$ as the control and treatment dose indicators, respectively, a statistic analogous to $Z_e$ is

$$Z_\rho = \frac{\sum_{i=0}^{1}(x_i - \overline{x})\sum_{j=1}^{J_i} Y_{ij}}{\sqrt{\overline{Y}(1 - \overline{Y})\sum_{i=0}^{1}\sum_{j=1}^{J_i}(1 + N_{ij}\widetilde{\rho} - \widetilde{\rho})N_{ij}(x_i - \overline{x})^2}}$$

where $\overline{x} = \sum_{i=0}^{1}\sum_{j=1}^{J_i} N_{ij}x_i / \sum_{i=0}^{1}\sum_{j=1}^{J_i} N_{ij}$, $\overline{Y} = \sum_{i=0}^{1}\sum_{j=1}^{J_i} Y_{ij} / \sum_{i=0}^{1}\sum_{j=1}^{J_i} N_{ij}$, and $\widetilde{\rho}$ is a moment estimator (Srivastava and Wu, 1993; Yamamoto and Yanagimoto, 1992) of the constant intralitter correlation based on the β-binomial model:

$$\widetilde{\rho} = \frac{\frac{\sum_{i=0}^{1}\sum_{j=1}^{J_i}(Y_{ij} - N_{ij}\overline{Y})^2}{\overline{Y}(1 - \overline{Y})} - \left\{\sum_{i=0}^{1}\sum_{j=1}^{J_i} N_{ij} - \frac{\sum_{i=0}^{1}\sum_{j=1}^{J_i} N_{ij}^2}{\sum_{i=0}^{1}\sum_{j=1}^{J_i} N_{ij}}\right\}}{\left[\sum_{i=0}^{1}\sum_{j=1}^{J_i} N_{ij}(N_{ij}-1)\right]\left(1 + \frac{\sum_{i=0}^{1}\sum_{j=1}^{J_i} N_{ij}^2}{\left(\sum_{i=0}^{1}\sum_{j=1}^{J_i} N_{ij}\right)^2}\right) - \frac{2\sum_{i=0}^{1}\sum_{j=1}^{J_i} N_{ij}^2(N_{ij}-1)}{\sum_{i=0}^{1}\sum_{j=1}^{J_i} N_{ij}}}$$

(if $\widetilde{\rho} < 0$ or $\widetilde{\rho} \geq 1$ set $\widetilde{\rho} = 0$ or $\widetilde{\rho} = 1$, respectively.) Notice that if $x_0 = 0$ and $x_1 = 1$, $\overline{x}$ simplifies to $\sum_{j=1}^{J_1} N_{1j}x_i / \sum_{i=0}^{1}\sum_{j=1}^{J_i} N_{ij}$. The one-sided test rejects $H_0$ when $Z_\rho$ is greater than an upper-$\alpha$ critical point from a standard normal reference distribution.

Recent advancements in statistical theory and methodology have made it possible to generalize the β-binomial model discussed in the foregoing to allow for greater applicability. Instead of any specific distributional characterizations, only limited assumptions on the mean and variance of $R_{ij}$ are required. This can be viewed as a generalization of the ML estimation scheme, where the equations used to calculate the ML estimators are modified to take different types of variance structures into account (Fung et al., 1994; Lefkopoulou et al., 1989). These are known as generalized estimating equations (GEEs). Applied to heritable mutagenesis data for the simple case of testing $H_0 : p_0 = p_1$, the GEE test statistic is

$$Z_{\text{GEE}} = \frac{\sum_{i=0}^{1} (x_i - \bar{x}) \sum_{j=1}^{J_i} Y_{ij}}{\sqrt{\sum_{i=0}^{1} (x_i - \bar{x})^2 \sum_{j=1}^{J_i} (Y_{ij} - N_{ij} \bar{\bar{Y}})^2}}$$

where $\bar{x}$ and $\bar{y}$ are the same values as used in $Z_\rho$. The one-sided test rejects $H_0$ when $Z_{\text{GEE}}$ is greater than an upper-α critical point from a standard normal reference distribution.

In a comparative study of the performance of $Z_e$, $Z_l$, $Z_\rho$, and $Z_{\text{GEE}}$ for testing $H_0$, Piegorsch (1993) found that all four are generally stable when the β-binomial model is true. Pack (1986) recommends the likelihood-based $Z_l$ statistic in this case. It is unclear, however, whether the β-binomial model provides a proper fit to data from dominant lethal or other heritable mutagenesis experiments. Lockhart et al. (1992) expressed reservations that this was true with their dominant lethal database, although further study by Garren et al. (1994) has suggested that the β-binomial model may provide a reasonable fit in many instances. The latter study proposes a computer-intensive test for assessing goodness-of-fit of the β-binomial model. If this test were applied to a set of heritable mutagenesis data, and if it suggested that the β-binomial model is not an appropriate model, then only $Z_e$ or $Z_{\text{GEE}}$ would be recommended for use.

## V. SAMPLE SIZE AND POWER CONSIDERATIONS

An important issue in the experimental design of heritable mutagenesis studies is the question of sample size requirements (e.g., how many animals are needed to achieve study objectives?) To determine sample sizes with a specific statistical procedure, the following factors must be specified: (1) The level of significance of the test procedure (generally $\alpha = 0.05$ or $\alpha = 0.01$); (2) the magnitude of the difference, $p_1 - p_0$, that the experimenter hopes to detect; (3) the desired probability (statistical "power") to detect the difference in (2); and (4) the underlying variability of the endpoint of interest. Once these values have been specified, the required sample sizes can be determined.

It is not unusual for sample size tables associated with pairwise comparisons to require computer calculation (Whorton, 1981). This is true, for example, for the empirical test based on $Z_e$. For this, Generoso and Piegorsch (1993) have provided computer-generated powers over a range of sample sizes for performing two-sample empirical tests with proportion endpoints such as $R_{ij}$. These tables can be used to determine sample sizes for pairwise tests in dominant lethal experiments.

Even if no formal sample size or power calculations are carried out, an experimenter planning heritable mutagenesis studies should consider carefully whether or not the available resources are sufficient to detect the magnitude of chemically related effects that are likely to occur. Otherwise, a "negative" study outcome may merely be reflecting an insensitivity of the assay for detecting chemically related effects.

# VI. DISCUSSION

Although there is no single procedure that is accepted as most appropriate for evaluating heritable mutagenesis data, there are certain basic principles for planning the statistical evaluation of such studies. These include (1) the statistical methodology should use the appropriate experimental unit, which usually will be the litter; (2) in multiple-dose or multiple-group studies (not discussed herein), the statistical procedures should take multiple comparisons among the different groups into account (Bristol, 1993; Piegorsch, 1991); and (3) when possible, the statistical methodology should be relatively straightforward and comprehensible both to the statistician and the biologist, and should require as few underlying assumptions as necessary.

From these perspectives, simpler, distribution-free approaches, such as the empirical test using $Z_e$, rank-based methods (Lehmann, 1975), or perhaps the GEE statistic $Z_{GEE}$ are good choices for assessing treatment effects in heritable mutagenesis assays. Nevertheless, one should not automatically dismiss a methodological approach based solely on its computational complexity. Indeed, in the current environment of rapidly increasing computer sophistication, this complexity—once considered a hindrance to implementation—has become less critical. It is conceivable that ultimately certain complex methods may be demonstrated as superior to the simpler methods commonly in use today, especially those that can incorporate per-conceptus covariates (Zeger et al., 1988). Study of the usefulness and value of these methods is an ongoing effort in statistical research (Fung et al., 1994; Piegorsch, 1993).

# ACKNOWLEDGMENT

Thanks are due to Dr. M. D. Shelby of the U. S. National Institute of Environmental Health Sciences, for his helpful suggestions on this exposition.

# REFERENCES

Aeschbacher, H. U., L. Vuataz, J. Sotek, and R. Stalder (1977). Use of the beta-binomial distribution in dominant-lethal testing for "weak mutagenic activity," *Mutat. Res.*, 44, 369–390.

Bishop, J. B., and R. L. Kodell (1980). The heritable translocation assay: Its relationship to assessment of genetic risk for future generations, *Teratogenesis Mutagen. Carcinog*, 1, 305–322.

Bristol, D. R. (1993). One-sided multiple comparisons of response rates with a control. In *Multiple Comparisons, Selection, and Applications in Biometry* (F. M. Hoppe, ed.), Statistics: Textbooks and Monographs, Vol. 134, Marcel Dekker, New York, pp. 77–98.

Brooks, R. J. (1984). Approximate likelihood ratio tests in the analysis of beta-binomial data, *Appl. Stat.*, 33, 285–289.

Chen, J. J., and R. L. Kodell, (1989). Quantitative risk assessment for teratological effects, *J. Am. Stat. Assoc.*, 84, 966–971.

Crump, K. S., R. B. Howe, and R. L. Kodell (1991). Permutation tests for detecting teratogenic effects. In *Statistics in Toxicology* (D. Krewski, and C. Franklin eds.), Gordon and Breach, New York, pp. 349–377.

Epstein, S. S., E. Arnold, J. Andrea, W. Bass, and Y. Bishop (1972). Detection of chemical mutagens by the dominant lethal assay in the mouse, *Toxicol. Appl. Pharmacol.*, 23, 288–325.

Fung, K. Y., D. Krewski, J. N. K. Rao, and A. J. Scott (1994). Tests for trend in developmental toxicity experiments with correlated binary data, *Risk Anal.*, 14, 639–648.

Garren, S. T., R. L. Smith, and W. W. Piegorsch (1994). *Bootstrap Goodness-of-Fit Tests for the beta-Binomial Model*, Technical Report, Mimeo Series No. 2314, Department of Statistics, University of North Carolina, Chapel Hill, NC.

Generoso, W. M. (1973). Evaluation of chromosome aberration effects of chemicals on mouse germ cells, *Environ. Health Perspect.*, 6, 13–22.

Generoso, W. M., and W. W. Piegorsch (1993). Dominant lethal tests in male and female mice. In *Male Reproductive Toxicology* (R. E. Chapen and J. J. Heindel, eds.), Methods in Toxicology, Vol. 3, Academic Press, New York, pp. 124–141.

Generoso, W. M., A. G. Shourbaji, W. W. Piegorsch, and J. B. Bishop (1991). Developmental responses of zygotes exposed to similar mutagens, *Mutat. Res.*, 250, 439–446.

Green, S., and J. A. Springer (1973). The dominant-lethal test: Potential limitations and statistical considerations for safety evaluation, *Environ. Health Perspect.*, 6, 37–46.

Haseman, J. K. and D. G. Hoel (1974). Tables of Gehan's generalized Wilcoxon test with fixed point censoring, *J. Stat. Comput. Simul.* 3, 117–135.

Haseman, J. K., and L. L. Kupper (1979). Analysis of dichotomous response data from certain toxicological experiments, *Biometrics*, 35, 281–293.

Haseman, J. K., and E. R. Soares (1976). The distribution of fetal death in control mice and its implications on statistical tests for dominant lethal effects, *Mutat. Res.*, 41, 277–288.

Kodell, R. L., R. B. Howe, J. J. Chen, and D. W. Gaylor (1991). Mathematical modeling of reproductive and developmental toxic effects for quantitative risk assessment, *Risk Anal.*, 11, 583–590.

Lefkopoulou, M., D. Moore, and L. Ryan (1989). The analysis of multiple correlated binary outcomes: Applications to rodent teratology experiments, *J. Am. Stat. Assoc.*, 84, 810–815.

Lehmann, E. L. (1975). *Nonparametrics: Statistical Methods Based on Ranks*, Holden-Day, San Francisco.

Léonard, A. (1975). Tests for heritable translocations in male mammals, *Mutat. Res.*, 31, 293–298.

Lin, F. O., and J. K. Haseman (1976). A modified Jonckheere test against ordered alternatives when ties are present at a single extreme value, *Biom. Z.*, 18, 623–631.

Lockhart, A.-M., W. W. Piegorsch, and J. B. Bishop (1992). Assessing overdispersion and dose response in the male dominant lethal assay, *Mutat. Res.*, 272, 35–58.

Mantel, N. (1963). chi-Square tests with one degree of freedom, extensions of the Mantel–Haenzel procedures, *J. Am. Stat. Assoc.*, 58, 690–700.

Maxwell, W. A., and G. W. Newell (1973). Considerations for evaluating chemical mutagenicity to germinal cells, *Environ. Health Perspect.*, 6, 47–50.

Pack, S. E. (1986). Hypothesis testing with overdispersion, *Biometrics*, 42, 967–972.

Piegorsch, W. W. (1991). Multiple comparisons for analyzing dichotomous response data, *Biometrics*, 47, 45–54.

Piegorsch, W. W. (1993). Biometrical methods for testing dose effects of environmental stimuli in laboratory studies, *Environmetrics*, 4, 483–505.

Piegorsch, W. W., and J. K. Haseman (1991). Statistical methods for analyzing developmental toxicity data, *Teratogenesis Carcinog. Mutagen.*, 11, 115–133.

Piegorsch, W. W., A. C. Lockhart, B. H. Margolin, K. R. Tindall, N. J. Gorelick, J. M. Short, G. J. Carr, E. D. Thompson, and M. D. Shelby (1994). Sources of variability in data from a *lacI* transgenic mouse mutation assay, *Environ. Mol. Mutagen.*, 23, 17–31.

Risko, K. J., and B. H. Margolin (1988). *Random Effects in Binomial Data: Some Implications for Inference*, Technical Report, Department of Biostatistics, University of North Carolina, Chapel Hill, NC.

Russell, W. L., and E. M. Kelly (1982). Mutation frequencies in male mice and the estimation of genetic hazards of radiation in men, *Proc. Natl. Acad. Sci. USA*, 79, 542–544.

Russell, L. B., and M. D. Shelby (1985). Tests for heritable genetic damage and for evidence of gonadal exposure in mammals, *Mutat. Res.*, 154, 69–84.

Ryan, L. (1992). Quantitative risk assessment for developmental toxicity, *Biometrics*, 48, 163–174.

Selby, P. B., and W. H. Olson (1981). Methods and criteria for deciding whether specific-locus mutation-rate data in mice indicate a positive, negative, or inconclusive result, *Mutat. Res.*, 83, 403–418.

Shelby, M. D. (1988). Genetic toxicology of mammalian male germ cells. In *Physiology and Toxicology of Male Reproduction* (J. C. Lamb, and P. M. D. Foster, eds.), Academic Press, New York, pp. 203–224.

Shelby, M. D., J. B. Bishop, J. M. Mason, and K. R. Tindall (1993). Fertility, reproduction, and genetic disease: Studies on the mutagenic effects of environmental agents on mammalian germ cells, *Environ. Health Perspect.*, 100, 283–291.

Smith, D. M. (1983). Maximum likelihood estimation of the parameters of the beta-binomial distribution, *Appl. Stat.*, 32, 196–204.

Smith, D. M., and D. A. James (1984). A comparison of alternative distributions of postimplantation death in the dominant lethal assay, *Mutat. Res.*, 125, 195–206.

Srivastava, M. S., and Y. Wu (1993). Local efficiency of moment estimators in beta-binomial model, *Commun. Stat. Theory Methods*, 22, 2471–2490.

Vuataz, L., and J. Sotek (1978). Use of the beta-binomial distribution in dominant-lethal testing for "weak mutagenic activity," *Mutat. Res.*, 52, 211–230.

Whorton, E. B., Jr. (1981). Parametric statistical methods and sample size considerations for dominant lethal experiments: The use of clustering to achieve approximate normality, *Teratogenesis Carcinog. Mutagen.*, 1, 353–360.

Yamamoto, E., and T. Yanagimoto (1992). Moment estimators for the beta-binomial distribution, *J. Appl. Stat.*, 19, 273–283.

Zeger, S. L., K.-Y. Liang, and P. S. Albert (1988). Models for longitudinal data: A generalized estimating equation approach, *Biometrics*, 44, 1049–1060.

# 26
# Statistical Analysis of Long-Term Animal Cancer Studies

**Gregg E. Dinse**
*National Institute of Environmental Health Sciences*
*Research Triangle Park, North Carolina*

## I. INTRODUCTION

Long-term animal cancer studies are an extremely important tool for learning about tumorigenesis. To limit or reduce human exposure to potentially harmful agents, both manufacturers and regulatory agencies use animal experiments to assess possible hazards of chemicals in the environment, including those associated with foods, drugs, cosmetics, household supplies, commercial products, industrial waste, and occupational exposures. Researchers at government, academic, and private laboratories conduct carcinogenicity studies to gain insight about tumor onset, growth, and lethality. Solid results from well-run animal cancer studies provide valuable information for decision making and supplement the base of knowledge derived from human cancer studies.

As an example of a well-designed animal carcinogenicity experiment, which often serves as a standard with which other protocols are compared, consider the type of study conducted over the past two decades by the U. S. National Cancer Institute (NCI) and the U. S. National Toxicology Program (NTP). Generally, these studies involve both sexes of two rodent species, usually one strain of mice (e.g., B6C3F$_1$) and one strain of rats (e.g., Fischer 344). Exposures in most NCI/NTP studies begin when animals are 6–8 weeks of age and continue for two years, which corresponds to late middle age in these mice and rats, at which point all live animals are killed and necropsied. Some 2-year NCI/NTP bioassays incorporate interim sacrifices, which call for randomly selected subsets of the live animals to be killed and examined at intermediate times during the study. For each sex and species combination, current NCI/NTP studies usually include one control group and three chemically exposed groups. Exposures are administered through various routes, such as food, drinking water, gavage, inhalation, or skin application. Generally, control animals are untreated, although some studies incorporate a "vehicle" control group, in which the animals are administered a placebo or a sham treatment by the same route of exposure used for the treated animals. When investigating a single type of exposure, the treatment groups differ, theoretically, only in the dose level of exposure. After stratifying on weight, typically 50 animals are randomly assigned to each group, with an additional 10 animals per group if an interim sacrifice is planned. Chhabra et al. (1990) describe the current NCI/NTP study design and Huff and co-workers (1991) discuss why these studies are important, as well as many other aspects of general concern.

The NCI/NTP study design is well accepted and often serves as the foundation to which other protocols make slight modifications. Experiments conducted by researchers at laboratories within the government, the academic community, and the private sector may differ relative to factors that include (but are not limited to) the choice of animal species and strains, study length, number and size of groups, dose and duration of exposure, and number and timing of sacrifices. An obvious and important tradeoff exists between minimizing costs and maximizing information. Large, complex studies provide the potential for great scientific gains, but tend to exceed common cost constraints. For example, the $ED_{01}$ study (Cairns, 1980) involved almost 24,000 mice, investigated seven dose levels, incorporated eight interim sacrifice times, and ran for 33 months. Even so, this huge experiment did not answer all the hypothesized questions. At the opposite end of the spectrum, tight budgets can result in small experiments that run the risk of being deemed inadequate by the scientific community. A design resembling the one employed by the NCI/NTP is a reasonable compromise between more informative, but extremely rare, "mega-mouse" experiments, such as the $ED_{01}$ study, and small experiments that are more easily affordable, but vastly underpowered.

Regardless of which design is used, the most basic piece of information recorded for each animal is a binary response indicator of whether a tumor was found at a given organ site. Thus, the simplest and most straightforward analysis focuses on the group-specific proportions of animals with tumors. Descriptive group summaries are obtained by estimating tumor response rates for control and exposed animals. Similarly, control and treatment groups are compared for tumor response by using standard hypothesis-testing procedures for proportions. These tests can be applied pairwise to compare each exposed group with the control group. Alternatively, the procedure can use information from all animals to test for heterogeneity of tumor response across groups, or to test for an increasing (or decreasing) trend in tumor response with increasing levels of exposure.

A second piece of information typically recorded for each animal is the time at which the tumor response was observed. This observation time is measured from some initial event, such as birth, weaning, or the start of the exposure period. Thus, the observation time reflects the animal's age, possibly time-shifted by the length of some initial waiting period. If tumors are detectable in live animals, such as visible skin tumors or palpable mammary tumors, the observation times equal the detection times which, we hope, are good surrogates for the tumor onset times. The longer the lag between the actual onset and eventual detection of a tumor, the more the time to detection will overestimate the time to onset. Most tumors are occult (i.e., undetectable in live animals), however, and the response indicator is observed just at the time of death. Here, the observation time equals the death time, which usually does not correlate well with the tumor onset time, except for extremely lethal tumors that kill almost immediately.

Therefore, in addition to analyzing the marginal response distribution, a separate analysis can focus on the marginal survival distribution. Survival rates can be estimated for control and treated animals, and comparisons of the longevity in these groups can be made by applying standard survival techniques, either in the form of pairwise tests or overall tests for heterogeneity or dose-related trends. Alternatively, information on tumor response and observation time can be considered together to produce some combined outcome measure. For example, an analysis based on the conditional distribution of response, given observation time, focuses on the time-specific response rate which, under certain assumptions, is simply the tumor prevalence rate. Similarly, the conditional distribution of observation time, given tumor status, or the joint distribution of observation time and tumor status also provide frameworks on which analyses can be based. The best analysis of time and response data depends on many factors, including what assumptions are made and which endpoints are most important.

Although virtually any long-term carcinogenicity study collects data on observation time and tumor response, other concomitant information might also be recorded. For example, most studies provide tumor response indicators for a large list of organ sites. Generally, data are available on an animal's weight and cage location (e.g., row, column, and side of the housing rack), which could be important if the cages are not rotated (Lagakos and Mosteller, 1981). Assessments of tumor size, stage, and multiplicity could be useful. Occasionally, study designs require each tumor's role in causing death to be specified, but rarely are pathologists comfortable in making these determinations. One practical problem is that the form, amount, and reliability of this extra information vary greatly from one study to another. Also, the more data included in the analysis, the more complex the choices become on how best to incorporate that extra information.

In view of the difficulties involved with appropriately adjusting for observation times, not to mention additional information, a common question is why not base the analysis on the marginal response distribution? What do we gain by taking time into account? For now, let us ignore any other information and address the issue of how and when time adjustments are important. Basically, an analysis potentially can benefit from taking time into account whenever the comparison groups differ by some time-related factor. For example, suppose that the groups exhibit different survival patterns. Animals that live longer have a greater lifetime risk of developing a tumor; or put another way, animals that die early might never reach the age at which tumors typically occur. Thus, fewer treated animals will have tumors if exposure shortens survival than if exposure does not affect (or lengthens) survival. Under this circumstance, a carcinogenic exposure can appear less hazardous than it really is and a noncarcinogenic exposure can appear beneficial. We can be misled simply by not adjusting for the fact that exposed animals are at risk of developing a tumor for a shorter time period than are the control animals. Generally speaking, the unadjusted analysis is usually perfectly adequate, but not always. Ideally, all else being equal, a survival-adjusted analysis is preferable because it can be applied regardless of whether the conditions relating to differential survival are satisfied.

Many adjustments for survival effects have been proposed. One approach modifies the marginal response analysis so that the number at risk (i.e., the sample size) in a group with poor survival is adjusted downward to reflect the reduced risk of tumor onset associated with that group's survival patterns. Otherwise, an analysis typically adjusts for survival by focusing on some endpoint that is a function of both time and response, such as the age-specific proportion having the tumor (tumor prevalence), the time to tumor onset (tumor incidence), the time to death with the tumor, or the time to death from the tumor (tumor mortality). In theory, the endpoint is selected according to which aspects of the underlying tumor process are most important and most interesting. In practice, however, the choice of endpoint depends on how the study was designed, what additional data are available, and which assumptions seem reasonable. Examples of practical considerations include incorporation of sacrifices, collection of data on cause of death, and assumptions about tumor lethality, parametric models, or functional constraints.

This chapter reviews the statistical analysis of tumorigenicity data from long-term animal cancer studies based on typical designs used today and does not consider how to design better studies in the future. Not every method of analysis is discussed, nor are all issues of potential interest addressed. The basic analyses are outlined, however, along with a summary of the required assumptions and an explanation of the important advantages and disadvantages of the various approaches. I hope that the reader will be provided with sufficient information to gain a reasonable understanding of the usual analyses applied to tumor data collected in long-term carcinogenicity experiments. For detailed descriptions of many of these analyses (and others) from different perspectives, as well as several worked examples that illustrate the methods, see Peto et al., (1980), McKnight and Crowley (1984), Haseman (1984), Lagakos and Louis (1985), Gart et al. (1986), and McKnight (1988). Also, for an extensive guide to the literature (at least through 1981) related to carcinogenic risk assessment, see Krewski and Brown (1981).

The chapter is organized as follows. Basic assumptions, goals, and notation are described in Section II. The unadjusted analysis of lifetime tumor rates is discussed in Section III. For comparison purposes, Section IV outlines a survival-adjusted incidence analysis, based on the actual onset times, for tumors that are observable in live animals. Each of the remaining sections deals with a different special case in which the survival-adjusted analysis of incidence rates is possible, even when tumors are not observable until after death. These special cases correspond to assumptions about tumor lethality (Sec. V), individual data on cause of death (Sec. VI), additional data from random sacrifices (Sec. VII), and increased structure from parametric models or functional constraints (Sec. VIII). The chapter ends with a brief section of concluding remarks.

## II. ASSUMPTIONS, GOALS, AND NOTATION

The analyses described in this chapter focus on tumors at a single site of interest, without addressing the issue of multiple comparisons that would arise if these methods were applied repeatedly to many tumor sites within the same experiment. Furthermore, relative to the site of interest, tumors are assumed to be irreversible, and the number of tumors per animal is not taken into account. Animals without a tumor at that site are classified as *tumor-free,* whereas those with one or more tumors are classified as *tumor-bearing. Tumor onset* is defined as the stage of tumor development at which the lesion could first be detected microscopically, based on the invasive diagnostic techniques used for examinations at necropsy. If multiple tumors of interest are present, the tumor onset time refers to the time associated with the *first* tumor.

The objective of most carcinogenicity studies is to compare groups of exposed and unexposed animals relative to the most appropriate measure of tumor response possible, as well as to provide group-specific summaries of that response. In addition to pairwise comparisons of each exposed group with the control group and an overall test for heterogeneity across groups, usually the main goal is to test for a dose-related trend in tumor response. Typically, the hypothesis tests are supplemented by separate tumor response estimates for each group, presented together in a joint summary. Perhaps the greatest problem is that, frequently, the endpoints available for analysis are not equivalent to the endpoint on which the analysis should be based, thereby creating biases when one endpoint is used as a surrogate for another.

The primary basis of analysis for a carcinogenicity experiment should be the *tumor incidence rate,* which refers to the risk of tumor onset among animals that are alive and tumor-free (McKnight and Crowley, 1984; McKnight, 1988). This chapter describes tests and estimators that are used to compare and summarize various tumor response rates, along with discussions of the conditions under which these response rates coincide with the incidence rates and some guidance concerning possible biases that can arise when these conditions are not satisfied. Related issues of study design and conduct, as well as data collection and management, are not discussed here.

Suppose that, in addition to a single control group, there are $K \geq 1$ exposed groups. Let $N$ denote the total number of animals placed on study, with $N_k$ animals randomized to the $k$th group ($k = 0, 1, \ldots, K$). Let $d_0 < d_1 < \cdots < d_K$ denote the ordered dose levels, where the control value is assumed to be $d_0 = 0$. Often transforms of the actual dose levels are used, such as logarithms or equally spaced scores, in which case the $d_k$ represent the transformed values. Let $T$ be the time to natural death, as opposed to a death by sacrifice; a sacrifice results in a censored value of $T$. Suppose there are $J$ distinct natural death times: $t_1 < t_2 < \cdots < t_J$. Let $Y$ be an indicator of whether the tumor is present ($Y = 1$) or absent ($Y = 0$) at death. Similarly, let $Y(t)$ be a response indicator for any general time $t$, which is 1 if the tumor is present at time $t$ and zero otherwise. In practice, the values of $K$, $N$, $N_k$, and $d_k$ are treated as fixed, and the random variables $T$ and $Y$ are always observable. The indicator $Y(t)$, however, is not observable for $t < T$, except in special situations such as when tumors are palpable or visible in live animals or at times of sacrifice.

Although, collectively, the many existing analyses have focused on a variety of outcomes, the most relevant endpoint for assessing tumorigenesis is tumor incidence, preferably as a function of time. In the simplest case, the marginal distribution of $Y$ can be viewed as a lifetime incidence rate that does not adjust for the time at risk. Analyses based on the joint distribution of $T$ and $Y$ typically provide only indirect information about tumor incidence, unless certain assumptions are made. The general definition of tumor incidence depends on $Y(t)$, which usually is not observable before death.

One instructive way to view the problem is in terms of a competing risks framework. Each animal is subject to two competing risks: tumor onset or natural death without the tumor. That is, suppose all animals are tumor-free initially (at time 0) and at some time point either develop the tumor or die naturally without ever having developed the tumor. The transition intensities for the two competing risks are the tumor incidence rate and the tumor-free death rate, which can be expressed in terms of $T$ and $Y(\cdot)$ as follows:

$$\lambda(t) = \lim \, \mathrm{pr}\{Y(t + \varepsilon) = 1 \,|\, Y(t) = 0, \, T \geq t\} / \varepsilon \tag{1}$$

$$\beta(t) = \lim \, \mathrm{pr}\{t \leq T < t + \varepsilon \,|\, Y(t) = 0, \, T \geq t\} / \varepsilon \tag{2}$$

All limits are taken as $\varepsilon$ decreases to 0. Alternatively, define $X$ as the time to the first of the two competing events, tumor onset or natural death without the tumor. The transition intensities can be rewritten in terms of $X$ and $Y(\cdot)$ as event-specific hazards:

$$\lambda(t) = \lim \, \mathrm{pr}\{t \leq X < t + \varepsilon, \, Y(X) = 1 \,|\, X \geq t\} / \varepsilon \tag{3}$$

$$\beta(t) = \lim \, \mathrm{pr}\{t \leq X < t + \varepsilon, \, Y(X) = 0 \,|\, X \geq t\} / \varepsilon \tag{4}$$

Once an animal develops a tumor, say at time $x$, the risk of death at time $t$ is

$$\alpha(t\,|\,x) = \lim \, \mathrm{pr}\{t \leq T < t + \varepsilon \,|\, T \geq t, \, Y(t) = 1, \, X = \chi\} / \varepsilon \tag{5}$$

where $t \geq x > 0$. Some analyses involve a simplified version of this conditional death rate:

$$\alpha(t) = \lim \, \mathrm{pr}\{t \leq T < t + \varepsilon \,|\, T \geq t, \, Y(t) = 1\} / \varepsilon \tag{6}$$

which can be considered as an average rate of death among all animals having the tumor (McKnight and Crowley, 1984).

The analysis should focus on estimating the tumor incidence rate in the $k$th group, say $\lambda_k(t)$, as well as testing the null hypothesis of equal tumor incidence rates,

$$H_\lambda: \, \lambda_1(t) = \lambda_2(t) = \cdots = \lambda_K(t), \tag{7}$$

against the alternative hypothesis that not all tumor incidence rates are identical (i.e., group heterogeneity), or that tumor incidence rates increase with dose (i.e., a positive trend). The pairwise comparison of a particular treatment group with the control group can be viewed as a special case of testing $H_\lambda$ when $K = 2$.

## III. LIFETIME TUMOR RATES

The most basic analysis focuses on the lifetime tumor rates, comparing the group-specific proportions of animals that develop the tumor during the study period. Ignoring group membership for a moment, let $P$ denote the lifetime risk of tumor onset, which is just the probability mass function for the marginal distribution of $Y$:

$$P = \text{pr}\{Y = 1\} \tag{8}$$

Alternatively, the lifetime tumor rate can be expressed in terms of the tumor incidence rate $\lambda$, and the tumor-free death rate $\beta$, by rewriting $P$ as a function of $X$ and $Y(\cdot)$:

$$P = \text{pr}\{X \le T^*, \ Y(X) = 1\} = \int_0^{T^*} \lambda(x) S_\lambda(x) S_\beta(x) \, dx \tag{9}$$

where $T^*$ is the time at which the study ends and $S_\lambda$ and $S_\beta$ are "pseudo"-survivorship functions defined for notational convenience in the following manner:

$$S_\lambda(t) = \exp\{-\int_0^t \lambda(u) \, du\} \quad \text{and} \quad S_\beta(t) = \exp\{-\int_0^t \beta(u) \, du\} \tag{10}$$

Henceforth, the subscript $k$ is appended to a term to indicate membership in a particular dose group. For example, $\lambda_k(t)$ denotes the tumor incidence rate in the $k$th group.

The standard nonparametric estimate of $P_k$ is the group-specific sample mean:

$$\hat{P}_k = \frac{\sum y_{ik}}{N_k} \tag{11}$$

where $y_{ik}$ is the observed value of $Y$ for the $i$th animal in the $k$th group, and the summation is over all $i$ from 1 to $N_k$. The null hypothesis of equal lifetime tumor rates is given by:

$$H_P: P_1 = P_2 = \cdots = P_K \tag{12}$$

which in general neither implies, nor is implied by, the hypothesis of equal incidence rates, $H_\lambda$. Usually pairwise comparisons are based on Fisher's exact test, an overall assessment of group heterogeneity is based on an omnibus chi-squared ($\chi^2$) test, and dose-related increases are judged on the basis of the linear trend test of Cochran (1954) and Armitage (1955). See Haseman (1984) and Gart et al. (1986) for a review of these tests and some worked examples based on data from real carcinogenicity studies.

Each of these tests assumes that all animals in the same group are subject to the same lifetime risk of developing the tumor. As the risk of tumor onset clearly increases with age, this underlying assumption is violated if some animals die earlier than others. These tests are described as unadjusted, as they do not adjust for survival effects when deaths occur at various times. If some animals die before the end of the study, but the mortality patterns are similar across dose groups, the unadjusted tests will remain valid (Gart et al., 1979), although possibly less powerful than analogous survival-adjusted tests (Ryan, 1985). Although unadjusted procedures often provide the correct interpretation, even when dose-specific survival patterns differ (see Table 3 of Gart et al., 1979), in some cases differential mortality can cause an unadjusted test of $H_P$ to produce biased inferences about tumor incidence. For example, suppose that exposure is toxic and thus causes the tumor-free death rates to increase with dose. As $P$ is a decreasing function of $\beta$, the Cochran–Armitage trend test (appropriate for assessing $H_P$) will tend to reject $H_\lambda$ less often than desired, which could result in a true carcinogen being missed.

One simple way to adjust for survival within this framework is to modify the number of animals at risk by reducing the denominator of each lifetime tumor rate. Rather than giving equal weight to all animals, less weight is assigned to those dying early without a tumor. For example, Gart et al. (1979) suggest assigning a weight of zero to any animal dying without the tumor at a time before the first death with the tumor, while assigning all other animals a weight of 1. Extending this idea, Bailer and Portier (1988) assign a weight of 1 to animals dying with the tumor and otherwise assign a weight proportional to a fixed power of the time on study, where the choice of the time exponent depends on the assumed shape of the tumor incidence curve. Bieler and Williams (1993) propose a variance correction for the Bailer–Portier procedure. Often the survival adjustment made by these methods is helpful, but generally an analysis that focuses on tumor incidence rates is preferable to one that focuses on lifetime tumor rates.

## IV.  OBSERVABLE TUMORS

The remainder of this chapter is devoted to survival-adjusted methods. Various factors complicate survival adjustments in the analysis of tumor incidence data from animal cancer studies. For example, as most tumor types are occult (i.e., unobservable in live animals), tumors typically are discovered only after death, and thus, tumor onset times are censored. Tumor lethality further confuses the survival adjustment procedure. If animals with the tumor die at a different rate than those without the tumor, then deaths from natural causes informatively censor tumor onset times. Most failure–time analyses, however, assume that the censoring mechanisms are noninformative (Lagakos, 1979). Thus, without direct observations on tumor onset times, survival adjustments usually are accomplished by restricting tumor lethality, requiring cause-of-death data, incorporating multiple sacrifice times, assuming parametric models, or imposing functional constraints. Primarily for purposes of comparison and illustration, this section concentrates on the analysis of observable tumors, such as visible skin tumors or palpable mammary tumors.

The best way to analyze tumor incidence data is to focus on the onset times directly. This approach adjusts for differential survival and tumor lethality, while avoiding the need for parametric models, functional restrictions, sacrifices, or cause-of-death data. If the event times are observable, most analyses employ standard nonparametric techniques, such as the survival estimator of Kaplan and Meier (1958), the logrank test (Mantel, 1966; Cox, 1972; Peto and Peto, 1972), and the modified Wilcoxon test (Gehan, 1965; Efron, 1967; Mantel, 1967; Breslow, 1970; Peto and Peto, 1972). For a discussion of these methods, see Tarone and Ware (1977) and Kalbfleisch and Prentice (1980).

Nonparametric analyses typically treat event times as discrete random variables. In this section only, let $t_j$ be the $j$th largest observed time of tumor onset (rather than death). If we treat $X$ as a discrete random variable, then the usual nonparametric estimate of the tumor incidence rate at time $t_j$, say $\lambda_j$, can be expressed as:

$$\hat{\lambda}_j = \frac{\#\{X_i = t_j,\ Y_i(X_i) = 1\}}{\#\{X_i \geq t_j\}} \tag{13}$$

where $\#\{A\}$ denotes the number of animals experiencing event $A$ and $\{X_i, Y_i\}$ is the value of $\{X,Y\}$ for the $i$th animal. In this case, $\hat{\lambda}_j$ is simply the number of animals developing the tumor at time $t_j$ divided by the number of animals at risk of developing the tumor at time $t_j$ (i.e., alive and tumor-free just before $t_j$).

Some analyses assume that all animals eventually would develop the tumor in the absence of death. Within this latent-variable framework, let $U$ denote the potential time to tumor onset. The Kaplan–Meier estimate of $Q(t) = \text{pr}\{U \geq t\}$, the survivorship function for the latent variable $U$, is a simple function of the tumor incidence estimates in Eq. (13):

$$\hat{Q}(t) = \prod (1 - \hat{\lambda}_j) \tag{14}$$

where the product is over the set $\{j : t_j < t\}$. The times to tumor onset and times to death (either natural or sacrificial) without the tumor provide uncensored and right-censored observations on $U$, respectively. Note, however, that $Q(t)$ usually has no interpretation outside the hypothetical latent-variable, competing-risks setting.

Various tests have been proposed for comparing multiple groups relative to failure time distributions, all of which require some further notation. Within the $k$th group, let $O_{jk}$ be the observed number of animals developing a tumor at time $t_j$ and let $R_{jk}$ be the number of animals at risk of developing a tumor at time $t_j$ $(j = 1, \cdots, J; k = 0, 1, \cdots, K)$:

$$O_{jk} = \#\{X_{ik} = t_j, Y_{ik}(X_{ik}) = 1\} \quad \text{and} \quad R_{jk} = \#\{X_{ik} \geq t_j\} \tag{15}$$

Under the null hypothesis of no dose effect on tumor incidence rates, $H_\lambda$, the associated expected counts and variance terms are given by:

$$E_{jk} = R_{jk} \left[ \frac{O_{j+}}{R_{j+}} \right] \quad \text{and} \quad V_{jkm} = \left[ \frac{O_{j+}(R_{j+} - O_{j+})}{R_{j+} - 1} \right] \left[ \frac{R_{jk}}{R_{j+}} \right] \left[ a_{km} - \frac{R_{jm}}{R_{j+}} \right] \tag{16}$$

where the plus signs indicate summations over all $K + 1$ groups and $a_{km}$ is an indicator that equals 1 if $k = m$ and 0 otherwise. For each $k$, create group-specific summaries for the observed counts, expected counts, and variance terms:

$$O_k = \sum O_{jk}, \quad E_k = \sum E_{jk}, \quad V_{km} = \sum V_{jkm} \tag{17}$$

where the summations are over all $J$ distinct tumor onset times. Let $D^T = (d_1, \ldots, d_K)$ be the K-vector of dose levels, let $O^T = (O_1, \ldots, O_K)$ be the K-vector of observed counts, let $E^T = (E_1, \ldots, E_K)$ be the K-vector of expected counts, and let $V$ be the $K \times K$ matrix of variance terms with $(k,m)$-element $V_{km}$ $(k = 1, \ldots, K; m = 1, \ldots, K)$. Note that these arrays do not include the summary terms from the control group $(k = 0)$.

The usual test for heterogeneity of groups is based on the statistic:

$$\chi_H^2 = (O - E)^T V^{-1} (O - E) \tag{18}$$

which is distributed asymptotically as $\chi^2$ on $K$ degrees of freedom under $H_\lambda$. Often the test for a dose related trend in incidence rates is based on the logrank statistic:

$$\chi_T^2 = \frac{\left[ D^T (O - E) \right]^2}{D^T V D} \tag{19}$$

which also is distributed asymptotically as $\chi^2$ under $H_\lambda$, but on a single degree of freedom. Finally, a test for departures from linearity can be based on the statistic:

$$\chi_D^2 = \chi_H^2 - \chi_T^2 \tag{20}$$

which is distributed asymptotically as $\chi^2$ on $K - 1$ degrees of freedom under the null hypothesis that tumor incidence rates increase linearly with dose.

For details on these and other related analyses see, for example, Tarone (1975), Tarone and Ware (1977), Kalbfleisch and Prentice (1980), and Gart et al. (1986). The main point is that standard estimators and tests that are appropriate for summarizing and comparing censored failure–time distributions in the ordinary survival analysis setting can be applied directly to the onset times when tumors are observable. The remaining sections deal with the typical situation in which tumors are occult and, consequently, other methods must be used to overcome the complications created by the tumors being unobservable. In particular, without direct observations on times to tumor onset, one must record more information, make additional assumptions, or focus on different endpoints. The methods described in the next section are based on assumptions about tumor lethality.

## V. TUMOR LETHALITY

If the presence of tumors at the organ site of interest do not alter the risk of death, then those tumors are classified as nonlethal. Alternatively, tumors that increase the risk of death are classified as lethal. In fact, tumors conceivably can be protective if they lessen the risk of death, although such instances are rare and are not considered here. The degree of lethality is often characterized, at least qualitatively, by how much the tumor's presence hastens the animal's demise. For example, tumors that result in short post-onset survival periods are referred to as rapidly lethal. The appropriateness of a lethality-based analysis depends on where tumors fall along the lethality spectrum. The next section deals with data on cause of death, which in a sense allow tumor lethalities to vary across animals. The current section assumes that lethality is an intrinsic property of all tumors at the site of interest and does not change on an individual animal basis.

Rather than focusing on an unobservable outcome, such as tumor onset, one of the earliest methods for analyzing data on both tumor response and survival concentrated instead on an observable endpoint, the combined event of death with a tumor present (Gart et al., 1979). Let $h(t)$ denote the unconditional hazard rate for "death-with-tumor":

$$h(t) = \lim \operatorname{pr}\{t \leq T < t + \varepsilon, \ Y(T) = 1 | T \geq t\} / \varepsilon \tag{21}$$

The same failure–time analysis described in the previous section is applied, except that the time to death with tumor is substituted for the tumor onset time. Here, the failure time is uncensored if a tumor is present at death and right-censored otherwise, and typically deaths due to sacrifice are not distinguished from natural deaths. The techniques of Kaplan and Meier (1958) can be used to estimate $h_j$, the discrete analog of $h(t_j)$:

$$\hat{h}_j = \frac{\#\{T_i = t_j, \ Y_i(T_i) = 1\}}{\#\{T_i \geq t_j\}} \tag{22}$$

and a log-rank statistic can be used to test the null hypothesis that dose groups do not differ in the distribution of time to death with tumor:

$$H_h: \ h_1(t) = h_2(t) = \cdots = h_K(t) \tag{23}$$

Note that the hypothesis $H_h$ neither implies, nor is implied by, the hypothesis $H_\lambda$.

Life table analyses based on Kaplan–Meier estimates and log-rank tests are reasonable when tumors are rapidly lethal. As tumor lethality increases, $h(t)$ converges to $\lambda(t)$, $\hat{h}_j$ more accurately estimates $\lambda_j$, and a test of $H_h$ provides a better test of $H_\lambda$. The greater the lethality, the shorter the time from tumor onset to death, and the better surrogate time to death with tumor is for time to tumor onset. The main problem is that life table analyses perform worse as lethality decreases, especially as the mortality patterns become more disparate; tests of $H_h$ can yield biased conclusions about tumor incidence rates when the post-onset survival times are relatively long. The bias is in the opposite direction of the bias in the unadjusted analysis, and Gart et al. (1979) characterize this effect as an overadjustment for survival. For example, suppose that exposure is toxic and causes treated animals to die sooner than controls. Nonlethal tumors will be discovered earlier in the exposed groups, and we might falsely conclude that the exposure is carcinogenic, even if the underlying tumor incidence rates are identical across groups. Thus, a life table test applied to data on nonlethal tumors will reject too often (Lagakos, 1982).

In view of these concerns, Hoel and Walburg (1972) propose an analysis that is appropriate for nonlethal tumors. Their analysis focuses on tumor prevalence, which is the expected proportion of animals having the tumor among those alive at that time:

$$\pi(t) = \text{pr}\{Y(t) = 1 | T > t\} \tag{24}$$

In general, the tumor prevalence rate is a function of the tumor incidence rate, $\lambda(t)$, the tumor-free death rate, $\beta(t)$, and the tumor-bearing death rate, $\alpha(t|x)$:

$$\{1 - \pi(t)\}^{-1} = 1 + \int_0^t \lambda(x) \exp\left\{\int_x^t \left[\lambda(u) + \beta(u) - \alpha(t | u)\right] du\right\} dx \tag{25}$$

If tumors are nonlethal, they do not affect the risk of death and thus $\alpha(t|x) \equiv \beta(t)$. Under this condition, $\pi(t)$ reduces to the following function of $\lambda(t)$ only:

$$\pi(t) = 1 - \exp\left\{-\int_0^t \lambda(u) du\right\} = 1 - S_\lambda(t) \tag{26}$$

which is of the form of a cumulative distribution function having hazard function $\lambda(t)$. Also, if tumors are nonlethal, the prevalence rate equals the time-specific response rate:

$$p(t) = \text{pr}\{Y(t) = 1 | T = t\} \tag{27}$$

which can be expressed in terms of $\lambda(t)$, $\beta(t)$, and $\alpha(t|x)$ as follows:

$$\{1 - p(t)\}^{-1} = 1 + \beta(t)^{-1} \int_0^t \lambda(x) \exp\left\{\int_x^t \left[\lambda(u) + \beta(u) - \alpha(t | u)\right] du\right\} \alpha(t | x) \, dx \tag{28}$$

Natural death acts as an unbiased sampling mechanism relative to the presence of nonlethal tumors, so animals that die are representative of those still alive (Lagakos and Ryan, 1985). Hoel and Walburg (1972) adjust for survival by partitioning the study period into intervals, using the intervals to stratify animals according to death times, assessing dose-specific response rates within intervals, and combining the results over intervals.

The natural estimate of the response rate for some time interval $I_j$ and dose $d_k$ is

$$\hat{p}_{jk} = \frac{\#\{T_{ik} \in I_j, Y_{ik}(T_{ik}) = 1\}}{\#\{T_{ik} \in I_j\}} \tag{29}$$

which is simply the observed proportion of animals having a tumor among those dying in the $j$th time interval and $k$th dose group. These empirical rates can fluctuate wildly when the numerators and denominators are small. As a result, analyses frequently constrain the response rates to be nondecreasing in time, which they should be when the tumors are strictly nonlethal and irreversible. Under this monotonicity restriction, the maximum likelihood estimate (MLE) of $p_k(t)$ is constant over time intervals, is of the same form as the $\hat{p}_{jk}$, and can be computed using the pool-adjacent-violators algorithm (Ayer et al., 1955; Hoel and Walburg, 1972). Regardless of how the intervals are determined, we can test the null hypothesis of equal tumor prevalence rates:

$$H_\pi: \pi_1(t) = \pi_2(t) = \cdots = \pi_K(t) \tag{30}$$

by comparing observed and expected counts within each interval and using the methods of Mantel and Haenszel (1959) to combine results over intervals. The test statistics are given by

Eqs. (18)–(20), except the observed counts ($O_{jk}$) are numbers of deaths with a tumor and the numbers at risk ($R_{jk}$) are the total numbers of deaths in $I_j$. As $\pi(t)$ is a one-to-one function of $\lambda(t)$ for nonlethal tumors, here a test of $H_\pi$ is equivalent to a test of $H_\lambda$.

Even if tumors are undeniably nonlethal, no consensus exists on the best choice of time intervals for estimating and comparing prevalence rates. Some analyses specify equal-width intervals, whereas others select intervals expected to contain roughly the same numbers of deaths. Differential mortality can cause problems in that time intervals within which all (most) of the deaths come from the same dose group make no (little) contribution to the interval-based test statistics. Peto et al. (1980) suggest using the time intervals created by applying the pool-adjacent-violators algorithm to the entire data set, combined over all dose groups. This technique has been criticized because different time intervals are generated for each tumor site investigated within the same experiment. Selwyn et al. (1985) propose a method that produces different intervals for each dose group to equalize the numbers of deaths per interval.

Approaching the problem from a different perspective, Dinse and Lagakos (1983) express the tumor response rate as a logistic function (Cox, 1970) of dose and time:

$$\log \left\{ \frac{p_k(t)}{1 - p_k(t)} \right\} = \mu + \theta d_k + \phi(t) \tag{31}$$

where $\mu$ is a constant, $\theta$ is the dose effect, and $\phi(t)$ is some function of time. Once $\phi(t)$ is specified, likelihood methods can be used to estimate and compare prevalence rates. Dinse and Lagakos avoid the arbitrariness of choosing time intervals at the expense of having to specify a particular form for $\phi(t)$. Note, however, that selecting a piecewise constant (step) function for $\phi(t)$ yields the Hoel–Walburg analysis, up to a finite population correction in the variance term. Despite its parametric nature, the logistic analysis is fairly robust and, for example, use of a linear function for $\phi(t)$ yields a test with operating characteristics that match or exceed those of the interval-based tests (Dinse, 1985). If the study incorporates at least one sacrifice time, the logistic prevalence analysis can be extended easily to estimate and to adjust for tumor lethality (Dinse, 1988a).

Similar to the problems that arise when a life table analysis is applied to nonlethal tumors, the use of a prevalence analysis when the tumors are lethal also can produce misleading results, except that the bias is in the opposite direction. Once again, suppose that exposure is toxic and causes the treated animals to die sooner than the controls. As the tumor response rate, $p(t)$, is a decreasing function of the tumor-free death rate, $\beta(t)$, a prevalence test oriented toward detecting an increase in $p(t)$ will not reject as often as a test appropriate for assessing $H_\lambda$ should reject. Thus, a prevalence test applied to data on lethal tumors will not reject often enough (Lagakos, 1982), which could result in a true carcinogen being missed or a noncarcinogen appearing protective.

In summary, one of the first ways of adjusting for survival in the analysis of animal tumorigenicity data involved a subjective assessment about tumor lethality. If the tumor type of interest was judged to be fairly lethal, the usual life table methods were used, and if the tumor type was deemed to be generally nonlethal, the newly developed prevalence methods were employed. What happens, though, if tumor lethality is felt to be constant, but at some intermediate level? If tumor lethality can be specified, then $\lambda(t)$ is identifiable (McKnight and Crowley, 1984), and appropriate estimators and tests can be derived (see, e.g., Lagakos and Louis, 1988). In general, however, tumor lethality is not known exactly and often both life table and prevalence methods are applied in the hope that the two procedures will give similar results. Unfortunately, Lagakos and Louis (1988) show that the significance levels produced by life table and prevalence analyses in this case need not bracket the $p$-value obtained by a test that incorporates a measure of the tumor's (unknown) lethality. Generally speaking, neither the hypothesis of equal prevalence rates, $H_\pi$, nor the hypothesis of equal rates of death with tumor, $H_h$, coincide exactly with the hypothesis of equal incidence rates, $H_\lambda$. Thus, an analysis that makes the extreme assumption that all tumors are strictly nonlethal or all tumors are rapidly lethal can yield misleading conclusions, and appropriate caution should be exercised. The next section discusses an alternative approach that relies on individual assessments of a tumor's effect on death for each animal, which in a sense eases the extreme lethality constraint, but introduces concerns about the availability and reliability of these individual assessments.

## VI. CAUSE OF DEATH

In general, a tumor might increase the risk of death, but not cause an animal to die immediately. Furthermore, even if most tumors at a given site are rapidly lethal, or most are nearly nonlethal, the assumption that all tumors can be characterized by one of these extremes might not be reasonable. This section discusses analyses that allow for a mix of lethal and nonlethal tumors at the same site.

Suppose that an individual context of observation (Peto, 1974; Peto et al., 1980) is specified for each tumor discovered. Occult tumors that do not alter longevity and are observed merely as the result of a death from an unrelated cause are classified as incidental. Occult tumors that affect mortality, either by directly causing death, or by indirectly increasing the risk of death from other causes, are classified as fatal (nonincidental). Note that death is a biased sampling mechanism relative to revealing fatal tumors, but unbiased relative to revealing incidental tumors. Information on context of observation commonly is referred to as data on cause of death.

The availability and reliability of cause-of-death data often is the subject of debate. Many pathologists do not feel comfortable making these assessments, at least not for every tumor found in every animal. Several investigations have shown that cause-of-death data are not always accurate (Kodell et al., 1982a; Lagakos and Ryan, 1985). Nevertheless, this section assumes that accurate cause-of-death data are provided, at least for a subset of the animals. By definition, a lethal tumor is observed in a fatal context and a nonlethal tumor is observed in an incidental context. Any tumor discovered in a randomly sacrificed animal is considered incidental.

Information on cause of death allows us to identify the tumor onset distribution and perform a survival-adjusted incidence analysis without lethality assumptions, parametric models, or random sacrifices. Let $C$ denote the cause of death, which indicates whether death was due to the tumor ($C = 1$) or other causes ($C = 0$). Deaths with the tumor present are partitioned into those due to the tumor itself (death with a fatal tumor) and those due to unrelated causes (death with an incidental tumor). The response-conditional, cause-specific rates of death with no tumor, an incidental tumor, and a fatal tumor are as follows:

$$\beta(t) = \lim \text{pr}\{t \le T < t + \varepsilon, \, C = 0 | T \ge t, \, Y(t) = 0\} / \varepsilon \tag{32}$$

$$\delta(t|x) = \lim \text{pr}\{t \le T < t + \varepsilon, \, C = 0 | T \ge t, \, Y(t) = 1, \, X = x\} / \varepsilon \tag{33}$$

$$\gamma(t|x) = \lim \text{pr}\{t \le T < t + \varepsilon, \, C = 1 | T \ge t, \, Y(t) = 1, \, X = x\} / \varepsilon \tag{34}$$

respectively. Thus, the death rate for tumor-bearing animals can be expressed as the sum of two cause-specific components: $\alpha(t|x) = \delta(t|x) + \gamma(t|x)$. By definition, an incidental tumor does not affect the risk of death, which implies that the death rate for animals with an incidental tumor is the same as the death rate for animals without the tumor:

$$\delta(t|x) \equiv \beta(t) \quad \text{for all} \quad t \ge x > 0 \tag{35}$$

Peto (1974) and Peto et al. (1980) describe a method that simultaneously compares groups relative to tumor prevalence and tumor mortality. Let $g(t)$ denote the tumor mortality rate, which is defined as the unconditional rate of death due to the tumor:

$$g(t) = \lim \text{pr}\{t \leq T < t + \varepsilon, \; Y(T) = 1, \; C = 1 | T \geq t\} / \varepsilon \tag{36}$$

The null hypothesis of equal tumor mortality rates is given by

$$H_g: \; g_1(t) = g_2(t) = \cdots = g_K(t) \tag{37}$$

which neither implies, nor is implied by, the null hypothesis of equal incidence rates, $H_\lambda$. Peto's method tests $H_\pi$ by applying a prevalence analysis to the subset of animals dying from other causes, tests $H_g$ by applying a life table analysis to all animals, and combines these components to obtain an overall assessment of group differences. The life table part of the analysis treats tumor deaths as uncensored events and deaths from other causes as censored events.

Extensions of Peto's analysis to the regression setting have been proposed (Dinse and Lagakos, 1983; Finkelstein and Ryan, 1987), based on a logistic model (Cox, 1970) for the prevalence component and a proportional hazards model (Cox, 1972) for the life table component. In fact, Lagakos and Louis (1988) show that the Peto test can be derived as a partial-likelihood score test under a specific dual model for the prevalence and mortality rates (see also, Finkelstein and Ryan, 1987; Burnett et al., 1989; McKnight and Wahrendorf, 1992). The validity of these cause-of-death methods, including Peto's, depends on the animals that die from other causes being representative of the live population relative to tumor response. Lagakos and Ryan (1985) and Archer and Ryan (1989a) show that this representativeness condition does not always hold. Furthermore, an analysis ideally should focus on tumor incidence, which means estimating $\lambda(t)$, rather than $\pi(t)$ and $g(t)$, and testing $H_\lambda$, rather than $H_\pi$ and $H_g$.

Within a parametric framework, Kodell and Nelson (1980) shift the focus to tumor incidence by postulating Weibull models for $\lambda(t)$, $\beta(t)$, and $\gamma(t)$, where $\gamma(t)$ is the marginal rate of tumor death among tumor-bearing animals (McKnight and Crowley, 1984):

$$\gamma(t) = \lim \text{pr}\{t \leq T < t + \varepsilon, \; C = 1 | T \geq t, \; Y(t) = 1\} / \varepsilon \tag{38}$$

Kodell et al. (1982b) propose a nonparametric estimate of the tumor onset distribution, under the assumption that tumor prevalence is a nondecreasing function. Dinse and Lagakos (1982) and Turnbull and Mitchell (1984) extend this analysis to allow nonmonotonic prevalences. All these approaches assume a latent-variable model with "potential" times to tumor onset, death due to the tumor, and death due to other causes for each animal. The time of death from other causes is assumed to noninformatively censor the times to tumor onset and tumor death. Under this model, the hazard rates for tumor onset and tumor death correspond to the incidence rate and the unconditional death rate given in Eq. (36), respectively. Thus, the associated survivorship functions are

$$S_\lambda(t) = \exp\{-\int_0^t \lambda(u) \, du\} \quad \text{and} \quad G(t) = \exp\{-\int_0^t g(u) \, du\} \tag{39}$$

If $\pi(t)$ is constrained to be monotone, Kodell et al. (1982b) show that its MLE is the Hoel Walburg estimate, the MLE of $G(t)$ is the Kaplan–Meier estimate for the tumor death times, and the MLE of $S_\lambda(t)$ is simply the product of the MLEs of $G(t)$ and $1 - \pi(t)$. If the monotonicity constraint is relaxed, the ML solution requires an iterative algorithm (Dinse and Lagakos, 1982; Turnbull and Mitchell, 1984). These same results can be derived without assuming a latent-variable model or noninformative censoring (Dinse, 1988b).

Pathologists often are reluctant to label every tumor as either definitely incidental or definitely fatal because classification errors can produce biases (Lagakos, 1982; Racine-Poon and

Hoel, 1984). Peto et al. (1980) suggest an expanded set of categories so that tumors also can be classified as probably incidental or probably fatal. In practice, though, the four categories often are reduced to two by combining definitely incidental and probably incidental tumors and combining definitely fatal and probably fatal tumors, at which point the usual analysis is applied to this newly formed dichotomy. Lagakos (1982) considers a single intermediate category to allow an unknown cause of death for some animals and proposes two ad hoc strategies: (1) relabel the unknowns as incidentals and fatals according to the proportions observed in those categories, or (2) relabel all unknowns as incidentals in the life table portion of Peto's analysis and then relabel all unknowns as fatals (i.e., exclude them) in the prevalence portion of Peto's analysis.

Alternatively, an analysis can formally account for uncertain contexts of observation. Racine-Poon and Hoel (1984) derive a modified Kaplan–Meier estimator for the tumor mortality distribution $G(t)$, which requires pathologists to assign a probability to each category of Peto's four-point cause-of-death scale. Dinse (1986) developed nonparametric prevalence and mortality estimators that use the data to estimate these probabilities. Within a latent-variable framework, Kodell and Chen (1987) estimate tumor onset and mortality rates from data with unknown causes of death. Dinse (1988b) generalized the analysis to allow various types of uncertainty, while avoiding the use of latent variables. In a similar manner, the Peto test can be modified so that it formally incorporates uncertainties, either in the form of a sensitivity analysis, or through probabilities estimated from the data in special cases (Lagakos and Louis, 1988; Archer and Ryan, 1989b).

## VII.  INTERIM SACRIFICES

The intentional killing (sacrificing) and examination of a random sample of healthy animals gives an unbiased snapshot (cross-sectional view) of the tumorigenic process. The proportion of animals having the tumor among those randomly sacrificed at time $t$ provides an unbiased estimate of the prevalence rate $\pi(t)$, just as $\hat{p}(t)$ does when all of the tumors are strictly nonlethal or incidental. Together with the usual observations on $T$ and $Y$, sacrifice data permit the analysis to focus on tumor incidence. The advantage is that no lethality assumptions, cause-of-death data, or parametric models are necessary. The survival adjustment improves with the number of sacrifice times, as well as with the number of animals killed at each sacrifice time, and thus the disadvantages are the extra expenses and complexities of a large experiment. In addition, the most appropriate timing of the sacrifices for detecting tumors at one site might not be ideal for another site, although these sorts of design issues are not considered here.

McKnight and Crowley (1984) state that without detailed knowledge of how tumor incidence affects the risk of death (e.g., lethality assumptions, cause-of-death data, or parametric models), sacrifice data are needed to identify $\lambda(t)$. They express the tumor incidence rate in terms of the prevalence rate, its derivative, and two death rates:

$$\lambda(t) = \frac{\pi'(t) + h(t) - \pi(t)f(t)}{1 - \pi(t)} \tag{40}$$

where $h(t)$ is the rate of death with tumor defined in Eq. (21) and $f(t)$ is the overall death rate:

$$f(t) = \lim \, \mathrm{pr}\{t \leq T < t + \varepsilon \,|\, T \geq t\} / \varepsilon \tag{41}$$

Lacking parametric assumptions or information on how tumors affect longevity, however, the prevalence rate is estimable only at the sacrifice times and thus the "resolution" of a nonparametric incidence analysis is limited by the number of sacrifice times.

For example, a nonparametric analysis of survival and sacrifice data generally is based on intervals with endpoints defined by the sacrifice times, in which case the amount of time adjustment increases with the number of sacrifice times. Most experiments include a final (terminal) sacrifice and occasionally studies incorporate one or two interim sacrifices, but rarely are studies designed with more than two interim sacrifices. Thus, an experiment with only a terminal sacrifice would have just one sacrifice-defined interval and, hence, would make no time adjustment. Even carcinogenicity studies with one or two interim sacrifices would yield very coarse nonparametric estimates of the prevalence function, not to mention its derivative, and thus the incidence function as well.

McKnight and Crowley (1984) described advantages of including multiple sacrifices, discussed identifiability issues, and proposed nonparametric estimators and tests that focused on tumor incidence. Dewanji and Kalbfleisch (1986) formalized these methods with an iterative ML analysis. Malani and Van Ryzin (1988) suggested a closed-form solution that coincides with the ML analysis when the data are well behaved, but can occasionally produce negative estimates of the incidences. Similar explicit estimators were proposed by Williams and Portier (1992a), who also derived explicit estimators under the constraint that the incidence rates are positive (Williams and Portier, 1992b). Based on a piecewise constant model for the transition intensities, Borgan and co-workers (1984) showed that multiple sacrifice data greatly increase efficiency.

Many other authors have dealt with survival–sacrifice experiments, but most have assumed parametric models or have not focused on tumor incidence rates. For example, Turnbull and Mitchell (1978) considered the simultaneous analysis of several diseases, but they used log-linear and logistic models to investigate tumor prevalence and lethality rates (see also, Mitchell and Turnbull, 1979; Berlin et al., 1979). In rare cases, such as the $ED_{01}$ study (Cairns, 1980), an experiment is large enough and has an adequate number of sacrifices to support a reasonable nonparametric analysis of tumor incidence rates, but this is clearly the exception, rather than the rule. In practice, the analysis should not depend on routinely having numerous sacrifice times.

## VIII.  PARAMETRIC MODELS AND FUNCTIONAL RESTRICTIONS

The previous sections have reviewed different approaches that permit the analysis of tumor incidence data. Extreme lethality assumptions seem unreasonable in general. Questions of availability and reliability plague analyses based on cause-of-death data. Enthusiasm for methods requiring an abundance of sacrifices usually is more than offset by practical concerns related to cost and complexity. Finally, this section describes the last of the various common alternatives, which involves postulating parametric models or imposing functional restrictions.

In the fully parametric setting, Kalbfleisch et al. (1983) suggest that the ML analysis is complicated, but feasible if the assumed models are identifiable. For example, Borgan and associates (1984) describe a special case in which the underlying intensity rates are piecewise constant. Without additional data, however, the modeling assumptions in a parametric analysis are untestable. The conclusions based on one model can differ greatly from those based on another. Thus, one must take care to select a sensible model, or at least a general model that is robust to misspecification.

A recent approach combines the benefits of parametric models and sacrifice data. Within a parametric framework, much information on tumor incidence can be gained by incorporating a few sacrifices. Likewise, relative to a nonparametric analysis, remarkably fewer sacrifices are needed owing to the increased structure provided by a parametric model. Portier (1986) proposes a semiparametric analysis in which the tumor incidence rate is assumed to follow a Weibull distribution (with scale parameter $b$ and shape parameter $c$):

$$\lambda(t) = bct^{c-1} \qquad (42)$$

but no parametric restrictions are placed on the conditional death rates (see also, Portier and Dinse, 1987; Dinse, 1988b). By reparameterizing in terms of more easily estimable quantities, Dinse (1988c) uses simple, flexible models to produce reasonable estimates of the incidence rate, the conditional death rates, and a measure of tumor lethality.

In a related approach, Ryan and Orav (1988) suggest modeling the death rate as a function of the tumor response indicator, as well as various covariates such as tumor size and histology. Under this model, the prevalence rates are identifiable and, thus, together with the rates of death with and without the tumor, so are the incidence rates.

Alternatively, rather than assuming parametric models for the actual components of the onset—death process, constraints can be placed on the way in which the components interact. For example, Dinse (1991) proposes the constant risk difference model, in which the difference between the death rates for animals with and without the tumor is assumed to be constant with respect to time:

$$\alpha(t \mid x) - \beta(t) = \Delta \tag{43}$$

Dinse (1991) also describes a constant risk ratio model, which assumes that the ratio of these death rates is constant with respect to time:

$$\frac{\alpha(t \mid x)}{\beta(t)} = \rho \tag{44}$$

Under either of these models, the tumor incidence rates and the tumor-free death rates are allowed to vary with each death time $t_j$, which yields a total of $2J + 1$ unknowns to be estimated in this nonparametric setting. Alternatively, we can assume parametric models for $\lambda(t)$ and $\beta(t)$. The MLEs and the operating characteristics of the likelihood-based test derived under the constant risk difference model appear very promising (Dinse, 1991, 1993, 1994). Lindsey and Ryan (1993) consider the constant risk ratio model in Eq. (44), but assume that the incidence rates and the tumor-free death rates are piecewise constant over a fixed set of time intervals.

## IX. DISCUSSION

Our understanding of the tumor onset and death process has evolved over time, as has our appreciation of which endpoints are important, what data must be collected, and how studies should be designed. In theory, the most appropriate analysis depends on all of these factors. In practice, statistical techniques must adapt to the current study designs and types of information commonly recorded in today's carcinogenicity experiments.

For example, the key outcome measure for assessing tumorigenesis is the time to tumor onset, which typically is characterized by the tumor incidence function. In the vast majority of organ sites, however, tumors simply are not observable in live animals; thus, the experiment provides no direct observations on the endpoint of primary interest. Consequently, one must focus on secondary endpoints, collect additional data, design studies differently, or make unverifiable assumptions. Although these possibilities were explored in the previous sections, we now briefly review each scenario individually.

If our goal is to estimate and to compare tumor incidence rates, an analysis oriented toward some other endpoint is unacceptable, unless a clear equivalence exists between tumor incidence and the other endpoint. The common alternatives, such as time-specific tumor prevalence, time to death with tumor, and time to death from tumor, suffer various shortcomings. Except in special situations, an analysis based on one of these other endpoints can produce biased inferences about tumor incidence. The best strategy, in general, is to focus on tumor incidence, if at all possible.

In a perfect world, with no budgetary limits, an ideal solution would be to design a large study with many interim sacrifices. Given enough sacrifice data, the analysis could focus on tumor incidence, without postulating parametric models or making assumptions about tumor lethality. Unfortunately, studies as expansive and expensive as this are rare; consequently, analyses that rely on an abundance of sacrifices will not routinely be applicable, regardless of how satisfying they are conceptually. In general, practical considerations in the real world will demand an approach that can be applied with few sacrifice times.

Assumptions about tumor lethality provide the simplest answer to the question of how to analyze time-specific tumor incidence rates. In this case, however, simplicity comes at the expense of sensibility. Most researchers would agree that the number of organ sites for which all tumors are strictly nonlethal or all tumors are immediately lethal must be very small indeed. Consequently, analyses that are based on either of these extreme lethality assumptions will produce biased inferences for tumor incidence when that lethality assumption is false. Techniques that rely on cause-of-death determinations experience similar problems. These approaches are sensitive to misclassification errors, and several investigations have shown that cause-of-death data can be unreliable.

The last resort seems to be the use of parametric models or functional constraints. Without sacrifice data, or other extraordinary information of some sort, the assumptions involved in a fully parametric analysis are untestable. Methods that rely on unverifiable assumptions generally are not considered reasonable. However, the increased structure of a parametric framework provides many benefits and should be explored further.

In conclusion, perhaps the most promising approach is based on a combination of some sacrifice data and some parametric structure. Although multiple sacrifice times are rare, most studies are terminated after a fixed time period, at which point all remaining animals are killed. In many cases, the data from this one terminal sacrifice can provide enough information about the overall tumorigenesis puzzle to allow a semiparametric analysis. That is, the data from the terminal sacrifice permit the incidence function to be identified when only some of the underlying transition rates are modeled parametrically or constrained in some way. For example, assuming a constant difference between the death rates for animals with and without the tumor is sufficient to provide an otherwise nonparametric analysis of the tumor incidence rates. In my opinion, this approach and other similar methods appear to be the most fruitful avenue for future research.

## ACKNOWLEDGMENTS

I am grateful to Joseph Haseman, James Huff, Ronald Melnick, and David Umbach for their constructive comments.

## REFERENCES

Archer, L., and L. Ryan (1989a). On the role of cause-of-death data in the analysis of rodent tumorigenicity experiments, *Appl. Stat.*, 38, 81–93.

Archer, L., and L. Ryan (1989b). Accounting for misclassification in the cause-of-death test for carcinogenicity, *J. Am. Stat. Assoc.*, 84, 787–791.

Armitage, P. (1955). Tests for linear trends in proportions and frequencies, *Biometrics*, 11, 375–386.

Ayer, M., H. Brunk, G. Ewing, W. Reid, and E. Silverman (1955). An empirical distribution function for sampling with incomplete information, *Ann. Math. Stat.*, 26, 641–647.

Bailer, A., and C. Portier (1988). Effects of treatment-induced mortality and tumor-induced mortality on tests for carcinogenicity in small samples, *Biometrics*, 44, 417–431.

Berlin, B., J. Brodsky, and P. Clifford (1979). Testing disease dependence in survival experiments with serial sacrifice, *J. Am. Stat. Assoc.,* 74, 5–14.

Bieler, G., and R. Williams (1993). Ratio estimates, the delta method, and quantal response tests for increased carcinogenicity, *Biometrics,* 40, 627–638.

Borgan, Ø., K. Liestøl, and P. Ebbesen (1984). Efficiencies of experimental designs for an illness–death model, *Biometrics,* 49, 627–638.

Breslow, N. (1970). A generalized Kruskal–Wallis test for comparing $K$ samples subject to unequal patterns of censorship, *Biometrika,* 57, 579–594.

Burnett, R., D. Krewski, and S. Bleuer (1989). Efficiency robust score tests for rodent tumorigenicity experiments, *Biometrika,* 76, 317–324.

Cairns, T. (1980). The $ED_{01}$ study: Introduction, objectives, and experimental design, *J. Environ. Pathol. Toxicol.,* 3, 1–7.

Chhabra, R., J. Huff, B. Schwetz, and J. Selkirk (1990). An overview of prechronic and chronic toxicity/carcinogenicity experimental study designs and criteria used by the National Toxicology Program, *Environ. Health Perspect.,* 86, 313–321.

Cochran, W. (1954). Some methods for strengthening the common $\chi^2$ tests, *Biometrics,* 10, 417–451.

Cox, D. (1970). *The Analysis of Binary Data,* Chapman & Hall, London.

Cox, D. (1972). Regression models and life-tables (with discussion). *J. R. Stat. Soc. B,* 34, 187–220.

Dewanji, A., and J. Kalbfleisch (1986). Non-parametric methods for survival/sacrifice experiments, *Biometrics,* 42, 325–341.

Dinse, G. (1985). Testing for a trend in tumor prevalence rates: I. Nonlethal tumors, *Biometrics,* 41, 751–770.

Dinse, G. (1986). Nonparametric prevalence and mortality estimators for animal experiments with incomplete cause-of-death data, *J. Am. Stat. Assoc.,* 81, 328–336.

Dinse, G. (1988a). A prevalence analysis that adjusts for survival and tumor lethality, *Appl. Stat.,* 37, 435–445.

Dinse, G. (1988b). Estimating tumor incidence rates in animal carcinogenicity experiments, *Biometrics,* 44, 405–415.

Dinse, G. (1988c). Simple parametric analysis of animal tumorigenicity data, *J. Am. Stat. Assoc.,* 83, 638–649.

Dinse, G. (1991). Constant risk differences in the analysis of animal tumorigenicity data, *Biometrics,* 47, 681–700.

Dinse, G. (1993). Evaluating constraints that allow survival-adjusted incidence analyses in single-sacrifice studies, *Biometrics,* 49, 399–407.

Dinse, G. (1994). A comparison of tumor incidence analyses applicable in single-sacrifice animal experiments, *Stat. Med.,* 13, 689–708.

Dinse, G., and S. Lagakos (1982). Nonparametric estimation of lifetime and disease onset distributions from incomplete observations, *Biometrics,* 38, 921–932.

Dinse, G., and S. Lagakos (1983). Regression analysis of tumour prevalence data, *Appl. Stat.,* 32, 236–248. Corrigenda (1984), 33, 79–80.

Efron, B. (1967). The two sample problem with censored data, *Proc. Fifth Berkeley Symp.,* 4, 831–853.

Finkelstein, D., and L. Ryan (1987). Estimating carcinogenic potency from a rodent tumorigenicity experiment, *Appl. Stat.,* 36, 121–133.

Gart, J., K. Chu, and R. Tarone (1979). Statistical issues in interpretation of chronic bioassay tests for carcinogenicity, *JNCI,* 62, 957–974.

Gart, J., D. Krewski, P. Lee, R. Tarone, and J. Wahrendorf (1986). *Statistical Methods in Cancer Research,* Vol. 3: *The Design and Analysis of Long-term Animal Experiments,* IARC Scientific Publications 79, International Agency for Research on Cancer, Lyon.

Gehan, E. (1965). A generalized Wilcoxon test for comparing arbitrarily single-censored samples, *Biometrika,* 52, 203–223.

Haseman, J. (1984). Statistical issues in the design, analysis and interpretation of animal carcinogenicity studies, *Environ. Health Perspect.,* 58, 385–392.

Hoel, D., and H. Walburg (1972). Statistical analysis of survival experiments, *JNCI,* 49, 361–372.

Huff, J., J. Haseman, and D. Rall (1991). Scientific concepts, value, and significance of chemical carcinogenesis studies, *Annu. Rev. Pharmacol. Toxicol.,* 31, 621–652.

Kalbfleisch, J., D. Krewski, and J. Van Ryzin (1983). Dose–response models for time-to-response toxicity data, *Can. J. Stat.,* 11, 25–49.

Kalbfleisch, J., and R. Prentice (1980). *The Statistical Analysis of Failure Time Data,* John Wiley & Sons, New York.

Kaplan, E., and P. Meier (1958). Nonparametric estimation from incomplete observations, *J. Am. Stat. Assoc.,* 53, 457–481.

Kodell, R., and J. Chen (1987). Handling cause of death in equivocal cases using the EM algorithm, *Commun. Stat. Theory Methods,* 16, 2565–2585.

Kodell, R., J. Farmer, D. Gaylor, and A. Cameron (1982a). Influence of cause-of-death assignment on time-to-death analyses in animal carcinogenesis studies, *JNCI,* 69, 659–664.

Kodell, R., and C. Nelson (1980). An illness-death model for the study of the carcinogenic process using survival/sacrifice data, *Biometrics,* 36, 267–277.

Kodell, R., G. Shaw, and A. Johnson (1982b). Nonparametric joint estimators for disease resistance and survival functions in survival/sacrifice experiments, *Biometrics,* 38, 43–58.

Krewski, D., and C. Brown (1981). Carcinogenic risk assessment: A guide to the literature, *Biometrics,* 37, 353–366.

Lagakos, S. (1979). General right censoring and its impact on the analysis of survival data, *Biometrics,* 35, 139–156.

Lagakos, S. (1982). An evaluation of some two-sample tests used to analyze animal carcinogenicity experiments, *Utilitas Math.,* 21B, 239–260.

Lagakos, S., and T. Louis (1985). The statistical analysis of rodent tumorigenicity experiments. In *Toxicological Risk Assessment,* 1, *Biological and Statistical Criteria* (D. Clayson, D. Krewski, and I. Munro, eds.), CRC Press, Boca Raton, FL, pp. 149–163.

Lagakos, S., and T. Louis (1988). Use of tumor lethality to interpret tumorigenicity experiments lacking cause-of-death data, *Appl. Stat.,* 37, 169–179.

Lagakos S., and C. Mosteller (1981). A case study of statistics in the regulatory process: the FD&C Red No. 40 experiments, *JNCI,* 66, 197–212.

Lagakos, S., and L. Ryan (1985). On the representativeness assumption in prevalence tests of carcinogenicity, *Appl. Stat.,* 34, 54–62.

Lindsey, J., and L. Ryan, (1993). A three-state multiplicative model for rodent tumorigenicity experiments, *Appl. Stat.,* 42, 283–300.

Malani, H., and J. Van Ryzin (1988). Comparison of two treatments in animal carcinogenicity experiments, *J. Am. Stat. Assoc.,* 83, 1171–1177.

Mantel, N. (1966). Evaluation of survival data and two new rank order statistics arising in its consideration, *Cancer Chemother. Rep.,* 50, 163–170.

Mantel, N. (1967). Ranking procedures for arbitrarily restricted observation, *Biometrics,* 23, 65–78.

Mantel, N., and W. Haenszel (1959). Statistical aspects of analysis of data from retrospective studies of disease, *JNCI,* 22, 719–748.

McKnight, B. (1988). A guide to the statistical analysis of long-term carcinogenicity assays, *Fundam. Appl. Toxicol.,* 10, 355–364.

McKnight B., and J. Crowley (1984). Tests for differences in tumor incidence based on animal carcinogenesis experiments, *J. Am. Stat. Assoc.,* 79, 639–648.

McKnight, B., and J. Wahrendorf (1992). Tumor incidence rate alternatives and the cause-of-death for carcinogenicity, *Biometrika,* 79, 131–138.

Mitchell, T., and B. Turnbull (1979). Log-linear models in the analysis of disease prevalence data from survival/sacrifice experiments, *Biometrics,* 35, 221–234.

Peto, R. (1974). Guidelines on the analysis of tumor rates and death rates in experimental animals [editorial], *Br. J. Cancer,* 29, 101–105.

Peto, R., and J. Peto (1972). Asymptotically efficient rank invariant test procedures, *J. R. Stat. Soc. A,* 135, 185–198.

Peto, R., M. Pike, N. Day, R. Gray, P. Lee, S. Parish, J. Peto, S. Richards, and J. Wahrendorf (1980).

Guidelines for simple, sensitive significance tests for carcinogenic effects in long-term animal experiments. In *Long-Term and Short-Term Screening Assays for Carcinogens: A Critical Appraisal,* IARC Monographs, Annex to Supplement 2, International Agency for Research on Cancer, Lyon, pp. 311–426.

Portier, C. (1986). Estimating the tumor onset distribution in animal carcinogenesis experiments, *Biometrika,* 73, 371–378.

Portier, C., and G. Dinse (1987). Semiparametric analysis of tumor incidence rates in survival/sacrifice experiments, *Biometrics,* 43, 107–114.

Racine-Poon, A., and D. Hoel (1984). Nonparametric estimation of the survival function when cause of death is uncertain, *Biometrics,* 40, 1151–1158.

Ryan, L. (1985). Efficiency of age-adjusted tests in animal carcinogenicity experiments, *Biometrics,* 41, 525–531.

Ryan, L., and E. Orav (1988). On the use of covariates for rodent bioassay and screening experiments. *Biometrika,* 75, 631–637.

Selwyn, M., A. Roth, and B. Weeks (1985). The weighted prevalence method for analyzing nonlethal tumor data. In *Proceedings of the Symposium on Long-Term Animal Carcinogenicity Studies: A Statistical Perspective,* American Statistical Association, Washington, DC, pp. 85–90.

Tarone, R. (1975). Tests for trend in life table analysis, *Biometrika,* 62, 679–682.

Tarone, R., and J. Ware (1977). On distribution-free tests for equality of survival distributions, *Biometrika,* 64, 156–160.

Turnbull, B., and T. Mitchell (1978). Exploratory analysis of disease prevalence data from survival/sacrifice experiments, *Biometrics,* 34, 555–570.

Turnbull, B., and T. Mitchell (1984). Nonparametric estimation of the distribution of time to onset for specific diseases in survival/sacrifice experiments, *Biometrics,* 40, 41–50.

Williams, P., and C. Portier (1992a). Analytic expressions for maximum likelihood estimators in a nonparametric model of tumor incidence and death, *Commun. Stat. A,* 21, 711–732.

Williams, P., and C. Portier (1992b). Explicit solutions for constrained maximum likelihood estimators in survival/sacrifice experiments, *Biometrika,* 79, 717–729.

# 27
# Risk Assessment for Nonquantal Toxic Effects

**James J. Chen, Ralph L. Kodell, and David W. Gaylor**
*National Center for Toxicological Research, Food and Drug Administration*
*Jefferson, Arkansas*

## I. INTRODUCTION

In quantitative risk assessment, the *risk* of a subject's experiencing a particular toxic effect is customarily defined as the statistical *probability* of the occurrence of such an effect. This characterization of risk in terms of probability originated with the mathematical modeling of carcinogenic effects associated with exposure to radiation and chemicals. In the case of *quantal* (binary: presence or absence) toxic responses such as cancer, the definition of an adverse health effect is self-evident, and the occurrence of such an effect can be observed on individual subjects. Hence, the modeled risk can be observed empirically. The same is true for traditional developmental toxic effects (malformations). By contrast, a clear-cut adverse effect for a quantitative (continuous) response, such as altered blood concentration of a toxicant, altered body weight or organ weight, or altered neurological function, is difficult both to define and to observe unequivocally. This partly explains why the widely accepted methods of risk assessment for quantal toxic endpoints have not carried over to quantitative responses. Although the risk of adverse quantal responses can be modeled easily in terms of the probability of occurrence of such effects, characterization of the risk of such responses in terms of probability of occurrence does not naturally follow.

The development of methods of risk assessment for continuous quantitative responses originated with the National Research Council (NRC, 1980) and with Crump (1984). Following a period of relative inactivity, interest in this problem has increased recently (Gaylor and Slikker, 1990; Stiteler and Durkin, 1990; Glowa, 1991; Chen and Gaylor, 1992; Kodell and West, 1993; West and Kodell, 1993). Some estimation methods are restricted to obtaining point estimates of the risk of quantitative effects, whereas others obtain statistical upper confidence limits on that risk. In cancer risk assessment, it is considered inadvisable to rely solely on model-based point predictions of risk for setting acceptable levels of exposure to carcinogenic substances, in light of the wide variability in the extrapolated predictions of various models that all fit well in the data range (FDA Advisory Committee on Protocols for Safety Evaluation, 1971; Office of Science and Technology Policy, 1985). Presently accepted methods of risk assessment for carcinogenic effects employ statistical upper confidence limits on the true excess risk above background risk. The present chapter discusses methods for obtaining both point estimates and statistical upper confidence limits on excess or additional risk for continuous quantitative toxic responses, using the familiar and customary framework of quantitative risk assessment for quantal effects.

## II. PRELIMINARIES

Let $y(d)$ be the quantitative response variable of an individual when exposed to dose $d$. For most continuous-type responses encountered in toxicology, either a normal or a lognormal distribution will adequately describe the data. In this paper, a normal distribution is assumed for the response variable $y(d)$, with mean $\mu(d)$ and variance $\sigma^2(d)$. Without loss of generality, let $c$ be a critical value for an abnormally low level of response, a level below which it is considered to be atypical. This level may or may not result in an adverse biological effect, but it represents a level that possibly should be avoided. Gaylor and Slikker (1990) suggested abnormal values are those that are far from the control mean and that occur with low probability in unexposed individual (i.e., the values in either the upper or lower tail). Thus, $c$ can be defined to be a response level equal to $\mu(0) - k\sigma(0)$, where $k$ is appropriately chosen to yield a specific low percentage point.

For exposure to a given dose $d$, the proportion of the individuals with response below the critical value $c = \mu(0) - k\sigma(0)$ is given by

$$P(d) = \Pr[y(d) \leq \mu(0) - k\sigma(0)]$$

$$= \Phi\left[\frac{\mu(0) - \mu(d) - k\sigma(0)}{\sigma(d)}\right]$$

where $\Phi$ is the standard normal cumulative distribution function, and $P(d)$ is the dose–response function representing the probability of an abnormal response. Note that $P(0) = \Phi(-k)$; and $P(d) = \Phi\{[\mu(0) - \mu(d)]/\sigma - k\}$ under a model of homogeneous variance, $\sigma^2(d) = \sigma^2$.

The function of interest from the risk assessment viewpoint is the additional risk,

$$R(d) = P(d) - P(0) \tag{1}$$

which measures the added response rate over the background response rate owing to the added dose, $d$. A *safe dose* is defined as the dose for which the additional risk satisfies

$$R(d) = \pi$$

where $\pi$ is a predetermined small number (e.g., $\pi = 10^{-4}$). To estimate an upper $100(1 - \alpha)\%$ confidence limit on the excess risk at dose $d = d^*$ is to determine a proportion $\pi^*$, with a probability or confidence of $100(1 - \alpha)\%$ that, at most, is a proportion $\pi^*$ of the population will be below $c$. This problem expressed mathematically is to determine a value $\pi^*$ such that

$$P[P(d^*) - \pi_0 \leq \pi^*] = 1 - \alpha$$

where $\pi_0 = P(0)$ is the proportion in the control for which $y(0) < c$. Conversely, the largest dose $d^*$ that satisfies the foregoing equation is the $100(1 - \alpha)\%$ lower confidence limit on the safe dose at given additional risk $\pi^*$.

As an alternative to determining directly a safe dose corresponding to a very small risk, Crump (1984) suggested using a benchmark dose, which is the lower confidence limit for a dose corresponding to 1–10% additional risk. A safe dose or allowable dose is then computed by applying a safety factor or uncertainty factor (e.g., 100) to the benchmark dose. The increased level of risk on which the benchmark is based would be near the lower limit of the experimental range that can be measured with reasonable accuracy (Crump, 1984), and the estimate of safe dose would be less model-dependent.

## III.   MAXIMUM LIKELIHOOD ESTIMATION

Consider an experiment of $g$ treatment groups, a control and $g - 1$ dose groups, with $m_i$ subjects in each group, $1 \leq i \leq g$ and $1 \leq j \leq m_i$. And let $y_{ij}$ be the response from the $j$th subject of the $i$th group. Suppose $y_{ij}$ is normally distributed, with the mean and variance given by

$$E(y_{ij}) = \mu(d_i) = \mu_i$$

and

$$\mathrm{Var}(y_{ij}) = \sigma^2(d_i) = \sigma_i^2$$

For estimation in and near the experimental dose–response range, assume the mean can be modeled by a polynomial in $d$ of degree $p < g$,

$$\mu_i = \beta_0 + \beta_1 d_i + \cdots + \beta_p d_i^p$$

The standard deviation can also be modeled by a link function, $\sigma_i = g^{-1}(\gamma, d)$, where $\gamma$ is a vector of parameters. For example, $g$ may be a constant function

$$g(\sigma_i) = \gamma$$

or an identity function

$$g(\sigma_i) = \sigma_i = \gamma_i$$

or an exponential–polynomial of degree $q < g$, i.e.,

$$\log(\sigma_i) = \gamma_0 + \gamma_1 d_i + \cdots + \gamma_q d_i^q$$

The identity function $g(\sigma_i) = \sigma_i$ is a nonparametric model in which separate standard deviations are estimated in each group. Estimation of the mean and standard deviation parameters can be obtained by the least-squares method if $g$ is a constant function, and by weighted least-squares if $g$ is an identity function. In general, the coefficient parameters can be estimated by using the maximum likelihood method. The log-likelihood function for the $N = \Sigma_i m_i$ samples is

$$LL = -1/2 \, \Sigma\Sigma \left[ \frac{(y_{ij} - \mu_{ij})^2}{\sigma_i^2} + \log(2\pi\sigma_i^2) \right]$$

The partial derivative of $LL$ relative to $\beta_k$ gives the estimating equations for $\beta_k$,

$$U(\beta_k) = \frac{\partial LL}{\partial \beta_k} = \left[ \Sigma\Sigma \frac{(y_{ij} - \mu_i)}{\sigma_i^2} \right] \left( \frac{\partial \mu_i}{\partial \beta_k} \right) \tag{2}$$

for $k = 1, 2, \ldots, p$. The partial derivative with respect to $\gamma_k$ gives the estimating equations for $\gamma_k$,

$$U(\gamma_k) = \frac{\partial LL}{\partial \gamma_k} = \left( \Sigma\Sigma \frac{s_{ij}^2 - \sigma_i^2}{\sigma_i^3} \right) \left( \frac{\partial \sigma_i}{\partial \gamma_k} \right) \tag{3}$$

for $k = 1, 2, \ldots, q$, where $s_{ij}^2 = (y_{ij} - \mu_i)^2$. The partial derivative of $U(\beta_k)$ with respect to $\gamma_k$ has expectation zero. Therefore, the parameters $\beta$ and $\gamma$ can be estimated by alternative iteration between $\mu_i$ and $\sigma_i$.

The maximum likelihood estimates (MLEs) of $\mu(d)$ and $\sigma(d)$ are

$$\hat{\mu}(d) = \hat{\beta}_0 + \hat{\beta}_1 d + \cdots + \hat{\beta}_p d^p$$

and

$$\hat{\sigma}(d) = g^{-1}(\hat{\gamma}_0, \ldots \hat{\gamma}_q; d)$$

where $\hat{\beta}$ and $\hat{\gamma}$ are the MLEs of $\beta$ and $\gamma$, respectively. The estimate of probability of an adverse effect at dose $d$ can be computed by substituting estimates of $\mu(d)$ and $\sigma(d)$ into Eq. (1),

$$\hat{R}(d) = \Phi\left\{ \frac{[\hat{\mu}(0) - \hat{\mu}(d) - k\hat{\sigma}(0)]}{\sigma(d)} \right\} - \Phi(-k) \tag{4}$$

Note that under the homogeneous standard deviation model, the estimate of the additional risk has the simpler form,

$$\hat{R}(d) = \Phi\left\{ \frac{[\hat{\mu}(0) - \hat{\mu}(d)]}{\hat{\sigma}} - k \right\} - \Phi(-k)$$

Since the operation between the expectation and $\Phi$ is not exchangeable, that is, $E[\Phi(x)] \neq \Phi[E(x)]$, the estimates $\hat{R}(d)$ in Eq. (4) will overestimate $R(d)$ at lower doses. Let $x$ be a random variable with mean $E(x)$ and variance $V(x)$. Expand $\Phi(x)$ in a Taylor series about $E(x)$,

$$\Phi(x) = \Phi[E(x)] + \phi[E(x)][x - E(x)] - 0.5E(x)\phi[E(x)][x - E(x)]^2 + \cdots$$

where $\phi$ is the standard normal density function. Taking the expectation, the second-order Taylor series approximation for the probability $\Phi[E(x)]$ is given by

$$\Phi[E(x)] = E[\Phi(x)] + 0.5E(x)\phi[E(x)]V(x)$$

Let $\hat{a}(d) = [\hat{\mu}(0) - \hat{\mu}(d)]$; the asymptotic distribution of $\hat{a}(d)$ is normal with mean

$$E[\hat{a}(d)] = \mu(0) - \mu(d)$$

and variance

$$V[\hat{a}(d)] = V[\Sigma_{i=1}\hat{\beta}_i d^i] = s_0^2(d)$$

Assuming $\hat{\sigma}(0)$ and $\hat{\sigma}(d)$ are constant, a second-order approximation for an estimate of the additional risk $R(d)$ is

$$\hat{R} = \Phi[\hat{m}(d)] + 0.5\hat{m}(d)\phi[\hat{m}(d)]V[\hat{a}(d)] / \hat{\sigma}^2(d) - \Phi(-k)$$

$$= \Phi[\hat{m}(d)] + 0.5\hat{m}(d)\phi[\hat{m}(d)][s_0(d) / \hat{\sigma}(d)]^2(d) - \Phi(-k) \tag{5}$$

where $\hat{m}(d) = [\hat{\mu}(0) - \hat{\mu}(d) - k\hat{\sigma}(0) / \hat{\sigma}(d)]$. The point estimate of safe dose at a given additional risk $\pi^*$ can be obtained by solving Eq. (5) reversely.

The assumptions that $\hat{\sigma}(0)$ and $\hat{\sigma}(d)$ are constant as well as the Taylor series approximation made in Eq. (5) to estimate the additional risk provide a simple method of correcting the bias caused by the nonlinearity of the $\Phi$ function. Simulation can be used to investigate the behavior of this approximation. A refinement may be to include the variance of $\hat{\sigma}(0)$ or $\hat{\sigma}(d)$, or both, in the approximation, or to use the higher orders of Taylor series. Note that, for large sample sizes, the variance $s_0^2(d)$ approaches 0, and the estimates of Eqs. (5) and (4) coincide; moreover, both estimates are unbiased asymptotically.

## IV. CONFIDENCE LIMIT

Procedures for obtaining upper confidence limits on additional risk (lower confidence limits on dose) were proposed by Chen and Gaylor (1992), Kodell and West (1993), and West and Kodell (1993). Three procedures are described in this paper: the likelihood ratio-based, asymptotic distribution of MLE, and bootstrap methods.

The likelihood ratio-based upper confidence limit on the additional risk at dose $d^*$ is defined to be the maximum value of $R(d^*)$, maximizing over $\beta = (\beta_0, \ldots, \beta_p)$ and $\gamma = (\gamma_0, \ldots, \gamma_q)$ that satisfies

$$-2[LL(\beta,\gamma) - LL(\beta,\gamma)] = \chi^2_{1,2\alpha}$$

Computational algorithms for calculating the confidence limits were given by Kodell and West (1993) and West and Kodell (1993).

The second approach to obtaining an upper confidence limit is based on the asymptotic distribution of the MLE.

1.  For the homogeneous standard deviation model, the distribution of $\hat{a}(d)$ is normal with mean $\mu(0) - \mu(d)$ and standard deviation $\sigma$. Assuming $\sigma$ is a constant, an approximate upper $100(1 - \alpha)\%$ confidence limit on the additional risk at dose $d$ can be obtained by

$$R_u(d) = \Phi\left\{\frac{[\hat{\mu}(0) - \hat{\mu}(d) + \hat{s}_o(d)z_{1-\alpha}]}{\hat{\sigma}} - k\right\} - \Phi(-k) \tag{6}$$

where $z_{1-\alpha}$ is the normal percentile.

2.  For the heterogeneous standard deviation model, the distribution of $\hat{\mu}(0) - \hat{\mu}(d) - k\hat{\sigma}(0)$ is asymptotic normal with mean $\mu(0) - \mu(d) - k\sigma(0)$ and variance

$$V[\hat{\mu}(0) - \hat{\mu}(d) - k\hat{\sigma}(0)] = V[\hat{a}(d)] + k^2V[\hat{\sigma}(0)] = \hat{s}^2(d)$$

Assuming $\hat{\sigma}(d)$ is a constant, an approximate upper $100(1 - \alpha)\%$ confidence limit is

$$R_u(d) = \Phi\left\{\frac{[\hat{\mu}(0) - \hat{\mu}(d) - k\hat{\sigma}(0) + \hat{s}(d)z_{1-\alpha}]}{\hat{\sigma}(d)}\right\} - \Phi(-k) \tag{7}$$

The third approach to obtaining upper confidence limits on additional risk is to use a bootstrap resampling of the original data with replacement using Monte Carlo techniques. The technique used in this paper is as follows:

1.  Compute the standardized residuals $e_{ij} = (y_{ij} - \hat{\mu}_i) / (stdr)_i$, where $(stdr)_i$ is the standard error of the residual for the $i$th group.
2.  Apply resampling with replacement to the standardized residuals $e_{ij}$, and construct a pseudoresponse variable $z_{ij} = \hat{\mu}_i + e_{ij}(stdr)_i$ for each group. This step is repeated 1000 times.

For each of these generated data sets of pseudoresponse variables, the MLEs of the parameters are obtained, and $R(d,\hat{\beta},\hat{\gamma})]$ is calculated using Eq. (5). The $(1000\alpha)$th largest value of $R(d,\hat{\beta},\hat{\gamma})]$ out of the 1000 would represent the bootstrap upper $100(1-\alpha)\%$ confidence limit on excess risk at $d*$.

A disadvantage of fitting the nonparametric model for the standard deviation is that the point estimates and the confidence limits can be estimated at only the experimental doses. The linear extrapolation method proposed by Gaylor and Kodell (1980) for quantal response is recommended for estimating the risks for nonexperimental doses. Let $r_i$ and $r_{i+1}$ be the additional risks at the experimental doses $d_i$ and $d_{i+1}$, respectively. The risk estimate $r_0$ at $d_0$, where $d_i < d_0 < d_{i+1}$, is obtained by

$$r_o = \frac{r_i + (r_{i+1} - r_i)(d_0 - d_i)}{(d_{i+1} - d_i)}$$

Conversely, the dose $d_0$ that corresponds to the excess risk $r_0$ is

$$d_o = \frac{d_i + (d_{i+1} - d_i)(r_o - r_i)}{(r_{i+1} - r_i)}$$

The upper confidence limit on risk or lower confidence limit on dose is computed similarly.

## A. Examples

Two examples are given. Both examples are for illustration purposes only; it is not intended to provide risk assessment of the two compounds. The first example considers the model with homogeneous standard deviation among treatment groups, and the second example considers the heterogeneous standard deviation.

The first example is from a 14-day dose–range-finding study on aconiazide conducted at the National Center for Toxicological Research (NCTR). The response variable is the body weight change in female rats. The data are listed in Table 1. The mean responses of the five groups are 10.40, 10.33, 8.48, 4.43, and –4.50 g for control, 100, 200, 500, 750 mg/kg per day, respectively. The mean body weight change decreases as dose increases. The no-observed-effect level (NOEL) is at 200 mg/kg per day.

The standard deviations for the five groups are 4.25, 2.67, 1.88, 3.29, and 2.93. The Bartlett test for homogeneity of variances was not significant ($p = 0.21$). Therefore, the homogeneous standard deviation model was fit in this example. Kodell and West (1993) assumed the quadratic (second-degree) polynomial for the mean model,

$$y(d) = \beta_0 + \beta_1 d + \beta_2 d^2 + \varepsilon$$

where $\varepsilon$ is a normal random variable, with mean 0 and a constant variance $\sigma^2$. The MLE estimates of the coefficients $\beta$ with the estimated standard errors for the fitted model are

$$\hat{\mu}(d) = 10.248 + 5.34 \times 10^{-4}d - 2.66 \times 10^{-5}d^2$$
$$\phantom{\hat{\mu}(d) = } (0.802) \quad (6.22 \times 10^{-3}) \quad (7.99 \times 10^{-6})$$

and the estimate of the common standard deviation $\sigma$ is 2.982.

Define the atypical values to be 3 standard deviations below the control mean, $k = 3$. The estimate of the additional risk for the NOEL, $d = 200$, is 0.0009, using Eq. (5). The upper 95% confidence limit on the excess risk is 0.0140, based on the asymptotic distribution of the MLE approach of Eq. (6), and is 0.0114, based on the bootstrap approach.

Conversely, the point estimate of the dose, corresponding to the additional risk level of

**Table 1**  Weight Gain or Loss (g)[a] in Female F344 Rats Treated with Aconiazide by Gavage Daily for 14 Days

| | Dose (mg/kg body weight) | | | | |
|---|---|---|---|---|---|
| | 0 | 100 | 200 | 500 | 750 |
| | 5.7 | 8.3 | 9.5 | 2.9 | −8.6 |
| | 10.2 | 12.3 | 8.1 | 5.6 | 0.1 |
| | 13.9 | 6.1 | 7.0 | −3.5 | −3.9 |
| | 10.3 | 10.1 | 7.8 | 9.5 | −4.0 |
| | 1.3 | 6.3 | 9.3 | 5.7 | −7.3 |
| | 12.0 | 12.0 | 12.2 | 4.9 | −2.2 |
| | 14.0 | 13.0 | 6.7 | 3.8 | −5.2 |
| | 15.1 | 13.4 | 10.6 | 5.6 | −1.0 |
| | 8.8 | 11.9 | 6.6 | 5.6 | −8.1 |
| | 12.7 | 9.9 | 7.0 | 4.2 | −4.4 |
| Mean | 10.40 | 10.33 | 8.48 | 4.43 | −4.50 |
| SD | 4.25 | 2.67 | 1.88 | 3.29 | 2.93 |

[a]The change in body weight is the final body weight on day 15 minus the initial weight on the day before the first treatment for each of ten rats in each dose group.

$\pi = 10^{-2}$ is 342 mg/kg per day. The 95% lower confidence limits on the dose are 178, 185, and 190 mg/kg per day using the likelihood ratio, MLE, and bootstrap approaches, respectively.

The second example is a study of dietary fortification with carbonyl iron. The response variable is the glucose level in black C5YSF1 mice. The data are listed in Table 2. The mean responses of the five groups are 75.83, 92.21, 97.23, 101.13, and 113.88 for control, 15, 35, 50, and 100 dg/kg per day (of iron), respectively. The mean level increases as dose increases. The lowest-observed-effect level (LOEL) is at 15 dg/kg per day. The standard deviations for the five groups are 11.36, 21.25, 20.56, 31.44, and 32.51. The Bartlett test for homogeneity of variances was significant ($p < 0.0001$). Therefore, a heterogeneous standard deviation model was assumed in this example.

The mean function is modeled as the quadratic polynomial and the standard deviation is modeled nonparametrically. The coefficient estimates of $\beta$ with the estimated standard errors are

$$\hat{\mu}(d) = 76.465 + 0.822d - 0.005d^2$$
$$(2.202) \quad (0.172) \quad (0.002)$$

The estimates of the means for the five groups are 76.47, 87.68, 99.17, 105.19, and 109.16, and the estimates of the standard deviations are 11.14, 21.29, 20.18, 30.80, and 30.60.

Again, define the atypical values to be 3 standard deviations above the control mean, $k = 3$. The point estimate of the additional risk for the lowest dose $d = 15$ is 0.146, from Eq. (5). The upper 95% confidence limits on the additional risk are 0.236, 0.262, and 0.248, using the likelihood ratio, MLE (see Eq. 7), and bootstrap approach, respectively.

Applying the linear extrapolation method to estimate the safe dose corresponding to the additional risk of 0.01, the point estimate is 1.027 and the lower confidence limit estimate is 0.605, by the likelihood ratio approach, and is 0.573, by the MLE approach.

An alternative standard deviation model is to use the quadratic exponential–polynomial. The

**Table 2** Glucose Level in C5YSF1 Black Mice Treated with Carbonyl Iron

| | Dose (dg/kg body weight) | | | | |
|---|---|---|---|---|---|
| | 0 | 15 | 35 | 50 | 100 |
| | 62 | 55 | 97 | 67 | 172 |
| | 64 | 94 | 96 | 76 | 123 |
| | 76 | 100 | 62 | 84 | 118 |
| | 59 | 98 | 114 | 104 | 133 |
| | 70 | 67 | 71 | 60 | 81 |
| | 70 | 106 | 84 | 110 | 97 |
| | 76 | 88 | 96 | 142 | 114 |
| | 90 | 64 | 87 | 113 | 97 |
| | 91 | 82 | 127 | 74 | 71 |
| | 80 | 108 | 131 | 124 | 70 |
| | 93 | 114 | 101 | 157 | 164 |
| | 80 | 124 | 98 | 142 | 130 |
| | 62 | 56 | 99 | 67 | 71 |
| | 63 | 97 | 64 | 76 | 128 |
| | 79 | 101 | 115 | 84 | 116 |
| | 56 | 101 | 73 | 104 | 133 |
| | 72 | 65 | 84 | 61 | 80 |
| | 70 | 106 | 96 | 112 | 97 |
| | 75 | 85 | 87 | 142 | 113 |
| | 91 | 63 | 125 | 108 | 94 |
| | 91 | 87 | 133 | 74 | 69 |
| | 79 | 110 | 99 | 121 | 71 |
| | 91 | 114 | | 154 | 165 |
| | 80 | 128 | | 143 | 126 |
| Mean | 75.83 | 92.21 | 97.23 | 104.13 | 113.88 |
| SD | 11.36 | 21.25 | 20.56 | 31.44 | 32.51 |

coefficient estimates of $\beta$ and $\gamma$ with the estimated standard errors for the fitted mean and standard deviation are

$$\hat{\mu}(d) = 76.820 + 0.853d - 0.005d^2$$
$$\phantom{\hat{\mu}(d) = } (2.411) \quad (0.187) \quad (0.002)$$

and

$$\log(\hat{\sigma}) = 2.521 + 0.026d - 0.0002d^2$$
$$\phantom{\log(\hat{\sigma}) = } (0.2553) \quad (0.013) \quad (0.0001)$$

The estimates of the means for the five groups are 76.82, 88.42, 100.16, 105.19, and 109.16, and the estimates of the standard deviations are 12.42, 17.69, 25.10, 29.83, and 30.42. This model appears to fit both means and standard deviations reasonably well.

The estimate of the additional risk for the low-dose group, $d = 15$, is 0.072 and the upper 95% confidence limit on the excess risk is 0.293, from Eq. (7). The bootstrap upper confidence limit estimate is 0.138.

Applying the linear extrapolation method to estimate the dose corresponding to the additional risk of 0.01, the point estimate is 2.083 and the lower confidence limit estimate is 0.512. By using the quadratic exponential–polynomial model to estimate the dose directly, the point estimate and the lower confidence limit are 6.091 and 0, respectively.

## B. Comparison with a Quantal Response Approach

It is of interest to compare the estimates obtained from a quantal analysis. The risk for the nonquantal response is defined to be the probability that the response on a quantitative scale for an individual will be below (or above) some critical level $c$. Assume that if a response is beyond the critical value, a biological quantal effect can be identified.

In the aconiazide example, the observed numbers of animals below the critical level $-2.75 = 10.40-4.25*3$ for the five groups were 0/10, 0/10, 0/10, 1/10, and 9/10. From the multistage model, using Global 86 (Howe and Crump, 1986), the maximum likelihood estimate of additional risk at the NOEL, $d = 200$, is 0.0080, and the 95% upper confidence limit is 0.056. Conversely, the maximum likelihood estimate of dose corresponding to the additional risk of $10^{-2}$ is 211, and the 95% lower confidence limit is 39.

Now, assume that $y(d)$ is normally distributed with a mean $10.248 + 5.34 \times 10^{-4}d - 2.66 \times 10^{-5}d^2$, and standard deviation 2.982. The probabilities that $y$ is less than or equal to $-2.75$ are 0., 0., 0., 0.0101, and 0.6988 for control, 100, 200, 500, and 750 ppm, respectively. If each group had contained 50 animals, then the expected numbers of animals that would be below or at $-2.75$ for the five groups are 0/50, 0/50, 0/50, 1/50, and 35/50. From the multistage model, the maximum likelihood estimate of the additional risk at $d = 200$ is 0.004, and the upper confidence limit is 0.0132. Conversely, the maximum likelihood estimate of safe dose corresponding to the additional risk of $10^{-2}$ is 243, and the lower confidence limit is 172. These numbers are very close to the numbers obtained in example 1. Thus, the response measured on a continuous scale provides more information than the binary classification of quantal response. The nonquantal method uses the data more effectively than the quantal method, since it takes five times as much quantal data to achieve the same results.

In the glucose example, the observed numbers of animals above the critical level $109.91 = 75.83 + 11.36*3$ for the five groups were 0/24, 5/24, 6/22, 11/24, and 13/24. From the multistage model, the maximum likelihood estimate of additional risks at the LOEL, $d = 15$, is 0.138, and the 95% upper confidence limit is 0.177. Conversely, the maximum likelihood estimate of safe dose corresponding to the additional risk of $10^{-2}$ is 1.013 and the 95% lower confidence limit is 0.771. These numbers are close to the numbers from the nonquantal method for the nonparametric standard deviation model with linear extrapolation.

Given this limited comparison, it appears that the efficiency of the quantal approach increases as the dose–response data become more linear. That is, the quantal approach provides better estimates for the approximately linear dose–response data (for risk) in example 2 than the highly nonlinear data in example 1.

## V. DISCUSSION

Three methods of computing confidence limits are the likelihood ratio, MLE, and bootstrap methods. The likelihood method has been studied by Kodell and West (1993) and West and Kodell (1993). Their simulation studies indicated that the likelihood ratio approach seemed to provide reasonably good coverage probabilities in both the homogeneous and heterogeneous standard deviation models. However, in their simulation the nonparametric standard deviation model was used; the performances based on fitting a parametric model (e.g., exponential–polynomial) or the linear extrapolation approach have not yet been studied.

The MLE approach described in this chapter assumes the standard deviation estimate $\hat{\sigma}(d)$ is constant. In the homogeneous standard deviation model, this approach performs well in terms of coverage probability. The MLE method is asymptotically equivalent to the noncentral *t*-distribution method given by Chen and Gaylor (1992). The MLE method, however, performs less well under the heterogeneous standard deviation model. In a simulation study, West and Kodell (1993) showed that the MLE method became very conservative if the variance of the $\hat{\sigma}(d)$ was included in the computation [i.e., $\hat{\sigma}(d)$ is treated as a random variable in Eq. (6) and (7)]. The confidence limit estimates computed from the likelihood ratio and MLE approaches did not attempt to correct the bias as being done in computing the point estimates. Whether use of an adjustment would improve the performance in the coverage probability requires further investigations.

The performance of the bootstrap approach depends on the point estimates of the additional risk and the safe dose. The bootstrap method can be improved by a better approximation for Eq. (5).

The additional risk for nonquantal responses is defined to be

$$R(d) = \Phi\left\{\frac{[\mu(0) - \mu(d) - k\sigma(0)]}{\sigma(d)}\right\} - \Phi(-k)$$

If the mean function $\mu(d)$ is a nondecreasing function of dose, then the additional risk will be nondecreasing under the homogeneous standard deviation model. However, this may not be true under the heterogeneous standard deviation model. That is, the additional risk may decrease as dose increases. Furthermore, the additional risk may be negative at small doses. These may be undesirable properties of the definition of adverse effect.

Ideally, the critical level should be based on a change that is toxicologically significant. The value used in the example was 3 standard deviations from the control mean. This value may be extreme; the number of observations beyond this value in the control group is likely to be zero for most of the experiments. Alternatively, $k$ may be chosen to be a level that corresponds to 1–10% tailed percentage points.

Under the linear mean and homogeneous standard deviation models, the dose–response model derived in this chapter is closely related to the probit model that is derived from the concept of a tolerance distribution. Assume that if the response reaches the critical level, an individual will respond quantally. Conversely, if the exposure is insufficient to reach the critical level, the quantal response will not occur. The tolerance distribution model assumes that each individual has its own tolerance to the dose, such that for a dose above the tolerance level, the individual responds quantally, and below that dose, there is no response. The relation between a quantal response and dose represents a cumulative distribution of tolerance, for which the tolerance of an individual is the dose level just insufficient for the quantal response to occur. Thus, the critical level and the tolerance level may have different interpretations, but may serve the same purpose.

## REFERENCES

Chen, J. J., and D. W. Gaylor (1992). Dose-response modeling of quantitative response data for risk assessment, *Commun. Stat. Theory Methods,* 21, 2367–2381.

Crump, K. S. (1984). A new method for determining allowable daily intake, *Fundam. Appl. Toxicol.,* 4, 854–871.

FDA Advisory Committee on Protocols for Safety Evaluation (1971). Protocols for safety evaluation: Panel on carcinogenesis report on cancer testing in the safety evaluation of food additives and pesticides, *Toxicol. Appl. Pharmacol.,* 20, 419–438.

Gaylor, D. W., and R. L. Kodell (1980). Linear interpolation algorithm for low dose risk assessment of toxic substances, *J. Environ. Pathol. Toxicol.,* 4, 305–312.

Gaylor, D. W., and W. L. Slikker (1990). Risk assessment for neurotoxic effects, *Neurotoxicology,* 11, 211–218.

Glowa, J. R. (1991). Dose–effect approaches to risk assessment, *Neurosci. Biobehav. Rev.,* 15, 153–158.

Howe, R. B., and K. S. Crump (1986). GLOBAL86: A computer program to extrapolate quantal animal toxicity data to low doses, prepared for the Office of Carcinogenic Standards, OSHA, U. S. Department of Labor, Contract 41USC252C3.

Kodell, R. L., and R. W. West (1993). Upper confidence limits on excess risk for quantitative responses, *Risk Anal.,* 13, 177–182.

National Research Council (1980). *Drinking Water and Health,* Vol. 3, Report of the Safe Drinking Water Committee, Board on Toxicology and Environmental Health Hazards, Assembly of Life Sciences, National Academy Press, Washington, DC.

Office of Science and Technology Policy (1985). Chemical carcinogens: A review of the science and its associated principles, U. S. Interagency Staff Group on Chemical Carcinogenesis, *Fed. Regist.,* 50, 10371–10442.

Stiteler, W. M., and P. R. Durkin (1990). Some statistical issues relating to the characterization of risk for toxic chemicals, Proceedings of the Workshop on Superfund Hazardous Waste: Statistical Issues in Characterizing a Site: Protocols, Tools, and Research Needs, Arlington, VA, February 21–22, 1990.

West, R. W., and R. L. Kodell (1993). Statistical methods of risk assessment for continuous variables, *Commun. Stat. Theory Methods,* 22, 3363–3376.

# 28

# Physiologically Based Pharmacokinetic Modeling of Phenanthrene

## I. Chu and Lung-fa Ku
*Health Canada*
*Ottawa, Ontario, Canada*

## I.  INTRODUCTION

Phenanthrene and its alkyl derivatives have been identified as major polycyclic aromatic hydrocarbons (PAH) in coal liquefaction products (Chu et al., 1988) and coprocessing products (Health Protection Branch, 1989). Phenanthrenes have also been found in automotive exhaust (Grimmer et al., 1977), sidestream cigarette smoke (Lee et al., 1976), and coal tar (Windolz, 1976). The carcinogenicity (IARC, 1983) and mutagenicity (LaVoie et al., 1983) of these compounds have been investigated, and some alkyl-substituted phenanthrenes have been mutagenic in *Salmonella typhimurium* TA98 and TA100. Studies from this and other laboratories have demonstrated that phenanthrene is readily metabolized in rats, guinea pigs, and rabbits to hydroxylated phenanthrenes and their conjugates (Chu et al., 1992; Chaturapit and Holder, 1978; Boyland and Sims, 1962). Because of their wide presence in the environment and their demonstrated biological effects, concern has been raised over their potential health hazards.

Although toxicity and metabolism of this PAH have been extensively investigated, there is no pharmacokinetic data available on this and other PAHs required for health hazard assessment. Recently, the application of physiologically based pharmacokinetic (PBPK) modeling has enabled the quantitative estimates of distribution and disposition of chemicals in tissues and organs, and cross-species extrapolations including different routes of administration (Andersen et al., 1987; for reviews see Dedrick, 1973; Hammelstein and Lutz, 1979). The PBPK models are different from the classic compartmental models, in that each compartment represents a well-defined physiological entity. Relying on the actual physiological parameters, such as body weight, cardiac output, blood flow rate, organ volumes, tissue/blood partition coefficients, and metabolism rates, PBPK models simulate the kinetics of chemicals in tissues and organs and, therefore, enable a better understanding of the complex dose–response relationship. The objective of the present work was to develop a physiologically based pharmacokinetic model for polycyclic aromatic hydrocarbons, and phenanthrene was selected as a model compound because of its wide presence in the environment and demonstrated biological effects.

## II.  MATERIALS AND METHODS

Phenanthrene, purchased from Aldrich Chemical Co. (Milwaukee, WI), was purified by recrystallization in ethanol to a purity of greater than 99%. The [9-$^{14}$C]phenanthrene was procured from Sigma Chemical (St. Louis, MO) and had a radiochemical purity and specific activity of greater than 99% and 10.4 mCi/mmol, respectively. The radiochemical purity was confirmed by thin layer chromatography (TLC) and radio-TLC methods. Other chemicals and solvents were of reagent grade obtained commercially.

Male Sprague–Dawley rats, weighing 300–330 g, were purchased from Charles River Laboratories (St. Constante, Quebec). The animals were acclimatized to laboratory conditions for 7 days before treatment. The jugular veins of the animals were cannulated with Silastic tubing (0.031 con id, 0.064 cm od, Dow-Corning, Toronto). Single IV doses of [$^{14}$C]phenanthrene at 0.7 mg/kg body weight (bw) or 7.0 mg/kg bw dissolved in a mixture of ethanol, saline, and Emulphor (1:8:1) were administered to groups of five rats through the cannula. Serial blood samples (0.2 ml) were withdrawn from the contralateral jugular vein at 10-min intervals up to 1 hr, then at hourly intervals up to 8 hr, and at 24, 48, and 72 hr after dosing. Approximately 0.1 ml of each sample was accurately measured and dissolved in 1.5 ml of 50:50 (v/v) mixture of isopropanol/Soluene-350 (Packard, Downers Grove, IL) and decolorized with 0.2 ml of 30% hydrogen peroxide. The decolorized samples were mixed with 10 ml Dimulume, and radioactivity was quantified with a Packard liquid scintillation counter (Model 2500 TR). The remaining samples were pooled according to the time point, and pooled samples were subjected to high-performance liquid chromatography (HPLC) analysis.

Tissue/blood partition coefficients for phenanthrene could not be determined by headspace gas chromatographic analysis because of its low volatility. As an alternative, concentrations of phenanthrene in blood and tissues were determined in rats administered the compound orally for up to 70 days for the high-dose groups and 77 days for the low-dose groups. Thus, two groups of 30 rats were administered phenanthrene with a 50 ppm or 500 ppm diet. Subgroups of three animals were sacrificed at week 5 to collect blood and tissues samples for analysis of phenanthrene. At week 10 another subgroup of three animals from each of the high- and low-dose groups on a phenanthrene-free diet for 2 days. Subsets of three animals were killed at 8 hr, 1 day, and 2 days, on the clean diet. At necropsy the animals were anesthetized with 3.0 ml/kg bw of pentobarbital (Somnotal) given intraperitoneally, and exsanguinated through the abdominal aorta. Blood and tissues, such as perirenal fat, liver, thigh muscle, and skin, were excised and analyzed using an HPLC fluorescence detection method previously described (Lawrence and Das, 1986).

## III.  EXPERIMENTAL DATA

### A.  Data From Intravenous Dose Experiments

Phenanthrene data are plotted in Fig. 1 and 2, and the mean values are listed in Table 1. The blood concentration data may be described by an exponential decay equation consisting of three exponential terms, commonly referred to as a three-compartmental model in the classic pharmacokinetic analysis. There were three time regions: $t < 1$, $1 < t < 8$, and $t > 8$ hr. The first region ($t < 1$ hr) had the steepest slope. The time constants were estimated to be 2.65, 0.12, and 0.04 hr$^{-1}$

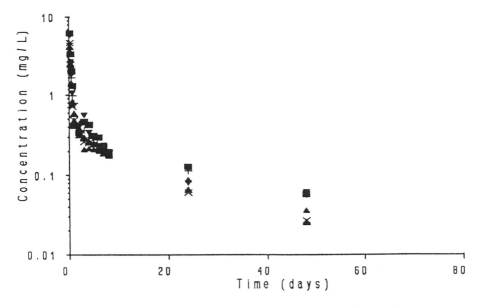

**Figure 1** Observed blood concentration (mg/L) for the high-dose (7 mg/kg) group.

for the three regions, respectively, in the high-dose group. In the low-dose group, they were 1.43, 0.13, and 0.02 hr$^{-1}$ for the three exponentials, respectively. The corresponding half-lives were 0.38, 8.56, and 28.09 hr for the high-dose, and 0.70, 7.83, and 41.65 hr for the low-dose groups.

The relation between the average blood phenanthrene concentrations in the high- and the low-dose groups is depicted in Fig. 3. The straight line in the figure had a slope of 1:10 which was the ratio of the dosage between the high (7 mg/kg) and the low dose (0.7 mg/kg). At $t = 30$ min, the ratio of the concentrations in blood were the same as the dosage ratio (1:10). At the

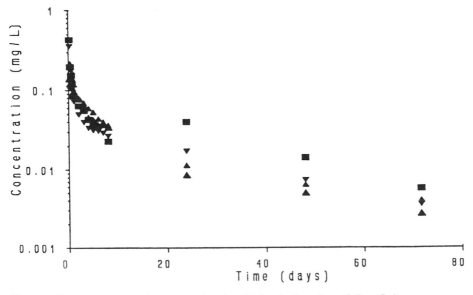

**Figure 2** Observed blood concentration (mg/L) for the low-dose (0.7 mg/kg) group.

**Table 1** Concentration of Phenanthrene in Blood (mg/L) Following Intravenous Administration

| | (Dose = 7 mg/kg bw, 6 rats) | | | (Dose = 0.7 mg/kg bw, 4 rats) | | |
|---|---|---|---|---|---|---|
| Time (hr) | Average | STD | STD % | Average | STD | STD% |
| 0.17 | 4.848 | 0.957 | 0.197 | 0.341 | 0.139 | 0.407 |
| 0.33 | 2.655 | 0.357 | 0.135 | 0.180 | 0.041 | 0.229 |
| 0.50 | 1.570 | 0.295 | 0.188 | 0.146 | 0.026 | 0.177 |
| 0.67 | 0.944 | 0.220 | 0.233 | 0.120 | 0.017 | 0.139 |
| 1.00 | 0.535 | 0.144 | 0.269 | 0.094 | 0.020 | 0.213 |
| 2.00 | 0.369 | 0.052 | 0.142 | 0.067 | 0.013 | 0.200 |
| 3.00 | 0.339 | 0.124 | 0.365 | 0.057 | 0.013 | 0.225 |
| 4.00 | 0.300 | 0.075 | 0.251 | 0.046 | 0.011 | 0.239 |
| 5.00 | 0.261 | 0.035 | 0.133 | 0.041 | 0.010 | 0.233 |
| 6.00 | 0.231 | 0.034 | 0.149 | 0.037 | 0.007 | 0.176 |
| 7.00 | 0.205 | 0.022 | 0.106 | 0.035 | 0.005 | 0.153 |
| 8.00 | 0.189 | 0.009 | 0.050 | 0.030 | 0.006 | 0.215 |
| 24.00 | 0.090 | 0.027 | 0.296 | 0.017 | 0.014 | 0.821 |
| 48.00 | 0.045 | 0.017 | 0.374 | 0.014 | 0.004 | 0.285 |
| 72.00 | | | | 0.006 | 0.001 | 0.220 |

time points earlier than 30 min, the concentration was high, and the concentration ratio became less than the dosage ratio. This might indicate that at high concentration, the phenanthrene might be retained in the blood proportionally more than for the low concentration owing to the saturation in the removal of the chemical. At $t > 30$ min, the ratios were very close to, or slightly higher than, the ratio of the dosage.

Figure 4 shows the relation between the average and standard deviation of data from both the high- and the low-dose groups. It shows that the standard deviation of the blood phenanthrene concentrations in rats is proportional to the level of the concentration, and is not dependent on

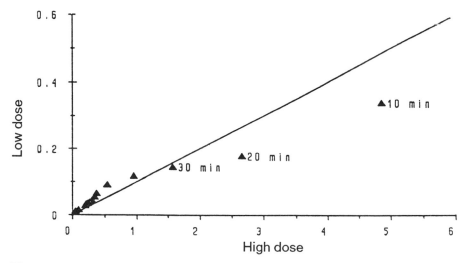

**Figure 3** Relation of blood concentration mg/L between high-dose and low-dose experiments.

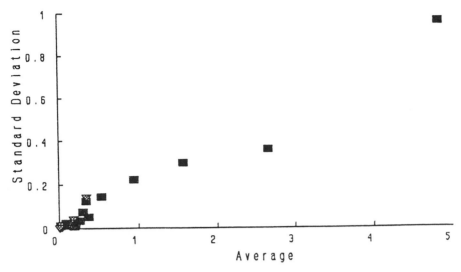

**Figure 4**  Relation between standard deviations and averages (■ high dose, ▼ low dose).

the administered dose. The regression coefficient of the standard deviation relative to the mean value was 0.186.

## B.  Data From Oral Dose Experiments

Blood and tissue phenanthrene data of the high (500 ppm) and the low (50 ppm) dose groups are shown in Figs. 5 and 6, respectively. Only the fat and blood data for the low-dose groups were available. Tables 2 and 3 display the mean and the range of phenanthrene concentrations in blood and tissues for the groups terminated at day 70 (high-dose) and at day 77 (low-dose).

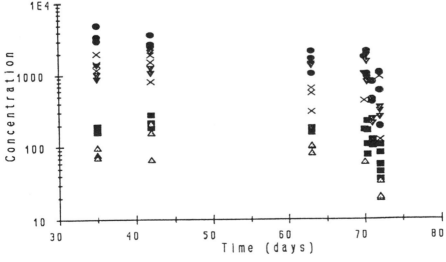

**Figure 5**  Average concentrations for high oral dose (500 ppm in diet) (■ = blood, ▼ = liver, ● = fat, ▲ = muscle, × = skin).

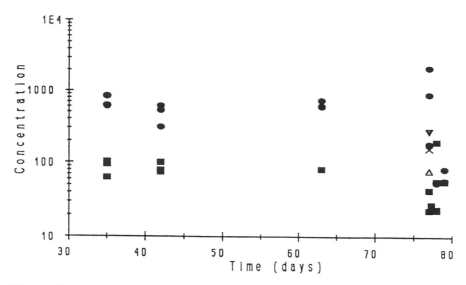

**Figure 6**  Same as Fig. 5 for low oral dose (50 ppm in diet).

At days 35, 42, and 63, the concentrations in blood were about 200 ng/ml for the high-dose and 100 ng/ml for the low-dose groups. This ratio of 2:1 was much smaller than the dosage ratio of 10:1. The ratio for fat of the two dose groups was about 4:1, which was higher than that for blood, but was still much smaller than the ratio of the dosage.

The difference between the highest and lowest fat phenanthrene concentrations at any sampling time between animals was about twofold. The only exception was for the high-dose group

**Table 2**  Concentration of Phenanthrene (µg/L) in Blood and Tissues of Rats Exposed Orally in the Diet[a]

| Time (days) | No.[b] | Blood | Liver | Fat | Muscle | Skin |
|---|---|---|---|---|---|---|
| | | | Average | | | |
| 35.0 | 3 | 179.3 | 1082.7 | 3818.6 | 82.5 | 1541.1 |
| 42.0 | 3 | 225.4 | 1474.0 | 2992.1 | 145.9 | 1427.8 |
| 63.0 | 3 | 168.0 | 1354.3 | 1627.7 | 95.5 | 498.5 |
| 70.0 | 1 | 169.3 | 1022.0 | 1782.0 | 60.9 | 427.0 |
| 70.3 | 4 | 141.1 | 1373.3 | 1369.3 | | |
| 71.0 | 4 | 110.2 | 224.0 | 557.1 | | |
| 72.0 | 6 | 62.8 | 300.3 | 622.0 | 24.6 | 665.5 |
| | | | Range | | | |
| 35.0 | 3 | 32.0 | 508.0 | 1966.1 | 26.1 | 825.3 |
| 42.0 | 3 | 91.1 | 1046.0 | 1153.3 | 146.4 | 1112.3 |
| 63.0 | 3 | 24.0 | 63.0 | 1105.7 | 22.4 | 340.9 |
| 70.0 | 1 | | | | | |
| 70.3 | 4 | 144.8 | 1060.0 | 1198.0 | | |
| 71.0 | 4 | 21.5 | 31.7 | 388.0 | | |
| 72.0 | 6 | 68.7 | 90.0 | 883.5 | 14.4 | 814.9 |

[a]Dose = 500 ppm.

[b]No., number of animals.

**Table 3** Concentration (µg/L) of Phenanthrene in Blood and Tissues of Rats[a]

| Time (days) | No.[b] | Blood | Liver | Fat | Muscle | Skin |
|---|---|---|---|---|---|---|
| | | | Average | | | |
| 35.0 | 3 | 92.3 | | 781.3 | | |
| 42.0 | 3 | 81.3 | | 585.7 | | |
| 63.0 | 3 | 78.9 | | 559.5 | | |
| 77.0 | 1 | 43.1 | 275.3 | 961.0 | 80.3 | 158.5 |
| 77.3 | 1 | 23.0 | | | | |
| 78.0 | 4 | 32.9 | | | | |
| 79.0 | 3 | 127.0 | | 66.1 | | |
| | | | Range | | | |
| 35.0 | 3 | 26.0 | | 240.7 | | |
| 42.0 | 3 | 38.0 | | 75.9 | | |
| 63.0 | 3 | 7.4 | | 429.5 | | |
| 77.0 | 1 | | | 1967.0 | | |
| 77.3 | 1 | | | | | |
| 78.0 | 4 | 33.7 | | | | |
| 79.0 | 3 | 139.6 | | 28.1 | | |

[a]Dose = 50 ppm.
[b]No., number of animals.

sacrificed at 70 days and the low-dose group at 77 days, for which the ratio was as large as 5:1. In general, the range was about half or equal to the average. Since samples were collected from different rats, this might be one of the reasons that the data had much larger variations than those of the intravenous data, for which serial blood samples were obtained from the same animals.

Tables 4 and 5 give tissue/blood concentration ratios that were used as initial estimates of

**Table 4** Concentration Ratios Between Tissue and Blood of Rats Fed High-Dose (500 ppm) Phenanthrene Diet

| Time (days) | No. | Liver/B | Fat/B | Muscle/B | Skin/B |
|---|---|---|---|---|---|
| | | Average | | | |
| 35.0 | 3 | 6.05 | 21.15 | 0.46 | 8.61 |
| 42.0 | 3 | 6.70 | 13.34 | 0.71 | 6.75 |
| 63.0 | 2 | 7.98 | 8.04 | 0.55 | 2.76 |
| 70.0 | 1 | 6.04 | 10.53 | | |
| 70.3 | 3 | 11.96 | 11.89 | | |
| 71.0 | 3 | 2.11 | 5.32 | | |
| 72.0 | 3 | 4.13 | 7.85 | 0.32 | 9.1 |
| | | Range | | | |
| 35.0 | 3 | 2.59 | 7.79 | 0.10 | 4.22 |
| 42.0 | 3 | 5.31 | 2.99 | 0.91 | 6.01 |
| 63.0 | 2 | 1.12 | 2.72 | 0.05 | 1.64 |
| 70.0 | 1 | | | | |
| 70.3 | 3 | 4.00 | 4.65 | | |
| 71.0 | 3 | 0.41 | 4.19 | | |
| 72.0 | 3 | 3.78 | 8.54 | 0.22 | 15.41 |

**Table 5** Concentration Ratio Between Tissue and Blood of Rats Fed Low-Dose (50 ppm) Phenanthrene Diet

| Time (days) | No. | Liver/B | Fat/B | Muscle/B | Skin/B |
|---|---|---|---|---|---|
| | | | Average | | |
| 35.0 | 3 | | 8.63 | | |
| 42.0 | 3 | | 7.47 | | |
| 63.0 | 3 | | 5.86 | | |
| 77.0 | 1 | 6.39 | 4.29 | 1.86 | 3.68 |
| 77.3 | 1 | | | | |
| 78.0 | 4 | | | | |
| 79.0 | 2 | | 1.31 | | |
| | | | Range | | |
| 35.0 | | | 4.52 | | |
| 42.0 | | | 3.58 | | |
| 63.0 | | | 3.45 | | |
| 77.0 | | | | | |
| 77.3 | | | | | |
| 78.0 | | | | | |
| 79.0 | | | 0.74 | | |

the partition coefficient for the model study. The concentration ratios between fat and blood from animals sacrificed after 42 days varied from 2 to 26 for the high dose, and 6 to 9 for the low dose. The average of all samples was 11, and half of them had values between 9 and 12. Phenanthrene in other tissues was analyzed only for the high-dose group. The ratio for liver varied from 2.4 to 9.8 and the average was 6. The ratio for muscle had the least variation of 0.2–1.2, the average being 0.5, and half of the samples had ratios between 0.4 and 0.5. The skin also showed a large variation of 2–17, with an average of 7; half of the samples had values between 6 and 9.

## IV. BASIC MODEL PARAMETERS

### A. Physiological Parameters

The tissue volume and blood flow in Table 6 are the same as those described by Leung et al. (1990). The cardiac output was as described by Arms and Travis (1988). The tissue volume and blood flow in the slowly perfused organs were separated into the muscle and the skin. It was assumed that 90% of the blood flow in the slowly perfused tissues was in the muscle and the remaining 10% in the skin; 70% of the tissue volume in the slowly perfused tissues was the muscle and the remaining 30% the skin.

### B. Partition Coefficients and Metabolic Constants

The partition coefficients were estimated by the ratio of tissue/blood concentrations in rats exposed to phenanthrene orally over 70 days. These values were used as a first approximation and are listed in Table 6. The value of $V_{max}$ and $K_m$ were determined to be 0.17 and 1.7 in vitro by incubation of phenanthrene with rat liver microsomes, using a standard method.

**Table 6** Physiological Parameters Used in Modeling

Body weight (bw) = 0.33 kg
Cardiac output (QC) = $14.1 \times \text{bw}^{0.75}$ (l/hr)

| Parameters[a] | Blood | Liver | Organs | Fat | Muscle | Skin |
|---|---|---|---|---|---|---|
| Volume | 0.050 | 0.050 | 0.040 | 0.110 | 0.497 | 0.213 |
| Volume (l) | | 0.017 | 0.013 | 0.036 | 0.164 | 0.070 |
| Blood flow | 1.0 | 0.250 | 0.510 | 0.050 | 0.171 | 0.019 |
| Blood flow (l/hr) | 6.139 | 1.535 | 3.131 | 0.307 | 1.050 | 0.117 |
| Partition coefficients | | 5.0 | 5.0 | 10.0 | 0.5 | 10.0 |
| Time constant (hr$^{-1}$) | | 18.600 | 47.439 | 0.846 | 12.802 | 0.166 |

Slowly perfused tissues

Volume = 0.71

|  |  | | | | Muscle | Skin |
|---|---|---|---|---|---|---|
| Ratio | | | | | 0.7 | 0.3 |

Blood flow = 0.19

| Ratio | | | | | 0.9 | 0.1 |

$V_{max} = 0.5$
$K_m = 1.78$

[a]Volume, fraction of body weight; blood flow, fraction of cardiac output; ratio, muscle (or skin)/slowly perfused tissue.

## V. MODELING OF INTRAVENOUS PHENANTHRENE DATA

By using the physiological parameters and biochemical data given in the preceding section, a PBPK model consisting of six compartments: blood, liver, richly perfused tissue, fat, muscle, and skin was constructed. A diagram of the model is shown in Fig. 7, and the equations for each compartment are given in Eqs. 1–6.

$$\text{Blood:} \quad \frac{d}{dt} C_b(t) = \left(\frac{1}{U_b}\right) \Sigma_i Q_i V_i(t) - \left(\frac{Q_b}{U_b}\right) C_b(t) + \left(\frac{1}{U_b}\right) Y_b(t) \tag{1}$$

$$\text{Liver:} \quad \frac{d}{dt} C_1(t) = \left(\frac{Q_1}{U_1}\right) [C_b(t) - V_1(t)] - \left(\frac{1}{U_1}\right) Z_1(t) \tag{2}$$

$$\text{Richly:} \quad \frac{d}{dt} C_r(t) = \left(\frac{Q_r}{U_r}\right) [C_b(t) - V_r(t)] \tag{3}$$

$$\text{Fat:} \quad \frac{d}{dt} C_f(t) = \left(\frac{Q_f}{U_f}\right) [C_b(t) - V_f(t)] \tag{4}$$

$$\text{Muscle:} \quad \frac{d}{dt} C_m(t) = \left(\frac{Q_m}{U_m}\right) [C_b(t) - V_m(t)] \tag{5}$$

$$\text{Skin:} \quad \frac{d}{dt} C_s(t) = \left(\frac{Q_s}{U_s}\right) [C_b(t) - V_s(t)] \tag{6}$$

$Q_i$ denotes the rate at which blood flows into and out of compartment $i$, $U_i$ denote the tissue volume of the compartment $i$. $C_b(t)$ is the concentration in arterial blood, $V_i(t)$ is the concentra-

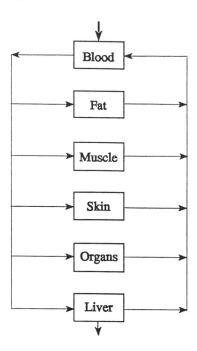

**Figure 7**  Six-compartments PBPK model.

tion in venous blood, and $Y_b(t)$ is the administered dose available for systemic circulation over time. $\Sigma_i$ denotes the summation excluding the blood compartment and

$$Q_b = \Sigma_i Q_i \tag{7}$$

The concentration in the venous blood is expressed as

$$V_i(t) = C_i(t) / P_i \tag{8}$$

where $P_i$ denotes the partition coefficient between tissue and blood; $Z_i(t)$ is the rate of metabolic removal, and the Michaelis–Menten removal mechanism is used:

$$Z_1(t) = \frac{V_{max}V_1(t)}{[K_m + V_1(t)]} \tag{9}$$

where $V_{max}$ is the maximum removal rate, and $K_m$ is the concentration at half the maximum removal rate.

## A.  The Basic Circulatory Model

In this model, the value of $V_{max}$ was initially set to 0.5 and the value of $K_m$ is 1.78. The prediction from the model and the observed data are plotted in Fig. 8. It showed that at $t < 8$ hr, the model prediction was generally slightly higher than the observed data for the low dose, but was much higher than the observed values for the high dose. The attenuation of the model concentration was faster than the observed data. This was especially obvious at $t > 8$ hr.

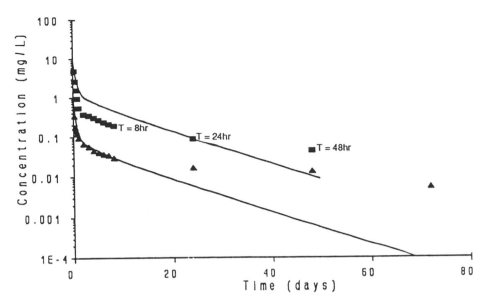

**Figure 8** Model (lines) and observed (symbols) data of intravenous high- (■) and low- (▲) dose experiments.

## B. The Refinement of Circulatory Model for the Low Dose

Since the model-fitting for low dose had a better result than that for the high dose, the low-dose model was further explored as discussed in the following sections.

### 1. Changes in $V_{max}$

The model used in the Michaelis–Menten excretion mechanism in the liver. With the partition coefficient of $P_1 = 5$, the time constant of liver, which could be expressed as $Q_1/P_1U_1$, was 0.31 min$^{-1}$. Therefore, the response of the liver was very fast. For the low-dose intravenous experiment, the venous concentration in liver reached its maximum of 0.74 at 0.04 hr. The concentration was much smaller than the Michaelis constant of 1.78. Therefore, the removal process was operating almost linearly at all times.

The rate of metabolic removal determined the overall slope of the concentration curve and had little effect on the shape of the curve. Therefore, by lowering the value of $V_{max}$, the attentuation rate would be decreased and, consequently, the concentration curve would rotate counterclockwise, as shown in Fig. 9 for $V_{max} = 1, 0.5$, and $0.25$. Therefore, very little improvement can be achieved by changing the $V_{max}$ alone, and $V_{max} = 0.5$ gives the best fit among the three values.

### 2. Changes in the Perfusion Rate of Skin

Skin had a very slow blood perfusion rate. For $P_s = 10$, the time constant of fat compartment is 0.166 hr$^{-1}$, which was the lowest among all of the compartments. Therefore, it largely controlled the shape of the concentration curve at a later time. By increasing the value of $P_s$, a larger portion of the substance would be stored initially in this compartment, which resulted in low phenanthrene concentrations in blood and other compartments. After the phenanthrene concentration

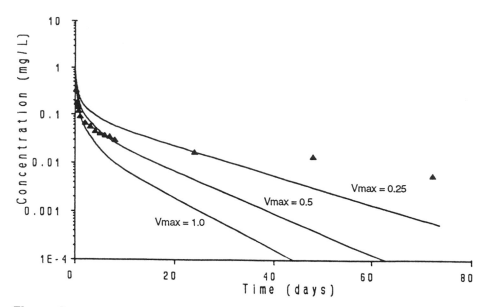

**Figure 9**   Intravenous dose model experiment by changing $V_{max}$.

in the skin compartment reached its maximum, the skin would start to reverse its role by releasing the substance.

The decrease in liver phenanthrene concentration would reduce the metabolic removal rate; therefore, the higher skin perfusion rate would result in more substance being retained in the body at any given time. Because of the small time constant of the skin compartment, the release

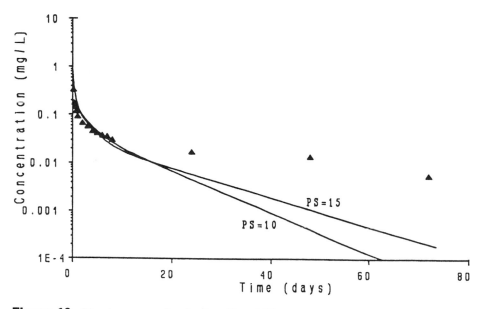

**Figure 10**   Blood concentration for $P_s = 10$ and 15.

of the substance from this compartment to others was also slower. Therefore, its removal by metabolism in the liver would also be slower. Consequently, the blood concentration will be higher than that obtained using $P_s = 10$, as illustrated in Fig. 10.

### 3. Change in Partition Coefficient of Fat/Blood

The other slow perfusion compartment was the fat, and laboratory data indicated that there was a large variation in the ratio of fat/blood concentration (see Tables 4 and 5). Therefore, the fat partition could be larger than 10, which was used in the previous models. It was expected that the increase in $P_f$ would produce the same result as that caused by changes in $P_s$, as shown in Fig. 11. Note that $P_f = 20$ also gives a much better fit for data below $t = 8$ hr.

## C. The Second-Order Metabolic Removal

The basic circulatory model failed to explain the slow rate of decrease in blood phenanthrene concentration when its values were low. To address this problem, the Michaelis–Menten removal function was modified to make it depend on the second order of the venous blood concentration, as shown in Eq. (10). The values of $V_{max}$ and $K_m$ obtained by fitting the high-dose and the low-dose data by the SIMUSOLV program (Mitchell and Gauthier Assoc. Concord, MA) were 4.455[0.073] and 1.569[0.049]. The values in the bracket are the standard deviations.

$$Z_1(t) = \frac{V_{max}V_1^2(t)}{(K_m + V_1^2(t))} \tag{10}$$

The result of the model is given in Fig. 12. It showed a good fit for the low-dose data, but the predicted concentrations were too low for the high-dose experiment. Since the rate of removal was determined by $V_{max}$ at high concentration and $V_{max} / K_m$ at low concentration, the

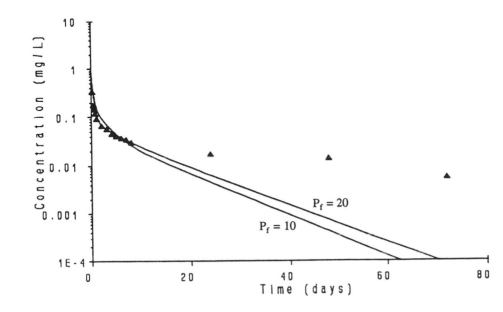

**Figure 11** Blood concentration for $P_f = 10$ and 20.

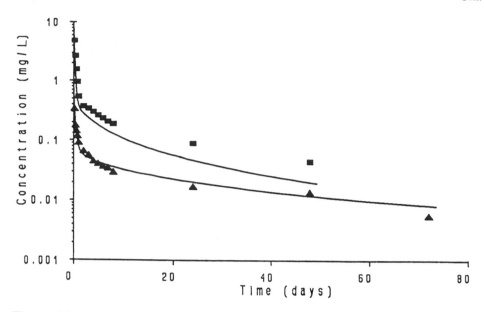

**Figure 12** Blood concentration for the high-dose and the low-dose intravenous model with second-order removal.

predicted value for the high dose could be raised by reducing $V_{max}$. At the same time, the value of $K_m$ should also be reduced to keep the ratio $V_{max} / K_m$ unchanged for the low dose. Figures 13 and 14 show this effect. The lower curve is the result from using the same $V_{max}$ and $K_m$ obtained previously. The middle and the upper curves are the result by reducing the parameters to 0.5 and 0.25 of their original values. Figures 13 and 14 show that the reduction in $V_{max}$ and $K_m$ to 0.5

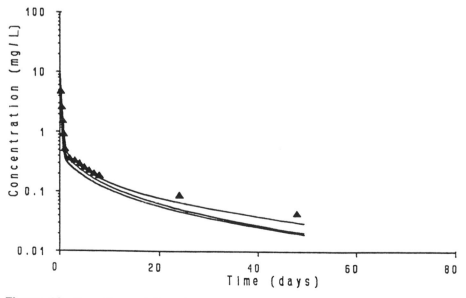

**Figure 13** Same $V_{max}$ and $K_m$ as in Fig. 12 (bottom curve); parameters reduced to 50% (middle curve) and 25% (upper curve).

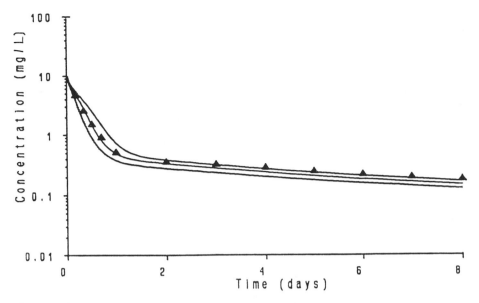

**Figure 14**  Same as Fig. 13 (with second order removal).

will improve the prediction for $t < 8$ hr. A further reduction to 0.25 improved fitting for $t > 8$ hr, but would overestimate the concentration for data $t < 1$ hr. Note that these changes in $V_{max}$ and $K_m$ did not have any significant effect on the prediction for the low dose.

## D.  The Saturation Input Model

The other mechanism that was investigated was the saturation in input. The model assumed that the amount of the dose initially available for circulation $Y_c$ was not equal to that administered into the body $Y_i$. This might occur when the dosage was high and where part of the dose was sequestered. These two are related by

$$Y_c = \frac{K_i Y_i}{(K_i + Y_i)} \tag{11}$$

At the low dose, $Y_c$ was almost equal to $Y_i$, but at the high dose, $Y_c$ was limited by $K_i$. This was a similar function used in the Michaelis–Menten removal mechanism.

The remaining compound $(Y_i - Y_c)$ was assumed to be released slowly as

$$\frac{d}{dt} Y_r(t) = (Y_i - Y_c) K_r (1 - e^{-\alpha t}) e^{-\beta t} \tag{12}$$

where $K_r$ is an integration constant which is

$$K_r = \frac{\beta(\alpha + \beta)}{\alpha} \tag{13}$$

Since the second-order removal model with $K_m = 0.442$ and $V_{max} = 1.116$ predicted a higher concentration than the data observed in the high-dose group, this saturation function was expected to produce some reduction in model prediction. Therefore, this model was used as a basis for adding the saturation on the input. The values of the parameters $K_i$,

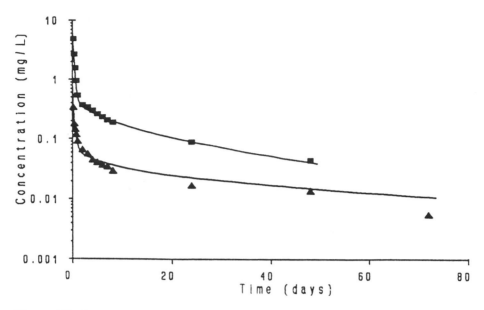

**Figure 15** Intravenous dose. Second-order removal and input saturation model.

$\alpha$ and $\beta$ were computed by the SIMUSOLV, using the high-dose data, and the results were 6.191[0.508], 2.469[0.097], and 0.094[0.005], respectively for $K_i$, $\alpha$, and $\beta$ (values in the brackets are the standard deviation]. The results of this model are plotted in Figs. 15 and 16. The same parameters were used to predict the low-dose data, and the results are plotted in the same two figures. It was obvious that this model produced a better fit to both the high- and the low-dose data.

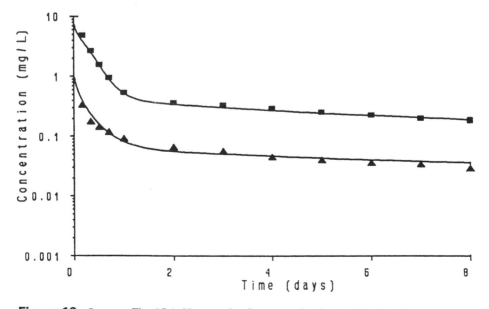

**Figure 16** Same as Fig. 15 (with second-order removal and saturation input).

## VI.  SUMMARY

Phenanthrene can be described by a six-compartment PBPK model consisting of liver, blood, fat, skin, muscle, and richly perfused tissue compartment. The modeling of a highly lipophilic compound, such as phenanthrene, necessitated a number of approaches different from those used in low molecular weight hydrocarbon solvents. Because of its low volatility, the tissue/blood partition coefficients of phenanthrene could not be determined by the headspace chromatography technique. The coefficients were estimated by the ratio of concentrations in tissues and blood of animals dosed with the compound to a steady state. This model prediction was improved by replacing the venous blood concentration in the Michaelis–Menten removal equation by its squares. The improvement was especially significant when the concentration was low. To improve the fitting of the predicted results to the observed data, it was further assumed that a saturation mechanism, which could be represented in an equation similar to the Michaelis–Menten equation, limited the immediate availability of the administered dose for circulation. The excess amount would be slowly released for circulation later. This modification improved the prediction for the high dose. The biological significance of the second-order term in a modified Michaelis–Menten equation was unknown, but the effect would make the curve similar to those caused by the existence of allosteric binding sites and increased affinity at high substrate concentrations (Roberts, 1977), a phenomenon that might have occurred to phenanthrene following dosing.

The present study provided one model whereby the pharmacokinetic behavior of phenanthrene may be described. There may be other models to describe the kinetic behavior of this compound. The usefulness of the modeling is that it prompts the investigator to refine the models so that they can better describe the kinetic process if the initial model fails to fit the observed data. Therefore, meaningful biological processes might be discovered through various modeling trials. Further work is being conducted to validate the model by examining phenanthrene at additional dose levels.

## REFERENCES

Andersen, M. E., H. J. Clewell, M. L. Gargas, F. A. Smith, and R. H. Reitz (1987). Physiologically based pharmacokinetics and risk assessment process for methylene chlorine, *Toxicol. Appl. Pharmacol.,* 87, 185–205.

Arms, A. D., and C. C. Travis (1988). Reference physiological parameters in pharmacokinetic modelling, U. S. EPA Final Report, EPA 600/6-88/004.

Boyland, E., and P. Sims (1962). Metabolism of polycyclic compounds, 21. The metabolism of phenanthrene in rabbits and rats: Dihydrodihydroxy compounds and related glucosiduronic acids, *Biochem. J.,* 84, 571–582.

Chaturapit, S., and G. M. Holder 91978). Studies on the hepatic microsomal metabolism of [$^{14}$C]phenanthrene, *Biochem. Pharmacol.,* 27, 1865–1871.

Chu, I., D. C. Villeneuve, M. Cote, V. E. Valli, and R. Otson (1988). The dermal toxicity of a medium-boiling (154–378°C) coal liquefaction product in the rat (Part 1), *J. Toxicol. Environ. Health,* 23, 193–206.

Chu, I., C. A. M. Suzuki, D. C. Villeneuve, and V. E. Valli (1992). Systemic toxicity of the heavy fraction of a coal coprocessing product in male rats following subchronic dermal exposure. *Fundam. Appl. Toxicol.,* 19, 246–257.

Dedrick, R. L. (1973). Animal scale up, *J. Pharmacokinet. Biopharm.,* 1, 435–461.

Grimmer, G., H. Bohnker, and A. Glaser (1977). Investigation on the carcinogenic burden by air pollution in man. XV. Polycyclic aromatic hydrocarbons in automobile exhaust gas—an inventory, *Zentralbl. Bakterol. Hyg. Abt. 1 Orig. B,* 164, 218–234.

Hammelstein, K. J., and R. J. Lutz (1979). A review of the applications of physiologically based pharmacokinetic modeling, *J. Pharmacokinet. Biopharm.,* 7, 127–145.

Health Protection Branch Report (1989). Analysis of coal coprocessing products.

[IARC] International Agency for Research on Cancer (1983). Polynuclear aromatic compounds. Monographs on the evaluation of the carcinogenic risk of chemicals to humans, Part I, 32, 419–430.

LaVoie, E. J., L. Tulley-Freiler, V. Bedenko, and D. Hoffmann (1983). Mutagenicity of substituted phenanthrene in *Salmonella typhimurium, Mutat. Res.,* 116, 91–102.

Lawrence, J. F., and B. Das (1986). Determination of nanogram/kilograms levels of polycyclic aromatic hydrocarbons in foods by HPLC with fluorescence detection, *Int. J. Anal. Chem.,* 23, 113–131.

Lee, M. L., M. Novotny, and K. D. Bartle (1976). Gas chromatography/mass spectrometric and nuclear magnetic resonance spectrometric studies of carcinogenic polynuclear aromatic hydrocarbons in tobacco and marijuana smoke condensates, *Anal. Chem.,* 48, 405–416.

Leung, H. W., D. J. Paustenbach, F. J. Murray, and M. E. Andersen (1990). A physiological pharmacokinetic description of the tissue distribution and enzyme-inducing properties of 2,3,7,8-tetrachlorodibenzo-*p*-dioxin in the rat, *Toxicol. Appl. Pharmacol.,* 103, 399–410.

Roberts, D. V. (1977). *Enzyme Kinetics,* Cambridge University Press, Cambridge, p. 192.

Windolz, M., ed. (1976). *The Merck Index,* 9th ed., Merck & Co., Rahway, NJ, p. 934.

# 29
# Biologically Based Cancer Modeling

**E. Georg Luebeck and Suresh H. Moolgavkar**
*Fred Hutchinson Cancer Research Center*
*Seattle, Washington*

## I. INTRODUCTION

Mathematical models of carcinogenesis serve a variety of useful purposes. Foremost, they provide a framework in which ideas about the mechanisms that lead to cancer can be discussed and further developed. Ultimately, one hopes that a better understanding of the carcinogenic process will lead to improved clinical therapies and more effective cancer prevention strategies. Mathematical cancer models have been used for analysis of experimental and epidemiological data and for quantifying the hazards of putative carcinogenic agents in our environment.

Several mathematical models have been developed over the past 40 years that are biologically motivated. They share much in common, but vary in details of their description and in degrees of mathematical sophistication (Nordling, 1953; Armitage and Doll, 1954). The basic tenet of these models is that malignant tumors arise from a single cell that has sustained a number of irreversible critical insults to its genome. Thus, the fundamental unit of description is the susceptible target cell together with its probability of malignant transformation.

The model that best embodies the multistage concept is the Armitage–Doll multistage model; Fig. 1 is a pictorial representation of this model. It has gained much popularity among risk assessors because it is intuitive, mathematically tractable, and yields age-specific tumor incidence curves that resemble the incidence patterns of many adult human carcinomas. Unfortunately, the Armitage–Doll model and approximations to it have been employed rather indiscriminately, often in situations that violate basic assumptions. This will be further discussed later in the chapter. However, the idea of a multistage nature of the carcinogenic process is well supported by modern laboratory observations (Land et al., 1983, Bishop, 1991; IARC, 1992).

It is important to identify the central aspects of carcinogenesis that should be modeled explicitly and those aspects that are peripheral or still poorly understood. New insights into the carcinogenic process were gained with the discovery of tumor suppressor genes, such as the *Rb*

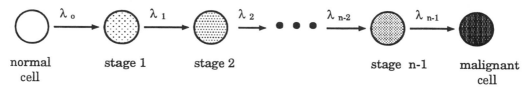

**Figure 1**  Armitage–Doll multistage model.

(retinoblastoma) gene and the *p*53 gene (Knudson, 1971; Hollstein et al., 1991; Levine et al., 1991). Both genes play important roles in the control of the cell cycle.

In 1971, Knudson showed that a two-mutation recessive oncogenesis model could explain both the sporadic and inherited form of the retinoblastoma childhood cancer. According to this model the sporadic form of this cancer is due to the somatic loss (or loss in function) of both copies of the *Rb* gene, whereas the hereditary form of the cancer is caused by a germ line transmission of a missing or defective copy of the *Rb* gene and the sporadic loss of the remaining copy.

For most adult cancers, the situation is less clear, and they do not seem to follow the recessive oncogenesis model just described. For instance, laboratory work suggests that a small number (three or four) of mutations are involved in colorectal carcinoma, implicating three tumor suppressor genes (*APC, p*53, and *DCC*) and one protooncogene (K-*ras*) (Fearon and Vogelstein, 1990). The difficulty in pinning down the exact number of rate-limiting steps is confounded by the problem of increasing genetic instability that accompanies tumor progression. Some mutational events may occur late in the development of a tumor and should not be considered rate-limiting or necessary for malignant conversion. In this context, the recent finding of a "mutator gene" on the long arm of chromosome 2 is of interest. The dysfunction of this gene seems to be responsible for a good fraction of familial colorectal cancers and causes a strong increase in genomic instability in tumor cells (Aaltonen et al., 1993).

Although earlier models of carcinogenesis, such as the Armitage–Doll model, were proposed to account for tumor incidence curves, new models were needed to explain the increasing number of systematic observations gathered from animal experiments that involve intermediate-stage lesions. In the last 20 years, much biological evidence has been gathered showing the importance of cell proliferation in the carcinogenic process. The Armitage–Doll model adequately describes the incidence of many human carcinomas (Cook et al., 1969; Renan, 1993). However, it is ill-suited for many experimental situations, for which the endpoints are intermediate, such as the appearance of preneoplastic lesions in the rat liver or the appearance of papillomas on mouse skin. A comprehensive description of these phenomena will necessarily have to include a description of the underlying growth processes that result in the *observable* lesions or tumors of interest.

The two-mutation clonal expansion model, as formulated by Moolgavkar and colleagues (Moolgavkar and Knudson, 1981; Moolgavkar et al., 1988), provides a minimalistic framework in which both aspects—the multistage nature of carcinogenesis, and the property of intermediate (initiated) cell populations to proliferate—are modeled explicitly. Growth of intermediate lesions is modeled as a stochastic birth and death process of the constituent cells. Cells are assigned probabilities to either divide into daughter cells, to die or differentiate, or to divide asymmetrically into one cell of the same lineage and one cell that has suffered another critical event on the pathway to cancer. A comprehensive review of stochastic models of carcinogenesis can be found in the book by Tan (Tan, 1991).

## II. THE ARMITAGE–DOLL MULTISTAGE MODEL

Despite that the Armitage–Doll model does not explicitly consider cell kinetics, it is still widely used for data analysis and in cancer risk assessment. The model has intuitive appeal and is mathematically straightforward. Here, we would like to review this model to introduce the key quantities that are used in time-to-tumor data analyses and to point out some of the potential pitfalls encountered in the common use of this particular model.

It has been observed that, for many human carcinomas, the age-specific incidence rate increases roughly as a power of age [i.e., $I(t) \cong ct^k$], and the Armitage–Doll model was originally proposed to explain this observation. The age-specific incidence rate is a measure of the rate of appearance of tumors in a previously tumor-free tissue. The appropriate statistical concept is that of the hazard function.

First, for the tissue of interest, let $T$ be a random variable representing the time to appearance of a malignant tumor. We define $P(t)$ as the probability that a malignant tumor has occurred by time $t$; that is, $P(t) = \text{Prob}[T \leq t]$. The hazard function $h(t)$, is then defined by

$$h(t) = \lim_{\Delta t \to 0} \frac{1}{\Delta t} \text{Prob}[t < T \leq t + \Delta t | T > t]$$

$$= \frac{P'(t)}{1 - P(t)}$$

and represents the rate of change in $P(t)$ conditional on there being no tumor present before time $t$. Obviously, $S(t) = 1 - P(t)$ is the probability of no tumor by time $t$, also termed the survival function.

Suppose that there are $N$ cells susceptible to malignant transformation in the tissue of interest, and let us assume that these cells are independent. Let $p(t)$ be the probability that a specific susceptible cell is malignant by time $t$. It can then be shown that the overall hazard is the sum of all the individual hazards; that is,

$$h(t) = \frac{Np'(t)}{1 - p(t)} \tag{1}$$

As seen in Fig. 1 a malignant tumor arises when a single susceptible cell sustains a number of critical insults (say $n$) that take it from a normal tissue cell to a malignant cell, which grows after a short lag time into a malignant tumor. The waiting time distribution for the cell to go from state $i$ to state $i + 1$ is assumed to be exponential with parameter $\lambda_i$. Let $p_i(t)$ be the probability that a cell is in stage $i$. Then Eq. (1) can be rewritten as $h(t) = Np'_n(t) / [1 - p_n(t)]$. If we now assume that malignancy (at the level of the cell) is a rare event [i.e., $p_n(t) \cong 0$], we may approximate the hazard function by $h(t) \approx Np'_n(t)$. In this case, Taylor series expansion (Moolgavkar, 1978, 1991) leads to the approximation

$$h(t) \approx Np'_n(t) = \frac{N\lambda_o \cdots \lambda_{n-1}}{(n-1)!} t^{n-1}[1 - \lambda t + f(\lambda,t)] \tag{2}$$

where $\lambda = \sum_{i=0}^{n-1} \lambda_i/n$ is the mean of the transition rates, and $f(\lambda,t)$ involves second and higher order moments of the transition rates.

Retention of only the first nonzero term in this series expansion leads to the Armitage–Doll approximation, namely

$$h(t) \approx \frac{N\lambda_o \cdots \lambda_{n-1}}{(n-1)!} t^{n-1} \tag{3}$$

Thus, with the two approximations made—(1) $p_n(t) \approx 0$ and (2) $|\bar{\lambda}t + f(\lambda,t)| \ll 1$—this model predicts an age-specific incidence curve that increases with a power of age that is one less than the number of distinct stages involved in malignant transformation.

Since the Armitage–Doll model does not allow for cell death, it is immediately clear that any susceptible cell eventually becomes malignant with probability 1. Furthermore, since the waiting time distribution to malignant transformation is the sum of $n$ exponential waiting time distributions, it follows that $h(t)$ is a monotone increasing function. Moreover, it can be shown that $h(t)$ has a finite asymptote: $\lim_{t \to \infty} h(t) = N\lambda_{min}$, where $\lambda_{min}$ is the minimum of the transition rates. Thus, the Armitage–Doll approximation, which grows without bound, becomes progressively worse with increasing age.

It is instructive, to rephrase the Armitage–Doll approximation in mathematical terms that involve the expectation of the occupancy in each stage. For this purpose, let $X_i(t)$ be a sequence of random variables associated with each cell, such that $X_i(t) = 1$ if the cell is in stage $i$ at time $t$ and zero otherwise. Since the probability $p_n(t)$ of a cell to become finally malignant obeys the Kolmogorov equation

$$p_n'(t) = \lambda_{n-1} p_{n-1}(t),$$

the hazard can also be written as

$$h(t) = \frac{Np_n'(t)}{1 - p_n(t)} \equiv N\lambda_{n-1} E[X_{n-1}(t) \,|\, X_n(t) = 0] \tag{4}$$

where $E$ denotes the expectation. In words, the hazard or incidence is proportional to the expected (or mean) number of cells in the penultimate stage, conditional on there being no cells that are malignant. When $p_n(t)$ is close to zero, or equivalently, the transition rates are small enough, the conditional expectation may be approximated by the unconditional expectation, and

$$h(t) \approx Np_n'(t) = N\lambda_{n-1} E[X_{n-1}(t)] \tag{5}$$

Thus, the Armitage–Doll approximation consists of replacing the conditional expectation of $X_{n-1}(t)$ by the unconditional expectation and, then, retaining only the first nonzero term in the Taylor series expansion of the unconditional expectation. Expressions similar to Eqs. (4) and (5) can also be written for the hazard function of the two-mutation model.

Obviously, for the Armitage–Doll model to hold, $\lambda$, and thus each $\lambda_i$, must be small enough. An example of how poorly this approximation may do is discussed in Moolgavkar (1978, 1991). In addition, in animal experiments, the probability of tumor may be too large for $p_n(t) \cong 0$ to hold, so that the approximation should be avoided altogether.

## A. Dose–Response Modeling

To model the action of environmental carcinogens, one or more of the transition rates can be made functions of the dose of the agent in question. Usually, the transition rates are modeled as linear functions of the dose, so that $\lambda_i = a_i + b_i d$. The assumption of first-order kinetics may be justified, at least for carcinogens that interact directly with DNA to produce mutations. Then, by using the Armitage–Doll approximation [see Eq. (3)], the hazard function at age $t$ and dose $d$ can be written as $h(t,d) = g(d)t^{n-1}$, where $g(d)$ is a polynomial in dose, and the probability of tumor is approximately given by $P(t,d) = 1 - \exp[-\tilde{g}(d)t^n]$. Note that $\tilde{g}(d)$ is a product of linear terms. It is in this form, called the linearized multistage model, that the Armitage–Doll model is commonly applied to the problem of low-dose extrapolation. Generally, the proportion of animals developing tumors at a specified age at each of three different dose levels is known. The linearized multistage model is fitted to the data and the estimated parameters used to extrapolate risk to lower doses. There are formally at least two problems with this procedure. First, as noted earlier, the Armitage–Doll approximation holds only when the probability of tumor is low, and this condition is not satisfied in the usual animal experiments used for risk assessment. Second, in the statistical analysis $\tilde{g}(d)$ is treated as a general polynomial, rather than a product of linear terms.

The foregoing discussion applies only when exposure to a carcinogen starts at birth or very early in life, and continues at the same constant level throughout the period of observation. With time-dependent exposures, the hazard function can no longer be couched in the form of Eq. (2). A starting point for the mathematical development is the set of Kolmogorov differential equations. However, the papers in the literature use approximation Eq. (3) as their starting point (see e.g., Whittemore, 1977; Day and Brown, 1980; Crump and Howe, 1984; Brown and Chu, 1987; Freedman and Navidi, 1989). This approximation is inappropriate unless one has reason to believe that each of the transition rates is small enough. The approximation is almost certainly inappropriate when applied to experimental data.

## III. TWO-MUTATION CLONAL EXPANSION MODEL

To account for the experimental observations in multistage carcinogenesis, biologically based cancer models need to be centered around the following points:

1. Cancer is a *multistep* process that involves the *clonal expansion* of intermediate and malignant cell populations.
2. Thus, model parameters should represent biological observables that can, at least in principle, be measured and tested by experiment (e.g., the number of normal target cells, cell kinetic rates, mutation rates, and so on). Parameters of interest are likely to be those that are affected by environmental agents.
3. The model should provide a unified framework of carcinogenesis in which both epidemiological and experimental data with intermediate endpoints can be analyzed.
4. The model should account for the observed phenomena in initiation–promotion (IP) experiments, such has the induction and promotion of enzyme-altered foci in the rat liver, or the occurrence of papillomas on mouse skin after painting with a promoter substance, such as 12-*O*-tetradecanoylphorbol-13-acetate (TPA).
5. The incorporation of time- and dose-dependent exposure patterns of carcinogens should not pose great mathematical difficulty.

The two-mutation clonal expansion model, as formulated by Moolgavkar and colleagues (Moolgavkar et al., 1988; Dewanji et al., 1989; Moolgavkar and Luebeck, 1990), presents a minimalistic framework that addresses (at least in part) all of these points. Slightly different versions of the model have been considered in the past by Neyman and Scott (1967), Kendall (1960), and more recently, by Portier and Kopp-Schneider (1991).

From a genetic point of view, the two-mutation clonal expansion model can essentially be seen as a mathematical generalization of the recessive oncogenesis model of Knudson (Knudson, 1971; Moolgavkar and Knudson, 1981), according to which the inactivation of both alleles of a specific tumor suppressor gene can lead to cancer. The main feature of the model is the transition of target stem cells into cancer cells through an intermediate, premalignant, stage in two rare rate-limiting mutational steps. The mutations are considered irreversible, although the possibility of cell death through apoptosis may effectively remove the mutation on the tissue level.

In the form that is currently used, the model takes explicit account of the growth kinetics of normal and intermediate cells. Growth of normal target cells is assumed to be deterministic. This is a reasonable assumption, because the number of normal cells is large and under tight homeostatic control. Intermediate or initiated cells are assumed to undergo a stochastic birth and death process because their numbers are small and, furthermore, the process of initiation has resulted in the loosening of homeostatic control. In the parlance of chemical carcinogenesis, the first rate-limiting event may be identified with initiation, clonal expansion of initiated cells with promotion; and the second rate-limiting event with progression or malignant conversion.

The assumptions required for the mathematical development can be summarized as follows: Let $X(t)$ be the number of normal target cells at time $t$. Then, initiated cells arise from normal cells according to an inhomogeneous Poisson process with intensity $\upsilon(t)X(t)$, where $\upsilon(t)$ is the first mutation rate. Intermediate cells then either divide with rate $\alpha(t)$, die (or differentiate) with rate $\beta(t)$, or divide into one intermediate and one malignant cell, with rate $\mu(t)$. Because of the presence of cell death, however, intermediate cells, or their clones, may become extinct before giving rise to malignant progeny. Further mathematical details can be found in references of Dewanji et al. (1989, 1991) and Moolgavkar and Luebeck (1990). Figure 2 is a graphic representation of the model.

The model has recently been extended to include the cell kinetics of malignant cells analogous to the kinetics of intermediate cells (Dewanji et al., 1991, Luebeck and Moolgavkar, 1994).

For the practical purpose of data analysis one often assumes that the occurrence of the first malignant cell will inevitably lead to a tumor after a certain lag time. This is an oversimplification that most likely leads to underestimation of the mutation rates. The problems and biases that can arise from this assumption have been studied in detail by Luebeck and Moolgavkar (1994).

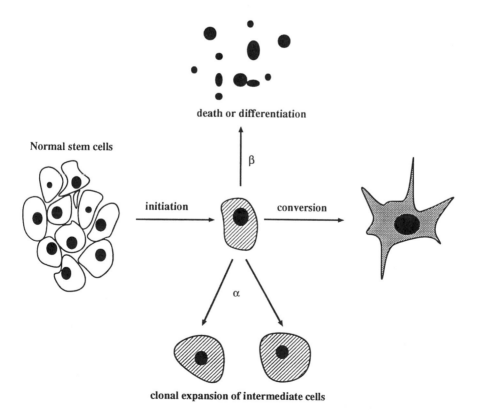

**Figure 2**  Pictorial representation of the two-mutation clonal expansion model.

It was found from computer simulations that the data analysis of tumor incidence data, within the framework of the two-stage model, was very insensitive to the use of a *lag time,* defined as the time between the occurrences of the first malignant transformation and the crossing of a viability threshold. In the simulations, viability was assumed when the probability of extinction of the tumor was less than $10^{-3}$. In the following, unless stated otherwise, we will assume that the tumor is synonymous with the first malignant cell in the tissue.

In contrast with the Armitage–Doll model, the two-mutation clonal expansion model also allows for environmental agents to influence cell proliferation. In general, both cell division rates $\alpha$ and cell death rates $\beta$ can be made functions of dose and time. Obviously, if an agent increases the net cell proliferation rate, $\alpha - \beta$, the pool of intermediate cells that are susceptible to malignant transformation will increase too and, thus, the cancer risk. However, there are distinct modes of action of so-called promoter carcinogens. An increase in $\alpha - \beta$ may come about through an increase in the cell division rate only. In this case, a corresponding increase in the second mutation rate is expected. On the other hand, when the increase in $\alpha - \beta$ originates from the decrease of cell loss (death or differentiation) no accompanying increase is expected in the transformation rate $\mu$.

It is useful to introduce the ratio of cell death rate and cell birth rate (i.e., $\beta / \alpha$). When both $\alpha$ and $\beta$ are constant in time and, when $\alpha > \beta$, this ratio equals the asymptotic probability of extinction; namely, the probability that a clone together with all its progeny ultimately becomes extinct. When $\alpha \leq \beta$ this probability is 1; that is, given long enough time, a clone will become extinct with certainty.

Interestingly, quantitative analyses of enzyme-altered foci in rat liver (Moolgavkar et al., 1990a; Luebeck et al., 1991) and of papillomas on mouse skin (Kopp-Schneider and Portier, 1992), all yield the result that $\beta / \alpha \cong 1$. This indicates that homeostatic control among intermediate cell populations remains very strong. In the mouse papillomas there is actually indication that homeostatic control is protective (i.e., $\alpha < \beta$). However, under the influence of the promoter, this protective effect seems to be abrogated. The finding that $\beta / \alpha \cong 1$ in these analyses underlines the importance of the stochastic nature of the underlying clonal expansion processes. An example is provided in Fig. 3. It shows ten processes that start off with one cell each. In this particular example only one out of ten expansions remains alive after 10 days.

Finally, the distinction between the *concepts* of initiation–promotion and the *action* of specific environmental agents must be kept clearly in focus. For example, although *promotion* is defined within the framework of the model as clonal expansion of initiated cells, an agent deemed to be a promoter may have other effects as well. It could cause hyperplasia of the normal

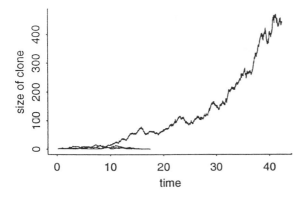

**Figure 3** Computer simulation of simple birth and death process ($n = 10$, $\alpha = 1$, and $\beta / \alpha = 0.9$).

tissue and, as pointed out earlier, indirectly increase the mutation rates. Other promoting agents may also induce enzyme systems that produce reactive oxygen species that are mutagenic (Cerutti, 1985).

For the analysis of epidemiological and experimental data in which the endpoint of interest is the appearance of malignant tumors, we need, as with the Armitage–Doll model, expressions for the hazard function and the probability of tumor. However, initiation–promotion experiments also often yield data on the number and size of intermediate lesions, such as the papillomas on the epidermis of the mouse or the enzyme-altered foci in the rat liver. These data provide important information on the cell kinetics of intermediate lesions. The next section introduces the essential mathematical expressions for the analysis of tumor incidence data.

Several analyses have employed an approximate solution to the two-stage model analogous to the Armitage–Doll approximation given in Eq. (5); that is, replacing the conditional expectation value for the number of intermediate cells by the unconditional one. Here we will not again belabor the problems associated with this approximation. However, it is worth pointing out that the use of the approximate hazard function, in our opinion, does not offer any real conceptual or computational advantages over the use of the exact hazard function. Later we shall see that the computation of the exact hazard can be couched as a recursive procedure in the case of piecewise constant model parameters.

## IV.  DATA ANALYSIS USING THE TWO-MUTATION MODEL

Depending on the nature of the data, different mathematical quantities need to be computed and employed. The discussions here will focus on model-fitting procedures using the maximum likelihood principle. In general, the likelihood expressions reflect the probability of the total observed outcomes of an experiment or a human study, properly adjusting for all the constraints and environmental factors that were present or that were built into the protocols of the experiments.

Often covariate information is available on an individual basis for a cohort of subjects, and the endpoint of interest is the appearance of tumors in members of the cohort. Here, the probability density of tumor (if the tumor is rapidly fatal or immediately diagnosed) or the probability of tumor (if the tumor is "incidental") and the survivor function are required to construct the likelihood. When aggregate data on groups of individuals are available, the hazard (incidence) function is required.

Some experimental data also provide information on the number and size of intermediate lesions, such as the enzyme-altered foci in the rat liver or the papillomas on the skin of the mouse. In this case, expressions for the number and size distributions of *nonextinct* lesions need to be derived. A complicating factor for the analysis of foci is that the data usually come from two-dimensional sectional observations on histological slides. Construction of the likelihood requires that the resulting stereological problem be addressed. Here, we will employ a simple method based on the Wicksell transformation (Wicksell, 1925).

### A.  The Probability of Tumor

We briefly describe the derivation of the quantities required for the model fitting of tumor (incidence) data. These quantities are the probability of tumor, the density function, and the hazard function. More details can be found in a recent paper (Moolgavkar and Luebeck, 1990). Let $Y(t)$, $Z(t)$, represent the number of intermediate and malignant cells, respectively, at time $t$ and let

$$\psi(y,z;t) = \sum_{j,k} P_{j,k}(t) y^j z^k$$

be the probability generating function with

$$P_{j,k}(t) = \text{Prob}\,[Y(t) = j, Z(t) = k \,|\, Y(0) = 0, Z(0) = 0]$$

Then the process $[Y(t),Z(t)]$ is Markovian, and $\Psi$ satisfies the Kolmogorov forward differential equation

$$\psi'(y,z;t) = \frac{\partial \psi(y,z;t)}{\partial t} = (y - 1)v(t)X(t)\psi(y,z;t)$$
$$+ \{\mu(t)yz + \alpha(t)y^2 + \beta(t) - [\alpha(t) + \beta(t) + \mu(t)]y\} \frac{\partial \psi}{\partial y} \tag{6}$$

with initial condition $\Psi(y,z;0) = 1$. $S(t) = \Psi(1,0;t)$ is the survival function and $P(t) = 1 - S(t)$ the probability of tumor for this model. As with the Armitage–Doll model the hazard (incidence) function is then given by Eq. (1)

$$h(t) = \frac{P'(t)}{1 - P(t)} = -\frac{\psi'(1,0;t)}{\psi(1,0;t)} \tag{7}$$

It follows immediately from the Kolmogorov equation that

$$\psi'(1,0;t) = -\mu(t) \frac{\partial \psi}{\partial y}(1,0;t)$$

and thus

$$h(t) = \mu(t)E[Y(t)\,|\,Z(t) = 0] \tag{8}$$

where $E$ denotes the expectation and where we have used the relationship

$$E[Y(t)\,|\,Z(t) = 0] = \frac{\partial \psi}{\partial y}(1,0;t)\,/\,\psi(1,0;t)$$

Two approaches can be used to obtain the exact solution to the two-mutation model. The first approach involves solving the characteristic equations associated with the Kolmogorov equation. The second approach is somewhat more general, and it is not described here, but can be found in Moolgavkar and Luebeck (1990). Specifically, the characteristic equations are

$$\frac{dy}{du} = -R(y,u) = -\{\mu(u)yz + \alpha(u)y^2 + \beta(u) - [\alpha(u) + \beta(u) + \mu(u)]y\}$$
$$\frac{dz}{du} = 0 \;(z \text{ is constant along characteristics}) \tag{9}$$
$$\frac{dt}{du} = 1 \quad \text{and} \quad \frac{d\psi}{du} = (y - 1)v(u)X(u)\psi$$

Now, the ordinary differential equation for $\Psi$ may be solved along characteristics to yield

$$\psi[y(t),z,t] = \psi_0 \exp \int_0^t [y(u,t) - 1]v(u)X(u)du \tag{10}$$

where $\Psi_0 = \Psi(y(0),z,0) = 1$ is the initial value of $\Psi$. We are interested in computing $\Psi(1,0;t)$ for any $t$, and thus we need to find the values of $\Psi$ along the characteristic through $(y(0),0,0)$ where $y(0)$ is the initial value of $y$ and $y(t) = 1$. Now, along the characteristic, $Y$ satisfies the differential equation $dy / du = -R(y,u)$ and this is just a Riccati equation that can be readily integrated in closed form if the parameters of the model are piecewise constant. To be precise, the Riccati equation for $y$ can be solved to yield a value for $y(u)$ for any $u$, with initial condition $y(t) = 1$. Note that $y$ depends on $u$ and $t$.

Thus, the survival function

$$S(t) = \psi(1,0;t) = \exp \int_0^t [y(u,t) - 1]v(u)X(u)du \tag{11}$$

where the explicit dependence of $y$ on $u$ and $t$ is acknowledged. The hazard function then is given by

$$h(t) = -\frac{\psi'(1,0;t)}{\psi(1,0;t)} = -\int_0^t v(u)X(u)y_t(u,t)du \tag{12}$$

where $y_t$ denotes the derivative of $y$ relative to $t$.

*1.  Solution for Piecewise Constant Parameters*

Assume there are $n$ intervals $[t_{i-1},t_i]$ with $i = 1,2,\ldots,n$, covering the time period $[t_0 = 0, t_n = t]$. Then the solution of Eq. (9), $y(u,t)$, can be computed recursively, starting from $u = t = t_n$ using the boundary condition $y(t,t) = 1$. For $u \in [t_{i-1},t_i]$ we have (see Moolgavkar and Luebeck, 1990)

$$y(u,t) = \frac{B_i - A_i \dfrac{y(t_i,t) - B_i}{y(t_i,t) - A_i} \exp\left[\alpha_i(A_i - B_i)(u - t_i)\right]}{1 - \dfrac{y(t_i,t) - B_i}{y(t_i,t) - A_i} \exp\left[\alpha_i(A_i - B_i)(u - t_i)\right]} \tag{13}$$

where $A_i$ $(B_i)$ are the lower (upper) root of the quadratic form: $\alpha_i x^2 - [\alpha_i + \beta_i + \mu_i]x + \beta_i$. The constant parameters $\alpha_i$, $\beta_i$, respectively, refer to cell division, cell death, and second mutation rate in the time interval $[t_{i-1},t_i]$. When $X(u)$ is constant over time, the time integral in Eq. (11) can be computed in explicit form. For $u \in [t_{i-1},t_i]$ we can rewrite the integrand $[y - 1]$ as

$$y(u,t) - 1 = \frac{C_i}{1 - r_i \exp\left[\delta_i(u - t_i)\right]} + (A_i - 1)$$

where $C_i = B_i - A_i$, $r_i = (y(t_i,t) - B_i) / (y(t_i,t) - A_i)$ and $\delta_i = \alpha_i(A_i - B_i)$. The survival function Eq. (11) can then be computed as

$$S(t) = \exp\left[-\sum_{i=1}^n H_i\right] \quad \text{with} \tag{14}$$

$$H_i = -vX \int_{t_{i-1}}^{t_i} [y(u,t) - 1]du \tag{15}$$

$$= -vX\left[(B_i - 1)(t_i - t_{i-1}) + \ln\left(\frac{1 - r_i}{1 - r_i \exp\left[-\delta_i(t_i - t_{i-1})\right]}\right)\Big/ \alpha_i\right] \tag{16}$$

The probability density function for developing a tumor at time $t$ is simply the time derivative of the tumor probability $P(t) = 1 - S(t)$ [i.e, $P'(t) = -S'(t)$].

The likelihood contribution of an individual in a study that monitors the incidence or appearance of a specific kind of malignant tumor can then be constructed as follows: Let $t_i$ be the time of observation at which the subject $i$ develops the tumor, dies (with or without tumor), or is lost to follow-up. Then subject $i$ contributes the term $L_i(t_i)$ to the entire likelihood which is given by $L = \prod L_i(t_i)$ with

$$L_i(t_i) = \begin{cases} P(t_i) & \text{if malignant tumor was incidental} \\ P'(t_i) & \text{if malignant tumor was fatal} \\ S(t_i) = 1 - P(t_i) & \text{if free of tumor} \end{cases}$$

If individual level information is not available, then the hazard function is needed. Since the derivative $y_i(u,t)$ in Eq. (12) is cumbersome to compute using the chain rule repeatedly, it is probably faster to compute the $P'(t)$ numerically with a midpoint formula. The hazard is then computed according to $h(t) = P'(t) / [1 - P(t)]$. For examples, see Moolgavkar et al. (1990b) and Moolgavkar and Luebeck (1990).

For many studies, one has to consider several different time intervals defined by a specific exposure pattern. On each of these intervals the parameters of the model can be assumed constant. The roots $A_i$ and $B_i$ of the quadratic polynomial [see Eq. (13)] on interval $i$ are functions of the parameters of the model and, accordingly, also of the exposure rate variables. There is no limitation on the number of intervals in the recursive scheme for the computation of the probability of tumor.

An example for which this scheme has been successfully applied is in an analysis of the Colorado Plateau uranium miners' cohort (Moolgavkar et al., 1993). It is the oldest and most completely studied cohort of underground miners who worked in the mines from 1950 to 1964. The cohort consists of 3346 miners with detailed information on the pattern of radon and cigarette exposure for each individual. This includes the ages at which exposure to radon and cigarette smoke began, the ages at which these exposures stopped, the cumulative exposure to radon in working level months (WLM), the number of cigarettes smoked per day, and the age at last observation or death.

With contiguous periods of smoking or radon exposure, there are up to five time intervals for the integration of the cumulative hazard. A summary of this analysis that also shows the patterns of exposure is shown in Fig. 4. Because there are very few unexposed miners, a simultaneous analysis of the miners cohort, together with the British doctors' cohort was conducted. Two distinct dose–response scenarios (referred to as model A and model B) were investigated. Let $d_s$ denote the rate of cigarette exposure in cigarettes per day and $d_r$ the rate of radon exposure on working level months (WLM) per month, then we assumed that

$$v(d_s, d_r) = a_0 + a_s d_s + a_r d_r$$

$$\mu(d_s, d_r) = b_0 + b_s d_s + b_r d_r$$

and

$$(\alpha - \beta)(d_s, d_r) = c_0 + c_{s1}(1 - \exp[-c_{s2} d_s]) + c_{r1}(1 - \exp[-c_{r2} d_r])$$

for the Colorado miners' data, and

$$(\alpha - \beta)(d_s) = e_0 + e_{s1}(1 - \exp[-e_{s2} d_s])$$

for the British doctors' data. For both data sets we assumed $X = 10^7$ and $\beta / \alpha = \text{constant}$ (i.e., independent of the level of exposure to radon or tobacco smoke). Preliminary analyses showed that $a_0 = b_0$ (i.e., the mutation background rates could be assumed to be equal) and $b_s = b_r \cong 0$; namely, the second mutation rate did not show a dose–response to either radon or cigarette smoke. Furthermore, a nonsigmoid saturation in the intermediate cell kinetics gave better fits to the data, explaining our choice for $\alpha - \beta$. Model A was then defined by the separate

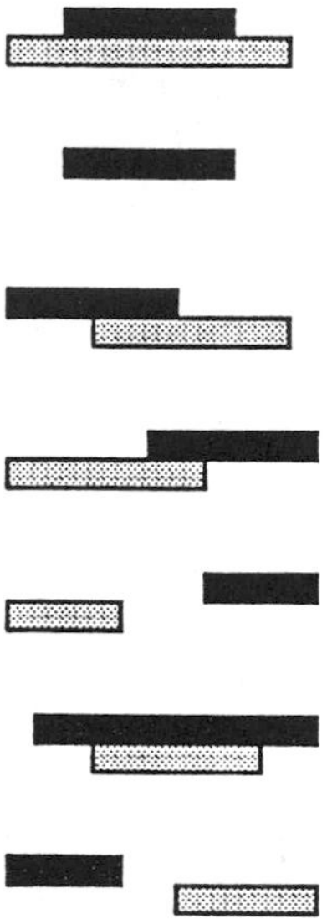

| Group | Exposure profile | No. of miners | No. of lung cancer deaths | | |
|---|---|---|---|---|---|
| | | | observed | Model A | Model B |
| I. No exposure | | 8 | 0 | .0084 | .0046 |
| II. Radon Tobacco smoke | | 2224 | 235 | 237.1 | 234.4 |
| III. Radon Tobacco smoke | | 477 | 13 | 16.04 | 12.03 |
| IV. Radon Tobacco smoke | | 116 | 15 | 15.25 | 16.02 |
| V. Radon Tobacco smoke | | 118 | 20 | 14.18 | 12.72 |
| VI. Radon Tobacco smoke | | 159 | 8 | 8.17 | 6.10 |
| VII. Radon Tobacco smoke | | 19 | 3 | 0.71 | 0.68 |
| VIII. Radon Tobacco smoke | | 11 | 0 | 0.53 | 0.40 |
| Total | | 3132 | 294 | 292.0 | 282.4 |

**Figure 4**  Schematic representation of patterns of exposure. Lengths of bars do not represent actual duration of exposure. In each category the number of miners, the observed number of lung cancer deaths, and the expected numbers generated by models A and B are shown.

treatment of the cell proliferation in the two cohorts, whereas model B assumed that $c_0 = e_0, c_{s1(2)} = e_{s1(2)}$, meaning equal dose–response to tobacco smoke for the cell proliferation in the two cohorts. The observed and expected number of tumors for the various exposure patterns are also shown in Fig. 4.

In conclusion we find no indication that radon and tobacco smoke interact on the level of the cell; that is, additional terms proportional to $d_s \times d_r$ in the foregoing parameter functions did not improve the fits significantly. Despite this, the relative risk of joint exposure is somewhere between additive and multiplicative. We also find no indication that radon or tobacco smoke affect the second mutation rate, consistent with findings in rats exposed to radon (Moolgavkar et al. 1990b). Perhaps most intriguing, however, is the prediction of an inverse dose–rate effect (i.e., protraction of a given total dose of radon increases the lifetime risk of tumor; for details see Moolgavkar et al., 1993).

## B.  Quantitative Analysis of Intermediate Lesions

We now discuss the analysis of data that are intermediate on the pathway to cancer. In many carcinogenesis studies, such as initiation–promotion experiments, intermediate lesions are detected and quantified according to their phenotype and size. It is believed that at least some of these lesions represent clones of initiated cells that are precursors to malignant tumors. Examples are provided by the papillomas in mouse skin painting experiments and the enzyme-altered foci (EAF) in rodent hepatocarcinogenesis. Here, we will focus on the latter example. Most of the mathematical results have been derived in Dewanji et al. (1989) and in Moolgavkar et al. (1990a). An application of the methods to mouse skin papillomas can also be found in Kopp-Schneider and Portier (1992). First, we discuss some of the consequences of explicitly considering cell division and cell death, rather than just the net rate of cell proliferation (i.e., the difference between division rate and death rate, $\alpha - \beta$). The sections that follow are meant to serve as an introduction to the statistical analysis of foci data, providing sufficient detail for the reader to carry out a quantitative analysis of such data.

## 1. *The Role of Cell Kinetics in Tumor Formation*

An important property of populations of cells undergoing cell division and cell death is that the population may become extinct. Thus, if the rate of cell death is greater than zero, then an initiated cell may die without giving rise to a detectable lesion, such as a papilloma on the skin or an altered focus in the liver. This conclusion may come as a surprise, because the irreversibility of initiation appears to be current dogma. However, we are not asserting here that individual initiated cells revert to normal, but rather, that initiation may be partially reversible on the level of the organ because initiated cells may die.

If the rates of cell division and death are constant (independent of time), then the probability that an initiated cell and all its progeny will die is given (asymptotically) by the ratio of the rate of death and the rate of cell division, $\beta / \alpha$. If the rate of death is larger than the cell division rate, then the (asymptotic) probability of extinction is 1. However, some foci may still become visible because of the stochastic nature of the clonal expansion process. In recent analyses of altered hepatic foci in rodent hepatocarcinogenesis experiments, it was concluded that most initiated cells (perhaps up to 90%) die without giving rise to altered foci (Moolgavkar et al., 1990a; Luebeck et al., 1991). Some preliminary data on GST-P positive cells appear to support this estimate (Satoh et. al., 1989; R. Schulte-Hermann, personal communication).

The mean number of initiated cells at any time depends on the rate of initiation and the net rate of intermediate cell division, $\alpha - \beta$. However, there is considerable stochastic variation around this mean number, and the actual number depends on $\alpha$ and $\beta$ individually, and not just on their difference. Furthermore, the distribution of the number of altered cells in foci also depends on $\alpha$ and $\beta$ individually. Thus, for a given value of $\alpha - \beta$, large values of $\alpha$ and $\beta$ lead to small numbers of large foci, and small values of $\alpha$ and $\beta$ lead to large numbers of small foci.

The number of *observed* intermediate foci depends on the rate of initiation as well as the growth kinetics of the initiated cells. Not only are there small unobservable foci in the tissue of interest, but many of them may simply not survive if cell death is greater than zero. As a matter of fact, in rapidly dividing cell populations cell death (apoptosis) or differentiation must almost balance the number of newly created cells to otherwise avoid an explosive growth of focal tissue, (i.e., $\beta / \alpha \sim 1$). The behavior of the number and size distribution is very sensitive to the parameter $\beta / \alpha$ under this condition.

Consider a hypothetical example. Suppose $\alpha - \beta = 0.01$ per cell per day, and suppose that one has the following two combinations of parameters: (1) $\alpha = 0.5$, $\beta = 0.49$, thus $\beta / \alpha = 0.98$; and (2) $\alpha = 0.1$, $\beta = 0.09$, hence, $\beta / \alpha = 0.90$. Both these combinations of parameters lead to $\alpha - \beta = 0.01$ and thus to the same mean number of initiated cells, provided that the rates of initiation are identical. However, with the first combination of parameters, 98% of initiated cells will ultimately become extinct, and, thus, one would expect to see a few large foci; with the second combination of parameters, 90% of initiated cells will ultimately become extinct, and one would expect to see a larger number of smaller foci. Moreover, the first combination of parameters carries a higher risk of malignant transformation than the second. This is because a high cell division rate implies a high mutation rate. Examples of the phenomenon described here are provided by promoters such as 4-dimethylaminoazobenzene (4-DAB) and the peroxisome proliferators, which lead to a small number of large foci, and others such as N-nitrosodiethanolamine (NDEOL) and phenobarbital (PB), which lead to a large number of small foci. By measuring labeling indices, it should be possible to confirm that division rates in foci associated with the former compounds are higher than the division rates in foci associated with the latter compounds. Some of the ideas developed in this section are depicted in Fig. 5.

### 2. Modeling Initiation and Promotion of Enzymes-Altered Foci

For completeness, a summary of the basic modeling ideas is provided here. Discussions of biochemical and physiological aspects and of the role of EAF in hepatotumorigenesis can be found in the literature (Emmelot and Scherer, 1980; Farber, 1980; Goldfarb and Pugh, 1981; Kunz et al., 1982; Goldsworthy et al., 1986; Buchmann et al., 1987; Pitot et al., 1987).

Let us assume that at time $s$, 1 ml of liver contains a number $X(s)$ of normal hepatocytes that transform into altered cells, with rate $\upsilon(s)$. The change in enzyme expression in transformed hepatocytes is considered a hereditary and irreversible trait of the altered cell. The number of initiated cells that arise from normal hepatocytes is then modeled as a Poisson distribution with mean $\int_0^t \upsilon(s)X(s)ds$.

Promotion is the clonal expansion of such altered cells and is mathematically described by a nonhomogeneous (time-dependent) birth–death process (Cox and Miller, 1972) with birth rate $\alpha(s)$ and death (or differentiation) rate $\beta(s)$. As before, this means that altered cells either divide into two altered cells with rate $\alpha(s)$ or die (or differentiate) with rate $\beta(s)$. The third possibility, namely, that altered cells divide asymmetrically into one altered and one further progressed (toward malignancy) cell, is not explicitly considered here. However, when simultaneous

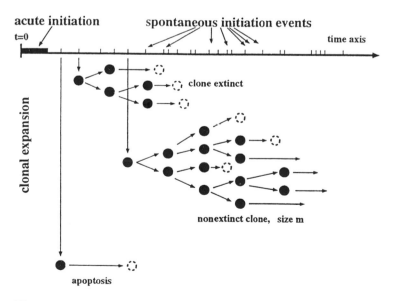

**Figure 5** Pictorial representation of initiation and promotion. Normal cells are initiated either spontaneously or by application of a chemical agent. These cells may either divide or undergo apoptosis. If all the cells in a focus undergo apoptosis, the focus becomes extinct. The probability of this occurring is high when the focus is small.

information on the occurrence of malignant tumors is available, the model can be extended to incorporate this information.

The parameter $\upsilon(s)$ is to be interpreted as the rate at which normal cells are altered to express a particular enzyme phenotype. It is conceivable that the initiated cell corresponds only to a subset of the particular phenotype in question, or that other phenotypes, not under study, can be transformed into malignancies as well. Thus, we simply view the enzyme alteration as a surrogate marker for initiation.

As formulated, the model does not yet distinguish killed cells from differentiated cells, or from cells that are quiescent; all are assumed absent from the proliferating (actively cycling) intermediate cell pool.

Programmed cell death (apoptosis) is important in altered foci (Bursch et al., 1984, 1985; Schulte-Hermann et al., 1990; Bursch et al., 1990) and has profound consequences. Some of these are discussed in earlier papers. One of the more important is that initiated or altered cells become extinct with high probability without giving rise to observable foci. In previous analysis of $N$-nitrosomorpholine (NNM)- and diethylnitrosamine (DEN)-induced foci (Moolgavkar et al., 1990a; Luebeck et al., 1991), we found that more than 90% of altered cells died without giving rise to foci.

The model yields mathematical expressions for the number of altered foci and their size distribution as a function of dose, age, and treatment time. A derivation of these expressions can be found in Dewanji et al, 1989 and in Luebeck and Moolgavkar, 1991, and their application to a typical IP protocol in Luebeck et al., 1991. General formulae and their relationship to cell kinetic parameters are given in what follows. The expected number of nonextinct foci at time $t$ is given by the integral

$$\Lambda(t) = \int_0^t \upsilon(s)X(s) \frac{1}{G(t,s) + g(t,s)} \, ds \tag{17}$$

and the probability, $p_m(t)$, of finding a nonextinct clone consisting of exactly $m$ cells at time $t$, is given by

$$p_m(t) = \frac{1}{\Lambda(t)} \int_0^t \upsilon(s)X(s) \frac{g}{G^2} \left( \frac{G}{G+g} \right)^{m+1} ds \tag{18}$$

where the functions $G$ and $g$ are defined by

$$g(t,s) = \exp\left[ -\int_s^t (\alpha(u) - \beta(u)) du \right] \tag{19}$$

and

$$G(t,s) = \int_s^t \alpha(u) g(u,s) du \tag{20}$$

The inverse function $g^{-1}(t,s)$ represents the expected size of a clone at time $t$ starting off with one cell at time $s$. The foregoing integrals can be explicitly computed when constant or piecewise constant parameters are assumed, a frequently made assumption (Kopp-Schneider, 1992; Luebeck et al., 1994). However, a more general case, discussed later, which is still explicitly tractable, allows us to model cell replication and death with exponential time dependence. The foregoing formulae are valid with arbitrary time-dependent parameters and, in general, may have to be evaluated numerically.

### 3.  *Gompertz Growth*

It has been noticed in continuous-labeling index (LI) experiments that measured LIs in foci are inconsistent with the assumption of foci growing exponentially (in the mean), presuming that DNA synthesis and apoptosis have constant rates. It seems that cellular responses to promoting agents are often more pronounced at the beginning of the treatment, accompanied by a spurt in focal cell replication that, as the treatment continues, may be slowed by adaptive responses (Schulte-Hermann et al., 1990). For instance, a significant slowing of exponential growth of EAF was observed in female Wistar rats initiated acutely with DEN and treated continuously with PB (Luebeck et al., 1991). Hence, we would like to relax the assumption of constant or piecewise constant parameters $\alpha$ and $\beta$. A straightforward generalization arises when $\alpha$ and $\beta$ are assumed to depend on time exponentially so that, beginning at some time $s$

$$\alpha(u) = \alpha_0 \exp\left[-a(u - s)\right], \quad \beta(u) = \beta_0 \exp\left[-a(u - s)\right] \tag{21}$$

Here $\alpha_0$, $\beta_0$ and $a$ are constants. These definitions imply that the ratio of cell death and cell birth rates, $\beta / \alpha$, is also a constant. If follows (Tan, 1986; Luebeck and Moolgavkar, 1991) that the resulting mean growth is Gompertz-like, following the curve

$$g^{-1}(u) \equiv \exp\left[(\alpha_0 - \beta_0)\{1 - \exp\left[-a(u - s)\right]\} / a\right] \tag{22}$$

When $a = 0$ then $\alpha - \beta =$ constant and the mean growth is exponential. Thus, the Gompertz model introduces one extra parameter $a$, which measures departures from exponentiality of the mean growth. When $a = 0$, mean growth is exponential; when $a > 0$, mean growth is gompertzian (subexponential); when $a < 0$, mean growth is superexponential. The hypothesis $a = 0$ can be tested using standard likelihood-based procedures, such as the likelihood ratio test.

In most carcinogenesis experiments initiation is induced by an acute exposure to a mutagenic carcinogen followed by an application of the promoter agent. Proper control groups need to be included to control for promoter-induced initiation in the absence of the primary initiator. Thus the initiation rate $\upsilon(s)$ is generally composed of an acute rate, say $\upsilon_0$, conveniently expressed by a Dirac delta-function, and a spontaneous background rate, say $\upsilon_1$. Once initiated, the cell will follow the stochastic birth and death process described earlier. The stochastic nature of the clonal expansions is also portrayed schematically in Fig. 5. The model is then fit to the observed number and size distribution of nonextinct foci seen at the various sacrifice times. This is the subject of the next section.

### 4.  *Statistical Analysis*

The number of nonextinct foci and their sizes were directly observable, Eqs. (17) and (18) would be sufficient to compute the overall likelihood of the experimental outcome. However, what is known is the number and the size (in terms of area or radius) of two-dimensional transections on particular histological slides stained for some enzyme marker activity. Hence, Eqs. (17) and (18) need to be translated into expressions describing the mean number of focal transections per unit area, say $n_2(t)$, and a probability density, $f_2^\xi$, of finding an observable transection of radius $y > \varepsilon$, respectively. Here $\varepsilon$ is a lower bound below which transections cannot be reliably detected.

To solve this problem, we use a formula developed by Wicksell (Wicksell, 1925) to relate the distribution of radii of three-dimensional spheres to the distribution of radii of transectional disks observed in two-dimensional sections. The Wicksell formula, however, requires the three-dimensional probability density function, $f_3(r)$, for finding a three-dimensional sphere of radius $r$, as input. Hence, we need to relate three-dimensional radii to the number of (actively cycling) cells in the foci, $m$.

If all cells in a spherically shaped focus are actively cycling (volume growth model) the number of cells can simply be inferred from the ratio of clone volume to cell volume: $m = r^3 / r_c^3$. However, there is some indication from pulse-labeling data that cell replication is inhomogeneous across individual foci, showing higher mitotic activity in the outer parts of the foci (A. Buchmann, personal communication), so that the relation between $m$ and $r$ may need modification.

After taking into account the Jacobian of the transformation ($m \rightarrow r$), which is given by the derivative $dm / dr$, Wicksell's formula can be written as

$$f_2^\varepsilon(y) = \frac{y}{\mu_\varepsilon} \int_y^\infty \frac{f_3(r)}{\sqrt{r^2 - y^2}} \, dr \tag{23}$$

where

$$f_3(r) = \frac{dm}{dr} \, p_{m = (r/r_c)^3}(t) \tag{24}$$

with $p_m$ given by Eq. (2) and with the (adjusted) mean radius, $\mu_\varepsilon$, given by

$$\mu_\varepsilon = \int_\varepsilon^\infty \sqrt{r^2 - \varepsilon^2} \, f_3(r) dr \tag{25}$$

Furthermore, the number of nonextinct transections (per unit area) is also assumed to be Poisson distributed with mean $n_2(t)$ and related to $\Lambda(t)$, its three-dimensional equivalent [see Eq. (17)], by means of

$$n_2(t) = 2\mu_\varepsilon \Lambda(t) \tag{26}$$

where $\Lambda(t)$ is given by Eq. (17). For more details, see Moolgavkar et al. (1990a).

If one also chooses to condition the analysis to foci that are smaller than a prescribed size, say radius $R$, then the foregoing formulae need to be modified accordingly. It can be shown that here $\mu_\varepsilon$ in the previous equations is simply replaced by $\mu_\varepsilon - \mu_R$, with $\mu_R$ defined like $\mu_\varepsilon$, correctly taking into account the new condition: $\mu_\varepsilon \leq r \leq R$. The values of $\varepsilon$, the smallest transection radius reliably detected, and of $R$, the largest size admitted, are in general determined by the experimenter.

The likelihood for the experimental data is constructed as a product of the contributions each animal makes. For each animal we have the Poisson probability of its section (area $A$) showing a total of $N_2 = n_2(t)A$ transections with radii between $\varepsilon$ and $R$ [see Eq. (26)] and the probability density $f_2^\varepsilon(y)$ that a particular transection is actually of size $y$ [see Eq. (23)]. The total likelihood is the product of the likelihood contributions made by each animal.

As an example we briefly discuss the analysis of an initiation and promotion experiment with DEN as initiator and a number of PCB congeners as promoters (Luebeck et al., 1991). The protocol is shown schematically in Fig. 6. There were two sacrifice points, the first 1 week after stop of promotion, the second, 8 weeks later. From the data, we were able to estimate the net cell proliferation parameter $\alpha - \beta$ during promotion and after promotion, together with the corresponding ratios $\beta / \alpha$, measuring the extinction of initiated cells. Focal transections were stained for two distinct marker enzymes (ATPase and GGT) on two adjacent sections. Three distinct phenotypes were defined according to whether foci were predominantly ATPase-negative (class 1), predominantly GGT-positive (class 2), or show both changes concomitantly (class 3). Table 1 lists the estimated parameters together with their Wald-based standard errors for class 1. All of the investigated PCB congeners were strong promoters.

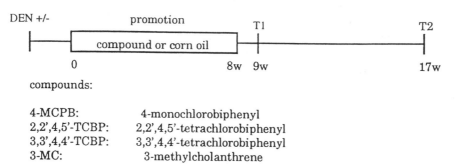

compounds:

4-MCPB:                4-monochlorobiphenyl
2,2',4,5'-TCBP:        2,2',4,5'-tetrachlorobiphenyl
3,3',4,4'-TCBP:        3,3',4,4'-tetrachlorobiphenyl
3-MC:                  3-methylcholanthrene

**Figure 6** Experimental protocol for the PCB experiment by Buchmann et al. (1991): DEN was administered for 10 consecutive days. Animals were killed at 9 or 17 weeks after the start of promoter treatment. See Luebeck et al. (1991) for more details.

## C. Joint Analysis of Premalignant and Malignant Lesions

In many experimental data sets, information is available both on malignant and benign tumors. If the benign tumors are known to lie on the pathway to malignancy, then it is important that they be considered in any analysis of the data. Currently, either the premalignant lesions are ignored, or they are thrown in with the malignant lesions. Both these procedures have obvious deficiencies. The first discards valuable information, and the second gives equal weight to premalignant and malignant lesions, which is clearly inappropriate. Recently, attempts are being made to quantify the appearance of "foci within foci"; that is, the appearance of small islands, presumably clonal, of cells within altered hepatic foci, characterized by a second phenotypic change. These foci within foci may represent the earliest stage of malignancy. The mathematical tools required for analyses of data in which information on both

**Table 1** Maximum Likelihood Estimates (MLE) and Standard Errors (SE) for the Listed PCB Compounds for ATPase Dominant Foci (class 1)

| | Estimates of promotion parameters | | | |
| | ATPase dominant | | | |
| Compound | $\alpha_1 - \beta_1$ | $\alpha_2 - \beta_2$ | $\beta_1 / \alpha_1$ | $\beta_2 / \alpha_2$ |
|---|---|---|---|---|
| Corn oil | $0.0286 \pm 0.0030$ | | $0.968 \pm 0.011$ | |
| 4-MCBP | $0.0433 \pm 0.0066$ | $-0.0021 \pm 0.0037$ | $0.965 \pm 0.013$ | $1.300 \pm 0.150$ |
| 2,2',4,5'-TCBP | $0.0592 \pm 0.0061$ | $0.0024 \pm 0.0026$ | $0.829 \pm 0.061$ | $0.998 \pm 0.002$ |
| 3,3',4,4'-TCBP | $0.0587 \pm 0.0056$ | $0.0214 \pm 0.0019$ | $0.769 \pm 0.077$ | $0.898 \pm 0.045$ |
| 3-MC | $0.0552 \pm 0.0061$ | $0.0090 \pm 0.0027$ | $0.872 \pm 0.044$ | $0.995 \pm 0.003$ |
| | Estimates of initiation parameters | | | |
| All | ATPase dominant | | $\upsilon_0 X$ | $\upsilon_1 X$ |
| | | | $5693 \pm 1800$ | $6.8 \pm 1.8$ |

On each of the time intervals, $I_1 = (0,t_1)$ during the treatment and $I_2 = (t_1,t_2)$ after the treatment ended until sacrifice the likelihood can be expressed in terms of the net proliferation parameters $\alpha_i - \beta_i$ and the ratios of cell death to cell division rates: $\beta_i / \alpha_i = 1,2$ (see Fig. 6). The parameter $\upsilon_0 X$ represents the number of cells altered by the DEN treatment per milliliter of liver and $\upsilon_1 X$ the number of spontaneously altered cells per milliliter per day during the experiment. $\alpha - \beta$ has units of $1 / day$, $\beta / \alpha$ is dimensionless.

premalignant and malignant lesions is available are currently being developed (Dewanji et al., 1991; de Gunst and Luebeck, 1994). However, a comprehensive discussion of these attempts would go beyond the scope of this chapter.

When one group of animals is monitored for premalignant lesions and another, independent, group for malignant lesions, the joint analysis is rather straightforward. We illustrate by means of an example.

### 1. Liver Foci and Carcinoma After Chronic Administration of N-Nitrosomorpholine

The data in this example are from an experiment in which a group of female Lewis rats were administered NNM in their drinking water in different concentrations (0, 0.1, 1, 5, 10, 20, 40, 80 ppm). The animals receiving the highest dose (80 ppm) were not considered further because of toxicity. Animals from each dose group were periodically killed, and their livers examined for ATPase-deficient foci, which were quantified according to the number of transections per section area, and the size of each transection. From each dose group some animals were followed until death, and their livers examined for the presence or absence of hepatocellular carcinoma. For the statistical analysis of the data, the malignant tumors were considered to be fatal. Among 107 animals followed in this way, there were 38 malignant tumors.

The analysis of the foci data follows Section IV.B, and was first reported in Moolgavkar et al., 1990a. For the joint analysis discussed here, we assume a linear dose–response in the net cell proliferation rate and the first mutation rate (i.e., $\alpha - \beta = a + b \times d$ and $\upsilon = \upsilon_0 + \upsilon_1 \times d$). The second mutation rate $\mu = \mu_0 + \mu_1 d$, but $\mu_1$ is estimated in this analysis to be zero. We assume that only surface cells undergo cell division while interior cells are resting. This last assumption needs elaboration: In the original foci analysis, all the cells in an ATPase-deficient focus were assumed to have the same probability of division [volume growth model: $m = (r / r_c)^3$]. In fact, there is probably a great deal of heterogeneity among the cells of a focus, and there is some limited evidence that, at least in large foci, cells close to the surface are more likely to divide (A. Buchmann, personal communication). We have made an attempt to incorporate heterogeneity by assuming that only cells on the surface of foci undergo division [$m = \pi(r / r_c)^2$]. This is undoubtedly an oversimplification, but it fits the data better than the assumption of homogeneity within foci. Each animal that's liver was examined for altered foci contributes to the likelihood as described in Section IV.B. Each animal that was followed until death makes one of two contributions to the total likelihood. If the animal had a malignant liver tumor, then the contribution is the density function for the time-to-tumor distribution derived from the two-mutation clonal expansion model, $P'(t)$. If the animal died without malignant tumor, then the contribution is the probability of no malignant tumor by the time of death derived from the same model, $1 - P(t)$. The total likelihood is the product of likelihood contributions from all animals, and is a function of all the parameters of the model. These parameters were estimated by maximizing the likelihood.

The results of the analysis are summarized in Table 2. They show that NNM affects the first mutation rate; that is, it increases the rate at which normal hepatocytes acquire the ATPase-deficient phenotype, and also increases the net proliferation rate of altered foci. However, no effect of NNM on the second mutation rate was observed. The asymptotic probability of extinction, $\beta / \alpha$, is high, 98.6%.

In a previous publication (Moolgavkar et al., 1990s), we had concluded that NNM was a strong initiator and a weak promoter. The joint analysis shown here (using the surface growth model) yields the same conclusion. Both, the rate of initiation and the net rate of proliferation of initiated cells, are consistent with a linear increase with dose of NNM. As noted earlier, the second mutation rate appears to be independent of dose of NNM. Moreover, the background rate

**Table 2**  Parameter Estimates and Their
95% Wald Confidence Intervals (CI) for the
N-Nitrosomorpholine (NNM) Example
Using the Surface Growth Model

| Parameter | Estimate | 95% CI |
|-----------|----------|--------|
| $a$ | 0.00543 | (0.0048,0.0062) |
| $b$ | 0.00018 | (0.00016,0.0002) |
| $\beta / \alpha$ | 0.986 | (0.982,0.990) |
| $\upsilon_0$ | 4.18 | (3.08,5.66) |
| $\upsilon_1$ | 8.06 | (6.74,9.65) |
| $\mu_0 \times 10^{10}$ | 8.0 | (5.70,11.2) |

Net cell proliferation rate defined as $\alpha - \beta = a + bd$,
and first transformation rate per milliliter liver de-
fined as $\upsilon = \upsilon_0 + \upsilon_1 d$, where $d$ is the dose in ppm.
Unit of time is days.

of the second mutation is estimated to be about $8 \times 10^{-10}$/cell per day. This appears to be far too low a number. One interpretation within the framework of the model is that only a small subset of ATPase-deficient foci is made up of truly initiated cells. Our estimate of the second mutation rate is based on the assumption that all ATPase-deficient cells are equally likely to go on to malignancy. Another explanation of this finding is that malignant cells also have a large probability of extinction, so that our estimate of the second mutation rate represents a lower bound only.

From the assumed linearity of the dose–response, a simple definition of initiation and promotion potencies can be given readily by the ratio of the slope and the corresponding intercept. This ratio is given per unit dose. For our NNM example we get (per ml liver)

$$\upsilon(d) = 4.18 + 8.06d$$

$\rightarrow$ initiation potency $= 1.93$ / ppm

and similarly for the net cell proliferation parameter $(\alpha - \beta)$

$$(\alpha - \beta)(d) = 0.00543 + 0.00018d$$

$\rightarrow$ promotion potency $= 0.033$ / ppm

From this result we conclude that NNM is a strong initiator, but a weak promoter. This does not mean, however, that the promotional effect of NNM is unimportant, since intermediate cell clones grow exponentially under the model, whereas newly initiated cells accrue only in linear fashion. Thus, sooner or later, the promotional effects will dominate the tumor risk.

## ACKNOWLEDGMENTS

The authors of this chapter were supported by grants from the National Cancer Institute and the U.S. Environmental Protection Agency.

# REFERENCES

Aaltonen, L. A., P. Peltomaki, F. S. Leach, P. Sistonen, L. Pylkkdnen, J. -P. Mecklin, H. Jdrvinen, S. M. Powell, J. Jen, S. R. Hamilton, G. M. Peterson, K. W. Kinzler, B. Vogelstein, and A. de la Chapelle (1993). Clues to the pathogenesis of familial colorectal cancer, *Science,* 260, 812–816.

Armitage, P., and R. Doll (1954). The age distribution of cancer and a multistage theory of carcinogenesis, *Br. J. Cancer,* 8, 1–12.

Bishop, J. M. (1991). Molecular themes in oncogenesis. *Cell,* 64, 235–248.

Brown, C., and K. Chu (1987). Use of multistage models to infer stages affected by carcinogenic exposure: Example of lung cancer and cigarette smoking, *J. Chron. Dis.,* 40 (Suppl.2), 171S–179S.

Buchmann, A., M. Schwarz, R. Schmitt, C. R. Wolf, F. Oesch, and W. Kunz (1987). Development of cytochrome P-450 altered preneoplastic and neoplastic lesions during nitrosoamine-induced hepato-carcinogenesis in the rat, *Cancer Res.,* 47, 2911–2918.

Buchmann, A., S. Ziegler, A. Wolf, L. W. Robertson, S. K. Durham, and M. Schwarz (1991). Effects of polychlorinated biphenyls in rat liver: Correlation between primary subcellular effects and promoting activity, *Toxicol. Appl. Pharmacol.,* 111, 454–468.

Bursch, W., B. Lauer, I. Timmermann-Trosiener, G. Barthel, J. Schuppler, and R. Schulte-Hermann (1984). Controlled death (apoptosis) of normal and putative preneoplastic cells in rat liver following with-drawal of tumor promoters, *Carcinogenesis,* 5, 453–458.

Bursch, W., N. S. Taper, B. Lauer, and R. Schulte-Hermann (1985). Quantitative histological and histochemical studies on the occurrence and stages of controlled cell death (apoptosis) during regression of rat liver hyperplasia, *Virchows Archiv. (Cell Pathol.),* 50, 153–166.

Bursch, W., B. Putz, G. Barthel, and R. Schulte-Hermann (1990). Determination of the length of the histological stages of apoptosis in normal liver and in altered hepatic foci of rats, *Carcinogenesis,* 11, 5, 847–853.

Cerutti, P. A. (1985). Prooxidant states and tumor promotion, *Science,* 227, 375–381.

Cook, P., R. Doll, and S. A. Fellingham (1969). A mathematical model for the age distribution of cancer in man, *Int. J. Cancer,* 4, 93–112.

Cox, D. R., and H. D. Miller (1972). *The Theory of Stochastic Processes,* Chapman & Hall, London.

Crump, K., and R. Howe (1984). The multistage model with a time-dependent dose pattern: Application to carcinogenic risk assessment, *Risk Anal.,* 4, 163–176.

Day, N., and C. Brown (1980). Multistage models and primary prevention of cancer, *JNCI,* 64, 977–989.

De Gunst, M. C. M., and E. G. Luebeck (1994). Quantitative analysis of two-dimensional clones in the presence or absence of malignant tumors, *Math. Biosci.,* 119, 5–34.

Dewanji, A., D. J. Venzon, and S. H. Moolgavkar (1989). A stochastic two-stage model for cancer risk assessment. II. The number and size of premalignant clones, *Risk Anal.,* 9, 179–187.

Dewanji, A., S. H. Moolgavkar, and E. G. Luebeck (1991). Two-mutation model for carcinogenesis: Joint analysis of premalignant and malignant lesions, *Math. Biosci.,* 104, 97–109.

Emmelot, P., and E. Scherer (1980). The first relevant cell stage in rat liver carcinogenesis: A quantitative approach, *Biochim. Biophys. Acta,* 605, 247–304.

Farber, E. and R. Cameron (1980). The sequential analysis of cancer development, *Adv. Cancer Res.,* 31, 125–226.

Fearon, E. R., and B. Vogelstein (1990). *Cell,* 61, 759–7676.

Freedman, D. A., and W. Navidi (1989). Multistage models for carcinogenesis, *Environ. Health Perspect.,* 81, 169–188.

Goldfarb, S., and T. D. Pugh (1981). Enzyme histochemical phenotypes in primary hepatocellular carcinomas, *Cancer Res.,* 41, 2092–2095.

Goldsworthy, T. L., M. H. Hanigan, and H. C. Pitot (1986). Models of hepatocarcinogenesis in the rat—contrasts and comparisons, *CRC Crit. Rev. Toxicol.,* 17, 61–89.

Hollstein, M., D. Sidransky, B. Vogelstein, and C. C. Harris (1991). *p*53 Mutations in human cancers, *Science,* 253, 49–53.

[IARC] International Agency for Research on Cancer (1992). Mechanisms of carcinogenesis in risk identification (H. Vainio, P. Magee, D. McGregor, and A. J. McMichael, eds.), IARC Scientific Publications No. 116, Lyon.

Kendall, D. G. (1960). Birth-and-death processes, and the theory of carcinogenesis, *Biometrika,* 47, 13–21.

Knudson, A. G. (1971). Mutation and cancer: Statistical study of retinoblastoma, *Proc. Natl. Acad. Sci. USA,* 68, 820–823.

Kopp-Schneider, A., and C. J. Portier (1992). Birth and death/differentiation rates of papillomas in mouse skin, *Carcinogenesis,* 13, 973–987.

Kopp-Schneider, A. (1992). Birth–death processes with piecewise constant rates, *Stat. Probability Let.,* 13, 121–127.

Kunz, W., G. Schaude, M. Schwarz, and H. Tennekes (1982). Quantitative aspects of drug-mediated tumor promotion in liver and its toxicological implications, *Carcinogenesis,* 7, 111–125.

Land, H., L. F. Parada, and R. A. Weinberg (1983). Cellular oncogenes and multistep carcinogenesis, *Science,* 222, 771–778.

Levine, A. J., J. Momand and C. A. Finlay (1991). The $p53$ tumour suppressor gene, *Nature,* 351, 453–456.

Luebeck, E. G., and S. H. Moolgavkar (1991). Stochastic analysis of intermediate lesions in carcinogenesis experiments, *Risk Anal.,* 11, 149–157.

Luebeck, E. G., S. H. Moolgavkar, A. Buchmann, and M. Schwarz (1991). Effects of polychlorinated biphenyls in rat liver: Quantitative analysis of enzyme-altered foci, *Toxicol. Appl. Pharmacol.,* 111, 469–484.

Luebeck, E. G., B. Grasl-Kraupp, I. Timmermann-Trosiener, W. Bursch, R. Schulte-Hermann, and S. H. Moolgavkar (1994). Growth kinetics of enzyme altered liver foci in rats treated with phenobarbital or α-hexachlorocyclohexane, *Toxicol. Appl. Pharmacol.,* 130, 304–315.

Muller, H. J. (1951). Radiation damage to the genetic material, *Sci. Prog.,* 7, 93–493.

Moolgavkar, S. H. (1978). The multistage theory of carcinogenesis and the age distribution of cancer in man, *JNCI,* 61, 49–52.

Moolgavkar, S. H. (1991). Stochastic models of carcinogenesis. In *Handbook of Statistics,* Vol. 8 (C. R. Rao and R. Chakraborty, eds.), Elsevier Science Publishers, Amsterdam, pp. 373–393.

Moolgavkar, S. H., and A. Knudson (1981). Mutation and cancer: A model for human carcinogenesis, *JNCI,* 66, 1037–1052.

Moolgavkar, S. H., and E. G. Luebeck (1990). Two-event model for carcinogenesis: Biological, mathematical and statistical considerations, *Risk Anal.,* 10, 323–341.

Moolgavkar, S. H., A. Dewanji, and D. J. Venzon (1988). A stochastic two-stage model for cancer risk assessment. I. The hazard function and the probability of tumor, *Risk Analy.,* 8, 383–392.

Moolgavkar, S. H., E. G. Luebeck, M. De Gunst, R. E. Port, and M. Schwarz (1990a). Quantitative analysis of enzyme-altered foci in rat hepatocarcinogenesis experiments I: Single agent regimen, *Carcinogenesis,* 11, 8, 1271–1278.

Moolgavkar, S. H., F. T. Cross, E. G. Luebeck, and G. E. Dagle (1990b). A two-mutation model for radon-induced lung tumors in rats, *Radiat. Res.,* 121, 28–37.

Moolgavkar, S. H., E. G. Luebeck, D. Krewski, and J. M. Zielinski (1993). Radon, cigarette smoke, and lung cancer: A reanalysis of the Colorado Plateau uranium miners' data, *Am. J. Epidemiol.,* 4, 204–217.

Neyman, J., and E. Scott (1967). Statistical aspects of the problem of carcinogenesis. *Fifth Berkeley Symposium on Mathematical Statistics and Probability.* University of California Press, Berkeley, CA, pp. 745–776.

Nordling, C. O. (1953). A new theory of the cancer inducing mechanism, *Br. J. Cancer,* 7, 68–72.

Pitot, H. C., T. L. Goldsworthy, S. Moran, W. Kennan, H. P. Glauert, R. R. Maronpot, and H. A. Campbell (1987). A method to quantitate the relative initiating and promoting potencies of hepatocarcinogenic agents in their dose–response relationships to altered hepatic foci, *Carcinogenesis,* 8, 10, 1491–1499.

Portier, C., and A. Kopp-Schneider (1991). A multistage model of carcinogenesis incorporating DNA damage and repair, *Risk Anal.,* 11, 535–543.

Renan, M. J. (1993). How many mutations are required for tumorigenesis? Implications for human cancer data, *Mol. Carcinog.,* 7, 139–146.

Satoh, K., I. Hatayama, N. Tateoka, K. Tamai, T. Shimizu, M. Tatematus, N. Ito, and K. Sato (1989). Transient induction of single GST-P positive hepatocytes by DEN, *Carcinogenesis,* 10, 11, 2107–2111.

Schulte-Hermann, R., I. Timmermann-Trosiener, G. Barthel, and W. Bursch (1990). DNA synthesis, apoptosis and phenotypic expression as determinants of growth of altered foci in rat liver during phenobarbitol promotion, *Cancer Res.*, 50, 5127–5135.

Tan, W. Y. (1986). A stochastic Gompertz birth–death process, *Stat. Probability Lett.*, 4, 25–28.

Tan, W. Y. (1991). *Stochastic Models of Carcinogenesis,* Statistics: Textbooks and Monographs, Vol. 116, Marcel Dekker, New York.

Whittemore, A. S. (1977). The age distribution of human cancer for carcinogenic exposures of varying intensity, *Am. J. Epidemiol.*, 106, 418–432.

Wicksell, D. S. (1925). The corpuscle problem, part I, *Biometrika,* 17, 87–97.

# PART VI
# USE OF HUMAN DATA AND ANIMAL TO HUMAN DATA EXTRAPOLATION

**Lynn Goldman**
*United States Environmental Protection Agency*
*Washington, D.C.*

Risk assessors need to make the best possible use of human and animal studies. Human data, when available and adequate, are preferable to experimental animal data. Use of human data obviates the need to consider interspecies differences. And human data often involve dosages and exposures that are much closer to "real-world" exposures. As with experimental animal toxicological studies, epidemiological and clinical studies of humans follow specific principles and methods. There are considerations and criteria that can be established to design a study, evaluate the findings, and provide guidance for assessing risks. These are described in this section, along with examples of chemicals for which human data have been useful as the basis for risk assessment. Some of these examples include lead, arsenic, selenium, and asbestos. Additional biological monitoring of chemicals in human tissues, and especially biological markers, are useful to support an overall health assessment.

Attention is also given to the consideration of other factors that may affect human health, such as environmental or metabolic breakdown products, which may contribute to toxicity of the parent compound, or chemical interactions, which can modify chemical toxicity. The resultant modifying effect could be synergism, antagonism, or additivity. Examples of chemicals that have metabolic or environmental breakdown products of health concern include the following: aldicarb: aldicarb sulfoxide; malathion: malaoxon; daminozide: 1,1-dimethyl hydrazine; metam sodium: methylisothiocyanate. Examples of chemical–chemical interactions include selenium and various other metals, such as cadmium and methylmercury. Although animal data constitute a large database for risk assessment, these data often have limitations and carry uncertainties. This section provides a discussion of the various issues surrounding the use of animal data for assessing human health risks. A consensus needs to be reached concerning interspecies scaling of body surface area. Interpretation of various toxicological findings in animals is still under debate. Risk assessors must consider the similarities and differences (physiological, biochemical, anatomical, and pharmacokinetic) between animals and humans;

interdose, interroute, and interspecies extrapolations; and how best to employ experimental data to assess risks that humans will encounter in everyday living.

A risk assessment is no better than the data that it comprises. Critical evaluation and approaches to make the most effective and valid use of data are key to the effective application of risk assessment to reduce risks to the public for health protection.

# 30
# Epidemiology: General Principles, Methodological Issues, and Applications to Environmental Toxicology

**Richard G. Ames**
*California Environmental Protection Agency*
*Berkeley, California*

## I. EPIDEMIOLOGY: A DEFINITION

*Epidemiology* has been defined as "the study of the distribution and determinants of disease and injuries in human populations" (Mausner and Bahn, 1974). This definition places epidemiology in contrast with clinical medicine; clinical medicine focuses on the observation and treatment of patients, whereas epidemiology focuses on the frequency and distribution of illness in society. The focus of epidemiology is on human health, not laboratory studies on animals.

Epidemiology is a method, or perspective, rather than a body of knowledge in its own right. In practice, epidemiology is highly integrative; many epidemiological studies are done by teams that include, in addition to epidemiologists, physicians, industrial hygienists, and toxicologists, because no person or discipline possesses the wide diversity of medical, statistical, environmental, and toxicological data or methods required for a successful study.

Epidemiology is a method with a mission: its goals include both disease prevention as well as understanding the nature, course, and causes of disease. Basic sciences, such as biology, chemistry, and the like, do not have such an action-orientation component to their discipline.

## II. RISK AND RISK FACTORS

The fundamental concept in epidemiology is *risk*. Epidemiologists look at diseases in terms of factors, called risk factors, that promote or protect against the occurrence of disease. The presence (or sometimes absence) of risk factors is associated with an increased likelihood that disease will develop. Hence, risk is a statistical measure of the increase in likelihood that disease will develop, given a specific exposure. A medical axiom states that not all persons exposed to an agent develop the disease. The looseness of association between agent and disease outcome on a case-by-case basis underscores the notion of statistical probability that characterizes risk. In the field of risk assessment, individual variations in response to an agent may be explained in terms of different individual sensitivity, based on differences in age, sex, genetic or biochemical factors, or other unidentified factors.

## III. EXPLORING RISK FACTORS

One goal of epidemiology is to understand the natural history of a disease and its causes. Epidemiologists start by searching for factors that place people at risk for getting the disease. Every finding presents another question: What is it about this risk factor that places the person at increased risk for getting the disease? Thus, explaining each identified risk factor becomes a process of exploring the associations in a search for risk factors that more and more closely approximate a cause for the disease.

Often epidemiologists start by exploring patterns and correlations of any kind, regardless of how loosely the factors seem to be tied to the disease. Age, sex, race, marital status, and the like, may be risk factors for a disease, although they do not necessarily cause the disease. As a case in point, the three original risk factors identified for acquired immune deficiency syndrome (AIDS) were the statuses: *hemophiliac, Haitian,* and *homosexual* (CDC, 1981a,b, 1982). Then, the question arose: What is it about these factors that is related to the disease? As we now know, the search progressed through blood transfusions (Ammann et al., 1983) and sexual practices, finally culminating in the identification of the human immunodeficiency virus (HIV) (Peterman, et al., 1985). A risk factor that is a true cause for a disease is called an *agent*. The finding of these three general risk factors, hemophiliac, Haitian, and homosexual, was the beginning of the inquiry process that narrowed the risk factors down until scientists could identify the agent causing the disease.

Many times epidemiologists move successively closer and closer toward understanding the causal nature of the relation between risk factors and the disease. At other times, hundreds of risk factors provide no explanation. Gastric cancer, for example, is a poorly understood disease: it appears to be related to everything, yet seemingly, it is explained by nothing (Mirvish, 1983).

## IV. ETIOLOGY

The search for the causes of disease is called *etiology*. Epidemiologists build a case for causality in roughly the same way that a lawyer builds a case for the guilt or innocence of the accused. *Biological plausibility* is one of the key elements in epidemiologists' search for cause: Does the purported explanation make sense biologically? Another key element in the search for causality is the *dose–response* relationship. If increased dose of an exposure factor is associated with increased level of response, that risk factor is more likely to be seen as a putative agent. Another key to establishing causality is a proper *time–order* relationship between the putative agent and the response. If the exposure to the agent occurs after the illness, one would not call that factor causal for that disease.

To prove causality, one must also exclude, in a convincing way, all other presumptive agents, as well as consider the range of potentially confounding factors. Excluding other possible causes is often accomplished by using control groups, or by measuring covariates and incorporating these measures into statistical analysis. To establish control over the unwanted effects of extraneous variables, epidemiologists often use regression analysis, analysis of covariance, and other statistical techniques. For conclusions to be convincing, sample size must be adequate.

Clearly, the attribution of causality in epidemiology is not an easy task. Establishing causality is made even more difficult because epidemiologists usually lack information on, or control over, exposure variables, since they frequently study events after they have occurred.

## V. THE EPIDEMIOLOGICAL PERSPECTIVE

Epidemiology, although relying on many aspects of research that are drawn from psychology, sociology, statistics, clinical medicine, and the basic sciences, is distinguished by a focus on risk factors, cofactors, agent–host–environment paradigms, and statistical methods, such as relative risks and odds ratios, that are uniquely its own. These unique concepts and methods will be explored in subsequent paragraphs.

## A. Cofactors

*Cofactors* are different from risk factors because cofactors do not cause a disease; however, their presence allows other risk factors to be operative. For example, if asbestos exposure leads to asbestosis, and asbestos exposure *plus cigarette smoking* leads to increased rates of asbestosis, but cigarette smoking by itself does not lead to asbestosis; cigarette smoking is then a cofactor for asbestosis. Cigarette smoking increases the probability that asbestos exposure will lead to asbestosis by inhibiting the lung clearance of asbestos fibers.

## B. The Epidemiological Paradigm

The *epidemiological paradigm* focuses attention on the interrelationships among agent, host, and environmental factors in the production of illness (Fig. 1). In theory, all risk factors exist in a

AGENT FACTORS

Chemicals in air, water, and food

Occupational exposures (asbestos)

Germs (<u>Cholera vibrio</u>)

Biological organisms (malaria protoza)

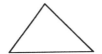

HOST FACTORS

High blood pressure

Genetic tags (Sickle cell)

Obesity

Demographic factors

ENVIRONMENT FACTORS

Temperature, wind

Diurnal variation

Amount of sunlight

Repetitive trauma

**Figure 1** The epidemiological paradigm.

state of interdependency. This interrelationship can make unraveling the causes of disease a very complex process. Examples of host, agent, and environmental risk factors are presented in Fig. 1.

## C.  Epidemiological Endpoints

Health may be viewed as a continuum from perfect health to death. We can identify measured or observed points along the continuum:

1. No apparent disease
2. Morbid preconditions: cholinesterase-inhibition, immune system deficiency, tumor latency
3. Early inapparent disease: methemoglobinemia from nitrate
4. Manifest disease (conditions that are clearly apparent): respiratory disease from air pollutants
5. Diseases in remission: malaria can go into remission
6. Mortality (death): death from lung cancer

States along this continuum are often not clearly defined. Individuals can move, almost imperceptibly at times, from states of good health to states of illness. A state of good health is a matter of cultural definition (Parsons, 1958). What is considered well in one culture or subculture may be considered ill health in another, or vice versa. States 2 through 5, various degrees of illness, are called *morbidity*. State 6, death, is called *mortality*. From an epidemiological perspective, morbidity and mortality are frequently analyzed using different sets of terms and statistics.

Intermediate outcomes, such as disability, can also be studied by epidemiologists. For example, Ames and Trent (1984) studied early retirement with disability among coal miners in relation to respiratory impairment. However, outcomes intermediate between morbidity and mortality appear to be studied more frequently by economists than epidemiologists.

## VI.  MEASUREMENT OF VARIABLES

Measurement of exposure and endpoint variables is a prerequisite for epidemiological analysis. *Measurement* has been defined as "the assignment of symbols to objects according to a set of rules" (Stevens, 1951). Measurement is always an indirect process. Concepts are defined and, then, a set of measurement operations is established. The empirical evidence that is actually measured always stands for some more highly conceptual quality.

Determining the weight of an item by balancing it against carob seeds on a balance-beam scale offers a measurement example dating from antiquity. Counting the number of carob seeds necessary to achieve balance was an effective measurement rule, since carob seeds are exceptionally uniform in weight from one seed to another. The measure of carat, used today to measure the weight of diamonds, stems from this early measurement procedure.

All measurement operations, be they measures of age, sex, race, disease, or cause of death, follow the same general procedure. A concept to be measured is defined. Then, measurement is defined as a set of operations necessary to apply symbols to objects to result in a measurement outcome, such as the counting of carob seeds necessary to achieve balance.

No measurement is ever perfect. The rules for assigning symbols to objects could be incorrect; or the rules could be correct, but applied imperfectly. Even overtly obvious measurements, such as classifying a person's sex, can be problematic, as was seen in one Olympic competition when some "women" athletes were disqualified on the basis of the application of a different set of rules, cytology rather than physical anatomy. Error is simply one component of measurement.

## A. Measuring Exposures

Measuring exposure variables often presents problems for epidemiologists. Many times, the occurrence of an exposure can only be inferred based on an individual's location at the time of an incident, or on job classification status. For example, in 1991, a Southern Pacific train derailed near the town of Dunsmuir, California, dumping 19,000 gallons of the pesticide metam sodium into the Sacramento river. The direction of the wind and the concentration of airborne pesticide or pesticide breakdown products may never be known. Individual exposures are even less certain. Possible exposures to contaminated river water is also unknown, although the incident occurred at night, when such contact would be less likely. In short, individual exposures were unmeasured. Any epidemiological study of the incident would have to rely on exposures that were inferred from the context of the spill incident.

Favorable measurement conditions exist when industrial hygienists can measure exposure; however, the epidemiologist would not have control over the conditions of the measurement process. Less favorable measurement conditions exist when the culpable agent is unknown, but being sought. The possibility exists, for example, that the agent could be misidentified. In the 1985 watermelon poisoning epidemic in California, which was quickly determined to be related to an improper and illegal use of Temik, the agent was aldicarb sulfoxide, a breakdown product of the active ingredient, aldicarb (Goldman et al., 1990). If the epidemiologists analyzing the poisonings had been looking for aldicarb residue in the melon samples, rather than aldicarb sulfoxide, the agent would have been misidentified, measurements would have been meaningless, and the analysis misdirected.

Some effects are not related to a single exposure; rather two or more exposures may work in conjunction with each other. Interaction is the extent to which two variables produce a different joint effect than would be expected given a knowledge of the effect of each variable by itself. Drug antagonism provides an example of interaction effects. Organophosphate pesticides and atropine are each lethal poisons; however, administering atropine to a person poisoned by organophosphates counteracts the effect of the organophosphate poison.

Confounding of effects is a measurement problem that is difficult to assess. Confounding exists when one cannot separate the effects of one variable from another; the epidemiologist is then left without a resolution of the importance of a variable of interest.

Sometimes measures are made on an aggregate level, and extrapolated to individuals, running the risk of an error in logic (Bogue, 1969; pp. 537–539). For example, if Native Americans were found to live in areas characterized by high rates of dental caries, and it was concluded that Native Americans had high rates of dental caries, this assumption would be based upon flawed logic.

In short, measuring exposure variables presents special problems to epidemiologists. An exposure may be unknown, or the degree of uncertainty about an estimated exposure may be large. Exposure measurements may be taken by other persons, or for different purposes than the study at hand, and thus be out of the epidemiologist's control. The exposure effect may result from interaction with another variable, or it may be impossible to distinguish one variable's effects from that of another. Or, the exposure measure may be extrapolated inappropriately to subjects. For all these reasons, exposure measurements may present problems of epidemiologists.

## B.  Measuring Mortality

Mortality is often measured using cause of death codes based on death certificate information. Causes of death are converted into International Statistical Classification of Diseases, Injuries, and Causes of Death (ICD) codes by nosologists, persons trained to code cause of death. The World Health Organization (WHO) revises the ICD codes at least every 10 years. Mortality can be analyzed by life table-based statistics. The 5-year survival function used to assess the efficacy of cancer treatments is an example of a life table-based mortality statistic.

## C.  Measuring Morbidity

Morbidity is usually measured in terms of rates of occurrence of a disease. A rate is a measure of some event, disease, or condition in relation to a unit of population, along with some specification of time (Mausner and Bahn, 1974). In addition to looking for causal relationships, epidemiologists measure the rate of occurrence of events with the goal of generalizing the rate to other populations or to the same population at another time period. A rate $R$ may be defined as,

$$R = \frac{\text{Events in time } t}{\text{Population at risk of event in time } t} \times 100 \text{ (or other factor)}$$

Not all populations are at risk of an event. For an infant mortality rate, defined as deaths at younger than 1 year of age, the population at risk of the event would be the population younger than 1 year old. Some diseases, such as measles, confer *immunity;* hence, persons who had measles at a prior time period would not be at risk during a subsequent time period. A *true rate* is established when the denominator is truly the population at risk of the event. Rates that do not fully meet the strict definition of a true rate, but that closely meet the definition, are called *quasi-rates.* A rate of airline fatalities based on millions of passenger miles as the denominator is an example of a quasi-rate.

   Both the numerator and the denominator are important in defining a rate. An error or change in definition in either numerator or denominator can change the nature of the rate and consequently its interpretation.

   Constructing meaningful rates can be challenging. Rates can be mathematically correct, but if the numerator and the denominator do not function together to capture the variable of interest, they may be lacking in interpretation. Because epidemiologists must convey information in an accurate and interpretable way, a thorough understanding of rates is important. Rates differ in underlying assumptions, the types of epidemiological study designs that support their use, and the interpretations that can be drawn from them. Several major classes of rates used in epidemiology are discussed in the following.

## VII.  INCIDENCE AND PREVALENCE RATES

*Incidence* is the rate of development of new cases of disease within a specified time period (usually 1 year). Incidence is important in epidemiology because it is related to etiology, the study of factors that cause disease. The time of disease onset relative to the time of exposure to the presumptive agent is critical to understanding the disease and disease process.

   *Prevalence* is the rate of disease cases that exist at one point in time. Prevalence rates are often used when planning for services, such as assessing the needs for hospitals, hospital beds, staff, resources, and the like. Prevalence, however, is not useful for understanding the etiology of a disease. These two concepts, incidence and prevalence, and the distinctions between them, are central to epidemiology and medical research generally.

## VIII. RELATIVE RISK

*Relative risk* (RR) is the major statistical tool used to measure risk when epidemiologists assess the etiology of a disease. It is defined as the disease incidence rate in the exposed population divided by the disease incidence rate in the unexposed population. Without incidence, one cannot directly measure relative risk, or assess causality. When data do not meet the assumptions required for relative risk, epidemiologists must estimate relative risk using the odds ratio (to be defined later). The type of study design determines the assumptions that can be made about appropriate measures of risk. A discussion of the basic epidemiological study designs, and the permissible statistics for each, follows.

## IX. EPIDEMIOLOGICAL STUDY DESIGNS

Listed now are some major types of epidemiological study designs. These are ideal designs. In practice, most studies are based on imperfect designs, or a combination of design types.

1. Prospective (or forward-looking) studies
2. Retrospective (or backward-looking) studies
3. Sample surveys (cross-sectional designs)
4. Outbreak investigations
5. Standardized mortality ratio (SMR) and proportional mortality ratio (PMR) studies
6. Experiments
7. Clinical trials
8. Life table-based studies

The following paragraphs provide a discussion of assumptions, strengths and weaknesses, and permissible statistics, associated with these study design types.

### A. Prospective Studies

Prospective studies follow a population over time for exposure status and disease incidence. A cohort design, defined in terms of a subpopulation experiencing a common event at one time point, is one type of prospective study. The atomic bomb survivors represent a cohort in which the possibility of radiation exposure from the A-bomb blast was the defining event. Mortality follow-up of A-bomb survivors focused on leukemia, since that was the disease of interest (Brill et al., 1962). Other examples of prospective studies include community health studies in which the population is enumerated and followed over time for exposure status and the development of disease, such as the Framingham Heart Disease Study (Dawber, 1980). Prospective designs allow incidence rates and relative risks to be computed and, thus, allow causality to be assessed. Disadvantages include the necessity of a larger sample size and a study period that often takes years.

### B. Retrospective Designs

Retrospective studies start with diagnosed cases of disease and work backward to recreate exposure status. Case–control studies are the most common type of retrospective study designs. Cases of a disease may be selected from a hospital, disease registry, or other reporting system.

Noncases are matched, usually by age and sex, and other potentially confounding variables to the cases; they become the controls. Case–control studies are used to determine what exposure statuses disproportionately characterize the cases as opposed to the controls.

The risk calculation from a case–control study is called an odds ratio. An odds ratio is an estimate of relative risk. Odds ratios greater than unity mean that the risk factor places the person at enhanced risk for getting the disease. Because the sample size in a retrospective study can be small, the study may be done quickly and cheaply. The lack of incidence data prevents the direct computation of relative risk and, hence, assessment of causality. Instead, relative risk must be estimated from the odds ratio. Odds ratios, in practice, are good estimates of relative risk.

An example of the calculation of the odds ratio compared with the calculation of relative risk is presented in Fig. 2. Each two-by-two data table is set up to present disease status on the top and exposure status on the side. The cells for "exposed-cases" or "exposed-ill" are placed in the upper left hand corners of each table.

In a case–control study, panel I, the odds ratio is computed as the product of the main diag-

**I. Retrospective design -- Case-control study**

|            | Disease |          |      |
|------------|---------|----------|------|
| Exposure   | Cases   | Controls |      |
| Exposed    | 30      | 42       | 72   |
| Non-exp.   | 5       | 63       | 68   |
|            | 35      | 105      | 140  |

Odds Ratio (OR) = 30 x 63 / 5 x 42  = 9.0

**II. Prospective design -- Cohort study**

|            | Disease |          |      |
|------------|---------|----------|------|
| Exposure   | Ill     | Not ill  |      |
| Exposed    | 30      | 42       | 72   |
| Non-exp.   | 5       | 63       | 68   |
|            | 35      | 105      | 140  |

Incidence rate in the exposed group  = 30/72 = 41.7%

Incidence rate in the unexposed group  =   5 / 68 = 7.4%

Relative Risk (RR) =   41.7 / 7.4   =   5.64

**Figure 2**  Sample data: Calculation of odds ratio versus relative risk.

onal divided by the product of the minor diagonal. In this example, $30 \times 63$ divided by $5 \times 42$ equals 9.0. Hence, the odds are 9 times greater for contracting the disease given the exposure.

In a prospective design, panel II, the relative risk is computed as the incidence rate in the exposed group divided by the incidence rate in the unexposed group. Here the incidence in the exposed group is 30/72, or 41.7%. The incidence in the unexposed group is 5/68, or 7.4%. The relative risk is 41.7/7.4, or 5.64. In other words, the risk is 5.6 times greater for contracting the disease in the exposed group compared with the unexposed group, given the exposure.

Note that the basic data are the same in both panels I and II, each representing data from different study design types. Differences lie in the assumptions that are made about the nature of the data which, in turn, lead to different permissible statistics; different statistics lead to different risk values, and possibly to different interpretations and conclusions. Therefore, the researcher must know the study design type to identify permissible statistics and data interpretations that can be defended to the scientific community.

## C. Sample Surveys

A sample survey is basically a cross-sectional study, at one time point, that cuts across many cohorts. Examples of surveys are the decennial censuses taken by the U. S. Census Bureau (100% enumeration), and certain sample surveys, such as many community health surveys. The sample survey is simple, inexpensive, and quick. The survey's primary disadvantage is that one cannot impute causality from a snapshot in time.

It is possible to produce a variant of the survey with an epidemiological orientation. In a study of acute symptoms and exposure to cotton defoliants, Scarborough and co-workers (1989) used a survey format to collect retrospective 2-week symptom incidence rates, so that relative risks could be computed. The epidemiological variations for this study included

1. A real control group was used; in essence, two surveys were done, one in exposed communities, and another in unexposed communities.
2. Retrospective recall was used to establish 2-week symptom incidence. This measurement stretched the assumptions underlying incidence rates to some degree.
3. The assumption that one could measure symptom incidence retrospectively in a 2-week period allowed the calculation of relative risk.

An unmodified cross-sectional survey would assume a count of existing cases of illness at one time point and, thereby, allow prevalence rates only.

## D. Outbreak Investigations

Epidemiologists frequently must undertake outbreak investigations with limited preparation owing to the immediate need for information. A first step often is the construction of an "epi-curve," a distribution of disease incidence plotted over time. Frequently, exposure measures are superimposed over the epi-curve. One goal of an outbreak investigation is to determine a culpable agent for a disease. Other goals include identification of the course of a disease, periods of infectivity, and the interactions of exposure factors with other variables.

An example of an outbreak investigation is the case in which a mysterious disease outbreak at the Bellevue–Stratford Hotel in Philadelphia was traced to microbial contamination of the air conditioning system (Fraser et al., 1977). The disease was subsequently name Legionnaires' disease in honor of the hotel's convention participants.

## E.  Standardized Mortality Ratio and Proportional Mortality Ratio Studies

Standardized mortality ratio (SMR) studies are often used when mortality records exist by cause of death. Death rates from a standard population are applied to the occupational subpopulation to compute an expected set of deaths for that workforce; this calculation is done for each category of the standardization variable, usually age. Then, the total observed deaths are divided by the total expected deaths to obtain the standardized mortality ratio.

Proportionate mortality ratio (PMR) studies are even less sophisticated than SMR studies. A ratio of the proportion of observed deaths by a selected cause of death in a workforce is formed against the proportion of deaths for that cause in a standard population. The PMRs are usually used in occupational mortality studies.

The SMR and PMR studies are quick and inexpensive; the disadvantages, however, are numerous. These studies lack sophistication and are imprecise; they are incapable of assessing causality, or even of ruling out potentially confounding factors. Such studies are used principally when other types of studies cannot be done.

## F.  Experiments

Experiments are the classic scientific design. A population is randomly divided into two similar subpopulations, one an experimental group, the other a control group. The experimental group is exposed to an agent, whereas the control group is given a placebo. Then, the outcomes of interest are measured. Outcome differences between the two groups are attributed to the exposure.

The advantages of experiments include the ability to assess causality, to define and measure the independent, or exposure, variable, and to control unwanted effects by randomizing subjects into experimental and control groups. Epidemiological experiments, however, raise ethical and moral questions relating to the experimental use of human subjects. Experiments are infrequently performed by epidemiologists.

## G.  Clinical Trials

Clinical trials are basically human experiments. Why then do clinical trials not fall under the same restrictions placed on experiments in general? The answer is that clinical trials are conducted to improve health directly. Some clinical trials are conducted on patients with a poor prognosis; much of AIDS treatment testing provides an example. Given an incurable disease, testing the efficacy of a new drug is considered legitimate and humanitarian. Drawbacks to clinical trials include the following: some tests are conducted in a charged atmosphere, many become unwieldy, as for example, multiple substudies each under a different director and, in the case of controversial tests, people are often reluctant to believe the results regardless of the outcome.

## H.  Life Table-Based Designs

Life tables are statistical models of stationary populations that present the population and mortality implications of a set of age-specific mortality rates (Bogue, 1969). Each column of the life table presents specific data, calculations, or functions. Insurance companies use life tables with a focus on the function $e_0$, the average expectation of life at birth, or the function $e_x$, the average expectation of life at age $x$. Cancer treatment efficacy studies, on the other hand, are based on the survival function $T_x$, and calculate the proportion of the treated population still alive in 5 years. Although life table analysis is a powerful statistical tool, 5-year survival may not be a good surrogate measurement for the concept "cure."

## X.  ANALYSIS

Analysis begins after the study design has been selected and measurements of the exposure, control, and disease outcome variables have been obtained. Analysis can focus on one variable at a time, descriptive epidemiology; two variables at a time, correlational analysis; or three or more variables at a time, analytic epidemiology.

Descriptive epidemiology characterizes an incident or a disease. Univariate statistics, such as percentage distributions, means, standard deviations, and the like, are used to present data. Major advances in epidemiology have been made through painstaking description.

Correlational studies relate one exposure measure to one health outcome measure. For example, plots of different types of leukemia against age, or an exposure variable, could be sufficient to show that the diseases likely have different etiologies.

Analytic epidemiology employs statistical tools, such as multiple linear regression analysis, that are capable of examining multiple exposure measures and one health outcome measurement. The inclusion of multiple exposure variables allows the calculation of regression effects that are adjusted for the effects of the other predictor variables, thereby allowing a way to control the unwanted effects of extraneous variables. Three or more variables considered together allows interpretation of relationships; the pitting of one explanation against another. Multivariate statistics, such as multivariate analysis of variance (MANOVA), are capable of assessing the effects of exposures measures on two or more health outcome measures considered jointly.

Interaction effects can be estimated in multiple regression and similar analysis by forming a new variable that is the product of two exposure variables. Given exposure variables $x_1$ and $x_2$, the interaction effect can be assessed by testing the new variable $x_3 = (x_1 \times x_2)$.

Major distinctions in analytic methods are made based on the level of measurement (nominal, ordinal, interval, and ratio). Simple categorization, such as measuring sex as "male" or "female," are called nominal scale measurements. Rankings are called ordinal level of measurement. Measurements of relationship between nominal or ordinal scale measures are called nonparametric statistics. Measures of relationship based on ratio scale measurements, the highest level of measurement, are called parametric statistics. Multiple linear regression, for example, extends the formula for a straight line to encompass several predictor, or exposure, variables. All variables, both exposure and outcome, should be interval level or higher in the regression model. Logistic regression is used where the health outcome is a nominal scale measurement, and the exposure measures are interval level or higher.

Parametric statistics are based on the applicability of the normal curve to assess probability of a relationship. The applicability of the normal curve is based on the logic of the central-limit theorem, which states that as sample size approaches infinity, the shape of the sampling distribution approaches normality (Hays, 1963). A sampling distribution is a theoretical curve based on an infinite number of samples of a given sample size. The importance of the appropriateness of normal curve-based statistics is that one can completely describe a normal curve from its mean and standard deviation. In tests of hypotheses based on the normal curve, the mean is assigned ($m = 0$ for the null hypothesis), and the standard deviation is estimated from the sample standard deviation. By using the area under the normal curve to represent unit probability, one can then measure probability of occurrence for an observed sample mean value given its distance from the theoretical mean value of zero (the null hypothesis). Parametric statistics, based on normal curve theory, are among the most powerful in the epidemiologists' arsenal.

Appropriate statistics are based on the assumptions that epidemiologists make concerning the nature of the variables measured, the levels of measurement, and the goal of the analysis.

Assumptions that cannot be defended lead to analyses that will be questioned, and perhaps rejected, by other scientists.

## XI.  APPLICATIONS TO ENVIRONMENTAL EPIDEMIOLOGY

To toxicologists, epidemiological findings of chemically induced human disease help to confirm experimental findings. Sometimes the reverse is true; epidemiological evidence provides the impetus for animal models, some of which have been more successful (e.g., thalidomide), and others less successful (e.g., arsenic). To risk assessors and risk managers, epidemiological findings have implications for judgments on the degree of appropriate health concerns relating to specific chemical exposures.

In the areas of toxicological risk assessment and regulatory decision-making for environmental chemicals, epidemiology has successfully identified the cause-and-effect relationship for a variety of chemicals and their health outcomes, such as those presented in Table 1.

Based on information from epidemiological studies, quantitative risk assessments have been made to characterize the risks of human chemical exposures, and regulatory actions have been taken to prevent excessive exposure and to minimize the associated health risks.

## XII.  SUMMARY

This overview of epidemiology presents some of the major epidemiological concepts and methodological issues involved in an epidemiological approach to understanding risks that may be associated with human exposure to environmental chemicals. Epidemiology, with its focus on risk factors and disease etiology, is simply one aspect of the study of environment and health. Laboratory analysis, clinical medicine, industrial hygiene, animal and human toxicology, and computer modeling, all help complete the picture. One hopes that this information will prove useful to scientists whose paths intersect epidemiology. An objective is that this

**Table 1**  Applications to Environmental Epidemiology

| Chemical agent | Health effects | Ref. |
| --- | --- | --- |
| Asbestos | Lung cancer | Blot, 1978; De Vos et al., 1993 |
|  | Mesothelioma | Ram and Lockey, 1982 |
| Arsenic | Skin cancer | Brown et al., 1989 |
|  | Kidney and lung cancer | Chen et al., 1992 |
| Selenium | Selenosis | Yang et al., 1989 |
| Nitrate | Methemoglobinemia | Kross et al., 1992 |
| DBCP | Reproductive | Kharrazi et al., 1980 |
| Vinyl chloride | Angiosarcoma | Monson et al., 1974 |
| Lead | Neurotoxicity | Bellinger et al., 1992 |
| Fluoride | Fluorosis | Vignarajah, 1993 |
| Chromium | Lung cancer | Braver et al., 1985 |
| Cadmium | Hypertension | Engvall and Perk, 1985 |
|  | Refuted by | Staessen and Lawwerys, 1993 |
| Mercury | Neurotoxicity | Ngim and Devathasaan, 1989 |
| Methylmercury | Neurotoxicity | Marsh et al., 1987 |
| Thalidomide | Birth defects | Mellin and Katzenstein, 1962 |

presentation can encourage further reading of the rich literature written by epidemiologists in their quest to understand disease, to mitigate harmful exposures, and to reduce the toll of injuries and disease in society.

# REFERENCES

Ames, R. G., and R. B. Trent (1984). Respiratory impairment and symptoms as predictors of early retirement with disability in U. S. underground coal miners, *Am. J. Public Health,* 74, 837–838.

Ammann, A. J., M. J. Cowan, D. W. Wara, et al. (1983). Acquired immunodeficiency in an infant: Possible transmission by means of blood products, *Lancet,* 1, 956.

Bellinger, D. C., K. M. Stiles, and H. L. Needleman (1992). Low level lead exposure, intelligence and academic achievement: A long-term follow-up study, *Pediatrics,* 90, 855–861.

Blot, W. J., J. M. Harrington, A. Toledo, et al. (1978). Lung cancer after employment in shipyards during World War II, *N. Engl. J. Med.,* 299, 620–624.

Bogue, D. J. (1969). *Principles of Demography,* John Wiley, New York, p. 551, ff.

Braver, E. R., P. Infante, and K. Chu (1985). An analysis of lung cancer risk from exposure to hexavalent chromium, *Teratogenesis Carcinog. Mutagen.,* 5, 365–378.

Brill, A. B., M. Tomonaga, et al. (1962). Leukemia in man following exposure to ionizing radiation: A summary of the findings in Hiroshima and Nagasaki, and a comparison with other human experiences, *Ann. Inter. Med.,* 56, 590.

Brown, K. G., K. E. Boyle, C. W. Chen, and H. J. Gibb (1989). A dose–response analysis of skin cancer from inorganic arsenic in drinking water, *Risk Anal.,* 9, 519–528.

[CDC] Centers for Disease Control and Prevention (1981a). Pneumocystis pneumonia—Los Angeles, *MMWR,* 30, 250.

[CDC] Centers for Disease Control and Prevention (1981b). Kaposi's sarcoma and pneumocystis pneumonia among homosexual men—New York City and California, *MMWR,* 30, 305.

[CDC] Centers for Disease Control and Prevention (1982). *Pneumocystis carinii* pneumonia among persons with hemophilia A, *MMWR,* 31, 365.

Chen, C. J., C. W. Chen, M. M. Wu, and T. L. Kuo (1992). Cancer potential in liver, lung, bladder, and kidney due to ingested inorganic arsenic in drinking water, *Br. J. Cancer,* 66, 888–892.

Dawber, T. R. (1980). *The Framingham Study: The Epidemiology of Atherosclerotic Disease,* Harvard University Press, Cambridge, MA.

De Vos, I. H., D. W. Lamont, D. J. Hole, and C. R. Gillis (1993). Asbestos and lung cancer in Glasgow and the west of Scotland, *Br. Med. J.,* 306, 1503–1506.

Engvall, J., and J. Perk (1985). Prevalence of hypertension among cadmium-exposed workers, *Arch. Environ. Health,* 40, 185–190.

Fraser, D. W., T. R. Tsai, W. Orenstein, W. E. Parkin, H. J. Beecham, R. G. Sharrar, J. Harris, G. F. Mallison, S. M. Martin, and J. E. McDade (1977). Legionnaires' disease: Description of an epidemic of pneumonia, *N. Engl. J. Med.,* 297, 1189–1197.

Goldman, L. R., D. F. Smith, R. R. Neutra, L. D. Saunders, E. M. Pond, J. Stratton, K. Waller, R. J. Jackson, and K. W. Kizer (1990). Pesticide food poisoning from contaminated watermelons in California, 1985, *Arch. Environ. Health,* 45, 229–236.

Hays, W. (1963). *Statistics,* Holt, Rinehart, & Winston, New York, pp. 238–242.

Kharrazi, M., G. Potashnik, and J. R. Goldsmith (1980). Reproductive effects of dibromochloropropane, *Isr. J. Med. Sci.,* 16, 403–406.

Kross, B. C., A. D. Ayebo, and L. J. Fuortes (1992). Methemoglobinemia: Nitrate toxicity in rural America, *Am. Fam. Physician,* 46, 183–188.

Marsh, D. O., T. W. Clarkson, C. Cox, G. J. Myers, L. Amin-Zaki, and S. Al-Tikriti (1987). Fetal methylmercury poisoning. Relationship between concentration in single strands of maternal hair and child effects, *Arch. Neurol.,* 44, 1017–1022.

Mausner, J. S., and A. K. Bahn (1974). *Epidemiology,* W. B. Saunders, Philadelphia.

Mellin, G. W., and M. Katzenstein (1962). The saga of thalidomide, *N. Engl. J. Med.,* 267:1184.

Mirvish, S. S. (1983). The etiology of gastric cancer, *JNCI,* 71, 631–647.

Monson, R. R., J. M. Peters, and M. N. Johnson (1974). Proportional mortality among vinyl chloride workers, *Lancet,* 2, 397.

Ngim, C. H., and G. Devathasan (1989). Epidemiologic study on the association between body burden mercury level and idiopathic Parkinson's disease, *Neuroepidemiology,* 8, 128–141.

Parsons, T. (1958). Definitions of health and illness in the light of American values and social structure. In *Patients, Physicians and Illness* (E. Gartly Jaco, ed.), Free Press, Glencoe, IL.

Peterman, T. A., D. P. Drotman, and J. W. Curran (1985). Epidemiology of the acquired immunodeficiency syndrome (AIDS), *Epidemiol. Rev.,* 7, 1.

Ram, W. N., and J. E. Lockey (1982). Diffuse malignant mesothelioma: A review, *West. J. Med.,* 137, 548.

Scarborough, M. E., R. G. Ames, M. J. Lipsett, and R. J. Jackson (1989). Acute health effects of community exposure to cotton defoliants, *Arch. Environ. Health,* 44, 355–360.

Staessen, J., and R. Lauwerys (1993). Health effects of environmental exposure to cadmium in a population study, *J. Hum. Hypertension,* 7, 195–9.

Stevens, S. (1951). Mathematics, measurement, and psychophysics. In *Handbook of Experimental Psychology* (S. Stevens, ed.), John Wiley & Sons, New York.

Vignarajah, S. (1993). Dental caries experience and enamel opacities in children residing in urban and rural areas of Antigua with different levels of natural fluoride in drinking water, *Commun. Dent. Health,* 10, 159–166.

Yang, G., S. Yin, R. Zhou, L. Gu, B. Yan, Y. Liu, and Y. Liu (1989). Studies of safe maximal daily dietary Se-intake in a seleniferous area in China. Part II: Relation between Se-intake and the manifestation of clinical signs and certain biochemical alterations in blood and urine, *J. Trace Elements Electrolytes Health Dis.,* 3, 123–130.

# 31

# Use of Epidemiological Data for Assessment of Low Levels of Lead as Neurotoxic and Developmental Toxicants

**Jerry J. Zarriello**
*Consultant*
*Tahoe City, California*

## I. INTRODUCTION

The relation between lead exposure and adverse health effects has been documented since antiquity. Today, despite their preventability, physicians and public health officials are still confronting overt and subtle clinical findings in lead-exposed persons. Lead has been reported to cause many adverse health effects, including neurotoxicity, male and female reproductive toxicity, developmental toxicity, nephrotoxicity, carcinogenicity, sideroblastic anemia, hypertension, cardiovascular disease, and death (USEPA, 1986a; ATSDR, 1988a; CDC, 1991; Goyer, 1993; Mushak and Crocetti, 1989). With scientific advances and improved data collection, there is more recognition of subtle effects (neurological, reproductive, and developmental) at lower levels of lead exposure than previously recognized. Lead exposures that were considered safe in the past are now considered hazardous. In 1975, the Centers for Disease Control (CDC) lowered the limit for blood lead to 30 µg/dl, in 1985 to 25 µg/dl, and in 1991 the level of concern was lowered to 10 µg/dl, with recent studies suggesting still lower limits.

## II. INTERACTION OF LEAD WITH OTHER CHEMICALS

Lead is chemically similar to calcium and is stored predominantly in the bone, but, unlike calcium, it is not considered to be an essential trace elements for humans and has no known physiological nor metabolic value (O'Flaherty et al., 1982). The toxicokinetics of lead in humans are affected by the metabolic and nutritional status of exposed subjects. Lead appears to inhibit the production of vitamin D, which is involved in cell differentiation, immunoregulation,

From data provided by the U. S. Food and Drug Administration (FDA), the following are the baseline values for average daily intake of lead by consumption of food, water, and beverages: 25.1 µg/day for 2-year-old children; 32.0 µg/day for adult males; and 45.2 µg/day for adult females (see Table 1). Increased exposure to lead through dietary intake by persons living in urban environments is estimated to be about 28 µg/day for adults and 91 µg/day for children, all of which can be attributed to atmospheric lead (dust). Atmospheric lead may also be added to food crops in the field or garden, during transport to market, during processing, and during kitchen preparation (USEPA, 1986a).

## B.  Water

The concentration of lead in surface water is highly variable, depending on the sources of pollution, the lead content of sediments, and the characteristics of the system (pH, temperature, and the like). Levels of lead in surface waters throughout the United States typically range between 5 and 30 µg/L, although levels as high as 890 µg/L have been monitored (USEPA, 1986a).

## C.  Tap Water Monitoring

The EPA has reported that lead concentrations in tap water in most households are between 7 and 11 µg/L, with the higher levels usually found in "first-draw" samples of water from the tap. In general, the amount of lead in the first-draw water is dependent on the age of the home, the type of plumbing used, and the amount of time the water was left standing in the pipes (USEPA, 1986b). For human exposure to lead from drinking water, see Table 1.

Lead in drinking water is more bioavailable and is absorbed more completely than lead in food. Adults absorb 35–50% of the lead they drink, and the absorption rate for children may be greater. The lead contamination of drinking water most often occurs in the distribution system, but can also occur at five points in or near the plumbing: lead connectors, lead service lines or pipes, lead soldered joints in copper plumbing, water fountains, coolers, brass faucets, and other fixtures containing lead. Acidic water, with low mineral content, can also leach large amounts of lead from lead pipes and solder (ATSDR, 1988b). An estimated 16% of household water supplies had lead concentrations greater than the proposed standard of 20 µg/L in 1991; the standard of 15 µg/L was established on June 7, 1991 under the Lead and Copper Rule, Section 40CFR 141.80 (USPEA, 1991).

Typically, lead pipes are found in residences built before the 1920s. However, pipes made of copper, soldered with lead, came into general use in the 1950s and are the major source of water contamination in homes and facilities such as schools. The Safe Drinking Water Act restricts lead in pipes and plumbing solder but a loophole allows faucets to be up to 8% lead, and recent studies have shown that a major portion of the lead in drinking water can be traced to the faucet. Test results obtained by the National Research Defense Council found lead in first-draw drinking water at levels up to 250 times the legal limit (*Amicus J.*, 1993).

## D.  Paint

Flaking paint, paint chips, and weathered powdered paint, which are most commonly associated with deteriorated housing stock in urban areas, are major sources of lead exposure for young children residing in these houses, particularly for children with pica (Bornschein et al., 1986; USEPA, 1986a). Lead concentrations of 1000–5000 µg/cm$^2$ have been found in chips of lead-based paint pigments, suggesting that consumption of a single chip of paint would provide greater exposure than any other source of lead (USEPA, 1986a).

The largest risk factor appears to be the age of housing; the prevalence and concentration of lead in paint is proportional to the age of the housing unit. It is estimated that 5 million tons of lead have been applied to houses in the United States and that between 40 and 50% of currently occupied housing may contain lead-based paint on exposed surfaces (Chisolm, 1986). In the Western U. S. census region, an estimated 80% of the privately owned housing units built before 1980 contain lead-based paint (USHUD, 1990). To reduce the effect of this significant source of lead contamination, the amount of lead allowed in paint was lowered by law to 1% in 1971 and 0.06% in 1977. Lead paint, however, remains the most substantial existing source of lead exposure; although the content of lead in paint has been reduced, high-content lead paint remains on the interior or exterior surfaces of 57 million American homes and is still being used in industrial, military, and marine applications.

In 1988, it was estimated that 560,000 California children younger than 6 years of age resided in housing units built before 1950 that probably contained high levels of lead in the paint (ATSDR, 1988a). Roughly one in six American children have blood lead concentrations above 10 μg/dl, the most recent CDC level of concern.

To reduce the amount of exposure from deteriorating leaded paint, paint is commonly removed from homes by burning (gas torch or hot air gun), scraping, or sanding. Unfortunately, these activities result, at least temporarily, in higher levels of exposure for the residents. In addition, those persons involved in the paint removal process can be exposed to such excessive levels that lead poisoning may occur (Rabinowitz et al., 1985; Fischbein et al., 1981; Chisolm, 1986; Feldman, 1978). In a report by Schlag and Flessel (1993), 5 of 28 lead abatement workers (18%) had blood lead concentrations greater than 40 μg/dl. The mean blood lead concentration was 24 μg/dl, and ranged from 11 to 45 μg/dl. The mean in the unexposed comparison group was 7 μg/dl, with no blood lead level exceeding 11 μg/dl. The workers' mean free erythrocyte protoporphyrin (FEP) was 28 μg/dl, which was also significantly higher than the mean of 19 μg/dl in the comparison group.

The burning of lead-painted wood in incinerators, home stoves, and fireplaces is also a source of lead exposure. Lead fumes and ash contaminates the home, and when contaminated ashes are disposed of in the yard or garden, further contamination occurs (CDC, 1991).

## E.  Tobacco

Lead is also present in cigarette smoke at a concentration that corresponds to approximately 2.5–12.2 μg/cigarette; about 2–6% of this lead may be inhaled by the smoker (USEPA, 1986a).

## F.  Ceramics

Ceramic tableware and leaded crystal glass are potential sources of lead. Lead-glazed pottery can release large amounts of lead into food and drink, especially imported ceramics from Mexico, China, Korea, Italy, and Spain. The U. S. Food and Drug Administration (FDA, 1991) has reduced the guidelines for levels of lead leaching from ceramic ware.

## G.  Medicines and Cosmetics

Various lead compounds are the major ingredients in traditional medicines such as Azarcon, Alarcon, Greta, Abli Goli (used by Hispanics) and Pay-loo-ah (used by Southeast Asians) for gastrointestinal upset or diarrhea (Bose et al., 1983; Baer et al., 1987). Substantial quantities of lead and other metals are also found in cosmetics such as surma (used by Hindus) and kohl (used by Moslems) for decorative or medicinal purposes around the eyes and may contain up to 60% lead. Exposure to these substances in the United States is due to imports from Arab cultures, the

Indo–Pakistan subcontinent, China, and Latin America. These products are frequently brought to recent immigrants by friends and relatives from their homelands (CDC, 1991). Recently, two cases of childhood lead poisoning have been identified in California in which the source of lead was imported cosmetics used as an eyeliner [California Childhood Lead Poisoning Prevention Program (CCLPPP), 1994].

## H. Calcium Supplements

Calcium supplements may also be a potential source of lead. The measured lead levels in five categories of calcium supplements (dolomite, bonemeal, refined and natural source calcium carbonate, and calcium chelates) ranged from 0.03 to 8.83 µg/g. Daily ingestion rates indicate that about 24% of the products exceed the FDA's "provisional" total tolerable daily intake of lead for children aged 6 years and under. Dolomite, bonemeal, and natural sources for the production of mineral supplements are suspect (Bourgoin et al., 1993).

## I. Hobbies

Many hobbies can result in substantial exposure to lead. For example, molten lead is used in casting, ammunition, and in making fish weights and toy soldiers; and lead solder is used in making stained glass. Leaded glazes and frits are used in making pottery; and artists' paints may also contain lead (CDC, 1991).

## J. Wine

A program to reduce consumers' exposure to lead foil capsules that cover the outside rim and cork of some wine bottles was announced by the FDA in September 1991. On November 25, 1992, the FDA published a proposed regulation that would prohibit the use of tin-coated lead foil capsules on wine bottles. Of table wines tested, 3–4% contained lead concentrations of more than 300 parts per billion (ppb), which could be harmful to consumers (DHHS, 1991b).

## V. LEAD EXPOSURE ASSESSMENT

Individuals who are sufficiently exposed to a lead source as to cause a change in some systemic quantitative measure may be identified as having a toxicologically active lead burden. Most of the exposure data are in terms of internal exposure, usually measured in vivo as blood lead levels of urinary coproporphyrins and δ-aminolevulinic acid. However, data reported as blood lead levels reflect exposure over the previous 1–3 months and are not accurate measures of the total body burden of lead. The total body lead burden has not been accurately measured.

A complete assessment of exposure in sensitive populations requires a knowledge of all sources of exposure. The aggregate impact of multiple small lead sources must be considered in assessing health risks. In 1982–1983, the average baseline intake of lead by 2-year-old children, adult females, and adult males was estimated to be 46.6, 37.5, and 50.6 µg/day, respectively, These baseline values (see Table 1) reflect minimum levels of exposure during normal daily living and are based on individuals who live and work in a nonurban environment, eat a normal diet of food, engage in normal mouthing behavior (in the case of children), and have no habits of activities that would tend to increase lead exposure. Additional exposure above baseline levels is common, however. Some of the more important additional lead exposures occur from residence in an urban environment, residence near stationary sources (e.g., smelters), ingestion of produce from family gardens grown in contaminated soil, renovation of homes containing lead-based paint, pica, interior lead paint dust, occupational exposure, secondary occupational exposure, smoking, and wine consumption. The highest and most prolonged lead exposures are found among workers in the lead smelting, refining, and manufacturing industries (USEPA, 1986a). Inhalation usually contributes a greater proportion of the dose for occupationally exposed groups, and ingestion contributes a greater proportion of the dose for the general population, especially infants and children.

## VI. POPULATIONS AT RISK TO HEALTH EFFECTS OF LEAD

Everyone is susceptible to the adverse health effects of lead, but at least three population groups at increased risk can be identified: preschool-aged children (particularly low-income and minority children), pregnant women and their fetuses, and males between 40 and 59 years of age who are occupationally exposed to lead. Overexposure to lead is still a major problem among workers in the United States.

### A. Preschool-Aged Children

Children are particularly susceptible to the toxic effects of lead, and the thresholds of blood concentrations for neurofunctional measures are lower in children. Since the toxic effects of lead poisoning may be silent, the vast majority of childhood cases go undiagnosed and untreated. The Agency for Toxic Substances and Disease Registry (ATSDR) reported that 17.7% of American children had blood lead levels (BLL) above 15 μg/dl (ATSDR, 1988a). There were 12 million children living in lead-painted houses and 6 million children living in homes built before 1940 when paint with the highest concentration of lead was used. A disproportionate number of poor and black children were affected (BLL > 15 μg/dl): black children living in poor communities (55%); white children living in poor communities (24%); and white children living in higher socioeconomic status (SES) areas (7%). The age of the housing, not the geographic location, is the best predictor for the presence of lead-based paint (USHUD, 1990).

The CDC (1991) suggests that the reason children are more vulnerable than adults when exposed to lead may be partly attributable to the following factors: (1) Ingestion is the major route of exposure for children owing to their hand-to-mouth behaviors, resulting in their ingestion of lead in soil, dust, paint chips, and so on. Pica is also a common behavior, especially between 2 and 4 years of age (Lin-Fu, 1973). (2) Children absorb substantially more lead from the gastrointestinal tract than adults (40–50% vs. 10%), especially when they are younger than 2 years of age, and children have increased metabolic rates, resulting in a proportionately greater intake of lead through food (Ziegler et al., 1978). In addition, they have a faster resting inhalation rate and tend to be mouth breathers while at play, resulting in less airborne inorganic lead particulate being trapped in the nasal passages (Cal EPA, 1993). (3) Children from economically disadvantaged backgrounds are especially vulnerable because they are more likely to have diets deficient in elements, such as iron and calcium, that suppress lead absorption (Mahaffey, 1981), and frequently live in homes built before 1950 that contain high levels of lead in the paint. (4) Children may have a less-developed blood–brain barrier and, therefore, greater neurological sensitivity (Smith, 1989).

### B. Pregnant Women and Their Fetuses

(See Sec. VIII.A for further discussion on this topic.)

## C.  The Lead-Exposed Worker

The highest and most prolonged lead exposures are found among workers in the lead smelting, refining, and manufacturing industries. In all work areas, exposure is by inhalation and ingestion of lead-bearing dusts. Airborne dusts settle onto food, beverages, water, clothing, hands, and other objects, and may be transferred to the mouth. Good personal hygiene, appropriate housekeeping, and adequate ventilation have a major influence on the extent of exposure (CDHS, 1988).

Although occupational exposure is widespread, environmental monitoring data on levels of exposure in many occupations are not available. Lead exposure is most often monitored by biological testing (e.g., determination of urinary lead levels, blood lead levels, urinary coproporphyrin, or δ-aminolevulinic acid), rather than by monitoring the workplace environment for lead concentrations (USEPA, 1986a).

Pirkle et al. (1985), focusing on white males, aged 40–59 years, with blood lead levels in the range of 7–34 µg/dl, reported no evident threshold in which BLL was not significantly related to blood pressure. Sharp et al. (1988) also reported a positive relation between lead exposure and elevated blood pressure in San Francisco bus drivers. By using multiple regression analysis, systolic and diastolic pressures varied from 102 to 172 mm Hg and from 61 to 105 mm Hg, respectively. The blood lead level varied between 2 and 15 µg/dl. The effect on blood pressure is now identified as the critical effect of lead in adults. The Cal EPA (1993) estimates that, with a 1-$\mu g/m^3$ increase in ambient lead concentration, there would be a range of 8,260–90,100 cases of hypertension per million adults between 20 and 70 years. Given California's population of approximately 18 million adults between 20 and 70 years of age, there would be approximately 52,000 additional cases of hypertension caused by ambient lead exposure statewide for the year 1990–1991.

## VII.  EPIDEMIOLOGIC STUDIES OF LOW-LEVEL EFFECTS OF LEAD AS A NEUROTOXIC AGENT

The toxicology of lead has moved from measuring overt clinical and life–death outcomes to the measurement of graded levels of performance and measurements of the brain such as cognition, attention, perception, and behavior. Early studies supported the hypothesis that low levels of lead impair children's IQ (Needleman et al., 1979). By using dentine lead levels from first and second graders, two groups were classified: one group representing the 90th percentile (> 20 ppm) and one group representing the 10th percentile (< 6 ppm). These lead values were compared with a variety of neuropsychological parameters, and the dentine lead was treated as a continuous variable. The association of dentine lead and IQ, using the Wechsler Intelligence Scale for Children (WISC), remained significant. When these children were tested 5 and 11 years later, these effects were still evident (USEPA, 1984; Needleman et al., 1985; Schwartz, in press; Bellinger et al., 1984; Needleman and Gatsonis, 1990).

Neurodevelopmental effects were reflected in lowered mental development index (MDI) scores of 2–8 points with a 10 µg/dl increase in blood lead level, and childhood blood lead levels greater than 30 µg/dl were associated with deficits of the central nervous system function that can persist into early adulthood. Elevated lead levels also appear to be associated with non-adaptive classroom behavior, including lower class standing, increased absenteeism, lower vocabulary and grammatical reasoning scores, poor hand-eye coordination, longer reaction time, and slower finger tapping. The lead content of teeth shed at ages 6 and 7 was also associated with reading disability and an increase in dropout rate from high school (Needleman et al., 1990).

There have been concerns over some of the early cross-sectional studies in their measurement of exposure and effect, and the control of confounding variables (Cal EPA, 1993). Failure to consider the home environment as an important confounder in lead's effect on intelligence was one concern, and statistical power was lost in Needleman's early research, since the middle of the distribution of lead levels were excluded from the study. However, in a subsequent reanalysis of the data by Schwartz (in press), who used a full sample, the reported effects were stronger than in the original analysis.

Many studies published since the Needleman et al. (1979) report are supportive of his conclusions. For instance, some studies reported that an inverse relation exists between reading scores and blood lead levels (Mayfield, 1983; Yule et al., 1981; Fulton et al., 1987; Silva et al., 1988); other studies, at higher lead exposures, indicated cognitive deficits in children's visual–spatial and visual–motor integration skills (McBride et al., 1982; Bellinger et al., 1991; Hansen et al., 1989; Winneke et al., 1987).

## A. Prospective Studies

Prospective studies allow measurement of temporal changes in outcome over time relative to prior exposure levels. Problems associated with prospective studies include high cost, loss of cases to follow-up, reduction of sample size, and reduced statistical power.

All five ongoing prospective studies in Boston, Cincinnati, Cleveland, and Port Pirie and Sydney (Australia) use blood lead levels to measure lead burden and the Wechsler Intelligence Scale for Children—Revised (WISC-R) after the age of 5 years to measure intelligence. Standardization of data was attempted, and the interim results from these studies have been published.

The Boston cohort (249 middle- and upper middle-class children) evidence shows that prenatal and postnatal exposure to lead may be associated with cognitive performance. The effects on intelligence were evident at prenatal blood lead levels as low as 6 µg/dl for children of lower socioeconomic status. Effects on intelligence in those with a cord blood of 10 µg/dl or greater persisted for 24 months for the cohort as a whole and up to 57 months for certain subgroups.

Higher postnatal blood lead levels at 24 months were significantly associated with lower full-scale IQ (FSIQ) and verbal IQ at the age of 10 years, and for each 10 µg/dl increase in blood lead levels, a decrease of almost 6 points on the FSIQ and 9 points on the Kaufman Test of Educational Achievement (KTEA) battery score was observed (Bellinger et al., 1989). These estimates included adjustments for maternal age, race, marital status, number of residence changes, and home observation measurement of environment (HOME) scores. At aged 10, using a child's maximum lead score, a smaller coefficient was found than when using the child's blood lead level at 24 months (Bellinger et al., 1992; Stiles and Bellinger, 1993).

The Cincinnati, Ohio, longitudinal study showed both an indirect and direct inverse association of prenatal lead and MDI score (Dietrich et al., 1986, 1987a,b; Bornschein et al., 1989). After adjusting for covariates, the 3- and 6-month MDI scores were significantly associated with maternal and cord blood lead levels. Neonatal blood lead levels (taken at 10 days) were significantly related to 6- and 12-month MDI scores (Dietrich et al., 1989). Males and children from the lower SES groups were more sensitive to lead's effects on the MDI score. The neonatal blood lead levels in these children from the poorest families were associated with poor performance on all the subscales of the Kaufman Assessment Battery for Children (K-ABC). The authors noted a weak relation between postnatal blood lead levels and performance on a K-ABC subscale that assesses visual–spatial and visual–motor integration skills (Dietrich et al., 1991). The mean blood lead level at 4 and 5 years was associated with the simultaneous processing subscale (SIM) ($p = 0.05$) and with near significant association with the nonverbal subscale of the K-ABC (Dietrich et al., 1992). The adjusted regression model revealed a significant inverse association between lead levels at 5 and 6 years and the full-scale intelligence quotient (FSIQ); a decrement of 3.3 points FSIQ per 10 μg/dl increase in blood lead was reported. Significant associations between lead levels at ages 3, 4, 5, and 6 and mean lifetime blood lead levels and performance IQ (PIQ) were also reported (Dietrich et al., 1993a,b).

In the Cleveland cohort study, the neurodevelopment effects of lead and alcohol could not be differentiated. The observed deficits could not be determined to be related to the independent effect of alcohol, the interactive effects of alcohol and lead, or the independent effects of lead. Also, many of the pregnant alcoholics were lost for follow-up studies (Cal EPA, 1993).

The Port Pirie, South Australian cohort study demonstrated that postnasal lead levels were inversely associated with MDI scores (Vimpani et al., 1985). The mean blood lead level at 6 months (14.4 μg/dl) was strongly inversely related to MDI performance at 24 months after adjustment for HOME score. A child's MDI at 24 months was calculated to be 1.6 points lower for every 10 μg/dl rise in blood lead level at 6 months. One-third of the children had levels about 25 μg/dl during the first 4 years of life. By using the integrated average General Cognitive Index (GCI) scores of the McCarthy Scales of Children's Abilities (MSCA), and incorporating multivariate analysis, the general cognitive scores declined 7.2 points as blood lead levels increased from 10 to 30 μg/dl at the age of 4 years (McMichael et al., 1988). The results of the analysis and those of an earlier analysis of children at the age of 2 years (Wigg et al., 1988) suggest that increased exposure to lead results in a developmental deficit, not just a developmental delay. Four hundred ninety-four children were tested at aged 7 using WISC-R after using a multivariate analysis incorporating many factors in the children's lives. The tests revealed a postnatal relation between blood lead and intelligence that persisted, especially with blood lead levels at 15 months and 4 years. With an increase of blood lead level from 10 to 30 μg/dl, the IQ dropped from 4.4 to 5.3 points. The authors concluded that low-level exposure to lead was inversely associated with neuropsychological development through the age of 7, and that strong correlations of FSIQ at aged 7 and McCarthy's GCI at aged 4, demonstrate that the same children had decrements in intelligence caused by their lead exposure (Baghurst et al., 1992).

In the Sydney, Australia cohort study, maternal and cord blood lead levels were tested at time of delivery, and the children's blood was tested every 6 months thereafter until the age of 4 and again at aged 5 years. Bayley's MDI was administered at ages 6, 12, and 24 months, and the McCarthy's GCI at 3, 4 and 5 years. Unadjusted bivariate correlations between maternal or cord blood lead levels (8.1 and 9.1 μg/dl, respectively) were neither both negative nor significant (Cooney et al., 1989a,b). However, there was a critical problem with the methodology of this study. The contamination of capillary samples by environmental lead resulted in high estimates of blood lead levels in the first 2 years of the study. Venous and capillary samples differed by as much as 10 μg/dl, with capillary samples being higher. At 24 months, 50% of the samples were still capillary (Cal EPA, 1993). If the precision of measurement of exposure is not sufficient for the detection of small relationships, the bias may be towards type II error. Measurement error can contribute to risks of both type I and II error.

## B.  Methodological Difficulties

Three of these five prospective studies of the neurodevelopmental effects of lead in children demonstrated an inverse relation between lead and intelligence (Boston, Cincinnati, and Port Pirie). The prenatal blood lead levels that showed an effect on intelligence seemed to decline by the age of 2–4 years, but the postnatal effect of blood lead level was present in all three prospective studies after the age of 4.

Comparisons of the lead effects on the neurodevelopment of children between the studies is difficult because the epidemiologist must address the methodological problems (including many major aspects of the design and analyses) and eliminate the risk of chance and confounding variables or bias. Some of the methodological difficulties in these prospective studies have been identified:

1. Confounders, although attempts were made to control them, are the most controversial issue. The exposure to lead may have been the proxy for many other variables (Cal EPA, 1993). One confounder not usually discussed is the toxic effects of the cooccurrence of heavy metals. Lewis et al. (1992) studied prenatal exposure to heavy metals (cadmium, mercury, lead, cobalt, silver, nickel, and chromium) by examining the amniotic fluid at 16–18 weeks of gestation. He found that these metals cooccurred in the amniotic fluid. By following the children born to these women, a toxic score risk was derived that negatively related to the children's performance on the McCarthy Scales of Children's Abilities and positively related to the number of childhood illnesses.

2. Mismeasurement or omission of explanatory factors can skew results. For instance, iron deficiency, which can also reduce MDI scores, was not measured directly (Lozoff et al., 1991).

3. There were also significant variations between the study populations. Some studies included, others excluded, single or alcoholic mothers, and some study populations had higher SES than others (Cal EPA, 1993; Dietrich et al., 1986).

4. In assessing the persistence of effect, two of the three prospective studies found a relation between prenatal blood lead levels and intelligence, with the effect disappearing by age 57 months. Dietrich et al. (1986) states that the association was not significant at 24 months. Bellinger et al. (1987) found an effect of lead on MDI and GCI at 24 months, but none at 57 months. In those children with cord blood lead levels of 10 µg/dl or higher and with equivalent levels at 24 months, the decrement persisted. In the three cohorts (Boston, Cincinnati, and Port Pirie), the effects were apparent again at age 5, 6.5, 7, and even 10 years, when using the WISC-R. These differences in persistence may be explained by the measure of effect. Bayley's MDI was used to age 3 years but, after age 3 to age 5, intelligence was measured by using differing IQ scales that also differ from Bayley's MDI. The results become more consistent when all cohorts studied used an identical intelligence scale (WISC-R) (Cal EPA, 1993).

5. The measures of intelligence may not be sufficiently sensitive to capture some of lead's effects on intelligence, or the measures may be ill-suited for ethnic minorities who speak a foreign language and lack the linguistic skills needed for the standardized tests. Grant and Davis (1989) found that classroom performance measures were more sensitive than IQ scales. The most persistent lead effects were the more general measures of classroom performance, such as probability of graduation. Needleman et al. (1990) found that children in the higher-lead level group were less likely to graduate from high school and were 2 or more years behind in reading level. These analyses were adjusted for several potential confounders, such as SES and maternal IQ, but the authors were not able to adjust the HOME score (Cal EPA, 1993).

6. The lack of statistical power may also cause differences in study results. Large sample sizes are necessary to detect small effects of lead on intelligence. Cohn (1977) states that a sample of 400 or more would be needed to detect an increase of 1%, with power of 0.80, at an alpha of 0.05, one-tailed. Four of the five prospective studies under discussion began with smaller samples and, therefore, would have had difficulty detecting a small, but significant, effect. Sample sizes were also noted to decline by attrition in these longitudinal studies, making power of detection of effect decline further over time (Cal EPA, 1993).

7. The file drawer bias was examined, but was not considered a problem based on Rosenthal procedure calculations and the method of Iyengar and Greenhouse (Rosenthal, 1984; Iyengar and Greenhouse, 1988). File drawer bias may result " . . . from the failure of some investigators to report their results and/or the failure of journals to publish some results submitted" (Gatsonis and Needleman, 1992).

8. There is also a potential family advantage or catch-up effect. Parents in higher SES groups and better-educated parents may have an ability to overcome deficits in intelligence caused by lead, but this phenomenon was not observed in the studies (Cal EPA, 1993).

## C. Metanalysis

*Metanalysis* is defined as "the application of statistical procedures to collections of empirical findings from individual studies for the purpose of integrating, synthesizing, and making sense of them" (Wolf, 1986). Needleman and Gatsonis (1990) performed a metanalysis of 24 studies of childhood exposure to lead in relation to IQ. Only 12 of the studies that employed multiple regression analyses, with IQ as the dependent variable, and nonlead covariables were selected for a quantitative, integrated review or metanalysis. The other studies were excluded for one or more reasons (small samples; inclusion of subjects with clinical lead poisoning; overcontrol of factors that reflect exposure to lead; inadequate quantitative information; inability to calculate the coefficient of lead in a multiple regression model; or poor measurement of covariates, such as socioeconomic factors, and parental education and intelligence). The 12 studies selected for final metanalysis were placed in two groups: the blood lead group (seven studies) and the tooth lead group (five studies).

Methods of measuring IQ also differed across the studies. The WISC-R scales were used in eight studies, the Stanford Binet scales in two, and British Ability Scales and McCarthy Scales in the remaining two studies. All studies selected controlled for age and socioeconomic status, and several included many other factors including maternal IQ, HOME inventory, sex, birth weight, and parental education (Needleman and Gatsonis, 1990).

It is a difficult task to assess the significance of the lead burden, even if all covariates of interest are available. The authors concluded that, taken together, these studies suggest that a 1 μg/dl increase in blood lead level results in a 0.24 point decrease in IQ. The metanalysis of these studies demonstrated a strong inference that low-dose lead exposure is causally associated and negatively correlated with covariate-adjusted psychometric deficits and that low-level lead exposure is neurotoxic.

Needleman and Gatsonis' metanalysis has only strengthened the general conclusion that lead is negatively associated with cognitive performance. Studies of associations between lead and IQ across a range of study designs and populations suggest that the association is probably not due to bias or imperfect covariate factors (Schwartz, in press).

Thacker et al. (1992) reviewed 40 reports from five longitudinal studies, Boston, Port Pirie, Sydney, Cincinnati, and Cleveland, and concluded that an inverse relation between prenatal and postnatal exposure to lead and the MDI in unadjusted analysis was shown in all five studies. However, after adjustment was made for confounding, no statistically significant relation was seen between blood lead levels and the MDI in the Cleveland and Sydney studies; statistical differences remained in studies from Boston, Cincinnati, and Port Pirie. Efforts to pool the data with metanalytic techniques were unsuccessful because report data were inconsistent. However, Thacker et al. (1992) state that the weight of evidence from this and other studies suggest an inverse relation of lead on the intelligence of children.

Schwartz (in press) states that his analysis represents a second type of metanalysis.

He focused on gaining insights into the role that confounding variables played in the consistent negative correlations between lead exposure and IQ. To rule out the possibility that the consistent negative correlation between lead and IQ found in essentially all studies is due to confounding variables, he assigned weights (the inverse of the estimated variance of the effect estimate) to each study. Schwartz examined the Boston, Cincinnati, and Port Pirie prospective studies and five cross-sectional studies. The full-scale IQ was regressed against age, race, children's stress score, father's and mother's occupational status, HOME score, mother's time working outside the house, marital status, gestational age, birth weight, mother's alcoholic drinks per week during pregnancy, otitis media history, birth order, and the Hollingshead four-factor SES scale. The blood lead level at 24 months was regressed against the same variables. A nonparametric smoothed curve was fit into the relation between the two sets of residuals to show the adjusted relation between full-scale IQ and blood lead. He found a highly significant association between lead exposure and children's IQ ($p = 0.001$). An increase in blood lead level from 10 to 20 µg/dl was associated with a decrease of 2.6 IQ points and a highly significant association between blood lead levels and full-scale IQ in school-aged children. The cross-sectional and longitudinal study results were quite similar. This consistency suggests that the use of this outcome is important for epidemiological as well as for public policy formulation.

Primate research also demonstrated that low levels of exposure (11–15 µg/dl), compared with a control group with blood levels of 3–5 µg/dl, resulted in behavioral impairment, such as attention deficits, learning disabilities, short-term memory problems, and decrements in discrimination and reversal tasks (Rice, 1985, 1992). Rice states that these findings provide evidence that the behavioral deficits observed in monkeys at the lowest blood levels examined are comparable with deficits observed in children, that the monkey's behavioral deficits correlate with lead exposure in children and are, in fact, the result of lead exposure. (Schwartz, in press) concluded that the experimental animal protocols, with no confounding variables, make it reasonable to assume that the strong inverse association between lead exposure and decreased IQ are causal.

The California EPA has developed estimates of the change in health effects associated with increases in ambient lead concentration. It is estimated that an increase of 1 µg/m3 of ambient lead concentration will result in a mean decrease in IQ points of 1.26–1.37 per child between birth and 10 years (Cal EPA, 1993).

To put this issue in perspective, the California Medical Association's Pediatric Lead Poisoning Technical Advisory Committee recently concluded that:

> while this drop in IQ points would not be clinically noticeable for individuals of average IQ, the implications of shifting the bell-shaped IQ distribution curve to the left for the entire population are serious in terms of increasing the proportion of children with very low IQs and decreasing the proportion with very high IQs. For society at large, this shift of the IQ curve ultimately results in higher special education costs, lower lifetime earnings and taxes paid, and a decrease in the number of adults prepared for the high tech jobs of the future (Ehling, 1993).

The California EPA has determined that both the level of concern for lead and the LOAEL for effects of lead on intelligence is 10 µg/dl. This is also the concern level for hypertension in adult males. This level of concern is consistent with EPA, the CDC, and the ATSDR. The biological or toxicologic effect may actually occur at levels lower than 6–7 µg/dl. Schwartz (in press) finds a continuum of lead effects down to 1 µg/dl, with no absolute threshold identified.

## VIII.  EPIDEMIOLOGICAL STUDIES OF REPRODUCTIVE AND DEVELOPMENTAL EFFECTS FROM LEAD EXPOSURE

### A.  Female Reproductive Effects

Early reports indicated that lead at high doses was associated with adverse reproductive and developmental outcomes. Goyer and Rhyne (1973) reported that severe lead intoxication may be associated with sterility, abortion, stillbirths, and neonatal morbidity and mortality from exposure in utero. The possible effect of lead exposure on the fetus was determined to be of concern as a public health issue and for the development of fetal protection policies in industry (Rom, 1976).

Recent studies of the effects of lead on the growth and development of fetuses and children examined the outcomes of stature, growth rates, birthweights, gestational age, and congenital anomalies. Since these effects may occur at low blood lead levels, large segments of the population may be involved: 4,460,000 U. S. women of childbearing age and 403,200 pregnant women were reported to have blood lead levels of 10 µg/dl or more (ATSDR, 1988b).

Lead crosses the placenta, with no metabolic barrier to the uptake of lead in the fetus, and is readily diffused to the fetus. It can also be mobilized from the mother's bone to the developing fetus, but the timing and amount of fetal lead transferred is uncertain. Lead may cross the placenta at different times and at different rates during pregnancy, and it has been detected in the human fetal brain as early as 13 weeks (Ernhart, 1992).

Lead may also appear in mother's milk during lactation (Bonithon-Kopp et al., 1986). Higher blood lead levels have been found in menopausal women than in premenopausal women, with the highest levels in the menopausal women who had never been pregnant (Silbergeld et al., 1988). Lead appears to be mobilized from bone during menopause and pregnancy (Silbergeld, 1991).

Higher blood lead levels have also been found in pregnant women than in nonpregnant women living near a lead smelter, indicating that blood lead levels in pregnant women may be higher than population averages (Zaric et al., 1987). Another study showed a statistically significant increase in blood lead levels in women 6 months after giving birth, but no significant increase during pregnancy (Ernhart and Greene, 1992). It has been estimated that the umbilical cord blood lead concentrations were 85–90% as high as the mother's blood lead concentration (ATSDR, 1990; Mahaffey, 1992).

A significant correlation was found between maternal lead levels and preterm delivery. Mothers with blood lead levels above 14 µg/dl have more than a fourfold relative risk of premature delivery, compared with mothers with blood lead levels below 8 µg/dl (McMichael et al., 1986).

Prenatal lead exposure (measured by maternal blood levels at the end of the first trimester) indicated an indirect relation between maternal blood levels and reduced birth weight; and reduced birth weight was associated with lower MDI scores (Dietrich et al., 1986, 1987a,b; USEPA, 1990). The National Research Counsel (NRC; 1993) stated that birth outcome measures, early physical growth measures, and early measures of infant development can be viewed as potentially reflecting the fetal toxicity of lead. It should also be noted that the USEPA (1989) and the International Agency for Research on Cancer (IARC; 1987a,b), based on animal studies, have identified lead as a reproductive toxicant and a probable carcinogen (class 2B).

Some researchers have concluded that, although the health effects of lead exposure depend on many factors, such exposure appears to be particularly dangerous to the unborn and young children, in whom it is believed to cause premature births, low birth weights, decreased mental ability, decreased IQ scores, and reduced growth (ATSDR, 1990). Borella et al. (1986) concluded that definitive conclusions cannot be drawn about the relation between maternal lead exposure and difficulty in conceiving, spontaneous abortion, or congenital anomalies. They found that abortion specimens did not indicate that lead accumulated in the fetus during the critical period of organogenesis, and neonatal behavior measures showed little evidence of the effect of low levels of prenatal lead exposure on infant behavioral measures. Ernhart (1992) found no evidence of a persisting effect on the cognitive development, language, or psychomotor performance of children, and no evidence for early effects consistent within the Boston, Cincinnati, Cleveland, Port Pirie, and Sydney studies. She concluded that there is little new information for an association of low fetal lead exposure and intrauterine growth retardation, and no sound evidence that prenatal low-lead exposure causes an increase of malformation in the neonate. Several studies have been unable to associate teratogenicity with cord blood lead levels (Needleman et al., 1984; Ernhart et al., 1986; McMichael et al., 1986). Ernhart recommends that more studies be performed before any definite conclusions be made.

Other studies, exploring relations between lead levels and elevations in blood pressure, found no link between cord blood lead and the toxemia of pregnancy (Rabinowitz et al., 1987; Angell and Lavery, 1982). Evidence of neonatal polycythemia ranges from 2.5 to 20% of newborns. Since lead is carried almost entirely in the erythrocytes and polycythemia has been related to developmental abnormalities, polycythemia may be a confounder when studying fetal lead exposure and adverse child developmental effects (Gross et al., 1973; Delaney-Black et al., 1989).

## B. Male Reproductive Effects

In males, an increase in blood lead is associated with gametotoxicity, including asthenospermia, hypospermia, increases in the percentage of teratospermia, and reduced levels of zinc, acid phosphatase, and citric acid. The data suggest that male reproductive effects may occur at blood levels at the 30–40 µg/dl range or lower (Telisman et al., 1990). The duration of exposure of smelter workers was invariably associated with endocrine testicular function; workers who were employed for more than 3 years had decreases in serum testosterone, steroid-binding globulin, and free-testosterone index. The mean blood lead concentrations were higher than 60 µg/dl (Rodamilans et al., 1988).

## C. Early Developmental Effects in Children

The epidemiological evidence illustrates that lead disturbs physical development in the fetus and child at low blood lead levels. The studies of birth weight, gestational age, postnatal growth, and postnatal status show some consistency. A significant drop in birthweight was found in the 13- to 18-µg/dl group, compared with the 7- to 12-µg/dl group, suggesting a level of effect at 13–18 µg/dl or lower (Bornschein et al. 1989).

One study using National Health and Nutrition Examination Survey II (NHANES II, 1976–1980) data showed small but significant reductions in early childhood growth (height, weight, and chest circumference), with no apparent threshold across a BLL range of 5–35 µg/dl. Of 2695 children aged 6 months to 7 years, after controlling for significant variables, 1.5% showed a decrease in mean height; at 25 µg/dl, a reduction in height appeared to have occurred in 3% of the children (Delaney-Black et al., 1989). Growth retardation was reported in another group of children with blood lead levels above 30 µg/dl compared with a control group from ages 24 months to 42 months (Angle and Kuntzelman, 1989). Schwartz et al. (1986) found that the three milestones of growth in the children under 7 years of age were inversely related to BLL: height ($p < 0.0001$), weight ($p < 0.001$), and chest circumference ($p < 0.026$).

Some animal and human studies demonstrate that the pituitary–thyroid endocrine system may be impaired by lead in a manner that may be related to its effect on growth. Lead may also impair the iodine-concentrating mechanism (Sandstead et al., 1970). Other studies showed decreased thyroid-stimulating hormone (TSH) release in response to thyrothropin-releasing hormone (TRH). This interference in pituitary–thyroid functioning may relate to correlation between lead exposure and growth (Huseman et al., 1987).

## IX. LEAD AS A NEUROLOGICAL AND NEURODEVELOPMENTAL TOXICANT

### A. Mechanism of Action

Lead neurotoxicity is not fully understood; there are many gaps in our information. Although there is no doubt about the causal relation between high exposure to lead and encephalopathy, it has been more difficult to prove causal relation between low levels of exposure and milder neurological disorders. It is known that the toxicological effects of lead disturb critical physiological, biochemical, and molecular events, including signal transmission processes (e.g., the release of neurotransmitters from presynaptic nerve endings), gene expressions and mitochondrial function, but these functional disturbances are not accompanied by gross structural changes (Goering, in press; NRC, 1993; Goldstein, 1992).

Goldstein (1992), discusses cellular and biochemical systems, including (1) synaptogenesis, (2) the blood–brain barrier, and (3) second-messenger metabolism. These are further discussed in the following.

### 1. Synaptogenesis

In describing the developmental neurobiology of lead toxicity, Goldstein (1992) stated that neuron proliferation and migration are considered to be complete before birth, whereas synaptic development is most active from 2 to 5 years. At aged 2–5 years, interconnections are double the number of synaptic contacts present at maturity. A pruning process occurs with a net reduction in the density of dentritic arborizations. These synaptic connections are crucial for learning, memory, and behavior and, unfortunately, coincide with the age of greatest vulnerability to the detrimental effects of lead (Cooper et al., 1984; Atchison and Narahasi, 1984).

The neural cell adhesion molecule (NCAM) is a complex of three polypeptides that regulate many neurodevelopmental processes, including neuronal fiber outgrowth and synapse formation (Edelman, 1986). The sialic acid content determines the strength of interactions between NCAMs and adjacent cells. Chronic lead exposure decreases the rate of NCAM desialylation and may induce dyssynchrony in rat cerebellar development to cause gross clinical changes manifested by reduced fine motor skills (Cookman et al., 1987; NRC, 1993).

### 2. Blood–Brain Barrier

The blood–brain barrier consists of the capillary endothelium and astrocyte sheath together and has potentially vulnerable sites for the toxic action of lead in the brain (Goldstein, 1984). High levels of lead may cause acute lead encephalopathy primarily due to severe capillary damage in the blood–brain barrier. Specific transporters are present to mediate passage across the endothelial barrier. These active transport pumps on the endothelium of the brain's surface remove molecules that might disrupt neuronal activity and transport them against a concentration gradient from the brain to the blood. Failure of this mechanism leads to brain edema or at lower levels of lead exposure, to synaptic dysfunction (Bressler and Goldstein, 1991). The endothelial cells in the microvessels of the nervous system that form the blood–brain barrier have a continuous belt of tight junctions that seal intimately opposed endothelial cells together (Brightman and Reese, 1969). This junction limits the free diffusion of molecules, such as plasma proteins and monovalent cations. To allow entry of essential nutrients, transport carriers for glucose and essential amino acids facilitate entry of these solutes into the brain, whereas active transport pumps for ions, neurotransmitters, and organic acids provide transfer of selected molecules across the barrier and against a concentration gradient (Betz et al., 1988; Betz and Goldstein, 1978). Astrocytes do not perform as a physical barrier in the brain, but play an important role in inducing and maintaining the blood–brain barrier. Injury to the astrocyte by lead may be the mechanism for disruption of the blood–brain barrier (Goldstein, 1988). Holtzman et al. (1984) found that lead-exposed rat pups' resistance to developing lead encephalitis by age 18–20 days was related to the formation of lead–protein complexes (inclusion bodies) in astrocytes that sequester lead away from mitochondria.

Subtle injury to the barrier affects the most energy-dependent aspects of the blood–brain barrier, such as the pumping of ions (K+, Na+, $Ca^{2+}$), organic acids, and neurotransmitters from brain to blood, interfering with homeostasis. Changes in the K+ level in the brain could interfere with the depolarization of nerve endings. Deficient pumping of amino acids and neurotransmitters by the endothelial cells would interfere with the efficiency of synaptic function. It would also lead to disturbance of calcium metabolism (Goldstein, 1992).

### 3. Second-Messenger Metabolism

Lead interferes with dopaminergic and cholinergic neurotransmission. A *neurotransmitter*, derived from amino acids, is defined as a chemical that is selectively released from a nerve terminal by an action potential, which interacts with a specific receptor on an adjacent postsynaptic neuron structure, and elicits a specific physiological response. Several intracellular second-messenger systems transform the stimulus of neurotransmission into a more lasting change in neuronal activity, which is important for the development of new memories and new neural nets that underlie learning. Modification of intracellular proteins by enzymes that alter their charge and form plays a key role in the process. Many hormonal systems including the neurotransmitters activate protein kinases to produce this effect. At the synaptic junction, when the postsynaptic neuron is occupied by a neurotransmitter, it is postulated that certain metabolic events are triggered. The immediate response is the opening of ion channels that allow movement of sodium, potassium, and chloride ions, thereby allowing the postsynaptic neuron to depolarize and generate an action potential to start the same mechanism in the next circuit neuron. The sensitivity of this mechanism depends on the amount of neurotransmitter (i.e., acetylcholine, dopamine, or other) released at the presynaptic terminal and on the degree of response at the postsynaptic neuron, and it is dependent on the state of phosphorylation of many neuronal proteins (Hemmings et al., 1989). The continued use of a given pathway leads to more efficient function and the development of established circuits.

According to Goldstein (1992), several second-messengers activate the several classes of protein kinases. The major second messengers include cyclic-AMP (cAMP) which is formed from the large intracellular adenosine triphosphate (ATP) pool when the transduction protein links to the receptor site, and to adenylate cyclase, the enzyme that converts ATP to cAMP (Northrop, 1989). The level of cAMP is a balance between the formation by adenylate cyclase and its degradation by phosphodiesterase. The cAMP binds to specific protein kinases that phosphorylate regulatory proteins. In certain cell systems, lead inhibits adenylate cyclase and stimulates phosphodiesterase, resulting in a lower level of cAMP and a decrease in the phosphorylation of protein substrates of cAMP–protein kinase (Nathanson and Bloom, 1975; Goldstein and Ar, 1983).

Calcium is another intracellular second messenger that has been reviewed in detail (Pounds, 1984). The concentration of calcium inside the cell is 10,000-fold less than in the interstitial space. Calcium enters the cell through the opening of specific channels and, when in the cell, directly activates certain enzymes or binds to a regulatory protein, such as calmodulin (Cheung,

1984). When calcium combines with binding sites on calmodulin, it is able to activate other enzymes and pump systems, including protein kinases, and also provides the regulatory mechanism by which phosphodiesterase can break down cAMP. Lead has been demonstrated to substitute for calcium in the activation of protein kinase C enzyme activity (Markovac and Goldstein, 1988a,b). Lead mimics calcium and exhibits a greater affinity for the calmodulin-binding sites than calcium (Goldstein, 1992), and it causes activation of the enzymes normally controlled by the level of intracellular calcium (Richardt et al., 1986). This lead–calmodulin combination may cause inappropriate activation of phosphodiesterase and the breakdown of cAMP, leading to less cAMP–protein kinase activity, causing disruption of neuronal function. Lead inhibits $Ca^{2+}$ entry when calcium channels are open owing to depolarization (Simons and Pocock, 1987). Cytoplasmic $Ca^{2+}$ signals are received by a variety of $Ca^{2+}$ receptor proteins, including calmodulin, protein kinase C, calcimedins, parvalbumins, troponin C, and others. Protein kinase C activates other protein kinases and other phosphatases. Protein kinase C-mediated responses at the synaptic junction are typically of longer duration than calmodulin-mediated responses, and some investigators speculate that it may be related to memory storage (Routtenberg, 1986).

Lead has diverse and complex actions on the neurotransmitters, on second-messenger metabolism, and on cellular and molecular processes, and there is evidence that low levels of lead exposure produce a disrupted and less efficient neurological system.

## B.  Clinical Levels of Health Concern

The neurodevelopmental effects of lead toxicity are of special concern in child development and of great public health significance. The central nervous system is principally involved in children and the peripheral nervous system in adults (Chisolm and Barltrop, 1979; Piomelli et al., 1984). Table 2 summarizes the benchmarks for key lead-induced health effects in children and adults.

There is a wide variation in individual susceptibility to lead intoxication and, in general, the number and severity of symptoms increases with increasing BLL, but overt clinical symptoms may begin in some individuals at a BLL of 40 µg/dl or less; in others, symptoms may not appear until 100 µg/dl. The principal neuropathological effect of acute encephalopathy, often fatal, occurs in children at blood lead levels of 80 µg/dl or higher. Acute encephalopathy results in severe interstitial edema of the brain, which is related to an increase in proteinaceous transudate from permeable capillary endothelium and intercapillary spaces in which blood vessels are surrounded by lead containing edemic fluid (Bressler and Goldstein, 1991). These changes in endothelial function may be mediated by the effects of lead on astrocytes, possibly through altering calcium homeostasis or by activation of protein kinase C (Gebhart and Goldstein, 1988). The pathological effects of lead are a consequence of toxicity to neurons and neurotransmitters.

Lead also impairs peripheral nerve conduction in children at levels as low as 30 µg/dl. Significant electroencephalographic (EEG) differences between normal children with high and low dentine lead concentrations have been observed by using new, sensitive techniques of quantitative spectral analyses and topographic mapping (Burchfiel et al., 1992). The spontaneous resting EEG of children with high lead values had higher percentages of low-frequency delta (0.5–3.5 Hz) activity and reduced percentages of alpha (8.0–12.0 Hz) activity. Changes in brain wave patterns have been observed with a blood lead level as low as 15 µg/dl. Qualitatively, these are EEG changes seen in acute lead toxicity and are common findings in a variety of toxic encephalopathies. Reduced auditory function has also been observed in children with blood lead levels as low as 4–6 µg/dl and was observed at frequencies of 400, 1000, 2000, and 4000 Hz. Children with BLL of 25 µg/dl had an average of 3-dB hearing loss compared with children with BLL of 5 µg/dl (Schwartz and Otto, 1987).

**Table 2**  Summary of Lowest Observed Lead-Induced Health Effects in Adults and Children

| Blood lead level (BLL) (μg/dl) | Health effect |
|---|---|
| > 100 | Adults: Encephalopathic signs and symptoms |
| > 80 | Adults: Anemia |
| | Children: Encephalopathic signs and symptoms, chronic nephropathy (e.g., amino-aciduria) |
| > 70 | Adults: Clinically evident peripheral neuropathy |
| | Children: Colic and other gastrointestinal (GI) symptoms |
| > 60 | Adults: Female reproductive effects, CNS symptoms (i.e., sleep disturbances, mood changes, memory and concentration problems, headaches) |
| > 50 | Adults: Decreased hemoglobin production, decreased performance on neurobehavioral tests, altered testicular function, GI symtoms (i.e., abdominal paid, constipation, diarrhea, nausea, anorexia) |
| | Children: Peripheral neuropathy |
| > 40 | Adults: Decreased peripheral nerve conduction, chronic nephropathy |
| | Children: Reduced hemoglobin synthesis and vitamin D metabolism |
| > 25 | Adults: Elevated erythrocyte protoporphyrin levels in males |
| 15–25 | Adults: Elevated erythrocyte protoporphyrin levels in females |
| | Children: Decreased intelligence and growth |
| > 10[a] | Adults: Elevated blood pressure (males aged 40–59 years) |
| | Fetus: Preterm delivery, impaired learning, reduced birth weight, impaired mental ability |
| ≤ 10[b] | Children: Both the level of concern and the lowest observed adverse effect level (LOAEL) for the effects of lead on intelligence has been determined to be 10 μg/dl |

*Source:* Adapted from CDC, May 1, 1992, p. 288.
[a]Safe BLLs have not been determined for fetuses or children.
[b]Both biological and toxicologic effects may occur at levels as low as 6–7 μg/dl; Scwartz (in press) finds a continuum of lead effects down to 1 μg/dl. No absolute threshold has been identified.

Lead is known to interfere with the synthesis of heme, a component of hemoglobin, which may result in sideroblastic anemia and may also play a role in the neurological effects of lead. Heme is also a constituent of cytochrome P-450 and electron transfer cytochromes, and the impairment of P-450 may result in an increased vulnerability to the harmful effects of other toxic chemicals. Decrements in heme synthesis have been observed at blood levels as low as 10 μg/dl, but the significance of effects at this level are unknown (ATSDR, 1990; USEPA, 1986a). A relation between iron deficiency and a reduction of MDI scores has also been demonstrated (Lozoff et al. 1991).

The dose–response curve for neurobehavioral effects in adults is based on the Sepplainen study in which motor nerve conduction velocity was examined in individuals occupationally exposed to lead. They were noted to have slower motor conduction velocities in one or more peripheral nerves as their blood lead levels increased (Sepplainen et al., 1979).

The toxicity of lead is a function of both dose and duration of exposure. Once absorbed, lead is found in all tissue, but eventually 90% of the body burden is bound to bone. Tissue lead levels can be measured by analyzing teeth, bone, or blood. Teeth and bone more accurately reflect the total body burden of lead. Most of an absorbed dose is excreted by the kidney. The single best diagnostic test for lead exposure is the blood lead level (BLL), and the method of choice is the anodic stripping voltammetry, with strict attention to contamination control, as well as quality assurance and quality control in a certified laboratory (NRC, 1993). The BLL generally reflects recent exposure and provides an in vivo measure of exposure. Indirect measures of long-term exposure are elevated erythrocyte protoporphyrin or zinc protoporphyrin levels, which indicate that lead has had an effect on the hematopoietic system. Rabinowitz and Needleman (1982) state that measurement of lead and biological indicators of lead toxicity may correlate with specific and differing patterns of ultradian and circadian rhythmicity.

## X. SUMMARY AND CONCLUSION

Risk assessment of lead exposure is based on human epidemiological evidence of adverse effects. Children, pregnant women and their fetuses, and the lead-exposed worker have been identified as sensitive subpopulations.

There is no safety margin between the concern level and exposure level of lead and there is no safe level of intake for lead; any level of lead intake carries an incremental health risk.

Although significant progress in prevention and abatement has been accomplished, further reduction or elimination of the risks of lead to human health are necessary. Silbergeld (1990) states, "Lead poisoning is poorly treatable and best prevented . . . [It] is one of the most common and preventable pediatric health problems today." Universal screening to aid in its early identification, prevention, and treatment should be initiated (CDC, 1991).

National estimates indicate that 3 million children had blood lead levels exceeding 15 µg/dl and 234,000 had levels exceeding 25 µg/dl in 1984. National health objectives have since been promulgated " . . . to reduce the prevalance of blood lead levels exceeding 15 µg/dl and 25 µg/dl among children aged 6 months through 5 years to no more than 500,000 and zero, respectively, by the year 2000 and to consider the year 2000 objective an interim step toward the year 2010 objective of eliminating all elevated blood lead levels in the United States" (USDHHS, 1991a).

## REFERENCES

*Amicus J.* (1993). 15, 52.

Angell, N. F., and J. P. Lavery (1982). The relationship of blood lead levels to obstetric outcome, *Am. J. Obstet. Gynecol.,* 142, 40–46.

Angle, C. R., and D. R. Kuntzelman (1989). Increased erythrocyte protoporphyrins and blood lead—a pilot study of childhood growth patterns, *J. Toxicol. Environ. Health,* 26, 149 156.

Atchison, W. D., and T. Narahashi (1984). Mechanism of action of lead on neuromuscular junctions, *Neurotoxicology,* 5, 267–282.

[ATSDR] Agency for Toxic Substances and Disease Registry (1988a). The nature and extent of lead poisoning in children in the United States: A report to Congress, U. S. Department of Health and Human Services, Atlanta, GA.

[ATSDR] Agency for Toxic Substances and Disease Registry (1988b). Toxicological profile for lead, U. S. Public Health Service. Atlanta, GA.

[ATSDR] Agency for Toxic Substances and Disease Registry (1990). Toxicological profile for lead, U. S. Public Health Service, Atlanta, GA.

Baer, R. D., J. Garcia de Alba, L. M. Cueto, A. Ackerman, and S. Davison (1987). Lead as a Mexican folk remedy: Implications for the United States. In *Childhood Lead Poisoning: Current Perspectives,* Proceedings of a national conference, December 13, 1987, Bureau of Maternal and Child Health, Health Resources and Services Administration, U. S. Department of Health and Human Services, Washington, DC. pp. 11–119.

Baghurst, P. A., A. J. McMichael, N. R. Wigg, G. V. Vimpani, E. F. Robertson, R. R. Roberts, and S. L. Tong

(1992). Environmental exposure to lead and children's intelligence at the age of seven years: The Port Pirie cohort study, *N. Engl. J. Med.,* 327, 1279–1284.

Bellinger, D. C., K. M. Stiles, and H. L. Needleman (1992). Low-level lead exposure, intelligence and academic achievement: A long-term follow-up study, *Pediatrics,* 90, 855–861.

Bellinger, D., A. Leviton, C. Waternaux, H. Needleman, and M. Rabinowitz (1989). Low level lead exposure, social class, and infant development, *Neurotoxicol. Teratol.,* 10, 497–503.

Bellinger, D., H. L. Needleman, R. Bromfield, and M. Mintz (1984). A follow up study of the academic attainment and classroom behavior of children with elevated dentine lead levels, *Biol. Trace Elem. Res.,* 6, 207–223.

Bellinger, D., J. Sloman, A. Leviton, M. Rabinowitz, H. L. Needleman, and C. Waternaux (1991). Low-level exposure and children's cognitive function in the preschool years, *Pediatrics,* 87, 219–227.

Bellinger, D., J. Sloman, A. Leviton, C. Waternaux, H. Needleman, and M. Rabinowitz (1987). Longitudinal analyses of prenatal and postnatal lead exposure and early cognitive development, *N. Engl. J. Med.,* 316, 1037–1043.

Betz, A. L., and G. W. Goldstein (1978). Polarity of the blood–barrier: Neutral amino acid transport into isolated brain capillaries, *Science,* 202, 225–230.

Betz, A. L., G. W. Goldstein, and R. Katzman (1988). Blood–brain CSF barrier. In Basic Neurochemistry, 4th Ed. (G. Siege, R. W. Albers, B. W. Agranoff, and P. Malinoff, eds.), Raven Press, New York.

Bonithon-Kopp, C., G. Huel, C. Grasmick, H. Sarmini, and T. Moreau (1986). Effects of pregnancy on the inter-individual variation in blood levels of lead, cadmium and mercury, *Biol. Res. Preg.,* 7, 37–42.

Borella, P., P. Picco, and G. Masellis (1986). Lead content in abortion material from urban women in early pregnancy, *Int. Arch. Occup. Environ. Health,* 57, 93–99.

Bornschein, R. L., J. Grote, T. Mitchell, P. A. Succop, K. N. Dietrich, K. M. Krafft, and P. B. Hammond (1989). Effects of prenatal lead exposure on infant size at birth. In *Lead Exposure and Child Development: An International Assessment* (M. A. Smith, L. D. Grant, and A. I. Sors, eds.), Kluwer Academic, Dordrecht, Netherlands, pp. 307–319.

Bornschein, R. L., P. A. Succop, K. M. Krafft, C. S. Clark, B. Peace, and P. B. Hammond (1986). Exterior surface dust lead, interior house dust lead and childhood lead exposure in an urban environment. In *Trace Substances in Environmental Health* (D. D. Hemphil, ed.), University of Missouri Press, Columbian, MO, pp. 322–332.

Bose, A., K. Vashistha, and B. J. O'Loughlin (1983). Azarcon por empacho—another cause of lead toxicity, *Pediatrics,* 72, 106–108.

Bourgoin, B. P., D. R. Evans, J. R. Cornett, S. M. Lingard, and A. J. Quattrone (1993). Lead content in 70 brands of dietary calcium supplements, *Am. J. Public Health,* 83, 115–1160.

Bressler, J. P., and G. W. Goldstein (1991). Mechanism of lead neurotoxicity, *Biochem. Pharmacol.,* 41, 479–487.

Brightman, M. W., and T. S. Reese (1969). Junctions between intimately apposed cell membranes in the vertebrate brain, *J. Cell Biol.,* 40, 648–654.

Burchfiel, J. L., F. H. Duffy, P. H. Bartels, and H. L. Needleman (1992). Low-level lead exposure: Effect on quantitative electroencephalography and correlation with neuropsychologic measures. In *Human Lead Exposure* (H. L. Needleman, ed.), CRC Press, Boca Raton, FL, pp. 209–242.

[CCLPPP] California Childhood Lead Poisoning Prevention Program (1994). CCLPPP Update, Winter, 1994, 6.

[CDHS] California Department of Health Services (1988). Department of Industrial Relations, Hazard evaluation system and information service medical guidelines 1, the lead-exposed worker, June, 1988, 1–6.

[Cal EPA] California Environmental Protection Agency (1993). Air Resources Board, Proposed identification of inorganic lead as a toxic air contaminant; Part B, health assessment: Technical Support Document (B. D. Ostro, J. Mann, J. F. Collins, R. J. Jackson, and G. Alexeeff, eds.), August, 1993.

[CDC] Centers for Disease Control (1975). Increase lead absorption and lead poisoning in young children: A statement by the Centers for Disease Control. U. S. Department of Health Education and Welfare, Atlanta, GA.

[CDC] Centers for Disease Control (1985). Preventing lead poisoning in your children, U. S. Department of Health and Human Services, U. S. Public Health Service, Center for Environmental Health, Chronic Diseases Division, Publication 99-2230, 7–19, Atlanta, GA.

[CDC] Centers for Disease Control (1991). Preventing lead poisoning in young children: A statement by the Centers for Disease Control—October 1991, CDC, U. S. Department of Health and Human Services, Atlanta, GA.

[CDC] Centers for Disease Control (1992). Department of Health and Human Services. U. S. Public Health Service. *MMWR,* May 1, 1992, p. 288.

Cheung, W. Y. (1984). Calmodulin: Its potential role in cell proliferation and heavy metal toxicity, *Fed. Proc.,* 43, 2995.

Chisolm, J. J., Jr. (1986). Removal of lead paint from old housing: The need for a new approach, *Am. J. Public Health,* 76, 236–237.

Chisolm, J. J., Jr., and D. Barltrop (1979). Recognition and management of children with increased lead absorption, *Arch. Dis. Child.,* 54, 249–262.

Cohn, J. (1977). *Statistical Power Analysis for the Behavioral Sciences,* Academic Press, New York.

Cookman, G. R., W. B. King, and C. M. Regan (1987). Chronic low-level lead exposure impairs embryonic to adult conversion of neural cell adhesion molecule, *J. Neurochem.,* 49, 399–403.

Cooney, G. H., A. Bell, W. McBride, and C. Carter (1989a). Neurobehavioral consequences of prenatal low level exposures to lead, *Neurotoxicol. Teratol.,* 11, 95–104.

Cooney, G. H., A. Bell, W. McBride, and C. Carter (1989b). Low-level exposures to lead: The Sydney lead study, *Dev. Med. Child Neurol.,* 31, 641–649.

Cooper, G. P., J. G. Suszkiw, and R. S. Manalis (1984). Heavy metals: Effects on synaptic transmission, *Neurotoxicology,* 5, 247–266.

Delaney-Black, V., B. W. Camp, L. O. Lubchenco, C. Swanson, L. Roberts, P. Gaherty, and B. Swanson (1989). Neonatal hyperviscosity associated with lower achievement and IQ scores at school age, *Pediatrics,* 83, 662–667.

Dietrich, K. N., K. M. Krafft, M. Bier, P. A. Succop, O. Berger, and R. L. Bornschein (1986). Early effects of fetal lead exposure: Neurobehavioral findings at 6 months, *Int. J. Biosoc. Res.,* 8, 151–168.

Dietrich, K. N., K. M. Krafft, R. L. Bornschein, P. B. Hammond, O. Berger, P. A. Succop, and M. Bier (1987a). Low level fetal lead exposure effect on neurobehavioral development in early infancy, *Pediatrics,* 80, 721–730.

Dietrich, K. N., K. M. Krafft, R. Shukla, R. L. Bornschein, and P. A. Succop (1987b). The neurobehavioral effects of early lead exposure. In *Toxic Substances and Mental Retardation: Neurobehavioral Toxicology and Teratology.* Monographs of the American Association on Mental Deficiency (S. R. Schroeder, ed.), No. 8, American Association on Mental Deficiency, Washington, DC, pp. 71–95.

Dietrich, K. N., K. M. Krafft, M. Bier, O. Berger, P. A. Succop, and R. L. Bornschein (1989). Neurobehavioral effects of foetal lead exposure: The first year of life. In *Lead Exposure and Child Development. An International Assessment.* (M. A. Smith, L. D. Grant, and A. I. Sors, eds.), Kluwer Academic, Dordrecht, Netherlands, pp. 320–331.

Dietrich, K. N., P. A. Succop, O. G. Berger, P. B. Hammond, and R. L. Bornschein (1991). Lead exposure and the cognitive development of urban preschool children: The Cincinnati lead study cohort at age 4 years, *Neurotoxicol. Teratol.,* 13, 203–211.

Dietrich, K. N., P. A. Succop, O. G. Berger, and R. Keith (1992). Lead exposure and the central auditory processing abilities and the cognitive development of urban children: The Cincinnati lead study cohort at age five years, *Neurotoxicol. Teratol.,* 14, 51–56.

Dietrich, K., O. Berger, P. Succop, P. Hammond, and R. Bornschein (1993a). The developmental consequences of low to moderate prenatal and postnatal lead exposure: Intellectual attainment in the Cincinnati lead study cohort following school entry, *Neurotoxicol. Teratol.,* 15, 37–44.

Dietrich, K., O. Berger, and P. Succop (1993b). Lead exposure and the motor developmental status of urban 6-year-old children in the Cincinnati prospective study, *Pediatrics,* 91, 301–307.

Edelman, C. M. (1986). Cell adhesion molecules in the regulation of animal form and tissue pattern, *Annu. Rev. Cell Biol.,* 2, 81–116.

Ehling, R. L. (1993, unpublished). Childhood lead poisoning in California, Presentation at Health Officers Association Meeting, November 17, 1993, California Department of Health Services, pp. 1–4.

Ernhart, C. B. (1992). A critical review of low level prenatal lead exposure in the human: I. Effect on the fetus and newborn, *Reprod. Toxicol.*, 6, 9–19.

Ernhart, C. B., and T. Greene (1992). Postpartum changes in maternal blood lead concentrations, *Br. J. Ind. Med.*, 49, 11–13.

Ernhart, C. B., A. W. Wolf, M. J. Kennard, P. Erhard, H. F. Filipovich, and R. J. Sokol (1986). Intrauterine exposure to low levels of lead: The status of the neonate, *Arch. Environ. Health,* 41, 287–291.

Feldman, R. G. (1978). Urban lead mining: Lead intoxication among deleaders, *N. Engl. J. Med.,* 298, 1143–1145.

Fischbein, A., K. E. Anderson, S. Sassa, R. Lilis, S. Kon, L. Sarkozi, and A. Kappas (1981). Lead poisoning from 'do-it-yourself' heat guns for removing lead-based paint: Report of two cases, *Environ. Res.,* 24, 425–431.

Fulton, M., G. Raab, G. Thomson, D. Laxen, R. Hunter, and W. Hepburn (1987). Influence of blood lead on the ability and attainment of children in Edinburgh, *Lancet,* 1, 1221–1226.

Gatsonis, C. A., and H. L. Needleman (1992). Recent epidemiologic studies of low-level lead exposure and the IQ of children: A meta-analytic review. In *Human Lead Exposure* (H. L. Needleman, ed.), CRC Press, Boca Raton, FL, pp. 243–255.

Gebhart, A. M., and G. W. Goldstein (1988). Use of an in vitro system to study the effects of lead on astrocyte–endothelial cell interactions: A model for studying toxic injury to the blood brain barrier, *Toxicol. Appl. Pharmacol.,* 94, 191–206.

Goering, P. L. (in press). Lead–protein interactions are a basis for lead toxicity, *Neurotoxicology,* 41(2).

Goldstein, G. W. (1984). Brain capillaries: A target for inorganic lead poisoning, *Neurotoxicology,* 5, 167–172.

Goldstein, G. W. (1988). Endothelial cell–astrocyte interactions: A cellular model of the blood–brain barrier, *Ann. N. Y. Acad. Sci.,* 529, 31–39.

Goldstein, G. W. (1992). Developmental neurobiology of lead toxicity. In *Human Lead Exposure* (H. L. Needleman, ed.), CRC Press, Boca Raton, FL, pp. 125–136.

Goldstein, G. W., and D. Ar (1983). Lead activates calmodulin sensitive processes, *Life Sci.,* 33, 1001–1006.

Goyer, R. A. (1993). Lead toxicity: Current concerns, *Environ. Health Prospect.,* 100, 177–187.

Goyer, R. A., and B. C. Rhyne (1973). Pathologic effects of lead, *Int. Rev. Exp. Pathol.,* 12, 1–77.

Grant, L. D. and J. M. Davis (1989). Effects of low-level lead exposure on paediatric neurobehavioural development: Current findings and future directions. In *Lead Exposure and Child Development* (M. A. Smith, L. D. Grant, and A. I. Sors, eds.), Kluwer Academic, Dordrecht, Netherlands, pp. 49–115.

Gross, G. P., W. E. Hathaway, and H. R. McGaughey (1973). Hyperviscosity in neonate, *J. Pediatr.,* 82, 1004–1012.

Hansen, O., A. Trillingsgaard, I. Beese, T. Lyngbye, and P. Grandjean (1989). A neuropsychological study of children with elevated dentine lead level: Assessment of the effect of lead in different socioeconomic groups, *Neurotoxicol. Teratol.,* 11, 205–213.

Hemmings, H. C., A. C. Nairn, T. L. McGuiness, R. L. Huganir, and P. Greengard (1989). Role of protein phosphorylation in neuronal signal transduction, *FASEB J.,* 3, 1583–1589.

Holtzman, D., C. DeVries, H. Nguyan, J. Olson, and K. Bensch (1984). Maturation of resistance to lead encephalopathy: Cellular and subcellular mechanisms, *Neurotoxicology,* 5, 97–124.

Huseman, C. A., C. M. Moriarity, and C. R. Angle (1987). Childhood lead toxicity and impaired release of thyrotropin-stimulating hormone, *Environ. Res.,* 42, 524–533.

[IARC] International Agency for Research on Cancer (1987a). Lead and lead compounds. Overall evaluation of carcinogenicity, IARC Monograph Evaluation of Carcinogen Risks Humans: An updating of IARC monographs Vol. 1–42 (Suppl. 7), 230–232.

[IARC] International Agency for Research on Cancer (1987b). Lead and lead compounds. Genetic and related effects, IARC Monograph Evaluation of Carcinogen Risks Humans: An updating of selected IARC monographs from Vols. 1–42 (Suppl. 6), 351–354.

Iyengar, S., and J. Greenhouse (1988). Selection and the file drawer problem, *Stat. Sci.*, 3, 109–135.

Lewis, M., J. Worobey, D. S. Romsay, and M. K. McCormack (1992). Prenatal exposure to heavy metals: Effect on childhood cognitive skills and health status, *J. Pediatr.*, 89, 1010–1014.

Lin-Fu, J. S. (1973). Vulnerability of children to lead exposure and toxicity, *N. Engl. J. Med.*, 289, 1229–1233; 1289–1293.

Lozoff, B., E. Jiminez, and A. W. Wolf (1991). Long-term development outcome of infants with iron deficiency, *N. Engl. J. Med.*, 324, 687–694.

Mahaffey, K. R. (1981). Nutritional factors in lead poisoning, *Nutr. Rev.*, 39, 353–362.

Mahaffey, K. R. (1992). Exposure to lead in childhood: The importance of prevention [editorial], *N. Engl. J. Med.*, 327, 1308–1309.

Mahaffey, K. R., and J. L. Annest (1986). Association of erythrocyte protoporphyrin level and iron status. In the Second National Health and Nutrition Examination Survey, 1976–1980, *Environ. Res.*, 41, 327–338.

Markovac, J., and G. W. Goldstein (1988a). Lead activates protein kinase C in immature rat brain microvessels, *Toxicol. Appl. Pharmacol.*, 96, 14–23.

Markovac, J., and G. W. Goldstein (1988b). Picomolar concentrations of lead stimulate brain protein kinase C, *Nature*, 344, 71–73.

Mayfield, S. (1983). Language and speech behaviors of children with undue lead absorption: A review of the literature, *J. Speech Hear. Res.*, 26, 362–380.

McBride, W. G., B. P. Black, and B. J. English (1982). Blood lead levels and behaviour of 400 preschool children, *Med. J. Aust.*, 2, 26–29.

McMichael, A. J., G. V. Vimpani, E. F. Robertson, P. A. Baghurst, and P. D. Clark (1986). The Port Pirie cohort study: Maternal blood lead level and pregnancy outcome, *J. Epidemiol. Commun. Health*, 40, 18–25.

McMichael, A. J., P. A. Baghurst, N. R. Wigg, G. V. Vimpani, E. F. Robertson, and R. J. Roberts (1988). Port Pirie cohort study: Environmental exposure to lead and children's abilities at age of four years, *N. Engl. J. Med.*, 319, 468–475.

Mushak, P. (1992). The monitoring of lead exposure. In *Human Lead Exposure* (H. R. Needleman, ed.), CRC Press, Boca Raton, FL, pp. 45–64.

Mushak, P., and A. F. Crocetti (1989). Determination of numbers of lead-exposed American children as a function of lead source: Integrated summary of a report to the U. S. Congress on childhood lead poisoning, *Environ. Res.*, 50, 210–229.

Nathanson, J. A., and F. E. Bloom (1975). Lead-induced inhibition of brain adenylate cyclase, *Nature*, 255, 419.

[NHANES II] National Health and Nutrition Examination Survey II (1976–1980).

[NRC] National Research Council (1993). Measuring lead exposure in infants, children and other sensitive populations, Committee on Measuring Lead in Critical Populations, Board of Environmental Studies and Toxicology, Commission on Life Sciences. National Academy Press, Washington, DC.

Needleman, H. L., and C. A Gatsonis (1990). Low-level lead exposure and the IQ of children. A meta-analysis of modern studies, *JAMA*, 263, 673–678.

Needleman, H. L., C. Gunnoe, A. Leviton, R. Reed, H. Peresie, C. Maher, and P. Barrett (1979). Deficits in psychologic and classroom performance of children with elevated dentine levels, *N. Engl. J. Med.*, 300, 689–695.

Needleman, H. L., M. Rabinowitz, A. Leviton, S. Linn, and S. Schoenbaum (1984). The relationships between prenatal exposure to lead and congenital anomalies, *JAMA*, 251, 2956–2959.

Needleman, H. L., S. K. Geiger, and R. Frank (1985). Lead and IQ scores: A reanalysis [letter], *Science*, 227, 701–704.

Needleman, H. L., A. Schell, D. Bellinger, A. Leviton, and E. N. Alfred (1990). The long term effects of childhood exposure to lead at low dose: An eleven year follow-up report, *N. Engl. J. Med.*, 322, 82–88.

Northrup, J. K. (1989). Regulation of cyclic nucleotides in the nervous system. In *Basic Neurochem*, 4th Ed. (G. J. Siegal, B. W. Agranoff, R. W. Albers, and P. B. Molinoff, eds.), Raven Press, New York, p. 349.

O'Flaherty, E. J., P. B. Hammond, and S. I. Lerner (1982). Dependence of apparent blood lead half-life on the length of previous lead exposure in humans, *Fundam. Appl. Toxicol.*, 2, 49–54.

Papanek, P. J., W. C. Gilbert, and S. A. Frangos (1992). Occupational lead exposure in Los Angeles County: An occupational risk surveillance strategy, *Am. J. Ind. Med.*, 21, 191–208.

Piomelli, S., J. F. Rosen, J. J. Chisolm, Jr., and J. W. Graef (1984). Management of childhood lead poisoning, *J. Pediatr.*, 105, 523–532.

Pirkle, J. L., J. Schwartz, J. R. Landis, and W. R. Harlan (1985). The relationship between blood lead levels and blood pressure and its cardiovascular risk implications, *Am. J. Epidemiol.*, 121, 246–258.

Pounds, J. G. (1984). Effect of lead intoxication on calcium homeostasis and calcium-mediated cell function: A review, *Neurotoxicology*, 5, 295–332.

Rabinowitz, M. B., and H. L. Needleman (1982). Temporal trends in the lead concentrations of the umbilical cord blood, *Science*, 216, 1429–1431.

Rabinowitz, M., A. Leviton, and D. Bellinger (1985). Home refinishing: Lead paint and infant blood levels, *Am. J. Public Health*, 75, 403–404.

Rabinowitz, M., D. Bellinger, A. Leviton, H. Needleman and S. Schoenbaum (1987). Pregnancy hypertension, blood pressures during labor, and blood levels, *Hypertension*, 10, 447–451.

Rice, D. C. (1985). Chronic low-level lead exposure from birth produces deficits in discrimination reversal in monkeys, *Toxicol. Appl. Pharmacol.*, 77, 201–210.

Rice, D. C. (1992). Behavioral impairment produced by developmental lead exposure: Evidence from primate research. In *Human Lead Exposure* (H. L. Needleman, ed.), CRC Press, Boca Raton, FL, pp. 137–152.

Richardt, G., G. Federolf, and E. Habermann (1986). Affinity of heavy metal ions to intracellular $Ca^{2+}$-binding proteins, *Biochem. Pharmacol.*, 35, 1331–1335.

Rodamilans, M., M. J. Martinez Osaba, J. To-Figueres, F. Rivera Fillat, J. M. Marques, P. Perez, and J. Corbella (1988). Lead toxicity on endocrine testicular function in an occupationally exposed population, *Hum. Tocicol.*, 7, 125–128.

Rom, W. N. (1976). Effects of lead on the female and reproduction: A review, *Mt. Sinai J. Med.*, 43, 542–552.

Rosen, J. F., R. W. Chesney, A. J. Hamstra, H. F. DeLuca, and K. R. Mahaffey (1980). Reduction in 1,25-dihydroxyvitamin D in children with increased lead absorption, *N. Engl. J. Med.*, 302, 1128–1131.

Rosenthal, R. (1984). *Meta-analytical Procedures for Social Research*, Sage Publications, Beverley Hills, CA, pp. 37–38.

Routtenberg, A. (1986). Synaptic plasticity and protein kinase C, *Prog. Brain Res.*, 69, 211–214.

Sandstead, H. H., D. N. Orth, K. Abe, and J. Steil (1970). Lead intoxication: Effect on pituitary and adrenal function in man, *Clin. Res.*, 18, 76–81.

Schlag, R., and P. C. Flessel (1993). Lead exposure associated with paint removal from Victorian style houses in San Francisco Bay Area, California Department of Health Services, Berkeley, CA.

Schwartz, J. (in press). Low level lead exposure and children's IQ: A meta-analysis and search for a threshold, Environmental Epidemiology Program, Department of Environmental Health, Harvard School of Public Health, Boston, MA.

Schwartz, J., and D. Otto (1987). Blood lead, hearing threshold and neurobehavioral development in children and youth, *Arch. Environ. Health*, 42, 153–160.

Schwartz, J., C. Angle, and H. T. Pitcher (1986). Relationships between childhood blood-lead levels and stature, *Pediatrics*, 77, 28–288.

Seppalainen, A. M., S. Hernberg, and B. Kock (1979). Relationship between blood lead levels and nerve conduction velocities, *Neurotoxicology*, 1, 313–322.

Sharp, D. S., J. Osterloh, C. E. Becker, B. Bernard, A. H. Smith, J. M. Fisher, B. L. Syme, and T. Johnson (1988). Blood pressure and blood lead concentrations in bus drivers, *Environ. Health Perspect.*, 78, 131–137.

Silbergeld, E. K. (1990). Towards the twenty-first century: Lessons yet to learn, *Environ. Res.*, 86, 191–196.

Silbergeld, E. K. (1991). Lead in bone: Implications for toxicology during pregnancy and lactation, *Environ. Health Perspect.*, 91, 63–70.

Silbergeld, E. K., J. Schwartz, and K. Mahaffey (1988). Lead and osteoporosis: Mobilization of lead from bone in postmenopausal women. *Environ. Res., 47*, 79–94.

Silva, P. A., P. Hughes, S. Williams, and J. M. Fald (1988). Blood lead, intelligence, reading attainment and behaviour in eleven year old children in Dunedin, New Zealand, *J. Child Psychol. Psychiatry, 29*, 43–52.

Simons, T. J. B., and G. Pocock (1987). Lead enters adrenal medullary cells through calcium channels, *J. Neurochem., 48*, 383–389.

Smith, M. (1989). The effects of low-level lead exposure on children. In *Lead Exposure and Child Development: An International Assessment,* Proceedings from international workshop on effects of lead exposure on neurobehavioral development; September, 1986, Edinburg, United Kingdom (M. A. Smith, L. D. Grand, A. I. Sors, eds.), Kluwer Academic, Dordrecht, Netherlands, pp. 1–45.

Stiles, K. M., and D. C. Bellinger (1993). Neuropsychological correlates of low-level lead exposure in school-age children: A prospective study, *Neurotoxicol. Teratol., 15*, 27–35.

Telisman, S., P. Cvitkovic, M. Gavella, and J. Pongracic (1990). Semen quality in men with respect to blood lead and cadmium levels, In *International Symposium on Lead and Cadmium Toxicology,* Peking, People's Republic of China, August 18–21, 1990, pp. 29–32.

Thacker, S. B., D. A. Hoffman, J. Smith, K. Steinberg, and M. Zack (1992). Effect of low level body burdens of lead on the mental development of children: Limitations of meta-analysis in a review of longitudinal data, *Arch. Environ. Health, 47*, 336–346.

U. S. Department of Health and Human Services (DHHS), Public Health Service. (1991a). *Health People 2000: National Health Promotion and Disease Prevention Objectives,* DHHS Publication No. (PHS) 91-50212, U. S. Government Printing Office, Washington, DC.

U. S. Department of Health and Human Services (DHHS), Public Health Service. (1991b). *FDA Consumer Magazine, 25*(6), 25–31, Office of Public Affairs, Rockville, MD.

U. S. Department of Housing and Urban Development (HUD) (1990). *American Housing Survey for the United States, 1989,* Office of Policy Development and Research, U. S. Department of Commerce, Bureau of the Census.

U. S. Environmental Protection Agency (EPA) (1984). Comment on issues raised in the neuropsychological effects of low-level lead exposure, Office of Policy and Analysis.

U. S. Environmental Protection Agency (EPA) (1986a). *Air Quality Criteria for Lead.* EPA-600/08-83/028aF-dF, (June, 1986), Environmental Criteria and Assessment Office, Office of Research and Development, Research Triangle Park, NC.

U. S. Environmental Protection Agency (EPA) (1986b). Reducing lead in drinking water: A benefit analysis, EPA Report EPA-230-09-86-019, Office of Policy Planning and Evaluation, Washington, DC.

U. S. Environmental Protection Agency (EPA) (1989). Evaluation of the potential carcinogenicity of lead and lead compounds. In *Support and Reportable Quality Adjustments Pursuant to CERCLA (Comprehensive Environmental Response, Compensation and Liability Act),* Section 102 EPA 600/8-89/045A, Office of Health and Environment Assessment, Washington, DC, NTIS PB89-18136.

U. S. Environmental Protection Agency (EPA) (1990). Air quality criteria for lead: Supplement to the 1986 addendum, Office of Research and Development. EPA/600/8-90/049F.

U. S. Environmental Protection Agency (EPA) (1991). EPA establishes maximum containment level goals, national primary drinking water regulations for level of lead and copper in drinking water, *Fed. Regist.,* (June 7), 56, 26460–26564.

U. S. Food and Drug Administration (FDA) (1991). New guidance on lead in ceramicware, DHS Message No. N. 1113-03, Nov. 5 and 12.

Vimpani, G. V., N. R. Wigg, E. F. Robertson, A. J. McMichael, P. A. Baghurst, and R. J. Roberts (1985). The Port Pirie cohort study: Blood level concentration and childhood developmental assessment. In *Lead Environmental Health—The Current Issues* (L. J. Goldwater, L. M. Wysocki, and R. A. Volpe, eds.), Duke University Press, Durham, NC, pp. 139–146.

Wigg, N. R., G. V. Vimpani, A. J. McMichael, P. A. Baghurst, E. F. Robertson, and R. R. Roberts (1988). Port Pirie cohort study: Childhood blood lead and neuropsychological development at age two years, *J. Epidemiol. Commun. Health, 42*, 213–219.

Winneke, G., W. Collet, U. Kraemer, A. Brockhaus, T. Ewert, and C. Krause (1987). Three- and six-year follow-up studies in lead-exposed children. In *Procedures of 6th International Conference on Heavy Metals in the Environment* (S. Lindberg and T. Hutchinson, eds.), CEP Consultants, Edinburgh, p. 60.

Wolf, F. M. (1986). Meta-analysis, quantitative methods for research synthesis, Sage University Paper, p. 5.

Yule, W., R. Lansdown, I. B. Millar, and M. A. Urbanowicz (1981). The relationship between blood lead concentrations, intelligence and attainment in a school population: A pilot study, *Dev. Med. Child Neurol.*, 23, 567–576.

Zaric, M., D. Prpic-Majic, K. Kostral, and M. Pissek (1987). Exposure to lead and reproduction. In *Summary Proceedings of a Workshop: Selected Aspects of Exposure to Heavy Metals in the Environment. Monitors, Indicators, and High Risk Groups,* April, 1985, Washington, DC: National Academy of Sciences; Yugoslavia: Council of Academies of Sciences and Arts, pp. 119–126. (Cited in ATSDR 1990).

Ziegler, E. E., B. B. Edwards, R. L. Jensen, K. R. Mahaffey, and S. J. Fomon (1978). Absorption and retention of lead by infants, *Pediatr. Res.*, 12, 29–34.

# 32
# Issues in Data Extrapolation

**Joseph P. Brown and Andrew G. Salmon**
*California Environmental Protection Agency*
*Berkeley, California*

## I. INTRODUCTION

The objective of data extrapolation in environmental toxicology is to predict more accurately the delivered effective doses, at relative low environmental exposures, from data obtained at higher exposures in experimental animal and in human epidemiological studies. Extrapolations may be required between doses (e.g., from applied dose to absorbed or metabolized dose, and to the dose reaching the target tissue) in an experimental animal, between routes of exposure (e.g., inhalation to oral), between species (e.g., rodent to human), or any combinations of these. Although many advances have been made in data extrapolation through the use of various mechanistic (e.g., kinetic) and statistical models, there remain significant areas of uncertainty in extrapolation of data as applied to chemical risk assessment. Although data extrapolations have been applicable to mostly carcinogen risk assessment, where assumptions of low-dose linearity and absence of threshold are often made, they may also be useful for noncancer toxic effects through incorporation of data variability and the slope of the dose–response relation (e.g., benchmark dose; Kimmel, 1990). This chapter will focus on some of the problems frequently encountered in data extrapolations for cancer and noncancer risk assessments.

## II. INTERDOSE EXTRAPOLATIONS

### A. Extrapolation Procedures

Armitage and Doll developed a mathematical model that proposed multiple "stages" or successive mutational events to describe the age-dependence of human cancers. This model was later used to explain the time and dose relationships for tumor incidence seen in animal carcinogenicity experiments, and computer software was developed by Crump and colleagues to fit a dose–response equation to these data. This "multistage model" was adopted by the

*601*

U. S. Environmental Protection Agency (USEPA) and, subsequently, by many other regulatory agencies, to provide numerical risk estimates that could be extrapolated to risks from potential exposures of humans to carcinogens. The model predicts that there is no dose at which the risk falls to zero; in other words, there is no "threshold." At low doses the relation between dose and carcinogenic response is linear, although at higher doses (such as those in animal carcinogenicity experiments), the response curve may become steeper. Since there is no threshold according to this model, this leads to the conclusion that there is no such thing as a *safe dose* of a carcinogen (i.e., a dose that carriers no risk). However, if the dose is low enough, the risk may be considered trivial for practical purposes. Several aspects of the multistage model remain uncertain or controversial, but it has stood up to over 30 years of scientific scrutiny.

Several commentators have questioned whether high-dose exposures used in animal tests should be used to develop linear relation between low doses and predicted responses, but no convincing alternatives have been proposed. Experimental data appear to support the assumption of a linear relationship. For example, in aflatoxin-exposed rats, there is a linear relation between the tumor incidence rate and the amount of chemically modified DNA measured over the entire observable range. Similarly, there is a linear relation between aflatoxin dose and the amount of DNA that has been modified by the binding of aflatoxin metabolites. This is illustrated in Fig. 1, which is based on data from Lutz (1986), Wild et al. (1986), and Garner et al. (1988).

The dose required for the lowest observable tumor response is higher than typical human exposures, but the dose required to produce observable DNA modifications is well within the range of human dietary exposures. Although this does not prove the linearity assumption, it is supportive.

## B. Pharmacokinetic Dose Modeling

For many years toxic effects in experimental animals, particularly cancer, have been assumed to be proportional to the applied dose, often expresses as the average daily dose (mg/kg per day) for the experimental lifetime of the animal. Recently, a more in-depth understanding of the biochemical and biological mechanism of the carcinogenic process has cast doubt on the validity of such simple assumptions. The dose–response relations for many chemical carcinogens studied in animal bioassays may show significant nonlinearities owing to progressive saturation of toxifying or detoxifying metabolic or other processes that play a role in carcinogenic processes. The use of simple applied dose estimates in quantal dose–response extrapolation programs, such as the linearized multistage model (LMS), will often require discarding one or more of these

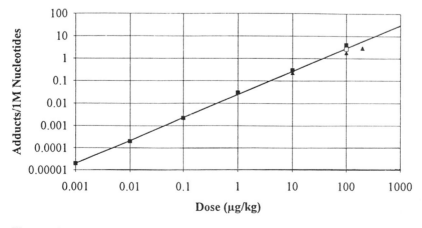

**Figure 1**   Aflatoxin $B_1$ binding to DNA in the rat.

higher-dose estimates to achieve acceptable fit of the multistage model to the quantal tumor incidence data. Often this lack of fit is due to inaccurate dose estimates for the measured responses (e.g., tumor formation; Whittemore et al., 1986). This situation has led many risk assessors to seek better estimates of dose that are more closely correlated to actual effects seen in the test animal. As a corollary, such investigation may also lead to better rationales for dose selection for cancer bioassay and other toxicity studies. To determine and evaluate alternative measures of dose, pharmacokinetic methods and models are often applied.

## C. Descriptive (Classic) Pharmacokinetic Models

The simplest descriptive models treat the body as a single homogeneous entity. The blood plasma is often the central reference compartment, and the rate of change in concentration in this compartment is assumed to reflect the change in concentration in other parts of the body. The simple one-compartment model is useful for chemicals that are rapidly distributed throughout the body. Other chemicals that are more slowly distributed may require more complicated models, with additional peripheral compartments.

These descriptive models predict the disposition of a chemical in the animal body with time, the concentration in body fluids, the rate of distribution to tissues, and the rate of elimination by excretion or metabolism. It should be emphasized that such information says nothing about toxic effects per se. However, several numeric quantities can be obtained that may prove useful as dose metrics: for example, the area under the blood plasma concentration times time curve (AUC), the peak plasma or peripheral compartment concentration, and the mean residence time (MRT) or the time it takes to eliminate 62.3% of the administered dose.

Such simple kinetic models are most applicable to reversible toxic effects and are much less applicable to toxic processes that involve long-lasting or permanent damage to tissues, cellular and subcellular structures (e.g., carcinogenesis, teratogenesis, mutagenesis, or necrosis; Monro, 1992).

## D. Pharmacokinetics and Reactive Metabolites

The realization that many carcinogens are biotransformed, and their reactive metabolites can form adducts with DNA (Wogan & Gorelick, 1985; Poirer & Beland, 1987), stimulated the further development of pharmacokinetic models to include relevant metabolic processes. When available data allowed, the newer models were constructed as physiologically based, pharmacokinetic (PBPK) models for which model compartments and flows were defined to represent actual body organs, such as liver, kidneys, fat, muscle, or other tissues. Such models, when they include Michaelis–Menten metabolic parameters ($V_{max}$, $K_m$) and DNA-binding constants, can predict metabolized or biologically effective doses as a function of exposure level (e.g., Gehring et al., 1978; Dunn, 1983; Corley et al., 1990; Rietz et al., 1990). In addition to basing dose metrics on the total generation or binding of metabolites, Reitz et al. (1990) proposed a model in which cell damage and repair were also affected by the *rate* of delivery of a cytotoxic metabolite. Such a model could help explain both toxicity and carcinogenicity that show dose rate dependency (e.g., butadiene; Melnick et al., 1990).

Table 1 lists a selection of dose metrics or surrogate doses employed in the assessment of risks for various chemicals. According to Bailer and Hoel (1989), risks estimates based on the total metabolite internal dose metric usually leads to a safe dose estimate that is less than 1 order of magnitude smaller than estimates based on the administered dose. Conversely, potency values based on internal doses would generally be greater by a similar degree. Whether or not this relationship is observed depends on the degree of low-dose linearity of the internal dose–response relation. Cox and Ricci (1992) have observed that, in squamous cell carcinoma, induced

**Table 1** Interdose Extrapolation in Risk Assessment

| Chemical | Route/species | Toxic endpoint | Dose metric | Ref. |
|---|---|---|---|---|
| Vinyl chloride | Inhalation/rat | Liver tumors | Amount metabolized (μg/4 hr) | Gehring et al., 1978 |
| Methylene chloride | Inhalation/mouse | Liver and lung tumors | AUC (mg/L) hr area under concentration time curve<br>Milligrams metabolized per liter of respective tissue (GST-dependent) | Andersen et al., 1987 |
| Chloroform | Inhalation, gavage/mouse | Liver tumors | μmol/L liver per day<br>% liver cells killed per day | Reitz et al., 1990 and erratum (1991) |
| Trichloroethylene | Inhalation, gavage/mouse | Liver tumors | Average amount metabolized (mg/kg-d)<br>Average amount TCA metabolite formed (mg/kg-d)<br>Average area under the plasma concentration curve for TCA (AUCTCA) | Allen and Fisher, 1993 |
| Butadiene | Inhalation/mouse | Lung and heart tumors, lymphomas | Metabolized dose (mg/kg-d)<br>Average area under the blood concentration curve for epoxide metabolite (AUCBMO); (mg/kg-d)<br>Continuous internal dose (mg/kg-d) | Hattis and Wasson, 1987<br>Johanson and Filser, 1993<br>USEPA, 1985<br>Brown et al., 1992 |

| Compound | Route/species | Endpoint | Dose measure | Reference |
|---|---|---|---|---|
| Benzene | Gavage/mouse | All squamous cell carcinomas | Total metabolized dose (mg/kg-d); Total hydroquinone (HQ) conjugate metabolites; Total muconic acid (MA) metabolite; AUC hydroquinone glucuronide (HQG); AUC MA all (mg/kg-d); Internal dose (Michaelis–Menten function) | Cox and Ricci, 1992; Medinsky et al., 1989 |
| Ethylmethane sulfonate | IP/mouse | Teratogenicity | Picomole 7-ethyl guanine per micromole guanine | Bailer and Hoel, 1989 |
| Methylnitrosourea | | | Picomole $O^6$-ethyl guanine per micromole guanine | Bochert et al., 1991 |
| Acetoxymethylmethyl nitrosamine | | $ED_{10}$, $ED_{50}$, $ED_{90}$ | | |
| Diethylnitrosamine | Drinking water/rats | $GGT^+$ foci per cubic centimeter liver | Picomole $O^4$-ethyl deoxythmidine per micromole dT | Swenberg et al., 1987 |
| Cigarette smoke | Inhalation/human | Lung cancer | Picomole 4-aminobiphenyl per microgram hemoglobin; Femtomole $^{32}$P per microgram DNA in peripheral blood cells; Femtomole benzo[a]pyrene adduct microgram per peripheral blood | Perera et al., 1987; Bryant et al., 1987; Phillips et al., 1986; Perera et al., 1987 |
| N-Nitrosamines | Oral/human | Esophageal cancer | Femtomole $O^6$ methyldeoxyguanosine per microgram esophageal DNA | Umbenhauer et al., 1985 |
| Ethylene oxide | Inhalation/human | Lung cancer | Picomole ethylene oxide adduct per microgram hemoglobin | Calleman et al., 1978; Tornqvist et al., 1986 |

by gavage administration of benzene in mice, the internal dose–response relation is cubic or quadratic-cubic for total metabolite or related dose metric, yielding much lower potencies and higher safe doses. A further discussion of the usefulness of biological markers in dosimetry and risk assessment can be found in Perera (1987).

## E.  Dose Assessment

Descriptive PBPK models that can fairly accurately predict the kinetics and disposition of parent toxicant following defined-dosing regimens can also be used in the reverse process of assessing exposure based on body fluid, tissue, and excreta analysis and some knowledge of the route(s) and time of exposure. This approach may be particularly useful if the test agent is somewhat volatile, unpalatable, or presents other uncertainties with ad libitum administration in drinking water or animal feed (Yuan, 1993).

## III.  INTERROUTE EXTRAPOLATIONS

The uptake of an environmental toxicant by dermal, oral, or respiratory routes, is not expected to be the same, since the corresponding membrane barriers, along with their physicochemical environments, are structurally different from one another. However, once the chemical is introduced into the general vascular system, its disposition or metabolic fate is expected to be the same, regardless of its route of entry.

It is often necessary to extrapolate from data obtained by one route of exposure to risks resulting from exposure by another route (e.g., inhalation to oral). Occasionally, such situations raise questions of biological relevance or route specificity of a given toxic endpoint of concern. When dealing with carcinogens it is usually assumed that, if an agent is active by one route, it is at least potentially active by all routes. There are exceptions, and occasionally, the carcinogenic potency by one route may be so low that it is virtually noncarcinogenic (Collins et al., 1992).

## A.  Inhalation–Oral

Oberdorster (1990) provides a detailed analysis of route-to-route extrapolation for inhalation and ingestion of cadmium compounds. A systemic dose of cadmium ($\mu g$) resulting from inhalation or ingestion is dependent on a number of factors. For inhalation the dose is determined by the air concentration (AC; $\mu g/m^3$), the volume inhaled daily ($V$; m3/day); the deposition fraction in the lung $d$; the respiratory tract absorption fraction $r$; and the mechanical lung clearance fraction $m$.

The ingested dose depends on food concentration (FC; $\mu g/g$), the amount of food ingested daily (g/day), and the intestinal absorption fraction $i$. Thus, the air and food concentrations resulting in equivalent systemic doses are related by the following expressions:

$$AC(\mu g/m^3) = \frac{FCAi}{Vd(r + mi)} = \frac{FCAi}{Vd(v + i)}$$

$$FC(\mu g/g) = \frac{ACVd(r + mi)}{Ai}$$

In these expressions it is assumed that cadmium mechanically cleared from the lungs is available for intestinal absorption. If all the foregoing parameters are known for the given cadmium compound, one could estimate an equivalent inhaled dose concentration for a known orally ingested dose or vice versa. For many compounds some of these parameters may not be known with sufficient accuracy to allow such extrapolations. Even in the case provided by Oberdorster, certain compounds of cadmium may differ widely in lung absorption versus mechanical clearance (e.g., CdO, 90% absorbed vs. CdS, 90% cleared). Nevertheless, using Cd-specific route-specific dosimetries, as just outlined, Obendorster shows that for Cd-induced kidney damage, 1 μg/m3 of inhaled Cd is equivalent to about 20 μg Cd ingested per day. However, for lung tumors induced by Cd, 1 μg/m$^3$ inhaled is equivalent to about 1000 μg ingested per day. Oberdorster notes that if the target organ is the same as the uptake organ (e.g., lung), then calculation of an equivalent exposure based on equal target organ dose from separate exposure routes may not be meaningful, since the administered dose reaches the target cells in the target organ from different sites (e.g., epithelial or interstitial). In such cases, more complex mechanisms may be involved in the toxic mechanism of action (e.g., contact site carcinogenicity).

## B. Dermal–Oral

The skin permeability of environmental contaminants, particularly from soil and water media, has been investigated by numerous authors. Maibach et al. (1971) showed that the anatomic location of dermal exposure is an important factor in the uptake of pesticides such as malathion. According to Scheuplein and Blank (1971), the stratum corneum layer of the epidermis has about 1000 times more diffusive resistance for low molecular weight electrolytes than do the underlying skin layers. Degrees of hydration of the stratum corneum and lipid solubility of the chemical permeant can significantly affect skin permeability. The effective diffusion coefficient through the stratum corneum is on the order of $10^{-13}$–$10^{-14}$ m$^2$/sec for low molecular weight compounds and $10^{-15}$–$10^{-17}$ m$^2$/sec for higher molecular weight compounds. In addition to physicochemical properties of the toxicant, the permeability may be significantly affected by the skin's metabolic capabilities. Skin metabolism of topically applied xenobiotics, although much less per gram of tissue than liver metabolism, may be comparable with the activity of metabolizing enzymes in the lung (Bronaugh, 1990).

Various arithmetic models of skin permeability usually account for the dependence of toxicant permeation on its water solubility, octanol/water partition coefficient, diffusivity in water and lipid phases, air/water partition coefficient, and molecular weight. A number of these models, as well as a new fugacity-based model, are described by McKone and Howd (1992). Dermal pharmacokinetic models have also been employed to simulate dermal uptake of environmental toxicants; these models appear to give predictions similar to observations in whole-animal models with trichloroethylene (TCE) and tetrachloroethylene (PCE) (Brown and Hattis, 1989; Bogen et al., 1992).

## C. Multiroute Models

Physiologically based pharmacokinetic (PBPK) models, based on the work of Ramsey and Anderson (1984), are usually developed to emphasize a particular exposure route. Oral models may seek to simulate in greater detail the ingestion, intestinal absorption, metabolism, and excretion processes, through a compartmentalized gastrointestinal tract and even a compartmentalized liver (Frederick and Chang-Mateu, 1990). Dermal PBPK models attempt to describe the rates of all physical and biological processes associated with dermal exposure to a given chemical. These models usually incorporate the volume and concentration of the chemical in the dosing solution, the rate of penetration of the chemical into the skin from the dosing solution, the rate of evaporation of a volatile chemical from the skin, some differentiation of the various skin layers, the rates of metabolism in various skin layers, and the rate of penetration into the underlying blood circulation or perfused skin layer (Frederick and Chang-Mateu, 1990). Dermal PBPK and descriptive models may vary significantly in complexity, from those that are highly theoretical in their portrayal of the dermal absorption and metabolism process, to those that are more empirical (Rabovsky and Brown, 1993). Frederick and Chang-Mateu (1990) have used oral and dermal PBPK models to estimate a dermal dose of ethylacrylate (delivered dose in milligrams per kilogram of tissue per day versus concentration in externally applied dosing solution) equivalent to an oral dose resulting in a $1 \times 10^{-5}$ forestomach cancer risk in the rat. The authors assumed that skin and the stomach were equally sensitive to the same delivered dose of ethylacrylate (in this case 0.017 mg/kg tissue per day). It may be argued that different tissue types, organs and so forth, may respond quite differently to similar delivered doses of parent toxicant or relevant metabolites, depending on rates of detoxifying metabolism, differential binding or repair of macromolecular targets or receptors, or other ill-defined and poorly understood factors that control 'susceptibility' to carcinogen exposure. This would seem to be true with 1,3-butadiene, for which PBPK analyses have not provided significant insight into the species- and tissue-specificity of its carcinogenic activity (Johanson and Filser, 1993). Notwithstanding such difficulties, the delivered dose-modeling methodology represents a rational approach to route-to-route extrapolation. Most PBPK models emphasize a single exposure route, but such models can relatively easily be constructed to accommodate multiple routes of exposure. Such multiroute models are particularly valuable in assessing typical human exposures to volatile organic chemicals during activities, such as showering, bathing, swimming, and such. Delivered doses from lifelike exposure scenarios can be compared with those from animal bioassays by using single exposure routes and with experimental data from human exposures (blood, urine, exhaled air) (Chinery and Gleason, 1993).

## D. Dermal–Inhalation

The ability to extrapolate between dermal and other routes of absorption requires a quantitative measure of skin penetration (i.e., a permeability constant) and a way to compare exposure concentration to an internal measure of dose. McDougal and Clewell (1990) reviewed data on 11 volatile organic chemicals and developed a method for interroute comparisons of internal doses. They assumed that distribution and elimination of a chemical would be the same at the same blood concentration, regardless of route of entry. Also, it was assumed that no significant metabolism takes place in the lung or the skin. Comparing the input for each route provides the means to extrapolate from systemic exposures to the toxicants. The input for inhalation ($I_{inhal}$) is the product of the alveolar ventilation ($Q_{alv}$) rate and the concentration in air ($C_{air}$). The input for dermal exposure ($I_{derm}$) is the product of the permeability constant ($P$), the area exposed ($A$) and the air concentration ($C_{air}$)

$$I_{inhal} = Q_{alv}C_{air} \tag{1}$$

$$I_{derm} = PAC_{air} \tag{2}$$

The ratio of air concentrations that give the same intake can be obtained by combining Eqs. (1) and (2):

$$R_{d/i} = \frac{Q_{alv}}{PA} \tag{3}$$

If dermal absorption is enough to reduce inhalation, Eq. (3) is modified as follows:

$$R_{d/i} = \frac{Q_{alv} + PA}{PA} \tag{4}$$

For compounds with permeability constants, ranging from isoflurane (0.03) to styrene (1.75), the human ratios ($R_{d/i}$) ranged from 1180 to 18, respectively. For the rat, with a larger ratio of surface area to alveolar ventilation rate, the ratios would range from 448 to 10, respectively. Assumptions that metabolism is insignificant at the tissue of entry (e.g., lung, skin) may not always hold and need to be evaluated on a case-by-case basis.

## IV.  INTERSPECIES EXTRAPOLATIONS

The objective of interspecies extrapolations is to obtain accurate estimates of toxicologically equivalent doses in a larger species (usually human) from toxicity data in smaller experimental species (usually rodents). Since the elimination rates of many toxic chemicals are proportional to a power of body weight, allometric scaling (e.g., the 0.75 power of body weight) has most frequently been employed to achieve interspecies extrapolations. Although such procedures are usually successful in estimating kinetically equivalent doses (O'Flaherty, 1989), on occasion, they may fail to account for important differences in qualitative or quantitative aspects of metabolism and toxic responses in target tissues and organs. This pharamacodynamic aspect of interspecies scaling introduces uncertainty that can justify a more conservative approach to simple body weight power scaling. Alternatives to interspecies scaling would include human kinetic models (e.g., PBPK), if sufficient human kinetic data exist, or the use of human toxicity data and epidemiology.

## A.  Allometric Scaling

O'Flaherty (1989) has examined the rationale for using kinetically equivalent doses for interspecies conversion of toxicity data. Kinetically equivalent doses are those that produce either equal concentrations in plasma or at receptor sites, or equal total doses (concentration × time). In the absence of differences in dynamics, kinetically equivalent doses would produce the same magnitude of toxic effects across species. A large number of anatomical, physiological, and metabolic variables are related to a fractional power of body weight (Mordenti, 1986). Kleiber (1947, 1975) suggested that (body weight)$^{3/4}$ be adopted as the measure of metabolic body size, and that, in animals for which organ and metabolic pool sizes are directly proportional to body weight, the total amount of chemical energy in the body mass is proportional to body mass. The turnover rate of chemical energy equals the metabolic rate divided by the total amount of chemical energy. Since metabolic rate is proportional to (body weight)$^{3/4}$, and the body chemical energy content is proportional to body weight, then the turnover rate is inversely proportional to (body weight)$^{1/4}$. Studies with a number of drugs have indicated that the turnover time is more closely proportional to (body weight)$^{-0.2}$ (Boxenbaum, 1982; Dedrick, 1973; Dedrick et al., 1970). The use of (body weight)$^{3/4}$ to derive kinetically equivalent doses applies to adults of the test and target species. It has been suggested that scaling within a species (e.g., adult to child) is more effectively accomplished with (body weight)$^{2/3}$. This power is used to scale adult to pediatric drug doses.

Several factors affect the relation between applied or administered dose and the dose actually delivered to the target tissue or organ. These would include age, sex, route of administration, bioavailability, dose timing, and level of physical activity. Although many metabolic processes display allometric relationships with body weight, more often such relationships are unpredictable. Species-specific factors, such as tissue localization of metabolizing enzymes, pattern of metabolite formation, and efficiency of metabolism, may significantly affect the "delivered dose" and its relation to applied dose (O'Flaherty 1989).

The delivered dose may be measured in various ways, depending on the mechanism of action of the drug or toxicant. For drugs, the concentration at the receptor sites affecting drug action is the most appropriate measure. Concentration in the blood or blood plasma is used as a surrogate measure. Toxicants may have various mechanisms of action in addition to reversible receptor binding; for instance, irreversible covalent binding. A more appropriate measure for such agents is the total integrated dose or AUC. O'Flaherty (1989) evaluated tissue concentrations and AUCs as interspecies equivalent-delivered doses under a variety of simulated conditions for elimination kinetics of parent toxicant and metabolite(s). She concluded that dose conversions on the basis of (body weight)$^{3/4}$ were consistently realistic or conservative when the conversion was carried out from a smaller to a larger species. An exception occurred when first-order elimination and capacity-limited production of an active metabolite coexisted. At low concentrations of toxicant, to the extent that metabolism is flow-limited (rather than capacity-limited), it will appear to follow first-order kinetics, and dose conversion based on (body weight)$^{3/4}$ may be realistic or conservative even though metabolism and first-order excretion coexist. These conclusions of O'Flaherty apply to "kinetically equivalent" interspecies doses. Whether such doses are "toxicologically equivalent" depends on the toxic endpoint and mechanism of action. Specifically, "the mechanisms of action of irreversibly-acting compounds, and especially of carcinogens and mutagens, are rarely well characterized in more than one species."

The simulations conducted by O'Flaherty (1989) illustrate two "important considerations in choosing a dose conversion procedure: (1) the appropriate measure of delivered dose is dependent on the mechanism of action of the toxicant; and (2) different measures of delivered dose do not necessarily scale in the same way across species even when it is assured that kinetic parameters do."

The choice of scaling factor for interspecies extrapolation of cancer potency values (slope factors) derived from animal bioassay data has been the subject of considerable debate, and a sizable literature exists on the subject (Davidson et al., 1986). Regulatory agencies have usually employed conservative scaling, such as (body weight)$^{2/3}$, to adjust animal potencies to human equivalent. The EPA has proposed to adopt the less conservative (body weight)$^{3/4}$ scaling, based on arguments similar to the foregoing discussion (USEPA, 1992). However, there still exists considerable uncertainty about the appropriate interspecies scaling factor for carcinogens, or even if there is a single factor. For example, Dedrick and Morrison (1992) studied the carcinogenic potency of three alkylating agents (melphalan, chlorambucil, and cyclophosphamide) in rodents and humans. They employed two dose metrics: (1) the excess incidence of cancer per unit concentration ($nM^{-1}$) averaged over the lifetime of the host (i.e., AUC/2 or 70 years); and (2) the excess incidence of cancer per unit [$(mM \, min)^{-1}$] of total lifetime plasma exposure (AUC). Carcinogenic potencies were defined as $\ln 2/TD_{50}/(AUC/dose)$, where the $TD_{50}$ is the dose that reduces the fraction of tumorless subjects by one-half, and dose is in milligrams per kilogram. With the first metric, potencies ranged from 0.12 to 2.0 in mice; 0.044 to 0.23 in rats; and 2.4 to 141 in humans. The second dose metric was less variant: 0.041–1.9 in rodents and 0.064–3.8 in humans. Although it is difficult to generalize from so few compounds, it is clear that for these agents, scaling rodent potencies with body weight powers of 3/4 or 2/3 would grossly underestimate cancer potency for humans.

Watanabe et al. (1992) reanalyzed acute toxicity data on cancer chemotherapeutic agents compiled by Freireich et al. (1966) and Schein et al. (1970) and derived coefficients for allometric interspecies scaling of toxic doses. By using Monte Carlo sampling, they accounted for measurement errors when deriving confidence intervals and testing hypotheses. Two hypotheses were tested: first, that the allometric scaling power $b$ varies for the chemicals studied; second, that the same scaling power holds for all 25 chemicals in the data set. For the first hypothesis, in 95% of the cases $b$ fell in the range of 0.42–0.97 with a population mean of 0.74. Assuming that the second hypothesis is true, the maximum likelihood estimate of the scaling power is 0.74. For the best case assumption of measurement error, the 95% confidence bounds on the mean were 0.71 and 0.77. For the alternative case assumption of error, the confidence bounds are larger including 0.67 but not 1.00. The authors conclude that both surface area or (body weight)$^{2/3}$ and 0.75 power scaling are consistent with the data set. Another conclusion that might be drawn from this study is that the second hypothesis is false, and a single scaling power of "scaling law," applicable to all compounds, does not exist. Although these data refer to acute toxicity and not cancer per se, they illustrate the importance of considering uncertainty and the potential for heterogeneity in selection of a default scaling factor for cancer potency extrapolation. Also, with the ready availability of software capable of performing probabilistic calculations involving Monte Carlo or related sampling, the use of a scaling power distribution should be considered. Such a distribution could be centered on the default value of 0.75.

## 1. Allometric Scaling For Contact Carcinogenicity

Dawson et al. (1992) have evaluated a number of interspecies scaling techniques for extrapolating formaldehyde carcinogenicity data in rats to humans. Cancer induced in these animals by inhalation of formaldehyde is located primarily in the nasal passages, suggesting a specific mechanism involving contact with the respiratory epithelium. In humans, inhaled formaldehyde absorption and sites of induced carcinogenic action appear to involve a broader area of the lung and upper respiratory tract than in rats. From the studies of formaldehyde-induced binding of protein to DNA and the measurement of subsequent DNA–protein crosslinks (DPX) in nasal epithelium of rats and monkeys (Casanova et al., 1989, 1991), Dawson and Alexeeff (1995, unpublished) derived a series of contact scaling factors from the following relation:

$$F_c = \left[ \frac{(EV)_{ex}}{(EV)_{test}} \right] \left( \frac{W_{test}}{W_{ex}} \right)^{0.67 + i - n + j}$$

where

$F_c$ = contact scaling factor
$E$ = proportion of carcinogen absorbed into target tissue
$V$ = rate of inhalation of air (cm$^3$/sec)
$W$ = body weight, kg
ex = experimental species (e.g., rat)
test = test species (e.g., human)
$i$ = allometric exponent for thickness of the target tissue
$n$ = allometric exponent for coefficient of the detoxification process (−)
$j$ = allometric exponent for coefficient of the binding rate

For a target tissue of with a thickness exponent of $i = 1/3$ and detoxification processes based in body weight powers of 2/3 (0.67), 3/4, and 1 ($n = 1/3$, 1/4, 0), the scaling factors for the dose metric of tissue concentration of formaldehyde ($j = 0$) are 1.3, 0.81, and 0.20, respectively. If action is confined to the surface only ($i = 0$) then these factors become 8.5, 5.3, and 1.3, respectively. If the relevant dose metric is assumed to depend on DPX per DNA (i.e., $j = n$), rather than formaldehyde concentration, then the scaling factors are 0.20 ($i = 1/3$) and 1.3 ($i = 0$) (Dawson and Alexeeff, 1995). These scaling factors are lower than simple surface area scaling $[(280)^{1/3} = 6.5]$, but higher than default scaling using inhaled concentration and uptake as a dose metric (1.2) or other estimates (e.g., USEPA, 1991 draft). Although the human risk assessment here adopted the default interspecies scaling, the foregoing approach as outlined is interesting in that it reveals some of the issues and problems associated with employing dosimetry data in interspecies contact scaling. In this case, additional site-specific data on nasal absorption, biological variability in DPX measurements, binding versus tissue depth, observed versus allometrically estimated ventilation rates, and effects of high concentration on

DPX formation, all would reduce uncertainties involved in using a dosimetry-based contact scaling factor. Similar factors would, no doubt, influence the accuracy of such factors developed for other contact carcinogens.

## B.  Species Specificity

There are numerous examples of species differences in carcinogen metabolism, potency, or target sites. The model carcinogen 2-acetyl aminofluorene (AAF) shows considerable species differences relative to hepatic carcinogenicity. Rats are much more susceptible than mice or hamsters, whereas guinea pigs and monkeys are resistant. The differences are thought to be related to the relative rates of AAF transformation and clearance of reactive metabolites such as $N$-hydroxy-AAF, and binding to liver DNA. (Dybing and Huitfeldt, 1992).

2-Naphthylamine induces mainly carcinomas of the urinary bladder in humans, dogs, and rats, but seems to be much more potent in humans and dogs then in rats. Studies by Kadlubar et al. (1977) suggest that 2-naphthylamine is oxidized and glucuronidated in the liver and that the $N$-glucuronide is excreted in the urine. Few interspecies differences in metabolism of 2-naphthylamine were seen. However, the excreted glucuronide of $N$-hydroxy-2-naphthylamine was hydrolyzed to $N$-hydroxy-2-naphthylamine and, subsequently, converted to a reactive arylnitrenium ion in the urine of dogs and humans, which is acidic, in contrast with the neutral urine of rats. Also both dogs and humans hold acidic urine in their urinary bladders longer than rats. These factors are thought to influence the noted interspecies differences in bladder cancer potency.

Benzidine is a potent human urinary bladder carcinogen, whereas liver is the prime target organ in mice, rats, and hamsters. Benzidine is a weak bladder carcinogen in dogs and rabbits and is apparently noncarcinogenic in monkeys (Morton et al., 1980).

Polycyclic aromatic hydrocarbons (PAH) show several species differences when administered subcutaneously (SC) or topically (Slaga, 1988). Rats responded strongly to SC injection, but are insensitive to topical administration, whereas rabbits show the reverse response. Mice are very sensitive by either route of administration, whereas the hamster is moderately responsive, and the guinea pig is poorly responsive by either exposure route. Benzo[$a$]pyrene, dibenz[$a,h$]anthracene, and 3-methylcholanthrene apparently have no carcinogenic action in monkeys (Adamson and Sieber, 1983). Comparative in vitro data on DNA binding and overall PAH metabolism suggest that human tissues are more susceptible to PAH carcinogenicity than those of mice, rats, or hamsters; however, differences in dose–response curves for tumor induction and DNA binding (Ashurst et al., 1983) cast doubt on any simple relation between the total tissue dose and carcinogenic response.

$N$-Nitrosamines have exhibited carcinogenicity in all species examined, but also show marked species differences in organ selectivity and potency. $N$-Nitrosodimethylamine (NDMA) is a more potent liver carcinogen in rats than in mice and hamsters and exhibits low potency in guinea pigs (Slaga, 1988). $N$-Nitrosodimethylamine appears equally potent for guinea pig and rat liver. Such species differences in nitrosamine carcinogenicity are thought to be due to routes and rates of metabolism to reactive metabolites, such as alkyldiazonium ions, and to the differential repair of specific DNA adducts (Lijinsky, 1983; Slaga, 1988).

Aflatoxin $B_1$ is a potent liver carcinogen in rats, but less potent in monkeys and hamsters, and essentially noncarcinogenic in mice by the oral route. The metabolic activation of aflatoxin $B_1$ involves oxidation to the 2,3-epoxide, which interacts with the N-7 position of guanine in DNA. Comparative in vitro studies of aflatoxin metabolism in liver fractions from rats, mice, monkeys, and humans showed that human and monkey liver were the most active in total aflatoxin conversion, but no consistent correlation of metabolism with carcinogenicity was observed. On the other hand, a good correlation was found with covalent binding of aflatoxin $B_1$ to DNA in liver slices, with the binding pattern of rat > hamster > mouse correlating directly with carcinogenic potency in these species. The rate of binding of aflatoxin $B_1$ to human liver DNA ranked between hamster and mouse (Booth et al., 1986).

Vinyl chloride (VC) is a known liver carcinogen in humans. It is metabolized by cytochrome P-450 oxidation to vinyl chloride oxide, which binds to DNA, whereas a rearrangement produce, chloroacetaldehyde, binds to protein (Guengerich et al., 1981). Marked interspecies differences in vinyl chloride metabolism are exhibited when the clearance rate was expressed on a body weight basis, with mice and rats metabolizing VC about 5 and 12 times faster than humans, respectively. This would indicate that humans would be less sensitive than these rodents to the carcinogenic effects of VC, a conclusion supported by Allen et al. (1988). When the clearance rate is expressed in terms of body surface area, however, mice, rats, and humans have similar values. On this basis, humans should be as sensitive as rodents to VC carcinogenicity. According to Gold et al. (1989), mice are about three times less sensitive than rats to VC carcinogenicity on a body weight basis, whereas a difference of two times could be expected if the data were based on surface area or (body weight)$^{2/3}$.

Arsenic is a known human carcinogen by the inhalation and oral exposure routes, causing lung and skin cancer, respectively (IARC, 1980). Recent epidemiological studies also indicate a link between chronic inorganic arsenic exposure from drinking water and several internal cancers (e.g., lung, liver, kidney, or bladder; Chen and Wang, 1990; Bates et al., 1992). Arsenic is the only confirmed human carcinogen lacking an animal model. There is only a single study, in mice, reporting adenomas of the skin, lung, peritoneum, and lymph nodes in animals dosed orally over a period of 6 months (Knoth, 1966). Ishinishi et al. (1989) and Pershagen et al. (1984) have demonstrated marginal increases in the incidence of lung tumors in hamsters given arsenic trioxide by intratracheal instillation. Although the overall metabolic pathways of arsenic disposition are similar in all mammals yet studied, there are significant differences in kinetics and excreted metabolite patterns. Arsenic is much more acutely toxic in humans than in rodents; there is evidence for a nutritional role of arsenic in some animal species, but not in humans (USEPA, 1988).

1,3-Butadiene (BD) is a probable human carcinogen that shows large species differences in potency and target sites in mice and rats. Mice exposed by inhalation to air concentration of BD ranging from 6.25 to 625 ppm for 6 h/day for 2 years developed cancers of the heart, hematopoietic system, lung, forestomach, and ovary. Highly significant increases in lung tumors were observed at 6.25 ppm and above versus concurrent controls (Melnick et al., 1990). By contrast, rats exposed to 1000 and 8000 ppm BD for 2 years showed significant increases in thyroid follicular cell adenoma and carcinoma, testis Leydig cell adenoma and carcinoma, pancreatic exocrine adenomas, and mammary fibroadenomas and carcinomas. Whether based on most sensitive site or sum of significant tumor sties, the mouse cancer potencies were about 30 times the rat potencies. This difference was about 200 times when the potencies are based on surface area, rather than body weight. Although the metabolism of BD is similar in rats and mice, it was observed, in early kinetic studies, that mice are capable of producing internal steady-state concentrations of the principal mutagenic BD metabolite, butadiene monoxide (BMO), that are 1.5- to 3-fold higher than those in rats (Filser and Bolt, 1984; Kreiling et al., 1987). It was thought that this might explain the higher sensitivity of the mouse to BD carcinogenicity. However, more recent pharmacokinetic work by Johanson and Filser (1993) casts serious doubt on a relatively simple metabolic–kinetic explanation of the pronounced interspecies differences. In view of such large differences in rodent target sites and potency, there has been much discussion about the appropriate species from which to extrapolate human risk. Regulatory agencies have usually chosen the most sensitive species, sex, target site, and so on (USEPA,

1985; Cal EPA, 1992); here, the female mouse lung. Two papers have reported the comparative metabolism and disposition of BD in monkeys and rodents (Sun et al., 1989; Dahl et al., 1990). The normalized uptake values for BD were 3.3, 0.46, and 0.52 µmol/hr per 10 ppm/kg in mouse, rat, and monkey, respectively. When these values were expressed in terms of surface area or (body weight)$^{2/3}$, the resulting values were 0.99, 0.35, and 0.94 µmol/hr per 10 ppm/kg$^{2/3}$. Thus, monkey and mouse appeared more similar in this comparison than monkey and rat. Also limited human epidemiology from occupational exposure is consistent with qualitative risk estimates based on mouse data for similar tumor types (i.e., lymphatic) (Cal EPA, 1992).

In addition to the foregoing examples cited, many more can be found in the literature (Allen et al., 1988; Gold et al., 1992; and Dybing and Huitfeldt, 1992). It is clear that accurate interspecies extrapolation of carcinogenic effects is seriously compromised by such large and common interspecies differences. These differences often cannot be fully accounted for by metabolic–pharmacokinetic corrections. Other factors that may determine cancer sensitivity include differences in host immune response, expression of oncogenes, DNA repair efficiency, and tissue–cell production or detoxification of carcinogenic metabolites. Extrapolations between species needs to be performed on a case-by-case basis, taking available dynamic and kinetic data into account. Often conservative assumptions, as noted earlier, will need to be employed to deal with the remaining uncertainties.

# REFERENCES

Adamson, R. H., and S. M. Sieber (1983). Chemical carcinogenesis studies in nonhuman primates. In *Organ and Species Specificity in Chemical Carcinogenesis* (R. Langenbach, S. Nesnow, and J. M. Rice, eds.), Plenum Press, New York, pp. 129–156.

Allen, B. C., R. S. Crump, and A. M. Shipp (1988). Correlation between carcinogenic potency of chemicals in animals and humans, *Risk Anal.*, 8, 531–544.

Allen, B. C., and J. W. Fisher (1993). Pharmacokinetic modeling of trichloroethylene and trichloroacetic acid in humans, *Risk Anal.*, 13, 71–86.

Andersen, M. E., H. J. Clewell, M. L. Gargas, F. A. Smith, and R. H. Reitz (1987). Physiologically based pharmacokinetics and the risk assessment process for methylene chloride, *Toxicol. Appl. Pharmacol.*, 87, 185–205.

Ashurst, S. W., G. M. Cohen, S. Nesnow, J. DiGiovanni, and T. J. Slaga (1983). Formation of benzo[a]-pyrene/DNA adducts and their relationship to tumor initiation in mouse epidermis, *Cancer Res.*, 43, 1024–1029.

Bailer, A. J., and D. G. Hoel (1989). Metabolite-based internal doses used in a risk assessment of benzene, *Environ. Health Perspect.*, 82, 177–184.

Bates, M. N., A. H. Smith, and C. Hopenhayn-Rich (1992). Arsenic ingestion and internal cancers: A review, *Am. J. Epidemiol.*, 135, 452–476.

Bochert, G., T. Platzek, U. Rahm, and D. Neubert (1991). Embryotoxicity induced by alkylating agents: 6. DNA adduct formation induced by methylnitrosourea in mouse embryos, *Arch. Toxicol.*, 65, 390–395.

Bogen, K. T., B. W. Colston, and L. K. Machicao (1992). Dermal absorption of dilute aqueous chloroform, trichloroethylene, and tetrachloroethylene in hairless guinea pigs, *Fundam. Appl. Toxicol.*, 10, 30–39.

Booth, S. C., H. Bosenberg, R. C. Garner, P. J. Hertzog, and K. Norpoth (1981). The activation of aflatoxin B$_1$ in liver slices and in bacterial mutagenicity assays using livers from different species including man. *Carcinogenesis*, 2, 1063–1068.

Boxenbaum, H. (1982). Interspecies scaling, allometry, physiological time, and the ground plan of pharmacokinetics, *J. Pharmacokinet. Biopharm.*, 10, 201–227.

Bronaugh, R. L. (1990). Metabolism in skin. In *Principles of Route-to-Route Extrapolation for Risk Assessment* (T. R. Gerrity and C. J. Henry, eds.), Elsevier, New York, pp. 185–191.

Brown, H. S., and D. Hattis (1989). The role of skin absorption as a route of exposure to volatile organic compounds in household tap water: A simulated kinetic approach, *J. Am. Coll. Toxicol.*, 8, 839–851.

Brown, J. P., M. A. Marty, J. F. Collins, A. G. Salmon, D. A. Holtzman, J. K. Mann, D. C. Lewis, and G. V. Alexeeff (1992). Health effects of 1,3-butadiene, Technical Support Document. Proposed Identification of 1,3-Butadiene as a Toxic Air Contaminant, Part B, Office of Environmental Health Hazard Assessment, Air Resources Board, California Environmental Protection Agency, Sacramento, CA.

Bryant, M. S., P. L. Skipper, S. R. Tannenbaum, and M. Maclure (1987). Hemoglobin adducts of 4-amino biphenyl in smokers and non-smokers, *Cancer Res.*, 47, 602–608.

[Cal EPA] California Environmental Protection Agency (1992). *Arsenic Recommended Public Health Level for Drinking Water.* Office of Environmental Health Hazard Assessment. Berkeley, CA.

Calleman, C. J., L. Ehrenberg, B. Jansson, S. Osterman-Golkar, D. Segarback, K. Svensson, and C. A. Wachtmeister (1978). Monitoring and risk assessment by means of alkyl groups in hemoglobin in persons occupationally exposed to ethylene oxide, *J. Environ. Pathol. Toxicol.*, 2, 427–442.

Casanova, M., D. F. Deyo, and H. d'A. Heck (1989). Covalent binding of inhaled formaldehyde to DNA in the nasal mucosa of Fischer-344 rats: Analysis of formaldehyde and DNA by high-performance liquid chromatography and provisional pharmacokinetic interpretation, *Fundam. Appl. Toxicol.*, 12, 397–417.

Casanova, M., K. T. Morgan, W. H. Steinhagen, J. I. Fueritt, A. Pofp, and H. d'A. Heck (1991). Covalent binding of inhaled formaldehyde to DNA in the respiratory tract of rhesus monkeys: Pharmacokinetics, rate-to-monkey interspecies scaling, and extrapolation to man, *Fundam. Appl. Toxicol.*, 17, 408–428.

Chen, C. -J., and C. -J. Wang (1990). Ecological correlation between arsenic levels in well water and age-adjusted mortality from malignant neoplasms, *Cancer Res.*, 50, 5470–5474.

Chinery, R. L., and A. K. Gleason (1993). A compartmental model for the prediction of breath concentration and absorbed dose of chloroform after exposure while showering, *Risk Anal.*, 13, 51–62.

Collins, J. F., J. P. Brown, P. R. Painter, I. S. Jamai, L. A. Zeise, G. V. Alexeeff, M. J. Wade, D. M. Siegel, and J. J. Wong (1992). On the carcinogenicity of cadmium by the oral route, *Regul. Toxicol. Pharmacol.*, 16, 57–72.

Corley, R. A., A. L. Mendrala, F. A. Smith, D. A. Staats, M. L. Gargas, R. B. Conolly, M. E. Andersen, and R. H. Reitz (1990). Development of a physiologically based pharmacokinetic model for chloroform, *Toxicol. Appl. Pharmacol.*, 103, 512–527.

Cox, L. A., Jr., and P. F. Ricci (1992). Reassessing benzene cancer risks using internal doses, *Risk Anal.*, 12, 401–410.

Dahl, A. R., W. E. Becktold, J. A. Bond, R. F. Henderson, J. L. Mauderly, B. A. Muggenburg, J. D. Sun, and L. S. Birnbaum (1990). Species differences in the metabolism and disposition of inhaled 1,3-butadiene and isoprene, *Environ. Health Perspect.*, 86, 65–69.

Davidson, I. W. F., J. C. Parker, and R. P. Beliles (1986). Biological basis for extrapolation across mammalian species, *Regul. Toxicol. Pharmacol.*, 6, 211–237.

Dawson, S. V., and G. V. Alexeeff (1995). Interspecies scaling using respiratory tract dosimetry for formaldehyde inhalation, (unpublished data).

Dawson, S. V., J. F. Collins, G. V. Alexeeff, et al. (1992). Cancer risk assessment for airborne formaldehyde, Technical Support Document, Final Report on the Identification of Formaldehyde as a Toxic Air Contaminant, Part B Health Assessment, Office of Environmental Health Hazard Assessment, Air Resources Board, California Environmental Protection Agency, Sacramento, CA.

Dedrick, R. L. (1973). Animal scale-up, *J. Pharmacokinetic. Biopharm.*, 1, 435–461.

Dedrick, R. L., K. B. Bischoff, and D. S. Zaharko (1970). Inter-species correlation of plasma concentration history of methotrexate. (NSC-740), *Cancer Chemother. Rep.*, 54, 95–101.

Dedrick, R. L., and P. F. Morrison (1992). Carcinogenic potency of alkylating agents in rodents and humans, *Cancer Res.*, 52, 2464–2467.

Dunn, B. P. (1983). Wide-range linear dose–response curve for DNA binding of orally administered benzo[a]pyrene in mice, *Cancer Res.*, 43, 2654–2658.

Dybing, E., and H. S. Huitfeldt (1992). Species differences in carcinogenic metabolism and interspecies extrapolation. In *Mechanism of Carcinogenesis in Risk Identification* (H. Vainio, P. N. Magee, D. B. McGregor, and A. J. McMichael, eds.), International Agency for Research on Cancer, Lyon, pp. 501–522.

Filser, J. G., and H. M. Bolt (1984). Inhalation pharmacokinetics based on gas uptake studies. VI.

Comparative evaluation of ethylene oxide and butadiene monoxide as exhaled reactive metabolites of ethylene and 1,3-butadiene in rats, *Arch. Toxicol.,* 55, 219–223.

Fischer, J. W., and B. C. Allen (1993). Evaluating the risk of liver cancer in humans exposed to trichloroethylene using physiological models, *Risk Anal.,* 13, 87–95.

Frederick, C. B., and I. M. Chang-Mateu (1990). Contact site carcinogenicity: Estimation of an upper limit for risk of dermal dosing site tumors based on oral dosing site carcinogenicity. In *Principles of Route-to-Route Extrapolation for Risk Assessment* (T. R. Gerrity and C. J. Henry, eds.), Elsevier, New York, pp. 237–270.

Freireich, E. J., E. A. Gehan, D. P. Rall, L. H. Schmidt, and H. E. Skipper (1966). Quantitative comparison of toxicity of anticancer agents in mouse, rat, hamster, dog, monkey, and man. *Cancer Chemother. Rep.,* 50, 219–244.

Garner, R. C., I. Dvorackova, and F. Tursi (1988). Immunoassay procedures to detect exposure to aflatoxin B, and benzo[a]pyrene in animals and man at the DNA level, *Arch. Occup. Environ. Health,* 60, 145–150.

Gehring, P. J., P. G. Watanabe, and C. N. Park (1978). Resolution of dose–response toxicity data for chemicals requiring metabolic activation: Example—vinyl chloride, *Toxicol. Appl. Pharmacol.,* 44, 581–591.

Gold, L. S., N. B. Manley, and B. N. Ames (1992). Extrapolation of carcinogenicity between species: Qualitative and quantitative factors, *Risk Anal.,* 12, 579–588.

Gold, L. S., T. H. Slone, and L. Bernstein (1989). Summary of carcinogenic potency and positivity for 492 rodent carcinogens in the carcinogenic potency database, *Environ. Health Perspect.,* 79, 259–272.

Guengerich, F. P., P. S. Mason, W. T. Stott, T. R. Fox, and P. G. Watanabe (1981). Roles of 2-haloethylene oxides and 2-halo acetaldehydes derived from vinyl bromide and vinyl chloride in irreversible binding to protein and DNA, *Cancer Res.,* 41, 4291–4298.

Hattis, D., and J. Wasson (1987). *A Pharmacokinetic/Mechanism-Based Analysis of the Carcinogenic Risk of Butadiene,* U. S. National Technical Information Service No. NTIS/PB 88-202817, MIT Center for Technology, Policy and Industrial Development, CTPID 87-3.

[IARC] International Agency for Research on Cancer (1990). Some metals and metallic compounds, IARC Monographs on the evaluation of the carcinogenic risk of chemicals to man: Vol. 23, IARC, Lyon.

Ishinishi, N., A. Yamamoto, A. Hisanaga, and T. Inamasu (1989). Tumorigenicity of arsenic trioxide to the lung in Syrian golden hamsters by intermittent instillations, *Cancer Lett.,* 21, 141–147.

Johanson, G., and J. G. Filser (1993). A physiologically based pharmacokinetic model for butadiene and its metabolite butadiene monoxide in rat and mouse and its significance for risk extrapolation, *Arch. Toxicol.,* 67, 151–163.

Kadlubar, F. F., J. A. Miller, and E. C. Miller (1977). Hepatic microsomal N-glucuronidation and nucleic acid binding of N-hydroxyarylamines in relation to urinary bladder carcinogenesis, *Cancer Res.,* 37, 805–814.

Kimmel, C. A. (1990). Quantitative approaches to human risk assessment for non-cancer health effects, *Neurotoxicology,* 11, 189–198.

Kleiber, M. (1947). Body size and metabolic rate, *Physiol. Rev.,* 27, 511–541.

Kleiber, M. (1975). Metabolic turnover rate: A physiological meaning of the metabolic rate per unit body weight, *J. Theor. Biol.,* 53, 199–204.

Knoth, W. (1966). Arsenic treatment, *Arch. Klin. Exp. Dermatol.,* 227, 228–234.

Kreiling, R., R. J. Laib, J. G. Filser, and H. M. Bolt (1987). Inhalation pharmacokinetics of 1,2-epoxy butane-3 reveal species differences between rats and mice sensitive to butadiene induced carcinogenesis, *Arch. Toxicol.,* 61, 7–11.

Lijinsky, W. (1983). Species specificity in nitrosamine carcinogenesis. In *Organ and Species Specificity in Chemical Carcinogenesis* (R. Langenback, S. Nesnow, and J. M. Rice, eds.), Plenum Press, New York, pp. 63–75.

Lutz, W. K. (1986). Quantitative evaluation of DNA binding data for risk estimation and for classification of direct and indirect carcinogens, *J. Cancer Res. Clin. Oncol.,* 112, 85–91.

Maibach, H. I., R. J. Feldmann, T. H. Milby, and W. F. Serat (1971). Regional variation in percutaneous penetration in man, *Arch. Environ. Health,* 23, 208–211.

McDougal, J. N., and H. J. Clewell (1990). Dermal to inhalation extrapolation for organic chemicals. In *Principles of Route-to-Route Extrapolation for Risk Assessment* (T. R. Gerrity and C. J. Henry, eds.), Elsevier, New York, pp. 313–317.

McKone, T. E., and R. A. Howd (1992). Estimating dermal uptake of organic chemicals from water and soil: I. Unified frugacity-based models for risk assessments, *Risk Anal.,* 12, 543–557.

Medinsky, M., P. J. Sabourin, G.Lucier, L. S. Birnbaum, and R. F. Henderson (1989). A toxicokinetic model for simulation of benzene metabolism, *Exp. Pathol.,* 37, 150–154.

Melnick, R. L., J. E. Huff, B. Chou, and R. Miller (1990). Carcinogenicity of 1,3-butadiene in C57BL/6 x C3HF1 mice at low exposure concentrations, *Cancer Res.,* 50, 6592–6599.

Monro, A. (1992). What is an appropriate measure of exposure when testing drugs for carcinogenicity in rodents? *Toxicol. Appl. Pharmacol.,* 12, 171–181.

Mordenti, J. (1986). Man versus beast: Pharmacokinetic scaling in mammals, *J. Pharm. Sci.,* 75, 1028–1040.

Morton, K. C., F. A. Beland, F. E. Evans, N. F. Fullerton, and F. F. Kadlubar (1980). Metabolic activation of N-hydroxy-N,N-diacetylbenzidine by hepatic sulfotransferase, *Cancer Res.,* 40, 751–757.

Oberdorster, G. (1990). Equivalent oral and inhalation exposure to cadmium compounds: Risk estimation based on route-to-route extrapolation. In *Principles of Route-to-Route Extrapolation for Risk Assessment* (T. R. Gerrity, C. J. Henry, eds.), Elsevier, New York, pp. 217–235.

O'Flaherty, E. J. (1989). Interspecies conversion of kinetically equivalent doses, *Risk Anal.,* 9, 587–598.

Perera, F. (1987). The potential usefulness of biological markers in risk assessment, *Environ. Health Perspect.,* 76, 141–145.

Perera, F. P., R. Santella, H. K. Fischman, A. R. Munshi, M. Poirier, D. Brenner, H. Mehta, J. Van Ryzin (1987). DNA adducts, protein adducts and sister chromatid exchange in cigarette smokers and nonsmokers, *JNCI,* 79, 449–456.

Pershagen, G., G. Nordberg, and N. E. Bjorklund (1984). Carcinomas of the respiratory tract in hamsters given arsenic trioxide and/or benzo-a-pyrene by the pulmonary route, *Environ. Res.,* 34, 227–241.

Phillips, D. H., A. Hewer, and P. L. Grover (1986). DNA adducts in human bone marrow and peripheral blood leukocytes, *Carcinogenesis,* 7, 2071–2075.

Poirier, M. C., and F. A. Beland (1987). Determination of carcinogen-induced macromolecular adducts in animals and humans, *Prog. Exp. Tumor Res.,* 31, 1–10.

Rabovsky, J., and J. P. Brown (1993). Malathion metabolism and disposition in mammals, *J. Occup. Med. Toxicol.,* 2, 131–168.

Ramsey, J. R., and M. E. Andersen (1984). A physiological model for the inhalation pharmacokinetics of inhaled styrene in rats and humans, *Toxicol. Appl. Pharmacol.,* 73, 159–175.

Reitz, R. H., A. L. Mendrala, R. A. Corley, O. F. Quast, M. L. Gargas, M. E. Andersen, D. A. Staats, and R. B. Conolly (1990). Estimating the risk of liver cancer associated with human exposures to choloform using physiologically based pharmacokinetic modeling, *Toxicol. Appl. Pharmacol.,* 105, 443–459.

Schein, P. S., R. D. Davis, S. Carter, J. Newman, D. R. Schein, and D. P. Rall (1970). The evaluation of anticancer drugs in dogs and monkeys for the prediction of qualitative toxicities in man. *Clin. Pharm. Ther.,* 1, 3–40.

Scheuplein, R. J., and I. H. Blank (1971). Permeability of the skin. *Physiol. Rev.,* 51, 702–747.

Slaga, T. J. (1988). Interspecies comparisons of tissue DNA damage, repair, fixation, and replication, *Environ. Health Perspect.,* 77, 73–82.

Sun, J. D., A. R. Dahl, J. A. Bond, L. S. Birnbaum, and R. F. Henderson (1989). Metabolism of inhaled butadiene to monkeys: Comparison to rodents, *Exp. Pathol.,* 37, 133–135.

Swenberg, J. A., F. C. Richardson, J. A. Boucheron, F. H. Deal, S. A. Belinsky, M. Charbonneau, and B. G. Short (1987). High to low dose extrapolation: Critical determinants involved in the dose response of carcinogenic substances, *Environ. Health Perspect.,* 76, 57–63.

Tornqvist, M., S. Osterman-Golkar, A. Kautianen, S. Jensen, P. B. Farmer, and L. Ehrenberg (1986). Tissue doses of ethylene oxide in cigarette smokers determined from adduct levels in hemoglobin, *Carcinogenesis,* 7, 1519–1521.

Umbenhauer, D., C. P. Wild, R. Montesano, R. Saffhill, J. M. Boyle, N. Huh, V. Kirsten, J. Thomale,

M. F. Rajensky, and S. H. Lu (1985). $O^6$-Methyldeoxyguanosine in oesophageal DNA among individuals at high risk of oesophageal cancer, *Int. J. Cancer,* 36, 661–665.

[USEPA] U. S. Environmental Protection Agency (1992). Draft report: A cross-species scaling factor for carcinogen risk assessment based on equivalence of mg/kg$^{3/4}$/day, *Fed. Regist.,* 57, 24152–24173.

[USEPA] U. S. Environmental Protection Agency (1991). Formaldehyde risk assessment update, Office of Toxic Substances, Washington DC.

[USEPA] U. S. Environmental Protection Agency (1988). Special report on ingested arsenic: Skin cancer; nutritional essentiality, EPA/625/3-87/013, Washington, DC.

[USEPA] U. S. Environmental Protection Agency (1985). Mutagenicity and carcinogenicity assessment of 1,3-butadiene, Office of Health Hazard and Environmental Assessment, EPA/600/8-85/004F, Washington, DC.

Watanabe, V., F. Y. Bois, and L. Zeise (1992). Interspecies extrapolations: A reexamination of acute toxicity data, *Risk Anal.,* 12, 301–310.

Whittemore, A. S., S. C. Grosser, and A. Silvers (1986). Pharmacokinetics in low dose extrapolation using animal cancer data, *Fundam. Appl. Toxicol.,* 7, 183–190.

Wild, C. P., R. C. Garner, R. Montesano, and F. Tursi (1986). Aflatoxin $B_1$ binding to plasma albumin and liver DNA upon chronic administration to rats, *Carcinogenesis,* 7, 853–858.

Wogan, G. N., and N. J. Gorelick (1985). Chemical and biochemical dosimetry exposure to genotoxic chemicals, *Environ. Health Perspect.,* 62, 5–18.

Yuan, J. (1993). Modeling blood/plasma concentration in dosed feed and dosed drinking water toxicology studies, *Toxicol. Appl. Pharmacol.,* 119, 131–141.

# 33
# Metam: Animal Toxicology and Human Risk Assessment

**Lubow Jowa**
*California Environmental Protection Agency*
*Sacramento, California*

## I. INTRODUCTION

On July 14, 1991, a chemical release from a train derailment in the Upper Sacramento River resulted in the killing of fish and other aquatic wild life for miles downstream, and affected the well-being of a neighboring community (DiBartolomeis et al., 1994). The released chemical was metam (also known as metam sodium, the formulated product) used for decades throughout the world as a soil fumigant. Although not the most widely used soil fumigant, metam shows potential for broader use as other soil fumigants, such as methyl bromide or Telone, are banned or designated restricted-use materials. In addition, the potassium salt of metam is marketed as a water biocide for use in sugar processing and cooling towers; however, its use (in tonnage) is less than that of the sodium salt.

Metam is usually available as a formulation of 32.7% of the product in water, which is stable at a self-buffered pH of about 10. Once the product is diluted with additional water, as in the spill into the river, the pH decreases and metam rapidly decomposes. Resulting products consist primarily of methylisothiocyanate (MITC), $H_2S$, and elemental sulfur (Howd, 1992). It is the MITC, produced as the result of metam breakdown, that is considered to be the direct agent of pesticidal activity.

In the light of anticipated more extensive use of metam, it is imperative that toxicity data on this product are available, and that there is an understanding of how the data should be extrapolated to real-life situations. The present chapter represents a compilation of the health effects data on metam. For human health assessment, metam is used here as a case sample for directing attention to the evaluation of birth defects data seen in experimental animals as it relates to human exposure, and to consider the breakdown products as contributors to toxicity in humans following initial exposure to the parent compound.

## II.  BIOKINETICS OF METAM IN THE RAT

The biokinetics of metam was investigated in single-dose administration studies (Hawkins, 1987). The [$^{14}$C]metam, at doses of 10 or 100 mg/kg, was given to five CrL:COBS(SD) CD rats of each sex, and labeled metam products were periodically sampled in blood, urine, feces, and expired air for up to 7 days. Results showed rapid and complete absorption. Plasma concentrations reached a maximum level in 1 hr and dropped to near background levels at 240 h. At the low dose (10 mg/kg), about 25% of the radioactivity was eliminated through the urine in 8 hr; by 168 hr, 55% was eliminated. At 100 mg/kg dose, about 18% of the label was excreted within 8 hr, and 40% within 168 hr. Within 24 hr, expired air was about 1% MITC, 15% carbon disulfide ($CS_2$)/carbonyl sulfide (COS), and 17% carbon dioxide ($CO_2$) at 10 mg/kg. At 100 mg/kg, expired air was about 24% MITC, 18% $CS_2$/COS, and 6% $CO_2$. Negligible amounts of labeled products were expired from 24 to 72 hr at either dose.

Approximately 2% of the labeled products associated with metam were retained by the tissues after the seventh day. The thyroid had the highest mean concentration of labeled products among all the sampled tissues. Significant concentrations of metabolites were also found in the liver, kidneys, and lungs.

In summary, exhalation and excretion of products through the urine are major routes of elimination for metam metabolites. With higher doses, an increase in both COS/$CS_2$ and MITC concentrations in the expired breath occurs, with a corresponding decrease in urinary elimination of these products. This suggests that the metabolic pathways for elimination by urinary excretion are saturated, and elimination of circulating metam products by exhalation is favored.

The breakdown of metam as characterized by these studies is summarized in Fig. 1. Metam degrades to either $CS_2$ or MITC in the stomach, accelerated by the stomach pH. The $CS_2$ is metabolized primarily by the liver to $CO_2$.

Glutathione conjugation with MITC was suggested as the source of the major metabolite found in the urine, identified as *N*-acetyl-*S*-(*N*-methylthiocarbamoyl)-1-cysteine, by mass spectrometry. This metabolite accounted for 21% of the excreted dose. Precursors of this metabolite were found in the liver and kidney within 30 min after treatment. No evidence for glucuronide or sulfate conjugates of the metabolites of metam were found.

Therefore, two different metabolic pathways appear to contribute to elimination of metam following administration by the oral route: one by $CS_2$ metabolism and the other by MITC conjugation. The MITC and $CS_2$ are nonenzymatically produced from metam in the stomach, then are absorbed and metabolized by the liver to MITC–glutathione conjugates or $CO_2$. At higher administered doses, saturation of the metabolic processes for both MITC and $CS_2$ occurs, resulting in exhalation of unmetabolized product.

## III.  GENERAL TOXICITY

### A.  Acute Toxicity

Metam is classified by the U. S. Environmental Protection Agency (USEPA) as slightly toxic by oral, dermal, and respiratory routes of exposure to rats. Oral and dermal median lethal doses (LD$_{50}$s) were greater than 1000 mg/kg for rats (Morgan, 1985; Northview, 1987a). Animals receiving fatal oral doses were reported to have symptoms of depression, piloerection, ptosis, lacrimation, and yellowish, darkened skin, with anogenital stains. Gross necropsy revealed darkened or spotted lungs, spotted thymuses, darkened stomach mucosa, gas in the intestines and stomach, darkened spleens, pale and rough liver, and darkened adrenals (Morgan, 1985; Deenihan, 1985; Northview, 1987a,b,c).

In respiratory exposures to aerosol droplets, LC$_{50}$s were estimated to be above 4.7 mg/L

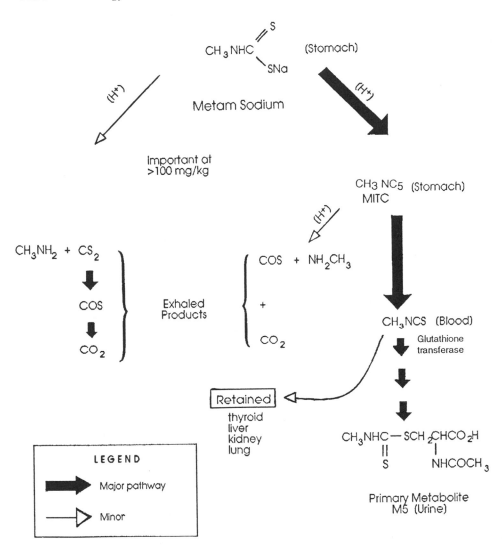

**Figure 1** Metabolism of metam sodium (metam) and its metabolite methylisothiocyanate (MITC).

(Miller, 1979; Rothstein, 1987). Significant symptoms noted in the respiratory studies included dyspnea, ataxia, and noisy respiration. On gross examination, focal lesions were noted in the lung, giving a mottled appearance.

In studies conducted in the former Soviet Ukraine, metam produced a slightly different pattern of effects and at lower doses than in the American and European studies (Nesterova, 1969). However, no experimental details were provided, and the results were questionable. Single intragastric doses of carbathion (metam) were administered to white mice, albino rats, and cats. Oral $LD_{50}$s were estimated to be 146.5 mg/kg for white mice and 450 mg/kg for albino rats. Cats died at 100 mg/kg and had toxic signs at 50 mg/kg. Clinical toxicity was reported to include reduced motor activity, tremor, and muscular fibrillation and incoordination in all animals, whereas doses above the $LD_{50}$ produced spasmodic twitching of limbs. Profuse salivation was the predominant symptom in cats at lower doses. A dermal $LD_{50}$ of 650 mg/kg was also determined for rats.

In a second study conducted in the former Soviet Ukraine (Baran et al., 1969), oral $LD_{50}$s of 200 and 450 mg/kg were determined for mice and rats, respectively. The major effects seen at death in these animals were parenchymal dystrophy and necrosis of liver cells. As with the previous study, lethality occurred at lower doses, and the toxic signs reported were different from those produced in the European and United States studies.

## B. Dermal Sensitivity and Irritation

In irritancy studies conducted on the eye and skin, metam showed strong skin, but not eye, irritation in rabbits (Morgan, 1985; Northview, 1987b). In the Soviet study (Nesterova, 1969) metam was not irritating to the skin if it was washed off after an hour. A summary of the acute effects is given in Table 1.

A modified Buehler test was performed using Vapam Technical (32.7% metam) applied to guinea pigs (Mutter, 1987). First, two primary dermal irritation studies were performed applying Vapam and MITC to the skin of guinea pigs for 3 days. Signs of irritation (erythema and edema) were observed at 30, 10, and some 3% metam doses, and at 0.5% MITC. The 1.0% metam- and 0.1% MITC-treated animals were unaffected; therefore, these doses were selected for the Buehler test.

In the Buehler test, a solution of 1% Vapam Technical (32.7% metam) was used for ten induction applications (three times per week) on the right flank of ten guinea pigs. Positive (0.1% dinitrochlorobenzene) and negative controls (vehicle) were treated in a similar fashion. No apparent systemic effects, or changes in body weight, general appearance, or behavior were noted in the Vapam or negative control animals. A slight erythemic reaction was seen by the third week in some Vapam-tested animals. Following the induction phase, a series of challenge doses were applied to the left flank of the guinea pigs, including 0.1 and 1% Vapam, and 0.1% MITC to the Vapam-induced groups. The negative controls received three challenge doses of 1% Vapam. The 1% Vapam and 0.1% MITC produced mild, but persistent, erythema and edema in the Vapam-induced groups, but the 0.1% Vapam did not produce any significant reactions.

**Table 1**  Acute Toxicity Summary of Metam

| Exposure route | Animal (sex) | Dose or classification | Ref. |
|---|---|---|---|
| $LD_{50}/LC_{50}$ studies | | | |
| Oral | Rats (M) | 1294 mg/kg | Morgan, 1985 |
| | (F) | 1428 mg/kg | |
| | Rats (M) | 1415 mg/kg | Northview, 1987a |
| | (F) | 1350 mg/kg | |
| Dermal | Rabbits | 1012 mg/kg | Morgan, 1985 |
| | Rabbits (M) | 3500 mg/kg | Deenihan, 1987 |
| | (F) | 2100 mg/kg | |
| Inhalation | Rats (M) | > 4.7 mg/L (4 hrs) | Miller, 1979 |
| | Rats | > 5.4 mg/L (4 hrs) | Rothstein, 1987 |
| Irritation studies | | | |
| Eye | Rabbits | Mild irritant | Morgan, 1985 |
| | Rabbits | Nonirritant | Northview, 1987b |
| Dermal | Rabbits | Severe | Morgan, 1985 |
| | Rabbits | Corrosive | Northview, 1987c |

Furthermore, when the negative controls were challenged for a second time, one induction dose of 1% Vapam was sufficient to produce a sensitization response.

Contact dermatitis has been reported in agricultural workers exposed to metam (Jung and Wolf, 1979; Jung, 1979; Schubert, 1978). The authors of these reports suggest that the principal allergen in the positive cases of dermatitis was MITC, since "older" (probably hydrolized) metam solutions provoked a better response than freshly prepared formulations (Schubert, 1978).

## IV.  ORAL STUDIES

## A.  Rats

An 11-day, oral dose range-finding study was performed in rats (Cave, 1991a). Metam (32.8 g/L) was administered daily by gavage at doses of 20, 50, and 200 mg/kg to groups of four Alpk:ApfSD (Wistar) rats of both sexes for 11 consecutive days. No mortalities were noted during the treatment period. Increased salivation, and reduced body weight gain and food consumption was observed in the 50- and 200-mg/kg dose groups in a dose-related fashion. Ulceration of nonglandular areas of the stomach was noted in animals in the 200-mg/kg dose group and in two females in the 50-mg/kg group. An increase was noted in the organ/body weight ratios for the liver and kidney in the 200-mg/kg dose group.

In a second study, oral gavage dosing was replaced by administering metam in the drinking water, to eliminate side effects, such as gastric ulceration, observed in the 11-day study (Cave, 1991a). Metam (Cave, 1991b), was administered at concentrations of 0, 0.018, 0.089, or 0.44 mg/ml, for 90 days, to groups of 12 rats per sex in drinking water buffered at pH 9 (Allen, 1991). The estimated mean daily doses were 1.7, 8.1, and 26.9 mg/kg for males, and 2.5, 9.3, and 30.6 mg/kg for females, based on the initial concentrations of metam and the volume of water consumed by the groups. Because of the instability of metam in water, the concentration of metam after 24 hr was greater than 70% at 0.32 mg/ml and higher, but only 30–40% for concentrations lower than 0.089 mg/ml. The MITC concentrations were not determined (even though it is the major breakdown product of metam in water).

Absolute body weights were reduced for both sexes in the highest-dose groups, and were marginally reduced for females at middose (Allen, 1991). Body weight gain at middose was significantly reduced for females, but only marginally so for males. Food and water consumption were reduced, particularly in the high-dose group. Water consumption was also slightly reduced for females at 0.089-mg/ml dose.

Gross necropsy and histological examination revealed no significant treatment effects, except for changes to the olfactory epithelium (Allen, 1991). There was an increase in the kidney organ/body weight ratios for females at the high dose. Histopathology of the olfactory epithelium and Bowman's glands were noted in both sexes at the high dose, with greater severity in females. The changes comprised prominent or vacuolated Bowman's gland or ducts, and disorganization and vacuolation of the olfactory epithelium. The authors suggested that these changes were due to the systemic effect of metam, rather than inhalation of volatilized products from drinking water, since the most affected tissue was toward the posterior portion of the nasal cavity. No changes were noted in the respiratory epithelium.

For clinical findings, a decrease in urine specific gravity and a decrease in urine volume was observed (Allen, 1991). In males, there was a slight dose-related reduction in urine pH. Urinary protein was decreased at the high dose, but slightly elevated at middose. All of these changes may have resulted from decreased food and water intakes. One death in a female rat may have been treatment-related, because marked cystitis was noted.

Plasma urea and triglyceride levels increased significantly from controls in the 0.44-mg/ml female group. In males, there were significant decreases at the high dose for only alanine transaminase (ALT), aspartate transaminase (AST), plasma glucose, and alkaline phosphatase (ALP) values. Significant decreases in red blood cell counts for males were noted at the mid- and high doses, whereas all dosed females were affected. Hematocrits were reduced in all treated males and females. The red blood cell counts and hematocrits showed very shallow dose–response curves, without significant trends.

In a 2-year study (Rattray, 1994), metam was administered to Hsd/Ola:Wistar Tox rats (50 per sex per dose) at 0, 0.019, 0.056, and 0.19 mg/ml in drinking water. This was equivalent to a mean dose of 1.5, 4.3, and 12.5 mg/kg for males and 2.7, 6.8, and 16.8 mg/kg for females. Reduced hindlimb function and thinness were observed in males at 0.19 mg/ml at the conclusion of the experiment. Clinical effects observed included body weight reduction for both sexes at the 0.19-mg/ml dose. Water consumption was reduced at all doses, whereas food intake was reduced at 0.056 mg/ml and higher. Decreases in hemoglobin were noted at 0.056 mg/ml and higher. Males at 0.056 mg/ml and higher, and females at 0.19 mg/ml had lower hematocrit and RBC count. Plasma levels of triglycerides, ALT, AST, and phosphorus were decreased in females at 0.19 mg/ml. At this dose, both sexes had decreases in urine volume, and males also had a decrease in urine pH. There was a significant increase in rhinitis, hypertrophy of Bowman's glands, hyperplasia or degeneration of olfactory epithelium, atrophy and adenitis of Steno's gland, and respiratory epithelial hyperplasia at 0.19 mg/ml, results consistent with previous observations. Furthermore, there were significant increases in the incidences of hemangiosarcomas and meningiomas at 0.056 mg/ml, but not higher. However, the incidence of hemangiomas was actually higher in the control group than any of the dose groups. Unfortunately, the incidences of these tumors in historical controls were not provided for an interpretation of the significance of these findings.

## B. Mice

Metam was administered in drinking water at concentrations of 0, 0.018, 0.088, 0.35, or 0.62 mg/ml to groups of 15 C57/10JfAP/Alpk mice of each sex for 90 days (Whiles, 1991). Five mice of each sex and group were scheduled for an interim kill on the 28th of the study. The mean daily dosages for this study were 2.7, 11.7, 52.4, and 78.7 mg/kg for males and 3.6, 15.2, 55.4, and 83.8 mg/kg for females. Decomposition of metam over a period of 24 hr in drinking water may have reduced the intended concentrations by as much as 20%, for the highest, and 70% for the lowest, concentrations.

Significant decreases in food consumption and body weight were evident at 0.62 and 0.35 mg/ml for both sexes (Whiles, 1991). At termination, body weights for animals dosed at 0.62 mg/ml were 11–13% lower, and at 0.35 group, they were 7–8% lower than controls. No other dose level was affected. Water consumption was reduced in males at 0.62 mg/ml, with a slight reduction in consumption at 0.35 mg/ml during the first 4 weeks of the study. Water consumption in females was reduced significantly at 0.35 mg/ml and 0.62 mg/ml, but was reduced only slightly at 0.088 mg/ml (with a slight recovery).

On termination, significant decreases in hemoglobin were noted in males at 0.35 mg/ml and higher, and in females at 0.088 mg/ml and higher (Whiles, 1991). Hematocrit and red blood cell levels were decreased in both sexes at 0.62 mg/ml and at 0.088 and 0.35 mg/ml in females. No dose–response relationship was evident among these parameters. Mean red blood cell volume was increased in both sexes at 0.62 mg/ml.

There was an increased ratio of liver/total body weight in treated males at greater than

0.088 mg/ml and in females at 0.35 mg/ml and greater (Whiles, 1991). Kidney/body weight and adrenal/body weight ratios were also increased for both sexes at 0.35 mg/ml and higher. Cystitis was reported in male mice at 0.62 mg/ml. Urinary bladder lesions were reported at 0.088, and 0.35, and 0.62 mg/ml for females. However, there was no evident dose–response relationship among these parameters, except for liver- and kidney/body weight ratios.

In a 2-year study (Horner, 1994), C57BL/10JfCD-1 Alpk mice were given 0.19, 0.074, or 0.23 mg/ml (55 per sex per dose) for 104 weeks. The mean daily dose received was 1.9, 7.2, or 28.9 mg/kg for males, and 2.6, 9.6, or 31.2 mg/kg for females. Decreased body weights and food consumption (sporadically) were observed at 0.23 mg/ml in males. Water consumption was initially decreased in males and females at the 0.23 mg/ml, than recovered and increased. At 0.23 mg/ml there was increased mean cell hemoglobin value in both sexes; females had decreased RBC count at this dose. Decreases in organ weights were observed for epididymus and kidney in males at dose levels of 0.074 mg/ml and above. Liver weights were increased at 0.074 mg/ml and higher in both sexes, and kidney weights were increased in females at the same dose levels. Signs of urinary bladder inflammation were evident: epithelial hyperplasia, mononuclear cell infiltration, eosinophilic–hyaline cytoplasmic inclusions, submucosal inflammatory cell infiltration, and submucosal hyalinization (at 0.074 mg/ml and higher for both sexes). Increases in hepatic fat vacuolization were evident at 0.23 mg/ml in both sexes. Increases in hemosiderosis was reported in females at 0.23 mg/ml. Angiosarcoma of the urinary bladder was increased in both sexes at 0.23 mg/ml. One transitional cell carcinoma and one transitional cell papilloma, two rare tumors of the bladder, were also reported at the high dose.

## C. Dogs

In a subchronic range-finding study in beagle dogs, groups of one dog per sex were given 0, 2.5, 10, or 25 mg/kg per day in gelatin capsules (Brammer, 1992a). Because the dogs regurgitated the capsules at 25 mg/kg per day, this dose was reduced to 15 mg/kg per day. An additional two dogs were added to the 15- mg/kg per day dose groups. After 3–4 weeks, two male dogs at 15 mg/kg per day were euthanized because of weight loss and clinical signs of jaundice. Females did not show these marked effects. The remaining dogs were dosed through the ninth week.

Animals dosed with 15 mg/kg per day of metam exhibited up to 40% body weight reductions (Brammer, 1992a). Decreased liver weight of 50–60% was also observed in the euthanized animals. Histopathological examination of these livers showed marked hepatitis, hepatocellular necrosis, slight to moderate hepatocellular pigmentation, and lymphocyte infiltration. The surviving dogs at 15 mg/kg per day had minimal to slight periportal inflammation, lymphocyte infiltration, and minimal to slight hepatocyte pigmentation. Dogs at 10 mg/kg per day had minimal to slight periportal inflammation, with inflammatory cell infiltration, and slight to moderate hepatocyte pigmentation. Renal cortical tubular degeneration and cast formation of moderate severity were also noted in a male and female dog at 15 mg/kg per day.

Clinical chemistry results paralleled those seen following histopathological evaluation. Male dogs at 15 mg/kg per day exhibited increased bilirubin, ALP, ALT, and AST levels, which are indicative of liver injury. In one dog, increases in plasma urea and creatinine were observed, suggesting renal damage. Prothrombin time was increased in the sacrificed animals, and there was an increase in platelet counts for females dosed with 10 or 15 mg/kg per day. Significant increases in ALT and ALP and a minimal increase in AST were observed in male and female dogs at 10 mg/kg per day. At 2.5 mg/kg per day a time-dependent increase in ALT was observed in a female dog.

In a 90-day toxicity study (Brammer, 1992b), beagle dogs (four dogs per sex per dose) were administered metam in capsules at doses of 0, 1, 5, or 10 mg/kg per day. Clinical signs included postdosing emesis at the two highest doses, and increased salivation associated with dosing at the highest dose. Decreased body weight and food consumption also occurred at 5 and 10 mg/kg per day. There were slight decreases in red blood cell parameters at 5 and 10 mg/kg per day, and prothrombin time was increased at 10 mg/kg per day. There were increases in plasma enzymes AST, ALP, ALT, γ-glutamyltransferase (GGT), or total bilirubin. These changes were indicative of liver damage and increased in incidence and severity with dose, occurring at all treatment levels. Two dogs at 10 mg/kg per day, one male and one female, were sacrificed near the end of the treatment period owing to poor clinical condition. Necropsy findings included abnormal liver coloration and texture at 5 and 10 mg/kg per day, with jaundice also present in the sacrificed animals. Histologically, severe hepatitis, composed of hepatocyte degeneration, and necrosis, inflammation, and increased pigmentation and biliary proliferation, was present in all animals at 10 mg/kg per day. Less severe changes were present at 5 mg/kg per day, and one female at 1 mg/kg per day had bile duct proliferation and inflammatory cell infiltration. Other treatment-related changes, included a minimal to slight increase in the number of mitoses of the urinary bladder epithelial cells in several animals at 5 and 10 mg/kg per day. A single occurrence of thymic atrophy, and of immature testis and prostate that occurred at the 10 mg/kg per day (males) may not have been treatment-related.

Finally, concluding the series of studies on the dog (Brammer, 1994), a 1-year exposure study was performed. Four beagle dogs of each sex, were dosed with 0, 0.05, 0.1, or 1.0 mg/day daily in gelatin capsules. No overt clinical signs were observed, except for salivation with dosing, at all doses. Significant elevation of plasma ALT and histopathology was observed in the liver of one female of the 1-mg/kg dose group, which paralleled the liver histopathology seen in previous studies, but was of reduced severity. One male of the same dose group had slightly less than 8% depression in body weight. There was no clear trend in inhibition of body weight gain in any of the dose groups. However, there was an increase in ALT for the 1-mg/kg per day female dose group and a slight trend in the other dose groups. Alkaline phosphate was elevated in both sexes at 1 mg/kg per day, whereas plasma triglycerides decreased in females.

## V.  OTHER TOXICITY

### A.  Inhalation Toxicity

Groups of 18 adult CD (Sprague–Dawley) rats of both sexes were exposed in chambers to Vapam Technical mist generated by nebulizers at cumulative mean concentrations of either 0, 6.5, 45, or 160 mg/m$^3$ for 6 hr per day, 5 days per week, for a total of 65 days (Knapp, 1983). Concentrations of MITC were monitored in these exposure chambers and did not exceed 0.7, 2.2, and 5.7 mg/m$^3$, respectively.

No significant systemic toxicities or treatment-related deaths were observed. Body weight and food consumption were decreased in the high-dose animals. Reduced amounts of total serum proteins, including albumin, occurred at all dose levels of females. A significant decrease in the level of serum albumin and an increase in liver weight, suggesting some hepatic dysfunction, were noted in females exposed to 160 mg/m$^3$. This level of metam also produced a noticeable change in the nasal passages, including mild hyperplasia of the mucigenic epithelium and lymphocytic rhinitis. Although gastric erosion was noted, it was attributed to treatment-related stress by the investigators.

Histopathological examination of the kidneys of male rats exposed to 45 mg/m$^3$ revealed microscopic lesions. However, it was not clear that these observations were treatment-related, since similar effects were not seen in rats exposed to 160 mg/m$^3$, nor in treated female rats.

## B.  Dermal Toxicity

Metam fluid (42%) was diluted in 0.8% aqueous hydroxypropylmethyl cellulose gel and applied to the skin of White Russian rabbits at 0 (vehicle), 31.25, 62.5, or 125 mg/kg per day, continuously for 21 days (Leuschner, 1979). Five rabbits per sex per dose had approximately 10% of their body covered with a nonocclusive dressing over intact or abraded skin. Animals at 62.5-mg/kg dose group showed slight to moderate reversible erythema and edema, corresponding to Draize stage 1–2. The 125-mg/kg dose groups showed more severe skin injury, corresponding to stage 2–3, which is marked epidermal dermatitis. All skin changes were reversed after a 3-week observation period. No intolerance reaction was observed after challenge doses of the same concentrations administered 21 days after skin treatments. No significant differences among food and water intake, clinical chemistry parameters, clinical observation, or histological assessments were noted.

## C.  Developmental Toxicity

Metam was administered to pregnant Wistar rats (25 per group) by oral gavage on days 6–15 of gestation at dose levels of 0, 10, 40, or 120 mg/kg per day (Hellwig and Hildebrand, 1987). Maternal toxicity, as evidenced by reduced body weight, reduced weight gain, and reduced food intake, was observed in the 40- and 120-mg/kg per day groups. Significantly decreased numbers of live fetuses (resulting from increased embryolethality, mostly early postimplantation loss) were observed at 10 and 120 mg/kg per day, and preimplantation loss was increased in the 40-mg/kg per day group (Hellwig and Hildebrand, 1987). In addition to embryolethality, 2 cases of meningocele (a neural tube closure defect) in 261 fetuses (0.8%) in 1 of 22 litters (5%) were observed with a maternal dose of 120 mg/kg per day, and in 12 cases out of 291 fetuses (4%) in 7 of 24 litters (29%) at 240 mg/kg per day in a dose range-finding study that preceded the main study. Although only two cases of meningocele and one case of microphthalmia were observed in the high-dose group, there was zero incidence of meningocele in historical controls.

In a recent study conducted in rats, mated female Alpk:APfSD rats (24 per dose) were given metam at 0, 5, 20, or 60 mg/kg by gavage on days 7–16 of gestation (Pearson, 1993). Clinical signs, salivation, stains around mouth, subdued behavior, and urinary incontinence, were more prevalent at doses of 20 and 60 mg/kg. There was a decrease in food consumption and body weight of dams at doses of 20 and 60 mg/kg, and a decrease in fetal weights at 20 and 60 mg/kg. Preimplantation loss was significantly higher at 60 mg/kg. An increase in skeletal anomalies was noted at doses of 20 mg/kg and higher, and severe malformations were noted at 60 mg/kg. There was one case of meningocele and anophthalmia, and two cases of microphthalmia.

In a Soviet study, an unknown quantity of white female rats, weighing 180–200 g, were treated with 0, 4.5, or 90 mg/kg per day carbathion (metam) from the beginning of their pregnancy until their 20th day (Chegrinets et al., 1990). Carbathion was diluted in water and administered to the rats in a periodic fashion on a daily basis. Although not specified in the study, the route of administration was assumed to be oral gavage. There was a significant increase in postimplantation, but not preimplantation, deaths at 90 mg/kg per day. The fetal body lengths and weights in this dose group were significantly less than controls. In addition, there was a significant increase in edema found in various organs and tissues and one case of hydrocephalus. Nine cases of umbilical hernia were also observed. There were no reported malformations. However, there was an increase in the number of delayed ossifications, 75% in the high-dose group, when compared with 12.5% in the controls. No significant increases in weight, length, or other identifiable changes or defects were noted for the low-dose group.

In an earlier Soviet study (Nesterova, 1969), rats dosed with 22 mg/kg before and through pregnancy and for 1 month after parturition, showed no significant differences in number of progeny, mean body weight, and length from control rats. On gross examination, young rats exhibited no pathological changes.

Metam was also administered to artificially inseminated female Himalayan rabbits (15 per group) by oral gavage at dose levels of 0, 10, 30, or 100 mg/kg per day on days 6–18 postinsemination (Hellwig, 1989). Reduced food intake and weight gain were observed in dams at 100 mg/kg per day. At 100 mg/kg per day, a significant increase in embryolethality (early postimplantation deaths) and a statistically significant trend toward the same effect at 30 mg/kg per day were observed (Hellwig, 1989). Two cases of neural tube defects out of 48 fetuses (4%) in 2 of 14 litters (14%) were reported at the maternal dose of 100 mg/kg per day.

In another study (Hodge, 1993), 20 mated New Zealand white females were administered metam at doses of 0, 5, 20, or 60 mg/kg by gavage. Food consumption and body weights were significantly reduced at the 20- and 60-mg/kg doses. Some clinical signs, including blood stains were evident at the 60-mg/kg dose. Postimplantation loss, early intrauterine deaths, and total litter resorptions were increased at 60 mg/kg. The incidence of skeletal variants increased at the 20-mg/kg dose, and the increase was significant at the 60-mg/kg dose. There were two fetuses with cleft palate and one fetus with meningocele at 60 mg/kg.

## D.  Immunotoxicological Studies

The immunotoxicity of metam (Vapam) was assessed in female B6C3F1 mice (6–10 weeks of age) by oral or dermal administration at a dose of 300 mg/kg per day orally or 150, 225, or 300 mg/kg per day, dermally (Pruett et al., 1992). Each experimental group included six mice in the oral study and five in the dermal study.

The greatest effects noted with oral administration of metam were decreases in thymus weight and cellularity at all time points and a decrease in lymphocyte numbers. There were transient behavioral changes throughout the study. An oral dose of 300 mg/kg per day of metam was near the "maximum tolerated dose" for up to 14 days, during which there was a 10% decrease in body weight. The body weight decrease was greater at 10 days of exposure (23%). The decrease in body weight may contribute to some immunological changes secondary to generalized toxicity, but some of the changes occurred after the 3- and 5-day treatments (and in other experiments in this report) were accompanied by less than 10% decrease in body weight; therefore, these are not considered likely to be secondary to generalized toxicity. Body weight, thymus weight, and lymphocyte numbers rebounded to higher values after 14 days, suggesting the induction of compensatory or detoxification mechanisms.

The changes in bone marrow and spleen parameters following oral administration at 300 mg/kg per day may also represent homeostatic mechanisms to compensate for lymphocyte loss by increased hemopoiesis. Among the depletion of all thymocyte subpopulations, CD4+CD8+ cells were depleted to the greatest extent.

Humoral immune response by splenocytes from mice treated at 300 mg/kg per day was suppressed when stimulated in vitro (IgM, SRBC) but not in vivo, and antibody production (all isotypes) in vivo was not affected. The number of IgM antibody-forming colonies (AFC) was increased significantly at 150 and 225 mg/kg per day, but not at 300 mg/kg per day. Lymphocyte responses to T- and B-cell mitogens and allogeneic lymphocytes were not affected.

After dermal administration of metam to mice, significant decreases in thymus weight and selective depletion of CD4+CD8+ subpopulations at 300 mg/kg per day were seen, and the suppressed natural killer cell activity at 200 and 300 mg/kg per day was consistent with the effect seen after oral administration.

In a different study by the same group (Padget et al., 1992), the immunotoxicity of metam was compared with two other dithiocarbamates: sodium diethyl dithiocarbamate (DEDC) and disodium ethylene-bis(dithiocarbamate) (EDB). These compounds were administered in doses ranging from 150 to 1000 mg/kg per day for 7 days to female B6C3F1 mice. At sacrifice, measurements were made of thymus and spleen weights and of natural killer cell activity. In addition, direct measurement of cytotoxicity of these compounds was made toward splenocytes and thymocytes in vitro.

Significant loss of thymic weight was observed in mice following 200, 225, or 300 mg/kg per day of metam. Spleen weight increased only marginally at 225 and 300 mg/kg per day. Natural killer cell activity was suppressed at doses of 150, 225, and 300 mg/kg per day, all of which confirmed the results of the previous study (Pruett et al., 1992)]. Very high doses of either EBD and DEDC (over 600 mg/kg per day) were required to affect either spleen or thymus weight, and neither affected splenic natural killer cell activity. Thus, the lack of change in natural killer cell activity from dosing with EBD and DEDC is probably not associated with splenomegaly. When relative cytotoxic potencies were compared in vitro among the three compounds, they were all comparably toxic. This result is in direct contrast with the apparent higher toxicity of metam over the other compounds in vivo, and may be the result of the different metabolites formed from each compound. In particular, MITC is not formed by hydrolysis from either EBD or DEDC as it is with metam.

## E. Neurotoxicity

An acute neurotoxicity study was performed in SD Crl:CDBR rats (12–16 per sex per dose) administered metam in one dose of 0, 50, 750, or 1500 mg/kg by gavage (Lamb, 1993). Animals were monitored for up to 2 weeks. There was a significant decrease in body weight gain at doses of 750 and 1500 mg/kg in both sexes. There was an increase in clinical signs, such as gait alterations, high carriage hypoactive, hypothermia, ptosis, and decreased defecation and urination at doses of 750 and 1500 mg/kg. Mortality was 31 and 19% for high-dose males and females, respectively. There was an increase in effects in the functional observational battery at 750- and 1500-mg/kg doses. Locomotor activity was affected significantly in both sexes at all doses on the same day as dosing, but exhibited normal motor activity, subsequently. Body temperature was depressed at 750- and 1500-mg/kg doses, and remained depressed for up to 7 days.

Twelve male and female rats were given metam by drinking water at 0, 0.0.2, 0.06, and 0.2 mg/ml for 13 weeks (Allen, 1994). Delivered mean doses were estimated to be 6, 14.7, mg/kg for males and 3.3, 8.4, and 17.8 mg/kg for females. These animals were monitored for clinical status, overall appearance, and measures for neurological function. The functional neurologic battery consisted of quantitative assessment of landing foot splay, sensory perception, and muscle weakness and changes in respiration. At 0.2 mg/ml, food and water consumption and body weight were reduced in both sexes. Water consumption was reduced also in the 0.06-mg/ml males and the 0.02-mg/ml females. No evidence for metam effects was seen on clinical, behavioral, or neurological status of the animals, although there was a high background rate of neuron necrosis and nerve fiber degeneration.

## F. Genotoxicity Studies

Metam was evaluated for its genotoxicity in in vivo and in vitro assays. Responses observed were mostly negative, with a suggestion for potential chromosomal aberration in human lymphocyte culture in one study. The studies are summarized in Table 2.

**Table 2**  Genetic Toxicity Studies for Metam

| Test type | Strains/cell treatment | Results | Ref. |
|---|---|---|---|
| Ames | *Salmonella typhimurium* TA1535, 1537, 1538, 92, 98, 100 (+/− S9) | Negative | BASF, 1987a |
| Ames | *S. typhimurium* TA 1535, 1537, 1538, 98, 100 (+/− S9) | Negative | Gentile et al., 1982 |
| Yeast | *Sacchromyces cerevisiae* strain D4 (+/− S9) | Negative | BASF, 1987a |
| HGPRT | Chinese hamster ovary 1 mg/kg per day (+/− S9) | Equivocal (potential positive with S9) | BASF, 1987b |
| Human lymphocyte cytogenetics | Human lymphocytes | Aberrant chromosomes, gaps | BASF, 1987c |
| Mammalian cytogenetics | Chinese hamsters treated with 0, 150, and 300 mg/kg sacrificed at 6, 24, 48 h | Polyploidy at all dose levels occurrence as soon as 6 h | BASF, 1987d |
| *Rec* assay | *Bacillus subtilis* H17 and M45 (+/− S9) | Equivocal | Hazleton, 1987a |
| Unscheduled DNA synthesis | Primary rat hepatocyte culture | Negative | Hazleton, 1987b |

## VI.  TOXICOLOGY: FROM ANIMALS TO HUMANS

## A.  Toxicity: Metam Versus Breakdown Products

The existing experimental studies on metam demonstrate that the most consistent and prominent toxic effects by any route of exposure include loss of body weight, which may be dependent on decreased food and water consumption, and irritation of exposed areas. Metam appears to be both a dermal irritant and sensitizer in humans. However, these irritant and sensitizing effects may be the result of conversion of metam to MITC, itself a strong irritant. The lack of significant irritation to the eye, or the nonirritancy of metam when applied to the skin, then washed off (Nesterova, 1969), indicate that metam does not immediately react with exposed surfaces. Some evidence for immunotoxicity is available, but data are limited to high doses.

With long-term administration, metam exposure was associated with hepatic, renal–urinary, hematological, and olfactory system toxicity. In all three species tested, rat, mouse, and dog, changes in urinary morphology and function were noted. Mice, the most sensitive species to these changes, exhibited higher incidences of angiosarcoma of the bladder and the appearance of two rare bladder tumors. Dogs were very sensitive to the hepatotoxicity induced by metam. At very low doses, 1.0–10 mg/kg per day, metam was associated with mild to severe liver injury. Depression in red blood cell counts and hematocrits was seen in rodent species, but its association with long-term toxicity is unknown. Damage to the olfactory epithelium did not appear to result from direct irritation by exhaled MITC, but from blood-borne metabolites or from metabolites produced by the olfactory epithelium.

The marked hepatoxic effects present in the dog studies were in contrast with the general lack of liver damage in most of the rodent studies. This may be due to the different methods used for dose administration. The dogs were dosed by capsule and thus received metam in a bolus, whereas rodents generally received the compound in a more gradual manner by their drinking water. The bolus dose might initially produce higher blood levels of metam or its metabolites, possibly leading to hepatocyte disruption and clinical signs of liver disease. Species differences in the biotransformation of metam could also be involved, but studies comparing enzymatic or microsomal function after metam administration have not been reported. Also unknown is the potential for permanent scarring of the liver after metam-induced cell death.

It is incontrovertible that metam causes fetal loss and specific birth defects. Evidence from five studies in two species shows an increased fetal loss and potential for a rare defect, meningocele, are associated with oral intakes of metam. Therefore, metam should be considered a developmental toxicant.

There is little evidence that would indicate the mechanism of toxicity of metam, particularly how it induces death. Nesterova (1969) suggested that the effects of metam may result from a reaction with sulfhydryl groups on proteins, which then leads to disruption of cellular respiration. Although, this explanation may be adequate for the interpretation of the localized irritant effects, it does not provide an adequate explanation for the observed teratogenic or hepatotoxic effects.

The experimental results described in the foregoing indicate that metam is predominantly converted in vivo to MITC by a nonenzymatic process. The MITC is more toxic than metam in both shorter- and longer-term exposures. Besides being a strong skin irritant and sensitizer, MITC exposure produces eye and gastric irritation, significant inhibition of body weight gain, lower food consumption, decreased red cell counts and increased white cell counts, fatty changes in the liver and increases in liver weight, and decreased sperm counts (OEHHA, 1992). However, the toxicity profile of MITC does not correspond well with that of metam, except in the areas of weight loss, skin and stomach irritation and, perhaps, liver pathology.

Orally administered metam can also produce significant amounts of $CS_2$ in the stomach, (catalyzed by its low pH). Therefore, some of the observed toxicities seen with oral doses of metam in experimental animals (but not with MITC administration), may be mediated by the formation of $CS_2$. Unfortunately, the toxicity of carbon disulfide does not correspond well with metam either. Carbon disulfide is known for its neurotoxicity and cardiovascular effects reported in humans, effects that are entirely absent from the metam toxicity profile (ATSDR, 1992). However, carbon disulfide toxicity has not been studied well in experimental animals. Carbon disulfide is known to reversibly inhibit cytochrome P-450 enzymes; and thus may modulate toxicities of other metam metabolites, notably MITC (Masuda, 1986).

The differences in the toxicity profiles for metam and MITC compounds could also be due to the substantially higher experimental doses of administered metam, when compared with doses of administered MITC. The results of dermal, inhalation, and oral studies indicate that animals were more able to tolerate higher doses of metam than MITC. MITC is much more irritating and inhibiting to normal feeding behavior than metam (OEHHA, 1992). Maximum doses administered to animals were typically three times higher for metam than for MITC. It is possible that some reported effects observed with metam administration were due to MITC, as the result of higher internal doses of MITC achieved from metabolism of metam than from direct administration of MITC.

## B.  Human Health Implications and Risk Assessment

Metam itself is relatively nonvolatile. However, inhalation of contaminated air was the most significant source of exposure following the metam spill because of the rapid conversion in the river of metam to its volatile and more toxic breakdown product MITC. This conversion should be considered in future risk assessments. In this toxic spill, eye irritation, headache, and respiratory effects were the most common complaints in effected individuals. It was likely that these individuals were exposed to the more volatile MITC and $CS_2$ than the parent compound metam. Eye irritation (no lacrimation) was the most sensitive endpoint based on an effect level of 70 ppb of MITC in air in a rat study (Nesterova, 1969), but this effect was not reported with metam. Additional data are being developed for evaluating the odor threshold and ocular irritation of MITC.

In experimental animal studies, oral administration of metam was associated with fetal loss and a potential for a neural tube defect, meningocele. Neural tube defects are the most common birth defect in humans, but the defects observed with metam in rats and rabbits are rare in these animal species. The possibility that MITC might have contributed to this effect was considered, but cannot be validated. The concern may not exist when exposures to humans are based on long-term, low-level exposures, but acute or short-term exposures following a chemical spill can lead to high-level exposures. Although estimated human inhalation exposures relating to the metam spill were generally below the reference level of 720 ppb for developmental toxicity of MITC, based on the worst-case exposure estimates and the teratogenic potential of metam, an advisory was issued for pregnant women who were in the affected areas to seek medical consultation and be administered the alpha-fetoprotein (AFP) test (DiBartolomeis, 1994). Blood testing at 14–16 weeks of gestation can detect neural tube defects.

Experience gained from toxicological risk assessment of the metam spill underlines the importance of identifying any breakdown products and major ingredients in the original formulation, in addition to the parent compound. Furthermore, in this case sample, metam itself was not specifically identified as a hazardous material under federal Department of Transportation criteria and there was no placard carried with the derailed train involved. Therefore, there was a delay in identifying the content of the tank car. Moreover, information on toxicity and physical and chemical property should be readily available to permit an adequate assessment. This information has to be assembled from diverse sources during the response period to the toxic spill in the process of risk assessment. The information presented here provides a toxicological base for metam and some guidance for risk assessment in the future.

## ACKNOWLEDGMENTS

The author is grateful to Earl Meierhenry and Marilyn Silva, Department of Pesticide Regulation, Cal/EPA, for their help in obtaining and summarizing studies, and review of the manuscript.

## REFERENCES

Allen, S. L. (1991). Metam-sodium: 90 day drinking water study in rats. Final Report, ICI Central Toxicological Laboratory, Study No. CTL/P/3213, Oct. 21.

Allen, S. L. (1994). Metam sodium: Subchronic neurotoxicity study in rats, Zeneca CTL., Report No. CTL/P/4334, May 5.

ATSDR (1992). The toxicological profile for carbon disulfide, Agency for Toxic Substances and Disease Registry, TP-91/09.

Baran, N. A., Y. A. Moreinis, and Y. A. Troitski (1969). Nekotoriye daniye po gigiyenicheskoy oschinke i beologecheckoy chenosti peschevch producktov posle obrabotki karbotion. [Some data on the hygienic assessment and biological value of food products following carbathione treatment], *Vopr. Ratsion. Pitan.*, 5, 37–41.

BASF (1987a). Report on the study of metam-sodium in the Ames test, BASF Aktiengesellschaft, FRG, Project No. 40/IM0232/85, June 15.

BASF (1987b). Report on the study for gene mutations in vitro of metam-sodium in Chinese-hamster ovary cells (HGPRT locus) with and without metabolic activation, BASF Aktiengesellschaft, FRG; Project No. 40/IM0232/85, Aug. 3.

BASF (1987c). Report on the in vitro cytogenetic investigations in human lymphocytes with metam-sodium, BASF Aktiengesellschaft, FRG, Project No. 30MO232/8574, Mar. 9.

BASF (1987d). Cytogenetic study in vivo of metam-sodium in Chinese hamster, bone marrow chromosome analysis. Single oral administration, BASF Aktiengesellschaft, FRG, Project No. 10 MO232/85116, Aug. 3.

Brammer, A. (1992a). Metam: Range finding oral toxicity study in dogs, Report No. CTL/T/2778, ICI Central Toxicology Laboratory, April 7.

Brammer, A. (1992b). Metam-sodium: 90-day oral dosing study in dogs, ICI Americas Report No. CTL/P/3679, Nov. 11.

Brammer, A. (1994). Metam-sodium: One-year oral toxicity in dogs, Zeneca CTL., Report No. CTL/P/4196, May 23.

Cave, D. A. (1991a). Metam-sodium: 11 day oral dosing study in rats, ICI Central Toxicology Laboratory. Report No. CTL/T/2727, Jan. 16.

Cave, D. A. (1991b). Metam-sodium: 90 day drinking water study in rats, Interm Report, ICI Central Toxicology Laboratory, Study No. CTL/P/3213, Oct. 21.

Chegrinets, G. Y., V. E. Karmazin, I. Y. Rybchinskaya, R. P. Petrova, and G. I. Leonskaya (1990). Yzuchenia vliyania karbateona na embriohenez byelikh kris. [Study of the influence of carbathion on embryogenesis of white rats], *Gig. Sanit.,* 5, 40–41.

Deenihan, M. J. (1985). Acute dermal toxicity of Vapam in rabbits, Northview Pacific Laboratories Inc., Berkeley CA, Report No. X6J034G, Jan. 7 and May 7.

DiBartolomeis, M. J., G. V. Alexeef, A. M. Fan, and R. J. Jackson (1994). Regulatory approach to assessing health risks of toxic chemical releases following transportation accidents, *J. Hazard. Mater.,* 39, 193–210.

Gentile, J. M., G. J. Gentile, J. Bultman, R. Sechriest, E. D. Wagner and M.J. Plewa (1982). An evaluation of the genotoxic properties of insecticides following plant and animal activation, *Mutat. Res.,* 101, 19–29.

Hawkings, D. B. (1987). The biokinetics and metabolism of $^{14}$C-metam in the rat, Vols 1–3, Addendum and Amendment, Huntingdon Research Centre, GB, BASF Report No. 88/0030, Nov. 12.

Hazleton (1987a). Report on the mutagenicity test on metam-sodium in the *rec*-assay with *Bacillus subtilis,* Hazleton Biotechnologies, The Netherlands; HBC Study No. E-9642-0-404, Mar. 27.

Hazleton (1987b). Report on the mutagenicity test on metam-sodium in the rat primary hepatocyte unscheduled DNA synthesis assay, Hazleton Laboratories America, Inc., HLA Study No. 9735-0-447, July 1.

Hellwig, J., and B. Hildebrand (1987). Report on the study of the prenatal toxicity of metam-sodium in rats after oral administration (gavage), BASF Aktiengesellschaft, FRG, Project No. 340232/8569, Mar. 25.

Hellwig, J. (1989). Report on the study of the prenatal toxicity of metam-sodium (aqueous solution) in rabbits after oral administration (gavage), BASF Aktiengesellschaft, FRG, Project No. 38R0232/8597, July 15.

Hodge, M. C. E. (1993). Metam sodium developmental toxicity study in the rabbit, Zeneca Central Laboratory, Cheshire, U.K., Report No. RB0623, Sept. 6.

Horner, S. A. (1994). Metam sodium: Two-year drinking study in mice, Zeneca CTL., Report No. CTL/P/4095, Apr. 20.

Howd, R. (1992). Chemistry, environmental fate, and monitoring in evaluation of health risks associated with the metam spill in the upper Sacramento River, Office of Environmental Health Hazard Assessment, Cal/EPA, Draft, Sec. B.

Jung, H. -D., and F. Wolff (1979). Berufliche Kontaktdermatitiden durch Nematin (Vapam) in der Landwirtschaft [Study of contact dermatitis from nematin (Vapam) in agriculture], *Dtsch. Gesuntheitwes.,* 25, 495–498.

Jung, H. -D. (1979) Arbeitsdermatosen durch Pestizide (Occupational dermatosis from pesticides), *Dtsch. Gesundheitwes.,* 34, 1144–1148.

Knapp, H. I. (1983). Subchronic inhalation study with Vapam Technical in rats. Environmental Health Science Center, Stauffer Chemical, Farmington, CT, Study T11006, Aug. 31.

Lamb, I. C. (1993). An acute neurotoxicity study of metam sodium in rats, WIL Research Laboratories, Inc., WIL-1880 09, Sept. 27.

Leuschner, F. (1979). 3-weeks-toxicity of metam-sodium fluid (methyl-dithio carbamic sodium) lot BAS

00500N—called for short "metam-sodium fluid"—during local administration in rabbits, Laboratorium fuer Pharmacologie und Toxikologie, BASF, FRG; Document 79/0140, Feb. 12.

Masuda, Y., M. Yasoshima, and N. Nakayama (1986). Early, selective and reversible suppression of cytochrome P-450-dependent monoxygenase of liver microsomes following the administration of low doses of carbon disulfide in mice, *Biochem. Pharmacol.*, 35, 3941–3947.

Miller, J. L. (1979). Acute inhalation study of Vapam Technical in albino rats, Northview Pacific Laboratories Inc., Berkeley CA, Report T-6457, June 1.

Morgan, R. L. (1985). Acute toxicity test battery for Vapam Technical, Stauffer Chemical Co., Richmond CA, Report T11494, Jan. 17.

Mutter, L. C. (1987). Dermal sensitization test with Vapam Technical. Final report, T-12378, Richmond Toxicology Laboratory, Richmond, CA, Apr. 24.

Nesterova, M. F. (1969). Standards for carbathion in working zone air, *Gig. Sanit.*, 34(5), 33–37.

Northview (1987a). Acute oral toxicity of Vapam in rats, Northview Pacific Labs Inc., Berkeley, CA, Report No. X6J034G, Jan. 7, and Oct. 7.

Northview (1987b). Primary skin irritation in rabbits, Northview Pacific Labs, Berkeley, CA, Report No. X6J34G, Jan. 7.

Northview (1987c). Primary eye irritation of Vapam in rabbits, Northview Pacific Labs, Berkeley, CA, Report No. X6J34, Jan. 7.

OEHHA (1992). Evaluation of the health risks associated with the metam spill in the upper Sacramento River. External review draft. Office of Environmental Health Hazard Assessment, California Environmental Protection Agency, Sept. 21.

Padgett, E. L., D. B. Barnes, and S. B. Pruett (1992). Disparate effects of representative dithiocarbamates on selected immunological parameters in vivo and cell survival in vitro in female B6C3F1 mice, *J. Toxicol. Environ. Health*, 37, 559–571.

Pearson, F. J. (1993). Metam sodium developmental toxicity study in the rat. Zeneca Central Laboratory, Cheshire, U.K., Report No. CTL/P/4052, Oct. 5.

Pruett, S. B., D. B. Barnes, Y. C. Han, and A. E. Munson (1992). Immunological characteristics of sodium methyldithiocarbamate, *Fundam. Appl. Toxicol.*, 18, 40–47.

Rattray, N. J. (1994). Metam sodium: Two-year drinking study in rats, Zeneca CTL., Report No. CTL/P/4139, May 23.

Rothstein, E. C. (1987). Acute inhalation toxicity in rats of metam labelled Vapam, Leberco Testing, Inc., Roselle Park, NJ, Report No. U6J005G, Feb. 12.

Schubert, H. (1978). Contact dermatitis to sodium *N*-methyldithiocarbamate, *Contact Dermatitis*, 4, 370–382.

Whiles, A. J. (1991). Metam-sodium: 90 day drinking water study in mice with a 28 day interim kill, ICI Central Toxicology Laboratory, Study No. CTL/P/3185, Sept. 26.

# 34
# Effects of Chemical–Chemical Interactions on the Evaluation of Toxicity

**Amy L. Yorks and Katherine S. Squibb**

*University of Maryland at Baltimore*
*Baltimore, Maryland*

## I. INTRODUCTION

The last two decades have seen great strides in our ability to assess the health risks of chemicals present in our air, water, and food. Our ever-growing scientific databases are increasing our understanding of the dose–response toxicity of individual chemicals and are permitting better predictions of health effects. However, we are now reaching the point at which we can, and must, increase the complexity of our calculations and incorporate chemical–chemical interactions into our risk assessment analyses.

Although single-compound exposures are possible, in most instances, contaminant chemicals are present in our environment as mixtures. Some of these mixtures are relatively well defined, such as coke oven emissions and diesel exhaust. Other mixtures, such as those released from old disposal sites, are highly variable, complex, and largely undefined. As there is a considerable body of literature indicating that chemical–chemical interactions occur, factors that influence the toxicity of the chemicals in mixtures must be better understood if they are to be effectively incorporated into our health risk assessments (EPA, 1986).

In theory, there are many ways in which one chemical could alter the toxicity of another. As indicated in Table 1, two chemicals could directly interact to form a new compound, or there may be changes in the intestinal absorption of the chemicals. Absorption could be decreased through competition for membrane-binding sites, or increased by the induction of a transport process. Plasma transport, tissue accumulation, and elimination processes could also be altered through competition or interference mechanisms. Cellular metabolism and intracellular effects may be modified either directly through competition for receptor- or enzyme-binding sites, or indirectly by the induction of metabolizing enzymes or other detoxification mechanisms, such

**Table 1**  Mechanisms by Which Chemicals Can Interact in Biological Systems to Alter Toxicity

Formation of new compounds
    Reactions between chemicals in the exposure media or in the digestive tract before absorption
Changes in intestinal absorption
    Competition for membrane-binding sites
    Induction of proteins that facilitate absorption
Altered plasma transport
    Competitive binding to transport proteins
Altered excretion patterns
    Competition for secretory pathways
    Altered metabolism of compounds to forms more or less easily excreted
Altered cellular toxicity
    Competitive binding to essential ligands in catalytic and regulatory proteins
    Metabolism by biotransformation enzymes to more or less toxic forms
    Competitive binding to or induction of metallothionein
    Changes in cellular glutathione concentrations
    Alterations in DNA repair enzymes

as metal-binding proteins or cellular glutathione levels (Dixon and Nadolney, 1987; Goldstein et al., 1990a; Davis, 1980).

Because of these interactions, it is not surprising that the net toxicity of a group of chemicals often cannot be predicted accurately by summing the toxicity of its individual components (Dixon and Nadolney, 1987). Chemicals can interact in additive, synergistic, or antagonistic fashions. *Additive* refers to a response equaling the sum of individual effects, whereas *synergism* is a response that is greater than additive. On the other hand, some chemical–chemical interactions can lead to a decrease in toxicological activity (this process serves as the basis of antidotal treatment) (Dixon and Nadolney, 1987). In this instance, the response is less than that shown by each chemical and is referred to as *antagonistic* (Goldstein et al., 1990a).

Although the problem of chemical–chemical interactions in risk assessment is relatively easily defined, its solution (with over 70,000 chemicals being manufactured and sold by more than 115,000 industries and firms) is extremely complex (Dixon and Nadolney, 1987). The following sections will review examples of the types of chemical–chemical interactions that have occurred in laboratory studies. We hope that this overview will serve as a catalyst for a greater research effort in this area. If risk assessments are to be successfully applied to chemical mixtures, we must understand the basis for the effects that occur when multiple chemicals are present.

## II.  ORGANIC–ORGANIC CHEMICAL INTERACTIONS

### A.  Biotransformation Enzymes

The toxicity of most organic chemicals is influenced by the action of mixed-function oxidases (MFOs) and phase II biotransformation enzymes that catalyze their metabolism to more hydrophilic forms in preparation for excretion. Because the synthesis of many of these enzymes is increased by the chemicals they metabolize, multiple mechanisms may be involved in the chemical interactions involving these enzyme systems (Kedderis, 1990). For example, an inhibition of toxicity can occur when the metabolism of one chemical to its more toxic form is prevented by the preferential metabolism of another compound, or when one chemical induces an MFO enzyme system that can catalyze the transformation of a second chemical to a less toxic form. On the other hand, enhancement of toxicity can occur when the enzyme that bioactivates a chemical is previously induced in a cell by exposure to a second compound. Thus, the toxicity of each individual chemical, in each situation, will depend on which biotransformation enzymes have been induced, the relative affinity of each chemical for the available enzymes, and the relative toxicity of the metabolized forms of the chemicals compared with the parent compounds.

There are numerous examples of chemical interactions in experimental animals that have their genesis in biotransformation. Chemicals such as piperonyl butoxide and proadifen (SK&F 525A), which inhibit MFO enzymes, decrease the hepatic toxicity of compounds, such as acetaminophen, bromobenzene, and cocaine, that require activation for toxicity (Mitchell et al., 1973; Reid et al., 1971; Thompson et al., 1979). Increased toxicity can also occur when MFO enzymes are inhibited if a compound is normally converted by these enzymes to a less toxic form. This appears to be the basis for the increased nephrotoxicity of cyclosporine that occurs following cotreatment with compounds such as ketoconazole, methyltestosterone, and erythromycin (Ferguson et al., 1982; Moller and Ekelund, 1985; Jensen et al., 1987).

The induction of specific biotransformation enzymes can also increase or decrease the toxicity and carcinogenicity of organic chemicals by altering their metabolism (Kedderis, 1990). Phenobarbital induction of MFO enzymes increases the acute hepatotoxicity of acetaminophen, 2-acetylaminofluorene, and cocaine (Mitchell et al., 1973; Peraino et al., 1971; Thompson et al., 1979), but decreases the acute lethality of parathion (Mourelle et al., 1986). Argus and co-workers (1978) have reported that the hepatocarcinogenicity of dimethylnitrosamine is increased by β-naphthoflavone, but is decreased by pregnenolone-16α-carbonitrile, presumably owing to the different enzymes induced by these compounds. Also, the nephrotoxic effects of chloroform and carbon tetrachloride are potentiated by ketonic solvents, such as acetone, 2-butanone, and 2-hexanone (Raisbeck et al., 1990).

Many studies have reported that coexposure to chlorinated aromatic hydrocarbons can alter the toxicity of other chemicals (Goldstein et al., 1990b; Kedderis, 1990). Chlorinated aromatic hydrocarbons, such as polychlorinated biphenyls, tetrachlorodibenzo-*p*-dioxin, and polybrominated biphenyls (PCBs, TCDD, and PBBs), are known to be effective inducers of cytochrome P-450 mixed-function oxidase enzymes, which is probably the basis for their effects. Shelton and co-workers (1984) observed that coadministration of PCBs with the well-known carcinogen aflatoxin $B_1$ inhibited the induction of hepatocellular carcinomas in rainbow trout. In in vitro studies, livers from fish treated with PCBs were less efficient in converting aflatoxin $B_1$ to a mutagenic compound, suggesting that the effect of the PCB exposure was to alter the metabolism of the aflatoxin to a less carcinogenic form. Interactions with halogenated hydrocarbons have also been observed, and indicate that there are differences between the chlorinated aromatic compounds. Kluwe and co-workers (Kluwe and Hook, 1978; Kluwe et al., 1979) found that the nephrotoxicity of carbon tetrachloride was greater in animals cotreated with PBBs, but less in animals cotreated with TCDD or PCB (Kluwe and Hook, 1980). Thus, the metabolic activation or detoxification reactions induced by TCDD and PCBs appear to differ from those induced by PBBs.

## 1. Time–Sequence Effects

As studies continue, the complexity of the interactions that can occur between organic chemicals because of changes in biotransformation enzyme systems becomes even more evident. As one might expect, the sequence and timing of the administration of two chemicals can significantly alter their interactive effects (Plaa and Vezina, 1990). Studies by Pessayre and co-workers (1982) have shown that rats treated with trichloroethylene and carbon tetrachloride showed few or no adverse effects when dosed with each agent alone, but when both solvents were administered simultaneously, extensive centrilobular necrosis was exhibited. When dosing was staggered, however, administration of a nonhepatotoxic dose of trichloroethylene 5 hr before the carbon tetrachloride showed enhanced liver injury, whereas the inverse of this process, also at 5-hr increments, resulted in no liver injury (Plaa and Vezina, 1990). Thus, the sequence of exposure is important in determining the interactive effects that occur.

In addition, the timing of the multiple-chemical exposures and the doses used can affect the outcome of an interaction study (Plaa and Vezina, 1990). Plaa and Hewitt (1982), for example, demonstrated that the magnitude of hepatotoxicity caused by chloroform varied over 100-fold when a second chemical, 2,5-hexanedione, was administered 10 versus 50 hr before the chloroform. Also, MacDonald and co-workers (1982) have shown that, whereas low doses of acetone enhanced the toxicity of haloethanes, such as trichlorethane, high-doses reduced toxicity. Thus, nonlinear or biphasic response curves for individual chemicals will lead to nonlinear and biphasic interactive effects that must be considered in predictive studies.

## B.  Promotors

One of the most classic examples of chemical interactions is the relation that exists between initiators and promoters in the carcinogenic process. The first step in carcinogenesis is the interaction of an electrophilic compound with nucleophilic sites, such as nitrogen and oxygen atoms, in DNA. This binding can result in mispairing during DNA replication, eventually causing mutations in specific gene sequences, which results in transformed cells. These alterations in DNA are additive and irreversible, but in many instances they do not produce tumors unless a promotor is present. The effects of promotors, unlike those of initiators, are reversible and nonadditive within a cell. Promotor chemicals are incapable of initiating carcinogenesis (i.e., irreversibly altering the original DNA), but they increase the chance that preneoplastic cells will develop into neoplastic lesions and, thereby, increase the carcinogenicity of an initiating chemical (Silberhorn et al., 1990). Promotors appear to act through a variety of mechanisms, including the stimulation of cell division and alterations in immune surveillance systems.

In the previous section, we reviewed mechanisms by which P-450 mixed-function oxidase-inducing chemicals could alter the carcinogenicity of a compound by altering its metabolism. There is also evidence that mixtures of PCBs, as well as individual congeners, can cause promotion of hepatocellular carcinomas in animals when given at appropriate doses for extended periods (Silberhorn et al., 1990). The PCB mixtures with a high chlorine content are more potent in promoting the induction of neoplastic nodules and hepatocellular carcinomas by benzene hexachloride than mixtures with less chlorination. The promotional activity of PCBs has also been demonstrated in experimental azo dye hepatocarcinogenesis, in which rats given Kanechlor 400 after treatment with 3′-methyl-4-dimethyaminoazobenzene exhibited a greater incidence of hepatic tumors (Kimura et al., 1976 as cited in Pelissier et al. 1992).

Pelissier and co-workers (1992) have found that phenoclor DP6, a French commercial PCB mixture, exerts a promoting effect in aflatoxin $B_1$ (AFB$_1$)-initiated rats. This promotion occurred even after only short periods of exposure to the PCB mixtures. Pelissier et al. (1992) suggest that PCBs may interfere with cellular defense mechanisms that protect against oxygen free radical damage in cells by inhibiting Se-glutathione peroxidase and superoxide dismutase activities in target cells.

Bailey and co-workers (1987) have used rainbow trout in experiments examining the initiation, promotion, and inhibition of cancers induced by AFB$_1$. Dietary treatment of trout with the compounds indole-3-carbinol (I3C), β-naphthoflavone (BNF), or the PCB complex, Aroclor 1254, before and during exposure to AFB$_1$, showed a variety of effects, ranging from inhibition to promotion, depending on the relative timing of the initiator and modulator exposures (Bailey et al., 1987). Results from these experiments indicated that the magnitude of the carcinogenic response did not appear to depend critically on the dose of the carcinogen, but rather, on the dose of the modulator compound (Bailey et al. 1987).

Rojanapo et al. (1993) have shown that DDT, an organochlorine insecticide, markedly inhibits hepatocarcinogenesis (both benign and malignant liver tumors) when it is given to rats at the start of $AFB_1$ exposure. Administering DDT in the middle or after $AFB_1$ treatment results in a significant enhancement of hepatocarcinogenesis, however. The DDT exhibited a maximal tumor-promoting effect when given either 1 or 3 weeks after completion of the $AFB_1$ treatment, increasing the number of animals bearing liver carcinomas as well as the number of carcinomas per animal. These experiments, which show that DDT can be a promotor for $AFB_1$ hepato-carcinogenesis, have implications in the cause of human hepatocellular carcinoma in African and Asian countries (Rojanapo et al., 1993).

It is clear from the foregoing discussion that not only are interrelationships between initiators and promotors important determinants of the final outcome of carcinogen exposure, but they are also very complex. One important aspect of these studies is that it is not necessary for exposures to occur simultaneously for one chemical to affect the carcinogenicity of another.

## III.  METAL–METAL INTERACTIONS

Humans rarely come into contact with simply one toxic metal. Metal contamination reflects natural, as well as anthropogenic, sources in which many metals occur in association with one another. Multiple exposure of humans to toxic metals can arise from metal-based pigments in paints, metal-smelting processes, emissions from coal-fired power plants, and other industrial processes (Mahaffey et al., 1981; Goyer, 1991). Although, historically, studies of metal toxicity have primarily focused on acute responses to high doses of metal exposure, technological advances and society's growing health awareness have redirected our attention to lower-dose, long-term effects of metals for which interactions between multiple metals may become even more important (Schubert et al., 1978; Goyer, 1991).

The toxic effects of metals arise from a wide variety of metal–ligand interactions that can interfere with normal cellular metabolic and regulatory processes. Many essential metal ions, such as $Ca^{+2}$, $Cu^{+2}$, and $Zn^{+2}$, play important roles in cells as components of metalloenzymes and DNA-binding proteins, and as activators of regulatory proteins. Toxic metals may interfere with the normal binding of essential metals to cellular ligands, or may interact with protein –SH, –COOH, or $–NH_3$ groups that are required for normal receptor or enzymatic activity (Squibb and Fowler, in press). The following discussion will be divided into toxic metal–toxic metal interactions and toxic metal–essential metal interactions, for both of these are extremely important in understanding the factors that influence the toxicity of metals.

### A.  Toxic Metal–Toxic Metal Interactions

When more than one toxic metal is present in a cell, the occupation of the critical receptor sites by these metals becomes competitive. Since occupation of the sites by the less toxic metal can partially block the binding of the more toxic metal, it is possible to have a protective effect exerted by one metal on another. Studies by Schubert and co-workers (1978) have demonstrated this effect. They observed that pretreatment of mice with lead (Pb) reduced mortality in mice subsequently administered mercuric chloride. However, these same investigators found that synergistic effects are also possible. When pretreatment occurred with mercury (Hg), far less Pb was needed to saturate or exceed a critical level of the remaining critical sites, leading to an increased sensitivity to lower doses of Pb (Schubert et al., 1978). Factors determining the combined effects of these metals include the intrinsic affinity of the individual metals for the critical binding sites and the relative concentrations and distribution of the metals within the target organ sites (Schubert et al., 1978).

Studies by Yanez and co-workers (1991) have demonstrated interactive effects of other toxic metals on median lethal dose ($LD_{50}$) values. In rats exposed to arsenic (As) and cadmium (Cd), 24-hr $LD_{50}$ values were decreased when Cd and As were administered simultaneously, compared with those obtained for the individual metals. Results indicated that As had a greater effect on the $LD_{50}$ values for Cd than vice versa. Additional studies by this group indicated that As decreased hepatic concentrations of Cd, whereas Cd increased As concentrations in heart tissue.

Recent studies, using more sensitive measures of toxicity, have also shown interactions of toxic metals. Studies of the nephrotoxic metals, Pb, Cd, and As, by Mahaffey and co-workers (Mahaffey and Fowler, 1977; Fowler and Mahaffey, 1978; Mahaffey et al., 1981; Fowler et al., 1987) have shown that combinations of these metals modified the toxicity of each individual metal and produced unique porphyrinuria patterns. Blood hemoglobin and hematocrit levels were decreased with Pb–Cd and Cd–As combinations, whereas specific effects of Pb on enzymes involved in heme synthesis were reduced by coexposure with Cd (Mahaffey and Fowler, 1977). In vitro studies with δ-aminolevulinic acid dehydratase (ALAD), the rate-limiting enzyme in the heme pathway, have shown that addition of Cd at low concentrations (100 $\mu M$ Cd) can reverse Pb-induced inhibition of this enzyme (Jacobson and Turner, 1980).

The urinary excretion of porphyrins resulting from effects of Pb and As on heme enzyme activities are also altered by multiple metal exposures. The increase in urinary aminolevulinic acid (ALA) resulting from Pb exposure was significantly decreased by Cd–Pb exposure, whereas Pb–As exposure produced an additive effect on coproporphyrin excretion (Fowler and Mahaffey, 1978).

The observed effects of Cd on the toxicity of Pb appear to be due, at least in large part, to reductions in blood and tissue Pb concentrations (Mahaffey et al., 1981; Mahaffey and Fowler, 1977). The number of nuclear inclusion bodies produced by Pb in the kidneys of treated rats was markedly decreased by coexposure to Cd (Mahaffey and Fowler, 1977), which is consistent with the decreased concentration of Pb in this tissue. More recent studies by Mistry and co-workers (1985, 1986) suggest that a low molecular weight renal Pb-binding protein (PbBP), which appears to mediate the translocation of Pb into the nucleus, may be an important site of Pb–Cd interaction within renal proximal tubule cells. Cadmium is an effective competitor for the metal-binding sites on the protein, and is able to displace Pb bound to the protein. This competition may lead to a decrease in Pb accumulation in cells that are able to synthesize the PbBP (Fowler, 1992).

Although minimal data exist, results from human studies also suggest that Cd influences the nephrotoxicity of Pb exposure. In a cohort study of men exposed to Pb and Cd, a low prevalence of renal disease was shown (Greenberg et al., 1986). The 38 men in the study were industrial workers exposed to the two nephrotoxins for 11–37 years. Greenberg and his co-workers (1986) concluded that the study clearly indicated that there was no additive effect of the combined metals and suggested that there was actually a moderation of kidney damage.

Mercury (Hg) is another highly toxic metal of environmental importance that has been studied relative to its interactions with other metals. Mercury–selenium (Se) interactions have been reported in rats treated with mercuric chloride and sodium selenate alone and in combination (Carmichael and Fowler, 1979). Nephrotoxic effects of Hg were reduced in animals receiving Se, apparently owing to the formation of unique crystalloid inclusion bodies that were present only in tissues of rats exposed to both elements.

Beattie and co-workers (1990) have studied the cytotoxicity of Cd and Hg in primary hepatocyte cultures. Lactate dehydrogenase (LDH) release by cells exposed to both Cd and Hg was greater than the sum of the LDH release observed with each metal individually. The mechanisms of this effect is unknown. Although membrane interactions of the metals are quite likely, intracellular effects may also play a role. Recent studies by Blazka and Shaikh (1992) in rat hepatocytes have shown that Hg inhibits the uptake of Cd and enhances Cd efflux in these cells, causing a decrease in the accumulation of Cd. Other sulfhydryl-binding metals also altered Cd uptake, as did organic —SH blockers, indicating that Cd uptake occurs primarily through a process involving —SH ligands. Cadmium and other sulfhydryl-binding agents, however, did not affect Hg uptake by the cells, suggesting that Hg and Cd do not share uptake pathways (Blazka and Shaikh, 1991, 1992).

A second mechanism by which Cd may decrease the toxicity of Hg is through the induction of metallothionein (MT), a low molecular weight metal-binding protein that is induced by Cd exposure (Kagi and Schaffer, 1988). Magos and co-workers (1974) have shown that, although pretreatment of rats with Cd increased the renal uptake of Hg, there was a less toxic effect of Hg on this organ. This is consistent with the belief that one of the primary functions of MT is to serve as a detoxification protein for sulfhydryl-binding metals, such as Hg and Cd in cells (Vallee and Maret, 1993). Whether MT is involved in reducing the renal toxicity of Hg following exposure to other compounds is uncertain. Nephrotoxic doses of sodium chromate, administered 7 days before $HgCl_2$ administration, decreased the tubular effects of the Hg (Tandon et al., 1980). Although Cr does not directly induce MT synthesis in cells, it is possible that higher renal concentrations of MT were present because of the stress effects and cellular regeneration produced by the Cr exposure. Other studies have shown that subtoxic doses of potassium dichromate, which presumably did not induce MT, caused an enhancement of the effects of $HgCl_2$ on renal cell transport of organic ions (Bagget and Berndt, 1984).

The chemotherapeutic agent cisplatin (*cis*-diamminedichloroplatinum) is another metal compound whose toxicity is influenced by intracellular concentrations of MT (Waalkes, 1993). Naganuma et al. (1993) found that bismuth subnitrate reduced the renal toxicity of cisplatin in rodents by increasing the synthesis of MT in normal renal tissue, but not in tumor tissue. Studies with cancer patients have supported this finding and demonstrate the benefits of using bismuth treatment in a regimen with cisplatin treatments of humans with renal, pulmonary, and urogenital tumors to decrease the renal toxicity of the cisplatin (Saijo et al., 1993; Kondo et al., 1993).

## B. Toxic Metal–Essential Metal Interaction

Essential metal ions are those that are required for normal biological functions. Ions, such as $Zn^{+2}$ and $Cu^{+2}$, for example, are required as cofactors for many metalloenzymes; Fe plays an important role in oxidation–reduction reactions as an integral component of the heme moiety in cytochrome P-450 mixed-function oxidase enzymes; and Ca ions serve as a second-messenger system, binding to and, thereby, activating many intracellular regulatory proteins. Although some of these trace elements may themselves become toxic if exposure becomes too high, our interest in them in this chapter is on their interactions with known toxic metals when they themselves are present at nontoxic concentrations.

Because essential and toxic metal ions share many similar chemical characteristics, it is not surprising that they compete within biological systems for specific protein- and DNA-binding sites. Cadmium, Hg, and As(III) are active sulfhydryl-binding metals that show interactions with essential metals that also bind sulfhydryl groups, such as zinc (Zn) and copper (Cu) (Fig. 1). Other toxic metals, such as Pb, will bind SH groups under some circumstances, but also interact with COOH groups in a manner similar to Ca. Most interactions that have been seen in experimental systems generally follow these chemical principles. In addition to relative binding

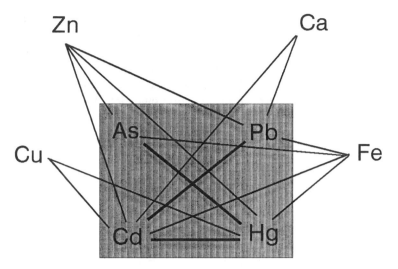

**Figure 1** Toxic metal–essential metal interactions.

affinities, however, one also has to consider the ionic radius of these elements. Studies have shown that $Cd^{+2}$, for example, can replace $Ca^{+2}$ in many of its binding sites owing to its similar ionic size (Jacobson and Turner, 1980).

The competitive binding of metals to macromolecules can influence their intestinal absorption, plasma transfer, tissue uptake, intracellular binding, and site-specific toxic effects. The following discussion cites examples of such interactions. Although many have been studied in some detail, one can imagine that we are just beginning to reveal the tip of the iceberg in this area of research.

### 1. Absorption and Tissue Accumulation

The intestinal absorption and tissue accumulation of most toxic metals are influenced, to a large extent, by the concentration of essential trace metals present in one's diet (Elsenhans et al., 1991; Iturri and Pena, 1986; Shukla et al., 1990; Mahaffey and Rader, 1980a). The intestinal uptake of Cd, for example, is significantly increased under conditions of Fe, Zn, and Ca deficiency (Flanagan et al., 1978; Bremner, 1978; Hamilton and Smith, 1978; Hamilton, 1978; Foulkes, 1985; Hoadley and Johnson, 1987). A deficiency of Ca, Mg, and Fe also increases Pb absorption (Chisholm, 1980; Six and Goyer, 1972; Flanagan et al., 1979; Elsenhans et al., 1991; Cerklewski, 1983), and dietary Zn alters Pb toxicity, as evidenced by decreased Pb absorption, lower blood and tissue Pb levels, and decreased inhibition of the Pb-sensitive enzyme ALAD (Cerklewski and Forbes, 1976) under conditions of elevated Zn exposure.

The mechanisms underlying these effects are undoubtedly multiplistic. Some of these interactions occur through competition of the metal ions for membrane transport systems, in a manner similar to that described by Blazka and Shaikh (1992) for Cd. These investigators have found that Cd uptake by rat hepatocytes occurs through an SH-containing transport process that is inhibited by concomitant exposure to Cu, Fe, and Zn. Thus, the relative extracellular concentrations of these ions will be an important determinant of Cd uptake and accumulation. In vivo studies of hepatic Cd, Cu, and Zn uptake and accumulation suggest that influx and efflux of metal ions are both important determinants of final tissue metal concentrations (Suzuki et al., 1991).

Indirect mechanisms can also affect the intestinal absorption of metals. When an animal is

Ca-deficient, homeostatic mechanisms involving 1,25-dihydroxycholecalciferol (a metabolite of vitamin $D_3$) stimulate Ca absorption by increasing the synthesis of a low molecular weight Ca-binding protein (CaBP) in intestinal cells. Because Cd absorption can also occur by this CaBP system, Ca-deficient conditions will increase Cd as well as Ca absorption (Washko and Cousins, 1976). Studies have also shown that, although different mechanisms are involved in Ca and Pb uptake in intestinal cells, Pb absorption is stimulated by 1,25-dihydroxycholecalciferol (Mahaffey and Rader, 1980b), suggesting that low dietary Ca levels will also increase the absorption of Pb.

### 2. Interactions Involving Metallothionein

As with toxic metal–toxic metal interactions, low molecular weight metal-binding proteins, such as metallothionein (MT) play an important role in mediating the interactions of essential metals, such as Zn and Cu, with toxic sulfhydryl-binding metals, such as Cd and Hg. Zinc and copper, in addition to Cd, are potent inducers of MT synthesis (Cherian and Chan, 1993). Many studies in whole animals and cell culture systems have demonstrated that induction of MT synthesis by pretreatment with Zn significantly decreases the toxicity and carcinogenicity of Cd (Probst et al., 1977; Webb, 1979; Goering and Klaassen, 1984; Waalkes et al., 1989). Goering and Klaassen (1984) have reported that Zn pretreatment increased the amount of Cd associated with MT intracellularly and decreased the amount bound to the endoplasmic reticulum and the nucleus. Manganese (Mn) pretreatment also produced tolerance to Cd lethality owing to increased binding of Cd to cytosolic MT (Goering and Klaassen, 1985). Although Mn is not known to directly induce MT, other factors that alter MT synthesis, such as cytokines or steroid hormones (Cherian and Chan, 1993) may have been involved. Thus, excess concentrations of essential metals, such as Zn and Cu, can decrease the toxicity of Cd and Hg. In addition to this, studies by Nomiyama and Nomiyama (1986) have demonstrated that Cd and Hg toxicity can be increased under conditions of Zn deficiency, presumably because of the low intracellular MT levels present when tissue Zn concentrations are low.

Increased levels of ZnMT in cells may also serve to protect sensitive enzymes from toxic effects of Pb. In in vitro studies, Goering and Fowler (1987) demonstrated that ZnMT is able to restore ALAD activity by chelating Pb from the enzyme and replacing Zn in the active site. This finding is consistent with the proposed role of MT as a protein that donates Zn to apoenzymes (Vallee and Maret, 1993) and raises an interesting question about the ability of ZnMT to restore the activity of metal-poisoned enzymes as well as protect them from toxic metal interactions (Fowler, 1989).

In addition to mediating cellular toxicity in target organs, MT in intestinal cells alters the absorption of metals from dietary sources. Richards and Cousins (1975) have proposed that MT regulates Zn absorption by chelating Zn ions in intestinal cells, preventing their transfer across the basal membrane into the circulatory system. This proposed function of MT is supported by the observation that intestinal MT concentrations are inversely proportional to Zn absorption (Bremner, 1993). The binding of Cd ions to MT in the intestine similarly decreases Cd absorption. Foulkes (1991) has demonstrated that pretreatment of animals with Zn at levels that increase mucosal MT content causes a decrease in Cd transport across the intestinal lumen.

### 3. Glutathione

In the absence of sufficient intracellular MT concentrations, glutathione (GSH) can efficiently accept the role of defense against toxic metal injury (Suzuki and Cherian, 1989). Glutathione is a cysteine-containing tripeptide that is involved in numerous cell processes, including the detoxification of both organic and inorganic compounds (Smith and Rush, 1990). It can protect a cell against the toxicity of metal ions by binding the metals and decreasing their interaction with other cellular ligands. Suzuki and Cherian (1989) have reported that GSH depletion in rats increased the nephrotoxicity of Hg and, in mice, increased the lethality of Cd. Since exposure to both organic and inorganic compounds can decrease GSH levels, this may be an important, general means by which one chemical can influence the toxicity of another.

*4. Carcinogenicity*

There is a considerable body of literature demonstrating that essential metal ions can alter the carcinogenicity of toxic metals (Kasprzak, 1990). As early as 1974, Sundermann and co-workers reported that coadministration of Mn dust with nickel subsulfide decreased the development of sarcomas at the injection site. Continued work in this area has shown that Ca, Mg, Mn, Zn, or Fe can alter the carcinogenicity of Ni, Cd, and Pb, either through direct interaction at the site of administration or by systemic interactions that are as yet poorly understood (Kasprzak, 1990).

## IV.  METAL–ORGANIC INTERACTIONS

An increasingly important area of investigation in the study of chemical interactions is the effect of metal ions on organic chemical toxicity and carcinogenicity. Naganuma et al. (1991) have reported that pretreatment of mice with zinc, bismuth, and cadmium will provide protection against the cardiotoxicity of doxorubicin (Adriamycin), a free radical-generating antitumor drug. The mechanism of this protection appears to be the induction of MT in heart tissue by these metal ions. These results support the hypothesis that MT plays a role in controlling oxidative stress by acting as a free radical scavenger (Shiraishi et al., 1982; Thornalley and Vasak, 1985). They also suggest that metals regulating MT synthesis can influence the free radical-mediated chemical toxicity of other chemicals, such as paraquat and carbon tetrachloride (Naganuma et al., 1991).

A second mechanism by which metals can influence the toxicity of organic carcinogens is through effects on DNA repair (Rossman, 1981a). Snyder (1990) has reviewed evidence that relatively low concentrations of metals, such as Hg, Ni, As, and Zn, can retard dimer removal and strand break resealing in mammalian cells following UV irradiation. This may occur through direct effects on the activities of DNA repair enzymes, or may be mediated by reduction in cellular glutathione to levels below those required for normal DNA repair (Snyder, 1990). In vitro studies have found that sulfhydryl group-reacting metals (Cd, Zn, Hg, and Pb) can inhibit the activity of human $O^6$-methylguanine-DNA methyltransferase, a DNA repair enzyme responsible for removing alkyl groups adducted to guanine bases in DNA (Bhattacharyya et al., 1988). Studies by Rossman (1981b) have also shown that arsenite can enhance UV mutagenesis, by inhibiting the excision repair process in *Escherichia coli*. The mechanism by which this occurs is unknown, but such an effect provides a possible explanation for the apparent cocarcinogenic effects of As exposure (Leonard and Lauwerys, 1980).

Although evidence, such as that discussed in the foregoing, suggests that many metal ions may act as promotors of the carcinogenic process, Waalkes and co-workers (1991, 1993) found that Cd exposure suppresses the development of tumors caused by organic carcinogens. Cadmium, given orally or by injection, inhibited diethylnitrosamine-induced tumors in mice, regardless of the exposure interval or sequence of exposure. Injected Cd also inhibited spontaneous liver tumor formation in B6C3F1 mice. The mechanism of this effect is not entirely clear, but Waalkes et al. (1993) suggest that it may be due to a lack of MT in, and, therefore, an increased susceptibility of, tumor cells to Cd cytotoxic effects.

## V. CONCLUSIONS

Assessment of the health impacts of chemicals present in our environment is a pressing problem. Although we have made progress in recent years by establishing "safe" concentrations and exposure conditions for many individual chemicals, related information for the same chemicals present in mixtures is, for the most part, unavailable. Our challenge now is to accurately evaluate the risk posed by multiple chemical exposures. This will occur only with a solid understanding of the mechanisms of toxicity of chemical agents and the factors that control their absorption, metabolism, and elimination.

## REFERENCES

Argus, M. F., C. Hoch-Ligeti, J. C. Arcos, and A. H. Conney (1978). Differential effects of beta-naphthoflavone and pregnenolone-16α-carbonitrile on dimethlynitrosamine-induced hepatocarcinogenesis, *JNCI*, 61, 441–449.

Baggett, J. McC., and W. O. Berndt (1984). Interactions of potassium dichromate with the nephrotoxins, mercuric chloride and citrinin, *Toxicology*, 33, 157–169.

Bailey, G., D. Selivonchick, and J. Hendricks (1987). Initiation, promotion, and inhibition of carcinogenesis in rainbow trout, *Environ. Health Perspect.*, 71, 147–153.

Beattie, J. H., M. Marion, J. -P. Schmit, and F. Denizeau (1990). The cytotoxic effects of cadmium chloride and mercuric chloride in rat primary hepatocyte cultures, *Toxicology*, 62, 161–173.

Bhattacharyya, D., A. M. Boulden, R. S. Foote, and S. Mitra (1988). Effect of polyvalent metal ions on the reactivity of human $O^6$-methylguanine–DNA methyltransferase, *Carcinogenesis*, 9, 683–685.

Blalock, T. L., and C. H. Hill (1988). Studies on the role of iron in the reversal of cadmium toxicity in chicks, *Biol. Trace Elem. Res.*, 17, 247–257.

Blazka, M. E., and Z. A. Shaikh (1991). Differences in cadmium and mercury uptakes by hepatocytes: Role of calcium channels, *Toxicol. Appl. Pharmacol.*, 110, 355–363.

Blazka, M. E., and Z. A. Shaikh (1992). Cadmium and mercury accumulation in rat hepatocytes: Interactions with other metal ions, *Toxicol. Appl. Pharmacol.*, 113, 118–125.

Bremner, I. (1978). Cadmium toxicity. Nutritional influences and the role of metallothionein, *World. Rev. Nutr. Diet.*, 32, 165–197.

Bremner, I. (1993). Involvement of metallothionein in the regulation of mineral metabolism. In *Metallothionein III* (K. T. Suzuki, N. Imura, and M. Kimura, eds.), Birkhauser Verlag, Boston, pp. 111–124.

Bremner, I., and J. K. Campbell (1980). Microelement interactions of zinc, copper, and iron in mammalian species. In *Micronutrient Interactions: Vitamins, Minerals, and Hazardous Elements* (O. A. Levander and L. Cheng, eds), New York Academy of Sciences, New York, pp. 319–332.

Carmichael, N. G., and B. A. Fowler (1979). Effects of separate and combined chronic mercuric chloride and sodium selenate administration in rats: Histological, ultrastructural and x-ray microanalytical studies of liver and kidney, *J. Environ. Pathol. Toxicol.*, 3, 399–412.

Cerklewski, F. L. (1983). Influence of maternal magnesium deficiency on tissue lead content of rats, *J. Nutr.*, 113, 1443–1447.

Cerklewski, F. L., and R. M. Forbes (1976). Influence of dietary zinc on lead toxicity in rats, *J. Nutr.*, 106, 689–696.

Cherian, M. G., and H. M. Chan (1993). Biological functions of metallothionein—a review. In *Metallothionein III* (K. T. Suzuki, N. Imura and M. Kimura, eds.), Birkhauser Verlag, Boston, pp. 87–110.

Chisolm, J. J. (1980). Lead and other metals: A hypothesis of interaction. In *Lead Toxicity* (R. L. Singhal and J. A. Thomas, eds.), Urban Schwarzenberg, Baltimore, pp. 461–482.

Davis, G. K. (1980). Microelement interactions of zinc, copper, and iron in mammalian species. In *Micronutrient Interactions: Vitamins, Minerals, and Hazardous Elements* (O. A. Levander and L. Cheng, eds.), New York Academy of Sciences, New York, pp. 130–139.

Dixon, R. L., and C. H. Nadolney (1987). Problems in demonstrating disease causation following multiple exposure to toxic or hazardous chemicals. In *Environmental Impacts on Human Health* (S. Draggan, J. J. Cohrssen, and R. E. Morrison, eds.), Praeger Publishers, New York, pp. 117–138.

Elsenhans, B., K. Schumann, and W. Forth (1991). Toxic metals: interactions with essential metals. In *Nutrition, Toxicity, and Cancer* (I. R. Rowland, ed.), CRC Press, Boca Raton, FL, pp. 223–258.

[EPA] United States Environmental Protection Agency (1986). Guidelines for the health risk assessment of chemical mixtures, *Fed. Regist.*, 51, 4014–34025.

Faux, S. P., J. E. Francis, A. G. Smith, and J. K. Chipman (1992). Induction of 8-hydroxydeoxyguanoside in *Ah*-responsive mouse liver by iron and Aroclor 1254, *Carcinogenesis*, 13, 247–250.

Ferguson, R. M., D. E. R. Sutherland, R. L. Simmons, and J. S. Najarian (1982). Ketoconazole, cyclosporin metabolism, and renal transplantation, *Lancet*, 2, 882–883.

Flanagan, P. R., J. S. McLellan, J. Haist, M. G. Cherian, M. J. Chamberlain, and L. S. Valberg (1978). Increased dietary cadmium absorption in mice and human subjects with iron deficiency, *Gastroenterology*, 74, 841–846.

Flanagan, P. R., D. L. Hamilton, J. Haist, and L. S. Valberg (1979). Interrelationships between iron and lead absorption in iron-deficient mice, *Gastroenterology*, 77, 1074–1081.

Forth, W. (1970). Absorption of iron and chemically related metals in vitro and in vivo; the specificity of an iron-binding system in the intestinal mucosa of the rat. In *Trace Element Metabolism in Animals* (C. F. Mills, ed.), Churchill Livingstone, Edinburgh, pp. 298–310.

Foulkes, E. C. (1985). Interactions between metals in rat jejunum: Implications on the nature of cadmium uptake, *Toxicology*, 37, 117–125.

Foulkes, E. C. (1991). Role of metallothionein in epithelial transport and sequestration of cadmium. In *Metallothionein in Biology and Medicine* (C. D. Klaassen and K. T. Suzuki, eds.), CRC Press, Boca Raton, FL, pp. 171–182.

Foulkes, E C. (1993). Metallothionein and glutathione as determinants of cellular retention and extrusion of cadmium and mercury, *Life Sci.*, 52, 1617–1620.

Fowler, B. A. (1989). Biological roles of high affinity metal-binding proteins in mediating cell injury, *Comments Toxicol.*, 3, 27–46.

Fowler, B. A. (1992). Mechanisms of kidney cell injury from metals, *Environ. Health Perspect.*, 100, 57–63.

Fowler, B. A., and K. R. Mahaffey (1978). Interactions among lead, cadmium, and arsenic in relation to porphyrin excretion patterns, *Environ. Health Perspect.*, 25, 87–90.

Fowler, B. A., A. Oskarsson, and J. S. Woods (1987). Metal- and metalloid-induced porphyrinurias. In *Mechanisms of Chemical-Induced Porphyrinopathies* (E. K. Silbergeld and B. A. Fowler, eds.), New York Academy of Sciences, New York, pp. 178–179.

Goering, P. L., and B. A. Fowler (1987). Kidney zinc–thionein regulation of delta-aminolevulinic acid dehydratase inhibition by lead, *Arch. Biochem. Biophys.*, 253, 48–55.

Goering, P. L., and C. D. Klaassen (1984). Zinc induced tolerance to cadmium hepatotoxicity, *Toxicol. Appl. Pharmacol.*, 74, 299–307.

Goering, P. L., and C. D. Klaassen (1985). Mechanism of manganese-induced tolerance to cadmium lethality and hepatotoxicity, *Biochem. Pharmacol.*, 34, 1371–1379.

Goldstein, R. S., W. R. Hewitt, and J. B. Hook, eds. (1990a). *Toxic Interactions.* Academic Press, San Diego.

Goldstein, R. S., C. -H. Kuo, and J. B. Hook (1990b). Biochemical mechanisms of xenobiotic-induced nephrotoxicity. In *Toxic Interactions* (R. S. Goldstein, W. R. Hewitt, and J. B. Hook, eds.), Academic Press, New York, pp. 262–298.

Goyer, R. A. (1991). Toxic Effects of Metals. In *Casarett and Doull's Toxicology* (M. O. Amdur, J. Doull, and C. D. Klaassen, eds.), McGraw-Hill, New York, pp. 623–680.

Greenberg, A., D. K. Parkinson, D. E. Fetterolf, J. B. Puschett, K. J. Ellis, J. Wielopolski, A. N. Vaswani, S. H. Cohn, and P. J. Landrigan (1986). Effects of elevated lead and cadmium burdens on renal function and calcium metabolism, *Arch. Environ. Health*, 41, 69–76.

Hamilton, D. L. (1978). Interrelationships of lead and iron retention in iron-deficient mice, *Toxicol. Appl. Pharmacol.*, 46, 651–661.

Hamilton, D. L., and M. W. Smith (1978). Inhibition of intestinal calcium uptake by cadmium and the effect of a low calcium diet on cadmium retention, *Environ. Res.*, 15, 175–184.

Hoadley, J. E., and D. R. Johnson (1987). Effects of calcium on cadmium uptake and binding in the rat intestine, *Fundam. Appl. Toxicol.*, 9, 1–9.

Iturri, S. J., and A. Pena (1986). Heavy metal-induced inhibition of active transport in the rat small intestine in vitro: Interactions with other ions, *Comp. Biochem. Physiol.*, 84, 363–368.

Jacobson, K. B., and J. E. Turner (1980). The interaction of cadmium and certain other metal ions with proteins and nucleic acids, *Toxicology*, 16, 1–37.

Jacobson, J. L., H. E. B. Humphrey, S. W. Jacobson, S. L. Schantz, M. D. Mullin, and R. Welch (1989). Determinants of polychlorinated biphenyls (PCBs), polybrominated biphenyls (PBBs), and dichlorodiphenyl trichloroethane (DDT) levels in the sera of young children, *Am. J. Public Health*, 79, 1401–1404.

Jensen, C. W., S. M. Flechner, C. T. Van Buren, O. H. Frasier, D. A. Cooley, M. I. Lorber, and B. D. Kahan (1987). Exacerbation of cyclosporine toxicity by concomitant administration of erythrombin, *Transportation*, 43, 263–270.

Jones, H. S., and B. A. Fowler (1980). Microelement interactions of zinc, copper, and iron in mammalian species. In *Micronutrient Interactions: Vitamins, Minerals, and Hazardous Elements* (O. A. Levander and L. Cheng, eds.), New York Academy of Sciences, New York, pp. 309–318.

Kagi, J. H. R., and A. Schaffer (1988). Biochemistry of metallothionein, *Biochemistry*, 27, 8509–8515.

Kasprzak, K. S. (1990). Metal interactions in nickel, cadmium and lead carcinogenesis. In *Biological Effects of Heavy Metals*, Vol. 2 (E. C. Foulkes, ed.), CRC Press, Boca Raton, FL, pp. 173–189.

Kasprzak, K. S., L. Marchow, and J. Breborowicz (1973). Pathological reactions in rat lungs following intratracheal injection of nickel subsulfide and 3,4-benzpyrene, *Res. Commun. Chem. Pathol. Pharmacol.*, 6, 237–245.

Kedderis, G. L. (1990). The role of the mixed-function oxidase system in the toxication and detoxication of chemicals: Relationship to chemical interactions. In *Toxic Interactions* (R. S. Goldstein, W. R. Hewitt, and J. B. Hook, eds.), Academic Press, New York, pp. 31–60.

Kluwe, W. M., and J. B. Hook (1978). Polybrominated biphenyl-induced potentiation of chloroform toxicity, *Toxicol. Appl. Pharmacol.*, 45, 861–869.

Kluwe, W. M., and J. B. Hook (1980). Effects of environmental chemicals on kidney metabolism and function, *Kidney Int.*, 18, 648–655.

Kluwe, W. M., C. L. Hermann, and J. B. Hook (1979). Effects of dietary polychlorinated biphenyls and polybrominated biphenyls on the renal and hepatic toxicities of several chlorinated hydrocarbon solvents in mice, *J. Toxicol. Environ. Health*, 5, 605–615.

Kondo, U., K. Yamagata, M. Satoh, N. Immura, and M. Akitmoto (1993). Clinical use of a bismuth compound as an adjunct in chemotherapy with *cis*-DDP against human urogenital tumors. In *Metallothionein III* (K. T. Suzuki, N. Imura, and M. Kimura, eds.), Birkhauser Verlag, Boston, pp. 269–278.

Leonard, A., and R. R. Lauwerys (1980). Carcinogenicity, teratogenicity and mutagenicity of arsenic, *Mutat. Res.*, 75, 49–62.

MacDonald, J. R., A. J. Gandolfi, and I. G. Sipes (1982). Acetone potentiation of 1,1,2-trichloroethane hepatotoxicity, *Toxicol. Lett.*, 13, 57–69.

Magos, L., M. Webb, and W. H. Butler (1974). The effect of cadmium pretreatment on the nephrotoxic action and kidney uptake of mercury in male and female rats, *Br. J. Exp. Pathol.*, 55, 589–594.

Mahaffey, K. R., and B. A. Fowler (1977). Effects of concurrent administeration of dietary lead, cadmium and arsenic in the rat, *Environ. Health Perspect.*, 19, 165–171.

Mahaffey, K. R., and J. I. Rader (1980a). Metabolic interactions: Lead, calcium and iron, *Ann. N.Y. Acad. Sci.*, 355, 285–297.

Mahaffey, K. R., and J. I. Rader (1980b). Microelement interactions of zinc, copper, and iron in mammalian species. In *Micronutrient Interactions: Vitamins, Minerals, and Hazardous Elements* (O. A. Levander and L. Cheng, eds.), The New York Academy of Sciences, New York, pp. 285–297.

Mahaffey, K. R., S. G. Capar, B. C. Gladen, and B. A. Fowler (1981). Concurrent exposure to lead, cadmium, and arsenic, *J. Lab. Clin. Med.*, 98, 463–481.

Mistry, P., G. W. Lucier, and B. A. Fowler (1985). High affinity lead-binding proteins from rat kidney cytosol mediate cell-free nuclear translocation of lead, *J. Pharmacol. Exp. Ther.*, 232, 462–469.

Mistry, P., C. Mastri, and B. A. Fowler (1986). Influence of metal ions on renal cytosolic lead-binding proteins and nuclear uptake of lead in the kidney, *Biochem. Pharmacol.*, 35, 711–713.

Mitchell, J. R., D. J. Jollow, W. Z. Potter, D. C. Davis, J. R. Gillette, and B. B. Brodie (1973). Acetaminophen-induced hepatic necrosis. I. Role of drug metabolism, *J. Pharmacol. Exp. Ther.*, 187, 185–194.

Moller, B. B., and B. Ekelund (1985). Toxicity of cyclosporine during treatment with androgens, *N. Engl. J. Med.*, 313, 1416.

Mourelle, M., K. Giron, J. L. Amezcua, and L. Martinez-Tabche (1986). Cimetidine enhances and phenobarbitol decreases parathion toxicity, *J. Appl. Toxicol.*, 6, 401–404.

Naganuma, A., M. Satoh, and N. Imura (1991). Effect of preinduction of metallothionein synthesis on toxicity of free radical generating compounds in the mouse. In *Metallothionein in Biology and Medicine* (C. D. Klaassen and K. T. Suzuki, eds.), CRC Press, Boca Raton, FL, pp. 305–310.

Naganuma, A., M. Satoh, and N. Imura (1993). Utilization of metallothionein inducer in cancer therapy. In *Metallothionein III* (K. T. Suzuki, N. Imura, and M. Kimura, eds.), Birkhauser Verlag, Boston, pp. 256–278.

Nomiyama, K., and H. Nomiyama (1986). Aggravated toxicities of cadmium chloride and mercury (II) chloride in zinc deficient rats, *Acta Pharmacol. Toxicol.*, 59(Suppl. 7), 75–78.

Parizek, J., and J. Kalouskova (1980). Microelement interactions of zinc, copper, and iron in mammalian species. In *Micronutrient Interactions: Vitamins, Minerals, and Hazardous Elements* (O. A. Levander and L. Cheng, eds.), New York Academy of Sciences, New York, pp. 347–360.

Pelissier, M. A., C. Frayssinet, M. Boisset, and R. Albrecht (1992). Effect of phenoclor DP6 on enzyme-altered foci and lipid peroxidation in livers of aflatoxin $B_1$-initiated rats, *Food Chem. Toxicol.*, 30, 133–137.

Peraino, C., R. J. M. Fry, and E. Staffeldt (1971). Reduction and enhancement by phenobarbitol of hepatocarcinogenesis induced in the rat by 2-acetylaminofluorene, *Cancer Res.*, 31, 1506–1512.

Pessayre, D., B. Cobert, V. Descatoire, C. Pegott, G. Babanay, C. Fungk-Brentano, M. Delaforge, and D. Larrey (1982). *Gastroentrology*, 83, 761–772.

Petering, H. G. (1980). Microelement interactions of zinc, copper, and iron in mammalian species. In *Micronutrient Interactions: Vitamins, Minerals, and Hazardous Elements* (O. A. Levander and L. Cheng, eds.), New York Academy of Sciences, New York, pp. 298–308.

Plaa, G. L., and W. R. Hewitt (1982). In *Advances in Pharmacology and Therapeutics II*, Vol. 5 (H. Yoshida, Y. Hagihara, and S. Ebashi, eds.) Pergamon, Oxford, pp. 65–75.

Plaa, G. L., and M. Vezina (1990). Factors to consider in the design and evaluation of chemical interaction studies in laboratory animals. In *Toxic Interactions* (R. S. Goldstein, W. R. Hewitt, and J. B. Hook eds.), Academic Press, New York, pp. 3–30.

Pruessman, R. (1990). Mechanisms of chemical carcinogenesis. In *Biochemistry of Chemical Carcinogens* (R. C. Garner and J. Hradec, eds.), Plenum Press, New York, pp. 25–35.

Probst, G. S., W. F. Bousquet, and T. S. Miya (1977). Correlation of hepatic metallothionein concentrations with acute cadmium toxicity in the mouse, *Toxicol. Appl. Pharmacol.*, 39, 61–69.

Raisbeck, M. F., E. M. Brown, S. Kanchanapangka, and W. R. Hewitt (1990). Ketonic potentiation of haloalkane-induced nephrotoxicity. In *Toxic Interactions* (R. S. Goldstein, W. R. Hewitt, and J. B. Hook, eds.), Academic Press, New York, pp. 321–366.

Rao, P. V., S. A. Jordan and M. K. Bhatnagar (1989). Ultrastructure of kidney of ducks exposed to methylmercury, lead, and cadmium in combination, *J. Environ. Pathol. Toxicol. Oncol.*, 9, 19–44.

Reid, W. D., B. Christie, G. Krishna, J. R. Mitchell, J. Moskowitz, and B. B. Brodie (1971). *Pharmacology*, 6, 41–55.

Richards, M. P., and R. J. Cousins (1975). Mammalian Zn homeostasis: Requirement for RNA and metallothionein synthesis, *Biochem. Biophys. Res. Commun.*, 64, 1215–1223.

Rimerman, R. A., D. R. Buhler, and P. D. Whanger (1977). Metabolic interactions of selenium with heavy metals. In *Biochemical Effects of Environmental Pollutants* (S. D. Lee, ed.), Ann Arbor Science Publishers, Ann Arbor, MI, pp. 377–396.

Roch, M., and J. A. McCarter (1986). Survival and hepatic metallothionein in developing rainbow trout exposed to a mixture of zinc, copper, and cadmium, *Bull. Environ. Contam. Toxicol.*, 36, 168–175.

Rojanapo, W., P. Kupradinum, A. Tepsuwan, and M. Tanyakaset (1993). Effect of varying the onset of exposure to DDT on its modulation of AFB$_1$-induced hepatocarcinogenesis in the rat, *Carcinogenesis,* 14, 663–667.

Rossman, T. G. (1981a). Effects of metals on mutagenesis and DNA repair, *Environ. Health Perspect.,* 40, 189–195.

Rossman, T. G. (1981b). Enhancement of UV-mutagenesis by low concentrations of arsenite in *E. coli,* *Mutat. Res.,* 91, 207–211.

Saijo, N., K. Miura, and K. Kasahara (1993). The role of metallothionein for the reduction of adverse effect of cisplatin and the induction of resistance to cisplatin. In *Metallothionein III* (K. T. Suzuki, N. Imura, and M. Kimura, eds.), Birkhauser Verlag, Boston, pp. 279–291.

Sandstead, H. H. (1980). Microelement interactions of zinc, copper, and iron in mammalian species. In *Micronutrient Interactions: Vitamins, Minerals, and Hazardous Elements* (O. A. Levander and L. Cheng, eds.), New York Academy of Sciences, New York, pp. 282–284.

Sato, M., M. Sasaki, and H. Hojo (1993). Induction of metallothionein synthesis by oxidative stress and possible role in acute phase response. In *Metallothionein III* (K. T. Suzuki, N. Imura, and M. Kimura, eds.), Birkhauser Verlag, Boston, pp. 125–140.

Schubert, J., E. J. Riley, and S. A. Tyler (1978). Combined effects in toxicology—a rapid systematic testing procedure: Cadmium, mercury, and lead, *J. Toxicol. Environ. Health,* 4, 763–776.

Shelton, D. W., J. D. Hendricks, R. A. Coulombe, and G. S. Bailey (1984). Effect of dose on the inhibition of carcinogenesis/mutagenesis by Aroclor 1254 in rainbow trout fed aflatoxin B$_1$, *J. Toxicol. Environ. Health,* 13, 649–657.

Shiraishi, N., K. Utsumi, S. Morimoto, I. Joja, S. Iida, Y. Takeda, and K. Aono (1982). Inhibition of nitroblue tetrazolium reduction by metallothionein, *Physiol. Chem. Phys.,* 14, 533–537.

Shukla, A., K. N. Agarwal, and G. S. Shukla (1990). Effect of latent iron deficiency on the levels of iron, calcium, zinc, copper, manganese, cadmium and lead in liver, kidney and spleen of growing rats, *Experientia,* 46, 751–752.

Silberhorn, M., H. P. Glauert, and L. W. Robertson (1990). Carcinogenicity of polyhalogenated biphenyls: PCBs and PBBs, *CRC Crit. Rev. Toxicol.,* 20, 439–496.

Six, K. M., and R. A. Goyer (1972). The influence of iron deficiency on tissue content and toxicity of ingested lead in the rat, *J. Lab. Clin. Med.,* 79, 128–136.

Smith, P. F., and G. F. Rush (1990). The role of glutathione in protection against chemically induced cell injury. In: *Toxic Interactions* (R. S. Goldstein, W. R. Hewitt, J. B. Hook, eds.), Academic Press, New York, pp. 87–114.

Snyder, R. D. (1990). Modulation of DNA repair by metals. In *Biological Effects of Heavy Metals,* Vol. 2. (E. C. Foulkes, ed.), CRC Press, Boca Raton, FL, pp. 77–93.

Squibb, K. S., and B. A. Fowler (in press). Protein interactions with detrimental metal ions. In *Handbook on Metal–Ligand Interactions in Biological Fluids* (G. Berthon, ed.).

Stott, W. T., and R. O. Sinnhuber (1978). Trout hepatic enzyme activation of aflatoxin B$_1$ in a mutagen assay system and the inhibitory effect of PCBs, *Bull. Environ. Contam. Toxicol.,* 19, 35–41.

Sundermann, F. W., Jr., T. J. Lau, and L. J. Cralley (1974). Inhibitory effect of manganese upon muscle tumorigenesis by nickel subsulfide, *Cancer Res.,* 34, 92.

Suzuki, C. A. M., and M. G. Cherian (1989). Renal glutathione depletion and nephrotoxicity of cadmium-metallothionein in rats, *Toxicol. Appl. Pharmacol.,* 98, 544–552.

Suzuki, K. T., S. Kawahara, H. Sunaga and E. Kobayashi (1991). Discriminative uptake of cadmium, copper and zinc by the liver. In *Metallothionein in Biology and Medicine* (C. D. Klaassen and K. T. Suzuki, eds.), CRC Press, Boca Raton, FL, pp. 197–208.

Tandon, S. K., L. Magos, and J. R. P. Cabral (1980). Protection against mercuric chloride by nephrotoxic agents which do not induce thionein, *Toxicol. Appl. Pharmacol.,* 52, 227–236.

Thompson, M. L., L. Shuster, and K. Shaw (1979). Cocaine-induced hepatic necrosis in mice—the role of cocaine metabolism, *Biochem. Pharmacol.,* 28, 2389–2395.

Thornalley, P. J., and M. Vasak (1985). Possible role for metallothionein in protection against radiation-induced oxidative stress. Kinetics and mechanism of its reaction with superoxide and hydroxyl radicals, *Biochim. Biophys. Acta,* 827, 36–44.

Vallee, B. L., and W. Maret (1993). The functional potential and potential functions of metallothioneins: A personal perspective. In *Metallothionein III* (K. T. Suzuki, N. Imura, and M. Kimura, eds.), Birkhauser Verlag, Boston, pp. 1–27.

Waalkes, M. (1993). Medical implications of metallothionein. In *Metallothionein III* (K. T. Suzuki, N. Imura, and M. Kimura, eds.), Birkhauser Verlag, Boston, pp. 243–253.

Waalkes, M. P., S. Rehm, C. W. Riggs, R. M. Bare, D. E. Devor, L. A. Poirier, M. L. Wenk, and J. R. Henneman (1989). Cadmium carcinogenesis in Wistar [Crl:(WI)BR] rats: Dose–response effects of zinc on tumor induction in the prostate, in the testes and at the injection site, *Cancer Res.,* 49, 4282–4288.

Waalkes, M. P., B. A. Diwan, C. M. Weghorst, R. M. Bare, J. M. Ward, and J. M. Rice (1991). Anticarcinogenic effects of cadmium in B6C3F1 mouse liver and lung, *Toxicol. Appl. Pharmacol.,* 110, 327–335.

Waalkes, M., B. A. Diwan, T. P. Coogan, C. M. Weghorst, J. M. Ward, J. M. Rice, M. G. Cherian, and R. A. Goyer (1993). The tumor suppressive activity of cadmium. In *Metallothionein III* (K. T. Suzuki, N. Imura, and M. Kimura, eds.), Birkhauser Verlag, Boston, pp. 303–314.

Washko, P. W., and R. J. Cousins (1976). Metabolism of $^{109}$Cd in rats fed normal and low-calcium diets, *J. Toxicol. Environ. Health,* 1, 1055–1066.

Webb, M., ed. (1979). *The Chemistry, Biochemistry and Biology of Cadmium,* Elsevier North-Holland, Amsterdam.

Whanger, P. D., J. W. Ridlington, and C. L. Holcomb (1980). Microelement interactions of zinc, copper, and iron in mammalian species. In *Micronutrient Interactions: Vitamins, Minerals, and Hazardous Elements* (O. A. Levander and L. Cheng, eds.), New York Academy of Sciences, New York, pp. 333–346.

Yanez, L., L. Carrizales, M. T. Zanatta, J. J. Mejia, L. Batres, and F. Diaz-Barriga (1991). Arsenic–cadmium interaction in rats: Toxic effects in the heart and tissue metal shifts, *Toxicology,* 67, 227–234.

# PART VII
# RISK ASSESSMENT: STATUTORY REQUIREMENTS AND RESOURCE NEEDS

**Yi Y. Wang and Anna M. Fan**
*California Environmental Protection Agency*
*Berkeley, California*

One of the most important shifts in environmental policy since the 1980s has been the acceptance of the role of risk assessment in decision making. Risk assessment, in combination with risk management and risk communication, has been used as an important tool for establishing standards and as a subject of research by many United States and international scientific and regulatory organizations in environmental protection, consumer product safety, and worker and public health protection in the past 15 years.

Risk assessments are typically performed to evaluate and characterize actual or potential chemical contamination situations and to set exposure limits for chemicals in environmental media, such as air, food, and drinking water. The former would fulfill the general responsibilities to protect the public as such contamination situations arise. The latter often involve establishing regulatory standards required by law and subsequent enforcement actions. The need for risk assessment may be assumed in any process of chemical evaluation, or it may actually be required by law in setting environmental standards. Sometimes the approaches to be used (e.g., the endpoints to be considered and the uncertainty factors used) and aspects to be considered (e.g., the chemicals to be considered) are also specified in the law. This section discusses the major environmental and related laws that govern the use of risk assessment directly or indirectly to fulfill the statutory requirements.

Some of the major laws include the federal Clean Air Act; Clean Water Act; Safe Drinking Water Act; Comprehensive Environmental Response, Compensation, and Liability Act; Federal Insecticide, Fungicide, and Rodenticide Act; Food, Drug, and Cosmetic Act; and Toxic Substances Control Act. Different states have also developed local laws and regulations. The many laws governing environmental regulation introduced during the last three decades signal the increased emphasis being put on environmental and public health protection.

Inherent in the risk assessment process is the need to have access to data (animal, human, research, or testing) that are needed for evaluation on which basis judgments are made. The electronic databases (e.g., Toxline), resource agencies (i.e., U. S. Environmental Protection Agency; California EPA), and special programs and data banks that compile such information and contribute to data availability on toxicology and environmental health, with the subject content, are presented here. These resources are the cornerstone of risk assessment, without which risk assessment on toxic substances cannot be performed.

Depending on the database, the following information can be obtained for each chemical of interest: physical and chemical properties, general toxicology citations (with titles, authors, journal, year of publication, and abstract), use and occurrence, specific subject citations (e.g., mutagen- or teratogen-related), or an overall survey on several pertinent areas (e.g., Hazardous Materials Data Bank). Some organizations (e.g., Agency for Toxic Substances and Disease Registry) provide toxicology summaries, fact sheets, brochures, and specific technical reports. Access and availability can be by electronic communication, on-line and off-line printout, telephone, and mail-in request. The in-house library, electronic communication and document acquisition support is indispensable to a successful risk assessment program.

# 35

# Environmental Laws and Risk Assessment

**Denise D. Fort**
*University of New Mexico*
*Albuquerque, New Mexico*

## I. INTRODUCTION

Environmental agencies rely on risk assessment in their implementation of environmental statutes, guided by statutory and regulatory mandates, scientific principles, agency policies, and case law. The role played by risk assessment and risk management policies in federal environmental law is discussed in this chapter.

Those who are primarily interested in the science of risk assessment may want to gain a general sense of how federal environmental laws operate. For this purpose, major federal environmental laws are summarized to provide the reader an overview of the regulatory framework that has been created to address selected environmental problems. Instances of how these statutes employ concepts of risk are presented. Notably, the statutes selected are directed primarily at human environmental health, not at the protection of natural resources nor other areas of environmental concern. The discussion focuses on the responsibilities of the Environmental Protection Agency (EPA), as the principal agency with responsibility for environmental health, but risk assessment practices of other federal agencies are also noteworthy. These include the Food and Drug Administration (FDA), the Occupational Safety and Health Administration (OSHA), and the Consumer Products Safety Commission.

## II. RISK ASSESSMENT AND RISK MANAGEMENT IN ENVIRONMENTAL REGULATION

Risk assessment challenges both science and law. Regulatory agencies are called on by federal statutes to make fundamental decisions about how stringently health risks are to be controlled in the face of the substantial benefits that may result from industrial and other waste-generating activity. Although Congress expresses a set of goals in an environmental statute, it is a regulatory agency that will decide what concentration of a pollutant makes water unsafe for drinking, or a hazardous waste site remediation concluded. The uncertainty of the scientific judgments inherent in risk assessments cannot obviate the regulator's need for a numeric limit to apply to a particular discharger, typically expressed in parts per million (ppm) or billion (ppb). The process of determining these limitations is the focus of intense scrutiny because of the legal and financial consequences that follow from the selection of that limit. The consequences may also be manifested in lives lost or adverse health consequences if risks are inadequately controlled.

The number of chemicals in use and the rate at which new ones are introduced suggest why risk assessment is difficult to successfully utilize in environmental decision-making. The National Research Council (NRC) reported that 70,000 chemicals are used commercially (NRC, 1983, citing Fishbein, 1980). The volume of toxics released into the environment is another indicator of the challenge confronting society; the 1987 Toxics Release Inventory stated that 10.4 billion tons of toxic pollutants were released by manufacturers (Gaines, 1990). In light of these numbers, the regulatory process proceeds excruciatingly slowly; one author suggests that a regulatory agency cannot regulate more than a few controversial chemicals a year. (Applegate, 1992). The number of chemicals in use and the lack of scientific certainty about their risks leaves society in a difficult position; it is neither feasible to stop generating pollutants nor to forego regulation until scientific certainty obtains.

A key report of the National Academy of Sciences (1983) propounded the distinction between risk assessment and risk management, distinguishing between the determination of risk from exposures to hazardous materials and the policies that society applies to manage those risks. Although the attempt to characterize this distinction as the difference between science and policy cannot always be maintained, it is a useful way to view the process under federal law.

Environmental statutes rarely specify how Congress intends risk to be approached. Statutes do not spell out how risk assessments are to be performed, nor the use to be made of them. Furthermore, the language chosen by Congress to express what is to be regulated, and under what standard, varies from statute to statute. Typically, environmental statutes require the administrative agency to examine "the existence, extent, and cause of harm to health and the environment before taking action" on a particular substance (Flournoy, 1991). The use made of this information depends on the mandate contained within a particular statute or regulation.

Several different approaches can be identified in how statutory schemes approach risk management. Essentially, regulation can be driven solely by health concerns, reflect a balancing of health effects against costs of regulation, or be established by available technology.

The pre-1990 air toxics regulations are an excellent example of a regulatory scheme driven by health concerns. The pre-1990 statute had identified *hazardous air pollutant* as a pollutant that "may be reasonably anticipated to result in an increase in mortality or an increase in serious irreversible, or incapacitating reversible, illness." The administrator was directed to establish emission standards "at the level which in his judgment provides an ample margin of safety to protect the public health from such hazardous air pollutant." [42 U.S.C. § 7412 (1983), amended by 42 U.S.C. § 7412 (1983 and West Supp. 1992)]. This led, one author charged, to a failure "to distinguish the separate functions of the target and predicate by making the stringent target level of regulation automatically follow the very low threshold for listing" (Applegate, 1992). The EPA's attempt to substitute technological feasibility for a health-driven standard was rejected in the *Vinyl Chloride* case [*NRDC v. U.S. EPA,* 824 F.2d 1146 (D.C.Cir.1987)]. The air toxics provision was unsuccessful by any measure: EPA regulated seven substances in 14 years under this section (Flournoy, 1991). Significantly, as is discussed later in this chapter, Congress has now changed this provision of the Clean Air Act in response to how poorly regulation under it had proceeded.

The regulatory approach incorporated in the Safe Drinking Water Act represents a balancing of public health and cost. Under the act, the distinction between public health considerations and what is both technologically and economically feasible is made explicit. Maximum contaminant level *goals* are to be "set at the level at which no known or anticipated adverse effects on the health of persons occur and which allows an adequate margin of safety." In contrast, the enforceable *regulations* are to be set "as close to the maximum contaminant level as is feasible," [42 U.S.C.A. § 300g-1(b)(4), 1991].

Available technology can be relied on in regulation development in lieu of exclusive reliance on either health or cost considerations. Under this approach the regulatory question becomes the practical one of how much pollution can be reduced under known technology, while still allowing the activity to continue. The merits of technology-based regulation have been severely criticized, primarily because it removes the incentives for further reductions of pollution and freezes technology at some arbitrary point. On the other hand, technology-based regulation continues to be used as a more practical means of regulation than strictly health-based standards.

The Clean Water Act illustrates this evolution in regulatory methods. The act initially required EPA to identify a list of toxic substances and formulate standards dictated by the environmental effects of the substance. This rule-making moved at a protracted pace, and the Natural Resources Defense Council brought suit to compel EPA action. The case was ultimately settled, with EPA agreeing to a different approach than the toxics-by-toxics approach of the statute [*Citizens for a Better Environment v. Gorsuch,* 718 F.2d 1117 (D.C. Cir. 1983); see Houck, 1991]. Instead, EPA agreed to promulgate standards for toxics as it promulgated industrial category standards, so that toxics would be approached along with other pollutants from industrial facilities. The significance of this approach was that technological feasibility, not health concerns, would determine toxic standards.

As depicted by these examples, Congress has played a less than clear role in determining what constitutes "acceptable" risk. On the one hand, environmental statutes do not contain explicit direction on how many excess cancers are to be avoided through regulation of a substance. On the other hand, Congress has acted when risk-based regulation has not been implemented by the administrative agencies, as it did in the instance of air toxics, and explicit debate over whether environmental statutes "overregulate" or "underregulate" is a common one. (This debate is occurring as Congress considers the reauthorization of the Superfund statute, discussed later, for which the cleanup standards have been criticized as overly expensive in view of the risks involved.) Congress can determine these questions under its powers to make laws, but the wisest allocation of powers among Congress, the courts, and the executive branch is another matter. The proper location of the discretion to determine "acceptable risk" in a democratic society is a richly fascinating question. These questions are explored in Rosenthal, et al. (1992).

## III. THE FUTURE OF RISK ASSESSMENT

Risk-based controls on toxic substances continue to be the source of lively debate by policy makers and those in academia. The current approaches can be criticized for many of the reasons implied here: the slowness of agencies, the expense of the process, and the exclusion of the public through the device of labeling policy judgments "scientific." Hornstein has developed a comprehensive critique of the role played by risk analysis in environmental policy-making (Hornstein, 1992, 1993).

The most radical criticism is directed at the efficacy of regulating, rather than banning, toxics. Barry Commoner, a well-known environmental critic, characterizes risk-based regulation as "a return to the medieval approach to disease, when illness and death itself was regarded as a debit on life that must be incurred in payment for original sin. Now we have recast this philosophy into a more modern form: some level of pollution and some risk to health is the unavoidable price that must be paid for the material benefits of modern technology" (Commoner, 1988). In contrast, he cites the banning of PCBs and DDTs as instances when actual pollution levels have been dramatically reduced.

Widespread bans on toxic chemicals do not seem to be an immediate prospect, although the prohibition of certain substances is likely to continue. Ironically, even this approach is likely to rely on risk assessments, and the delays, scientific uncertainties, and political questions they entail.

Pollution prevention, however, is also based in questioning of risk based regulation, and has become a watchword in environmental policy. As an alternative to controlling the release of pollutants, adherents of pollution prevention might seek to prevent their use, searching, for example, for changes in production methods to prevent the use of toxic agents. Examples of industries that have succeeded in reducing releases of these agents far below any regulatory requirement abound, and policymakers have been searching for means of furthering its use. The Pollution Prevention Act of 1990 [42 U.S.C.A. §§ 13101-13109 (West, 1993)], contains a congressional endorsement of the hierarchy of pollution prevention, declaring that

> pollution should be prevented or reduced at the source whenever feasible; pollution that cannot be prevented should be recycled in an environmentally safer manner, whenever feasible; pollution that cannot be prevented or recycled should be treated in an environmentally safe manner whenever feasible; and disposal or other release into the environment should be employed only as a last resort and should be conducted in an environmentally safe manner [42 U.S.C. 13101 (b) (West, 1993)].

Pollution prevention as a basis for environmental policy deemphasizes risk-based regulation by discouraging the use of toxic chemicals entirely. Nonetheless, pollution prevention approaches assume familiarity with the risks posed by different chemicals and, to that degree, relies on risk assessment. Pollution prevention may lessen the magnitude of the use made of toxic agents, but it is unlikely to remove enough of them from our lives to make risk assessments unnecessary.

A second challenge to the prominence of risk assessment is more fundamental. Risk assessment has been a critical component of regulatory schemes in the United States because the protection of human health from environmental pollutants is the central theme of most environmental legislation. Trends in environmental policy suggest that this emphasis may change. One trend comes out of the changing perception of the environmental crisis; another out of the questions raised by the fragmented approach environmental statutes take to environmental protection.

Ecosystem health, both as a means of protecting human health and as an important end in itself, has been given new importance by environmental policymakers (see USEPA Science Advisory Board, 1990). The protection of ecological systems is a more comprehensive goal than the regulation of effluent and emission streams from individual dischargers, and regulatory approaches are being rethought to reflect that comprehensive approach. The protection of rivers, for example, is no longer viewed as primarily a problem of regulating point source discharges to the stream, but rather, as one of managing land uses, water supplies, and disturbances that affect the functioning of the stream. In that context, chemical water analyses are not the singular measure of environmental protection.

The new emphasis on ecological systems has also resulted in the use of risk assessment to protect species other than the human. The greatest risk presented by toxics in certain settings may be to nonhuman species and regulatory policies are beginning to reflect those concerns. The EPA is working to develop a framework for "ecological risk assessment," in which the agency will assess the ecological costs of actions as it now does the human health costs. (*Environ. Rep.,* 1992, p. 1717).

Environmental policies need to address the fundamental causes of environmental degradation, such as population increases, the increasing consumption of natural resources, and the generation of pollutants and greenhouse gases. These policies will need to address developmental and equity issues on a global basis, the choice of energy and transportation technologies, land use planning, and the preservation of biological diversity. The second aspect of the evolving role for risk assessment lies in how regulatory policies are formulated to address these enormous challenges.

Fragmented pollution programs have been decried as incapable of achieving the goals that the nation has set for itself in environmental protection. "Integrated pollution control" has been offered as an answer to the failings of fragmented programs. In one sense, the term is used to refer to the oft-cited phenomenon in which an air pollution problem is transformed into a solid waste disposal problem (the use of scrubbers generating sludge) as an unexamined consequence of regulatory policies. In another sense, "it includes physical, economic and sociopolitical interactions at a level of global planning [footnotes omitted]." (Wilson and Harris, 1992).

As the world grapples with a burgeoning population, resource shortages, and environmental refugees, environmental management must move far beyond determining what level of smokestack emissions pose dangers to human health. Risk assessments narrowly focused on human health risks from cancer may be of limited relevance to the pressing issues of managing environmental crises. "Risk based priority setting," is offered as a means to direct society's attention to the most important risks to the environment (Wilson and Harris, 1992, p. 3). Even here, the use of any form of risk analysis to determine environmental priorities has subjected to criticism for many of the reasons health-oriented risk assessment has been criticized. (Hornstein, 1992). The allure of quantifying risks to provide policy direction has been felt in Congress and is reflected in current developments there [S.110, 103d Congress, 1st Sess. (1993); Risk Assessment: Strengths and Limitations of Utilization for Policy Decisions, H.R. Doc. No. 53, 102nd Cong., 1st Sess. (1991)].

As the scientific basis for risk assessment is refined, the use made of it in environmental law will change to reflect new scientific understanding. Risk assessment will continue to play a role in environmental law because it will be necessary to determine what substances cause cancer in humans, but it may also be used to aid in comparisons of ecological risks and the trade-offs in different courses of societal action.

## IV. OVERVIEW OF FEDERAL ENVIRONMENTAL STATUTES

The remainder of the chapter provides an overview of some of the major federal statutory schemes that address environmental protection. This is an overview of these provisions; the statutes, regulations, and case law should be consulted for more precise descriptions. State laws are not described here. Many states have adopted their own versions of these federal laws, and may administer the federal law under authority delegated from EPA. States have also adopted innovative approaches to pollution in separate environmental statutes; these statutes are too numerous to discuss here, but are important to consider.

Environmental law has been changing since its creation, as new policies are devised by federal agencies, courts interpret the laws, and Congress revises them. Many of the major federal statutes described here are subject to reauthorization in the near future, and they may emerge substantially altered.

## A.  Water

*1.   The Clean Water Act [33 U.S.C.A. §§ 1251-1387 (1986; West Supp., 1992)]*

Water pollution and air pollution were the first areas in which Congress acted to protect the environment, although state and local regulation predated congressional action. Water pollution was identified as a major public health risk in the 19th century because of the dangers of waterborne contaminants. The utilization of public sewer systems led to marked improvements in public health. In the mid-20th century an increasing recognition that state and local governments were not effectively regulating polluters led to a growing federal role, first in providing federal funding and finally culminating in the Clean Water Act as we now know it.

The Clean Water Act and other pieces of federal legislation must all address, in some fashion, the relationship between the federal and state governments. The predominant model of environmental legislation is reflected in this act; a controlling federal framework is established under which technological standards and scientific criteria are promulgated at the federal level, although a substantial role is retained by state governments in the standard setting function. State governments can administer the permitting provisions of the act, provided that their programs are approved as being equivalent to the federal program [33 U.S.C.A. § 1342(b), (c) (1986; West Supp., 1992)]. In virtually all pieces of legislation, federal standards function as a floor, not a ceiling for the states. This means that states are free to regulate more stringently than the national government has, without danger of preemption by more lenient federal standards. The federalism reflected in the Clean Water Act and other acts demonstrates the national commitment to clean water, while allowing, or more frequently, encouraging, state administration of programs.

The Clean Water Act has as its goal the elimination of discharges of pollutants and the protection of rivers so that they are swimmable and fishable [33 U.S.C.A. § 1251 (1986; West Supp., 1992)]. It applies to "waters of the United States," which through court decisions has been determined to encompass all waters that reach navigable waters, wetlands, intermittent streams, and essentially, all waters in which there is a federal interest (under the Commerce Clause) [33 U.S.C.A. § 1362 (1986; West Supp., 1992); Quivira Mining Co. v. U.S.E.P.A., 765 F.2d 126 (10th Cir. 1985)].

In all environmental regulation schemes, lawmakers must decide whether to specify a level of environmental quality to be achieved in a given environmental medium, such as the air or water, or whether to regulate the effluent from specific facilities, regardless of the condition of the receiving medium. (In fact, statutes can and do use both approaches, but a tension between the ultimate goal and the controls on a particular discharger are always present). Congress initially directed states to set standards for their rivers and streams, with pollution limits expected to follow from those standards.

In 1972, Congress tried the alternative approach. Industries were classified and required, according to various timetables, to meet the effluent limits that the best of their class could meet [33 U.S.C.A. § 1311 (1986; West Supp., 1992)]. Those dischargers that could not meet effluent limits could be required to close. Additionally, states were to continue to designate stream standards, so that additional measures to meet the stream standards could be required.

The effluent limitations imposed under the act, by requiring use of the "best available technology economically achievable," pushed industries to utilize new technologies to control pollution. The focus of rule-making under the act is the technical feasibility of achieving the effluent limits. The resulting regulations have been criticized for becoming quickly outdated as technology progresses.

States are also required to formulate water quality standards that reflect the state's desired water quality for bodies of water. The standards contain both "designated uses" for streams, such as swimming or livestock watering, and specific, usually numerical, criteria for maximum pollution [33 U.S.C.A. § 1313 (1986; West Supp., 1992)].

Effluent limits, water quality standards, and water quality criteria are brought together when a discharger applies for a permit to discharge. The linchpin of the Clean Water Act is the National Pollutant Discharge Elimination System (NPDES), under which permits are required for all point source dischargers [33 U.S.C.A. § 1342 (1986; West Supp., 1992)]. The term *point source* is intended to encompass sources such as pipes and outfalls [33 U.S.C.A. § 1362(14) (1986; West Supp., 1992)]. Through a permit, an individual discharger is required to comply with effluent limits established for categorical sources. State standards and criteria can be met by imposing limitations in a permit that are tailored for those requirements.

Sewage treatment plants (referred to in environmental law as publicly owned treatment works, or POTWs) play a major role in water pollution control. It was a major step forward, accomplished at great cost, to provide sewage treatment to most domestic users. The POTWS were subjected to a requirement of secondary treatment in 1972. Ironically, they have been a source of noncompliance with pollution standards in many instances.

In the eastern United States, industrial activity has occurred along the banks of rivers, with direct discharge made into rivers. In the western United States, it is much more common for discharges to be made into sewage treatment plants and from the plants into waterways. This is significant for industrial dischargers, because discharges to POTWs do not have to have NPDES permits. Additionally, discharges to POTWs are exempt from the Resource Conservation and Recovery Act's provisions under the domestic sewage provision [42 U.S.C.A. § 6903(27) (1983; West Supp., 1992)]. These discharges can be significant, because POTWs are designed to treat domestic wastes, not industrial wastes. Some jurisdictions are required to have "pretreatment" programs, in which discharges to POTWs are regulated, but there are many questions about how well these programs are administered.

Another provision in the act has attempted to get at toxic pollution from another perspective. The so-called toxic hot spots provision required that states identify areas that did not meet water quality standards because of the presence of toxic substances. The states are then to identify the responsible point source dischargers and apply additional effluent limitations to them [33 U.S.C.A. § 1314 (West Supp., 1992)].

Despite 20 years of progress under the Clean Water Act framework, much remains to be done before the act's goals are met. The population and affluence of the United States continue to grow, with resulting pressure on streams, rivers, and estuaries. The act has been most effective with certain types of point source pollution. Nonpoint source pollution, that is, pollution from nondiscrete sources, such as seepage, runoff, and groundwater, is still not regulated by the act, although it accounts for most of the impairment of the nation's waters. Thus far, Congress has urged states to control nonpoint pollution [33 U.S.C.A. § 1329 (West Supp., 1992)], but compliance has been mixed. The regulation of nonpoint source pollution requires different types of regulatory actions than technology-based effluent limits and permits, however, and land use controls will need to be utilized, along with best management practices and other controls on those who cause runoff.

## 2. The Safe Drinking Water Act [42 U.S.C.A. §§ 300f to 300j-26 (1991)]

The Safe Drinking Water Act (SDWA) was enacted in 1974, with a major amendment made to it in 1986. The SDWA requires EPA to set maximum levels for contaminants in water delivered to users of public water systems. Although it provides for promulgation of health-based "goals," and is intended to eliminate all exposure to toxic agents in drinking water that may have an adverse effect on the health of persons, its regulations take feasibility into account.

*Public water system* is defined in the SDWA as "a system for the provision to the public of piped water for human consumption, if such system has at least fifteen service connections or regularly serves at least twenty-five individuals" [42 U.S.C.A. § 300f(4) (1991)]. The EPA was authorized to publish a list of all contaminants that "may have any adverse effect on the health of persons and which is known or anticipated to occur in public water systems" [42 U.S.C.A. § 300g-1(b)(3)(A) (1991)]. *Contaminant* is defined as "any physical, chemical, biological, or radiological substance or matter in water" [42 U.S.C.A. § 300F(6) (1991)].

The SDWA is an interesting statutory model because it recognizes a distinction between public health goals and regulatory limits. Under the act, EPA publishes both maximum containment level *goals* (MCLG), and maximum contaminant levels (MCLs). Each MCLG "shall be set at the level at which no known or anticipated adverse effects on the health of persons occur and which allows an adequate margin of safety" [42 U.S.C.A. § 300g-1(b)(4) (1991)]. Under the national primary drinking water regulations (NPDWR), EPA sets the levels that water must achieve, the maximum contaminant level (MCL). *Maximum contaminant level* means "the maximum permissible level of a contaminant in water which is delivered to any user of a public water system" [42 U.S.C.A. § 300f(3) (1991)]. The MCLs are to be "as close to the maximum contaminant level goal as is feasible" [42 U.S.C.A. § 300g-1(b)(4) (1991)]. In this context, *feasible* means "feasible with the use of the best technology, treatment techniques and other means which [EPA] finds, after examination for efficacy under field conditions and not solely under laboratory conditions, are available (taking cost into consideration)" [42 U.S.C.A. § 300g-1(b)(5) (1991)]. The regulations must specify an MCL for each contaminant that has had a MCLG published for it, *if* "it is economically and technologically feasible to ascertain the level of such contaminant in water or public water systems" [42 U.S.C.A. § 300f(1)(C)(i) (1991)]. If it is not feasible to ascertain the contaminant level, the regulations must specify an appropriate treatment technique [42 U.S.C.A. § 300f(1)(C)(ii) (West, 1991)].

In addition to national primary drinking water regulations, SDWA also authorizes EPA to publish national secondary drinking water regulations (NSDWR), which are defined as regulations that specify the maximum contaminant level that is required to protect the public welfare. Such regulations may apply to any contaminant in drinking water "which may adversely affect the odor or appearance of such water and consequently may cause a substantial number of people . . . to discontinue its use," or "which may otherwise adversely affect the public welfare" [42 U.S.C.A. § 300f (West, 1991)].

The SDWA empowers states to have the primary enforcement responsibility for public water systems if the state: (1) has adopted drinking water regulations and variances that are no less stringent than the national regulations of SDWA; (2) has adopted and is implementing adequate procedures for the enforcement of such state regulations; (3) will keep the necessary records and make the necessary reports; and (4) has adopted and can implement an adequate plan for the provision of safe drinking water under emergency circumstances [42 U.S.C.A. § 300g-2 (West, 1991)]. When a state has this primary enforcement responsibility, EPA is required to notify the state when EPA has found a violation of national primary drinking water regulations. If the state fails to take appropriate enforcement action, EPA is authorized to commence a civil action against the violator. Owners or operators of public water systems must notify their customers of the violations [42 U.S.C.A. § 300g-3 (West, 1991)].

A state with primary enforcement responsibility may grant a variance to a public water system for various reasons, but the state must find that the variance will not result in an unreasonable risk to health [42 U.S.C.A. § 300g-4 (West, 1991)]. A state may also exempt a public water system from any requirement as to a maximum contaminant level or any treatment technique requirement, or both, of an NPDWR if the state finds that (1) "due to compelling factors (which may include economic factors), the public water system is unable to comply with such contaminant level or treatment requirement"; (2) the system was in operation on the effective date of such contaminant level or treatment technique requirement; and (3) the granting of the exemption will not result in an unreasonable risk to health [42 U.S.C.A. § 300g-5 (West, 1991)].

States with primary enforcement responsibility are authorized to enforce the prohibition that "any pipe, solder, or flux, which is used . . . in the installation or repair of any public water system, or [in] any plumbing in a residential or nonresidential facility providing water for human consumption which is connected to a public water system shall be lead-free" [42 U.S.C.A. § 300g-6(a)(1) (1991)]. *Lead-free* is defined as solders and flux containing not more than 0.2% lead, and as pipes and pipe fittings containing not more than 8.0% lead [42 U.S.C.A. § 300g-6 (West, 1991)].

Although groundwater is the primary source of drinking water for many Americans, especially in the western United States, there is no comprehensive national groundwater law. The SDWA, however, does establish a program to regulate underground injection of wastes. These sources may be endangered "if such injection may result in the presence in underground water which supplies or can reasonably be expected to supply any public water system of any contaminant, and if the presence of such contaminant may result in such system's not complying with any [NPDWR] or may otherwise adversely affect the health of persons" [42 U.S.C.A. § 300h(d) (West, 1991)]. Specifically excluded from this authorization is the underground injection of brine or other fluids that are brought to the surface in connection with oil or natural gas production or natural gas storage operations, or any underground injection for the secondary or tertiary recovery of oil or natural gas [42 U.S.C.A. § 300h(b)(2) (1991)].

The EPA is authorized to designate an area within a state as an area in which no new underground injection wells may be operated until an underground injection control program is in place if EPA finds that "the area has one aquifer which is the sole or principal drinking water source for the area and which, if contaminated, would create a significant hazard to public health" [42 U.S.C.A. § 300h-3(a)(1) (West, 1991)].

The EPA may also take action if a contaminant that is present in or is likely to enter a public water system or an underground source of drinking water may present "an imminent and substantial endangerment to the health of persons," when state and local authorities have not acted to protect their health [42 U.S.C.A. § 300i(a) (West, 1991)].

Few people would argue with the need for safe and healthful drinking water, but the SDWA presents the tension between preventing health risks and paying the costs of control in a stark fashion. Because its regulatory targets are usually local governments that may plead lack of resources to comply with the regulations, the environmental and economic costs are more uniformly distributed than they are when the regulatory target is a major corporation, or when the environmental costs fall on those who receive no economic benefits.

The costs involved in compliance are indeed major. For example, EPA regulations require communities with unfiltered drinking water to install filtration systems unless EPA approves an alternative watershed protection plan. New York City officials claim that a filtration system would cost the city 4 billion dollars (Percival et al. 1992). On a smaller scale, the same costs face municipal governments throughout the nation.

## B. Air

*1. The Clean Air Act [42 U.S.C.A. §§ 7401-7671q (1983; West Supp., 1992)]*
The Clean Air Act of 1970 was a major initiative by Congress to reduce air pollution in the United States. As with the Clean Water Act, Congress built on earlier federal and state programs, gradually increasing the federal role. Since that time, experience with the successes and shortcomings of each statutory scheme has led to refinement of the act, with Congress acting in 1990 to comprehensively revise it.

The architecture of the act, as established in 1970, was based on national ambient air quality standards, which were promulgated by EPA pursuant to congressional directives. The statute directs the administrator of the EPA to publish a list of pollutants that "may reasonably be anticipated to endanger public health or welfare" [42 U.S.C.A. § 7408(a)(1) (West, 1983)] and to then prescribe national standards for these pollutants. In so doing Congress distinguished between "primary" and "secondary" standards. *Primary standards* are "requisite to protect the public health" and contain "an adequate margin of safety"; *secondary standards* are set "to protect the public welfare from any known or anticipated adverse effects associated with the presence of such air pollutant in the ambient air" [42 U.S.C.A. § 7409(b)(2) (West, 1983)].

The approach used in the Clean Air Act is noteworthy because its scope is national. The primary standards do not require EPA to balance nonhealth considerations against health concerns [*Lead Industries Assn., Ins. v. EPA,* 647 F.2d 1130 (D.C.Cir. 1981)]. The EPA has not, however, interpreted the statute to require it to set primary standards such that no health effects will be felt. Primary air quality standards have been promulgated for six pollutants: particulate matter, sulfur dioxide, nitrogen oxide, carbon monoxide, ozone, and lead [40 CFR part 50 (1992)].

Standards are not self-implementing. The sources of air pollution are myriad, from large industrial facilities to lighter fluid. Automobiles present different challenges than do coal-fired power plants. Furthermore, although the Clean Air Act represents a substantial assertion of federal concern over air pollution, it reserves a major role for state governments. It is the states, through their own implementation plans, that identify how they will bring and maintain their regions in compliance with the national standards. Most recently, the conviction of some economists that market approaches could result in more efficient environmental programs has been incorporated into parts of the act, so that conventional "command and control" regulations are joined by market incentive programs. Major features of regulatory approaches under the Act are sketched in the following.

*Key Regulatory Features.*   The Clean Air Act relies in part on national emission standards, comparable to those of the Clean Water Act. One such set of standards is the new source performance standards (NSPS) that are applicable to stationary sources of pollution. The statute defines *NSPS* as "a standard for emissions of air pollutants which reflects the degree of emission limitation achievable through the application of the best system of emission reduction which (taking into account the cost of achieving such reduction and any nonair quality health and environmental impact and energy requirements) the Administrator determines has been adequately demonstrated" [42 U.S.C.A. § 7411(a)(1) (1983; West Supp., 1992)]. The NSPS are determined by the "achievable" degree of emission reduction, which is based on reference to a system that has been "adequately demonstrated." Additionally, EPA must take costs, nonair quality health effects, and environmental and energy impacts "into account" in setting the standard. The requirement that costs be considered means that economically healthy industries may be subjected to stricter standards than would a weaker sector. (Novick, 1992).

The scope of the problems presented by hazardous air pollutants was not well known when the Clean Air Act was adopted in 1970. Although Congress directed EPA to promulgate standards for air toxics, the program was a virtual failure. This, in no small part, was due to the problems of relying on risk assessment in a regulatory statute; the required studies, the opportunities for appeal, and what EPA and others believed to be an overly stringent statutory standard set by Congress, all contributed to EPA inaction.

In 1990, Congress was faced with widespread concern over hazardous air pollutants and the need to reform an administrative scheme that had failed to address more than a few of these pollutants. Noteworthy of Congress's 1990 approach was the list it provided of 189 hazardous air pollutants. Although this list could be amended through administrative action, that it was provided through congressional and not administrative action was a measure of congressional frustration with the pace of administrative action.

The approach chosen by Congress to regulate these pollutants was to direct EPA to promulgate emission standards based on technical achievability, on a source category basis. (This is analogous to how Congress was to approach toxics in water). The statute directs, in part, that "(e)missions standards promulgated under this subsection and applicable to new or existing sources of hazardous air pollutants shall require the maximum degree of reduction in emissions of the hazardous air pollutants subject to this section (including a prohibition on such emission, where achievable) that the Administrator, taking into account the cost of achieving such emission reduction, and any non-air quality health and environmental impacts and energy requirements, determines is achievable for new or existing sources . . . " [42 U.S.C.A. § 7412(d)(2) (1983; West Supp., 1992)]. These standards are referred to as "maximum available control technology," or MACT. The EPA is no longer required to set standards based solely on health effects, and may consider the costs of regulation as well.

The act, however, provides for an analysis of health effects from this approach after 6 years. Significantly, Congress has explicitly called on EPA to give it risk assessment information. The EPA is to prepare a report to Congress on "(A) methods of calculating the risk to public health remaining, or likely to remain, from sources subject to regulation under this section . . . . (B) The public health significance of such estimated remaining risk and the technologically and commercially available methods and costs of reducing such risks; (C) the actual health effects with respect to persons living in the vicinity of sources, any available epidemiological or other health studies, risks presented by background concentrations of hazardous air pollutants, any uncertainties in risk assessment methodology or other health assessment technique, and any negative health or environmental consequences to the community of efforts to reduce such risks; and (D) recommendations as to legislation regarding such remaining risk" [42 U.S.C.A. § 7412(f) (1983; West Supp., 1992)].

Following receipt of this report, Congress may act in response to the information and recommendations contained in it. If it does not, however, the administrator is directed, within an additional time period, to reconsider the standards promulgated by the agency and to ensure that "an ample margin of safety" is provided. This language marks a return to the stringent, pre-1990 approach of the act. The provision is also significant in specifying that EPA must act under this section where the emissions limits for human carcinogens adopted earlier "do not reduce lifetime excess cancer risks to the individual most exposed to emissions from a source in the category or subcategory to less than one in one million" [42 U.S.C.A. § 7412(f)(2) (1983; West Supp., 1992)].

Another notable feature of the new approach to hazardous pollutants is found in section 42 U.S.C.A. § 7412(i)(5) (1983; West Supp., 1992), that permits existing facilities to, in effect, act quickly to reduce emissions in exchange for which a temporary variance of compliance with MACT standards will be granted.

Pollution from mobile sources, such as automobiles and trucks, is another major component of the United States' air pollution problem. There are two key features in the revised act addressing vehicle pollution: emissions standards for vehicles and fuel content requirements. Emissions standards have a turbulent history; given the reliance of the United States on automobiles, technological feasibility has been the effective standard, and this has, of necessity, been determined by legislators over the protests of manufacturers. The 1990 amendments further tightened emissions standards for automobiles, light duty and heavy duty trucks, and diesel engines [42 U.S.C.A. § 7521 (1983; West Supp., 1992)]. The amendments also defined, and under specified situations, required, the use of reformulated and oxygenated fuels.

In certain types of nonattainment areas, compliance with the stricter California emission limits are required.

Stratospheric ozone depletion is one of the more serious problems facing the world. In the 1990 revisions of the Clean Air Act, Congress addressed the United States' contribution to the problem. Ozone depleting substances are identified as class I or class II substances, with class I substances having a greater harmful effect on the ozone layer. Numerical ratings reflecting a relative ozone depletion potential are to be assigned by the administrator. The production of class I substances is to be generally phased out by the year 2000 [42 U.S.C.A. § 7671(c) (West Supp., 1992)]. Class II substances, with their lower potential for ozone depletion, are to be phased out over a more prolonged schedule [42 U.S.C.A. § 7671(d) (West Supp., 1992)]. The administrator is given the discretion under certain circumstances to regulate more stringently [42 U.S.C.A. § 7671(e) (West Supp., 1992)]. Reflecting the regulatory innovations found within the act, production "allowances" can be traded among producers, provided a net environmental benefit results [42 U.S.C.A. § 7671(f) (West Supp., 1992)]. Recycling and disposal requirements are also established for some of the existing sources of ozone depletion, such as appliances and motor vehicle air conditioners [42 U.S.C.A. §§ 7671g, 7671h (West Supp., 1992)].

Acid rain is the source of long-standing concern and controversy, primarily among states in the Northeast and Midwest, and with Canada. Because the effects of acid deposition can be felt outside the state where the dischargers are located, important principles of transboundary pollution are raised. When Congress acted in 1990, it took as its purpose the reduction over a 1980 baseline of 10 million tons of sulfur dioxide and 2 million tons of nitrogen oxides.

One of the means of forcing these cutbacks represents a change from the "command and control" regulatory approach typically used in environmental statutes. "Allowances" to emit 1 ton of sulfur dioxide are issued to facilities of a certain type. The number of allowances will be reduced in the year 2000, with the decrease in allowances effectuating the 10 million tons reduction. (This is the concept behind the allowances; the actual scheme is far more complicated.) These allowances can then be sold or transferred as the holders wish, thereby encouraging a market in which pollution reductions (the saved allowances) can be sold. Profits can be made by reducing pollution.

States and substate regions share in responsibility for air pollution abatement and prevention through a key mechanism of the act, the State Implementation Plan (SIP) [42 U.S.C.A. § 7410 (1983; West Supp., 1992)]. Here, the actual air quality of a region determines what steps a state must take to move the area toward attainment or keep it in attainment status. Although the state formulates the plan, it is subject to public comment and approval by EPA. The SIP is to contain an inventory of sources, an identification of control strategies, which can include land use-type reviews (reviewing indirect sources of air pollution), and a showing of the ability to implement the plan, among other items.

Nonattainment areas, of which the Los Angeles area is the most extreme case, have proved to be far more difficult to bring into compliance than earlier legislation assumed. Nationally, the progress made in reducing individual pollutants varies, but continuing population growth and growth in the use of automobiles indicate that urban areas will always be hard pressed to meet national standards. Congress intended that states achieve compliance with national standards, but the "hammers" to be applied to the states have proved politically difficult to use, and a frustrating relationship, often marked by litigation among cities, environmentalists, industries, state and federal regulators, has resulted.

The 1990 amendments represent the latest attempt by Congress to bring cities into compliance with the federal standards. The act now categorizes areas by the severity and nature (type of pollutant for which the area is in noncompliance) of their problem: marginal, moderate, serious, severe, or extreme, with different compliance dates for each category. Progressively more stringent regulatory measures are required of these areas. These measures range from upgrading inspection and maintenance programs for automobiles, to transportation control measures. Additionally, the twin strategies of fuel formulation and emissions tightening described in the foregoing are part of the national program for attainment.

## C. Hazardous Wastes

*1. The Resource Conservation and Recovery Act*
*[42 U.S.C.A. §§ 6901-6992k (1983; West Supp., 1992)]*

The Resource Conservation and Recovery Act (RCRA) grew out of Congressional concern with solid waste disposal problems. This concern later broadened to include hazardous waste. Although hazardous wastes might seem remote from common garbage, the history of wastes has shown that the province of "safe," conventional wastes is small indeed, and that virtually all forms of waste require some management to prevent environmental contamination. Both RCRA and the Superfund program might be understood as primarily concerned with groundwater contamination because that is the medium most affected by waste sites. Although, as noted earlier, there is no single comprehensive federal groundwater statute, these two programs constitute a major federal commitment to preventing groundwater contamination from specified sources.

There are three distinct programs under RCRA, related to hazardous waste, solid waste, and underground storage tanks.

*Hazardous Wastes.* The RCRA addresses the hazardous waste problem through regulations that control these wastes "from cradle to grave." It regulates those who generate, transport, and treat, store, or dispose of wastes. The statutory scheme is based on a definition of solid waste, of which hazardous waste is one type. The statute defines *hazardous waste* as a waste "which because of its quantity, concentration, or physical, chemical, or infectious characteristics may (A) cause, or significantly contribute to an increase in mortality or an increase in serious irreversible, or incapacitating reversible, illness; or (B) pose a substantial present or potential hazard to human health or the environment when improperly treated, stored, transported, or disposed of, other otherwise managed" [42 U.S.C.A. § 6903(5) (1983; West Supp., 1992)]. The EPA was directed to identify criteria to develop a list of hazardous wastes and the characteristics of hazardous waste, which it has done through regulation [40 C.F.R. part 261 (1992)]. Exemptions were statutorily created [42 U.S.C.A. § 6921 (1983; West Supp., 1992)].

Those who produce hazardous waste (generators) are brought under the act, initiating its regulatory controls. Regulations address record-keeping, labeling practices, container use, information to be given subsequent holders of the wastes, manifest requirements (the manifest is a form that provides information on the wastes and its transportation), and information to be given to regulatory entities [42 U.S.C.A. § 6922 (1983; West Supp., 1992)]. Transporters are also regulated under this act.

Facilities that treat, store, or dispose (TSDs) of wastes are subject to comprehensive regulation under RCRA. Record-keeping and financial assurances requirements are imposed. A permitting system is used to implement the act. Lengthy regulations and lengthy permits spell out a myriad of requirements that a facility must meet. These regulations are not intended to be static; as new technologies are developed "minimum technological requirements" are to be revised [42 U.S.C.A. § 6924 (1983; West Supp., 1992)].

The disposal of hazardous wastes on land was the particular target of the 1984 amendments to the act. Deadlines were imposed for the phaseout of land disposal (ibid.), which have resulted in the closing of many facilities around the country. In this respect the act represented a gamble that sufficient facilities would be available to handle the nation's waste.

The RCRA also requires corrective action and financial assurances at TDSFs which are permitted under the act (ibid.). The corrective action provisions provide for cleanups to be carried out under RCRA regulations and under the terms of the facility's permit.

*Nonhazardous Solid Waste.* Nonhazardous wastes are the province of state regulatory decisions under RCRA. The act contains a number of policies to encourage regional facilities for solid wastes, resource recovery, and environmentally sound disposal methods. States are required to submit plans that will, among other features, lead to the use of "sanitary landfills," rather than "open dumps," and funds were provided for various forms of assistance in reaching the act's objectives. States were directed to institute permits for solid waste management facilities that might receive hazardous waste from households or small-quantity generators [42 U.S.C.A. § 6945(c)(1)(B) (1983; West Supp., 1992)]. The permits are to ensure compliance with federal criteria, including requirements for groundwater monitoring, location criteria for new facilities, and corrective action [42 U.S.C.A. § 6949(c) (1983; West Supp., 1992)].

*Underground Storage Tanks.* Gasoline stations are ubiquitous in the industrialized world. It was relatively recently that their tanks were discovered to be susceptible to leaks, with the potential to contaminate vast amounts of water and soil. Additionally, tanks can hold other potentially hazardous materials, with a similar contamination threat. The RCRA regulates certain tanks that contain "hazardous substances" and petroleum [42 U.S.C.A. § 6991 (1983; West Supp., 1992)].

The underground storage tank program (UST) contains requirements for notification of the location and other information concerning tanks, inventories by the states of tanks, regulations to detect leaks from the tanks, corrective action, closure, and financial responsibility. For new tanks "performance standards" are to be promulgated by EPA. Additionally, the administering agency is authorized, under certain circumstances, to undertake corrective action to "protect human health and the environment." In undertaking these actions, the agency is permitted to perform an *exposure assessment,* which is defined as

> an assessment to determine the extent of exposure of . . . individuals to petroleum from a release . . . based on such factors as the nature and extent of contamination and the existence of or potential for pathways of human exposure (including ground or surface water contamination, air emissions, and food chain contamination), the size of the community within the likely pathways of exposure, and the comparison of expected human exposure levels to the short-term and long-term health effects associated with identified contaminants and any available recommended exposure or tolerance limits for such contaminations [42 U.S.C.A. § 6991b(h)(10) (West Supp., 1992)].

The UST program follows the established pattern of providing a federal standard that states can meet if they wish to administer the programs themselves. Program authority can be withdrawn from a state by the administrator for failure to meet the requirements of the delegation [42 U.S.C.A. § 6991(c) (West Supp., 1992)].

*2. The Comprehensive Environmental Response, Compensation, and Liability Act*
*[42 U.S.C.A. §§ 9601-9657 (1983; West Supp., 1992)]*

Regardless of how effective society's efforts to regulate hazardous materials presently are, a long legacy of past mismanagement will require attention. The Comprehensive Environmental Response, Compensation, and Liability Act (CERCLA) is an attempt to deal with the waste sites that dot the nation. The principles under which liability is imposed, however, also establish public policies that should discourage the creation of future sites.

The CERCLA was initially adopted by Congress in 1980 and then amended by the Superfund Amendments and Reauthorization Act in 1986 (SARA). Its basic purpose was to create a means by which some types of hazardous wastes sites would be "cleaned up," either by the government or private parties, with the responsible parties paying the costs. Fundamental questions are still raised about this act a number of years after its adoption, and some of these concerns will be noted.

The act applies, inter alia, to *releases of hazardous substances,* which is defined to include wastes regulated under other named federal environmental statutes [42 U.S.C.A. § 9601(14) (1983; West Supp., 1992)]. Although the definition is encompassing, there are exclusions, including one for "petroleum . . . natural gas, natural gas liquids, liquefied natural gas, or synthetic gas usable for fuel . . . (ibid.).

The President is authorized under specified circumstances to act "whenever (A) any hazardous substance is released or there is a substantial threat of such a release into the environment, or (B) there is a release or substantial threat of release into the environment of any pollutant or contaminant which may present an imminent and substantial danger to the public health or welfare . . . " [42 U.S.C.A. § 9604 (1983; West Supp., 1992)]. The response is controlled under the National Contingency Plan, which contains "procedures and standards for responding to releases of hazardous substances, pollutants, and contaminants . . . " [42 U.S.C.A. § 9605 (1983; West Supp., 1992)]. In it, criteria are to be formulated for determining the highest priorities for action. The statutory language is instructive in the risks for which Congress was concerned:

> Criteria and priorities under this paragraph shall be based upon relative risk or danger to public health or welfare or the environment, in the judgment of the President, taking into account to the extent possible the population at risk, the hazard potential of the hazardous substances at such facilities, the potential for destruction of sensitive ecosystems, the damage to natural resource which may affect the human food chain and which is associated with any release or threatened release, State preparedness to assume State costs and responsibilities, and other appropriate factors . . . (ibid.).

From these criteria, the National Priorities List is promulgated, that identifies sites for remedial actions.

The process for sites that are remediated through CERCLA is as follows: sites are brought to EPA's attention, formally reviewed and scored through the hazard ranking system, high-ranking sites are placed on the National Priorities List, a remedial investigation and a feasibility study are conducted to identify options, a record of decision identifies the chosen option, a remedial design is prepared and, finally, the remedial action is undertaken. Various opportunities for comment by the public are afforded.

The liability provisions of CERCLA were intended to encompass all who have some connection to the mishandling of wastes. It imposes this liability on

> (1) the owner and operator of a vessel or a facility, (2) any person who at the time of disposal of any hazardous substance owned or operated any facility at which such hazardous substances were disposed of, (3) any person who by contract, agreement, or otherwise arranged for disposal or treatment, or arranged with a transporter for transport for disposal or treatment, of hazardous substances owned or possessed by such person, by any other party or entity, at any facility or incineration vessel owner or operated by another party or entity and containing such hazardous substances, and (4) any person who accepts or accepted any hazardous substances for transport to disposal or treatment facilities, incineration vessels or sites selected by such person, from which there is a release, or a threatened release which causes the incurrence of response costs, of a hazardous substance . . . [42 U.S.C.A. § 9607(a) (1983; West Supp., 1992)].

The act removes virtually all defenses and has been interpreted to impose liability on a strict, joint, and several basis [*U.S. v. R.W. Meyer, Inc.*, 932 F.2d 568 (6th Cir. 1991); *General Electric Co. v. Litton Industries Automation Systems, Inc.*, 920 F.2d 1415 (8th Cir. 1990); *U.S. v. Monsanto*, 858 F.2d 160 (4th Cir. 1988)]. This means that parties that are liable can be held responsible for all costs, regardless of their share of individual liability. These parties can pursue "contributions" from other potentially liable parties [42 U.S.C.A. § 9613 (1983; West Supp., 1992)]. Liability extends to the costs of removal or remediation, loss of natural resources, and any health assessment or health effects studies (ibid.). States and local governments can be liable under the act [*Pennsylvania Union Gas Co.*, 491 U.S. 1 (1989)].

The selection of cleanup standards, which determines to what standard the site should be remediated, has been highly controversial under the act. The 1986 reauthorization added a provision to address this issue [codified at 42 U.S.C.A. § 9621 (West Supp., 1992)], but it has continued to attract attention from congressional members. The statute expresses a preference for treatment that "reduces the volume, toxicity or mobility" of substances, and the transport of materials off-site is least favored (ibid.). The agency is directed to assess alternative treatment technologies for a site, and to "select a remedial action(s) that is protective of human health and the environment, that is cost effective, and that utilizes permanent solutions and alternative treatment technologies or resource recovery technologies to the maximum extent practicable" (ibid.).

The standards applicable to remediation of sites were also addressed by this provision. Controversy occurred over whether state standards should be applicable to CERCLA cleanups. Furthermore, the parties responsible for cleanups argued that what numeric standards do exist under state or federal statutory schemes were often not promulgated with superfund sites in mind, and were not relevant to the problems posed by such sites. In the 1986 reauthorization, Congress determined that federal standards from other statutory schemes and promulgated state standards would generally apply, in that the remedial action would have to achieve the levels of control found in a standard of this sort to the extent it is a "legally applicable or relevant and appropriate standard, requirement, criteria, or limitation" (ibid.).

The CERCLA has been criticized for the protracted process under which sites are remediated and the high costs associated with site assessments and remediation. The debate over the act is over the same questions that recur in any discussion of risk: Is the public attention directed to hazardous waste sites proportionate to the risk they present? Is the judgment of "experts" concerning risk considered credible by the public? How fairly are the benefits and risks of hazardous materials distributed by our society? One measure of public concern over hazardous wastes is provided by congressional appropriations for CERCLA: 8.5 billion dollars were appropriated in 1986 for the fund. Clearly, toxic risks have a strong hold on public concern and this must be taken into account by members of Congress as they review the act.

*3. The Emergency Planning and Community Right to Know Act of 1986*
*[42 U.S.C.A. §§ 11001 to 110050 (West Supp., 1992)]*

The reauthorization of CERCLA in 1986 gave rise to a new approach to preventing accidental toxic exposures. The Emergency Planning and Community Right to Know Act (EPCRA), built on statutory provisions providing information to workers about the presence of toxic substances in their environment, by mandating that this information would now be made available to citizens and emergency response officials. Even though the act contains regulatory provisions, its operative effect comes from a requirement that information be made available, with appropriate local action then presumed to follow. What is novel about this approach is that, rather than promulgating standards of safety for all the substances covered by the act, the statute provides the information to those who might have an interest in the facility, in the expectation that citizen action of some sort might follow.

The act applies to "extremely hazardous substances" possessed in quantities over a specified threshold [42 U.S.C.A. § 11002(a) (West Supp., 1992)]. After facilities subject to the act identify themselves, local emergency planning committees are to prepare emergency response plans [42 U.S.C.A. § 11003 (West Supp., 1992)]. Owners and operators of facilities must give notice of certain releases from the facilities [42 U.S.C.A. § 11004 (West Supp., 1992)]. "Material safety data sheets" (or lists of chemicals) must be made available to local emergency planning committees, the state emergency response committee, and the relevant fire department [42 U.S.C.A. § 11021 (West Supp., 1992)]. Additionally, information about inventories of chemicals must be submitted to those bodies [42 U.S.C.A. § 11022 (West Supp., 1992)].

One product of EPCRA is the Toxics Release Inventory (TRI), which has been a valuable source of information about toxic agents in the environment. Certain facilities are required to report

(i) Whether the toxic chemical at the facility is manufactured, processed, or otherwise used, and the general category or categories of use of the chemical.

(ii) An estimate of the maximum amounts (in ranges) of the toxic chemical present at the facility at any time during the preceding calendar year.

(iii) For each wastestream, the waste treatment or disposal methods employed, and an estimate of the treatment efficiency typically achieved by such methods for that wastestream.

(iv) The annual quantity of the toxic chemical entering each environmental medium [42 U.S.C.A. § 11023(g)(1) (West Supp., 1992)].

The toxic chemicals subject to the act were specified by Congress, as well as the criteria for adding to or deleting from the list. EPA publishes national data assembled from these individual inventories, which have been used for estimates of the volume of toxics released to various media and trends in releases.

## D.  Toxics and Pesticides

*1.  The Toxic Substances Control Act [15 U.S.C.A. §§ 2601-2671 (1982; West Supp., 1992)]*

The Toxic Substances Control Act (TSCA) was passed by Congress in 1976. In contrast with earlier environmental scheme that focused on "conventional" pollutants, it reflects Congress's growing awareness of toxic chemicals. In its findings, Congress stated that "human beings and the environment are being exposed each year to a large number of chemical substances and mixtures" [15 U.S.C.A. § 2601(a)(1) (1982)], and "among the many chemical substances and mixtures which are constantly being developed and produced, there are some whose manufacture, processing, distribution in commerce, use, or disposal may present an unreasonable risk of injury to health or the environment [15 U.S.C.A. § 2601(a)(2) (1982)].

Environmental statutes are generally directed toward a particular environmental medium (i.e., the air or water). The TSCA, in contrast, gives broad powers to EPA to regulate toxic substances before they enter the environment as waste. The statutory scheme might have become the preeminent authority for all types of toxic pollution; that it has never had this significance may be indicative of the difficulty of employing risk-based statutes for the implementation of environmental policy.

There are three controlling policies expressed in TSCA: (1) data should be developed, primarily by industry, on the health and environmental effects of these chemicals; (2) government should have the necessary authority "to regulate chemical substances and mixtures which present an unreasonable risk of injury to health and the environment," and "to take action with respect to these chemical substances and mixtures which are imminent hazards"; and (3) governmental authority should be exercised so as "not to impede unduly or create unnecessary economic barriers to technological innovation while fulfilling the primary purpose of [TSCA] to assure that such innovation and commerce in such [chemicals] do not present an unreasonable risk of injury to health and the environment" [15 U.S.C.A. § 2601(b) (1982)]. Thus, TSCA, like the Federal Insecticide, Fungicide, and Rodenticide Act (FIFRA) (discussed later), is a balancing statute. The EPA is authorized by TSCA to balance the risk posed by a chemical substance against the economic consequences of regulation of that chemical substance.

To achieve these policy goals, EPA is authorized to gather required toxicity data, and to regulate the manufacture and distribution of chemical substances. Congress exempted from the act, pesticides, drugs, food products, cosmetics, tobacco products, devices used for diagnosis or treatment, firearms, ammunition, and most nuclear materials [15 U.S.C.A. § 2602(2)(B) (1982; West, 1992)]. The EPA was left with the overwhelming task of reviewing each new chemical marketed (estimated at 1000 per year) (Rogers, 1988, p. 373), as well as determining if the over 60,000 "old" chemicals already in commerce (compiled in a list by EPA as required by TSCA) met the standard of no unreasonable risk of injury to health or the environment (Anderson, 1990). In 1991, approximately 23,000 chemicals had been added to the inventory database since 1979 (Outen and Hart, 1992).

The EPA is authorized to adopt a "testing requirement rule" that requires the manufacturer to test a chemical substance if EPA determines that (1) "there are insufficient data and experience upon which the effects of the manufacture, distribution in commerce, processing, use, or disposal of the [substance] on health or the environment can reasonably be determined or predicted" [15 U.S.C.A. § 2603(a)(1)(A)(ii) (1982)]; (2) testing of the substance is necessary to develop such effects data [15 U.S.C.A. § 2603(a)(1)(A)(ii) (1982)]; and *either* (3) "the manufacture, distribution in commerce, processing, use, or disposal of the [substance]" has the potential to "present an unreasonable risk of injury to health or the environment" [15 U.S.C.A. § 2603(a)(1)(A)(i) (1982)]; *or* (4) the chemical is manufactured in substantial quantities and there may be significant or substantial human exposure to the substance, and it enters or may reasonably to anticipated to enter the environment in substantial quantities [15 U.S.C.A. § 2603(a)(1)(B)(i) (1982)].

In a landmark case, *Chemical Manufacturers Assoc. v. EPA* [859 F.2d 977 (D.C. Cir. 1988)], the court determined that, at least for an existing chemical, "a test rule is warranted when there is a more-than-theoretical basis for suspecting that some amount of exposure occurs and that the substance is sufficiently toxic at that exposure level to present an 'unreasonable risk of injury to health'."

When EPA determines that a testing requirement rule is necessary, it must include the identification of the chemical substance or mixture, and standards for the development of test data for such substance [15 U.S.C.A. § 2603(b)(1) (West, 1982)]. The health and environmental effects for which standards for the development of such test data may be prescribed include carcinogenesis, mutagenesis, teratogenesis, behavioral disorders, cumulative or synergistic effects, and any other effect that may present an unreasonable risk of injury to health or the environment [15 U.S.C.A. § 2603(b)(2)(A) (West, 1982)]. The characteristics of substances for which such standards may be prescribed include persistence, acute toxicity, subacute toxicity, chronic toxicity, and any other characteristic that may present such a risk. The methodologies that may be prescribed in such standards include epidemiological studies, serial or hierarchical tests, in vitro tests, and whole-animal tests.

The Interagency Testing Committee (ITC), a group composed of representatives from eight federal agencies, is authorized by TSCA to recommend to EPA, on a semiannual basis, a list of chemicals (not to exceed 50 chemicals) to be given priority consideration for promulgation of a test rule by EPA. The ITC is to consider all relevant factors including (1) the quantities in which the substance will be manufactured; (2) the quantities in which the substance enters or will enter the environment; (3) the number of individuals who are or will be exposed to the substance in their workplace and the duration of such exposure; (4) the extent to which human beings are or will be exposed to the substance; (5) the extent to which the substance is closely related to a chemical substance that is known to present an unreasonable risk of injury to health or the environment; (6) the existence of data concerning the effects of the substance on health or the environment; (7) the extent to which testing of the substance may result in the development of test data on which the effects of the substance on health or the environment can be reasonably determined or predicted; and (8) the reasonably foreseeable availability of facilities and personnel for performing testing on the substance [15 U.S.C.A. § 2603(e) (West, 1982)]. The ITC, in making the list, is directed to give priority attention to those chemical substances that are known to cause or contribute to or which are suspected of causing cancer, gene mutations, or birth defects. The ITC, however, often lacks basic data needed to establish testing priorities (Percival et al., 1992).

Each year, the EPA must, within a year of the publication of that year's ITC list, initiate test rulemaking procedures or publish an explanation why such testing is not required. In 1990 the General Accounting Office (GAO) reported that the EPA and the ITC in 1980 had identified 2226 chemicals that they believed might be harmful, yet EPA had compiled complete test data for only six chemicals since the enactment of TSCA and had not finished assessing any of them. [GAO, EPA's Chemical Testing Program Has Made Little Progress 3 (April 1990); cited in Percival et al., 1992].

The EPA must be given 90 days premanufacture notice (PMN) before a new chemical substance is manufactured or imported, or an "old" chemical is put to a significant new use [15 U.S.C.A. § 2604(a) (West, 1982)]. The PMN must include any known information on the health and environmental effects of the chemical substance, as well as "insofar as is known . . . or insofar as reasonably ascertainable" (1) the common or trade name, the chemical identity, and the molecular structure of each chemical substance or mixture; (2) proposed category of use of the substance; (3) estimated production volume; (4) expected by-products; (5) disposal method; and (6) "the number of individuals exposed, and the reasonable estimates of the number who will be exposed, to such substances or mixtures in their place of employment and the duration of such exposure" [15 U.S.C.A. § 2607(a)(2) (West, 1982)]. Test data to evaluate the effect of methods of manufacturing, distribution in commerce, processing, use or disposal of a chemical substance on health or the environment are required if "in the possession or control" of the company required to submit a PMN [15 U.S.C.A. § 2604(d)(1)(B) (West, 1982)]. Also required in a PMN is any other data concerning the health and environmental effects of such substances "insofar as known to . . . or insofar as reasonably ascertainable" [15 U.S.C.A. § 2604(d)(1)(C) (West, 1982)].

Critics of TSCA point to these provisions as major weaknesses (see Hanan, 1992, Ruggerio, 1989). A manufacturer is not necessarily required to generate information on the potential toxicity of a substance, but is required only to supply whatever test data may be available, which may be inadequate to determine potential toxicity. However, testing and evaluation of the "new" chemical can be required of the manufacturer by EPA using test rules promulgated by EPA. If so, these data must be included with the PMN. However, fewer than half of all PMNs contain test data, and no toxicity information is available for more than three-quarters of all existing chemicals (Percival et al., 1992). A partial explanation for the paucity of test data may be that the information disclosure process required of manufacturers by TSCA may result in the inadvertent disclosure of trade secrets to competitors, despite statutory efforts to protect the confidentiality of data submitted.

If EPA does not act within 90 days to prohibit or restrict the manufacture of the new chemical substance, manufacture of the chemical substance may commence. However, as indicated, EPA may require testing of the new chemical substance under a promulgated test rule.

After review of the test results of either old or new chemicals, if EPA concludes that there is a "reasonable basis to believe [that the chemical substance] presents or will present an unreasonable risk of injury to human health or the environment," then EPA can prohibit or limit the manufacture of that chemical substance [15 U.S.C.A. § 2605(a) (West, 1982)]. The EPA received 10,842 PMNs and requests for PMN exemptions between 1979 and 1987; 183 PMNs were withdrawn in the face of regulatory action, whereas EPA accepted voluntary testing by manufacturers in an additional 149 cases and voluntary control actions by manufacturers in 45 cases. Only four PMNs resulted in prohibitions or restrictions actually being put into effect by the EPA. [EPA, Environmental Progress and Challenges: EPA's Update 126 (Aug. 1988), cited in Percival et al., 1992].

Section 2607(e) of TSCA requires manufacturers, importers, processors, and distributors who obtain information "which reasonably supports the conclusion that [the substance] presents a substantial risk of injury to health or the environment" to inform the EPA of such information [15 U.S.C.A. § 2607(e) (1982)]. The information need not conclusively indicate a substantial risk to be subject to the reporting requirement, nor is it subject to any economic test. Thus, "substantial risk" under section 2607(e) is not equivalent to "unreasonable risk," the TSCA threshold finding for regulation [Outen and Hart, (1992)]. Section 2607(c) of TSCA requires a manufacturer, processor or distributor of a substance to maintain records of "significant adverse reactions to health or the environment . . . alleged to be have been caused by the substance or mixtures" [15 U.S.C.A. § 2607(c) (1982)]. The EPA has defined *significant adverse reactions* for purposes of this section as "reactions that may indicate a substantial impairment of normal activities, or long-lasting or irreversible damage to health or the environment" [40 C.F.R. § 717.3(i) (1992)]. Under another important reporting section, TSCA can gain access to unpublished health and safety studies of chemical substances and mixtures in the possession of chemical manufacturers, importers, processors, and distributors [15 U.S.C.A. § 2607(d) (1982)]. *Health and safety study* is defined by the EPA as any study of effects of a chemical substance or mixture on health or the environment, including toxicological and epidemiological studies, clinical and ecological effects studies, studies of occupational exposure, studies based on environmental monitoring data, data on physical and chemical properties, bioconcentration, and other data that bear on the effects of a chemical on health or the environment [40 C.F.R. § 716.3 (1992)].

The TSCA has been used by Congress as the statutory home for its direct actions relative to especially notorious chemicals. Section 2605(e) of TSCA specifically authorized EPA to prohibit the manufacture, processing, or distribution in commerce of polychlorinated biphenyls (PCBs) [15 U.S.C.A. § 2605(e) (West, 1982)]. Title II of TSCA, Asbestos Hazard Emergency Response Act (AHERA), was added in 1986 and specifically deals with management of asbestos in public and private schools [15 U.S.C.A. §§ 2641-2656 (1982; West Supp., 1992)].

Title III of TSCA was added in 1989 and is known as the Indoor Radon Abatement Act. The goal of this act is that "air within buildings in the United States should be as free of radon as the ambient air outside of the buildings" [15 U.S.C.A. §§ 2661 (1982; West Supp., 1992)]. This act provides for a limited federal role in radon pollution, primarily limiting EPA to providing information and funding, but not prescribing mandatory regulations. (Generally, Congress and EPA have been reluctant to regulate indoor air pollution, although concentrations of indoor air pollutants may present greater health risks than those found outdoors.) It includes model construction standards and techniques, radon mitigation methods, technical and grant assistance to state radon programs, information generation and dissemination, and training of the public [15 U.S.C.A. §§ 2662-2671 (1982; West Supp., 1992)].

Civil penalties of up to 25,000 dollars per violation of TSCA per day can be assessed. Willful and knowing violations of TSCA can result in criminal penalties of 25,000 dollars per violation per day, in addition to civil penalties. Finally, courts may issue injunctions to immediately stop manufacture, importation, distribution, and use in the event of imminent and substantial human endangerment.

Environmentalists feel that TSCA's "action-forcing" provisions, which set deadlines and authorized citizens' suits, have not been as effective as similar provisions were in promoting the vigorous implementation of other major pollution control statutes (Anderson et al., 1990). Moreover, TSCA has been disappointing to its proponents, who do not believe that its testing and premanufacture review provisions have improved chemical product safety. There is controversy over whether TSCA successfully shifts the burden of proof for safety to the chemical manufacturer, whether Congress really intended EPA to screen thousands of chemicals, rather than control the few that present the greatest risk, and whether the test of "unreasonable risk" can be applied with a balanced emphasis on health protection and economic productivity.

On the other hand, because TSCA relies on a concept of balancing the risks and benefits of chemical use, TSCA rulemaking has been useful to EPA in developing the approach of maintaining a clear distinction between risk assessment and risk management. It is EPA's philosophy that maintaining this distinction leads to better public understanding of the regulatory process and the scientific predictions (and uncertainties) that support it (Outen and Hart, 1992). Furthermore, TSCA may have been more effective at reducing chemical risk than is immediately apparent because manufacturers work with EPA to reduce risk before submitting formal PMNs, and because manufacturers take steps to reduce the risks they are required to report in Section 8 substantial risk notices (Outen and Hart, 1992). Most observers can agree that the full regulatory powers of TSCA are formidable and have not been fully utilized.

## 2. The Federal Insecticide, Fungicide, and Rodenticide Act
*[7 U.S.C.A. §§ 136-136y (1980; West Supp., 1992)]*

The Federal Insecticide, Fungicide, and Rodenticide Act (FIFRA) regulates the sale and distribution of pesticides within the United States. It was first enacted in 1947, was amended in 1972 with the enactment of the Federal Environmental Pesticide Control Act, and has been occasionally amended since that time.

*Pesticide* is defined in FIFRA as "(1) any substance or mixture of substances intended for preventing, destroying, repelling, or mitigating any pest, and (2) any substance or mixture of substances intended for use as a plant regulator, defoliant, or desiccant . . ." [7 U.S.C.A. § 136(u) (1980; West Supp., 1992)]. *Pest* is defined in FIFRA as "(1) any insect, rodent, nematode, fungus, weed, or (2) any other form of terrestrial or aquatic plant or animal life or virus, bacteria, or other micro-organisms . . . which the Administrator declares to be a pest . . ." [7 U.S.C.A. § 136(t) (1980)].

The FIFRA is essentially a licensing statute. Section 3 of FIFRA requires that all pesticides be registered with the EPA, which may limit the distribution, sale or use in any state of any unregistered pesticide [7 U.S.C.A. § 136a (1980; West Supp., 1992)]. A pesticide will be registered if EPA determines that (1) "its composition is such as to warrant the proposed claims for it"; (2) "its labeling and other material required to be submitted" are in regulatory compliance; (3) "it will perform its intended function without unreasonable adverse effects on the environment"; and (4) "when used in accordance with widespread and commonly recognized practice it will not generally cause unreasonable adverse effects on the environment" [7 U.S.C.A. § 136a(5) (1980; West Supp., 1992)]. *Unreasonable adverse effects on the environment* is defined as "any unreasonable risk to man or the environment, taking into account the economic, social, and environmental costs and benefits of the use of any pesticide" [7 U.S.C.A. § 136bb (West, 1980)].

The FIFRA, thus, requires a balancing of the environmental costs and economic benefits of pesticides. Before a new pesticide can be registered, EPA must calculate the risks and benefits of use of the pesticide using data supplied by the registrant, as required in the registration statement. Congress has not, however, indicated what weight should be given the risks and benefits that EPA identify. (This is in marked contrast with the statutory provision governing pesticide residues in food, the Delaney cause [21 U.S.C. § 348(c) (1988)].

As part of the registration process, EPA classifies the pesticide for either "general" or "restricted" use. A pesticide will be given the *general* classification if EPA determines that the pesticide will not generally cause unreasonable adverse effects on the environment "when applied in accordance with its directions for use, warnings and cautions and for the uses for which it is registered . . . or in accordance with a widespread and commonly recognized practice" [7 U.S.C.A. § 136a(d)(1)(B) (1980; West Supp., 1992)]. The pesticide will be given a *restricted* use classification if, "without additional regulatory restrictions," and when applied as indicated above, it may cause unreasonable adverse effects on the environment, including injury to the applicator [7 U.S.C.A. § 136a(d)(1)(C) (1980; West Supp., 1992)]. If EPA further determines that "the acute dermal or inhalation toxicity of the [restricted use] pesticide presents a hazard to the applicator or other persons," the pesticide must be applied only by or under the supervision of a certified applicator [7 U.S.C.A. § 136a(d)(1)(C)(i) (1980; West Supp., 1992)].

Because many existing pesticides were registered when there was a paucity of data on long-term environmental effects of the use of the pesticide, EPA was directed in the 1972 amendment of FIFRA to reregister pesticides. This was a daunting task because more than 50,000 pesticides have been registered under FIFRA since 1947, most before 1972 (Percival et al., 1992). Perhaps it is not totally surprising, therefore, that the General Accounting Office (GAO) found in a 1986 study that none of the active ingredients in older pesticides had been fully tested and evaluated for health and environment effects; the potential toxicity of inert ingredients of pesticides had been almost completely ignored. [GAO, 1986, *Pesticides: EPA's Formidable Task to Assess and Regulate their Risks,* cited in Percival et al., (1992)].

The 1988 amendment to FIFRA [7 U.S.C.A. § 136a-1 (West Supp., 1992)] was a response to the slow progress of EPA in reregistering existing pesticides (Ferguson and Gray, 1989). It established a specific schedule for EPA to complete the reregistration of any pesticide first registered before November 1, 1984 [7 U.S.C.A. § 136a-1 (West Supp., 1992)]. In addition, it established a priority list for reregisteration of those pesticides containing active ingredients that (1) are in use on or in food or feed and may result in postharvest residues; (2) may result in residues of potential toxicological concern in potable ground water, edible fish, or shellfish; (3) have been determined . . . to have significant outstanding data requirements; or (4) are used on crops, including in greenhouses and nurseries, where worker exposure is most likely to occur [7 U.S.C.A. § 136a-1(c)(1) (West Supp., 1992)].

An important part of the reregistration process is the submission by the registrant or manufacturer of summaries of previous studies of the active ingredients that were included in support of the original registration. The data from these studies must be reformatted by the registrant as to "chronic dosing, oncogenicity, reproductive effects, mutagenicity, neurotoxicity, teratogenicity, or residue chemistry of the active ingredient . . . " [7 U.S.C.A. § 136a-1(e)(1)(C) (West Supp., 1992)].

The 1988 amendment shifted the burden of many of the costs and tasks of reregistration to the manufacturers [7 U.S.C.A. § 136a-1 (1980; West Supp., 1992)]. The 1988 amendment also shifted the responsibility for the cost of storage and disposal of canceled pesticides to the pesticide industry. Finally, the statute does provide for reimbursement under certain conditions to end users and registrants for economic losses if a pesticide's registration is canceled [7 U.S.C.A. § 136m (1980; West Supp., 1992)].

The FIFRA contains several pesticide registration cancellation provisions. The first provision requires EPA to cancel a pesticide's registration after the first 5 years the registration has been in effect (and at the conclusion of every subsequent 5-year period) "unless the registrant or other interested person with the concurrence of the registrant . . . requests . . . that the registration be continued in effect" [7 U.S.C.A. § 136d(a)(1) (1980; West Supp., 1992)].

The second cancellation provision allows EPA to propose the cancellation of a pesticides's registration if "it appears . . . that a pesticide or its labeling . . . does not comply with the provisions of [FIFRA] or, when used in accordance with widespread and commonly recognized practice, generally causes unreasonable adverse effects on the environment . . . " [7 U.S.C.A. § 136d(b)(1) (1980; West Supp., 1992)]. Actual cancellation occurs only after extensive administrative hearings.

The EPA may suspend the registration of a pesticide pending completion of these formal cancellation hearings if EPA determines an "action is necessary to prevent an imminent hazard" [7 U.S.C.A. § 136d(c)(1) (1980; West Supp., 1992)]. *Imminent hazard* is defined as a "situation which exists when the continued use of the pesticide . . . would be likely to result in unreasonable adverse effects on the environment or will involve unreasonable hazard to the survival of a species declared endangered or threatened . . . pursuant to the Endangered Species Act of 1973" [7 U.S.C.A. § 136(1) (1980; West Supp., 1992)]. The registration of the pesticide is not suspended until there has been an expedited hearing on the issue of whether an imminent hazard exists. However, if EPA determines that an emergency exists that does not permit EPA to hold a hearing before suspending the registration, a suspension may be put into effect immediately [7 U.S.C.A. § 136d(c)(3) (1980; West Supp., 1992)]. Obviously, a pesticide's existing registration normally is not canceled easily or quickly [see Lolley (1990) for a discussion of the difficulties involved].

Although EPA is directed not to make public information that, in its judgment, contains or relates to trade secrets or commercial or financial information obtained from a person (i.e., in a registration statement) or privileged and confidential, "any information concerning the effects of [a] pesticide on any organism or the behavior of [a] pesticide in the environment, including, but not limited to, data on safety to fish and wildlife, humans and other mammals, plants, animals, and soil, and studies on persistence, translocation and fate in the environment, and metabolism, shall be available for disclosure to the public" [7 U.S.C.A. § 136h (1980; West Supp., 1992)].

A state can be delegated the primary enforcement responsibility for pesticide use violations if its programs are as protective as EPA's. [7 U.S.C.A. § 136w-1(a) (1980; West Supp., 1992)].

Because pesticide use is supported by a powerful constituency of industry, agricultural associations, and much of the agricultural research community, Congress, in enacting FIFRA, has moderated EPA's duty to protect public health with extensive duties to consider the economic benefits of pesticide use. It thus illustrates the use of risk assessment in conjunction with economic analysis in determining regulatory decisions. Experience under the 1988 Amendments to FIFRA will be important in evaluating the practicality of reliance on risk assessment at EPA: will more money to perform risk assessments and more information from registrants enable the agency to effectively administer a statute in which risk assessment is of crucial importance?

## V. CONCLUSION

Risk assessment plays a major role in each of the environmental schemes described in the foregoing. Society is rarely willing to regulate or prohibit a substance, regardless of the costs involved, although there are exceptions in which a regulatory agency has done just that. The economic consequences of determinations made pursuant to these statutes are so pronounced to the regulated community, and of such concern to affected citizens, that risk assessment will remain at the center of environmental controversy for the foreseeable future, despite the increasing emphasis on broader objectives for environmental management.

## ACKNOWLEDGMENT

The author gratefully acknowledges the assistance of Barry Goldstein, Ph.D., a law student at the School of Law, University of New Mexico.

## REFERENCES

Anderson, F. R., D. R. Mandelken, and A. D. Tarlock (1990). *Environmental Protection: Law and Policy*, Boston, Little, Brown & Co.

Applegate, J. S. (1990). Worst things first: Risk, information, and regulatory structure in toxic substances control, *Yale J. Regul.*, 9, 277–353.

Atcheson, J. (1991). The department of risk reduction or risky business, *Environ. Law*, 21, 1375–1412.

Commoner, B. (1988). Failure of the environmental effort, *Environ. Law Rep.*, 18, 10195–10199.

*Environmental Reporter* (1992). Approach to ecological risk shifting to EPA from organisms to ecosystems, 23, 1717–1718.

Ferguson, S., and E. Gray (1989). 1988 FIFRA amendments: A major step in pesticide regulation, *Environ. Law Rep.*, 29, 10007.

Fishbein, L. (1980). Potential industrial and mutagenic alkylating agents. In *Safe Handling of Chemical Carcinogens, Mutagens, Teratogens, and Highly Toxic Substances*, Vol. 1 (D. B. Walters, ed.), Ann Arbor Science, Ann Arbor), MI, pp. 329–363.

Flournoy, A. C. (1991) Legislating inaction: Asking the wrong questions in protective environmental decisionmaking, *Harvard Environ. Law Rev.*, 15, 327–391.

Gaines, S. E. (1990). Science, politics, and the management of toxic risks through law, *Jurimetrics J.*, 30, 271–321.

Hanan, A. (1992). Pushing the environmental regulatory focus a step back: Controlling the introduction of new chemicals under the Toxic Substances Control Act, *A. J. Law Med.*, 18, 395.

Hornstein, D. T. (1992). Reclaiming environmental law: A normative critique of comparative risk analysis, *Columbia Law Rev.*, 92, 562–633.

Hornstein, D. T. (1993). Lessons from federal pesticide regulation on the paradigms and politics of environmental law reform, *Yale J. Regul.*, 10, 369.

Houck, O. A. (1991). The regulation of toxic pollutants under the Clean Water Act, *Environ. Law Rep.*, 21, 10528–10560.

Lolley, M. (1990). Carcinogen roulette: The game played under FIFRA, *Md. Law Rev.*, 49, 975.

National Research Council (1983). *Risk Assessment in the Federal Government: Managing the Process*, National Academy Press, Washington, DC.

Novick, S. M., D. W. Stever, and M. G. Mellon, eds. (1992). Environmental Law Institute Release No. 8, July.

Outen, R. P., and K. M. Hart (1992). Toxic chemicals. In *Law of Environmental Protection*. Vol. 3 (S. M. Novick, S. W. Stever, and M. G. Mellon, eds.), Clark Boardman Callaghan, New York, 1992, pp. 15-1–15-47.

Percival, R. V., A. S. Miller, C. H. Schroeder, and J. P. Leape (1992). *Environmental Regulation: Law, Science, and Policy,* Little, Brown & Co., Boston.

Reed, P. D., P. H. Wyckoff, G. B. Forte, R. A. Penna, L. E. Tunick, R. A. Weissman, M. A. Law, N. D. Shutler, and J. P. C. Fogarty (1992). In *Law of Environmental Protection,* Vol 2 (S. M. Novick, D. W. Stever, and M. G. Mellon, eds.), Clark Boardman Callaghan, New York, pp. 11-1–11-243.

Rosenthal, A., G. Gray, and J. Graham (1992). Legislating acceptable cancer risk from exposure to toxic chemicals, *Ecol. Law Q.,* 19, 269.

Rodgers, W. H. Jr. (1989). *Environmental Law: Pesticides and Toxic Substances.* Vol 3, West Publishing, St. Paul.

Ruggerio, C. (1989). Referral of toxic chemical regulation under the Toxic Substances Control Act: EPA's administrative dumping ground. *Boston Coll. Environ. Affairs Law Rev.,* 17, 85.

USEPA Science Advisory Board (1990). *Reducing Risk: Setting Priorities and Strategies for Environmental Protection,* Washington, DC.

Wilson, P. S., and T. K. Harris (1992). Integrated pollution control: A prologue, *Environ. Law,* 22, 1–21.

# 36
# Resource Agencies with Information on Toxic Substances' Health Effects

**Hanafi Russell, Todd Miller, and Yi Y. Wang**
*California Environmental Protection Agency*
*Berkeley, California*

Information about hazardous substances is given in many textbooks, handbooks, fact sheets, material safety data sheets (MSDSs), and collected in many guides and databases. Not so readily accessible, however, is a directory of resource agencies that can provide information or assistance concerning the health effects or emergency handling of hazardous substances.

This chapter contains the names, addresses, and descriptions of such organizations and programs. The resources have been divided into two groups: national and California. There is some overlap between them (e.g., U.S. Environmental Protection Agency listed under "national" has addresses and phone numbers for regional offices in California). The listing of California-based resources has been retained for this chapter because of the wealth of programs that can serve as models for providing information useful to other parts of the world. The agencies generally appear alphabetically, with some modifications to emphasize area of interest (e.g., occupational programs appear alphabetically by their key word "occupational"). An index is also provided for each section.

The information presented here is updated from a California Environmental Protection Agency (Cal/EPA) report entitled *The Toxics Directory* (4th ed., 1994). This directory not only lists resource agencies, but also literature and electronic databases on toxic substances and their health effects. Scientific staff involved in risk assessment and other activities have provided recommendations for what they consider the most important resources and references on each subject for inclusion in the directory. To inquire about this directory, write to the Office of Environmental Health Hazard Assessment, Pesticide and Environmental Toxicology Section, 2151 Berkeley Way, Berkeley, CA 94704-1011.

# NATIONAL RESOURCES ON TOXICS

## Agency for Toxic Substances and Disease Registry (ATSDR)

1600 Clifton Road, N.E.
Atlanta, Georgia 30333
(404) 639-6360 24 hour, Emergency Response

Region IX Office (California)
75 Hawthorne (H-1-2)
San Francisco, CA 94105
(415) 744-2194

ATSDR coordinates those provisions of the Comprehensive Environmental Response, Compensation, and Liability Act of 1980 (CERCLA) which relate to the public health and worker safety and health and which are carried out through appropriate components of the Public Health Service. Specifically, the agency is charged with protecting the public health from exposure to hazardous substances. The agency arranges for program support to ensure adequate response to public health emergencies declared under the authority of CERCLA.

For incidents in California contact U.S. Environmental Protection Agency Region IX offices first, if you are unable to contact anyone at Region IX, then contact the Atlanta 24 Hour Emergency number.

The 24-hour number is used by both the Centers for Disease Control and the Agency for Toxic Substances and Disease Registry. It is therefore important for the caller to indicate that the incident involves hazardous materials and toxic wastes.

## Air Risk Information Support Center (Air RISC)

Office of Air Quality Planning and Standards (MD-13)
Air RISC
U.S. EPA
Research Triangle Park, NC 27711

Air RISC Hotline
(919) 541-0888
Monday–Thursday, 8:00 AM to 5:00 PM, EST
Friday, 8:00 AM to 4:00 PM, EST

The Air Risk Information Support Center (Air RISC) provides, in a timely fashion, technical assistance and information relative to health, exposure, and risk assessments for toxic and criteria air pollutants. The EPA has worked with the State and Territorial Air Pollution Program Administrators (STAPPA), the Association of Local Air Pollution Control Officials (ALAPCO), and EPA regional offices in the design and development of the Air RISC to ensure that the Center will be useful for State and local agencies as well as EPA Regional Offices. The primary goal of Air RISC is to provide health, exposure, and risk information for state and local air pollution control agencies and EPA Regional Offices and, where needed, assist in reviewing and interpreting that data.

## American Cancer Society

National headquarters:
1599 Clifton Road NE
Atlanta GA 30329
(404) 320-3333

California Division Office
1710 Webster Street, Suite 210
P.O. Box 2061
Oakland, CA 94604
(510) 893-7900 (See telephone book for local chapter)

Offers public and professional education on cancer prevention, detection, diagnosis, and treatment. Has printed information on subjects including carcinogens in the workplace and on nutrition and cancer. Patient services are available.

## American Lung Association

National headquarters:
1740 Broadway
New York, NY 10019
(212) 315-8700

American Lung Association of California:
424 Pendleton Way (State Office)
Oakland, CA 94621
(510) 638-5864 (638-LUNG)

American Lung Association of Los Angeles County:
5858 Wilshire Blvd., Suite 300
Los Angeles, CA 90036
(213) 935-5864 (935-LUNG)
Also see phone directory for other local associations.

The Lung Association is a voluntary health agency that focuses on education about occupational and environmental causes of lung disease. It also promotes research into causes, treatments and cures for lung diseases.

## Americans for Nonsmokers' Rights

2530 San Pablo Ave.; Suite J
Berkeley, CA 94702
(510) 841-3032

Information available on environmental tobacco smoke. Promotes rights of nonsmokers. Conducts lobbying nationally at all levels of government.

## Asbestos Hotline

Office of Toxic Substances (TS-799)
U.S. EPA
401 M Street, SW
Washington, DC 20460
(202) 554-1404

The Asbestos Hotline provides technical information concerning asbestos abatement problems in schools and gives referrals to other asbestos programs. Information specialists answer questions about compliance with regulations and funding sources for asbestos removal or encapsulation.

## Bio-Integral Resource Center (BIRC)

P.O. Box 7414
Berkeley, CA 94707
(510) 524-2567

BIRC offers practical information on the least toxic methods of managing pests and land resource problems. Its interdisciplinary staff and nationwide network of advisors and associates have designed integrated pest management programs for community groups, public agencies, and private institutions throughout the U.S. and Canada. BIRC offers two publications to its members. The first, "Common Sense Pest Control Quarterly," informs readers about alternatives for managing insect, weed, rodent, and plant-disease pests found in the home, on the human body, on pets, and in the garden, workplace, and community. The "IPM Practitioner," BIRC's second publication, provides valuable information on the latest in integrated pest management for pest control professionals, farmers, and managers of community facilities. All of BIRC's publications, including a 715 page resource book, "Common Sense Pest Control," are available by mail order. Send $1 to receive a listing of publications.

## Cancer Information Service

Office of Cancer Communication
National Cancer Institute
NCI Building 31, Room 10A1B
Bethesda, MD 20892
1-800-4-CANCER (1-800-422-6237)
Monday–Friday, 9:00 AM to 7:00 PM
All phone calls are automatically routed to the nearest Cancer Information Service office. In California, it is the UCLA Johnson Comprehensive Cancer Center.

Responds to questions about cancer and related diseases, including causes, diagnosis, treatment and prevention. Provides the latest information on cancer, including occupational cancer; treatment; medical referral, including referrals to low cost clinics; medical consultation; referrals to patient support groups; and materials. Publications are available on request. Spanish-speaking staff are available during daytime hours at some locations. Some of the written materials are also available in Spanish.

## Center for Safety in the Arts

5 Beekman Street
New York, New York 10038
(212) 227-6220

Responds to questions relating to hazards in the arts (e.g., visual arts and performing arts). Distributes newsletters and publications on hazards relating to various arts and crafts. Makes referrals to doctors specializing in toxic-related illnesses. Provides qualified speakers to address hazards in the arts. National clearinghouse for information on hazards in the arts. Offers courses nationwide. Provides on-site consultation and inspection.

## Chemical Referral Center Chemical Manufacturers Association

Chemical Manufacturers Association
2501 M Street, N.W.
Washington, D.C. 20037
(800) 262-8200
Monday through Friday, 9:00 AM–6:00 PM, EST

Provides a means for the public to obtain access to non-emergency health and safety information concerning chemicals.

## Chemical Transportation Emergency Center (CHEMTREC)

Chemical Manufacturers Association
2501 M Street, N.W.
Washington, D.C. 20037
(800) 424-9300 (24 hours a day)
(202) 887-1100 (for Chemical Manufacturers Association)

*\*\*\*For Chemical Emergencies Only involving spills, leaks, fires, or exposures to chemicals\*\*\**

Provides immediate and comprehensive initial emergency response information for first responders involved in responding to or operating at the scene of hazardous material emergencies. CHEMTREC also notifies manufacturers and shippers of incidents involving their products so appropriate follow-up action and assistance can be rendered. CHEMTREC can also activate mutual aid programs such as the Chlorine Emergency Plan (CHLOREP) for chlorine emergencies and the Phosphorus Emergency Response Team (PERT) for phosphorus emergencies.

## Chevron/Ortho Emergency Information Center

1003 W. Cutting Blvd., Suite 120
Richmond, CA 94804-0054
(800) 457-2022 or (510) 233-3737
24 hours a day

Ortho Consumer Services Dept.
P.O. Box 5047
San Ramon, Ca 94583-0947

The Chevron Emergency Information Center (CEIC) provides health and spill clean-up advice to members of the medical community and consumers concerning all of the products and chemicals produced and marketed by the various Chevron operating companies and Valent USA. Most of the inquiries received at CEIC concern the ORTHO consumer pesticide products.

The emergency response technicians answer all incoming CEIC inquiries and provide consultation and advice in those cases involving minor exposure to products having a low degree of toxicity and irritation potential.

Situations involving either potential extensive exposure, signs and symptoms of illness, or inquiries from physicians or other members of the medical community are referred to one of the 14 toxicologists that rotate through an "on-call" status. Attending physicians are provided with information concerning product composition, results of toxicology studies, clinical findings and medical management. The service includes all of the products and chemicals produced and marketed by the various Chevron operating companies and Valent USA.

## Citizen's Clearinghouse for Hazardous Wastes, Inc.

PO Box 6806
Falls Church, VA 22040
(703) 237-2249

Provides citizen groups, individuals and municipalities with information needed to understand and resolve their chemical waste problems. They offer an extensive list of publications including books, fact packs, manuals, bibliographies, action bulletins, Everyone's Backyard (magazine), and Environmental Health Monthly.

## Consumer Product Safety Commission, U.S.

(800) 638-CPSC (Nationwide toll free hotline)

National headquarters:
4330 East West Highway
Bethesda, MD 20814-4408
Attn. Office of the Secretary
(301) 504-0800

600 Harrison Street, Room 245
San Francisco, CA 94107
(415) 744-2966

4929 Wilshire Boulevard, Suite 320
Los Angeles, CA 90010
(213) 251-7464

Provides information on health and safety effects related to consumer products. Has direct jurisdiction over chronic and chemical hazards in consumer products.

## Control Technology Center (CTC)

Office of Air Quality Planning and Standards, MD-10
U.S. Environmental Protection Agency (U.S. EPA)
Research Triangle Park, NC 27711

Control Technology Center (CTC) Hotline
(919) 541-0800
Monday through Friday, 8:00 AM to 5:00 PM, EST

The Control Technology Center (CTC) supports state and local agencies and EPA regional offices in implementing air pollution programs for both toxic and criteria air pollutants by providing engineering guidance and support on air pollution control technology. Support is supplied to others on a cost reimbursement basis. In addition, the CTC has a bulletin board operating through the Office of Air Quality Planning and Standards (OAQPS) Technology Transfer Network (TTN) Bulletin Board System. The bulletin board system is open to all.

## Emergency Planning and Community Right-to-Know Information Hotline

SARA Title III Hotline
Office of Solid Waste and Emergency Response (OS-120)
U.S. EPA
401 M Street, S.W.
Washington, DC 20460
(800) 535-0202
(703) 412-9877 FAX: (703) 412-3333
Monday through Friday, 8:30 AM to 7:30 PM, EST

The Emergency Planning and Community Right to Know Information Hotline is operated under the guidance of the Office of Solid Waste and Emergency Response and the Office of Pollution Prevention and Toxics. The Hotline can answer questions from manufacturers, government agencies, and the general public regarding the Emergency Planning and Community Right-to-Know Act (known as EPCRA, or SARA Title III). This law establishes requirements for Federal, State, and local governments and industry regarding emergency planning and community right-to-know reporting on hazardous and toxic chemicals.

## Environmental Action Foundation

Wastes and Toxic Substances Project
6930 Carroll Avenue, 6th Floor
Takoma Park, MD 20912
(301) 891-1100

An independent, tax-deductible organization founded in 1970 to promote environmental protection through research, public education, organizing assistance and legal action. Offers technical assistance and organizing expertise to community groups and public officials. Services include information packets, up-to-date information on state waste management plans and contacts with activists across the country. Work is currently focused on toxics, community right to know, energy, solid waste and The Energy Conservation Coalition. Publishes Environmental Action Magazine and several informational publications.

## Environmental Protection Agency, U.S.

EPA Headquarters
401 M Street, SW
Washington, DC 20460
(202) 260-2090—EPA program locator number
(202) 260-2080—Public Information Center

(919) 541-2777—Library Services, North Carolina
(202) 260-5921—EPA Headquarters Library
(202) 260-8909—Exposure Assessment Group
(800) 426-4791—Safe Drinking Water Hotline

EPA has 10 regional offices serving the country. The following phone numbers are for Region IX. Some other nationwide hotline services offered by EPA have been listed separately in this section.

REGION IX (California, Nevada, Arizona, Hawaii, Guam, and Pacific Trust Territories)

75 Hawthorne St.
San Francisco, Ca 94105
General Information—(415) 744-1500

Responds to information requests on acute and chronic health effects of hazardous materials. Basic function is to provide information on Environmental Protection Agency regulations and programs. Archives available for reference use on wide range of issues: air and water pollution, toxic substances including PCBs and asbestos, pesticides, radiation, and so on.

Library—(415) 744-1500

Information on current spills:
Emergency Response Section
(415) 744-2000 (24-hour number)

Information in situations on which legal action is pending.
Regional Counsel Office
(415) 744-1365

Freedom of Information Officer
(415) 744-1586
Information on past incidents and responses by EPA in the agency's files

Asbestos information phone referral
(415) 744-1690. See description under Asbestos Hotline (listed separately) for more asbestos numbers.

ACCESS EPA

The Office of Information Resources Management in the U.S. Environmental Protection Agency (EPA) has available ACCESS EPA, a series of directories that provide contact information and descriptions of services offered by libraries, databases, information centers, clearinghouse, hotlines, dockets, records management programs, and related information sources. EPA produced the series, which is updated annually, to improve access to environmental information provided by EPA and other public sector organizations. The series includes one consolidated volume, entitled ACCESS EPA ($21), and the following seven directories.:

Public Information Tools ($8);
Major EPA Dockets ($7);
Clearinghouses and Hotlines ($7);
Records Management Programs($7);
Major EPA Environmental Databases ($8);
Libraries and Information Services ($8); and
State Environmental Libraries ($8).

The consolidated volume of ACCESS EPA is available through the Government Printing Office (GPO): New Orders, Superintendent of Documents, P.O. Box 371954, Pittsburgh, PA 15250-7954
Telephone (202) 783-3238
FAX (202) 512-2250, Publications
FAX: (202) 512-2233, Subscriptions

All eight titles are available from the National Technical Information Service (NTIS): NTIS, Sills Building, 5285 Port Royal Road, Springfield, VA 22161; telephone (703) 487-4650; fax (703) 321-8547.

## Food and Drug Administration, U.S.

National Headquarters
200 C Street, S.W.
Washington, D.C. 20204

San Francisco District
Federal Office Building, Room 536,
50 United Nations Plaza
San Francisco, CA 94102
(415) 556-2062 (same for emergency answering service after hours)

District Office:
Los Angeles District
1521 West Pico Boulevard
Los Angeles, CA 90015
(213) 252-7586 (for emergency after hours (213) 245-0290)

Inspects manufacturing plants and warehouses, collects and analyzes samples of foods, drugs, import cosmetics and therapeutic devices for adulteration and misbranding. Responsibilities also extend to sanitary preparation and handling of foods, and waste disposal on interstate carriers and enforcement of the Radiation Control Act as related to consumer products. Epidemiological and other investigations are conducted to determine causative factors or possible health hazards involved in adverse reactions or hazardous materials accidents. Investigators are located in resident posts in major cities through the state. Analytical laboratories are located in the two district offices.

## Lead Poisoning Prevention information line

1-800-LEAD-FYI (1-800-532-3394)

By calling the toll-free number, citizens can request a Spanish or English language information package describing how to help protect children from lead poisoning.

## National Air Toxics Information Clearinghouse (NATICH)

National Air Toxics Information Clearinghouse
Pollutant Assessment Branch
Office of Air Quality Planning and Standards (MD-13)
U.S. EPA
Research Triangle Park, NC 27711

(919) 541-0850
Monday through Friday, 7:30 AM to 5:00 PM, EST

The National Air Toxics Information Clearinghouse assists federal, state, and local agencies in exchanging information about air toxics and the development of air toxics programs. The core of the Clearinghouse is the NATICH data base which contains all of the information collected from federal, state, and local agencies. This information is generally organized according to agency, pollutant, and emission source. The data base report is updated once a year and is available on hardcopy. NATICH also publishes other material on an annual basis, and special reports.

## National Health Information Clearinghouse (NHIC)

U.S. Public Health Service
P.O. Box 1133, ODPHP
Washington, DC 20013-1133
(800) 336-4797
Monday through Friday 9:00 AM to 5:00 PM, EST

Publishes a series of resource guides, one of which is a listing of selected federal health information clearinghouses and information centers. Helps the general public and health professionals locate health information through identification of health information resources and an inquiry and referral system. Health questions are referred to appropriate health resources that, in turn, respond directly to inquirers. Does not provide medical advice, diagnosis, or physician referrals.

## National Institute for Environmental Health Sciences (NIEHS)

Dr. Anne Sassaman (Director)
Division of Extramural Research and Training
P.O. Box 12233
104 T.W. Alexander Drive
Research Triangle Park, NC 27709
(919) 541-7723

NIEHS is the principal federal agency for biomedical research on the effects of chemical, physical, and biological environmental agents on man's health and well being. Such research is very diverse; it includes but is not limited to:

- studies of the extent and consequences of exposure of population groups to environmental pollutants;

- the effects of toxic substances on biochemical processes and body organs;

- pharmacodynamics of chemical substances in the body;

- molecular, biochemical and physiological mechanisms of toxicity of chemical and physical factors; and

- development and validation of test methods for health hazard assessment of environmental chemicals.

# National Institute for Occupational Safety and Health (NIOSH)

Headquarters:
1600 Clifton Road
Atlanta, GA—30333 Mail Stop D-32
(404) 639-3691

Western Region:
California, Nevada, Arizona, Hawaii, Guam, American Samoa, Pacific Trust Territories (formerly Region IX) residents contact:
Federal Office Building, Rm 1185
1961 Stout Street
Denver, CO 80294
(303) 844-6166

Division of Surveillance and Field Studies
Alice Hamilton Laboratories (DSHEFS)
55 Ridge Avenue
Cincinnati, OH 45213
(513) 841-4382

NIOSH conducts research on various safety and health problems, provides technical assistance to the Occupational Safety and Health Administration (OSHA), and recommends standards for OSHA's adoption. NIOSH investigates toxic substances and develops criteria for the use of such substances in the workplace. While conducting its research, NIOSH may make workplace investigations, gather testimonies from employers, and measure and report employee exposure to potentially hazardous materials. It may also require employers to provide medical examinations and tests to determine the incidence of occupational illness among employees. When such examinations and tests are required by NIOSH for research purposes, they may be paid for by NIOSH rather than the employer.

Publications Dissemination
4676 Columbia Parkway
Cincinnati, Ohio 45226
(513) 533-8326

Many NIOSH documents and those published by other federal agencies are also available from the National Technical Information Service (NTIS) or the Government Printing Office as follows:

NTIS
5285 Port Royal Road
Springfield, VA 22161 (Write to establish deposit account $25.00 minimum.)
(703) 487-4780 Research Services—Call to check for availability of document.
(703) 487-4650 Call to order documents.

Government Printing Office
Washington, D.C. 20402
(202) 783-3238

## National Pesticide Medical Monitoring Program

c/o Sheldon Wagner, M.D.
Oregon State University
Department of Agricultural Chemistry
Agricultural and Life Sciences
Room 1007
Corvallis, OR 97331-7301
(503) 757-5086

Under contract to the U.S. Environmental Protection Agency, Dr. Wagner provides basic and clinical information on the toxicology of pesticides. (Emergency calls for acute treatment information should be directed to poison control centers.) Dr. Wagner also provides laboratory analysis of pesticides and metabolites in human tissue.

## National Pesticide Telecommunications Network

Texas Tech University Health Sciences Center
School of Medicine
Department of Preventive Medicine
Lubbock, TX 79430
(800) 858-7378 (toll-free, 24-hours)

Provides information on pesticide toxicity, health effects, residue data, efficacy, etc. Referral services available. Specific information is available on such pesticides as herbicides, fungicides, insecticides, and rodenticides.

## National Response Center

U.S. Coast Guard Headquarters
2100 2nd Street, S.W. Room 2611
Washington, D.C. 20593
(800) 424-8802 (toll-free, 24-hours)

Functions in accordance with the National Contingency Plan to provide for coordinated pollution response by federal and state government agencies. The National Response Center receives initial reports of oil and chemical spills and rapidly passes the information to the predesignated federal on-scene coordinator for action. Technical information such as hazard assessments and movement forecasting is available to federal on-scene coordinators through the National Response Center. The National Response Center also provides support to the National Response Team (representatives of 14 federal agencies which plan for and provide guidance during major oil and hazardous substance spills). The 14 agencies are the Environmental Protection Agency, U.S. Coast Guard (Department of Transportation), Department of Agriculture, Department of Commerce, Department of Defense, Department of Energy, Department of Health and Human Services, Department of the Interior, Department of Justice, Department of Labor, Department of State, the Federal Emergency Management Agency, Nuclear Regulatory Commission and Research and Specific Program. The National Response Team meets monthly to discuss and review matters pertinent to the U.S. response posture.

## National Toxics Campaign Fund

1168 Commonwealth Ave.
Boston, MA 02134
Tel: (617) 232-0327
Fax: (617)232-3945

West Coast Regional Organizer
1912 F Street, Suite 100
Sacramento, CA 95814
Tel: (916) 446-3350
Fax: (916) 446-3394

Los Angeles Organizer
5450 Slauson Avenue, Suite 204
Culver City, CA 90230
Tel: (213) 953-8201
Fax: (213) 953-8203

The National Toxics Campaign Fund (NTCF) is a grassroots-based organization encompassing a network of over 1,500 community, state and regional groups, which undertakes environmental research, education, and organizing. Fueled by the commitment of citizens who have been most directly poisoned by toxic chemicals, NTCF also educates and involves the broader public to support groundbreaking pollution prevention measures.

## Natural Resources Defense Council (NRDC)

71 Stevenson Street
Suite 1825
San Francisco, CA 94105
(415) 777-0220

The Natural Resources Defense Council is a nonprofit membership organization dedicated to the protection of public health and the environment. The council has worked extensively to protect children's health and to control a variety of environmental threats to health, including pesticides. Publications and reports are available on children, pesticides in food, selected individual compounds, and pesticide regulatory issues.

## Occupational Safety and Health Administration, U.S. Department of Labor

Office of Administrative Services (Headquarters)
200 Constitution Avenue, North West, Room N-3101
Washington, D.C. 20210
(202) 219-4667

OSHA Region IX
71 Stevenson Street, Suite 420
San Francisco, CA 94105
(415) 744-6670

Enforces national occupational health and safety standards. In states such as California that have their own programs, federal OSHA may only have jurisdiction for federally owned properties and services and for maritime activities.

## Pesticide Education Center

P.O. Box 420870
San Francisco, CA 94142-0870
(415) 391-8511

The Pesticide Education Center works with community groups, workers, individuals, and others harmed by or concerned about risks to their health from exposure to pesticides used in agriculture, the home and garden, and other environmental and industrial uses. Its goal is to provide critical information about pesticides so that the public can make more informed decisions and choices. The PEC provides information, curricular materials, and help with seminars and workshops on a nationwide basis.

## Reasonably Available Control Technology (RACT)/ Best Available Control Technology (BACT)/ Lowest Achievable Emission Rate (LAER) Clearinghouse

Emission Standards Division
Office of Air Quality Planning and Standards (MD-13)
U.S. EPA
Research Triangle Park, NC 27711
(919) 541-2736
Monday through Friday, 8:00 AM to 4:30 PM, EST

The Reasonably Available Control Technology (RACT)/Best Available Control Technology (BACT)/Lowest Achievable Emission Rate (LAER) Clearinghouse assists federal, state, and local agencies in exchanging information about RACT, BACT and LAER determinations as established under the Clean Air Act. The Clearinghouse also provides information to non-government groups interested in control technology applications.

## Resource Conservation and Recovery Act (RCRA)/ Comprehensive Environmental Response, Compensation, and Liability Act (CERCLA) Hotline

RCRA/CERCLA Hotline
c/o Booz, Allen, and Hamilton
1725 Jefferson Davis Highway
Arlington, Virginia 22202
1-800-424-9346 or (703) 412-9810
Monday through Friday, 8:30 AM to 7:30 PM, EST

The Resource Conservation and Recovery Act (RCRA)/Comprehensive Environmental Response Compensation and Liability Act (CERCLA) Hotline. It is operated under the guidance of the U.S. Environmental Protection Agency's (EPA) Office of Solid Waste and Emergency Response. The primary function of the RCRA/CERCLA Hotline is to assist the public and regulated community in understanding EPA regulations and policy under the RCRA/CERCLA (Superfund) and Underground Storage Tank (UST) programs. Hotline specialists answer regulatory and technical questions, and can respond to requests for documents on virtually all aspects of the RCRA, CERCLA, and UST programs.

## Safe Drinking Water Hotline

(800) 426-4791

This is a public information service operated by the U.S. Environmental Protection Agency.

## Sierra Club

730 Polk Street (National Office)
San Francisco, CA. 94109
(415) 776-2211

Founded in 1892, the Sierra Club is one of the leading environmental protection organizations in the United States. Its goal is to prevent the exhaustion of our natural resources and assure that a decent quality of life is available to future generations. It also has interests in preventing toxic contamination of air, land and water. Over the past few years, the Sierra Club has been part of a number of domestic and overseas hazardous waste and toxics management efforts. It has been extensively involved in the reauthorization of the Resource Conservation and Recovery Act (RCRA). The club has many local chapters, and produces numerous publications.

## Teratogen Information System (TERIS)

Department of Pediatrics
RES 207, CDMRC WJ-10, Box 38
University of Washington
Seattle, WA 98195
(206) 543-2465

TERIS is an automated system for the identification, assessment, storage, and retrieval of published information regarding the teratogenicity of drugs and other environmental agents. The system summarizes 896 agents, including 200 of the most-frequently prescribed drugs. The summaries are derived primarily from information obtained in human investigations, but animal studies are used to amplify and clarify the analysis. Each summary includes a rating of the risk of teratogenic effects in the children of women exposed to the agent under usual conditions during pregnancy. In addition, TERIS provides an updated version of Shepard's Catalog of Teratogenic Agents which provides information on more than 2100 agents.

The Teratogen Information System is designed to assist physicians and other health professionals in counselling pregnant patients who have concerns about possible effects of environmental agents on their developing babies. The agent summaries comprise only part of a comprehensive pregnancy risk evaluation which must also include obtaining information on the patient's state of health, previous and current pregnancy history, and family history.

TERIS can be used throughout the U.S. in an on-line version that is accessible by terminal and modem over ordinary telephone lines. TERIS is also available in a hard disk version for industry-standards MS-DOS microcomputers. (For further information contact Janine E. Polifka, Ph.D., at (206) 543-2465).

## Toxic Substances Control Act (TSCA) Assistance Information Service

TSCA Assistance Information Service
Office of Toxics (TS-799)
Pollution Prevention and U.S. EPA
401 M Street, SW
Washington, DC 20460
(202) 554-1404
Monday through Friday, 8:30 AM to 5:00 PM, EST
FAX (202) 554-5603

The Toxic Substances Control Act (TSCA) Assistance Information Services provides information on TSCA regulations to the chemical industry, labor and trade organizations, environmental groups, and the general public. The TSCA Assistance Information Service can direct inquiries to the appropriate EPA personnel and handle requests for certain publications related to management of toxic substances.

## White Lung Association

National Headquaters:
3030 Barclay St.
Baltimore, MD 21218
(410) 243-5864

Southwestern Region
3917 Linden Ave
Long Beach, CA 90807
(310) 305-6406

A volunteer organization dedicated to the protection of the worker and general public from asbestos through legislation, procurement of compensation, education, and other efforts. Provides information including referrals to physicians and attorneys who are versed in the problems of asbestos.

# INDEX

## CALIFORNIA RESOURCES ON TOXICS

### Air Quality Management Districts and Air Pollution Control Districts, California

The air quality management districts and air pollution control districts regulate stationary sources of air pollution, including factories, dumps, and industrial sites. Mobile sources of air pollution, such as cars, trucks, and buses are exempt from their jurisdiction and are regulated in California by the state Air Resources Board. The districts have the authority to grant permits, enforce emission regulations, issue violation notices, and impose civil penalties on companies or individuals who violate air quality regulations. They maintain networks of air monitoring stations. Jurisdiction, by law, is largely limited to ambient (outdoor) air. The districts do enforce several EPA regulations on hazardous air pollutants, however, including demolition and disposal of asbestos.

### Air Resources Board, California

P.O. Box 2815
Sacramento, CA 95812
(916) 322-2990

The Air Resources Board (ARB) and the local air pollution control and air quality management districts work together to preserve and enhance the air quality in California. The ARB has publications on air pollution and air toxics.

### Art Hazards Program

Office of Environmental Health Hazard Assessment
601 North 7th Street, Room 307/276
P.O. Box 942732
Sacramento, CA 94234-7320
(916) 445-6900

California's Education Code requires the state to develop a list of art and crafts materials which cannot be purchased or ordered for use in kindergarten or grades one through six because they contain toxic substances. This office can answer questions on and provide copies of the art and crafts materials list.

### Asbestos Hotline

Office of Toxic Substances (TS-799)
U.S. EPA
401 M Street, SW
Washington, DC 20460
(202) 554-1404

The nationwide Asbestos Hotline provides technical information concerning asbestos abatement problems in schools and gives referrals to other asbestos programs. Information specialists answer questions about compliance with regulations and funding sources for asbestos removal or encapsulation. Some California sources for information and assistance on asbestos are as follows:

(415) 744-1690—EPA Region IX referral line (Recorded message with different services listed).

(415) 744-1093—EPA Region IX also has information on asbestos inspection and management plans for schools under the Asbestos Hazard Emergency Response Act (AHERA) and on abatement funding under the Asbestos School Hazard Abatement Act (ASHAA).

(916) 445-2360—Office of the State Architect has a program for identification and abatement of hazardous asbestos conditions in state-owned buildings.

(415) 703-5501—Cal/OSHA, for information on asbestos in the workplace. (see also Occupational Safety and Health, California Division of, in this section for phone numbers and locations of area offices).

(415) 703-5501—Cal/OSHA for a list of licensed asbestos certified contractors. There is a charge for this list, currently $30, make a check out to: The State of California, D.O.S.H., and send it to:

Asbestos Contractors List
D.O.S.H.
P.O. BOX 420603
San Francisco, CA 94142
ATTN. O.C.C.U.

(916) 255-3900—California Licensing Board for information on how contractors can become licensed asbestos contractors.

(800) 638-2772—U.S. Consumer Product Safety Commission for information on consumer products containing asbestos.

## Birth Defects Monitoring Branch, California

California Department of Health Services
Division of Environmental and Occupational Disease Control
5900 Hollis Street, Suite A
Emeryville, CA 94608
(510) 540-3091

The California Birth Defects Monitoring Branch (CBDMB) conducts an ongoing birth defects registry and cluster identification and investigation program. The registry includes all children born to residents of the following California counties: Fresno, Kern, Kings, Los Angeles, Madera, Merced, San Francisco, San Joaquin, Santa Clara, Shasta, Siskiyou, Stanislaus, and Tulare, who have a birth defect represented by one or more of over 500 diagnostic codes. Cases are identified and data abstracted by CBDMP field staff. The cluster investigation system responds to public inquiries regarding birth defect clusters or suspected birth defects from exposure to environmental agents including chemicals, infections, dietary factors, drugs, medication, occupational exposures, etc. California clinicians and other community members are encouraged to report suspected clusters of birth defects to the CBDMV.

## Bureau of Home Furnishings

3485 Orange Grove Avenue
North Highlands, CA 95660

Inquiries about furniture or bedding:
Sacramento: (916) 574-2040
Los Angeles:(213) 897-4408

Inquiries about thermal insulation:
Sacramento: (916) 574-2046

The bureau provides free brochures on product flammability and how to purchase water beds, furniture, mattresses, etc., and how to deal with custom upholsterers. Publications are also available in Spanish.

The bureau enforces California statutes and regulations governing upholstered furniture, bedding, and thermal insulation industries. Oversees guarantees, warranties and advertising for thermal insulation, waterbeds and furniture that contain filling materials (for example, sofas, pillows, quilts). For registering complaints call or write to request a complaint form. The form used by the Department of Consumer Affairs, Division of Consumer Services, also is acceptable.

## California Environmental Protection Agency, Office of the Secretary

555 Capitol Mall, Suite 235
Sacramento, CA 95814
(916) 445-3846 (General Information)
(916) 324-9670 (Communications Office)
(916) 324-9667 (Enforcement)
(916) 323-2520 (External Affairs)
(916) 322-7315 (Legislation)
(916) 322-5844 (Regulatory Reform)
(916) 327-1848 (Help Desk)

In July 1991, the California Environmental Protection Agency (Cal/EPA) was created to coordinate the State's environmental quality programs and assure that there is a cabinet level voice for environmental protection. As a result the reorganization process, Cal/EPA consists of:

> Office of the Secretary
> Air Resources Board
> Department of Pesticide Regulation
> Department of Toxic Substance Control
> Integrated Waste Management Board
> Office of Environmental Health Hazard Assessment
> State Water Resources Control Board and Regional Water Quality Control Boards

These programs represent the basic components of the State's environmental protection efforts, but more programs may be included in the future. The Cal/EPA programs are individually described elsewhere in this section. See also, the Hazardous Materials Data Management Program, Cal/EPA.

## California Institute for Rural Studies

P.O. Box 2143
Davis, CA 95617
(916) 756-6555

The institute is a nonprofit, public interest organization specializing in contemporary problems and concerns of rural California. Takes interest in examining questions of pesticide use, worker health and safety, and resource use issues. Educational materials include 2 slide shows— a 15-minute one, "Pesticides: A Guide for Farmworkers" and a 22-minute one, "Clean Water: Who Needs It?" These come with a cassette tape sound track in Spanish or English. Also available is a guidebook for California farmworker agencies that includes information on how to handle a poisoning case, the symptoms of pesticide illness, workers' legal rights, etc.

The CIRS Rural Toxics Project provides direct support (advice and referrals) for individuals who have been adversely affected by exposure to agricultural chemicals. This program also organizes technical assistance for farmers who are seeking to reduce or eliminate the use of toxic chemicals in growing crops.

## Cancer Surveillance Section

California Department of Health Services
601 N. Seventh St.
P.O. Box 942732
Sacramento, CA 94234-7320
(916) 327-4663
Hours: 8:00 AM–5:00 PM

Operates the California Tumor Registry (CTR), which is a statewide population-based cancer reporting and surveillance system. Data collected through ten regional registries will enable the Department of Health Services to monitor the occurrence of cancer among the entire population of the state. Each year the CTR collects data on an expected 120,000 cancer cases a year diagnosed throughout the state. Mandatory cancer reporting was initiated on a staggered basis, the first registries reporting data effective January 1, 1987, and the last registry effective July 1, 1988. Non-confidential data are made available on request to universities, health departments, and the public on magnetic tape which will be updated annually. Access to confidential data by qualified researchers is possible upon review and approval of a detailed study proposal by the Human Investigation Review Committee of the State of California or its designee.

## Childhood Lead Poisoning Prevention Branch

California Department of Health Services
5801 Christie Ave., Ste., 600
Emeryville, CA 94608
(510) 450-2445

The California Childhood Lead Poisoning Prevention Branch (CLPPB) provides technical assistance and educational materials to local health departments and health care providers on the identification, treatments, and environmental management of childhood lead poisoning. Since lead poisoning is a reportable condition, this program maintains a surveillance system that assists local health departments in efficiently following up cases and determining the magnitude and causes of identified cases. Conducting research on medical, epidemiological, abatement, and environmental issues are a program mandate. CLPPB also works with the DHS Air and Industrial Hygiene Laboratory on a laboratory proficiency assurance program.

## Citizens for a Better Environment—California

501 Second Street, Suite 305
San Francisco, CA 94107
(415) 243-8373

CBE is a California organization that seeks to reduce human exposure to toxic chemicals in the urban environment. It works through technical research, watch dogging government agencies and industry, public information and participation and responsible legal action. Current concerns in California include toxics in San Francisco Bay, state hazardous materials policy and environmental racism. Publishes Environmental Review and various reports.

## Communicable Disease Control, Division of

California Department of Health Services
2151 Berkeley Way, Room 708
Berkeley, CA 94704
(510) 540-2566 (days)
(510) 540-2308 (nights, weekends, holidays)

This Branch is responsible for the surveillance of infectious diseases of public health importance in California. The Branch also provides consultation and assistance to local health departments, other agencies, and physicians on the diagnosis and public health control and management of infectious disease problems. In addition, the Branch consults on public health aspects of food borne diseases caused by natural biological toxins such as paralytic shellfish poisoning (PSP), possible mushroom poisoning, and botulism. The Branch collaborates with poison control centers in the management of these food borne toxin diseases.

## Consumer Affairs, California Department of

Consumer Assistance Office
400 R Street, Suite 1040
Sacramento, CA 95814
(916) 445-1254

The California Department of Consumer Affairs' Division of Consumer Services educates and informs consumers about their rights and responsibilities in the marketplace, and protects consumers from deceptive or fraudulent business practices.

The Division of Consumer Assistance Office: Assists consumers with complaints by advising them on steps toward resolving marketplace problems.

General Complaints
Main Office
(See above)

Consumer Infoline
(800) 344-9940

Provides California consumers with a variety of pre-recorded consumer information.

The department's consumer booklets cover a variety of subjects, including sales tactics, landlord-tenant relations, and auto repair. To obtain a copy of the publications list, send a stamped, legal-size envelope to:

Publications List
400 R Street
Sacramento, CA 95802

## Consumer Protection Offices

State, county, and some city governments have consumer protection offices located in the state attorney general's and local district attorney's offices. The staff in these offices can help consumers resolve complaints, furnish information and helpful publications, or provide other services. Because most offices require that complaints be in writing, the consumer might save time by writing, rather than calling, with the initial complaint. (See also Dept. of Consumer Affairs)

## Cooperative Extension, University of California
## Division of Agriculture and Natural Resources

Each county in California is served by the University of California Cooperative Extension, with offices in 57 of the Counties. Sometimes called the Farm and Home Advisors Office, it is staffed by farm, home, marine, forest, and 4-H youth development advisors who are academic employees of the University. They bring together the resources of the University and apply them to the needs of local areas. The advisors are often able to help with information on the uses and hazards of pesticides for home, farm, and forest use. The advisors are supported by Cooperative Extension specialists and other University researchers. Statewide specialists are located at the Berkeley, Davis, and Riverside campuses of the University of California and at the Kearney Agriculture Center in Parlier. Several special services should be mentioned:

*The Office of Pesticide Information and Coordination* provides liaison between the University of California Division of Agriculture and Natural Resources and the various state agencies which regulate pesticides. The Pesticide Impact Assessment Program generates benefit assessment data on registered pesticides. For both of these programs contact:

M.W. Stimmann
Statewide Pesticide Coordinator
Environmental Toxicology
University of California
Davis, CA 95616
(916) 752-7011

U.C. Cooperative Extension also produces pesticide education and safety training materials in both the English and Spanish languages and has a full-time Extension Toxicologist who is available to provide information to members of the public:

A. Craigmill
Extension Toxicologist
Environmental Toxicology
University of California
Davis, CA 95616
(916) 752-2936

*The Center for Pest Management Research and Extension* serves as a clearing house for pest management information in UC, helping to identify emerging issues and recommend short and long term research and extension priorities.

Center for Pest Management Research and Extension
Robert K. Washino, Director
University of California
Davis, CA 95616
(916) 752-5274

*The Statewide Integrated Pest Management Project* was created by the California Legislature to develop and promote the use of integrated, ecologically sound pest management programs. A wide variety of information is available in publications and on-line data systems, also conducts extensive programs in pesticide applicator training.

IPM Project
F.W. Zalom, Director
University of California
Davis, CA 95616
(916) 752-8350

## Drinking Water and Environmental Management, Division of

California Department of Health Services
2151 Berkeley Way, Room 458
Berkeley, CA 94704
(510) 540-2158

Headquarters: 601 North Seventh Street
P.O. Box 942732
Sacramento, CA 94234-7320
(916) 323-6111

Collects and evaluates water quality information on drinking water in California. Provides assistance to local health departments, water purveyors, and the general public on issues related to water quality, water supply, and water treatment. Advises state and regional water quality control boards on public health protection of water supplies. In cooperation with the Hazard Identification and Risk Assessment Branch, develops state drinking water standards and insures compliance with drinking water standards by water purveyors.

Other regional and/or district offices are as follows:

Santa Rosa—50 D Street, Suite 205, 95404-4752, (707) 576-2145
Sacramento—8455 Jackson Road., Room 120, 95826, (916) 387-3126
Redding—415 Knollcrest Drive, Suite 110, 96002, (916) 224-4800
Fresno—5545 E. Shields Avenue, 93727, (209) 297-3883
Stockton—State Bldg. 31 E. Channel Street, Room 270, 95202, (209) 948-7697
Santa Barbara—530 E. Montecito St., Room 102, 93105, (805) 963-8616
Santa Ana—28 Civic Center Plaza, Room 325, 92701, (714) 558-4410
Los Angeles—1449 West Temple Street, Room 202, 90026, (213) 620-2980
San Diego—State Bldg., 1350 Front Street, Room 2050, 92101, (619) 525-4159
San Bernardino—1836 S. Commercenter Circle, Suite B, 92408, (909) 383-4328

## Emergency Medical Services Authority, California

1930 9th Street, Suite 100
Sacramento, CA 95814
(916) 322-4336
FAX # (916) 324-2875

The Emergency Medical Services Authority has developed general guidelines for the medical management of hazardous materials victims in the field and hospital emergency departments. The "Hazardous Materials Medical Management Protocols" are available to health professionals. Training courses are jointly offered with the University of California Hazardous Substances Programs and the California Specialized Training Institute (CSTI) for personnel involved in or planning for the emergency medical response to hazardous materials incidents. This training covers such topics as site safety, triage and medical management of patients, and limiting secondary contamination. CSTI and the University of California at Davis Extension should be contacted directly to register. The EMS Authority also manages the Regional Poison Control Centers Program.

## Emergency Services Warning Center, Office of (California)

2800 Meadowview Road
Sacramento, CA 95832
(916) 262-1800 General information
(800) 852-7550 24 hours a day,
(916) 391-7715 for radiation emergencies

Serves as the central notification point for hazardous materials incidents throughout the State. Notifies other State agencies which are qualified to give technical assistance and information regarding hazardous materials incidents. (See chart on inside of back cover for notification information flow).

## Environmental Health Investigations Branch

California Department of Health Services
5900 Hollis Street, Ste., E
Emeryville, CA 94608
(510) 540-3657

The Environmental Health Investigations Branch (EHIB) assists local governments and regulatory agencies in investigating health problems that may be related to chemicals or other non-infectious agents in the environment. For example, EHIB has investigated unusually high numbers of cancer cases or other rare illnesses that have occurred in some neighborhoods where there may have been exposures to toxic substances. EHIB also responds to other concerns about possible long-term health effects from exposure to agents in the environment, such as effects from a chemical spill, food contamination, or new medical technologies. The staff, which includes physicians, scientists, and health educators, provides information to the public, and training and technical assistance on environmental health issues for local governments, regulatory agencies, health care providers, and non-governmental organizations.

EHIB is overseeing the conduct of studies on the possible health effects of exposure to electromagnetic fields (EMF) generated by electric power lines and electric appliances. The studies are focused on childhood cancers and spontaneous abortions. The section has also produced educational materials, sponsored training on EMF for local health staff, and worked with the Public Utilities Commission, Energy Commission, and others in developing public policy regarding the complex EMF issues. In late 1991, funding for this activity was terminated. However, there is a possibility that the program may be reinstated at a later date.

## Environmental Health Division

California Department of Health Services
601 North Seventh St.
P.O. Box 942732
Sacramento, CA 94234-7320
(916) 322-2308

Responds to information inquiries on all environmental health effects. Coordinates activities involving State Food and Drug, Radiological Health, and Environmental Management.

## Exposure Assessment and Molecular Epidemiology Section

California Department of Health Services
Division of Environmental and Occupational Disease Control
5900 Hollis Street, Suite E
Emeryville, CA 94608
(510) 540-3657, FAX (510) 540-2673

This section assesses human exposure to environmental, chemical, and physical agents. Exposure assessment is needed for the toxicological characterization of risk or the interpretation of environmental epidemiological results. The National Priority List Health Assessments Unit of this section reviews existing historical, environmental, and epidemiological information about Superfund sites in the state. This unit assesses the potential health consequences, further needed information, and necessary public actions related to each site. The Exposure Field Investigation Team carries out exposure field investigations and provides technical guidance to laboratories and regulatory agencies. They also assess measurements taken by others to estimate human exposures and provide training to county personnel on exposure assessment.

## Fetal Alcohol Syndrome/
## Fetal Alcohol Effects Prevention Assistance Program

California Urban Indian Health Council, Inc.
3637 Marconi Ave.
Sacramento, CA 95821
(916) 484-4353

The California Urban Indian Health Council (CUIHC) Fetal Alcohol Syndrome/Fetal Alcohol Effects Prevention Assistance Program (FAS/FAE) is available to provide workshop training upon request to health care professionals who want to learn more about FAS/FAE. Technical assistance is also provided to help local agencies establish referral and treatment networks with Indian Health Clinics and other agencies throughout the State of California. Assistance will also be given in designing and implementing public awareness campaigns about FAS/FAE. FAS/FAE Community Education Material are available at cost.

## Food and Drug Branch

California Department of Health Services
601 North Seventh Street
Sacramento, CA 94234-7320
(916) 445-2263

Regional Offices:
2151 Berkeley Way, Room 610
Berkeley, CA 94704
(510) 540-2261

8455 Jackson Road, Suite 120
Sacramento, CA 95826
(916) 387-3125

1449 W. Temple St., Rm. 224
Los Angeles, CA 90026
(213) 620-2965

Responsible for public protection programs for food, drugs, medical devices, cosmetics, hazard-ous household products, and cancer quackery. Programs are designed to prevent manufacture, distribution and sale of adulterated, misbranded or falsely advertised products. Activities include but are not limited to investigation of complaints, routine inspection of facilities, licensing of a variety of manufacturers, and preparation of materials relevant to court actions. State Food and Drug is headquartered in Sacramento and has 10 district offices. Food and drug investigators are located throughout the state and may be called into service at any time.

## Hazard Evaluation System and Information Service (HESIS)

California Departments of Health Services and Industrial Relations
Divison of Environmental and Occupational Disease Control
2151 Berkeley Way, Annex 11, 3rd Floor
Berkeley, CA 94704
For workplace hazard information, please write. For other business, call (510) 540-2115.

Reviews and evaluates information on health effects of toxic substances in the workplace only. Provides early warning of newly identified occupational health hazards, so that workers, employers, health professionals and government agencies can take action to reduce exposures. Responds to inquiries concerning the health effects of toxic substances in the workplace, safe work practices, health and safety controls, and methods for monitoring workers' health. Inquiries must be work-related. Occasionally provides planning assistance and speakers for occupa-tional health training programs. Staff includes toxicologists, physicians, a health educator, and industrial hygienists.

## Hazardous Materials Data Management Program

California Environmental Protection Agency
555 Capitol Mall, Sutie 235
Sacramento, CA 95814
(916) 327-1848 or (916) 327-1849

The Hazardous Materials Data Management Program in the California Environmental Protection

Agency (Cal/EPA) collects, manages and distributes toxic information in California. The Office has the following features:

Help Desk: A central location for obtaining assistance and referrals on any hazardous substance-related question.

Guide to Toxic Databases: Document that lists existing hazardous substances databases, summarizes their purpose and content, and tells who to contact for further information.

Facility Inventory: A database that combines facility identification and information from various programs which regulate facilities handling hazardous substances at federal, state, and local levels of government.

Toxic Chemical Release Inventory: Under section 313 of the Emergency Planning and Community Right-To-Know Act (Title III of the Superfund Amendments and Reauthorization Act of 1986), facilities are required to file a Toxic Chemical Release Form with the United States Environmental Protection Agency and the California Environmental Affairs Agency, on any release to air, water and land as well as discharges to publicly-owned treatment works and transfers to off-site locations. Summaries of the information reported, as well as copies of the forms, may be obtained from the "Help Desk."

Chemical Cross-Index (List of Lists): Under contract, the University of California, Davis compiled a cross-index of hazardous chemicals regulated by various state and federal agencies. The cross-index shows, for each chemical, whether or not the chemical is regulated under each of 14 programs.

The *Guide to Hazardous Substances Reporting Requirements* describes the current structure of state, federal, and local environmental regulatory agencies, and lists appropriate contacts. Over 40 state and federal environmental reporting forms are illustrated, along with specific regulatory program contact information, filing criteria, filing frequency, and due dates for the reports. The relevant local business plan form, a list of helpful telephone numbers and possible sources of financial assistance are included.

Copies of the guide, which costs $30, may be ordered by writing to the Hazardous Materials Data Management Program at the above address.

## Indoor Air Quality Branch, California

California Department of Health Services
Divison of Environmental and Occupational Disease Control
2151 Berkeley Way
Berkeley, CA 94704
(510) 540-2469

California has established the first state program devoted entirely to addressing indoor environmental problems in private residences, schools, offices, and public buildings. The California Indoor Air Quality Section is responsible for promoting, coordinating, and conducting research aimed at understanding the determinants of healthful indoor environments. The ultimate goal is to assess the nature and magnitude of potential hazards within the state so that health risks can be evaluated rationally.

## Labor Occupational Health Program (LOHP)

School of Public Health
University of California, Berkeley
2515 Channing Way
Berkeley, CA 94720
(510) 642-5507

Provides training sessions, publications, films, slide shows and technical assistance on occupational health and safety issues. Allows use of their extensive resource library with information available on hazard identification, toxicology, industrial hygiene, health and safety organizing, standards and regulations, ergonomics and VDT training, hazardous waste and toxic cleanup, training sessions on AIDS in the workplace, etc. Hazard awareness and waste training is available in both Spanish and English.

## Labor Occupational Safety and Health (LOSH) Program

Center for Labor Research and Education
University of California, Los Angeles
1001 Gayley Ave., 2nd Floor
Los Angeles, CA 90024
(310) 794-0369, or (310) 794-0390

Offers training courses for workers, union members, and health professionals on health and safety as requested; large conferences on current issues in occupational health; a quarterly newsletter, "Workers Connection"; brochures on health and safety topics (some in Spanish); technical and research assistance; and student interns specializing in occupational safety and health. Provides educational, audio visual, and written materials as well.

## Laboratory Accreditation Program, Environmental

California Department of Health Services
2151 Berkeley Way, Annex 2
Berkeley, CA 94704-1101
(510) 540-2800

Accreditation as a certified environmental laboratory in California is provided to applicant private and public laboratory facilities in the areas of drinking water, wastewater, and hazardous waste testing, and for pesticide residues in food. Other areas of certification are available, such as bulk asbestos testing and shellfish sanitation. Lists of laboratories certified to conduct drinking water, wastewater, or hazardous waste testing is available from the program. Lists are also available for bulk asbestos testing, bioassay testing (wastewater and hazardous waste), and radiochemistry. Special lists can be produced, but are charged at the rate of $0.25/page.

## Local health agencies, county and city

Local health agencies frequently serve as a good information or referral source especially on hazards particular to their jurisdictions. They may also provide help to local citizens. Their general duties in respect to toxic substances are as follows: Local directors of environmental health are frequently involved in emergency and regulatory actions relative to toxic substance control. These actions might include inspection programs for underground storage or generation of hazardous materials, emergency response, and implementation of community right-to-know ordinances. Local health officers have broad authority and responsibility to protect the health and safety of the public within their jurisdictions. This authority includes powers to take action in emergency and nonemergency situations involving toxic chemicals.

## Local Government Commission, Inc.

909 12th Street, Suite 205
Sacramento, CA 95814
(916) 448-1198

The Local Government Commission, a nonprofit organization, serves both cities and counties and is directed toward promoting cooperative efforts among all levels of government. It is involved in developing and implementing local solutions to problems of state and national significance. In particular, the commission assists elected officials, government staff, and citizens in their efforts to design comprehensive local policies which prevent public exposure to hazardous and toxic materials. The commission can provide technical information, model policies, and strategic guidance on a wide variety of local programs to address the toxics problem (e.g., zoning ordinances; household hazardous waste collection; sanitary, building, and fire code amendments; and sewer use ordinances.) Publications include: "Household Hazardous Waste: Solving the Disposal Dilemma" (a handbook); "Low Cost Ways to Promote Hazardous Waste Minimization: A Resource Guide for Local Governments"; "Reducing Industrial Toxic Wastes and Discharges: The Role of POTW's (Publicly Owned Sewage Treatment Works)"; "Minimizing Hazardous Wastes: Regulatory Options for Local Governments"; and "Making the Switch, Alternatives to Using Toxic Chemicals in the Home."

## Medical Waste Management Program

California Department of Health Services
601 North 7th Street
P.O. Box 942732
Sacramento, CA 94234-7320
(916) 322-2042

The Medical Waste Management Program of the California Department of Health Services administers the Medical Waste Management Act (the Act) which stipulates how medical waste is to be contained, stored, transported, and treated (rendered non-infectious). This office responds to inquiries regarding appropriate handling of medical waste, inspects medical waste generators, permits medical waste treatment facilities and enforces the act in the 24 counties and 1 city for which the state Department of Health Services is the local enforcement agency. In the remaining 34 counties and 3 cities the local health jurisdiction serves as the enforcement agency. The counties and city for which this office is the local enforcement agency are:

Alpine, Amador, Butte, Calaveras, Fresno, Glenn, Imperial, Inyo, Kings, Lake, Los Angeles, Mariposa, Mendocino, Mono, Nevada, Placer, Plumas, Riverside, San Benito, San Luis Obispo, Sierra, Solano, Sutter, Yolo, and the City of Berkeley.

## Occupational and Environmental Health, Center for, Davis

University of California
Division of Occupational/Environmental and Epidemiology
Institute of Toxicology and Environmental Health
Old Davis Road
Davis, California 95616
(916) 752-3317

The goal of the Center is to increase understanding of the causes of human health problems due to occupational and environmental hazards and to work towards reducing morbidity and mortality from these hazards through research and educational and clinical service. Research activities are concentrated in the area of epidemiology, toxicology and occupational medicine.

## Occupational and Environmental Health, Center for, UCLA

University of California, Los Angeles
School of Public Health
10833 Le Conte Avenue, Room 41, 230 CHS
Los Angeles, CA 90024-1772
(310) 206-6920

The UCLA Center for Occupational and Environmental Health (COEH) is housed in the School of Public Health and embodies faculty and staff from the Schools of Public Health, Nursing, and Medicine and the Institute of Industrial Relations. The mission of COEH is to train occupational health professionals, conduct research on occupational and environmental health, provide community outreach through continuing education, clinical services, and technical consultation. The Center is equipped with elaborate laboratory facilities to conduct toxicity tests and to identify and quantify organic compounds.

Recently, the COEH has expanded its efforts to include environmental health research and training. The COEH is one of the three participating units (the other two are the School of Engineering and Architecture & Urban Planning) in the UCLA Toxics Reduction Group. COEH also has active collaborations in occupational and environmental health research and training with scientists in Latin America and Asia. Special activities are underway in Mexico, Taiwan and Indonesia.

The Occupational Health Clinical center and the Labor Occupational Safety and Health Program (LOSH) are integral parts of the COEH, which offer consultative services and educational opportunities to the community. See separate listings for detailed program descriptions.

## Occupational and Environmental Medicine Clinic, UC Davis

University of California, Davis Medical Center
Professional Building, Suite I
4301 X Street, Suite 1
Sacramento, CA 95817
(916) 734-2715

Clinic for medical evaluation of work related illness and injury, both industrial and agricultural. Screening of working populations, medical surveillance programs, workplace evaluation, and medico-legal consultation and/or referral available. Hours are Thursday afternoons from 1 to 5 PM.

## Occupational Health Center, UC Irvine

University of California
19722 MacArthur Blvd.
Irvine, CA 92715
(714) 856-8640

The Occupational Health Center (IOHC) is headquartered at the University of California campus in Irvine. The center provides professional education, research and community services.

IOHC's professional education includes specialties in industrial hygiene, occupational epidemiology, occupational health nursing, occupational and environmental medicine, occupational and environmental toxicology, and occupational and environmental health education. IOHC's community services include consultative assistance to nurses and physicians working in occupational health engineering, industrial hygiene and safety evaluation, diagnosis of referred patients either by individual occupational medicine physicians or through the UCI Occupational Medicine Clinics, toxicity information, a resource center for published materials, a classroom space for community groups concerned with occupational health issues, environmental community health information, research into causes of occupational disease and cancer, and involvement with a regional tumor registry.

Eligibility requirements: For professional programs, check with IOHC; medical services at UCI available only through referral.

Bilingual services: Spanish

College of Medicine
Irvine, CA 92717
(714) 856-7438

## Occupational Health Clinic at UCSF and San Francisco General Hospital

San Francisco General Hospital Bldg. 9, Room 109
1001 Potrero Avenue
San Francisco, CA 94110
(415) 206-5391

Provides consultation, diagnoses, and treatment of occupational and environmental health problems by referral and appointment. Medical surveillance of lead, asbestos, and other worksite problems. Industrial hygiene services and worksite evaluations.

## Occupational Health Clinical Center, UCLA

Center for Health Sciences
UCLA School of Medicine
10833 Le Conte Avenue
Los Angeles, CA 90024-1736
(310) 206-2086

Provides California employers and workers with convenient access to the resources of UCLA

Medical Center. Full range of services which include access to all UCLA Medical Center Services, the Occupational Medical Branch, independent medical examinations, occupational lung disease, occupational back pain program, and occupational medical seminars.

## Occupational Lead Poisoning Prevention Program

California Occupational Health Branch
California Department of Health Services
2151 Berkeley Way, Annex 11, 3rd Floor
Berkeley, CA 94704
(510) 540-3448 (leave message)

The Occupational Lead Posioning Prevention Program (OLPPP) maintains a registry of laboratory-reported cases of work-related lead poisoning in California adults. Periodic analysis identifies patterns of lead poisoning among individual industries and population groups. The program provides follow-up to occupational lead poisoning cases, to identify and control sources of lead exposure, and to investigate whether workplace lead exposures may result in take-home exposure and lead poisoning in household members. OLPPP develops educational materials and provides training about the hazards of lead to workers, employers, and health professionals. The program also makes recommendations for the prevention of lead poisoning. Legislation passed in 1991 established OLPPP, and provided for funding of the program through an annual fee assessed on lead-using industries.

## Occupational Medicine Branch, UCLA

Center for the Health Sciences, Room 37-131
University of California
1099 Heyburn Avenue, Suite 344
Los Angeles, CA 90024-7027
(310) 206-2086

Clinical evaluation of occupational and environmental illness and injury. Medical surveillance of worker populations, worksite walk through surveys, applied research, and preventive and medico-legal consultative services are available. On-site worker training and medical testing can be arranged.

## Occupational Medicine Clinics, UC Irvine

University of California at Irvine
19722 Mac Arthur Blvd.
Irvine, CA 92715
(714) 856-8640

Services and programs include patient evaluation and diagnosis, toxicity information, medical referral, and medical treatment.

## Occupational Safety and Health (Cal/OSHA), California Division of

The Cal/OSHA Program has four independent cooperating components. Two which pertain here are the following. Also see units listed below.

## THE DIVISION OF OCCUPATIONAL SAFETY AND HEALTH (DOSH)

Enforces occupational safety and health standards and regulations.

Headquarters
455 Golden Gate Ave., Room 5202
San Francisco, CA 94102
(415) 703-4341

Regional Offices
Anaheim—2100 E. Katella, Suite 125, Anaheim, CA 92806 Tel: (714) 939-8611
Los Angeles—3550 West 6th Street, Room 413, Los Angeles, CA 90020 Tel: (213) 736-4911
Sacramento—2424 Arden Way, Suite 125, Sacramento CA 95825 Tel: (916) 263-2803
San Francisco—1390 Market Street, Suite 822, San Francisco CA 94102 Tel: (415) 557-8640

District offices are located in the following cities: Anaheim/Santa Ana, Bakersfield, Concord, Covina, Fresno, Los Angeles, Modesto, Oakland, Pico Rivera, Redding, Sacramento, San Bernardino, San Diego, San Francisco, San Jose, San Mateo, Santa Rosa, Torrance/Long Beach/South Bay, Van Nuys, Ventura.

Field offices are located in the following cities: Chico, Eureka, Salinas, Santa Fe Springs, Stockton, Ukiah.

## THE CAL/OSHA CONSULTATION SERVICE

Provides free on-site consultation to employers and advice and information on occupational safety and health to employers and employee groups. The consultation service is not involved in Cal/OSHA enforcement activities.

Headquarters
455 Golden Gate Ave., Room 5246,
San Francisco 94102
(415) 703-4050

Area Offices
Downey—10350 Heritage Park Drive, Santa Fe Springs, CA 90670, (310) 944-9366
Fresno—1901 N. Gateway Blvd. Suite 102, Fresno, CA 93727, (209) 454-1295
Sacramento—2424 Arden Way, Suite 410, Sacramento, CA 95825, (916) 263-2855
San Diego—7827 Convoy Court, Suite 406, San Diego, CA 92111, (619) 279-3771
San Mateo—3 Waters Park Drive, Room 230, San Mateo, Ca 94403, (415) 573-3864

Units
In addition, Cal/OSHA has the following units, all located in its headquarters (note that descriptions follow the list):

Public Information—(415) 703-4981
Audio Visual Library—(415) 703-4050
Occupational Carcinogen Control—(415) 703-3631
Research and Standards Development—(415) 703-5501
Right to Know—(415) 703-4511

Cal/OSHA PUBLIC INFORMATION is a source for all Cal/OSHA publications, which include fact sheets on general and specific job health and safety standards and issues. All Cal/OSHA publications are available at any local Cal/OSHA office or by calling (415) 703-5281.

AUDIO VISUAL LIBRARY provides VHS videotapes free of charge to those in California interested in promoting safety and health on the job. Tapes may be selected from a list of all tapes available through the Unit. The tapes are available without charge; the user need only pay return postage charges. For tape service information write to this unit at 455 Golden Gate Ave. Room 5246, San Francisco, call (415) 703-4050, or FAX (415) 703-5131.

MEDICAL UNIT responds to inquiries on all regulatory aspects of workplace exposure to toxic substances. Determines whether adverse health effects are being caused by a workplace exposure and, if so, formulates corrective action. Example of problems handled include tight or sick building syndrome and ergonomic work problems. There are 3 offices, San Francisco (415) 557-8640, Los Angeles (213) 736-4927, and Sacramento (916) 263-2793.

OCCUPATIONAL CARCINOGEN CONTROL UNIT (OCCU) maintains a list of all industries using regulated carcinogens (22 at present) and provides information regarding employee exposures to carcinogens in California. All employers who work with asbestos on jobs greater than 100 square feet of surface area must have a special registration. Also contractors must be certified by the Contractors State License Board. (415) 703-5501

RESEARCH STANDARDS DEVELOPMENT UNIT develops health standards in conjunction with advisory committees. (415) 703-5501.

RIGHT TO KNOW UNIT (aka HAZARD COMMUNICATION) reviews material safety data sheets (MSDSs) for accuracy and assists employers or employees in obtaining MSDSs from companies that refuse to give them out. (415) 703-4511.

## Occupational Safety and Health, Santa Clara Center for

760 North First Street
San Jose, CA 95112
(408) 998-4050

Provides information on health effects of toxic substances, including health and safety information on the electronics industry. Provides health and safety advocacy information and movie and slide show rentals on occupational safety and health. Permits public use of library resources. Distributes newsletter and conducts workshops and trainings on specific occupational hazards, especially for workers of limited literacy and those for whom English is a second language.

## Office of Environmental Health Hazard Assessment (OEHHA)

Main office:
601 North 7th Street, Room 307/276
P.O. Box 942732
Sacramento, CA 94234-7320
(916) 324-7572

Address for sections listed below:
2151 Berkeley Way, Annex 11
Berkeley, CA 94704

Air Toxicology and Epidemiology Section, (510) 540-3324
Pesticide and Environmental Toxicology Section, (510) 540-3063
Reproductive and Cancer Hazard Assessment Section, (510) 540-2084, (916) 324-7572

The Office of Environmental Health Hazard Assessment (OEHHA) of the California Environmental Protection Agency is responsible for identifying the adverse effects of chemicals in the environment, and assessing the health risks associated with exposures to environmental contaminants. The department includes the following sections:

The Air Toxicology and Epidemiology Section assesses toxic air contaminants and pollutants for the development of regulatory standards and health advisories. This section also reviews risk assessments of air emissions from industrial facilities.

The Pesticide and Environmental Toxicology Section assesses the risks of environmental contaminants in food, water, and some consumer items, as well as the risks of community and worker exposure to pesticides. This section also educates health professionals and the public about health effects of environmental toxicants. A list of publications is available.

The Reproductive and Cancer Hazard Assessment Section recommends which chemicals to include on the lists of Proposition 65 carcinogens and reproductive toxicants. It also develops guidelines that the State uses in determining which chemicals should be treated as carcinogens and reproductive toxicants, and in assessing their risks.

## Pesticide Regulation, California Department of

1020 N Street, Room 100
Sacramento, CA 95814
(916) 445-4300

This department of the California Environmental Protection Agency is charged with ensuring the safe use of pesticides, protecting human health and the environment, and providing adequate tools and alternatives for pest managment. The Department of Pesticide Regulation (DPR) is the primary agency charged with assessing and mitigating the environmental and human health impacts of pesticide use. DPR oversees pesticide registration and the safety of the pesticide workplace, and enforces state and federal pesticide laws. DPR consists of six branches, five of which are pertinent here. These units are headquartered in Sacramento with various branch offices located throughout the state, as listed below.

PESTICIDE ENFORCEMENT BRANCH
1020 N Street Room 300
Sacramento, CA 95814
(916) 445-4038

Enforces EPA and Departmental laws and regulations and label requirements concerning pesticide use throughout the state. Enforces pesticide residue regulations pertaining to food. Conducts a program of testing raw commodities intended for human consumption for pesticide residue levels. Oversees local enforcement by county agricultural commissioners.

Branch Offices:
727 Allston Way
Berkeley, CA 94710
(510) 540-2910

169 E. Liberty Ave.
Anaheim, CA 92801-1014
(714) 680-7903

2895 N. Larkin, Suite B
Fresno, CA 93727
(209) 445-5401

PESTICIDE REGISTRATION BRANCH
1020 N Street, Room 332
Sacramento, CA 95814
(916) 445-4400

INFORMATION SYSTEMS

1020 N Street, Room 445-4130
P.O. Box 942871
Sacramento, CA 94271-0001
(916) 654-1353

Responsible for all pesticide registration actions and a repository of registrant information supporting registration of all pesticides.

WORKER HEALTH AND SAFETY BRANCH
1020 N Street, Room 200
Sacramento, CA 95814
(916) 445-4222

Evaluates potential workplace hazards of pesticides. Evaluates pesticide exposure studies submitted by registrants and conducts its own studies to evaluate potential risks from exposure to pesticides. Recommends measures designed to provide a safer environment for workers who handle or are exposed to pesticides. Provides medical advice and assistance on pesticide exposures.

ENVIRONMENTAL MONITORING AND PEST MANAGEMENT BRANCH
1020 N Street, Room 161
Sacramento, CA 95814
(916) 324-4100

Monitors the environment (air, water and soil) to determine the environmental fate of currently registered pesticides, and identifies and recommends chemical, cultural and biological alternatives for managing pests.

Branch Office:
Statewide Air Pollution Center, Trailer 14
University of California, Riverside
Riverside, CA 92521
(714) 787-4683

MEDICAL TOXICOLOGY BRANCH
1020 N Street, Room 234
Sacramento, Ca 95814
(916) 445-4233

Medical Toxicology Branch has two major functions: review of toxicology studies and preparation of risk assessments. Data are reviewed for chronic and acute health effects for: new active ingredients and new products containing already registered active ingredients; label amendments on currently registered products which include major new uses; and for reevaluation of currently registered active ingredients. The results of these reviews as well as exposure information from other branches are used in the conduct of health risk characterizations.

## Poison Control Centers

Regional Poison Control Centers are staffed around-the-clock by clinical pharmacists with doctor of pharmacy degrees and specially trained registered nurses with professional certification as poison center specialists. Additional consultative support from a staff of on-call physician toxicologists certified in medical toxicology with primary specialties in internal, emergency, laboratory, or occupational medicine are immediately available. The staff provide the public, physicians, and other health care providers with information and consultation on poisoning emergencies involving household products, industrial chemicals, mushrooms and other plants, foods, and drug reactions or overdoses. Referrals for the diagnosis and treatment of poisonings are also given. The centers are a resource for the education of both the public and health professionals, and most have health educators. They are researching the epidemiology, prevention, and treatment of poisonings. The centers maintain extensive hazardous materials and poisoning library with computerized databases, have access to chemical laboratories for toxicological analyses to meet the needs of the public, health professionals, first responders, and government agencies for emergency information on the toxic and hazardous properties of chemical substances. They are an important part in the hazardous material spill response system. A state program coordinating the regional poison control centers is operated under the Emergency Medical Services Authority, listed separately.

A list of Regional Centers and the counties each serves follows

FRESNO COMMUNITY HOSPITAL
Fresno Regional Poison Control Center
P.O. Box 1232
Fresno, CA 93715-1232
(800) 346-5922
(209) 445-1222

Counties served under the Fresno Regional Poison Control Center are Fresno, Kern, Kings, Mariposa, Madera, Merced, and Tulare.

LOS ANGELES REGIONAL DRUG AND POISON INFORMATION CENTER
Drug and Poison Control Information Center
1925 Wilshire Blvd.
Los Angeles, CA 90057-1465
(800) 777-6476 (Public)
(213) 222-3212 (Public)
(800) 825-2722 (Physicians)
(213) 222-8086 (Physicians)
(213) 226-4194 (Fax)

Counties served under the Los Angeles Regional Drug And Poison Information Center are Inyo, Los Angeles, Mono, Orange, Riverside, San Bernardino, Santa Barbara, and Ventura.

SAN FRANCISCO BAY AREA REGIONAL POISON CONTROL CENTER
San Francisco General Hospital
1001 Potrero Avenue
San Francisco, CA 94110

(800) 523-2222
(415) 206-6600
(415) 821-8513 (Fax)

Counties served under the San Francisco Bay Regional Poison Control Center are Alameda, Contra Costa, Del Norte, Humboldt, Marin, Mendocino, Napa, San Francisco, San Mateo, and Sonoma.

SANTA CLARA VALLEY MEDICAL CENTER
Regional Poison Control Center
751 South Bascom Ave.
San Jose, CA 95128
(800) 662-9886
(408) 299-5112
(408) 286-2344 (Fax)

Counties served under the Santa Clara Valley Regional Poison Control Center are Monterey, San Benito, Santa Clara, Santa Cruz, and San Luis Obispo.

UNIVERSITY OF CALIFORNIA DAVIS MEDICAL CENTER
Poison Control Center
2315 Stockton Blvd.
Sacramento, CA 95817
(800) 342-9293
(916) 734-3692
(916) 724-7796 (Fax)

Counties served under the UCD Poison Control Center are Alpine, Amador, Butte, Calaveras, Colusa, El Dorado, Glenn, Lake, Lassen, Modoc, Nevada, Placer, Plumas, Sacramento, San Joaquin, Shasta, Sierra, Siskiyou, Solano, Stanislaus, Sutter, Tehama, Trinity, Tuolumne, Yolo, and Yuba.

UNIVERSITY OF CALIFORNIA SAN DIEGO MEDICAL CENTER
San Diego Regional Poison Control Center
225 Dickenson Street, H-925
San Diego, CA 92103-1990
(800) 876-4766
(619) 543-6000
(619) 692-1876 (Fax)

Counties served under the San Diego Regional Poison Control Center are Imperial and San Diego.

## Proposition 65 Implementation Office

(916) 445-6900

As the lead agency for the implementation of the Safe Drinking Water and Toxic Enforcement Act of 1986 (Proposition 65), the Office of Environmental Health Hazard Assessment (OEHHA) formulates policies and promulgates regulations relating to the Act; convenes meetings of a Scientific Advisory Panel responsible for identifying chemicals to be listed and reviewing risk assessments on listed chemicals; and compiles the list of chemicals known to the State to cause cancer or reproductive toxicity. These activities are carried out by OEHHA's Proposition 65 Implementation Office.

Technical and scientific activities in support of these functions are carried out by the Reproductive Cancer Hazard Assessment Section. (See Office of Environmental Health Hazard Assessment)

For more information, contact:
Office of Environmental Health Hazard Assessment
P.O. Box 942732
601 N 7th Street
Sacramento, CA 94234-7320

## Public Health Library, University of California, Berkeley

42 Warren Hall
University of California
Berkeley, CA 94720
(510) 642-2511

Hours when school is in session are
9:00 AM–9:00 PM Monday-Thursday
9:00 AM–5:00 PM Friday and Saturday
1:00 PM–5:00 PM Sunday
Please call for hours during intersession

Contains a collection of approximately 80,000 monographs and 2,100 journals to support the research needs of the students, faculty, staff of the UC Berkeley campus, the personnel of the Department of Health Services, and the general public.

## Radiologic Health Branch

California Department of Health Services
P.O. Box 942732
601 North Seventh St.
Sacramento, CA 94234
(916) 445-0931

Has general information on radiologic health effects and handling of materials. Makes referrals to consulting physicians and technicians. Offers hands-on help in emergency incidents. 24-hour emergency phone: (916) 445-0931.

## Radon Program, California

California Dept. of Health Services
Environmental Management Branch
P.O. Box 942732
601 North 7th Street
Sacramento, CA 94234-7320
(916) 322-2040
(800) 745-7236 (recording for leaving information requests)

The radon program (1) identifies radon levels in California, including homes and schools;

(2) assesses public health effects; (3) develops appropriate mitigation response measures; and (4) develops educational materials.

## Reproductive Epidemiology Section

California Department of Health Services,
Divison of Environmental and Occupational Disease Control
2151 Berkeley Way
Berkeley, CA 94704-1011
(510) 540-2669

The Reproductive Epidemiology Section investigates clusters of miscarriage and infertility. This group conducts long term studies to identify causes of impaired reproductive function in men and women, particularly looking for effects of such environmental exposures as environmental tobacco smoke, occupational solvent exposure and electro-magnetic radiation on fertility and pregnancy outcome.

## San Francisco Bay–Delta Aquatic Habitat Institute

180 Richmond Field Station
1301 South 46th Street
Richmond, CA 94804
(510) 231-9539

The San Francisco Bay–Delta Aquatic Habitat Institute conducts a research and monitoring program to evaluate the present and potential future effects of pollution on the beneficial uses of the waters of San Francisco Bay and the Sacramento–San Joaquin River Delta. The institute maintains an inventory of existing research and monitoring in the Bay–Delta and provides this information to all scientists, organization, and the public. The on-line system can be accessed without charge by modem.

## Structural Pest Control Board

California Department of Consumer Affairs
1422 Howe Avenue, Suite 3
Sacramento, CA 95825-3280

Provides licensing and regulation of structural pest control operators.

General information and complaints
(916) 263-2533 Sacramento
(415) 557-9114 San Francisco
(213) 897-7838 Los Angeles

Licensing information
(916) 263-2544

## Teratogen Information Services, California

U.C. San Diego Medical Center
Department of Pediatrics, 8446
200 W. Arbor Drive
San Diego, CA 92103-8446

(800) 532-3749
(619) 294-6084
Monday–Friday 9:00 AM–5:00 PM

The Teratogen Information Service provides information on the effects of drugs, medications, environmental exposures, infections, etc., on pregnancy to pregnant women and their health care providers.

## Tox-Center

266 El Portal
Palm Springs, CA 92264
(800) 682-9000 (in California only)
(619) 778-1077
(619) 323-6275
(619) 323-6289
24 hours a day service

The Tox-Center provides information from computerized databases on toxics to public safety agencies, industries, physicians, chemists, hospital emergency rooms, and also to individuals who are referred by poison control centers. Information can be faxed to the user. In conjunction with state and county agencies, the center has also developed protocols, which satisfy state requirements, for responding to spills, fires, and other emergencies involving hazardous materials.

## Toxic Substances Control, Department of

400 P Street, 4th Floor, Sacramento
P.O. Box 806
Sacramento, CA 95812-0806
(916) 324-1826

The Department of Toxic Substances Control provides the executive management and control of the state's toxic control program and provides the necessary focus and leadership to assure adequate protection to human health and the environment.

The department's core programs are: Site Mitigation, Hazardous Waste Management (this includes permitting and enforcement responsibilities) and External Affairs.

The overall goal of the Site Mitigation Program is to identify and clean up California sites where an uncontrolled release of hazardous substances has occurred. The program's emphasis is directed toward base closures, privatization of site cleanup, and cost recovery. (916) 255-2006

The Hazardous Waste Management Program combines the functions of permitting and enforcement for an integrated statewide approach to the management of hazardous waste. Waste classification, treatment standards, and recycling standards are also incorporated into the program to foster coordination of these distinct management elements. (916) 324-7193. This program also operates the Waste Alert Hotline (listed separately).

The Office of External Affairs focuses on pollution prevention, technology development, industry and small business assistance, industry and community relations, public participation and public education. (916) 324-2471

The department now has regional ombudspersons in each regional office. The ombudspersons are available to assist any outside interest with concerns, issues, and questions that the department is responsible to address.

The department has four regional offices

## Toxic Substances Research and Training Program, University of California Systemwide

University of California
Davis, CA 95616
(916) 752-2097

The Toxic Substances Research and Training Program supports long-term research and graduate education in toxics-related fields that will help provide the new concepts and scientific talent essential to solving the growing problems of toxic chemicals in our environment. The program also serves as a focal point of communication among researchers, industry, the government, and the public. A compendium of courses and research in the toxic substances field for the University of California is available on request.

## Toxics Coordinating Project

The California Toxics Coalition
c/o National Toxics Campaign Fund
1912 F Street, Suite 100
Sacramento, CA 95814
(919) 446-3350

A statewide coalition of environmental, labor, public health, victims, and community organizations and individuals. TCP's mission is to build a strong advocacy network to prevent the adverse impact of toxics on California's health, economy, and environment. The group's policy focus includes: (1) prevention of toxic pollution before it occurs, such as by supporting legislation to require industry to reduce the use of toxics in manufacturing; (2) expansion and use of right-to-know laws, which enable citizens and workers to become better informed about the presence of toxic chemicals in their area; (3) greater citizen participation in the formulation of toxics policies; and (4) the rights of those injured by toxic chemicals and the strict liability of polluters responsible for those damages. TCP was formed in 1985 by statewide toxics leaders representing key public interest constituencies. TCP brings together over 100 California-based organizations with a broad spectrum of issue, geographical, and tactical perspectives, ranging from grassroots neighborhood groups to large statewide organizations. TCP's newsletter, the "Toxics Watchdog," is published six times per year.

## Underground Storage Tanks (UST)

Contact address:
State Water Resources Control Board
P.O. Box 100
Sacramento, CA 95812-0100

General Information:
Office of Legislative and Public Affairs
(916) 657-2390

All 58 counties, by state law, have local "UST" programs. In addition, 49 cities operate independent urban UST programs within some counties.

Whereas these local agencies are responsible for permitting, inspecting and overseeing UST closures, the nine regional water quality control boards often take the lead in overseeing cases where releases from USTs affect, or threaten to affect, ground or surface water.

## Video Display Terminals Coalition

2515 Channing Way—2nd Floor
Berkeley, CA 94720
(510) 642-5507

Statewide coalition of VDT users, unions, health and safety professionals. Provides on-site training sessions, technical assistance, and publications on video display terminal health and safety issues. Extensive library with files open to public. Publishes quarterly newsletter, Video Views, containing updates on legislation, research technology, etc.

## Waste Alert Hotline

Department of Toxic Substances Control
400 P Street, 4th Floor
P.O. Box 806
Sacramento, CA 95812-0806
(800) 69-TOXIC or (800) 698-6942

This hotline is operated by the Hazardous Waste Management Program of the Department of Toxic Substances Control (see separate listing). It is for reporting suspected illegal hazardous waste managment activities such as "midnight dumping." Messages can be left at any time, but staff is available only during normal working hours. Anonymous calls are accepted. An informant reward option is available.

## Waste Information Service Hotline

California Integrated Waste Management Board
8800 Cal Center Drive
Sacramento CA 95826
1-800-553-2962 (Monday through Friday, 7:30 AM to 5:30 PM)

Provides information on reducing, reusing, recycling, and composting waste. Linked to an electronic database that includes the location of more than 2,600 recycling centers and contains information about upcoming household toxic "roundups" and collection facilities.

## Water Resources Control Board, State and Regional

901 P Street
P.O. Box 944213
Sacramento, CA 94244-2130
(916) 657-0768

The State Water Resources Control Board and nine regional water quality control boards work together to preserve California water. The law assigns overall responsibility for water rights and water pollution control to the State Water Board and directs the regional boards to plan and enforce water quality standards within their boundaries.

## Western Medical Center

1001 N. Tustin Avenue
Santa Ana, CA 92705
(714) 953-3339

Provides acute treatment for poisonings and spills. Furnishes complete decontamination services including a special decontamination facility which can simultaneously treat and decontaminate severely injured patients requiring stretchers. The facility is also capable of containing all drain water for testing and possible special disposal. Personnel are trained and equipped with protective gear to minimize the potential of secondary injuries. Hyperbaric oxygen is available for treatment of carbon monoxide poisoning.

## Workers Compensation Insurance Carriers

Workers compensation insurance companies often provide occupational health and safety services to policy holders for free or at reduced cost. Many have industrial hygiene consultants who can provide advice or on-site consultation and evaluation regarding chemical hazards.

# INDEX

# 37
# Resources for Toxicology Risk Assessment

**Po-Yung Lu and John S. Wassom**
*Oak Ridge National Laboratory\**
*Oak Ridge, Tennessee*

*Beneath the imposing structure of toxicological risk assessment lies the dingy basement of uncertainties, extrapolation factors, and elusive information* (Lu and Wassom, 1994).

## I. INTRODUCTION

Risk assessment can be viewed as a means of organizing and analyzing all available scientific information associated with probability. The purpose of this chapter is to review key information resources that can be used in conducting toxicological risk assessments. Before beginning an examination of these resources, we provide definitions of key words used in the text.

The following definitions are from the *American Heritage Dictionary.*

| | |
|---|---|
| *Information:* | Communication of knowledge |
| *Resource:* | An available supply that can be drawn upon when needed |
| *Toxicology:* | The study of the nature, effects, and detection of any substance that causes injury, illness, or death |
| *Risk:* | The possiblity of suffering harm or loss; danger; a factor, element, or course involving uncertain danger; hazard |
| *Assessment:* | Evaluation; appraisal. |

From these words and definitions, two words form the cornerstone of all discussions regarding risk assessment: *possibility* and *uncertainty*.

Over the past few years, toxicology as a science has evolved into a multidisciplinary field of study (Fig. 1) [see Casarett (1975) for an excellent treatise on this subject]; however, no easy

---

\*Managed by Lockheed Martin Energy Systems for the U.S. Department of Energy, under contract number DE-AC05-840R21400.

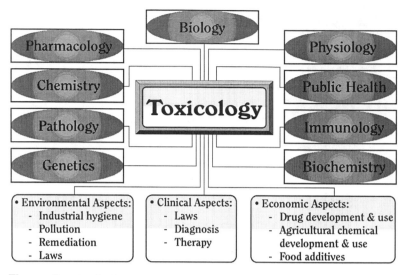

**Figure 1**  The disciplines of toxicology.

and quick means are available to assess the overall toxicity of a substance, whether it is chemical, physical, or biological. Risk assessment is not a precise science, and no magical methods, as yet, will provide ready-made, error-free risk evaluation. Every assessment is unique, and each combines knowledge of specific data parameters and other information with a liberal portion of sound reasoning. Those who perform risk assessments must use all available reliable data and information to make sound forecasts.

In 1983 and 1994, the National Research Council (NRC) defined four steps in assessing the toxicological risks of an agent (e.g., a chemical). Access to data and information may be necessary at any time during the risk assessment process, particularly for the first two steps. These steps are

1. Hazard identification
2. Dose–response evaluation
3. Human exposure evaluation
4. Risk characterization

For step one—identifying potential hazards posed by the agent—data and information must be reviewed on the toxicity, epidemiology, adsorption, distribution, metabolism, and excretion of the agent, as well as on the agent's mechanism of action. When the hazard has been identified, a dose–response evaluation must be made because the nature, severity, and risk of toxicity vary with dose. For each established form of toxicity (e.g., genotoxicity, carcinogenicity, or teratogenicity) caused by an agent, quantitative relationships should be established between an experimental dose and one that induces a toxicological effect. However, because of the lack of human data, extrapolation from animal studies is frequently required. This extrapolation should be done with a good scientific basis, creating further need for reliable sources of data and information. Determination of human exposure thus considers dose received, period of exposure, individual and population sensitivity, and population segments at risk of exposure. Finally, risk characterization can be established. The key to addressing these four steps effectively is the availability of required data and information.

## II. INFORMATION REQUIREMENTS FOR THE RISK ASSESSMENT PROCESS

Much attention is being given to the importance of computer applications in the study of modern biology and in data storage. Risk assessment practitioners should have a thorough working knowledge of the personal computer and its applications.

Another requirement in the risk assessment process is information access. With the emergence of computer networks such as Internet, the information access opportunities available to risk assessors have been expanded significantly. By using this international information highway, one may access databases from all over the world to cover a variety of subjects and scientific disciplines. Several excellent references will provide interested individuals with details about this information resource (see Sec. VI).

## III. INFORMATION RESOURCES AVAILABLE FOR USE IN TOXICOLOGICAL RISK ASSESSMENT

The foundation of all research studies and health risk assessments is data that are usually obtained from the peer-reviewed scientific literature. Experimental data needed to make a health risk assessment can be obtained from the primary toxicology literature, or from reliable, specialized information resources. For those who wish to do the searching themselves, we recommend a recent paper by Lu and Wassom (1993), which provides a guide to various sources that can be used to screen primary and secondary literature. Conversely, for those without the time or experience to conduct literature searches, we recommend that such searches be done by experienced individuals whose professional duties focus solely on searching toxicological literature. One organization specifically designed for this purpose is the Toxicology Information Response Center (TIRC).

The TIRC was organized at Oak Ridge National Laboratory (ORNL) in 1971 under the sponsorship of the National Library of Medicine (NLM). The center provides custom search services to the scientific, administrative, and public communities under a cost-recovery system. It has access to the expertise and information resources of ORNL, as well as on-line access to virtually all the world's scientific and technical databases (Table 1).

The TIRC can supply information on the toxic effects of chemicals; the amounts of chemicals released in specific locations or by specific companies; the environmental uptake and transport of chemicals; protective measures and cleanup procedures for hazardous chemicals; genetic, teratogenic, and carcinogenic effects of chemicals; regulatory standards; and properties and structural classification of chemicals.

Products available from TIRC range from customized bibliographies and formal reports, to the design of specialized databases. The TIRC staff works closely with the requestor to refine and clarify needs and develop a reasonable cost estimate based on per-hour staff charges, on-line use of copyright fees, and reproduction costs. Products can be provided in printed or electronic form. Requests may be directed to TIRC by mail, telephone, or fax.

Toxicology Information Response Center
Attention: Kimberly G. Slusher
Oak Ridge National Laboratory
1060 Commerce Park MS-6480
Oak Ridge, Tennessee 37830
Telephone: 615/576-1746 Fax: 615/574-9888
e-mail: slusherkg@iravx2.hsr.ornl.gov

**Table 1**  Sampling of National On-Line Information Systems Searched by TIRC

| Database name | Database name |
| --- | --- |
| AGRICOLA | Integrated Risk Information System (IRIS) |
| Aquatic Sciences and Fisheries Abstracts | Legal Resource Index |
| Aquatic Information Retrieval (AQUIRE) | LEGISLATE |
|   Data Base | LEXUS |
| Chemical Information System (CIS) | Medical Literature Analysis and Retrieval System |
| Chemical Regulations and Guidelines System |   (MEDLARS) |
|   (CRGS) | National Technical Information Service (NTIS) |
| Chemical Carcinogenesis Research Information | NEXUS |
|   System (CCRIS) | Occupational Safety and Health (NIOSHTIC) |
| Chemical Identification (ChemID) File | Pollution Abstracts |
| Chemical Abstracts On-line (CAS ONLINE) | PTS Newsletter Data Base |
| CHEMLINE | Registry of Toxic Effects of Chemical Substances |
| Congressional Information Service (CIS) |   (RTECS) |
| Defense Technical Information Center (DTIC) | Scientific and Technical Information Network |
| Dialog Information Service (DIALOG) |   (STN) |
| Energy Science and Technology | Toxic Chemical Release Inventory (TRI) |
| ENFLEX | Toxicology Literature from special sources |
| ENVIROLINE |   (TOXLIT and TOXLIT65) |
| Environmental Bibliography | Toxicology Information Online (TOXLINE) |
| Environmental Fate Data Bases | Toxicology Data Network (TOXNET) |
| Federal Research in Progress (FEDRIP) | Transportation Research Information Service |
| Federal Register Abstracts |   (TRIS) |
| Federal Register | Water Resources Abstract (WRA) |
| Integrated Technical Information System (ITIS) | WATERNET |

In response to the needs of individuals faced with the voluminous array of expanding environmental requirements and regulations, TIRC has expanded its services to include environmental regulation information. In addition to custom-computerized searches for specific regulations or analysis, TIRC provides analyses of U.S. Department of Energy orders, assessment of probable compliance issues, identification of treatment options, procedural options, expert identification, legislative tracking, and litigation history. Environmental regulatory products available from TIRC range from custom searches and analytical reports to the design of specialized databases, PC-expert systems, newsletters, and reference books.

To illustrate the nature and complexity of the types of questions that can be answered by TIRC, the following list is a sample of searches received and processed during the last few months.

Is the chemical dioxin a carcinogen?
Has the chemical ethylene oxide been shown to be teratogenic?
Does the chemical 1,3-butadiene induce point mutations?
On which regulatory lists is the chemical benzo[*a*]pyrene found?
What is the acceptable concentration of the chemical acrylamide in drinking water?
What is the slope factor, the reference dose, and the reportable quantity for the chemical ethylene glycol?
Have any QSAR studies been performed on the class of compounds called nitrosamines?
What transgenic animal models are available for the study of diabetes?

To address effectively the responsibilities associated with the risk assessment of chemicals, access to reliable toxicological information resources is needed. To provide some insight into such resources, descriptions and commentaries are given in this section for selected databases, information files, and publications dealing with genetic toxicology, carcinogenicity, and general toxicology. An excellent historical review on the development of several key databases (Waters, 1994) is described in the following sections.

## A.  U.S. Environmental Protection Agency Genetic Toxicology Database

The Genetic Toxicology (Gene-Tox) database is a product of the U.S. Environmental Protection Agency's (EPA's) Gene-Tox Program (Waters, 1994; Auletta et al., 1991). This program was initiated in 1979 at ORNL for conducting a systematic evaluation of selected short-term bioassays detecting genotoxic activity and presumptive carcinogenicity. Sponsored and directed by the Office of Testing and Evaluation within EPA's Office of Pesticides and Toxic Substances, the Gene-Tox Program was conducted and coordinated by the Environmental Mutagen information Center (EMIC) of the Biomedical and Environmental Information Analysis (BEIA) Section of ORNL. The Gene-Tox Program provides a resource for establishing standard genetic toxicology testing and evaluation procedures in the regulation of toxic substances.

At the end of 1991, peer-reviewed information on over 4600 different chemicals had been entered into the Gene-Tox database. This information represents evaluation of these compounds in 1 or more of 64 genetic toxicology and 9 cell transformation assays or test systems.

The Gene-Tox database is available on-line through NLM's Toxicology Data Network (TOXNET) system (Vasta and Casey, 1991). Information from the Gene-Tox database is also included in chemical records of the Hazardous Substances Data Bank (HSDB), and locator tags are placed with chemical records that are part of the Chemical Identification file and the Registry of Toxic Effects of Chemical Substances database (Hazard and Hudson, 1993). Information on accessing the Gene-Tox database may be obtained from the HSDB address shown on page 733.

In our opinion, the Gene-Tox database provides the best, and most reliable, means of acquiring an assessment of a chemical agent's genotoxicity. This resource is a suggested starting point when gathering information about the ability of a chemical to induce damage to the genome of different organisms. Answers to several types of questions, such as the following, are possible for chemicals evaluated by the Gene-Tox program.

What genetic toxicology data exist for a specific chemical?
For which chemicals have certain specific mutagenicity assays been conducted?
What chemicals or classes of chemicals are responsive (or unresponsive) in given test systems?
What are the best assay systems to use in determining genotoxicity of a specific chemical?
What assays are unlikely to give a good indication of the genotoxicity of a specific chemical?
What is the likelihood that an untested chemical will be genotoxic based on the known activity
    of chemicals that are structurally or functionally analogous?
How predictive of mammalian in vivo genotoxicity are the in vitro assay systems?
How predictive of heritable mutagenicity and of carcinogenicity are given assays?

## B.  International Agency for Research on Cancer Monographs

In 1971, the International Agency for Research on Cancer (IARC) initiated a program to evaluate the carcinogenic risk of chemicals to humans. The object of the program was to provide government authorities with expert independent scientific options concerning environmental carcinogenesis through the publication of critical reviews of carcinogenicity and related data.

The aim of IARC is to evaluate possible human carcinogenic risk from detailed review and analysis of pertinent literature.

The *IARC Monographs* summarize evidence for the carcinogenicity of individual chemicals and other relevant information on the basis of data compiled, reviewed, and evaluated by a working panel of experts. Priority is given to chemicals, groups of chemicals, or industrial processes for which at least some suggestion of carcinogenicity exists, either from evidence of human exposure or from observations in animals. Note that the inclusion of a particular compound in an IARC volume does not mean that it is carcinogenic. As new data become available on chemicals for which monographs have already been prepared, or as new principles for evaluation evolve, reevaluations may be made at subsequent IARC meetings. If the new evidence warrants, revised *IARC Monographs* are published.

More than 1000 chemicals, chemical groups, or other agents have been reviewed by IARC. As of October 1995, 62 volumes of the *IARC Monographs* and several supplements had been published. These volumes contain indexes both for chemical name and molecular formula as well as *Chemical Abstracts* Service (CAS) registry numbers. The monographs provide the best and most thorough review of chemical-induced cancer in animals. Carcinogenicity evaluations have not been made on all the chemicals reviewed because either the data were unavailable or the data were judged inadequate for evaluation. Specialized information files and databases developed at ORNL, such as the EMIC file and the Gene-Tox database, are used routinely by IARC in the production of its monographs. The *IARC Monographs* may be obtained by contacting any bookseller through the network of World Health Organization sales agents. These *monographs* also are distributed internationally to governmental agencies, industries, and scientists.

The monographs can be used as a quick reference source for information on the chemicals reviewed by IARC in the following areas:

1.  Chemical and physical data and analysis
2.  Production and use
3.  Occurrence
4.  Regulations and guidelines
5.  Carcinogenicity
      In experimental animals
      Human potential
6.  Adsorption, distribution, metabolism, and excretion
7.  Toxicity
8.  Genotoxicity
9.  Developmental/reproductive toxicity

## C.  Hazardous Substances Data Bank

The Hazardous Substances Data Bank (HSDB), formerly called the Toxicology Data Bank (Oxyman et al., 1976), was prepared by ORNL in the early 1970s under the sponsorship of NLM. It is a numerical and factual database composed of over 4300 comprehensive chemical records. These records contain about 150 different data elements grouped into 11 categories, as well as administrative information. The categories include pharmacological and toxicological data (e.g., $LD_{50}$ values), environmental and occupational information, manufacturing and use data, regulatory information, analytical methods, and information on the physical properties of each chemical. Substances selected for HSDB include high-volume production or exposure chemicals; drugs and pesticides exhibiting potential toxicity or adverse effects; and other substances subject to regulation under the provisions of the Comprehensive Environmental Response,

Compensation, and Liability Act (CERCLA) of 1980 (Superfund) and the Superfund Amendment Reauthorization Act (SARA) of 1986.

The information used in an HSDB record is selected mostly from secondary sources, such as standard reference books, handbooks, criteria documents, and monographs. The data extracted from secondary sources are reviewed quarterly by a scientific review panel (SRP) of experts convened by NLM. Members of the SRP are professional toxicologists, industrial hygienists, and environmental engineers from academia or industry. The SRP may select additional information from pertinent literature and develop it into consensus statements for on-line databases, such as Toxicology Information Online (TOXLINE). The additional information is then incorporated into an HSDB record to ensure that the record contains the most relevant and accurate information available. Records in HSDB are, in our opinion, the best on-line resources for obtaining information on the general toxicity of a chemical. Components included in the toxicology category of the HSDB database are shown in Table 2, which illustrates the type of information that this database can provide.

Readers can obtain further information on HSDB by contacting Specialized Information Service; Toxicology Information Program; National Library of Medicine; 8600 Rockville Pike; Bethesda, MD 20894.

## D. The U.S. Air Force Installation Restoration Toxicology Guide

The *U.S. Air Force Installation Restoration Toxicology Guide* (AFTG) was sponsored by the Harry G. Armstrong Aerospace Medical Research Laboratory and prepared by staff of the BEIA Section of ORNL. It is a peer-reviewed, five-volume document consisting of over 3500 pages that are devoted to a review of the toxicology of select chemical compounds.

One of the objectives of AFTG is to provide individuals responsible for managing and

**Table 2** Data Elements of Toxicity and Biomedical Effects of the Hazardous Substances Data Bank, National Library of Medicine

Toxicity summary
Toxic hazard rating
Antidote and emergency treatment
Medical surveillance
Toxicity excerpts
  Human toxicity excerpts
  Nonhuman toxicity excerpts
Toxicity values
  Human toxicity values
  Nonhuman toxicity values
  Ecotoxicity values
Minimum fatal dose level
Populations at special risk
Pharmacokinetics
  Absorption, distribution and excretion
Metabolism/metabolites
  Biological half-life
  Mechanism of action
  Interactions

implementing the U.S. Air Force Installation Restoration Program with information to evaluate health hazards associated with actual or potential contamination of drinking water supplies. Volumes 1 through 4 of AFTG contain information on 70 chemicals and complex mixtures that are of environmental concern to the U.S. Air Force. Volume 5 contains similar information on 7 metals and over 80 environmentally significant compounds containing these metals. Data summary sections that provide concise, easily accessible data useful to environmental engineers precede detailed environmental and toxicological review sections. These summaries include chemical names and synonyms; registry numbers; physicochemical data; information on reactivity and handling precautions; soil–water persistence; pathways of exposure; health hazard data; environmental standards and criteria; and state, federal, and European Economic Community regulatory status.

The toxicology review sections for each chemical in the AFTG include detailed information on acute, subchronic, and chronic toxicity data, as well as information on developmental toxicity, genotoxicity, and carcinogenicity. Environmental information for each chemical encompasses environmental fate and exposure pathways and fate and transport in soil and ground water. A section on biological monitoring for each metal-containing compound is included.

Components of AFTG are shown in Table 3. A review of these components will indicate the type of questions that AFTG material may be able to answer.

Information on AFTG may be obtained by contacting the National Technical Information Service, 5285 Port Royal Road, Springfield, VA 22161.

## IV. RECOMMENDED INFORMATION RESOURCES FOR CHEMICAL TOXICOLOGY AND REGULATION

Peer-reviewed or value-added databases, such as those previously described, offer the most expedient and comprehensible toxicology information resources for use by risk assessors and

**Table 3**  Components of the *U.S. Air Force Installation Restoration Toxicology Guide* (AFTG)

| |
|---|
| Synonyms |
| Reactivity |
| Physical and chemical properties |
| Persistence in soil |
| Exposure pathways |
| Health hazard data summaries |
|     Acute toxicity |
|     Chronic toxicity |
|     Teratogenicity, embryotoxicity, and reproductive effects |
|     Carcinogenicity |
|     Genotoxicity |
| Handling precautions |
| Air exposure limits |
| Water exposure limits |
| Reference dose |
| Regulatory status |
|     Federal |
|     State |
| Human and epidemiological studies |

others involved with chemical regulations. Most often, individuals who must assess the toxicity of chemicals are faced with tight schedules and must reach decisions quickly. These decisions must be supported by factual data, whenever possible, or with liberal applications of intuitive reasoning when the data are weak or nonexistent. We believe that the first tier in the data and information selection process should include the resources reviewed in this section, as summarized in Table 4, and should be supplemented with other resources from those listed in Table 1. Because of a lack of peer-reviewed toxicity information on most chemical substances, resources such as chemical structure analysis must be used to support intuitive reasoning. The next section discusses this approach.

**Table 4** Recommended Sources[a] for Accessing the Toxicology Literature

Genetic toxicology
  Recommended source for access to primary literature
    Environmental Mutagen Information Center files available through the NLM TOXNET system (over 90,000 records). This file covers literature published from 1968 to present.
  Recommended source for evaluated (peer-reviewed) data
    a. Gene-Tox through TOXNET system (over 4600 chemicals)
    b. International Agency for Research on Cancer Monograph, Supplement 7, 1987 (950 chemicals)
    c. Hazardous Substances Data Bank (over 4200 chemicals)
Teratology and reproductive and developmental toxicology
  Recommended source for access to primary literature
    Environmental Teratology Information Center files available through TOXNET for literature published from 1950 to 1989 (46,000 records); literature published since 1989 may be obtained from NLM's Developmental and Reproductive Toxicology file, also available on TOXNET
  Recommended source for evaluated (peer-reviewed) data
    Although several books and monographs are available summarizing experiments, no comprehensive peer-reviewed computerized database is publicly available through 1994. Evaluations of the teratogenicity and developmental and reproductive toxicology of compounds reviewed by IARC are available in the IARC monograph series (62 volumes); currently over 1000 chemicals have been reviewed.
Carcinogenicity
  Recommended source for access to primary literature
    No specific information file devoted solely to this area of research is available. Bibliographic information is scattered throughout numerous biological-oriented information files.
  Recommended source for evaluated (peer-reviewed) data
    a. IARC monographs (62 volumes covering over 1000 chemicals)
    b. Gene-Tox database available through the NLM TOXNET system (392 chemicals)
General toxicology
  Recommended source for access to primary literature
    NLM's TOXLINE and TOXLIT systems
  Recommended source for evaluated (peer-reviewed) data
    a. Hazardous Substances Data Bank available through the TOXNET system
    b. U.S. Air Force Installation Restoration Toxicology Guide, available through DTIC No. Vol. 1: ADA219797, Vol. 2: ADA214999, Vol. 3: ADA215001, Vol. 4: ADA215002, and Vol. 5: ADA238093 (Volumes 1–4 covers 70 organic chemicals and Volume 5 covers 6 metals with 87 environmentally significant metal-containing compounds)
    c. IARC monographs (described above)

[a]For details on accessing the information files, databases, or computer systems referred to in this table, contact the Toxicology Information Response Center; Oak Ridge National Laboratory; 1060 Commerce Park MS-6480; Oak Ridge, TN 37830.

## V.  THE ROLE OF CHEMICAL STRUCTURE–ACTIVITY RELATIONSHIPS IN TOXICOLOGICAL RISK ASSESSMENTS

A considerable amount of activity is focused on the way in which chemical structure influences biological activity, and attention is being given to studies to develop machine-based systems that will allow predictions of toxicological events from chemical structure. Several interesting techniques, models, and systems have been devised (Beauchamp, 1993; Ashby and Tennant, 1988; Rosenkranz and Klopman, 1988; Malacarne et al., 1993), but none of these has evolved into all-purpose systems for widespread application. Because structure–activity relationships (SAR) is an important component of the risk assessment process, this section contains a brief review of the SAR concept as it relates to toxicology.

The correlation of chemical structure with biological activity is rooted in the early history of the pharmaceutical sciences, when compounds with structures similar to known medicinal agents were selected tested for their efficacy in combating human disease. The principles of drug action that are based on chemical structure have been carried over to the toxicological sciences, for which structural characteristics of chemicals with known activity are compared with compounds for which activities are unknown. Such comparisons make it possible to predict the activity of a chemical for some specific toxilogical endpoint (e.g., mutagenicity and carcinogenicity).

Because the volume of toxicological literature has grown significantly over the years, an enormous information base on various toxicological endpoints is available for comparing chemical structure with untoward biological activity. The information resources reviewed in this chapter can serve as valuable resources in SAR studies for particular endpoints, such as genotoxicity, carcinogenicity, and reproductive toxicity. Several other worthwhile toxicology databases also can be used for SAR studies. These databases were reviewed comprehensively in a recently published paper (Lu and Wassom, 1993). Through the use of these information resources, the quality and the quantity of SAR predictions can be improved and increased. Additionally, new computer software and hardware that can be applied to SAR studies appears on the market with increasing frequency. These ingredients (i.e., information base, novel hardware and software) should make notable advancements possible in the use of SAR for toxicological risk assessment; however, these advancements have not matured to the point of practical application.

Even though the information base and technology for the efficient conduct of SAR studies have improved, individuals engaged in regulating chemicals must realize that no easy or completely effective method exists for predicting toxicological activity from chemical structure. The best and most efficient method is still the intuitive reasoning of a person knowledgeable in both chemistry and a given area of toxicology. Federal agencies [e.g., EPA and the Food and Drug Administration (FDA)] responsible for the regulation of chemicals and exposure to toxic substances employ the intuitive reasoning technique when using SAR in risk assessment studies. In evaluating chemicals under section 5 of the Toxic Substances Control Act, EPA convenes a structure–activity team composed of chemists, toxicologists, and environmental scientists. These individuals use their professional judgment to study a chemical structure and, then, compare it with data of structural analogues to render an assessment of potential health and environmental hazards (Auletta, 1993). Because of the lack of a sufficiently validated machine-aided method or procedure to augment human reasoning, application of SAR varies in the evaluation of chemical risks or the assessment of chemical hazard, and the contribution of SAR to chemical hazard assessment may not be fully realized.

As with the example cited for EPA, the SAR studies that are performed among federal agencies usually are approached through intuitive and deductive reasoning by responsible staff, much to the credit of the individual practitioners of this procedure. Although separating human reasoning from SAR practices will never be practical, total reliance on "personal views" should not be the primary method of choice. Most of the methods and models proposed for SAR work are too complicated, theoretical, or costly for practical use in day-to-day efforts to assess chemical hazards or risks. Furthermore, current machine predictions with computer models, artificial intelligence programs, or neural networks should be used only in categorizing chemicals for further study and assessment. This opinion is based on the fact that most of these models and approaches have not been validated thoroughly. However, the use of SAR is important in the risk assessment process. Success among current methods capitalizes on the human element when making inferences about the role that chemical structure plays in initiating a toxic effect.

## VI. FUTURE DIRECTIONS FOR INFORMATION RESOURCES AND ACCESS TO RISK ASSESSMENT

The future of risk assessment is linked proportionally to the future and well-being of data and information resources that endeavor to provide access to the scientific literature. Risk assessment is not a precise science; however, precision will come with the production and availability of quality data and information. Support of research to generate the needed data must continue and increase along with the activities to collect, analyze, evaluate, and store scientific information. Unfortunately, support of activities that strive to make the scientific literature available to users (risk assessors) has been curtailed severely over the last decade in favor of new-age informatics. In this matter, the focus is almost totally on software development to manipulate data, not to make data available and ensure data quality. A balance is needed among efforts to monitor scientific literature. Documents in a particular discipline must be selected, analyzed, and indexed; techniques, methods, and software are then developed to analyze and evaluate specialized data sets. This balance must be maintained to allow the information cycle (Fig. 2) to continue.

The future of risk assessment also will be linked with the much-acclaimed information super highway, which is currently provided by the Internet (Fig. 3). In ever-increasing numbers, databases and information files needed by the risk assessor are becoming available on Internet. Internet provides vast amounts of information and the means to communicate with colleagues anywhere. If risk assessors want to stay current in the 1990s and into the next century, familiarity with Internet is a must.

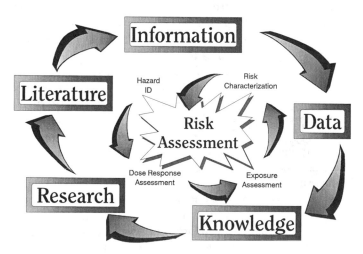

**Figure 2** Risk assessment paradigm and the information cycle.

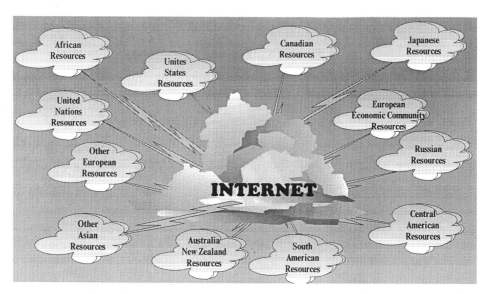

**Figure 3**   Internet: The network of networks.

Because of the importance and diversity of the Internet, we recommend several books now available on this subject, including the following:

Falk, B. (1994). *The Internet Roadmap,* SYBEX, Inc., San Francisco, CA, 263 pp.
Krol, E. (1992). *The Whole Internet User's Guide and Catalog,* O'Reilly and Associates, Sebastopol, CA, 376 pp.
LaQuey, T., and J. C. Ryer (1993). *The Internet Companion,* Addison-Wesley Publishing Co., Reading, PA, 196 pp.
Hahn, H. and R. Stout (1994). *The Internet Complete Reference,* Osborne McGraw-Hill, Berkeley, CA, 817 pp.

Another area that will play an ever-increasing role in the risk assessment process is the use of computer models and expert systems. Computer-assisted risk assessment will become more common as a result of the ability to link and integrate information from various databases and to use this assembled knowledge with computer models designed to assess the risk of a particular toxicological endpoint. Several models or systems have already been developed (Marnicio et al., 1991), and many more are under development. Because technical advancements in software and hardware development are being made at a fast pace, computer science experts should monitor these new developments for possible application to a particular type of risk assessment. Information is the fuel that powers a risk assessment model, and all models are only as good as the information used.

Sharing information is another "key resource" for risk analysis. Because toxic and hazardous wastes are found throughout the country, many chemicals are common to many waste sites, particularly at National Priority Listing sites. The lack of an expedient means to share information ensures that risk assessment is continually repeated for the same agent. A national risk analysis repository or clearing house is urgently needed to capture the procedures, models, and results of risk analysis performed on chemicals so that a common structure for risk assessments can be developed. A central segment of this proposed repository would be a section for searching and capturing all the relevant data and information resources. Users of this repository could benefit from what has been done by other investigators and reported in the literature; they could also review the toxicity evaluations or extrapolations of exposures reported directly to the repository. Note that basic toxicity information or toxicity summaries are independent of time and place. In addition, both the merits and pitfalls of earlier risk assessment efforts can be reviewed to minimize the repetition of problems or errors. A foundation for such a repository can be established from resources currently available. As previously stated, risk assessment is not a precise science; it will become more mature as it grows, with assistance from a resource such as the risk assessment repository.

## VII.  CONCLUSIONS

Risk assessment resides in the field of "trans-science" (Weinberg, 1971), thus making it difficult to derive quantitative risk estimates and extrapolate them to human health hazards. Generating a risk assessment requires the use of extrapolation factors that are not always based on scientific observations because of the lack of reliable data and information. Although uncertainties are involved in making sound toxicological risk assessments, legislative mandates and the intrinsic concern for the well-being of the human population dictate that health risk assessments be made. Although defining the risk extrapolation process may be overwhelming, progress toward a better understanding of this process and its implications for society will be made only through the meticulous use of available data and information to create risk assessment models that can be tested and evaluated. The intent of this chapter has been to review several key information resources that can offer great help in assessing toxicological risks and creating risk assessment models, thus making it possible to focus more directly on the problem at hand. A national data and information repository is critically needed to document the four steps in the risk assessment process for environmental agents. This resource would be an effective tool in eventually elevating risk assessment from the trans-science area and in evaluating the effectiveness of the risk assessment process.

The chapter has endeavored to present problems and solutions in acquiring toxicological data so that risk assessors can measure how much their assessments can be based on available data and how much has to be given over to speculation. Presently, risk assessment is anything but easy. Conducting thorough searches of the literature and applying extracted data and information to the risk assessment process will make the task of determining potential health risks more credible. The quote below illustrates the dilemma facing individuals who attempt to conduct genetic risk assessments. Similar statements can be made for all other toxicity endpoints.

> The main problem with current genetic risk assessment exercises is the concept that induced genetic damage will only provide increases in the types of adverse biological effects that occur spontaneously. The marked specificity of the genetic damage produced by such chemical mutagens as Aflatoxin $B_1$ and Acrylamide in experimental organisms has provided impetus for the acceptance of an alternative concept that the induced spectrum of adverse biological effects can be quite different from that occurring spontaneously. This new concept makes the overall problem of genetic risk assessment inherently more difficult, since risk management exercises will become agent specific (F. J. de Serres, 1994).

Accuracy and precision in making toxicological risk assessments on an agent-by-agent basis or any other basis will be determined largely by the quality and quantity of data available for analyses. Ideally, assessments using a diverse assemblage of data and information from epidemiological studies, laboratory testing, or SAR studies, should provide the best estimates of risk. Efficient and effective use of these critical information resources will be predicated on the availability of a good access map. This chapter has attempted to provide such a map.

## REFERENCES

Auletta, A. E., M. Brown, J. S. Wassom, and M. C. Cimino (1991). Current status of the Gene-Tox program, *Environ. Health Perspect.,* 96, 33–36.

Auletta, A. (1993). Structure activity relationships to assess new chemicals under TSCA. In *Proceedings of the Symposium to Access and Use of Information Resources in Assessing Health Risks From Chemical Exposure,* pp. 53–60.

Ashby, J., and R. W. Tennant (1988). Chemical structure, salmonella mutagenicity and extent of carcinogenicity as indicators of genotoxic carcinogenesis among chemicals tested in rodents by the U.S. NCI/NTP, *Muta. Res.,* 204, 17–115.

Beauchamp, R. O., Jr. (1993). Chemical substructure analysis in toxicology. In *Proceedings of the Symposium on the Access and Use of Information Resources in Assessing Health Risks From Chemical Exposure,* pp. 211–217.

Casarett, L. J. (1975). Origin and scope of toxicology. In *Toxicology, The Basic Science of Poisons* (L. J. Casarett and J. Doull, eds.) Macmillan Publishing, New York, pp. 3–25.

de Serres, F. J. (1994). Commentary on an unresolved problem: Effective genetic risk assessment of human exposure to mutagenic environmental agents, *Environ. Mol. Mutagen,* 23 (Suppl. 24), 7–10.

Hazard, G. J., Jr., and V. W. Hudson (1993). Chem-ID: Gateway to NLM Files, 206th Meeting of the American Chemical Society, August 1993.

Lu, P. Y., and J. S. Wassom (1993). Risk assessment and toxicology databases for health effects assessment. In *Proceedings of the Symposium on the Access and Use of Information Resources in Assessing Health Risks From Chemical Exposure,* pp. 179–194.

Malacarne, D., R. Pesenti, M. Paolucci, and S. Parodi (1993). Relationship between molecular connectivity and carcinogenic activity: A confirmation with a new software program based on graph theory, *Environ. Health Perspect.,* 101, 332–342.

Marnicio, R. J., P. J. Hakkinen, S. D. Lutkenhoff, R. C. Hertzberg, and P. D. Moskowitz (1991). Risk analysis software and databases: Review of Riskware '90 Conference and Exhibition, *Risk Anal.,* 11, 545–560.

National Research Council (1983). Risk assessment in the federal government: Managing the process, Committee on the Institutional Means for Assessment of Risks to Public Health, Commission on Life Sciences, NRC National Academy Press, Washington, DC.

National Research Council (1994). Science and judgment in risk assessment, Committee on Risk Assessment of Hazardous Air Pollutants, Commission on Life Sciences, NRC National Academy Press, Washington, D.C.

Oxyman, M. A., H. M. Kissman, J. M. Burnsides, J. R. Edge, C. B. Haberman, and A. A. Wykes (1976). The Toxicology Data Bank, *J. Chem. Inf. Comput. Sci.,* 16, 19–21.

Rosenkranz, H. S., and G. Klopman (1988). CASE, the Computer-Automated Structure Evaluation Method, correctly predicts the low mutagenicity for salmonella or nitrated cyclopenta-fused polycyclic aromatic hydrocarbons, *Muta. Res.,* 199, 95–101.

Vasta, B. M., and S. M. Casey (1991). Down-sizing: A case study of the National Library of Medicine's TOXNET system. *Manage. Technol. Q.,* 21, 11–15.

Waters, J. D. (1994). Development and impact of the Gene-Tox Program, genetic activity profiles, and their computerized data bases, *Environ. Mol. Mutagen.* 23 (Suppl. 24), 67–72.

Weinberg, A. M. (1971). Science and trans-science, *CIBA Found. Symp.,* 1, 105–122.

# 38
# Electronic Resources for Toxicology and Environmental Health

**Mary Ann Mahoney and Charleen Kubota**
*University of California at Berkeley*
*Berkeley, California*

There is an immense number of databases available to those searching for information about toxicology and environmental health hazards. The following is a selection of the databases that have proved to be the most useful. Included are only commercially available databases. Databases that are primarily regulatory have been excluded. The list is arranged by database vendor. Often, the same database is available from two or more vendors. The choice of vendor, and the order that they appear in this document, is very subjective—prime considerations are always cost and ease of searching software. There is only one major organizational division: online databases are separated from those that are in other formats, such as CD-ROM.

The databases described are of two general types, factual and bibliographic. Factual databases provide a profile of a specific chemical, drawing from the scientific literature. A typical record may provide a common chemical name, synonyms, trade names, CAS registry number, molecular formula, and molecular weight for a specific substance along with its physical/chemical properties, toxicity, environmental fate, regulatory status, and health and safety requirements. Bibliographic databases generate a listing by subject or author of journal articles, books, government reports, and published proceedings. Some databases also provide abstracts of the cited materials.

In addition to different types of databases, such as factual and bibliographic, databases also come in varied formats. Most of the databases on the list are available online. *Online* access means the searcher connects to the database, usually by modem, and is charged according to the length of the search session with an additional charge for each record that is displayed. Each vendor has its own price structure. With online databases, the searcher is charged for the information retrieved during the search session. If a database needs to be searched frequently, it might be cost-efficient to purchase the entire database. Databases are increasingly becoming available in CD-ROM format, and you can purchase some environmental toxicology databases as packages. Many are also available as magnetic tapes or computer diskettes. The Internet, an international network of networks, also provides access to many resources: actual documents, discussion groups, bulletin boards, and access to many databases. To search commercial databases through the Internet, you still need to establish an account with the vendor.

Once a bibliographic listing of relevant citations is compiled from the appropriate database, you may want to obtain some of the articles or reports. Check the resources and services of local libraries. Alternatively, many of these database vendors offer document delivery services and will supply requested materials for a fee.

This listing was originally prepared by the authors to update the listing in the *Toxics Directory: References and Resources on the Health Effects of Toxic Substances*: 4th ed., which may be purchased by mail order only from the California Department of General Services, Publications Section, P.O. Box 1015, North Highlands, CA 95660.

## ONLINE DATABASES

### *National Library of Medicine (NLM)*
**8600 Rockville Pike #38/4N-421**
**Bethesda, MD 20894**
**(800) 272-4787**
**Internet address: mms@nlm.nih.gov**

The following database descriptions are reproduced by permission of Medlars Management Services, National Library of Medicine.

CANCERLIT®
Coverage: 1963 to the present
Updates: Monthly
Data Type: Bibliographic
Availability: Online
Provider: U.S. National Cancer Institute
CANCERLIT® provides carcinogenicity, mutagenicity, tumor promotion, tumor inhibition information from more than 3,500 journals, monographic series, government reports, symposia, dissertations, books and theses as well abstracts of papers presented at meetings. Topics covered include: all aspects of experimental and clinical cancer therapy; information on chemical, viral, and other agents that cause cancer; mechanisms of carcinogenesis; biochemistry, immunology, physiology, and biology of cancer, and both in vivo and in vitro studies of growth factors and other agents that stimulate cell division, mutagens, and mutagen testing.

CHEMID
Data Type: Factual
Availability: Online
Provider: U.S. National Library of Medicine
A chemical dictionary/thesaurus containing about 200,000 records on chemicals of biomedical or regulatory interest. Records contain the following data fields: CAS® registry number, molecular formula, systemic name, synonyms, mixture, MESH heading, classification code (general use category from RTECS), note, and locator.

CHEMLINE®
Data Type: Factual
Availability: Online
Provider: U.S. National Library of Medicine
National Library of Medicine's chemical dictionary file developed in collaboration with Chem-

ical Abstracts Service. The file contains records for over 550,000 chemicals indexed in other NLM files (e.g., MEDLINE®, TOXLINE®, HSDB®). Records contain the following chemical identifiers: full nomenclature and synonyms; structural data on fragments; preferred, alternate replaced, and replacing Chemicals Abstracts registry numbers; molecular formula and other linear notation systems; and ring system information.

## CHEMICAL CARCINOGENESIS RESEARCH INFORMATION SYSTEM (CCRIS)
Data Type: Factual
Availability: Online
Provider: U.S. National Cancer Institute
National Cancer Institute's scientifically evaluated and fully referenced database containing carcinogenicity, tumor promotion and mutagenicity test results for over 1,000 chemicals.
Data are derived from primary literature, special reviews, and a wide range of NCI reports.

## DEVELOPMENTAL AND REPRODUCTIVE TOXICOLOGY (DART™)
Coverage: 1989 to the present
Updates: Monthly
Data Type: Bibliographic
Availability: Online
Provider: U.S. Environmental Teratology Information Center
DART is a bibliographic database that contains citations to publications concerning developmental and reproductive toxicology. DART primarily covers teratology (birth defects) information and is a continuation of ETICBACK (back file of the Environmental Teratology Information Center). DART contains citations to documents published since 1989. For older information, refer to ETICBACK. Approximately 2400-3600 citations will be added annually. Citations in DART are either derived from MEDLINE or created especially for this database. Many citations contain abstracts and all citations contain MeSH terms.

## ENVIRONMENTAL MUTAGEN INFORMATION CENTER (EMIC)
Coverage: 1991 to the present
Data Type: Bibliographic
Availability: Online
Provider: U.S. Environmental Mutagen Information Center
EMIC (Environmental Mutagen Information Center) is a bibliographic database that contains citations to literature concerning agents that have been tested for genotoxic activity. EMIC covers literature published since 1991. Older citations (1950–1990) are found in EMICBACK (the backfile for EMIC). Records in EMIC are either derived from MEDLINE or created especially for this database. Many records contain abstracts and MeSH terms and all records contain EMIC specialized indexing keywords and the names and CAS Registry Numbers of all chemicals. The database is produced by the Oak Ridge National Laboratory and is supported by the Environmental Protection Agency, the National Institute of Environmental Health Sciences and the National Library of Medicine.

## ENVIRONMENTAL TERATOLOGY INFORMATION CENTER BACKFILE (ETICBACK)
Coverage: Pre-1950 to 1987
Updates: Continued by DART
Data Type: Bibliographic
Availability: Online
Provider: U.S. Environmental Teratology Information Center
ETICBACK contains less current material than the Developmental and Reproductive Toxicology (DART) bibliographic database. This database includes citations to articles concerning teratol-

ogy and developmental toxicology and covers from pre-1950 to 1987. Citations contain complete bibliographic citations, Chemical Abstract Service registry numbers for chemicals, and specialized indexing keywords. The database is produced by the Environmental Mutagen, Carcinogen, and Teratogen Information Program of the Oak Ridge National Laboratory and is funded by the federal government. Current teratology information is found in Developmental and Reproductive Toxicology (DART).

GENE-TOX
Data Type: Factual
Availability: Online
Provider: U.S. Oak Ridge National Laboratory
GENE-TOX is an online database created by the U.S. Environmental Protection Agency (EPA) containing genetic toxicology (mutagenicity) data on over 4,000 chemicals. The database is the result of reviews by work panels of experts in the specific test systems of papers published in the open scientific literature. These reviews were themselves published in the "Reviews in Genetic Toxicology" section of *Mutation Research.* The database is structured into two subject categories: one for substance identification and the other for information on specific test systems. The information for each assay system is organized into data tabs and carries a **PEER REVIEWED** status tag. Each test system is referenced with an EMIC number and brief bibliographic citation for the original source paper and/or to the Gene-Tox panel report publication for the assay.

HAZARDOUS SUBSTANCES DATA BANK (HSDB®)
Updates: About 100 new chemicals added annually and 400+ existing records revised annually
Data Type: Factual
Availability: Online
Provider: U.S. Environmental Protection Agency
Detailed, scientifically reviewed, fully referenced profile for 4,300+ chemicals. Records have up to 144 data fields in 11 categories including substance identification, manufacturing/use information, chemical and physical properties, safety and handling, toxicity/biomedical effects, pharmacology, environmental fate/exposure potential, exposure standards and regulations, monitoring and analysis methods, additional references and express data category which allow retrieval of the most up-to-date information.

INTEGRATED RISK INFORMATION SYSTEM (IRIS)
Data Type: Factual
Availability: Online
Provider: U.S. Environmental Protection Agency
Environmental Protection Agency (EPA) database provides scientifically reviewed health risk assessment information on 600+ chemicals. Contains reference oral and inhalation reference doses, carcinogenicity assessment, U.S. regulatory actions and drinking water advisories. The information on IRIS is most useful if applied in the larger context of risk assessment as outlined by the National Academy of Sciences. IRIS supports the hazard identification and dose-response steps of the risk assessment process. The reference dose and carcinogenicity assessments on IRIS can serve as guides in evaluating potential health hazards and selecting a response to alleviate a potential risk to human health. It is important to note that the risk information on IRIS will be revised as additional health effects data become available and new developments in risk assessment methods arise. Health Risk Assessment information on a chemical is included in IRIS only after a comprehensive review of chronic toxicity data by work groups composed of U.S. EPA scientists. The information presented in the Noncarcinogenic Assessment and Carcinoge-

nicity Assessment categories represents a consensus reached in the review process. Other information in IRIS, such as the Drinking Water Health Advisories, have undergone reviews dictated by the responsible EPA Office. Users should be aware that Regulatory Action information (e.g., Clean Air Act Requirements) may not reflect the most recent EPA risk assessment data found elsewhere in the record and may take into account factors other than health effects. Background documentation with data definitions and explanations of the methods used to derive the values in IRIS are available from EPA.

MEDLINE®
Coverage: 1966 to the present
Updates: Weekly
Data Type: Bibliographic
Availability: Online
Provider: U.S. National Library of Medicine (NLM)
Comprehensive index to world medical and health literature. Especially useful for research toxicology of a particular chemical by using subheadings (adverse effects, poisoning, toxicity); for biological monitoring of a chemical apply subheadings analysis, blood, urine; for linking a disease to chemical exposure apply subheading chemical induced to name of disease; use subheading metabolism for absorption, distribution, excretion; and pharmacokinetics (1988–   ) for pharmacokinetics (mechanisms, dynamics and kinetics of exogenous chemical and drug absorption, biotransformation, distribution, release, transport, uptake and elimination as a function of dosage, extent and rate of metabolic processes).

REGISTRY OF TOXIC EFFECTS OF CHEMICAL SUBSTANCE (RTECS®)
Coverage: June 1971 to the present
Updates: Quarterly
Data Type: Factual
Availability: Online
Provider: U.S. National Institute for Occupational Safety and Health
Produced and maintained by the National Institute for Occupational Safety and Health (NIOSH). Provides basic toxicity data for 90,000+ potentially toxic chemicals, including acute and chronic toxicity data, carcinogenicity, mutagenicity and reproductive effects, chemical identifiers, exposure standards, NTP test status and status under various Federal regulations and programs. Selected Federal regulatory requirements and exposure levels are also presented. References are available for all data. RTECS is built and maintained by the National Institute for Occupational Safety and Health (NIOSH), which also periodically publishes paper and microfiche versions of the file.

TOXIC CHEMICAL RELEASE INVENTORY (TRI)
Coverage: 1987–
Updates: Annual
Data Type: Factual
Availability: Online
Provider: U.S. Environmental Protection Agency
The Toxic Chemical Release Inventory (TRI) is authorized under Section 313 of the Emergency Planning and Community Right-to-Know Act of 1986. EPA collects information on releases of over 300 listed chemicals and chemical categories from facilities in Standard Industrial Classification (SIC) codes 20 through 39 with 10 or more full-time employees. Information is collected on an annual basis and organized into a series of files based on reporting years, TRI87, TRI88, etc. While the data entry accuracy is checked, the information is entered

as the reporting facility submitted it on EPA Form R. Each chemical reported by a facility is treated as a separate submission.

TRI contains information on the annual estimated releases of toxic chemicals into the environment based upon data collected by the EPA. Includes facility identification, substance identification, environmental release of chemical, waste treatment, off-site waste transfer. Data includes names, addresses of public contacts of plant manufacturing, processing or using the reported chemicals, the maximum amount stored on site, the estimated quantity emitted into the air (point and non-point emissions), discharged into bodies of water, injected underground, or released to land, methods used in waste treatment and their efficiency, and data on the transfer of chemicals off-site for treatment/disposal.

TRIFACTS supplements the environmental release data on chemicals in the TRI series of files, with information related to the health and ecological effects, and safety handling of these chemicals. The data may be useful to workers, employers, and community residents. The data should be supplemented with technical literature to answer in-depth questions. In case of health emergencies, a physician or Poison Control Center should be consulted.

TOXLINE®

Coverage: Varies by subfile
Updates: Monthly
Data Type: Bibliographic
Availability: Online
Provider: U.S. National Library of Medicine
Toxicology Literature Online (TOXLINE) is the central database in a collection of bibliographic databases covering the pharmacological, biochemical, physiological, and toxicological effects of drugs and other chemicals. Covers the pharmacological, biochemical, physiological, environmental, and toxicological effects of chemicals and drugs. TOXLINE is comprised of references from major published secondary sources and from special literature collections. It provides comprehensive coverage of all areas of toxicology related to published studies of health effects in humans and animals and to chemical (especially pesticide) pollution in the environment and the related analytical methodology. Specialized information is included in the fields of teratology, neurotoxicity, mutation data, and poisonings.

TOXLINE® FILES:

| | |
|---|---|
| ANEUPL | Aneuploidy |
| BIOSIS | Toxicological Aspects of Environmental Health from Biological Abstracts |
| EMIC & ETIC | Environmental Mutagen and Teratology Information Centers |
| EIS | Epidemiology Information System from U.S. Food and Drug Administration |
| HMTC | Hazardous Materials Technical Center |
| ILO | International Labour Office |
| IPA | International Pharmaceutical Abstracts |
| NIOSH | NIOSHTIC |
| NTIS | National Technology Information Service Toxicology Document and Data Depository (TD3) |
| PESTAB | Pesticides Abstracts |
| PPBOB | Poisonous Plants Bibliography |
| TSCATS | Toxic Substances Control Act Test Submissions |
| TOXBIB | Toxicity Bibliography from MEDLINE |

## DIALOG Information Services, Inc.
### World-wide Headquarters
### 3460 Hillview Avenue
### P.O. Box 10010
### Palo Alto, CA 94303-0993
### (800) 334-2564
### (415) 858-3810
### (415) 858-7069 FAX

The following database descriptions are reproduced with permission of DIALOG Information Services, Inc.

AGRICOLA FILES, 10, 110
Coverage: 1970 to the present
Updates: Monthly
Data Type: Bibliographic
Provider: U.S. National Agricultural Library, Beltsville, MD
AGRICOLA is the database of the National Agricultural Library (NAL). This massive file provides comprehensive coverage of worldwide journal literature and monographs on agriculture and related subjects. Related subjects include: animal studies, botany, chemistry, entomology, fertilizers, forestry, hydroponics, soils, and more.

THE AGROCHEMICALS HANDBOOK FILE 306
Coverage: Current
Updates: Twice a year
Data Type: Factual, directory
Provider: The Royal Society of Chemistry, Cambridge, U.K.
The Agrochemicals Handbook provides information on the active components found in agrochemical products used worldwide. This information provides the identity of substances used in crop protection and pest control. For each of the substances found in the Agrochemicals Handbook, the following information is given: chemical name (including synonyms and trade names), CASR Registry Numbers, molecular formula, molecular weight, manufacturers' names, chemical and physical property, toxicity, mode of action, activity, health and safety, and much more.

ANALYTICAL ABSTRACTS FILE 305
Coverage: 1980 to the present
Updates: Monthly
Data Type: Bibliographic
Provider: The Royal Society of Chemistry, Cambridge
Analytical Abstracts is devoted to all aspects of analytical chemistry: any general application, inorganic chemistry, organic chemistry, pharmaceutical chemistry, environmental chemistry and more. The database contains references from approximately 1,300 journals which are core journals, as well as information gathered from conference papers, books, standards, and technical reports. Information found in a record from ANALYTICAL ABSTRACTS includes chemical names, including synonyms and/or trade names, CAS® Registry numbers, analyte and matrices information, and more.

AQUATIC SCIENCES AND FISHERIES ABSTRACTS FILE 44
Coverage: 1978 to the present
Updates: Monthly

Data Type: Bibliographic
Availability: Online
Provider: United Nations
Aquatic Sciences and Fisheries Abstracts (ASFA) is a comprehensive database on the science, technology, and management of marine and freshwater environments. The database corresponds to the print *Aquatic Sciences and Fisheries Abstracts,* Part 1: *Biological Sciences and Living Resources*; Part 2: *Ocean Technology, Policy, and Non-Living Resources*; and Part 3: *Aquatic Pollution and Environmental Quality.* ASFA includes citations to 5,000 primary journals, monographs, conference proceedings, and technical reports.

BIOSIS PREVIEWS® FILES 5, 55
Coverage: 1969 to the present
Updates: Weekly
Data Type: Bibliographic
Availability: Online
Provider: BIOSIS, Philadelphia, CA
BIOSIS PREVIEWS contains over 8.3 million citations from Biological Abstract (BA), Biological Abstracts/RRM (Reports, Reviews, Meetings (BA/RRM)), and BioResearch Index (Biol), the major publications of BIOSIS. Together, these publications constitute the major English-language service providing comprehensive worldwide coverage or research in the biological and biomedical sciences.

CA SEARCH® FILES 399, 308-313
Coverage: 1967 to the present
Updates: Every two weeks
Data Type: Bibliographic
Availability: Online
Provider: Chemical Abstracts Services, Columbus, OH
The CA Search database includes over 10 million citations to the literature of chemistry and its applications. CA Search is an expanded database that contains the basic bibliographic information appearing in the print *Chemical Abstracts.*

CANCERLIT® FILE 159 see NLM for database description

CHEMICAL SAFETY NEWSBASE FILE 317
Coverage: January 1981 to the present
Updates: Monthly
Data Type: Bibliographic
Availability: Online
Provider: The Royal Society of Chemistry, Cambridge, U.K.
CHEMICAL SAFETY NEWSBASE provides information on the hazardous and potentially hazardous effects of chemicals and processes encountered by workers in industry and laboratories. It also covers microbiological and radiation hazards encountered in the workplace. It is of interest to workers, safety officers, and all those concerned with health and safety management. The database includes information on: animals, microorganisms, and radiation; biological effects of chemicals; chemical reactions; emergency planning; fires and explosions; laboratory design, management, and practice; legislation and standards; occupational health and hygiene; safe practices and equipment; transportation and storage of chemicals; and waste management. Items on well-known hazards are not included unless new information is given. Chemical Safety

Newsbase corresponds to the print publications *Chemical Hazards in Industry* and *Laboratory Hazards Bulletin.*

CHEMSEARCH™ FILE 398
Coverage: 1957 to the present
Updates: Monthly
Data Type: Factual
Availability: Online
Provider: Chemical Abstracts Service, Columbus OH
CHEMSEARCH™ contains over 12 million chemical substances registered by Chemical Abstracts Service since 1957. It is the most comprehensive collection of organic and inorganic substances available on DIALOG. Each record in CHEMSEARCH™ contains identifying information about the chemical substance, such as CAS® Registry Number, molecular formula, CA Substance Index Name(s), synonyms, complete ring data, and other chemical substance information. Name searching is available, as well as substructure searching via nomenclature. The primary purpose of this file is to support specific substance searching for all substances cited in the CAS literature since 1957.

CHEMTOX® ONLINE FILE 337 (forthcoming file)
Coverage: Current
Update: Quarterly
Data Type: Factual
Availability: Online
Provider: Resource Consultants, Inc., Brentwood, TN
CHEMTOX ONLINE, a file of regulated toxic and hazardous substances, is a comprehensive collection of data on over 6,400 chemicals having physical and chemical properties that make them dangerous to individuals and/or the environment. Data coverage includes a chemical's physical, chemical, and toxicological properties; health, safety, and risk management aspects; first aid procedures; and regulatory status under various United States EPA (RCRA, EPCRA, CAA CWA, etc.) DOT (HM181), and OSHA regulations. In addition, a chemical's regulatory status on numerous state lists is included. Of special interest in the total integration of toxicity data, including carcinogenicity status as reported by IARC, NTP, OSHA ACGIH, and other agencies.

EMBASE (formerly Excerpta Medica) Files 72, 73
Coverage: June 1974 to the present
Updates: Weekly
Data Type: Bibliographic
Availability: Online
Provider: Elsevier Science Publishers, Amsterdam, The Netherlands
The Excerpta Medica database, EMBASE, is one of the leading sources for searching the biomedical literature. It consists of abstracts and citations to over 3,500 biomedical and pharmacological journals published throughout the world. EMBASE is known for its coverage of the drug-related literature.

ENVIRONLINE® FILE 40
Coverage: 1971 to the present
Updates: Monthly
Data Type: Bibliographic
Availability: Online

Provider: R. R. Bowker, a Reed Reference Publishing Company, New Providence, N.J.
ENVIROLINE covers the world's environmental information. Its comprehensive, interdisciplinary approach provides indexing and abstracting coverage of more than 5,000 international
primary and secondary source publications reporting on all aspects of the environment. Included
are such fields as: management, technology, planning, law, political science, economics, geology,
biology, and chemistry as they relate to environmental issues. Literature covered includes
periodicals, government documents, industry reports, proceedings of meetings, newspaper
articles, films, and monographs.

ENVIRONMENTAL BIBLIOGRAPHY FILE 68
Coverage: 1973 to the present
Updates: Bimonthly
Data Type: Bibliographic
Availability: Online
Provider: Environmental Studies Institute, Santa Barbara, CA
Environmental Bibliography covers the fields of general human ecology, atmospheric studies,
energy, land resources, water resources, and nutrition and health.

KIRK-OTHMER ONLINE FILE 302
Coverage: 4th edition of the Kirk-Othmer Encyclopedia of Chemical Technology
Update: Irregular
Data type: Factual, full text
Availability: Online
Provider: Wiley Electronic Publishing, New York, NY
Kirk-Othmer Online is an exhaustive and comprehensive treatise of applied chemical science
and industrial technology. File 302 covers methods and materials, as well as the latest scientific
advances in every branch of the useful arts of chemistry. The database is the online equivalent
to the *Kirk-Othmer Encyclopedia of Chemical Technology,* well known as the standard reference
work on any chemical topic or industry. File 302 provides access to a wide range of chemistry
subject areas, including: agricultural chemicals, energy, drugs, fibers and textiles, food, fossil
fuels, glass and ceramics, metals and metallurgy, semiconductors and electronic materials, and
more. All tabular materials in the hard copy is included and is searchable online.

MEDLINE® Files 152, 153, 154, 155 see NLM for database description

NATIONAL TECHNICAL INFORMATION SERVICE (NTIS) File 6
Coverage: 1964 to the present
Updates: Biweekly
Data type: Bibliographic
Availability: Online
Provider: National Technical Information Services (NTIS)
U.S. Department of Commerce, Springfield, VA
The NTIS database provides access to the results of U.S. government-sponsored research,
development, and engineering, plus analyses prepared by federal agencies, their contractors or
grantees. It is the means through which unclassified, publicly available, unlimited distribution
reports are made available for sale from agencies such as NASA, EPA, DOE, HUD, DOD
Department of Commerce, and some 600 other agencies. In addition, some state and local
government agencies now contribute their reports to the database.

NTIS also provides access to the results of government-sponsored research and development from countries outside the U.S. Organizations that currently contribute to the NTIS database include: the Japan Ministry of International Trade and Industry (MITI); laboratories administered by the United Kingdom Department of Industry; the German Federal Ministry of Research and Technology (BMFT); the French National Center for Scientific Research (CNRS); and many more.

OCCUPATIONAL SAFETY AND HEALTH (NIOSHTIC®) File 161
Coverage: 1973 to the present
Updates: Quarterly
Data Type: Bibliographic
Availability: Online
Provider: U.S. National Institute for Occupational Safety and Health, Cincinnati, OH
Occupational Safety and Health (NIOSHTIC®) is a product of the Technical Information Branch, a component of the National Institute for Occupational Safety and Health. It includes citations to more than 2,000 journal titles, as well as over 70,000 monographs and technical reports. NIOSHTIC covers all aspects of occupational safety and health.

POLLUTION ABSTRACTS FILE 41
Coverage: 1970 to the present
Updates: Bimonthly
Data Type: Bibliographic
Availability: Online
Provider: Cambridge Scientific Abstracts, Bethesda, MD
Pollution Abstracts is a leading resources for references to environment-related literature on pollution, its sources, and its control. Among the subjects covered by the Pollution Abstracts database are: air pollution, environmental quality, noise pollution, pesticides, radiation, solid wastes, water pollution, and more.

REGISTRY OF TOXIC EFFECTS OF CHEMICAL SUBSTANCES (RTECS®) FILE 336 see NLM for database description

TOXLINE® FILE156 see NLM for database description

## DIALOG/DATASTAR
**One Commerce Square**
**2005 Market Street, Suite 1010**
**Philadelphia, PA 19103**
**(800) 221-7754**
**(215) 587-4400**

The following database descriptions are reproduced by permission of Dialog Information Services, Inc.

ANALYTICAL ABSTRACTS see DIALOG for database description

BIOSIS PREVIEWS® see DIALOG for database description

CANCERLIT® see NLM for database description

CHEMICAL ABSTRACTS see DIALOG for database description

CHEMICAL SAFETY DATABASE see DIALOG for database description

ENVIROLINE® see DIALOG for database description

EXCERPTA MEDICA see DIALOG for database description

HAZARDOUS SUBSTANCES DATA BANK see NLM for database description

HSELINE—HEALTH & SAFETY
Coverage: 1977 to date
Updates: Monthly
Availability: Online
Producer: Health & Safety Executive, Sheffield UK
HSELINE is produced by the United Kingdom Health and Safety Executive (HSE) Library and Information services. The subject areas of this database include all aspects of health and safety at work. The database reflects HSE's wide subject interests and covers science, technology manufacturing industries, agriculture, production, occupational hygiene, safety, explosives, engineering, mining and nuclear technology. The references cover all the United Kingdom Health and Safety Commission and the Safety Executive's publications and also books, reports, translations, standard specifications, guidance, conference proceedings, decided cases, legislation in the UK and elsewhere relevant to health and safety at work. Approximately 250 national and international periodicals are abstracted.

KIRK-OTHMER ENCYCLOPEDIA OF CHEMICAL TECHNOLOGY see DIALOG for database description

MEDICAL TOXICOLOGY & HEALTH—DHMT
Coverage: October 1983 to the present
Updates: Weekly
Availability: Online
Producer: Department of Health, London
DHMT offers specialized information covering medical toxicology and environmental health, using the resources of the Department of Health Library in London. The DHMT database specializes in medical toxicology and environmental health. Areas covered include: chemicals in food, consumer products and the environment, health consequences of smoking, radiation and noise, pesticides, air and water pollution, industrial chemical, and radiation biology. Other subjects covered include: veterinary medicines, good laboratory practice, cosmetics and general toxicology. Articles indexed from about 2,000 mainly English-language journals are included, together with records of conference proceedings, reports, books, pamphlets, administrative circulars and other official publications. An important feature of the database is the inclusion of full details, including sources of supply, of DOH publications. Abstracts are available for documents added to the database from 1984.

MEDLINE® see NLM for database description

POLLUTION ABSTRACTS see DIALOG for database description

RTECS REGISTRY OF TOXIC EFFECTS OF CHEMICAL SUBSTANCES see NLM for database description

TOXLINE® see NLM for database description

**STN (Science and Technology Network)**
**c/o Chemical Abstracts Service**
**2540 Olentangy River Road**
**P.O. Box 3012**
**Columbus OH 43210-0012**
**(614) 447-3600**
**(800) 848-6538**
**FAX (614) 447-3751**
**Internet address: help@cas.org**

The following database descriptions are reproduced by permission of STN.

AQUATIC SCIENCES AND FISHERIES ABSTRACTS (AQUASCI) see DIALOG for database description

BIOSIS Previews®/RN see DIALOG for database description.
On STN, BIOSIS has been enhanced with CAS registry numbers for substances appearing in the title and added keyword fields.

CHEMICAL ABSTRACTS (CA) see DIALOG for database description.
While CA is available from many vendors, only STN has all the abstracts available online. TOXLIT on the NLM system has CA abstracts, but TOXLIT is only a subset of the entire CA database.

CAOLD
Coverage: 1957–1966, limited number prior to 1957
Updates: Intermittently
Data Type: Bibliographic
Availability: Online
Provider: Chemical Abstracts Service
CAOLD file contains records for Chemical Abstracts (CA) references 1957-1967, with a limited number of references prior to 1957. This file is only available through STN.

CApreviews®
Coverage: Current
Updates: Daily
Data Type: Bibliographic
Availability: Online
Provider: Chemical Abstracts Service
CApreviews contains information for records that will appear in the CA file. The information in CApreviews is available six to eight weeks before the full document record appears in the CA file. Once the reference appears in CA, it can no longer be searched in CApreviews®.

CHEMSAFE
Updates: Two times a year
Data Type: Factual
Availability: Online
Provider: Physikalisch-Technische Bundesanstalt, Bundesanstalt fuer Material forschung und-pruefung, and DECHEMA
Provides evaluated safety characteristics of 1,500 flammable substances and their mixtures and

more than 40 properties for gases, liquids, dusts, and hybrid mixtures. If possible, values are marked with a safety recommendation for the user. Database is in English.

CHEMICAL SAFETY NEWSBASE (CSNB) see DIALOG for database description

EMBASE see DIALOG for database description

HEALSAFE
Coverage: 1981 to the present
Updates: Quarterly
Data Type: Bibliographic
Availability: Online
Provider: Cambridge Scientific Abstracts
Health and Safety Science Abstracts file covers public health, safety, and industrial hygiene. Topics include aviation; aerospace; and environmental, nuclear, medical, and occupational safety. HEALSAFE corresponds to the printed *Health and Safety Science Abstracts.*

HAZARDOUS SUBSTANCES DATA BANK (HSDB®) see NLM for database description. On STN, HSDB® displays chemical structures, and data appear in a tabular format.

JICST-E
Coverage: 1985 to the present
Updates: Monthly
Data Type: Bibliographic
Availability: Online
Provider: The Japan Information Center of Science and Technology
JICST-E contains abstracts and indexes in English to scientific and technical information published in Japan. The JICST-E file provides access to toxicology and other health and safety reports from Japanese companies and research institutes.

MEDLINE® see NLM for database description

MSDS-CCOHS
Data Type: Factual
Availability: Online
Provider: Canadian Centre for Occupational Health and Safety
The MSDS-CCOHS file contains MSDSs for over 9,000 U.S. and Canadian products manufactured or used in Canadian workplaces. Data sheets are prepared and supplied by producers or distributors and contain product identification information, relevant addresses, emergency contacts, and full text of the material safety data sheet.

MSDS-OHS
Data Type: Factual
Availability: Online
Provider: Occupational Health Services, Inc.
The MSDS-OHS file contains occupational and safety data for over 90,000 substances, including approximately 74,000 mixtures. The file is available through a gateway with STN providing access to the file that is loaded at the remote host in Nashville, Tennessee. Each material data safety sheet includes occupational, environmental, and regulatory information, as well as names, CAS Registry Numbers, EPA numbers and RTECS numbers.

MSDS-PEST
Data Type: Factual
Availability: Online
Provider: Occupational Health Services, Inc.
The MSDS-PEST file contains material safety data sheets for over 1,100 pesticide and related chemicals including pesticide products and active ingredients registered with the EPA, inert ingredients and other chemicals used in the formulation of pesticides. This file is available through the same gateway as MSDS-OHS.

MSDS-SUM
Data Type: Factual
Availability: Online
Provider: Occupational Health Services, Inc.
The MSDS-SUM file contains occupational and health summaries, in lay terms, of 12,000 of the chemical substances found in the MSDS-OHS file. MSDS-SUM is available through the same gateway as MSDS-OHS.

NATIONAL TECHNICAL INFORMATION SERVICE (NTIS) see DIALOG for database description

POLLUTION ABSTRACTS (POLLUAB) see DIALOG database description

REGISTRY
Coverage: 1957 to the present
Updates: Weekly
Availability: Online
Provider: Chemical Abstracts Service
REGISTRY is a chemical structure and dictionary database of over 11.5 unique substances. The REGISTRY file contains records for all the substances cited in the CAS Registry System. All substance records contain a unique CAS REGISTRY Number® and index name. Substance records may also have synonyms, molecular formulas, alloy composition labels, polymer classes, nucleic acid and protein sequences, ring analysis data, and structure diagrams—all of which are displayable and searchable.

REGISTRY OF TOXIC EFFECTS OF CHEMICAL SUBSTANCES (RTECS®) see NLM for database description. On STN, RTECS® displays chemical structures, and data appear in a tabular format.

**The Chemical Information System (CIS)**
**A Division of PSI International, Inc.**
**810 Gleneagles Court, Suite 300**
**Towson, Maryland 21286**
**(410) 321-8440**
**(800) CIS-USER**
**FAX (410) 296-0712**

The following database descriptions are reproduced by permission of CIS.

AQUATIC INFORMATION RETRIEVAL (AQUIRE)
Updates: Last Update, September, 1993
Data Type: Factual
Availability: Online

Provider: U.S. Environmental Protection Agency
Aquatic Information Retrieval contains data on acute, chronic, bioaccumulative, and sublethal effects from experiments performed on freshwater and saltwater organisms. Each record contains experimental results from a single assay. Includes data on more than 5,200 chemical substances in 114,000 records.

CHEMICAL CARCINOGENESIS RESEARCH INFORMATION SYSTEM (CCRIS) see NLM for database description

CHEMICAL EVALUATION SEARCH & RETRIEVAL SYSTEM (CESARS)
Updates: Irregular
Data Type: Factual
Availability: Online
Provider: Michigan Department of Natural Resources
Chemical Evaluation Search & Retrieval System provides detailed information and evaluations on a group of chemicals of particular importance in the Great Lakes Basin. CESARS provides detailed, evaluated chemical profiles, including toxicity data and environmental fate, taken from primary literature for over 194 compounds.

CHEMICAL HAZARD RESPONSE INFORMATION SYSTEM (CHRIS)
Data Type: Factual
Availability: Online
Provider: U.S. Coast Guard
Chemical Hazard Response Information System provides information needed to respond to emergencies that occur during the transport of hazardous chemicals. Contains information on labeling, physical and chemical properties, health hazards, fire hazards, chemical reactivity, water pollution, and hazard classifications for over 1,200 chemicals.

CHEMICAL HAZARDS INFORMATION SYSTEM (CHEMHAZIS)
Data Type: Factual
Availability: Online
Chemical Hazards Information System contains information drawn primarily from data compiled by the National Toxicology Program (NTP). The NTP was established as a U.S. Department of Health and Human Service cooperative effort to coordinate and provide information about potentially toxic chemicals with potential for human exposure to regulatory and research agencies. The database contains information on 2,280 chemicals drawn from the literature and experimentally determined under the sponsorship of the NTP.

CLINICAL TOXICOLOGY OF COMMERCIAL PRODUCTS (CTCP)
Data Type: Factual
Availability: Online
Clinical Toxicology of Commercial Products is based on the fifth edition (1984) of the book of the same title by Drs. Gosselin, Smith and Hodge. It contains manufacturer, uses, and composition information for approximately 23,000 commercial products. For chemicals comprising a product, CAS Registry Numbers, concentrations, and indication of toxicity (if applicable) are given.

DERMAL ABSORPTION (DERMAL)
Data Type: Factual
Availability: Online
Provider: U.S. Environmental Protection Agency

Dermal Absorption contains data on toxic effects, absorption, distribution, metabolism, and excretion related to dermal application of chemicals. Data on toxic effects of chemical exposure through other routes, such as oral or inhalation, are included if they appear in articles along with dermal data. Dermal contains over 3,000 test records for 655 substances

EMERGENCY RESPONSE NOTIFICATION SYSTEM (ERNS)
Coverage: 1987 to the present
Data Type: Factual
Availability: Online
Provider: U.S. Environmental Protection Agency and U.S. Department of Transportation
Emergency Response Notification System provides data compiled on accidental release notification of oil and hazardous substances in the United States. The ERNS program is a cooperative data sharing effort between the U.S. EPA, and the U.S. Department of Transportation. The database contains more than 231,312 records of initial notifications. ERNS may be used to examine the characteristics of hazardous substance release notifications under the following categories: transportation accident, equipment failure, operator error, natural phenomenon, dumping, and unknown. Five statutes require release reporting and are included in ERNS: CERCLA, SARA, CWA, NCP and HMTA. Users may also search the database by the location of the spill.

ENVIRONMENTAL FATE (ENVIROFATE)
Data Type: Factual
Availability: Online
Provider: U.S. Environmental Protection Agency
Environmental Fate deals with environmental fate or behavior (transport and degradation) of chemicals released in the environment. Envirofate includes data on environmental transformation rates and on physical-chemical properties. Includes over 15,000 records on approximately 16,000 substances.

GASTROINTESTINAL ABSORPTION DATABASE (GIABS)
Updates: Last Update, October, 1988
Data Type: Factual
Availability: Online
Provider: U.S. Environmental Protection Agency
GIABS contains references to articles in the scientific literature on absorption, distribution, metabolism, or excretion of chemical substances in test animals or humans. Each record in the database deals with a specific experiment involving a specific chemical. At its most recent update (October, 1988), GIABS included 12,052 citations to a total of 4,941 unique literature references from 1967 to 1987; information on more than 3,100 unique chemicals is included.

GENE-TOX see NLM for database description

HAZARDOUS CHEMICALS INFORMATION AND DISPOSAL GUIDE (HAZINF)
Data Type: Factual
Availability: Online
Hazardous Chemicals Information and Disposal Guide is based on the *Hazardous Chemicals Information and Disposal Guide* by M.A. Armour, L. M. Browne, and G.L. Weir of the Chemistry Department of the University of Alberta. The database provides information necessary to assess and respond to hazards associated with chemical substances, particularly as they are

likely to arise in the laboratory. Contains detailed instructions on the safe handling and disposal of some 220 chemicals or classes of chemicals.

INTEGRATED RISK INFORMATION SYSTEM (IRIS) see NLM for database description

MATERIAL SAFETY DATA SHEETS (MSDSs: BAKER, MALLIN, CCOHS, and CROPPRO)
Data Type: Factual
Availability: Online
BAKER and MALLIN are collections of material safety data sheets prepared by the J. T. Baker Chemical Company of Phillipsburg, New Jersey, and Mallinckrodt, Inc. of St. Louis. BAKER contains 1,960 MSDSs and MALLIN contains 1,635 MSDSs. One chemical substance is covered in each sheet/record. Each sheet/record contains a variety of information on safe handling, storage, and disposal of the substance.
CCOHS is a collection of MSDSs provided by the Canadian Center for Occupational Health and Safety. Database as described in the STN section. Access to the CCOHS collection is by CIS "valet service" only. CROPPRO (Crop Protection Chemicals) is a database of MSDSs for various types of crop protection products such as insecticides, fungicides, and herbicides, with more than 1036 data records representing over twenty-five manufacturers. CROPPRO is based on two published volumes: *MSDS Reference for Crop Protection Chemicals* and *Turf & Ornamental Chemicals Reference*. Both books are from Chemical and Pharmaceutical Publishing Corp., a subsidiary of OVP of Paris. As with BAKER, MALLIN and CCOHS, records contain all of the standard MSDS data fields in a general MSDS format.

MERCK INDEX ONLINE (MERCK ONLINE)
Data Type: Factual, full text
Updates: Semi-annually
Availability: Online
The Merck Index Online includes all the monographs on chemical substances from the 11th printed edition plus 100 additional monographs that are not in that edition and a number of monographs revised since the eleventh edition appeared. Covers preparation, chemical and physical properties, principal pharmacological action and toxicity of substances. Full text is searchable online.

OIL AND HAZARDOUS MATERIALS/TECHNICAL ASSISTANCE DATA SYSTEM (OHM/TADS)
Data Type: Factual
Availability: Online
Provider: U.S. Environmental Protection Agency
Oil and Hazardous Materials/Technical Assistance Data System provides information for responding to emergency situations involving substances that have been designated as oils or hazardous materials by the EPA. Provides up to 126 different fields of information for 1,402 materials. Includes physical, chemical, biological, toxicological, and commercial data on these materials, with emphasis placed on their environmental effects and emergency response.

REGISTRY OF TOXIC EFFECTS OF CHEMICAL SUBSTANCES (RTECS®) see NLM for database description

TOXIC SUBSTANCES CONTROL ACT TEST SUBMISSIONS (TSCATS)
Updates: Quarterly
Data Type: Bibliographic

Availability: Online
Provider: U.S. Environmental Protection Agency
Toxic Substances Control Act Test Submissions includes information on unpublished health and safety studies submitted to U.S. EPA under the provision of the Toxic Substances Control Act. TSCATS presently includes over 49,899 citations on more than 6,454 chemical substances. Studies can be identified by CAS registry number, chemical name, by name of submitting organization, by study purpose, by observed effects, and by a variety of other entries. Copies of the studies (distributed on microfiche) can be ordered through the Chemical Information System and the National Technical Information Service.

## *CD Plus formerly BRS (Bibliographic Retrieval Services Online)*
**CD Plus Technologies**
**333 7th Avenue**
**New York, NY 10001**
**(800) 950-2035**
**(212) 563-3006**

The following database descriptions are reproduced by permission of CDP Plus/BRS.

BIOSIS PREVIEWS® see DIALOG for database description

CA SEARCH® see DIALOG for database description

CANCERLIT® see NLM for database description

COMPREHENSIVE CORE MEDICAL LIBRARY (CCML)
Coverage: Current and retrospective issues of journals and current editions of textbooks and reference works
Updates: Twice a week, textbooks updated with issuance of new edition
Data type: Bibliographic, full text
Availability: Online
The Comprehensive Core Medical Library database is a master library of medical information drawn from prominent reference works, textbooks and journals in the fields of emergency, internal and critical care medicine. The content of this medical information resources is conveyed in its entirety online. Coverage includes *JAMA: Journal of the American Medical Association.*

HAZARDLINE
Updates: Monthly
Data Type: Factual
Availability: Online
Provider: Occupational Health Services, Inc.
The HAZARDLINE database provides regulatory, handling, identification, and emergency care information for over 4,000 hazardous substances. The information in HAZARDLINE is gathered from regulations issued by state and U.S. government agencies, court decisions, books and journal articles, in order to assemble a comprehensive record for each substance.

MEDLINE® see NLM for database description

NTIS see DIALOG for database description

TOXLINE® see NLM for database description

**Questel Inc.**
**2300 Clarendon Blvd., Suite 1111**
**Arlington VA 22201**
**(703) 527-7501**
**(800) 424-9600**
**FAX (703) 527-9664**

CHEMICAL ABSTRACTS (CAS) see DIALOG for database description

CIS OCCUPATIONAL HEALTH AND SAFETY
Data Type: Bibliographic
Availability: Online
Provider: International Occupational Safety and Health Information Centre (CIS), International Labour Office (ILO). CIS Occupational Health and Safety provides international coverage of occupational health and safety documents.

MERCK ONLINE (MRCK) see CIS for database description

MEDLINE® see NLM for database description

**ORBIT**
**QUESTEL/ORBIT**
**8000 Westpark Drive**
**McLean, VA 22102**
**(800) 456-7248**
**(703) 442-0900**
**(703) 893-4632 FAX**

ANALYTICAL ABSTRACTS see DIALOG for database description

CHEMICAL ABSTRACTS see DIALOG for database description

CHEMICAL DICTIONARY
Coverage: 1957 to the present
Updates: Monthly
Data type: Dictionary
Availability: Online
Provider: Chemical Abstracts Service, American Chemical Society
See DIALOG for database description

CHEMICAL SAFETY NEWSBASE see DIALOG for database description

ENVIROLINE® see DIALOG for database description

HEALTH & SAFETY EXECUTIVE LINE
Coverage: 1977 to the present
Updates: Monthly
Data type: Bibliographic
Availability: Online
Provider: U. K. Health and Safety Executive
Contains more than 150,000 bibliographic references from journals, books, pamphlets, government publications, and conference proceedings. Covers occupational health and safety aspects of the following areas: manufacturing and process industries, agriculture, engineer-

ing, mines and quarries, nuclear technology, offshore oil industry, railway transportation, and hazardous substances.

NIOSHTIC see Dialog for description

NTIS see DIALOG for database description

## *National Pesticide Information Retrieval System (NPIRS)*
## Center for Environmental & Regulatory Information Systems
## 1231 Cumberland Avenue Suite A
## West Lafayette, IN 47906-1317
## (317) 494-6616

The following database descriptions are reproduced by permission of NPIRS.

MATERIAL SAFETY DATA SHEETS
Updates: Quarterly (CPCR); Annually (TOCR)
Data Type: Factual
Availability: Online
This database contains over 1,000 MSDSs from 29 chemical manufacturers of pesticides used in the protection of crops, turf, and ornamental plants. The database is an online version of *C&P Press' Crop Protection Chemicals Reference* (CPCR), and *Turf & Ornamental Chemicals Reference* (TOCR).

PESTICIDE DOCUMENT MANAGEMENT SYSTEM
Updates: Monthly
Data Type: Bibliographic
Availability: Online
Pesticide Document Management System provides an index of all citations to more than 260,000 studies submitted to EPA in support of pesticide registrations. One can search this database to obtain a list of all studies submitted by a specific company in support of registration of a specific pesticide.

PESTICIDE FACT SHEETS
Data Type: Factual
Availability: Online
Provider: U.S. Environmental Protection Agency
Pesticide Fact Sheets provides access to fact sheets for over 200 registered pesticides. These pesticide summaries are issued by the U.S. EPA's Office of Pesticide Program's Registration Division. Each fact sheet contains a description of the chemical, use patterns, toxicity information, environmental characteristics, a summary science statement, a summary of the regulatory position, a summary of major data gaps and a contact person at EPA.

PESTICIDE PRODUCT INFORMATION
Data Type: Factual
Availability: Online
Provider: U.S. Environmental Protection Agency
Pesticide Product Information contains key label information on more than 21,000 active pesticide products federally registered for use in the U.S., and more than 60,000 canceled and transferred products. There are about 1,700 active ingredients represented in the database, as well as more than 2,100 company registrants, and over 17,000 distributors and 130,000 currently

registered products by brand name. Thirty-six state regulatory agencies also provide information on all state registered pesticide products.

## PESTICIDE TOLERANCE INFORMATION
Updates: monthly
Data Type: Factual
Availability: Online
This database contains pesticide tolerances listed in the U.S. Code of Federal Regulations. Each entry shows the allowable ppm residue levels by chemical for raw agricultural commodities, processed food, and animal feed. This database covers more than 400 chemicals and about 1,200 commodities.

## STATE REGISTRATION REPORTS
Data Type: Factual
Availability: Online
Thirty-six state regulatory agencies submit product registration data for this database. For the states that participate, the following data is available: master state registration list, selected product lists, state pesticide registration cross reference list of products in brand name, EPA registration number or state registration number sequence, and state pesticide state registration number range for each registrant.

## OTHER FORMATS

### *SilverPlatter Information Inc.*
**100 River Ridge Drive**
**Norwood, MA 02062-5026**
**(800) 343-0064**
**(617) 769-2599**
**(617) 769-8763 fax**
**Internet address: info@silverplatter.com**

The following database descriptions are reproduced by permission of SilverPlatter Information, Inc.

### COMPACT DISC FORMAT

AGRICOLA see DIALOG for database description

BIOLOGICAL ABSTRACTS ON COMPACT DISC for database description

BIOLOGICAL ABSTRACTS/RRM ON COMPACT DISC see DIALOG for database description

CANCER-CD
Coverage: 1984 to the present
Updates: Quarterly
Data Type: Bibliographic
Availability: CD-ROM
Provider: Elsevier Science Publishers and the U.S. National Cancer Institute
Made up of references, abstracts and commentaries from the world's literature on cancer and related subjects.

CANCERLIT® see NLM for database description

CHEM-BANK
Updates: Quarterly
Data Type: Factual
Availability: CD-ROM
Provider: U.S. Environmental Protection Agency, National Institute for Occupational Safety and Health, National Library of Medicine provides three National Library of Medicine databases: IRIS (Integrated Risk Information System), RTECS (Registry of Toxic Effects of Chemical Substances), and HSDB (Hazardous Substances Data Bank), Chemical Information Service's OHMTADS (Oil and Hazardous Material-Technical Assistance Data) and CHRIS (Chemical Hazard Response Information System).

See NLM for IRIS, RTECS, and HSDB database descriptions and CIS for OHMTADS and CHRIS database descriptions.

EMBASE ON CD see DIALOG for database description

IARCancer Disc
Published since 1971, this database series focuses on the links between environmental chemical exposure and the development of human cancer and genetics defects. It contains evaluations of over 700 chemicals, complex mixtures and lifestyle factors.
Coverage: 1971 to the present
Data Type: Full text
Availability: CD-ROM
Provider: International Agency for Research on Cancer

INTERNATIONAL OCCUPATIONAL SAFETY AND HEALTH (CISDOC)
Updates: Quarterly
Data Type: Bibliographic
Availability: CD-ROM
Provider: International Occupational Safety and Health Information Centre (CIS), International Labour Office (ILO)
Provides citations and abstracts to worldwide literature pertaining to occupational health and safety.
See QUESTEL for database description

MEDLINE® (EXPRESS AND PROFESSIONAL) see NLM for database description

OSH-ROM
Coverage: 1960 to the present
Updates: Quarterly
Data Type: Bibliographic
Availability: CD-ROM
Provider: International Labour Office, U.K. Health and Safety Executive, U.S. National Institute for Occupational Safety and Health
OSH-ROM brings together four bibliographic databases. All of these databases together form a resource for researching international occupational health and safety issues: NIOSHTIC see DIALOG for description, HSELINE, from the Health and Safety Executive (U.K.) covering occupational health and safety issues in the United Kingdom. CISDOC from the International Occupational Safety and Health Information Centre, International Labour Organisation providing an international perspective on occupational health and safety and MHIDAS, from the United Kingdom Atomic Energy Authority, covering potential dangers in handling hazardous materials.

PEST-BANK
Updates: Quarterly
Data Type: Factual
Availability: CD-ROM
Provider: Center for Environmental and Regulatory Information System; Purdue Research Foundation
Covers approximately 27,500 currently registered U.S. pesticides used in agriculture, industry, and general commerce as well as data on over 35,000 canceled products. The information in PEST-BANK is developed by the Center for Environmental and Regulatory Information System (CERIS) from data supplied by the U.S. Environmental Protection Agency and state pesticide regulatory agencies. PEST-BANK records provide pesticide product names and synonyms registration dates and registering companies, active ingredients, composition and formulation, sites and pests for which the pesticide is registered, and permissible residue levels.

POL-TOX I: NLM, CSA, IFIS
Coverage: 1966 to the present
Updates: Quarterly
Data Type: Bibliographic
Availability: CD-ROM
Provider: Cambridge Scientific Abstracts, International Food Information Service (IFIS), U.S. National Library of Medicine
Offers single search access to seven pollution and toxicology databases; contains 10 years of coverage and over 800,000 citations to the world's pollution and toxicology literature. Pol-Tox I combines the entire TOXLINE subfile from the National Library of Medicine, the complete toxicology subset of the Food Science and Technology Abstracts from International Food Information Service, and five databases from Cambridge Scientific Abstracts including Pollution Abstracts, Toxicology Abstracts, Ecology Abstracts, Health and Safety Science Abstracts and portions of the Aquatic Sciences and Fisheries Abstracts. Topics covered include air, water, soil, noise and radiation pollution, environmental risks, food additives, pharmaceutical side effects, agrochemicals, and industrial chemicals.

POL-TOX II: EMBASE
Coverage: 1983 to the present
Updates: Quarterly
Data Type: Bibliographic
Availability: CD-ROM
Provider: Elsevier Science Publishers
Extracts pollution and toxicology citations from EMBASE (see Dialog for database description). Topics covered include chemical pollution and its effects on humans, animals, plants, and microorganisms, environmental impact of chemical pollution, waste water treatment and measurement, meteorological aspects of pollution, pharmaceutical toxicology, chemical teratogens, mutagens and carcinogens.

TOXLINE® ON SILVERPLATTER see NLM for database description

TOXLINE® PLUS
Coverage: 1985 to the present
Updates: Quarterly
Data Type: Bibliographic
Availability: CD-ROM
Provider: American Society of Hospital Pharmacists (ASHP), Biological Abstracts, Inc. (BIO-

SIS), Chemical Abstracts Service (CAS), National Chemicals Inspectorate (Sweden), U.S. National Library of Medicine

Combines the complete TOXLINE file (including BIOSIS, Chemical Abstracts, and International Pharmaceuticals Abstracts) with data from the National Chemicals Inspectorate. Covers adverse drug reactions, interactions of chemical substances with biological systems, environmental pollution, industrial medicine, occupational health, waste disposal, and hazardous materials management.

WASTEINFO
Coverage: 1973 to the present
Updates: Quarterly
Data Type: CD ROM

The world's literature on waste management is covered in WasteInfo. Provides nearly 20 years of reference to the world's literature on non-radioactive waste management. WasteInfo encompasses over 60,000 citations and abstracts. The database offers current information on waste treatment, disposal, recycling, and associated environmental hazards. Corresponding to the monthly print publication, *Waste and Environment Today,* WasteInfo covers all aspects of waste disposal and treatment, such as landfill, incineration, biological or chemical treatment, and separation techniques, aspects of waste recycling, impact of wastes on the environment, and waste management policy, guidelines, legislation and regulation.

## *CCINFO*
## Canadian Centre for Occupational Health and Safety
## 250 Main Street East
## Hamilton Ontario Canada
## L8N 1H6
## (800) 668-4284 or (905) 570-8094
## FAX (905) 572-2206

MSDS SERIES A1
MSDS Series A1 is a CD-ROM product that contains the CHEMINFO and MSDS databases:

CHEMINFO
Data Type: Factual
Availability: Online, CD-ROM, magnetic tape, (forthcoming on the Internet, Fall of 1994)
Provider: Canadian Centre for Occupational Health and Safety
Contains summarized occupational health and safety information on chemicals. Each chemical profile uses non-technical information to describe potential workplace hazards and control measures.

MATERIAL SAFETY DATA SHEETS (MSDS)
Data Type: Factual
Availability: Online, CD-ROM, magnetic tape, (forthcoming on the Internet, Fall of 1994)
Complete text of over 92,000 Material Safety Data Sheets on chemical products, exactly as contributed directly by over 500 manufacturers and suppliers. Each MSDS provides information on product hazards, emergency response and first-aid measures, as well as safe working procedures. Many new and updated MSDSs are added to the database each quarter. Records are in English or French as provided by contributors.

CHEM SOURCE SERIES A2
CHEM Source Series A2 is a CD-ROM product that contains thirteen different databases on

regulatory, transportation, environmental and health information for industrial chemicals. Some of these databases are highlighted below:

CHEMICAL EVALUATION SEARCH AND RETRIEVAL SYSTEM (CESARS)
Data Type: Factual
Availability: Online, CD-ROM, (forthcoming on the Internet, Fall of 1994)
Provider: Michigan Department of Natural Resources and the Ontario Ministry of the Environment Database as described in the CIS section.

CHEMINFO see CCINFO MSDS SERIES A1

MAXIMUM RESIDUE LIMITS IN FOODS
Availability: Online, CD-ROM, (forthcoming on the Internet, Fall of 1994)
Provides access to information on maximum residue limits of registered pest control products on agricultural commodities. These limits are set by Health and Welfare Canada in the Regulations under the Food and Drugs Act.

NEW JERSEY HAZARDOUS SUBSTANCE FACT SHEETS
Data Type: Factual
Availability: CD-ROM
Provides workers, employers, emergency responders and others with information on the hazards and safe use of industrial chemicals and environmental contaminants. Fact Sheets contain basic summarized information on the hazards, safe storage, handling, control measures, first aid, and emergency procedures for common chemicals. Hazardous Substance Fact Sheets are prepared by the Right To Know Program, New Jersey Department of Health. About 800 of these non-technical 6-page summaries are currently available.

OSH INTERDATA SERIES B2
OSH InterData Series B2 is a CD-ROM product providing access to five databases on international aspects of occupational health and safety. One of these databases is highlighted below:

CISILO
Provider: International Occupational Safety and Health Information Centre (CIS), International Labour Office (ILO)
Data Type: Bibliographic
Availability: Online, CD-ROM, (forthcoming on the Internet, Fall of 1994)
See Questel for database description

NIOSHTIC SERIES C1
NIOSHTIC Series C1 is a CD-ROM product that contains two databases, one of which is NIOSHTIC®. The other is a listing of NIOSH documents that can be ordered from NIOSH, the U.S. Government Printing Office or the National Technical Information Service (NTIS).

NIOSHTIC®
Provider: Technical Information Center, U.S. National Institute for Occupational Safety and Health
Data Type: Bibliographic
Availability: Online (in Canada only), CD-ROM, (forthcoming on the Internet, Fall of 1994)
See DIALOG for database description

RTECS SERIES C2
RTECS Series C2 is a CD-ROM product that contains the RTECS database.

REGISTRY OF TOXIC EFFECTS OF CHEMICAL SUBSTANCES (RTECS®)
Data Type: Factual
Availability: Online (in Canada only), CD-ROM, (forthcoming on the Internet, Fall of 1994)
Provider: U.S. National Institute for Occupational Safety and Health
See NLM for database description

NIOSH MANUAL OF ANALYTICAL METHODS
Data Type: Factual
Availability: Diskette for microcomputer
Provider: U.S. National Institute for Occupational Safety and Health
Electronic version of the third edition of the NIOSH Manual of Analytical Methods. Contains over 200 methods covering approximately 440 substances.

CHEMICAL HAZARD RESPONSE INFORMATION SYSTEM (CHRIS)
Data Type: Factual
Availability: Online, CD-ROM (expected Fall, 1994)
Provider: U.S. Coast Guard
See CIS for databases description

OIL AND HAZARDOUS MATERIALS/TECHNICAL ASSISTANCE DATA SYSTEM
Data Type: Factual
Availability: Online, CD-ROM (expected Winter, 1994)
Provider: U.S. Environmental Protection Agency
See CIS for database description

**Micromedex, Inc.**
**600 Grant Street**
**Denver CO 80203-3527**
**(303) 831-1400**
**(800) 525-9083**
**FAX (303) 837-1717**

Database descriptions are reproduced by permission of Micromedex.

MATERIAL SAFETY DATA SHEETS (MSDS)
Data Type: Factual
Updates: Quarterly
Availability: CD-ROM
Provider: Micromedex and U.S. Pharmacopeial Convention
Provides access to over 1,000 material data sheets issued by the U.S. Pharmacopeial Convention.

POISINDEX® SYSTEM
Provider: Micromedex
Data Type: Factual
Updates: Quarterly
Availability: CD-ROM
POISINDEX® identifies ingredients for hundreds of thousands of commercial, pharmaceutical

and biological substances. For each substance, information on clinical effects, toxicity, and treatment protocols are provided.

TOMES Plus® System (TOXICOLOGY, OCCUPATIONAL MEDICINE & ENVIRON-MENTAL SERIES)
TOMES Plus® System is a CD-ROM product that brings together fourteen different databases, including:

CHEMICAL HAZARD RESPONSE INFORMATION SYSTEM (CHRIS) see CIS for database description

HAZARDOUS SUBSTANCES DATA BANK (HSDB®) see NLM for database description

HAZARDTEXT™ Hazard Managements
Data Type: Factual
Updates: Quarterly
Availability: CD-ROM
Provider: Micromedex
HAZARDTEXT contains information for the safe handling of industrial chemicals, as well as for responding to hazardous chemical spills.

INTEGRATED RISK INFORMATION SYSTEM (IRIS) see NLM for database description

MEDITEXT™ Medical Managements
Data Type: Factual
Updates: Quarterly
Availability: CD-ROM
Provider: Micromedex
MEDITEXT provides information for the evaluation and treatment of persons acutely exposed to industrial chemicals.

NEW JERSEY FACT SHEETS see CCINFO for database description

NIOSH POCKET GUIDE TO CHEMICAL HAZARDS
Data Type: Factual
Availability: CD-ROM
Provider: Micromedex and U.S. National Institute for Occupational Safety and Health
Electronic version of the popular industrial hygiene guide of the same name

OIL AND HAZARDOUS MATERIALS/TECHNICAL ASSISTANCE DATA SYSTEM (OHM/TADS) see CIS for database description

REGISTRY OF TOXIC EFFECTS OF CHEMICAL SUBSTANCES (RTECS®) see NLM for database description

SARATEXT® Database
Data Type: Factual
Updates: Quarterly
Availability: CD-ROM
Provider: Micromedex

Provides information on the acute and chronic effects of the chemicals included on the SARA Title III Extremely Hazardous Substance List.

## REPROTOX™ SYSTEM REPRODUCTIVE HAZARD INFORMATION

Data Type: Factual
Updates: Quarterly
Availability: CD-ROM
Provider: Micromedex and Reproductive Toxicology Center, Columbia Hospital for Women
Provides summarized information on chemical and physical agents effects on human fertility, pregnancy and fetal development. Includes industrial and environmental chemicals as well as prescription, over-the-counter and recreational drugs. The reviews are designed primarily for use in counseling pregnant patients. Database contains more than 4,000 agents (as of 1992) with an average of 500 new agents added each year.

## REPROTEXT® REPRODUCTIVE HAZARD REFERENCE

Data Type: Factual
Updates: Quarterly
Availability: CD-ROM
Provider: Micromedex
Provides reviews on the health effects, including reproductive, carcinogenic and genetic effects, of over 600 chemicals and physical agents encountered in the workplace. Originally developed by Betty J. Dabney, Ph.D. and now maintained by the Micromedex TOMES Plus editorial board.

## SHEPARD'S CATALOG OF TERATOGENIC AGENTS

Data Type: Factual
Updates: Quarterly
Availability: CD-ROM
Provider: Micromedex and Thomas H. Shepard, M.D., University of Washington
Electronic version of Thomas H. Shepard's *Catalog of Teratogenic Agents*. Information on more than 2,000 teratogenic agents, including chemicals, food additives, drugs, viruses, and environmental pollutants.

## TERIS

Data Type: Factual
Updates: Quarterly
Availability: CD-ROM
Provider: Micromedex and University of Washington
Provides information on the teratogenic effects of more than 700 drugs and environmental agents.

## REPRORISK® SYSTEM

Data Type: Factual
Updates: Quarterly
Availability: CD-ROM
Provider: Micromedex and others
REPRORISK® System is a compilation of four reproductive risk information databases: REPROTEXT®, REPROTOX™, SHEPARD'S Catalog and TERIS. For database descriptions see the Micromedex TOMES Plus® System section.

**Reproductive Toxicology Center**
**Columbia Hospital for Women**
**2440 M Street N.W. Suite 217**
**Washington D.C. 20037-1404**
**(202) 293-5137**

REPROTOX
Data Type: Factual
Availability: Online, diskettes for microcomputer, CD-ROM
Updates: Diskettes and CD-ROM updated quarterly
Provider: Reproductive Toxicology Center, Columbia Hospital for Women
See Micromedex TOMES Plus® System for database description.

**National Technical Information Service (NTIS)**
**5285 Port Royal Road**
**Springfield, VA 22161**
**(703) 487-4650**
**FAX (703) 321-8547 or (703) 321-9038**
**Online ordering through FedWorld™: via modem by dialing**
**(703) 321-8020 or telnet via Internet to fedworld.gov**

The following database descriptions are reproduced by permission of NTIS.

AQUATIC INFORMATION RETRIEVAL (ACQUIRE)
Data Type: Factual
Availability: Magnetic tape
Provider: U.S. Environmental Protection Agency, Office of Science and Technology
See CIS for database description

ENVIRONMENTAL MONITORING METHODS INDEX (EMMI)
Data Type: Factual
Availability: Diskettes for microcomputer
Provider: U.S. Environmental Protection Agency
Environmental Monitoring Methods Index is a database on all EPA-regulated substances, methods for their analysis, and regulatory and office-based lists on which they appear. The EMMI database includes information on more than 2600 substances from over 50 regulatory and non-regulatory lists and more than 900 analytical methods. The database provides a cross-reference between substances and analytical methods and contains information on related laws and organizations and additional databases for further information.

GASTROINTESTINAL CHEMICAL ABSORPTION DATABASE (GIABS) March 1987
Updates: Last Update, March, 1987
Data Type: Factual
Availability: Magnetic tape
Provider: U.S. Environmental Protection Agency, Office of Science and Technology
See CIS for database description—database on CIS updated October 1988.

INTEGRATED RISK INFORMATION SYSTEM (IRIS)
Updates: Quarterly
Data Type: Factual
Availability: Diskettes for microcomputer
Provider: U.S. Environmental Protection Agency
See NLM for database description

NIOSH POCKET GUIDE TO CHEMICAL HAZARDS
Data Type: Factual
Availability: Diskettes for microcomputer
Provider: U.S. National Institute for Occupational Health and Safety
See Micromedex for database description

OIL AND HAZARDOUS MATERIALS/TECHNICAL ASSISTANCE DATA SYSTEM
(OHM/TADS)
Data Type: Factual
Availability: Diskettes for microcomputer
Provider: U.S. Environmental Protection Agency
See CIS for database description

ROADMAPS
Data Type: Factual
Availability: Diskettes for microcomputer
Provider: U.S. Environmental Protection Agency, Office of Pollution Prevention and Toxic
Substances
Roadmaps to Sources of Information on Chemicals Listed in the Emergency Planning and
Community Right-to-Know Act (also know as SARA Title III), Section 313, Toxic Release
Inventory, is a database of sources of information on the chemicals listed in Section 313 of the
Superfund Amendments and Reauthorization Act (SARA). This database is intended to assist
users of the Toxic Release Inventory data to perform exposure and risk assessments of these
chemicals. The Roadmaps system displays and/or prints information for the chemicals on health
and environmental effects, federal regulations and state air and water regulations, monitoring
data and state contacts.

TOXIC CHEMICAL RELEASE INVENTORY (TRI)

Coverage: 1987–
Updates: Yearly
Data Type: Factual
Availability: CD-ROM, magnetic tapes, and as diskettes for microcomputer
Provider: U.S. Environmental Protection Agency
See NLM for database description

TOXIC SUBSTANCES CONTROL ACT TEST SUBMISSIONS (TSCATS)
Data Type: Bibliographic
Availability: Magnetic tape
Provider: U.S. Environmental Protection Agency, Office of Science and Technology
See CIS for database description

**Chemtox System**
**8 West Franklin Avenue**
**Pennington, New Jersey 08534**
**(609) 737-9009**
**FAX (609) 737-3323**

CHEMTOX® DATABASE
Updates: Quarterly
Data Type: Factual
Availability: Diskettes for microcomputer, magnetic tape, CD-ROM
See DIALOG for database description

**Occupational Health Services, Inc.**
**11 West 42nd Street, 12th Floor**
**New York, NY 10036**
**(212) 789-3535**
**(800) 445-MSDS**
**FAX (212) 789-3646**

OHS MSDS ON DISC
Updates: Quarterly
Data Type: Factual
Availability: CD-ROM
Provider: Occupational Health Services, Inc.
Over 100,000 different chemical product Material Safety Data Sheets are included in this collection. OHS MSDS reports contain all the legally required information plus additional toxicological, regulatory, transportation, and environmental information. Texts of current CFRs for the regulations that apply to the chemicals are available on the disc. The CFR database is also searchable separately.

**Lewis Publishers**
**2000 Corporate Blvd., N.W.**
**Boca Raton FL 33431**
**(407) 994-0555**

The following product descriptions are reproduced by permission of Lewis Publishers.

EPA'S PESTICIDE FACT SHEET DATABASE
Availability: Diskettes for microcomputer
Provider: Mary M. Walker and Lawrence H. Keith
See NPIRS (National Pesticide Information Retrieval System) for database description

EPA'S SAMPLING AND ANALYSIS METHODS DATABASE
Availability: diskettes for microcomputer
Provider: Edited by Lawrence H. Keith, Radian Corporation and William Meuller and David Smith, U.S. Environmental Protection Agency
This database was compiled by EPA chemists. It provides access to sampling and analytical methods summaries for 150 EPA-approved methods. The database is divided into three

volumes: Industrial chemicals; Pesticides, Herbicides, Dioxins, and PCBs; Elements and Water Quality Parameters

INTEGRATED RISK INFORMATION SYSTEM (IRIS)
Coverage: Current
Updates: Quarterly
Data Type: Factual
Availability: Diskettes for microcomputer
Provider: U.S. Environmental Protection Agency, Adapted for publication by Lawrence H. Keith, Radian Corporation
See NLM for database description

PC ENVIRONMENTAL FATE DATABASES
Availability: Diskettes for microcomputer
Provider: Philip H. Howard, Syracuse Research Corporation
The DATALOG, CHEMFATE, BIOLOG, and BIODEG databases provide data for predicting the behavior of chemicals in the environment.

THE NATIONAL TOXICOLOGY PROGRAM'S CHEMICAL DATABASE VOLUMES 1–8
Availability: Diskettes for microcomputer
Provider: Lawrence Keith, Radian and Douglas B. Walters
This database is divided into eight volumes. It contains information on chemical and physical properties, standards and regulations, medical hazards and symptoms of exposure, medical first aid, personal protective equipment, hazardous properties and uses, and shipping classifications and regulations for 2,270 chemicals.

**DIALOG OnDisc**
**Dialog Information Services, Inc.**
**3460 Hillview Avenue**
**Palo Alto, CA 94304-0993**
**(800) 334-2564**
**(415) 858-3810**
**FAX (415) 858-7069**

COMPACT DISC FORMAT

KIRK-OTHMER ENCYCLOPEDIA OF CHEMICAL TECHNOLOGY see DIALOG for database description

MEDLINE® see NLM for database description

NTIS see DIALOG for database description

**Electronic Handbook Publishers, Inc.**
**P.O. Box 3571**
**Bellvue, WA 98009-3571**
**(206) 836-0598**

ELECTRONIC HANDBOOK OF RISK ASSESSMENT VALUES (EHRAV)
Updates: Monthly or quarterly
Data Type: Factual

Availability: Diskettes for microcomputer

This electronic handbook provides access to risk assessment values from the EPA's Integrated Risk Information system (IRIS) and the EPA's Health Effects Assessment Summary Tables (HEAST), including RfDs, RfCs, slope factors, unit risk factors, MCLs, AWQCs, and health advisories. The radionuclides toxicity values from HEAST as well as a chemical/physical properties database of more than 450 chemicals are also available in the handbook. The Electronic Handbook of Risk Assessment Values (EHRAV) contains more than 40,000 data entries for more than 700 chemicals.

# PART VIII
## RISK ASSESSMENT AND RISK MANAGEMENT

**Michael J. DiBartolomeis**
*California Environmental Protection Agency*
*Berkeley, California*

*Risk assessment,* as described in the context of this book, might be defined as a process using scientific data and judgment to evaluate the probability that some external threat (e.g., chemical pollutant) will adversely affect human health or the environment. *Risk management* might then be defined as a value-based process to determine what level of risk is significant, and to identify options and means to reduce or maintain risk below that level. Risk management considers risk along with other factors such as cost, benefit, public perception, technical feasibility of controls, and enforcement capabilities, to name a few.

Historically, risk assessment and risk management have been separated into two distinct steps; risk assessment being first followed by risk management. Recent debate, however, has proved that the line drawn between risk assessment and risk management is blurred, and the separation of the two steps may not be advantageous or even possible.

The separation model assumes that risk assessment should be based on the "best available science," with no consideration of management or social values in estimating risk. Under this model, significant risk is defined independently of the risk assessment, and "no significant risk" would be accomplished through management options that are developed after the results of the risk assessment are known. Critics of the separation model argue that risk assessment is not a pure science and value judgments are, and should be, an integral part of the process. Indeed, the distinction between objective science and subjective scientific judgment is often unclear and promotes debate among the involved parties. That is, what is considered science to one risk assessor, may be considered policy by another.

A fully integrated model would assume that risk assessment should combine scientific analysis and judgment with management and social values. Under this model, risk assessment results would include management considerations, such as costs, benefits, and other technical or social factors. Critics of the integrated model argue that risk assessment should remain pure, devoid of social input that might dilute the science. In addition, some argue that public health and the environment would be ill-served because the magnitude of a risk would be masked by factoring in management and social factors.

In practice, features of these two models are generally combined into some form of a hybrid model. A hybrid model allows interaction of risk assessors and risk managers throughout the process. In a hybrid application, a series of "checks and balances" are created allowing risk assessors and risk managers to communicate and thus share ideas, critique, and problem solving. Proponents of a hybrid model suggest that decisions resulting from early and frequent interaction of risk assessors and risk managers are more clearly understood and defensible. Critics of this model might argue that this type of interaction does not allow the opportunity for independent scientific and value-based evaluations from perspectives that serve public health, environmental, and business interests.

Risk assessment was evolved to aid in the evaluation of the safety of synthetic chemical use or the exposure to humans from chemicals contaminating the environment. As such, the current practice of risk assessment is best described in this context. However, the types of "threats" to human health and the environment are now considered more inclusive than just synthetic chemicals. For example, we now apply risk assessment to evaluate the safety of naturally occurring chemicals, plant and animal toxins, bioengineered microorganisms, and other categories of potential health hazards. The broadening of the application of risk assessment methods results in more complicated risk management issues and problems. This lends further justification to the belief that our decision-making process is multifaceted and must incorporate views from a variety of scientific disciplines and social perspectives.

In government, the manner in which risk assessment results are used in management decisions may vary depending on statutorily specified requirements relevant to the regulatory agency involved. Federal and state agencies have developed approaches for considering risk assessment and risk management issues. Regardless of the approaches adopted by any group or agency, the intent of the risk assessment and management process is to prevent overexposure of some threat to the public or the environment, and to minimize the associated risks. Risk assessment and risk management principles and methods are also used by the private sector, nonprofit organizations, and citizens' groups to feed information into their decision-making processes.

This section includes five chapters that describe the relation between risk assessment and risk management from different perspectives, concentrating on the roles, results, and effects of risk assessment as they relate to risk management and regulatory decision-making in environmental and public health. These are only examples of how risk assessment and risk management relate in practice, and they by no means attempt to include a survey of all relevant applications.

# 39
# Role of Risk Assessment in Regulatory Decision-Making for Biotechnology: EPA's Experience Under TSCA

**Ellie F. Clark**
*United States Environmental Protection Agency*
*Washington, D.C.*

## I. INTRODUCTION AND BACKGROUND

Microorganisms have provided humans with useful products for centuries. At the same time, humans have always worked to improve the efficacy of these products as well as to expand the uses to which they could be put. Recent advances in scientific knowledge have allowed scientists to speed up the development of new microbial products. Many of the beneficial new products represent improvements to traditional uses of microorganisms, whereas others represent expansion to new uses of microorganisms. Some of these traditional and new uses fall under the purview of the Toxic Substances Control Act (TSCA), which is administered by the U.S. Environmental Protection Agency (EPA). The EPA's regulation of microorganisms under TSCA provides an excellent illustration of how the basic concepts of risk assessment have been adapted and applied to the development of regulations for an emerging technology. This chapter will describe EPA's TSCA biotechnology program and discuss the role of risk assessment in the evolution of that program.

*Biotechnology* has been defined as "any technique that uses living organisms (or parts of organisms) to make or modify products, to improve plants or animals, or to develop microorganisms for specific uses" (U.S. Congress, 1987). This definition includes centuries' old uses of microorganisms, such as yeasts for baking and brewing, as well as the modern highly sophisticated manipulations involving recombinant DNA (rDNA) and cell fusion. Products developed from the less-sophisticated biotechnology techniques have been traditionally regulated, in general, by a variety of product-specific laws administered by different federal agencies. When products of the more-sophisticated biotechnology techniques began to be developed, concern was expressed that these new products might pose risks that are greater than, or significantly different from, the older products and, therefore, they might need to be regulated under a different framework.

To address the issues presented by the new biotechnology products, an interagency working group was formed under the White House Cabinet Council on Natural Resources and the Environment in 1984. This working group determined that the network of existing laws that regulated older biotechnology products could, with some modifications, also adequately regulate the newer biotechnology products. The results of the working group were presented in a proposed statement that was published on December 31, 1984, and finalized on June 26, 1986, as the "Coordinated Framework for Regulation of Biotechnology" under the auspices of the White House Office of Science and Technology Policy (OSTP) (OSTP, 1986). The announcement included descriptions of the regulatory and research policies of each of the federal agencies involved: EPA, the Food and Drug Administration (FDA), the National Institutes of Health (NIH), the National Science Foundation (NSF), the Occupational Safety and Health Administration (OSHA), and the U.S. Department of Agriculture (USDA). While the notice included individual agency statements, it also provided a framework for interagency coordination wherever possible.

EPA administers two statutes which can cover biotechnology products, depending on the specific uses of the products. Under the Federal Insecticide, Fungicide, and Rodenticide Act (FIFRA), EPA reviews and may register pesticide products. Under TSCA, EPA reviews chemical substances, with the exception of products covered by other federal statutes. In 1986 as part of the Coordinated Framework, EPA issued a policy statement which provided EPA's plans and rationale for addressing biotechnology products subject to FIFRA or TSCA. EPA was able to implement part of its biotechnology program for microbial products with the publication of the 1986 Policy Statement. To fully implement programs under both statutes, however, additional rulemaking was necessary. In September 1994, EPA's Office of Pesticide Programs (OPP) published final regulations for microbial pesticides under FIFRA (USEPA, 1994a). At the same time, on September 1, 1994, EPA's Office of Pollution, Prevention and Toxics (OPPT) published proposed rules to fully implement its biotechnology program under TSCA (USEPA, 1994b). OPPT will continue to operate under the 1986 Policy Statement until final rules have been published under TSCA.

## II.  EPA's BIOTECHNOLOGY PROGRAM UNDER TSCA

### A.  The Toxic Substances Control Act

The Toxic Substances Control Act (TSCA) was enacted in 1976 to identify and control chemical substances that present unreasonable risks of injury to human health or the environment. The TSCA definition of a chemical substance includes any organic substance of a particular molecular identity, including any combination of such substances occurring in whole or in part from a chemical reaction or occurring in nature (U.S. Congress, 1976). Therefore, this definition describes not only the nucleic acids that compose an organism's genetic material, but also the living organism as a whole, because it is a combination of substances of particular identities (OSTP, 1986). EPA has included living organisms in its definition of chemical substances since the development of its initial regulations under TSCA.

In order to identify potentially hazardous substances early, TSCA section 5 provides for EPA to require submission of a notification for new chemical substances prior to their initial manufacture for commercial purposes. The EPA has 90 days to determine whether additional controls should be imposed on the chemical substances. Notification is not triggered by a risk determination; however, risk is considered during the review process. Premanufacture notification (PMN) is required for new chemical substances that are defined in TSCA as substances not on the TSCA Inventory of Chemical Substances manufactured in the United States. TSCA required EPA to initially compile the Inventory; EPA keeps the Inventory current by listing each substance on the Inventory following EPA's review and the initiation of production of the substance by the manufacturer. Once a substance is listed on the Inventory, it is no longer new. The PMNs do not have to be submitted before subsequent uses, unless EPA determines that a use presents new risk concerns and issues a significant new use rule (SNUR) requiring additional reporting.

During the 90-day review period for a PMN, EPA must decide whether use of the chemical substance may present an unreasonable risk, as opposed to no risk at all. Although TSCA does not specifically define "unreasonable risk," the legislative history for the statute does give an indication of how Congress expected the term to be applied. The house report indicated that implementation of the no unreasonable risk standard required a balancing of the risks of the product against the benefits to be derived from the product. Congress recognized that scientific data would always possess some amount of uncertainty and should not be the sole determinant of a regulatory decision. Therefore, EPA must consider the weight of the evidence for both risks and benefits. When the likelihood and severity of risk are high, a no unreasonable risk finding is less likely to be made, and restrictions are more likely to be imposed. Alternatively, a higher level of risk will be acceptable if a product is shown to be very beneficial to society (USEPA, 1994b). Other uses of the TSCA "no unreasonable risk" standard will be discussed in the rulemaking section.

At the conclusion of the review, EPA may make one of three determinations. First, if EPA determines that use of the substance would not present an unreasonable risk, EPA will take no action. Production of the substance may begin at the end of the 90-day review period. Second, if EPA determines that there is insufficient information to make a determination and the substance may present an unreasonable risk, or its use may result in substantial exposure, EPA may issue a TSCA section 5(e) consent order to prohibit or limit production. The EPA generally negotiates a consent order with the submitter to restrict use of the substance until additional information is available. Third, if EPA finds that a substance presents or will present an unreasonable risk, EPA may use TSCA section 5(f) to issue an order or rule to restrict or prohibit production of the substance (OSTP, 1986).

Section 5(h) of TSCA provides EPA with mechanisms for exempting chemical substances from full reporting under certain circumstances. Sections 5(h)(3) and 5(h)(4) have been key to reducing reporting requirements for certain substances.

Section 5(h)(3) allows EPA to exempt from full reporting persons manufacturing or processing substances in "small quantities" only for research and development (R&D), if all employees are notified of any health risks posed by the substance. EPA is required by section 5(h)(3) to define "small quantities" by rule and is directed to determine what constitutes appropriate employee risk notification (U.S. Congress, 1976). As part of the New Chemicals Program, EPA developed an "R&D exemption" for traditional chemicals produced "only in small quantities solely for the purposes of research and development" (OSTP, 1986).

Under section 5(h)(4), EPA may exempt manufacturers of new substances from all or part of the full reporting requirements, if EPA determines that the substances will not present unreasonable risks of injury to human health or the environment (U.S. Congress, 1976). Section 5(h)(4) provides EPA with the flexibility to develop a variety of exemptions. EPA's utilization of this flexibility to develop proposed rules for its biotechnology program will be discussed in the rulemaking section.

## B.  The 1986 Policy Statement

Since 1986, EPA has been reviewing TSCA section 5 notices for microorganisms and continues to operate its biotechnology program under the policy statement made as part of the aforementioned interagency "Coordinated Framework for Regulation of Biotechnology" (OSTP, 1986). The biotechnology program was adapted from the New Chemicals Program established for traditional chemicals under TSCA section 5 during the late 1970s and early 1980s. Differences between the two programs are due to different risk concerns for microorganisms versus traditional chemicals.

Living microorganisms were reported to the original TSCA Inventory established in the late 1970s. However, in 1984, EPA clarified that living microorganisms were considered "chemical substances" and thus potentially subject to TSCA, just like traditional chemicals. Although plants and animals could also be chemical substances under TSCA , as a matter of policy, EPA has limited its current biotechnology program under TSCA to microorganisms. In the future, EPA will consider whether it would be appropriate to develop a program under TSCA section 5 to include transgenic plants and animals.

Figure 1 shows how potential submitters can determine if they might have reporting obligations under TSCA section 5. The first step is to determine whether a product is subject to TSCA jurisdiction. TSCA authorizes EPA to regulate any chemical substance except certain substances covered by other federal statutes. The specific TSCA exclusions most relevant to microorganisms are exclusions for (1) pesticides (but not pesticide intermediates), which are subject to FIFRA, and (2) foods, food additives, drugs, and cosmetics, and their intermediates, which are covered by the Federal Food, Drug, and Cosmetic Act (FFDCA). Any other environmental, industrial, or consumer uses of microorganisms could potentially be subject to TSCA. Certain microorganisms that are subject to TSCA, but are also known plant pests are regulated jointly by EPA under TSCA and the U.S. Department of Agriculture (USDA) under the Federal Plant Pest Act. If the microorganisms are not known to be plant pests, those used for TSCA purposes would be regulated solely by EPA. However, USDA would become involved if an EPA

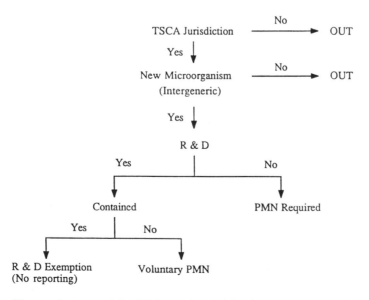

**Figure 1**  Determining TSCA section 5 obligations under the 1986 policy statement.

review determined that the microorganism had plant pest qualities. Uses of microorganisms that are subject to TSCA include specialty chemical production, nitrogen fixation, bioremediation, biosensors, biomass conversion, and mineral recovery. To date, the primary uses reviewed by EPA have been for microorganisms developed for enhanced nitrogen fixation, or for microorganisms used as intermediates to produce enzymes for use in laundry detergents.

The next step is to determine whether the product would be considered a "new" microorganism under TSCA section 5 (see Fig. 1). In the biotechnology program, new microorganisms trigger PMN reporting, just as new chemical substances do in the traditional chemicals program. When EPA originally established the TSCA Inventory, it considered naturally occurring substances to be implicitly included on the Inventory and, therefore, not new. No specific policy was outlined addressing what constitutes a new microorganism. Determining how the "naturally occurring" distinction should be interpreted for microorganisms has been a continuing challenge for EPA. Under the 1986 policy statement, EPA determined that new microorganisms would be intergeneric microorganisms not listed on the TSCA Inventory. Intergeneric microorganisms contain deliberate combinations of genetic material from source organisms in different taxonomic genera. Excluded from the definition of new microorganisms are naturally occurring microorganisms, genetically modified microorganisms other than intergenerics, and intergeneric microorganisms resulting from only the addition of well-characterized, noncoding regulatory regions (OSTP, 1986).

If a product is being manufactured for a TSCA use and is a new microorganism, it will be subject to some requirements under TSCA section 5. As Fig. 1 indicates, the specific TSCA section 5 reporting obligations for new microorganisms are determined by whether the microorganisms will be used for R&D activities, or will be manufactured for distribution in commerce. If a microorganism will be used for R&D activities that are contained, that use could qualify for the R&D or "small quantities" exemption developed under section 5(h)(3) for traditional chemicals. The 1986 policy statement indicates that a microorganism will be considered environmentally contained if it is used either in a laboratory that complies with the National Institutes of Health (NIH) guidelines or in a contained greenhouse, fermentor, or other contained structure. The latter are defined as buildings or structures that have roofs and walls. It is further suggested that these structures have certain features designed to minimize unintentional releases of microorganisms (OSTP, 1986). This is a broad definition that could include a variety of structures. Persons eligible for the R&D exemption must comply with the same requirements as those using the R&D exemption for traditional chemicals. The key feature is that there is no required reporting to EPA.

In 1986, EPA indicated that because microorganisms may reproduce and increase beyond the quantity initially released to the environment, they should not be eligible for the R&D exemption. Persons who are using new microorganisms in R&D activities involving release to the environment are encouraged to file a voluntary PMN with EPA before initiating such activities. If they do not file a voluntary PMN, they should, nevertheless, follow the requirements for the R&D exemption. EPA includes mandatory R&D release-reporting requirements in its proposed rule, which will be discussed in a later section.

Once use of new microorganisms has moved beyond the R&D stage, PMN submission is required before commencement of manufacture for distribution in commerce. TSCA requires PMN submitters to include all reasonably ascertainable information that would assist EPA in determining whether use of the new substance would pose an unreasonable risk to human health or to the environment. Because codified information requirements are not yet available specifically for microorganisms, EPA has prepared for submitters a "Points to Consider" document to assist them in preparing microorganism PMNs (USEPA, 1994c).

## C.  Risk Assessment and Risk Management of Microorganisms

The EPA used the risk assessment process developed under TSCA for traditional chemicals as the starting point for developing its risk assessment process for microorganisms. The same general formula is used for both types of assessments, that is, Risk = hazard × exposure. The assessment of genetically modified microorganisms under TSCA has been reviewed recently elsewhere (Sayre and Kough, 1993); therefore, only a few summary comments will be made here.

Generally, four individual scientific assessments are prepared during a workgroup PMN review of a microorganism. These include (1) a human health hazard assessment, (2) an environmental hazard assessment, (3) a construct analysis of the genetically modified microorganism, and (4) an exposure assessment (Sayre and Kough, 1993). These individual assessments are combined to develop an integrated risk assessment. At the same time, a marketing analysis has been prepared by the economist on the workgroup. The marketing analysis includes the economist's estimates of the microorganism's benefits based on information supplied in the PMN as well as independent economic research, when appropriate. The risk assessment and the marketing analysis are used to prepare a regulatory decision document. Following the balancing of potential risks and benefits presented by a PMN microorganism, EPA comes to one of the three regulatory decisions discussed in the previous section. These decisions are based on whether EPA has enough information to make a risk determination and whether EPA feels that use of the product may present an unreasonable risk (OSTP, 1986).

Two important characteristics of PMN microorganisms have dominated the process. First, since unlike chemicals, living microorganisms have the ability to reproduce and increase beyond the number initially released to the environment and thus may be able to transfer genetic information to other organisms, emphasis is placed on the examination of fate and effects of the microorganisms. For the types of microorganisms reviewed to date under TSCA, the particular emphasis has been on environmental effects, as opposed to human health effects (Sayre and Kough, 1993). Then, because TSCA section 5 excludes naturally occurring substances from PMN reporting, during the risk assessment the behavior of the genetically modified microorganism is compared with that of its naturally occurring parent microorganism. If data indicate that a PMN microorganism exhibits behaviors within a range expected for the naturally occurring parent microorganism, then uncertainty about use of the PMN microorganism is greatly reduced.

The two characteristics of PMN microorganisms discussed in the foregoing have had important effects on EPA's decisions to date. First, most of the PMN microorganisms have not been found to exhibit behaviors significantly different from the naturally occurring parents, and this has greatly reduced risk concerns. Second, fate of microorganisms in the environment has received considerable scrutiny during reviews, since the inability to survive and disseminate also lessens concerns for risk to the environment. For microorganisms used as intermediates in fermentation systems, the focus has been on unintended releases of microorganisms through exit ports or waste disposal. Where microorganisms have been intentionally released in field tests, the focus has been on whether the microorganisms could move beyond the test site and establish in the environment.

Since 1986, EPA has reviewed voluntary PMNs for 25 genetically modified microorganisms for use in small-scale field tests for R&D. Most of these reviews have been for sequential field tests conducted with the goal of developing a commercial product that would be a genetically modified bacterium with enhanced nitrogen fixation capabilities. Because these field tests were some of the earliest reviews of environmental releases of genetically modified microorganisms under TSCA, the reviews also significantly influenced the development of the TSCA biotechnology program and the proposed rules, which will be discussed in the next section.

For all of the voluntary PMNs, EPA used its authority under TSCA section 5(e) to negotiate consent orders to restrict use of the microorganisms to the specific field tests and to obtain additional data before allowing larger-scale uses of the microorganisms. In 1994 the company that had been field testing the bacteria with enhanced nitrogen fixation capabilities asked EPA to approve one of its strains for commercialization. If approved, this would be the first commercialization under TSCA of a genetically modified microorganism for intentional environmental release. EPA has also reviewed PMNs for commercial use of a variety of intergeneric microorganisms used as intermediates in specialty chemical production, primarily of enzymes. All of these have been mandatory PMNs for contained structure uses beyond the R&D stage. For all of the microorganisms used as intermediates to produce enzymes, no regulatory action has been taken, because EPA determined during the PMN reviews that their use would not present an unreasonable risk. Most of these microorganisms are in production and have been added to the TSCA inventory. The EPA's experience with both types of reviews has led to the development of many of the provisions in its proposed rule. The remainder of this chapter considers how risk assessment has affected the development of the proposed rule.

## III. DEVELOPMENT OF THE PROPOSED TSCA BIOTECHNOLOGY RULE

## A. Introduction

### 1. History of Proposed Rulemaking

The EPA could implement only part of its TSCA biotechnology program with the 1986 policy statement. To fully implement the program, EPA needed to employ the official rulemaking process, which requires publication of a proposed rule for public comment followed by promulgation of a final rule. Therefore, after publication of the 1986 policy statement, EPA began working toward this goal by developing a proposed rule to address TSCA uses of microorganisms. In 1988, EPA sent a proposed TSCA biotechnology rule to the Office of Management and Budget (OMB) for review before publication. The OMB sent the proposal to the OSTP's Biotechnology Science Coordinating Committee (BSCC) for consideration. Following unsuccessful negotiations during most of 1988, EPA withdrew the proposed rule from OMB (USGAO, 1992). On February 15, 1989, EPA published a notice in the *Federal Register* asking for comment on certain issues in the 1988 draft proposed rule (USEPA, 1989).

Following the close of the comment period in May 1989, EPA reviewed the public comments and began reconsideration of some of the key elements in the 1988 draft proposal. In June 1991, EPA made a draft of the new proposed TSCA biotechnology rule available to the public as part of its announcement of a meeting of its Biotechnology Science Advisory Committee to provide advice on certain scientific issues raised in the draft proposal (USEPA, 1991). After making additional revisions to the 1991 draft, on September 1, 1994, EPA published the proposed TSCA biotechnology rule for public comment (USEPA, 1994b). The development of the basic reporting mechanisms and exemptions in the 1994 proposal is the subject of this section.

### 2. Use of TSCA Section 5(h)(4)

One goal of the proposed rule is to tailor the basic TSCA section 5 PMN reporting process specifically to microorganisms. However, the basic PMN reporting process is just one part of the proposal. The EPA has taken advantage of the flexibility offered by TSCA section 5(h)(4) to develop a program for microorganisms that recognizes the differences in risk concerns for different uses of microorganisms and attempts to adjust the reporting requirements accordingly.

As noted earlier, TSCA section 5(h)(4) provides that EPA may exempt manufacturers of new substances from all or part of the full PMN reporting requirements, if EPA determines that the substances will not present unreasonable risks of injury to human health or the environment. This essentially requires EPA to make a generic risk assessment upfront about the substances it wishes to exempt. However, a balancing of risks and benefits is required, since EPA must determine whether a new substance will present an unreasonable risk, as opposed to no risk. Thus, EPA must weigh the potential harm that could result from allowing an activity to proceed without full PMN reporting against the gain in social and economic benefits from that activity. The EPA can develop a partial or a full exemption from reporting. Therefore, a more complete exemption from reporting can be developed for an activity that presents low risk and provides greater benefits (USEPA, 1994b). When EPA does not have sufficient information to allow a full exemption, it can develop a partial exemption that would consist of limited reporting requirements and a shortened review period, as well as compliance with specific eligibility requirements.

In the 1986 policy statement, EPA indicated its intent to use its TSCA section 5(h)(4) authority, when appropriate, to reduce the burden of PMN-reporting requirements (OSTP, 1986). Figure 2 shows how potential submitters would determine TSCA section 5 obligations under the 1994 proposed rules. A comparison with Fig. 1 indicates that the primary changes are the inclusion of exemptions from full reporting for R&D and commercial uses of certain micro-organisms. Although Fig. 2 appears to present submitters with a more complicated flowchart, it also shows how EPA has utilized its section 5(h)(4) authority both to provide regulatory relief and to tailor its section 5 program more appropriately to microorganisms. Three of the exemptions will be discussed to illustrate the use of risk assessment in regulatory development. In each example, EPA had to craft an exemption that successfully balanced the need to meet the no unreasonable risk standard of TSCA against the desire to provide a mechanism less costly than full reporting.

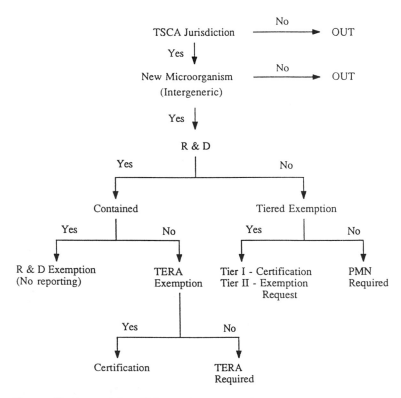

**Figure 2** Determining TSCA section 5 obligations under the proposed rule.

## B. Development of the Tiered Exemption

In the 1986 policy statement, EPA reminded readers that, although most of the agency's attention was focused on environmental releases of microorganisms, TSCA also required reporting for contained-structure uses of microorganisms at commercial scale. The EPA further stated its belief that many contained-structure uses of new microorganisms would present less risk than environmental releases of those same microorganisms. For that reason, EPA announced its intent to explore the use of TSCA section 5(h)(4) to create an exemption for contained-structure uses of new microorganisms (USEPA, 1994b).

An internal EPA workgroup evaluated a variety of alternatives for development of a contained-structure exemption. The tiered exemption that resulted from these deliberations illustrates how EPA was able to successfully develop criteria to define low-risk categories plus offer the submitter an option of no review or limited review, either choice representing a substantial benefit to the submitter. The tiered exemption provides specific criteria for the recipient microorganism, the introduced genetic material, and the conditions for manufacture and use of the microorganism. The recipient microorganism is the key to making the no unreasonable risk determination required by TSCA section 5(h)(4). If the recipient is a low-risk microorganism, then adding introduced genetic material meeting the specified criteria would not cause the new microorganism's behavior to be significantly different from that of the recipient parent. Additionally, the conditions of manufacture and use are designed to minimize releases of microorganisms from the structure, thereby providing a further reduction in potential risk. Although these criteria were developed to reduce risk to both human health and the environment, the emphasis is on human health, because the primary exposure to these microorganisms will be to workers in fermentation facilities.

The following six criteria were used to select candidates to be listed as recipient microorganisms eligible for the tiered exemption: (1) the microorganism can be clearly identified and classified; (2) the relation of the microorganism to known pathogens can be evaluated ; (3) the microorganism has a history of safe commercial use; (4) the microorganism's commercial uses indicate a potential for TSCA uses; (5) information is available on the potential for the microorganism to cause adverse effects on human health and the environment; and (6) information is available on the survival of the microorganism in the environment. From a review using the six evaluation criteria, EPA weighed the combination of responses before determining the candidate's eligibility. Initial candidates were chosen and a subset was selected for complete risk assessments by EPA staff. These risk assessments were placed in the public docket as support for EPA's TSCA section 5(h)(4) determination. The candidates listed in the 1994 proposed rule include the following: *Acetobacter aceti, Aspergillus niger, Aspergillus oryzae, Bacillus licheniformis, Bacillus subtilis, Escherichia coli* K-12, *Penicillum roqueforti, Saccharomyces cerevisiae,* and *Saccharomyces uvarum.*

To be eligible for the tiered exemption, the introduced genetic material must be limited in size, well characterized, free of certain toxin sequences, and poorly mobilizable. Introduced genetic material must be limited in size to those genes required to perform the intended function. Those genes must also be well characterized, meaning that their function as well as their phenotypic expression is known. These first two criteria serve to exclude extraneous and uncharacterized DNA, thereby improving the ability to predict the behavior of the new microorganism. The well-characterized criterion also helps assure that the introduced genetic material is free of certain toxin sequences that EPA listed in the 1994 proposed regulations. The toxins listed were all polypeptides with fairly high vertebrate toxicity. Other toxins were excluded because of their lower toxicity and their multigenic derivation. The three criteria combine to reduce risk concerns about behaviors, such as pathogenicity, that are of multigenic origin. The fourth criterion, that the introduced genetic material be poorly mobilizable, reduces the potential for transfer of the genetic material to other microorganisms. The EPA included this criterion, because no restrictions are being placed on the organisms that can serve as sources of the introduced genetic material.

The conditions under which the microorganisms are manufactured and used are what create a tiered exemption. For the tier I exemption, specific performance standards must be followed. Manufacturers who use the tier I exemption would be required to file a one-time certification statement with EPA 30 days before first commercial manufacture of their microorganism. The statement would certify that the manufacturer is complying with all of the tier I requirements. There would be no EPA review. For the tier II exemption, manufacturers would be asked to use the tier I standards as guidance for developing their conditions of manufacture and use. Manufacturers would then send EPA a tier II exemption request certifying compliance with the recipient microorganism and introduced genetic material requirements and describing their conditions of manufacture and use, which would be subject to a 45-day review by EPA.

The conditions of manufacture and use include requirements that the structure be designed and operated to contain the microorganism, access be limited to essential personnel, and general worker hygiene and protection practices be followed. The EPA is specifying that liquid and solid wastes containing microorganisms be inactivated to give a validated 6-log reduction in viable organisms, and that aerosols and exhaust gases be treated to give a 2-log reduction in viable organisms.

The EPA is prescribing specific standards to minimize the number of microorganisms released from a contained structure, because a diverse group of microorganisms will be eligible for the exemption and because the tier I exemption involves no EPA review. In addition, EPA is broadly defining a *structure* as a building or vessel that effectively surrounds and encloses the microorganism; so that a variety of structures could potentially be used under this exemption. Therefore, to make the no unreasonable risk finding for the tier I exemption, EPA must be assured that microbial emissions are minimized. Because EPA is not specifying performance standards for conditions of use in the tier II exemption, EPA is proposing a 45-day review. Not only is the review period abbreviated, but the information in a tier II exemption request would be limited to that which would allow EPA to determine whether the conditions of use would be appropriate for the microorganism.

Both the tier I and tier II exemptions provide benefits to EPA and the industry. EPA has focused on microorganisms that have been subject to TSCA reporting to guarantee that this exemption could be used after promulgation of final regulations. The EPA will also benefit by being able to focus its resources on organisms presenting greater risk as will industry from reduced reporting costs and decreased delays associated with reporting. The EPA believes its requirements for minimizing microbial emissions are within standard operating procedures for the microbial fermentation industry. However, the tiered exemption gives industry the opportunity to choose between the trade-offs offered by tier I, using EPA standards and no EPA review, versus tier II, using company standards and abbreviated EPA review. In both cases, EPA believes it has successfully achieved a balance of providing an exemption that reduces costs for both industry and EPA, while still meeting the no unreasonable risk standard. A further benefit is the flexibility offered by future expansion of the exemption. EPA indicated in the proposed rule that it is considering nominating other microorganisms as recipients eligible for the tiered exemption. It would be necessary for EPA to complete a risk assessment before each recipient is added to the list. Therefore, in the 1994 proposed rule EPA asked commenters to nominate additional candidate organisms and provide information to support a no unreasonable risk determination (USEPA, 1994b).

## C. Development of the TERA Process

The greatest difference between the TSCA section 5 programs for traditional chemicals and microorganisms is in the area of R&D. The TSCA section 5(h)(3) allows EPA to exempt from reporting R&D activities involving chemical substances produced in small quantities (U.S. Congress, 1976). What has often been overlooked is that this is a conditional exemption. TSCA gives EPA the authority to define "small quantities" and to impose controls on the R&D activities. EPA has used this authority to make supervision by a technically qualified individual (TQI) a requirement for eligibility for the exemption. Under the traditional chemicals program, most R&D is exempt when chemicals are used in small quantities solely for R&D. Although this definition is appropriate for discrete amounts of chemicals, it cannot be applied with the same expectations to living microorganisms, since microorganisms have the ability to reproduce and spread in the environment.

In 1986, EPA indicated that if the existing small quantities definition was applied to living microorganisms, many R&D releases of microorganisms would occur without EPA review. The EPA would review only microorganisms and uses that became commercial products. Because of the concern that some R&D releases could present significant risks, EPA stated its intent to change the R&D exemption to require reporting of R&D activities involving environmental releases of new microorganisms. EPA asked for voluntary PMN reporting of R&D releases until a final rule was promulgated (OSTP, 1986).

In the 1988 draft of the TSCA rule, the public got its first glimpse of EPA's proposal for an R&D reporting process. The EPA proposed the establishment of the TSCA Experimental Release Application (TERA) process, specifically tailored to reporting R&D activities involving environmental releases of new microorganisms. Of all the issues raised for public comment in EPA's 1989 *Federal Register* notice, TSCA oversight of R&D field tests of microorganisms proved to be the most controversial. For this reason, after an internal EPA workgroup reconsidered coverage of R&D releases, EPA held a 2-day meeting in September 1989 with interested parties to discuss major issues concerning TSCA oversight of R&D field tests. Although there was a diversity of opinion about what the actual process should be, many meeting participants felt that there should be some TSCA section 5 review of R&D field tests.

In developing the TERA process proposed in the 1994 proposal, EPA carefully considered the issues raised by public commenters as well as the experience gained in reviewing voluntary PMNs submitted for R&D field tests. The proposed TERA process would involve a 60-day review that would focus on information concerning the R&D activity for which approval is sought. This is in contrast to full reporting for commercialization, which requires information on all manufacture, processing, transport, use, and disposal activities involving a new microorganism. Unlike full reporting that mandates a 90-day review, the TERA process would allow a submitter to proceed at any time during the 60-day period upon EPA's determination that the R&D field test presented no unreasonable risk. The TERA process also includes a more flexible method for negotiating a legal agreement, thereby avoiding the delays involved in developing Consent Orders under TSCA section 5(e).

In establishing the TERA process, EPA is also proposing to use its authority under TSCA section 5(h)(4) to conditionally exempt from full reporting requirements R&D activities involving releases of new microorganisms to the environment. The exemption is conditional, because EPA believes that case-by-case review is needed to determine whether a microorganism used in environmental testing has the potential to establish in the environment and present an unreasonable risk and, thus, should be restricted in its use. EPA has proposed, therefore, that all R&D activities involving environmental releases be eligible for the abbreviated TERA process in lieu of full reporting. The EPA believes that the TERA represents a balance of EPA's need to review some information to make its no unreasonable risk finding against the flexibility and reduction in burden provided by the abbreviated review period, information requirements, and TERA agreement.

To propose the TERA process under section 5(h)(4), EPA must find that R&D activities reviewed under the TERA, in lieu of the full 90-day process, will not present an unreasonable risk. The EPA has been able to make that finding, since the same risk determination will be made at the conclusion of both the TERA and the full-reporting processes. Because the TERA review should reduce reporting costs by eliminating EPA procedures that are unnecessary for R&D, it should encourage innovation and beneficially affect organizations conducting R&D with new microorganisms (USEPA, 1994b).

## D.  Development of the TERA Exemption

Public comments received in 1989 recommended that a process for exemption from EPA review be developed in conjunction with any R&D reporting process. The "TERA exemption" is an outgrowth of the TERA process, but it also represents a synthesis of EPA's experience developing the R&D exemption and the tiered exemption as well as reviewing voluntary PMNs for R&D field tests.

In developing the TERA process for reporting R&D releases, EPA recognized that not every R&D test would need to be reviewed. EPA first developed the abbreviated TERA process and then examined ways to craft an exemption from TERA reporting. EPA took advantage of its success with the tiered exemption and focused on setting criteria for the recipient microorganism, the introduced genetic material, and the conditions of use. For candidate recipients, EPA had to look no further than its PMN reviews of microbial field tests. At the time this exemption was being developed, EPA had completed reviews of voluntary PMNs for six intergeneric strains of *Bradyrhizobium japonicum* and 13 intergeneric strains of *Rhizobium meliloti*. These microorganisms had been genetically modified for enhanced nitrogen fixation. Instead of conducting additional risk assessments, EPA relied on the risk assessments generated by its staff for the PMN reviews as well as the data received from the field tests of the intergeneric strains. Naturally occurring rhizobial strains have been used safely in agriculture for over 80 years. As with the tiered exemption, knowledge of a history of safe use with the recipient microorganism was an important component of the risk assessment.

The introduced genetic material had general requirements similar to the tiered exemption, that is, limited in size, well characterized, and poorly mobilizable. However, based on PMN review experience and knowledge of potential risks, EPA also limited the source of the introduced genetic material to the genera of *Bradyrhizobium* and *Rhizobium,* although any organism could serve as the source of antibiotic-resistance marker genes. Neither the recipients nor the introduced genetic material could have the capacity to produce rhizobitoxin or trifolitoxin. Borrowing from the R&D exemption, EPA required that the field tests be supervised by a TQI. Again, based on its reviews, EPA limited the test sites to 10-acres or less. The TQI was to assure that practices were in place to limit the spread of the organisms beyond the test site. Persons eligible for this exemption would be required to certify to EPA that they complied with the requirements of the exemption.

There would be no EPA review. This exemption would be field test-specific. Once a researcher planned to test on greater than 10 acres, a TERA would be required. Full reporting would be required before commercialization of the microorganisms. Since a significant degree of R&D field testing of rhizobia takes place in tests of less than 10 acres, this exemption can provide an important reduction in reporting.

The EPA is proposing this exemption under section 5(h)(4). Here, EPA was able to make the no unreasonable risk finding by using the framework established in the tiered exemption and proposing candidates for which it already had the necessary information. Like the tiered exemption, the TERA exemption also establishes a framework to which eligible candidates can be added by EPA, and the proposed rule encourages commenters to suggest additional candidates and provide information necessary to support exemptions from TERA reporting (USEPA, 1994b).

## E.  Concluding Remarks

The three proposed exemptions discussed in the foregoing provide ample illustration of the flexibility offered by TSCA section 5(h)(4) and the role played by risk assessment in the development of EPA's proposed TSCA biotechnology rule. The EPA is proposing other uses of section 5(h)(4) in this rule. Although it is not yet possible to predict a future publication date for the biotechnology rule, EPA will analyze the public comments received on the 1994 proposal and then begin to draft the final rule. Until the final rule is published, EPA will continue to operate its program under the 1986 policy statement and will continue to review PMNs. As EPA gains more experience through its reviews and as general scientific knowledge increases, EPA will continue to take advantage of the flexibility offered by TSCA section 5(h)(4) to tailor its TSCA biotechnology program to achieve an appropriate risk–cost balance.

## ACKNOWLEDGMENTS

The author gratefully acknowledges the assistance of the following individuals from the U.S. EPA who helped with editorial review of this manuscript: Lawrence Zeph, Robert Andrei, and David Giamporcaro.

## DISCLAIMER

The views expressed are those of the author and not of the U.S. Environmental Protection Agency or the U.S. government.

## REFERENCES

[OSTP] Office of Science and Technology Policy. (1986). Coordinated framework for regulation of biotechnology; announcement of policy and notice for public comment, *Fed. Regist.* 51, 23302–20093.

Sayre, P. G., and J. L. Kough (1993). Assessment of genetically engineered microorganisms under TSCA: Considerations prior to use in fermentors or small-scale field release. In *Environmental Toxicology and Risk Assessment* (W. G. Landis, J. S. Hughes, and M. A. Lewis, eds.), ASTM STP 1179, American Society for Testing and Materials, Philadelphia, pp. 65–79.

U.S. Congress (1976). Toxic Substances Control Act, and as amended, *U.S. Code, 15,* 2601 et seq.

U.S. Congress, Office of Technology Assessment (1987). *New Developments in Biotechnology: Ownership of Human Tissues and Cells—Special Report, OTA-BA-337,* U.S. Government Printing Office, Washington, DC.

[USEPA] U.S. Environmental Protection Agency (1989). Biotechnology; request for comment on regulatory approach, *Fed. Regist.* 54, 7027.

[USEPA] U.S. Environmental Protection Agency (1991). Microbial Products of Biotechnology; proposed regulation under the Toxic Substances Control Act, Chemical Control Division, EPA Office of Pollution Prevention and Toxics, Washington, DC (unpublished draft).

[USGAO] U.S. General Accounting Office (1992). *Biotechnology: Delays in and Status of EPA's Efforts to Issue a TSCA Regulation,* GAO/RCED-92-167, U.S. General Accounting Office, Washington, DC.

[USEPA] U.S. Environmental Protection Agency (1994a). 40 CFR Part 172, Microbial pesticides: Experimental use permits and notifications, final rule, *Fed. Regist.,* 59, 45600–45615.

[USEPA] U.S. Environmental Protection Agency (1994b). 40 CFR Part 700, et al. Microbial products of biotechnology; proposed regulation under the Toxic Substances Control Act: proposed rule, *Fed. Regist.,* 59, 45526–45585.

[USEPA] U.S. Environmental Protection Agency (1994c). *Points to Consider in the Preparation of and Submission of TSCA Premanufacture Notices (PMNs) for Microorganisms,* Chemical Control Division, EPA Office of Pollution Prevention and Toxics, Washington, DC (Unpublished).

# 40
# Risk Assessment for Risk Management and Regulatory Decision-Making at the U.S. Food and Drug Administration

**P. Michael Bolger, Clark D. Carrington, and Sara Hale Henry**

*United States Food and Drug Administration*
*Washington, D.C.*

One of the major responsibilities of the Center for Food Safety and Applied Nutrition (CFSAN) of the U.S. Food and Drug Administration (FDA) is to ensure that foods in U.S. commerce are safe to eat. The CFSAN, therefore, is charged with protecting the public from chemical hazards in foods. The FDA regulates food safety under the federal Food, Drug, and Cosmetic Act (FD&C Act).

## I. STATUTORY MANDATES

In 1958 Congress enacted the Food Additives Amendment to the FD&C Act. Currently, section 409 of the act provides that a food additive must be shown to be safe under its intended conditions of use before it is allowed for use in food. A food additive must be shown to serve a technical function in the food at levels of safe use. The FDA has been provided with authority to issue tolerances and regulations approving the use of food additives in or on food; the act requires preclearance evaluation of safety by the agency (Kokosi et al., 1989).

The FD&C Act also recognizes generally recognized as safe (GRAS) and "prior sanction" status for certain food ingredients, which technically are not considered food additives under the act. General recognition of safety must be based on the views of "experts" qualified by scientific training and experience to evaluate the safety of substances added to food. This recognition may be based on either a safe history of common use in food before 1958 or scientific procedures (Kokoski et al., 1989).

The Food Additives Amendment includes both direct (or secondary direct) and indirect food additives. *Direct additives* are substances added deliberately in finite amounts, for whatever technical purpose served, and remain in the food as consumed. *Secondary direct* food additives represent substances added to food or food components somewhere during manufacture or processing, but that are removed before the final product is consumed; only low levels of these substances, usually processing aids, might remain in the final food. *Indirect food additives* represent potential residues of substances that may become components of food because they migrate from food contact surfaces during production, manufacturing, packing, processing, preparing, treating, packaging, transporting, or holding the food, including sources of radiation (Kokoski et al., 1989).

In 1960, Congress enacted the Color Additives Amendments that required that color additives be shown to be safe for use in or on food, drugs, or cosmetics before being allowed by color additive regulation. The provisions of the FD&C Act and the regulations for color additives are very much the same as those for food additives (Kokoski et al., 1989).

The Delaney Anticancer Clause of the FD&C Act precludes the use of quantitative risk assessment for substances deliberately added to food and contains the proscription against the addition to food of substances determined to induce cancer in humans or animals. Unavoidable contaminants of foods are regulated under Section 402 or 406 of the act when the Delaney Clause is not applicable and for which FDA has the authority to set tolerances for substances that cannot be avoided by good manufacturing practices. Under Section 406, FDA is required to balance the benefits of the availability of food against the risk a contaminant in that food might pose to the public health. Risk assessment is a tool used by FDA to estimate the upper limit of risk posed by the contaminant.

The FDA has also found risk assessment to be a useful tool in estimating the risk from contaminants of food or color additives (impurities policy to be discussed later); and in estimating the risk from residues of animal drugs in animal food products (Sensitivity of Method guideline). Risk assessment is also used by FDA to help set priorities and to provide information for the urgency of a regulatory action.

The FDA published on April 2, 1982, an Advanced Notice of Proposed Rulemaking (ANPR) describing its impurities or constituents policy. The impurities policy represents a significant change for FDA in its general policy toward regulating carcinogenic chemicals in food and color additives. The impurities policy may be described as follows: if a food or color additive itself is found to induce cancer, it is clearly subject to the Delaney clause; however, if the additive itself is not a carcinogen, but a contaminant or constituent of the additive is found to be a carcinogen, the General Safety Clause applies. Under this clause, FDA will use risk assessment procedures, when appropriate, to determine the upper limit of risk to the consumer from the presence of the contaminant or constituent chemical. FDA continues to be concerned about carcinogenic contaminants that get into the food supply, but it believes that a reasonable scientific approach, taking into consideration new developments in science, may be used without compromising their mandate to protect public health. For example, on April 2, 1982, FDA approved for permanent listing D&C Green No. 6, which had not been shown to be carcinogenic in appropriate tests, even though it contains the carcinogenic impurity, *para*-toluidine. In this decision, FDA stated its belief that the upper limit of risk can be adequately estimated from animal data and applied to humans. The impurities policy survived legal challenge in the 6th Circuit Court of Appeals in a unanimous ruling in favor of FDA.

## II. THE NATIONAL RESEARCH COUNCIL REPORT ON RISK ASSESSMENT

The National Research Council's (NRC) report *Risk Assessment in the Federal Government: Managing the Process* (NRC, 1983) defines risk assessment as the "use of the factual base to define the health effects of exposure of individuals or populations to hazardous materials and/or situations." According to NRC, an ideal risk assessment should contain some or all of the following four steps:

*Hazard identification:* The determination of whether a particular chemical is or is not causally linked to particular health effects.

*Dose–response assessment:* The determination of the relationship between the magnitude of exposure and the probability of occurrence of the health effects in question.

*Exposure assessment:* The determination of the extent of human exposure before or after application of regulatory controls.

*Risk characterization:* The description of the nature—and often the magnitude—of human risk including attendant uncertainty.

The NRC notes that both scientific judgments and policy choices may be involved in selecting from among possible inferential bridges, and recommends the use of the term *risk assessment policy* to differentiate those judgments and choices from the broader social and economic policy issues that are inherent in risk management decisions. Controversy surrounding regulatory decisions has resulted from failing to distinguish risk assessment policy from risk management policy.

The NRC report points out that the term *risk assessment* is often given a very narrow meaning and becomes synonymous with quantitative risk assessment and heavy reliance on numerical results. But quantitative numerical estimates of risk are not always scientifically possible or feasible for reasons of policy.

The NRC report discusses the four steps of risk assessment, which are now summarized briefly.

Hazard identification involves determining whether exposure to an agent can cause an increase in the incidence of a health condition, such as cancer, birth defects, and other adverse health outcomes. This is seldom a simple question; data from mutagenicity studies may provide useful support for findings from epidemiological investigations or animal studies; comparing an agent's chemical or physical properties with those of known carcinogens also can provide some support.

Dose–response assessment is used to evaluate tests performed on laboratory animals. Several problems may arise here. The NRC report notes that animal carcinogenicity bioassays are rarely able to detect even a 1% increase in tumor incidence, and regulatory agencies often must deal with risks that are much lower (1:1 million or 1:1000). Several methods for low-dose extrapolation have been developed, but the current state of knowledge does not permit the determination of an optimal method; currently, regulatory agencies must make a risk assessment policy choice among various methods.

In quantitative risk assessments, regulatory scientists must compensate for size differences between animals and humans. Some methods for making this compensation may be used more frequently than others or may be preferred by certain regulatory agencies, but one single method has not been established as preferable to others by rigorous scientific evidence. The NRC report defines *exposure assessment* as the determination of the concentration of the chemical to which humans are exposed. Frequently, human exposure cannot be directly measured and must be estimated from incomplete or indirect data.

As described in the NRC report, risk characterization involves estimating the nature and often the magnitude of the public health problem. Scientific judgment and experience on the part of regulatory scientists are critical in this step. Such important considerations include, for example, the statistical and biological uncertainties in estimating the extent of health effects, how to describe those uncertainties to risk managers, which dose–response and exposure assessments to use, and which populations to choose as the primary targets for protection.

## III.  GUIDELINES FOR RISK ASSESSMENT

A second important set of principles for risk assessment of carcinogens is that assembled by the Office of Science and Technology Policy (OSTP), Executive Office of the President, entitled *Chemical Carcinogens: A Review of the Science and its Associated Principles* (1985). The federal interagency group that authored this set of guidelines included scientists from the National Center for Toxicological Research, Rood and Drug Administration, National Cancer Institute, Environmental Protection Agency, Consumer Product Safety Commission, National Institute of Environmental Health Sciences, and Food Safety and Inspection Service of the U.S. Department of Agriculture. In performing risk assessments, CFSAN follows the principles contained in this document.

The purpose of the OSTP document was (1) to articulate a view of chemical carcinogenesis that scientists generally hold in common and (2) to draw upon this common view to construct a series of general principles that can be used to establish guidelines for assessing carcinogenic risk. The document points out that, because of present gaps in understanding, the principles contain judgmental (science policy) decisions about unresolved issues, as well as statements of generally accepted fact. However, an attempt was made to distinguish clearly between these different types of information. The OSTP document does not suggest that one method of cancer risk assessment is better than another, but instead, tries to evaluate the effect on the scientific findings of the last decade on general assumptions or principles important to risk assessment.

The OSTP document points out that risk assessments by federal regulatory agencies are done in response to various forms of legislation. Some legislation calls for action in the presence of any risk; other legislation uses the concept of *reasonable risk,* often defined as a condition in which the risks outweigh the benefits (e.g., the Toxic Substances Control Act and the Federal Insecticide, Fungicide, and Rodenticide Act). Different legislation calls for a spectrum of responses from federal agencies that range from informing the public of risks, through restricted use, to a complete ban.

Part I of the OSTP document presents 31 principles relevant to the evaluation of the role of chemicals in carcinogenesis. These principles cover such topics as mechanism of carcinogenesis (including the application of the threshold principle in carcinogenesis), the role of short-term tests in determining carcinogenicity, interpretation of long-term animal bioassays, strengths and limitations of epidemiology studies and exposure assessments, and risk characterization (including the weight-of-evidence approach and recognition of the various important sources of uncertainty in risk assessment).

Part II of the OSTP document is divided into six chapters, each containing a discussion of current information in an area of science relevant to risk assessment. Discussions of recent advances in understanding the mechanisms of carcinogenesis, short-term testing and the relation between genetic toxicity and carcinogenicity, long-term animal bioassays and their importance in assessing cancer risks, the current state of epidemiological knowledge relating to human cancer, and recent advances and current problems in exposure assessment are included. The final chapter in Part II describes how the hazard and exposure elements discussed in the preceding five chapters are used as inputs into qualitative and quantitative cancer risk assessment.

Other guideline documents have been developed for specific areas of interest, such as exposure, carcinogenicity, reproductive toxicity, Superfund sites, among others, by the U.S. Environmental Protection Agency. These are discussed in other chapters in this book.

## IV. RISK ASSESSMENT PROCESS AT CFSAN

The Food and Drug Administration follows NRC guidelines contained in *Risk Assessment in the Federal Government: Managing the Process* (1983). At the Center for Food Safety and Applied Nutrition (CFSAN), the Cancer Assessment Committee (CAC) performs hazard identification with input from various scientific disciplines, such as chemistry, toxicology, pathology, epidemiology, and mathematics. The exposure assessment portion of the qualitative risk assessment is performed by chemists and experts in statistical modeling and dietary surveys. The Quantitative Risk Assessment Committee (QRAC) performs dose–response assessment, exposure assessment, and risk characterization.

The risk assessment process at CFSAN may be set in motion when industry files a food or color additive petition. In other cases, CFSAN management requests a risk assessment on a particular chemical compound, or additional scientific information compels a new risk assessment on a compound currently regulated by FDA. In addition, increasingly sophisticated analytical methodology may reveal a previously unrecognized contaminant of a food or food additive, and CFSAN management may request an assessment of possible consumer risk from the contaminant.

Experts within FDA (internal experts) independently evaluate all data relevant to each chemical under consideration. These include experts in pathology, toxicology, mathematics and statistics, food chemistry, and epidemiology. In the case of suspect carcinogens, these persons present and collectively discuss this information in CAC meetings. The Cancer Assessment Committee, therefore, serves as an additional internal peer review body for chemicals that involve possible carcinogenicity.

The Cancer Assessment Committee plays a central role in the risk assessment process at CFSAN. This standing committee, which was established in 1978, is made up of ten CFSAN experts in the various fields of expertise related to chemical carcinogenesis: pathology, toxicology, mathematics, and food chemistry and technology. The decisions of the Cancer Assessment Committee form the basis for the center's recommendations to FDA.

In addition to reviewing information presented by various scientific disciplines, the Cancer Assessment Committee may request additional information from internal and external experts, such as a review of available epidemiology data or a special review of mutagenicity data. The Cancer Assessment Committee may choose to postpone a final decision on the carcinogenicity of a compound pending the outcome of ongoing or anticipated animal or analytical experiments. In some cases, the Cancer Assessment Committee may request that CFSAN pathologists review slides from an animal bioassay. External scientific peer review is sometimes requested by the Cancer Assessment Committee when a particularly difficult or controversial scientific issue is involved.

The primary task of the Cancer Assessment Committee is to determine whether or not a substance that has been regulated or petitioned for regulation by CFSAN, or whether a substance that is a contaminant of food or cosmetics is a carcinogen. If a determination is made that a substance is a carcinogen, and if it is believed that a quantitative risk assessment may impinge on the regulation of the substance, the Cancer Assessment Committee informs the Quantitative Risk Assessment Committee (QRAC) of this decision.

The QRAC was formed in 1983; although quantitative risk assessments were performed under the auspices of the Cancer Assessment Committee before this, the QRAC was formed because of the increasing number of quantitative risk assessments needed by CFSAN. Given its evaluation of all relevant data on a substance, the Cancer Assessment Committee recommends to the QRAC the bioassays or epidemiological studies most appropriate for low-dose extrapolation. The Cancer Assessment Committee also recommends to the QRAC the tissue site(s), species, and sex most suitable for quantitative evaluation.

The QRAC then conducts a quantitative risk characterization. This portion of the risk assessment process is highly controversial, even among experts. Currently, the QRAC uses a linear-at-low-dose approach, similar to that described by Gaylor and Kodell (1980). The QRAC cannot determine the most probable expected human risk for any case because of the uncertainties and sources of error inherent in quantitative risk assessment using high-dose animal data. However, the QRAC believes that, in cases for which dose–response data are suitable, it can predict the upper limit of risk with a degree of confidence. Although details vary with particular cases, a generally acceptable level of risk (upper bound) is considered to be $10^{-6}$, or one additional human cancer over background in a population of 1 million. The QRAC reports to CFSAN management, who then uses this assessment as a partial basis for a decision on how to manage the risk.

The discussion until this point has been a presentation of the carcinogenic risk assessment process used by the FDA for contaminants or constituents of foods. However, risk assessment is not a process that should be confined to carcinogenic endpoints. Nor is it a static process, but rather an evolutionary one in which continual improvements will need to be made. The remaining discussion will focus on possible improvements that should be explored in the risk assessment process, particularly by more closely linking research and risk assessment and, not incidentally, better separating risk assessment and risk management.

## V.   THE RISK ASSESSMENT QUESTION VERSUS THE SAFETY ASSESSMENT QUESTION

There are two types of questions that a toxicologist may be asked. The first question—"Is it safe?"—is basically a "yes" or "no" question; it does not require, and need not be answered by use of a quantitative risk assessment. Rather, the toxicologist is asked to identify an acceptable or tolerable level of exposure to a compound that is thought to result in an inconsequential increase in risk. It does not communicate the elements of the risk (e.g., magnitude, heterogeneity, and uncertainty). The use of the no-observed adverse effect level–uncertainty factor approach is primarily designed to produce a decision, thereby answering the safety assessment question.

The second question—"How bad is it?"—is a request to the toxicologist to supply information specifically about the level of risk. There are at least two and usually three dimensions to this information that the decision maker will need: (1) The magnitude of the response or effect in an individual; (2) the extent of variability in the population of concern that may be expected (heterogeneity); and (3) the range of uncertainty associated with the prediction of the first two dimensions (the likelihood that other possible answers may also be correct). Although cancer risk assessment begins to address these questions, a great deal more can be done.

### A.   The Interplay Between Risk Assessment and Scientific Research

Although research is a process for developing knowledge, a risk assessment needs to provide a snapshot of current human knowledge. In other words, it is used to answer a question as well as it can be answered with the available knowledge. While risk assessment and scientific research can and should interact, this interaction will not occur without some deliberate planning. In particular, a rigorous description of uncertainty is needed to identify those areas for which information is most lacking and for which additional research would reduce the uncertainty.

Scientists are trained to generate facts through hypothesis testing. However, this training and the desire for certainty does not necessarily prepare an individual to make the best use of data in answering risk assessment questions. Scientists are frequently willing to dismiss a data set even though it may possess some predictive power (even if it is the only data set available). A statistical standard for evaluating whether or not a particular data set supports a particular hypothesis for acceptance in a scientific publication is not necessarily useful in the risk assessment process.

## B. The Value of Measuring Heterogeneity

Research study designs are often constructed to eliminate all variability to obtain a reproducible result. However, variability is often an inextricable part of the question the risk assessment must answer. In such circumstances, therefore, it is desirable to design an experiment that will provide some measure of the variability, rather than to eliminate it. For instance, taking great pains to ensure that all animals within an experimental group are identical makes the data less useful in predicting what will happen in a highly heterogeneous human population.

## C. Description of Uncertainty

In addition to identifying areas in which additional research is needed, description of uncertainty is essential in separating risk assessment from risk management. If the risk assessor does not communicate uncertainty to the "decision maker," then he or she has no choice but to manage the uncertainty in a manner deemed, by the assessor, to be appropriate for the situation. This obviously constitutes participation in the decision-making process.

There are many uncertainties in toxicological risk assessment for which descriptive techniques have not been developed. For instance, techniques for describing uncertainties associated with model selection, balancing mechanistic data versus empirical data, and categorical extrapolation (e.g., species extrapolation) are not encompassed by current statistical discipline. This occurs partly from a reticence to deviate from the application of probability theory; that is, uncertainties that cannot be ascribed to random variation are often considered to be too uncertain to describe.

We would suggest that any measure is better than no measure. In fact, the quality of a risk assessment cannot be evaluated (by an expert or anyone else) without some internal standard of certainty. By explicitly identifying what those standards are, a means of communicating uncertainty will be obtained. Furthermore, it will be possible to ensure that standards of uncertainty are consistently applied across risk assessments, thereby making them more comparable. Even a "bad" measure is an opportunity for improvement. Once a standard of uncertainty has been described explicitly, its usefulness can be publicly inspected and discussed.

As an example, we would suggest that the likelihood that a model is correct is proportional, in some way, to the degree to which it is able to describe the data. For instance, a model that provides a perfect fit should be considered more likely to be correct than one that does not. As a corollary, a prediction based on a data set that may be fitted equally well by a number of different models is less certain than one that fits much more closely by one and only one model. The CFSAN has generated a computer program that uses this principle to generate a continuous measure of uncertainty arising from model selection.

The product of a risk assessment is an answer, not a fact, and it should be the best available at the time. To separate risk assessment and risk management, and to provide an explicit means of evaluating the value of additional data, descriptions of uncertainty, magnitude of response, and heterogeneity need to be integral parts of the risk assessment answer.

## REFERENCES

Code of Federal Regulations (1988). Food additives. In *Food and Drugs,* Title 21, Parts 170–199, April 1, U.S. Government Printing Office, Washington DC.

Food and Drug Administration (1982). Policy for regulating carcinogenic chemicals in additives, advanced notice of proposed rulemaking, *Fed. Regist.,* 47, 14464.

Kokoshi, C.J., S. H. Henry, C. S. Lin, and K. B. Edelman (1989). Methods used in safety evaluation. In *Handbook of Food Additives* (A. L. Branen, P. M. Davidson, S. Salminen, eds.), Marcel Dekker, New York.

National Research Council (1983). *Risk Assessment in the Federal Government: Managing the Process.* National Academy Press, Washington, DC.

U.S. Office of Science and Technology Policy (1985). Chemical carcinogens: A review of the science and its associated principles, *Fed. Regist.,* 50, 10672–10442.

# 41
# Comparative Risk: Adding Value to Science

**Richard A. Minard, Jr.**
*Vermont Law School*
*South Royalton, Vermont*

## I.  BEYOND QUANTITATIVE RISK ASSESSMENT

Reviled by some as "antidemocratic" (Hornstein, 1992) and embraced by others as scientific and objective, the "comparative risk process" is becoming a widely used tool for guiding environmental policy: for deciding which environmental problems are most serious and which solutions will be most effective. The process remains controversial, even as it evolves in response to justified criticism. This paper will trace that evolution and demonstrate that the process is maturing into a practical tool that can help democratic governments make wiser environmental choices.

By the end of 1993, 25 states, plus Guam, numerous cities from Seattle to Atlanta, the federal government, the 10 regional offices of the U.S. Environmental Protection Agency (EPA), and cities and states across Eastern Europe and the developing world had turned to some form of the comparative risk process.* Comparative risk is gaining adherents because it provides a framework for bringing both more science and more public involvement into public policy. This combination can produce better policy and budget decisions on technical environmental issues, and it can help counter the pressures that come from crisis management and environmental fads. Just as important, the process can strengthen the badly frayed bond between people and their government (Minard et al., 1993).

---

*States and cities with EPA-supported comparative risk projects either completed, under way, or in advanced planning stages, as of November 1993 included: Washington, Colorado, Pennsylvania, Vermont, Louisiana, Michigan, Utah, Alabama, Hawaii, California, Maine, Florida, Arizona, Maryland, Texas, Kentucky, Tennessee, Missouri, New Jersey, Wisconsin, Minnesota, Alaska, New Hampshire, Guam, Seattle, Atlanta, Jackson, Miss., Baltimore, the Northern Ohio Region, Columbus, OH, Charlottesville, VA, and Houston. EPA has also supported projects on Native American reservations in Wisconsin and throughout the West. Oregon conducted a related "cross-media" risk project. Several other states and cities were preparing to announce projects at this writing (Northeast Center for Comparative Risk 1993).

Comparative risk can do the opposite, however. Some scientists argue that comparative risk is a technical tool that should empower them—the experts—to set the environmental agenda in a way that is rational, scientific, and wholly superior to any process corrupted by politics and public misperceptions. Senator Daniel Patrick Moynihan, D-NY, introduced legislation in 1991 (U.S. Senate Bill 2132) based on the assertion that "ranking of relative risks to human health, welfare, and ecological resources is a complex task, and is best performed by technical experts free from interests that could bias their objective judgment." The bill would have created two panels of experts to reshape EPA's activities based on their comparisons of risks. Fortunately, this "hard" version of comparative risk appears to be losing ground to more democratic versions.

This chapter will argue that the comparative risk process works. By examining the experience gained in several state and city projects, the paper will demonstrate that the process will have its biggest influence on public policy when projects are conceived as pragmatic, political tools, rather than abstract technical inquiries, and when they reach out to, rather than exclude, the public.

Implicit in these assertions is a definition of *risk* that extends well beyond those used in most quantitative risk assessments: A risk is any damage or potential damage to something people value.

The things people value may include human health, ecological health, economic well-being, environmental justice, aesthetic qualities in the environment, and even the quality of life of future generations. Environmental problems may pose serious risks to how a community functions as a social institution, or to individuals' spiritual relationships with the land, or to a culture's very sustainability.

Needless to say, describing risks to all of these values requires more than scientific analysis. Just as toxicology, epidemiology, and ecology can help people understand the biological and physical processes at work in the environment, so economics, public opinion polling, and the results of political elections can help measure the social and emotional effects of environmental problems. Taken together, this body of knowledge, systematically gathered and carefully articulated, can be a foundation for comparing problems, ranking risks, and setting priorities.

However, for those priorities to have any political consequence—and, hence, any environmental one—the comparative risk process must be designed from the start as a political process for change, rather than as a search for scientific truth. The power of comparative risk stems less from the quality of the scientists' technical analyses than from the scientists' ability to help the *decision-making public* answer its most fundamental questions: What problems are most serious? How best can we solve them?

This chapter will focus on how the basic techniques of quantitative risk assessment can and should be integrated into the demanding world of public policy, and on how comparative risk can help policy makers use risk assessments wisely. Rather than rehash the causes and consequences of the uncertainties inherent in risk assessments, the paper focuses on the importance of honestly confronting the value-laden choices that risk assessments may obscure.

To illustrate its major points, the paper starts with a few definitions and then follows a roughly chronologic path from EPA's internal, technically oriented projects in the mid-1980s to some of the states' highly public and socially responsive efforts of the early 1990s.

## II. THE WHY AND HOW OF COMPARATIVE RISK

The comparative risk process is a political response to three seemingly universal conditions:

1. Neither the public sector, the private sector, nor the public at large, has sufficient resources to eliminate all environmental problems at once.
2. Not all environmental problems are equally severe.
3. In a democracy, power flows from the people to their government. Eventually, the people will get what they ask for.

The first two conditions lead to the simple conclusion that government should direct its limited resources toward where they can do the most good. Any observer of government might rightly conclude that it is unlikely that, in fact, most governments are spending their resources where they could do the most good. The failure may not only be "where" but "how": Not only are governments typically failing to address the most serious problems, they also are failing to use the most appropriate techniques to reduce risks. Thus, even large increases in investments in environmental protection may buy less than they ought unless governments change their priorities and approaches. Most comparative risk projects to date have provided ample evidence to support these conclusions. [The introduction to EPA Region 6's "Comparative Risk Project Overview Report," for example, notes: "The percentage of resources [in Region 6's budget] which are committed to resolving the Region's combined ecological and human health problems in the high and moderate-high risk categories is 9.8 percent. Ninety percent of the Region's resources are utilized to address problems in the moderate-low to lowest risk categories" (U.S. EPA, Region 6, 1990).] In a sense, the comparative risk projects' results have defined the challenge:

> *Comparative risk* is a process to identify which environmental problems are most severe and which strategies for risk reduction will do the most good.

The third condition defines the context for setting priorities in a democracy: Government agencies and legislatures need the consent of the governed. In other words, it will ultimately be up to the public to decide which problems or risks are most "severe," and which solutions would do the most "good." Indeed, as noted in the definition of risk, it is up to the public to decide which criteria analysts should use to define and measure risk.

In America today, these decisions usually emerge in contradictory fragments from the chaotic, crisis-driven, inarticulate, short-sighted, and poorly informed world of elections, legislatures, and courts. New laws and programs rarely seem to have been created with a knowing regard for old laws and programs, let alone for the actual fate of chemicals and changes in the real global environment. Although the environment is interconnected, comprehensive, and long-term, America's environment policies are not. Nor do existing federal statutes provide any clear sense of priority: as then EPA Deputy Administrator Henry Habicht told a conference in November 1992, federal statutes create "dozens of number-one priorities" and bolster the greatest enemy of effective environmental protection: bureaucratic "compartmentalization" (Habicht, 1992).

A comparative risk project can help improve this situation by providing decision-makers with the best technical and social data available about a comprehensive set of environmental problems. Engaging in the process encourages decision-makers to look at the real, complex, physical world, rather than the compartmentalized world of specific bureaucratic programs. The process can encourage decision-makers to use the data in a fairly rigorous and systematic way.

The process of comparing and ranking environmental risks educates decision-makers about a wide range of problems and possible solutions, and thus makes it possible for them to make better-informed judgments about environmental priorities.

The strength of the comparative risk process is that it can be open to people without advanced degrees in science, law, or economics. Although generating and analyzing the data at the heart of a comparative risk project requires highly specialized skills, understanding and using that data to make decisions requires only an open mind and a habit of critical thinking. Judgment, after all, is in nearly everyone's domain. As this paper will demonstrate, lay bodies have made risk-ranking decisions that differ very little from the experts' opinions, except, perhaps, in how the decisions are perceived by the lay public.

Comparative risk projects have taken many different shapes and approaches, but all have followed a basic sequence:

1. Start-up: setting goals for the project; assigning responsibilities and deciding whom to involve and who is in charge; deciding on the role of the press and the public; defining risks; selecting analytical methods for estimating risks; selecting the environmental problems to analyze.
2. Risk analysis: finding the most useful and complete data; estimating risks; documenting risks.
3. Risk ranking: deciding which problems pose the most serious risks.
4. Goal setting: deciding which risks are most important to reduce, and by how much.
5. Strategic analysis: developing and analyzing possible risk-reduction strategies.
6. Implementation: deciding which strategies to adopt and implement.
7. Monitoring: determining the impact over time of the choices made as a result of the project.

One of the first challenges of any comparative risk project is to define what it means by risk. All comparative risk projects to date have looked at risks to human health and the health of ecosystems. A few early EPA projects also estimated and compared risks to "welfare," by which they meant the lost income or higher expenses caused by a pollution-induced illness, for example, or the lost market value of a crop or commercial fishing operation because of environmental degradation. Several of the more recent state and municipal projects have included risks to the "quality of life," including risks to aesthetics, outdoor recreation, peace of mind, the sense of community, fairness, and future generations (Vermont Agency of Natural Resources, 1991).

Note that every one of these definitions of risk flows from the public's values, not from the natural sciences, and many require further definition. Risks to human health, for example, are many and diverse, ranging from occasional itchy eyes to a lifetime of mental retardation or premature death from cancer. These risks are generally not evenly distributed: whereas whole populations may be exposed to some risks, only very small groups may be exposed to others. It is up to people—not some preprogrammed black box—to decide which types of health endpoints and exposure scenarios are most important or severe. Because these answers are based on values, not science, they will probably be different in different locations and at different times.

Some comparative risk projects and enthusiasts have ignored these values-related questions. Senator Moynihan's 1991 legislation, for example, concluded that "funds can only be used most effectively when they protect the largest number of people from the most egregious harm" (U.S. Senate Bill 2132, 1991). This definition ignores the possibility that in the interest of justice, acute risks to subpopulations might merit the nation's attention before moderate risks to many.

Although the importance of values was rarely mentioned in EPA's early work on comparative risk (or risk assessment), the agency did understand that environmental risks would differ across the nation. In a move that was relatively daring for a federal agency, EPA's Regional and State Planning Branch encouraged EPA's ten regional offices and numerous states to conduct their own comparative risk projects to set geographically specific priorities. This effort has led to the flowering of comparative risk in America today.

## III.  UNFINISHED BUSINESS: A PRODUCT OF SCIENCE AND NECESSITY

Comparative risk was born at the U.S. Environmental Protection Agency in the mid-1980s out of the highly technical and controversial discipline of risk assessment, the field that brought together toxicologists and epidemiologists to estimate the risks that environmental chemicals pose to human health.

The EPA has long struggled to win its policy battles on the merits: on scientific or technical grounds. (See Landy et al., 1990, for a thorough discussion of efforts in the 1970s to bring science to the forefront in decisions on ozone standards, cancer policy, and other issues. Note, also, the lack of attention the agency paid to engaging the public in decisions based on values.) Good science would win the agency credibility, and in the mid-1980s, EPA desperately needed credibility. The tenure of Administrator Anne Gorsuch Burford had made the public deeply suspicious of EPA. When William Ruckelshaus, the Agency's first administrator (1970–1973) returned to rescue EPA in 1983 and 1984, he set a tone that continued for a decade. In articles, speeches, and in deeds, he sought to strengthen the quality of EPA's science as well as the public's understanding of risk and involvement in risk management.

In a 1983 article in *Science,* Ruckelshaus wrote:

> We also need to strengthen our risk assessment capabilities. We need more research on the health effects of the substances we regulate. I intend to do everything in my power to make clear the importance of this scientific analysis at EPA . . . .
>
> Risk assessment at EPA must be based only on scientific evidence and scientific consensus. Nothing will erode public confidence faster than the suspicion that policy considerations have been allowed to influence the assessment of risk . . . .
>
> To effectively manage the risk, we must seek new ways to involve the public in the decision-making process. Whether we believe in participatory democracy or not, it is a part of our social regulatory fabric. Rather than praise or lament it, we should seek more imaginative ways to involve the various segments of the public affected by the substance at issue (Ruckelshaus, 1983).

Although Ruckelshaus overstates the objectivity of risk assessment, his call for putting good science in the hands of the public still rings true. [See Landy et al., 1990 for a thorough discussion of the impact of "conservative" assumptions on the interpretation of bioassays (Chapter 6, "Forging a Cancer Policy," pp. 172–203).] Nine months after his presentation to the National Academy of Sciences, from which the *Science* article was drawn, Ruckelshaus made an even more significant call for sharing technical information and decision-making authority with the public. In a speech at Princeton University he said that EPA should "expose to public scrutiny the assumptions that underlie our analysis," including "the stacking of conservative assumptions one on top of another" (*BNA Environ. Rep.,* 24 Feb 1984, p. 1829, quoted in Landy 1990, p. 253).

Two-and-a-half years after Ruckelshaus made his public pronouncements about risk and democracy, his successor, Lee M. Thomas, asked 75 EPA career staff people to conduct the first comparative risk project, assessing the relative risks posed by 31 pollution sources over which EPA had jurisdiction, including, for example, stationary sources of criteria air pollutants, municipal sewage treatment plant discharges, abandoned hazardous waste sites, and leaking underground storage tanks. The project's result, published in February 1987, was called *Unfinished Business: A Comparative Assessment of Environmental Problems.* Thomas modestly echoed some of Ruckelshaus' themes in his preface to the thick document:

> Their report—although subjective and based on imperfect data—represents a credible first step toward a promising method of analyzing, developing, and implementing environmental policy. That is why I am presenting it to the public as I have received it.
>
> In a world of limited resources, it may be wise to give priority attention to those pollutants and problems that pose the greatest risks to our society. That is the measure this study begins to apply. It represents, in my view, the first few sketchy lines of what might become the future picture of environmental protection in America (U.S. EPA 1987).

The project's technical work groups started by analyzing 31 problems for four types of risk: cancer risk; noncancer human health effects; ecological effects; and welfare effects.

The health risk analysis, like most of those that have followed, tried to use the basic techniques of site-specific risk assessments and scale them up to cover the entire population. The work group first broke each problem area down into a list of a few of the most serious "stressors"—chemical pollutants, or physical agents such as ultraviolet radiation. Then the team attempted to estimate human exposures to these stressors and the likely health risks each problem posed to the most exposed individuals and the population as a whole. When data were sparse or nonexistent, the analysts substituted their best professional judgment. Given the paucity of national exposure data or hazard assessments on most stressors, the team had to resort to judgment in almost all decisions.

The ecological risk analysis in *Unfinished Business,* like others that have followed, relied on analogous techniques to estimate the risks that stressors pose to the environment. Typically, the ecologic risk investigators attempt to estimate the exposure and likely consequences of the most pervasive or toxic stressors on various types of ecosystems. Most analysts define the effect in terms of damage to an ecosystem's structure or function. The spatial scale of the impact is considered, as is its reversibility—the time it would take the system to recover once the stressor is removed. These definitions of risk are necessarily broad because ecosystems are enormously complex and dynamic, and because the effects of most stressors over time are extremely difficult to measure and as yet not well understood. The ecologists working on *Unfinished Business* had to rely heavily on their own professional judgment.

The welfare team focused on the types of damage to which dollar figures could most easily be affixed: economic losses caused by damage to materials and crops, and health care costs. The introduction to *Unfinished Business* candidly recognizes that the analysis omitted "intangible characteristics that people often find just as important," such as equity, degree of voluntariness, and what economists call *existence value*—the value people place on having something around, even if they never plan to use it.

After estimating the risks, the *Unfinished Business* teams compared the risks and used their best judgment to rank the problems in order of the seriousness of the risks they posed. The work groups did not try to integrate the four rankings into a single list, nor did they suggest that the rankings ought to be taken up as a political priority list. They did, however, point out that the biggest risks in various categories (e.g., indoor air pollution and radon, global warming, ozone depletion) were generally not EPA budget priorities or even covered by EPA's statutory mandates. Moreover, the biggest risks tended to rank low in the public's ranking of risk, as revealed by opinion polls. EPA's most expensive programs (e.g., those addressing hazardous waste facilities and abandoned hazardous waste sites, and underground storage tanks) tended to address problems that the public ranked as high risks, even though the comparative risk teams ranked them medium to low (U.S. EPA, 1987).

The report did not change EPA policy overnight and it certainly did not change the public's perception of risks. Although *Unfinished Business* was a ground-breaking document, it had relatively little direct political impact, because it never really emerged from the EPA bureaucracy and technical staff. The tentativeness revealed by Thomas's suggestion that it "may be wise" to base priorities on risk delayed the impact of *Unfinished Business* until William Reilly took over EPA in 1989.

Reilly, like Ruckelshaus, constantly stressed the need for better science at EPA. During his term as administrator, he complained publicly about the lack of rational planning at the agency and its failure to address the most serious risks in an appropriate manner. In a special issue of the *EPA Journal* devoted entirely to a "debate on risk," Reilly explained why he believed risk should be the foundation for setting priorities:

> Each time a new issue appeared on the radar screen of public concern, we would unleash an arsenal of control measures in a style reminiscent of the old 'space invaders' video game . . . . The consequence of this approach is obvious to all our employees: For 20 years we have established goals on a pollutant-by-pollutant and medium-by-medium basis without adequately considering broader environmental quality objectives. Rarely have we evaluated the relative importance of pollutants or environmental media—air, land, and water. Nor did we assess the combined impacts on whole ecosystems and human health. Given the scatter-shot evolution of the Agency and its missions, we were seldom encouraged to look at the total loadings of pollutants deposited through different media from separate routes of exposure at various locations. We have seldom if ever been directed by law to seek out the best opportunities to reduce environmental risks, in toto, or to employ the most efficient, cost-effective procedures (Reilly, 1991).

By the time this article appeared in 1991, Reilly had already transformed the debate about risk. He had moved in two directions at once: from the top, and from the bottom.

Soon after the publication of *Unfinished Business,* EPA headquarters began recruiting other jurisdictions to conduct similar comparative risk projects. EPA's regional offices in New England, the Mid-Atlantic states, and the Pacific Northwest were the first to volunteer. They followed headquarters' model closely and produced similar results. The projects were careful in-house exercises that neither sought nor produced much external publicity. Although many within the regions and EPA headquarters dismissed both the validity and the usefulness of the process, some of EPA's most influential policy leaders found the work persuasive enough to encourage states to try comparative risk. Over the next two years, five states started projects with EPA's financial and technical support. The first group included Washington, Pennsylvania, and Colorado, and then Vermont and Louisiana (Minard et al., 1993).

In 1990, EPA's Regional and State Planning Branch directed each of the seven remaining EPA regions to conduct in-house comparative risk projects and to use them as the basis for their strategic plans. The regions complied and, in the process, explored several new approaches to comparing risks. Several of the regions strove to make the process as scientific as possible. Region 6, for example, used a computerized system to interpret the data and "rank" ecological risks, and a Geographic Information System to illustrate the results on maps. The regions generally perceived the process as a quest for technical answers and as an internal management tool. In most regions, staff scientists did the work with little if any involvement from state governments or the general public. Some regions never even publicly announced their results.

The regions' technical approach was a reasonable response to their culture and EPA's hierarchy. The projects' results were primarily intended to persuade teams of senior EPA managers—the scientists and appointees who had some discretionary control over the regional offices' budgets or who could influence the margins of EPA's overall strategic plan. Because the managers could exercise this minimal discretion without appealing to Congress, state legislatures, or local constituents, the regional projects could be effective while involving only a small cadre of well-trained professionals.

As the regions were doing their work, EPA's Science Advisory Board (SAB) agreed to Reilly's request to conduct a peer review of and follow-up to *Unfinished Business*. The result, a four-volume report called *Reducing Risk: Setting Priorities and Strategies for Environmental Protection,* was published with maximum public fanfare in September 1990. The SAB acknowledged many of the problems with the comparative risk method, but endorsed it as a valuable tool for setting priorities.

In the three years following the SAB report, the EPA has invested in or encouraged comparative risk projects in more than a dozen more states, as well as the cities of Seattle, Atlanta, Jackson, Mississippi, and Columbus, Ohio, as well as Guam, Bangkok, Poland, Bulgaria, and India. Other cities, counties, and regional governments, as well as nongovernment organizations at various levels, are now turning to comparative risk.

As a measure of the institutional acceptance of comparative risk, note that by the end of 1993, the National Governors' Association and the Carnegie Commission on Science, Technology, and Government had endorsed the tool (National Governors' Association, 1993; Carnegie Commission, 1993), the Western Governors' Association was sponsoring a multistate environmental project that included comparative risk methods (Western Governors' Environmental Policy Council, 1993), and three national organizations dedicated to improving the quality of state governments—the Council of Governors' Policy Advisors, the Council of State Governments, and the National Conference of State Legislatures—were introducing their members to the process.

Although comparative risk is becoming almost a standard tool of "good government," it is still controversial, evolving, and being practiced in many forms. The future of comparative risk will depend on how its practitioners resolve the critical issues of public involvement and public values. If the scientific priesthood clings to the myth that the process is scientific and thus exclusively theirs, it will die. A closer look at two projects—the Science Advisory Board's and the State of Vermont's—will help illuminate some of these issues.

## IV.  EPA'S SCIENCE ADVISORY BOARD: TO THE EDGE OF SCIENCE

*Reducing Risk* was the torch that William Reilly used to guide EPA in new directions. Three of the report's conclusions continue to be particularly powerful, framing the debate about comparative risk and defining the general approach:

1.  The report's first recommendation endorsed the policy choice inherent in comparative risk: "EPA should target its environmental protection efforts on the basis of opportunities for the greatest risk reduction" (U.S. EPA Science Advisory Board, 1990). The report also urges EPA to create risk-based budgets and risk-based strategic plans. The SAB specifically endorsed the comparative risk process, including its subjective components:

    > In order to set priorities for reducing environmental risks, EPA must weigh the relative risks posed by different environmental problems, determine if there are cost-effective opportunities for reducing those risks, and then identify the most cost-effective risk reduction options. This effort should build on the analytical process begun in *Unfinished Business* and in this report and its appendices.

However, the SAB recognizes that risk analyses always will be imperfect tools. No matter how much the data and methodologies are improved, EPA's decisions to direct specific actions at specific risks will entail a large measure of subjective judgment. Yet the SAB believes that relative risk data and risk assessment techniques should inform that judgment as much as possible.

2. "EPA should attach as much importance to reducing ecological risk as it does to reducing human health risk." Although the SAB did not formally compare remaining ecological risks and human health risks and decide which were most serious, its conclusion implied that EPA had paid too little attention to ecological threats.

3. "EPA—and the nation as a whole—should make greater use of all the tools available to reduce risk." The project's Strategic Options Committee showed that many of the most serious remaining environmental problems were not amenable to traditional command-and-control regulation. New tools, including market-based incentives, education, and the aggressive use of information, would need to be employed to help achieve the most risk-reduction at the lowest cost to society.

Reilly embraced these recommendations with gusto. In January 1991, he and several of the principals in the SAB project presented their conclusions at a formal hearing of the State Environmental and Public Works Committee. Reilly endorsed the report's call for risk-based priorities and pointedly showed the divergence between the SAB's "expert" ranking of environmental risks and the public's judgment, as revealed in a Roper opinion poll (Stevens, 1991). The SAB had reached conclusions similar to those in *Unfinished Business:* The highest risks to ecosystems included habitat alteration and the loss of biodiversity, global climate change, and ozone depletion; the highest human health risks included air pollution, indoor air pollution, drinking water contamination, and worker exposure. The SAB's risk list contrasts with the public's, which still put hazardous waste sites at the top.

Note, however, that the SAB report made no pretense of being the final answer or of having discovered the "scientific truth" about the nation's environment. The recommendations quoted in the foregoing were political suggestions on how EPA could make better decisions and be more effective.

Use more science, the SAB said, but do not expect science alone to resolve all of the nation's environmental policy issues. Do not even expect science to simplify the problem of setting priorities, the board concluded. (For more on how additional scientific information can make decision-making more complex, see Chap. 7 of Graham et al., 1988.)

Although the SAB's Ecology and Welfare Subcommittee had no intellectual or moral trouble dividing the nation's environmental problems into three ranked groups, the project's Human Health Subcommittee refused to do the same, despite the repeated requests of the project's cochairmen to offer some policy guidance to the EPA. The health subcommittee concluded that there were not enough exposure data to justify a ranking, and that answering critical value-laden questions about the relative severity of diseases would exceed their responsibilities as a technical committee. The health scientists did not believe that their expertise qualified them to make what are essentially political decisions. Instead of ranking the problems, the health subcommittee suggested only that some problems posing direct human exposure to toxicants might be worse than problems posing no such direct exposures:

Given the limitations in the taxonomy of the environmental problem areas in the UB [*Unfinished Business*] report and in the toxicity and exposure data on which their respective risk assessments were based, *it is not illogical* that those problem areas representing proximal human exposure situations were assigned the highest relative risk rankings for cancer and/or other adverse health effects in the report. Such problem areas included the following: criteria air pollutants, hazardous air pollutants, the application of pesticides . . . (U.S. EPA, Science Advisory Board, 1990b; emphasis added).

The health scientists declined to make the value judgments inherent in deciding which health effects were the most severe. The committee's report is clear about the challenge, however:

"To attempt a relative ranking in terms of severity (or significance) of such disparate health outcomes as birth defects in infants compared [with] paralysis in older persons requires consideration on many dimensions of the values we place on various members of society, families, and the utility of specific physical and mental functions for individuals and society. Such a comparison requires that the impact of each effect be scored for severity, a process necessitating selection of suitable measures and scales of severity, as well as appropriate weighting factors."

The health subcommittee ultimately recommended that lay people be involved in a process to rank various types of health effects: "One possible way to accomplish this is through the use of lay and professional focus groups meeting separately and then together. The process by which this is done, whatever it may be, the way in which the views of informed potential sufferers (and how they become informed) and of medically and technically trained experts are brought together is critical to developing severity factors or indices with any validity or credibility."

The subcommittee, when faced with huge gaps in essential technical data and little if any indication of the public's values, chose to withhold its judgment. Rather than ranking risks, the committee produced a model for ranking health risks when, in some distant age, all the data about exposures, toxicity, and public attitudes are known. Science could not answer the question that Reilly had asked, so the scientists on the committee chose to ask more questions and to recommend a politically based process to answer some of them.

The response to this problem in EPA's Region 6 could not have been more different. The region's *Overview* report notes that ranking various types of pollution-induced health problems requires the use of a "hazardous index" [sic] that gives different scores to different types of illnesses, but the lengthy volume offers no hints about what the index, is, where it came from, or the significance of the values choices that must be imbedded in the index. Instead, the report explains that science provided the answers:

> The Human Health workgroup had to find common ground upon which to compare and ultimately rank the 21 problem areas. This became very difficult in that different programs and media (air, land, and water) often had little in common from a regulatory data standpoint. Data bases were not compatible, nor were the problem area languages (MCL, NAAQS standards, restricted days, future vs. present/residual risks). Given these difficulties, workgroup members found that basic scientific approaches and adherence to the concepts provided by EPA risk assessment methodologies became the needed common ground. The Human Health workgroup believes that the rankings represent the risks in the Region (U.S. EPA, Region 6, 1990).

Many in EPA have embraced Region 6's comparative risk work as a model of clarity and sophistication. Supporters are justified in their respect for the project's thoroughness and attempts at intellectual rigor. The project probably does represent the best that the process can achieve when it is conducted by scientists for scientists, rather than for public decision-makers. Yet the *Overview* report's omission of any explanation of the source or implications of its severity index obscures the role of human values in making decisions about health risks. The approach betrays an unfortunate disconnection between the analysts and those whom the analysis would serve.

At nearly the same time that the SAB's health subcommittee and Region 6's work groups were reaching such different conclusions about the ability of science to compare health risks, the SAB's Ecology and Welfare Subcommittee was expeditiously sorting the nation's environmental problems into six ranked tiers of relative risk. How, when most people complained that ecological risk assessment was not nearly as advanced a science as health risk assessment, did the team come up with answers? The ecology subcommittee certainly did not have all the data it wanted. The debate about global climate change in 1990, for example, was still based on conflicting computer models. Experts could point to very few definitive studies to quantify either the extent of chemicals in the environment or the magnitude of the repercussions they were having on biological processes.

What the ecology committee did have, however, was a leader who understood his mission and who positively enjoyed making controversial decisions on behalf of the public. Bill Cooper, an aquatic biologist from Michigan State University, was fond of saying that his subcommittee could certainly make better decisions about ecological priorities than a bunch of lawyers could, so he and his colleagues took the plunge into the realm of risk-based policy.

The committee focused its analysis on the intensity of a problem's effect on an ecosystem's function and structure, emphasizing the spatial extent of the damage and the time it would take the system to recover once the stress was removed (U.S. Science Advisory Board, 1990a).

The "values issues" that had plagued the health subcommittee were simpler here, but not less important. The emphasis on recovery time, for example, reflects the value the committee placed on future generations; the emphasis on space reflects not only a technical assumption that all ecosystems are interrelated, but also a value placed on maintaining ecosystem health across the globe, not merely in a few nice places. Perhaps the strongest value represented in the analytical criteria and results was on the preservation of genetic diversity and the survival, in something approaching their natural state, of a diverse range of ecological communities. Maintaining that degree of diversity would be the best guarantor that ecosystems would be able to adjust to a broad range of unpredictable stresses.

The subcommittee's analysis of the nation's environmental problems was brief, general, easy to understand, and compelling. The localized, slow-moving problems caused by hazardous waste dumps dripping contaminants into the groundwater simply paled in comparison with the global distribution of airborne toxics, greenhouse gases, and ozone-depleting chemicals. Likewise, the dramatic and obvious destruction of rare habitats and the consequent permanent loss of species proved to be demonstrably more serious in ecological terms than most oil spills, which bacteria can obliterate in a short while.

The subcommittee's analysis was not quantitative in any sense of the word. The researchers did not estimate the precise number of acres of wetlands being destroyed each year. Nor did they try to push what data they did have through a formula or a computer program that would produce a numerical ranking of risk. Rather, the analysis and ranking process relied on a series of simpler comparisons that were captured in a series of tables. The first table sorted the problems by the spatial scale of the stress; the second sorted the risks by environmental media; and the third by recovery time. Finally, the members used their judgment to combine the three tables into a single ranked list. The report explains: "The synthesis rankings were derived qualitatively using expert judgment rather than a numerical metric based on the more detailed risk matrices discussed previously, as the Subcommittee decided that any specific quantitative or semi-quantitative methodology for combining risks assigned across scales and media . . . would not be defensible with present ecological risk assessment capabilities."

As this conclusion was coming off the presses, however, several of the EPA regions were finishing up their ecological risk estimates and rankings. Most started with data and criteria quite similar to the SAB's, but then assigned numerical values to the different pieces of information in a way that made it simple to calculate a risk score for each problem area. The higher the score, the higher the ranking. Many people argue that using an algebraic formula to rank problems is more rigorous and scientific than the SAB's discussion-based ranking. The formula's illusion of precision, however, is false. Moreover, the formula obscures the importance of judgment throughout the process. If the SAB committees pushed their analyses to the edge of science, some of the regions went one step beyond.

The Ecology and Welfare Subcommittee went on to propose a "welfare ranking" of the environmental problems. The subcommittee's approach boiled down to concluding that if a problem is bad for ecosystems it is bad for people, too. The group acknowledged that its membership included no economists or others with expertise in defining or measuring welfare effects, and it made no significant attempt to wrestle with equity issues or other social values. The subcommittee made several valuable points about the danger of using simplistic, short-term economic measures to quantify environmental damage, but on the whole, the SAB's welfare discussion has had little influence and rarely gets mentioned when EPA compares its "real risks" with the public's list of priorities, as when Reilly testified before the Senate Environment and Public Works Committee in January 1991. The committee received the recommendations warmly.

Three years later, however, EPA is still pumping most of its money and attention into Superfund and Congress has not given the agency authority to reorganize its management or its priorities. The agency has, however, redirected some of its limited discretionary funds in risk-based ways. Its regional offices have submitted strategic plans proposing small but significant resource shifts toward higher-risk problems. Some of the program offices have adopted the vocabulary of risk and risk-reduction.

Thus, the impact of the SAB's *Reducing Risk* report seems to have been both profound and puny. Because of the energy Reilly and his top management team invested in creating a climate within EPA for risk-reduction, pollution-prevention, cross-media analysis, and geographically specific protection strategies, the report seems to have changed how EPA thinks as an institution. Reilly succeeded in starting a debate about risk and priorities among policy makers and academics across the country.

The SAB report has not made much of a dent in how the general public thinks about environmental risks or priorities, however, and neither Congress nor the 1992 presidential candidates seemed to have noticed that the debate was supposed to have changed. The news media have not shifted their attention from the drama of hazardous waste and oil spills to the mundane destruction of wetlands and natural prairie communities. Most Americans have not heard the SAB's alarm about the great risks posed by the cumulative effects of their cars, energy consumption, and lifestyles. Instead, most Americans still think of "heavy industry" as the source of most environmental degradation, the bad guys who must be regulated and punished.

Clearly, Congress is unlikely to make substantial spending or policy shifts until the public catches up with the experts' opinions. State legislatures and city councils may be a bit faster to act.

## V.  COMPARATIVE RISK IN THE STATES: SCIENCE TO THE PEOPLE

One of the corollaries to EPA's goal of reducing the nation's worst risks first is that environmental risks are unlikely to be uniform across the country. Colorado has acid mine drainage to worry about; Louisiana has the loss of coastal wetlands; the East has the Midwest's sulfur and nitrogen oxides. Not only will the physical nature of the environmental problems differ from region to region, but so too may the public's values and, hence, their priorities for risk reduction.

Congress created EPA with strong regional offices precisely to ensure geographic sensitivity and decentralized management. Despite the tension that the structure has always created between Washington, the 10 regional offices, and the 50 states (not to mention Guam and Puerto Rico), EPA's focus on comparative risk has included an effort from headquarters to further decentralize control. Grants from headquarters have helped the states conduct their own comparative risk projects and, thereby, to set their own risk-based environmental agendas. In addition to cash to support the analysis, headquarters has held out the elusive carrot of "grant flexibility": the power to move EPA money destined for the state from one mandated program to another of higher risk.

Among the states that have undertaken comparative risk projects, Pennsylvania most closely followed the EPA regional model of conducting the study within an administrative agency far removed from the political process or public oversight. That insularity proved fatal: when the work groups completed their rankings, the state's political leaders refused to sign on. A draft report never saw the light of day. This failure contrasted with the enormous success of Washington State's project which featured an aggressively inclusive public process that culminated in a statewide environmental summit. The summit's open discussion of the comparative risk project's results created the momentum for several significant legislative initiatives (Minard et al., 1993).

Washington's politically tuned project set a pattern for the state and municipal projects that followed. Most state projects now involve not only state employees, but also public advisory boards and ordinary citizens. The best projects use town meetings, statewide environmental summits, the electronic media, public opinion polls, and the Governor's bully pulpit to reach out to residents and draw them into the risk analysis and ranking, and ultimately, into changing the environmental agenda.

The official leaders of the Vermont comparative risk project, for example, were a team of appointed commissioners and agency secretaries, but they put a lay board completely in charge of the risk analysis and ranking. Jonathan Lash, then secretary of the Vermont Agency for Natural Resources, knew that the only way to change Vermont's environmental agenda would be through changing the perceptions of the decision-making public: the legislators, interest group leaders, and ordinary voters. For the results of the analysis to have any political power they had to be credible to the public; and for members of the public to believe the results, they had to be in control. Good science could not survive a bad process.

The Vermont experiment worked, up to a point. The so-called Public Advisory Committee, composed of 20 Vermonters from all walks of life, did an extraordinary job. It made thoughtful decisions about the scope of the analysis and the criteria to use to measure the impact of environmental problems on Vermonters' "quality of life." The committee actively engaged interested members of the public in the discussion about values and technical issues. For example, in public forums and in a printed survey, the committee asked Vermonters what types of environmentally induced illnesses they wanted government to address first.* The committee studied the hundred of pages of technical information produced by the professionals who composed the project's three technical work groups. After about 10 months of work, the public committee spent two days discussing the analysis with the technical committee members, then

---

*The Vermont survey's respondents said that government should address health risks in this order: problems that may be fatal to people when they are young; problems that may cause permanent mental disabilities in children; problems that may cause long-term pain; problems that may be fatal to people when they are old; and problems that may cause many people to get sick for a while (Vermont Agency of Natural Resources, 1991).

another two days ranking the problems. The public members used their own judgment to fill in the data gaps and wrestle with the values choices.

The committee was unanimous on nearly all points, and clearly articulated the few disagreements it had about interpretation of data or weighting of values. It believed strongly in its work and urged the Agency of Natural Resources and the Department of Health to use its ranking of risks as a foundation for changes in state policy and spending.

The committee's ranking had only a modest effect on spending and policy decisions. The Department of Health, for example, found that because of the project, it had the public support it needed to focus more attention on radon and childhood lead poisoning. The Agency of Natural Resources initiated efforts to emphasize the preservation of biodiversity in Vermont, to bolster public information and education programs, to capitalize on EPA's offer of "grant flexibility" based on risk, and to create a pollution prevention division.

The project's political influence was sharply reduced, however, by the political upheaval that accompanied a gubernatorial election that switched the party in power, and eight months later, the subsequent death of the governor and another change of party. During both transitions, neither governor made it a priority to engage the public in a debate about environmental risks and the value of rethinking the state's agenda.

Although the Vermont project's political influence has been subtle, it still demonstrated several important points about the comparative risk process. The most important of these was that it is not dangerous to ask nonscientists to make risk-based decisions. The Public Advisory Committee's ranking of Vermont's environmental problems was very similar to the rankings generated by the project's technical work groups and consistent with results from other state and federal comparative risk projects. In other words, the public members demonstrated that a lay board's judgment could be sound. The committee proved wrong those scientists who argued that only scientists could rank problems without contaminating the results with bias, ignorance, or political opportunism.

State Toxicologist Dr. William Bress of the Vermont Department of Health put it this way in a note to his colleagues in other states: "My first impression . . . of the comparative risk process was that it was a huge waste of time . . . . I felt that I knew what the comparative risks for different problems were. Why should I spend many hours confirming something I already knew ? . . . My opinion of the process started to change after my first meeting of the citizens' committee. When I saw how they were using the data we supplied, I was pleasantly surprised. Groups of people from all walks of life were often ranking problems in the same order as I had. They came up with these rankings on their own . . . . Risks we had high on our [the Department of Health's] priority list are now a high priority to the public. This has resulted in shifting of funds and resources to these areas of concern. This might not have happened without going through this useful, although painful, process" (Bress, 1992).

Vermont's process also demonstrated that when given the chance to learn about environmental problems, ordinary citizens can and will change their minds. The advisory committee's final ranking was as far from the Vermont public's perception of risks as *Unfinished Business's* ranking was from the Roper Poll.

A third lesson from the Vermont project is that comparative risk should not disguise itself as hard science. The project's technical reports on human health and ecological risks were as quantitative as the data would permit. The health reports, for example, included individual and population cancer risks derived from EPA's cancer potency figures and a variety of exposure estimation techniques. The reports tried to pinpoint the sources of pollution and the range of exposures individuals might encounter in the state. All of these data made the reports the most comprehensive and quantitative that had ever been generated in Vermont. Nevertheless, the reports frankly discussed the gaps in both the data and the science of risk assessment and the resulting uncertainty inherent in many of these estimates.

When it came time to rank the problems, the Advisory Committee arrayed the health risk data on a fairly simple matrix that put the estimated size of the exposed population on one axis and the relative individual risk the exposures might pose on the other axis. This array helped the committee see the relationships between the risks posed by the problems, without conveying more precise risk estimates than the crude data would support. The project's honesty about uncertainty and the importance of subjective values seem to have made its findings more credible among its readers. The report's openness made it somewhat more difficult for critics to dismiss it as "unscientific" and hence worthless.

The Vermont project also showed that comparative risk can and should incorporate some of what *Unfinished Business* called those "intangible characteristics that people often find just as important" as the risk assessors' probabilities. After conducting a dozen public forums throughout the state, the advisory committee had heard enough to conclude that Vermonters' definition of risk included threats to fairness (such as involuntary risks of inequitable distributions of risk and benefits), sense of community, peace of mind, and future generations, as well as threats to their economic well-being, aesthetics, and recreational opportunities. Although the technical analysis of these risks was necessarily qualitative, it was systematic, thoughtful, and illuminating.

Most importantly, the quality of life analysis and ranking helped the advisory committee more precisely answer its driving question: "What problems pose the most serious risks to Vermont and Vermonters?" The health and ecological analysis of solid waste, for example, showed that landfills pose relatively low health and ecological risks; and the quality of life analysis showed that landfills pose relatively high risks to aesthetics and fairness (the risks are borne by the few who live nearby, while the benefits accrue to everyone in the region). Thus, solid waste ranked in the middle of the quality of life list. This moderate ranking pulled solid waste up one level from the lowest tier in the integrated ranking. That result reflects the "intangible" risks in a way that is both accurate and potentially useful for risk management purposes.

The quality of life analysis helped the public to see that the comparative risk project was not just a trick to force an unfeeling technocracy's rules down their throats. It also helped Vermonters better understand the nature of the environmental problems facing the state. The quality of life information strengthened the project's foundation for effective risk reduction efforts.

Risk reduction, after all, is the goal of environmental protection. At least it should be if the definition of risk is broad enough to include those intangibles that people want their government to promote or protect, including social justice and the well-being of future generations. The challenge of identifying and implementing the best possible risk-reduction strategies is made somewhat simpler if both the physical and social goals are clearly articulated in advance.

## VI.  RISK REDUCTION: FROM DATA TO ACTION

The usefulness of comparative risk has to be measured in terms of its ability to help decision-makers make and implement *better* decisions about the environment. In an ideal world where both the science and political processes were more advanced, perhaps comparative risk could lead to the *right* decision, the ideal set of policies and spending choices. In the face of uncertainty, however, no one should sell the process as a device to find perfect answers.

One of the unfounded complaints about comparative risk and EPA's emphasis on risk-based budgeting is that any changes driven by the risk rankings will only make the environment worse.

According to this view, EPA or a state environmental agency will spend money futilely trying to solve the highest risks (global climate change, for example) only after dropping the programs that are keeping the relatively low-risk problems (such as sewage treatment) under control. Taken to its extreme, the critique envisions people across America dying of cholera because EPA stupidly stopped spending money on sewage treatment systems.

Some critics take the same theme and add a paranoid conspiracy theory to it: the whole risk assessment and comparative risk business is a fraud designed to justify EPA's hidden agenda: dropping all of its controls on industry by fooling the public into believing that radon in their cellars is the real devil.

Both versions of this complaint rest on two false assumptions: that environmental programs are all or nothing; and that decision-makers are idiots or crooks.

Part of this perception has grown out of EPA's tendency to promote the ranked list of environmental problems as the most important product of comparative risk. If the list really were the most important product, then simple-minded managers *would* simply move money from the problems at the bottom of the list to the problems at the top. In reality, the rankings are just a shorthand, a reminder to decision-makers, the press, and the public that if their goal is to reduce environmental risks, they need to change their individual and collective spending and policies. A ranking of risks with habitat alteration at the top and Superfund sites at the bottom is so startling to most people that it tends to grab their attention.

The most important products of comparative risk are the complex collections of data that make the ranking possible, and the new perspectives on the problems that the project's participants share. By having worked through all the details, the participants should complete the process with a far more sophisticated understanding of the environment, the problems that threaten it, and the strategies available to reduce risks (Minard, et al., 1993). These people are not going to let risks from failed sewage systems get out of hand just because they were not at the top of the risk list.

Indeed, as long as the participants remain focused on reducing risks they will demand a constantly improving set of data and risk-reduction policies. They will develop better environmental monitoring systems to help them anticipate, prevent, or correct growing problems. They will develop and implement policies that reduce a wide range of risks at once. And if economic conditions demand spending cuts, at least the cuts will increase risks as little as possible. If the definitions of environmental risk include threats to social justice and future generations, a risk-based approach to problem solving can be socially constructive and forward-looking, contrary to the conclusions of some critics (see, e.g., Atcheson, 1991; Hornstein, 1992). A focus on risk should be an agent of constant change and adjustment.

Most importantly, if the project's participants have included a broad mix of public leaders and decision-makers—and, through the press, the general public as well—the process may have made the conventional wisdom considerably wiser. That seems to have happened in Washington State, and it created a potent political force for change. Comparative risk projects continue to demonstrate the truth behind the adage that public policy can be no more sophisticated than a public's understanding of a problem.

The technocratic approach to comparative risk not only ignores this law of public policy, but also exacerbates the problem by forgetting another post-Watergate fact of American life: the people do not trust their governments. Credible science, in the public's mind, is not synonymous with prestigious scientists. It is not enough for a comparative risk project to have been meticulous, systematic, and "scientific," if it has not also been open to the public and based on the public's values. And God help the technocracy that believes it can—or should—significantly change environmental priorities without first persuading legislatures, governors, Congress, and ultimately the voters, that the specific revisions are truly in the public's interest. Without securing that authority from the voters, the technocrats' policies will not long survive and only further discredit their agencies.

These political imperatives are all the more significant given the conclusions that most comparative risk projects are reaching. Command-and-control regulation of industrial polluters cannot go much further, at any reasonable social price, to reduce risks. The most serious risks in many parts of the country are those caused by the aggregation of many individuals' actions, particularly wasting energy, ignoring indoor air pollutants, and bulldozing natural habitats. The most effective strategies to address these problems will include pollution prevention techniques and market incentives to companies and individuals to change their behavior. By their nature, some of these approaches may be less predictable or certain to succeed than command-and-control methods, and they do not satisfy the public's desire to treat someone else as the enemy. It is a safe bet that Americans will agree to shoulder the costs of reducing risks only when they have decided that the evidence shows that the risks are serious.

The comparative risk process cannot bring instant wisdom or altruism to a population. It probably will not even create a "consensus." It certainly cannot prove scientifically that a ranked list of problems is the correct basis for public action; but comparative risk projects have started important debates about risk and policy. They have encouraged the debates' participants to marshal the best technical and social information available today to make decisions. Both the process and the results strengthen America's ability to make sound decisions about the environment.

## REFERENCES

Atcheson, J. (1991). The department of risk reduction or risky business, *Environ. Law,* 21, 1375–1412.

Bress, W. (1992). Unpublished written statement presented to attendees at a conference for comparative risk practitioners sponsored by the Northeast Center for Comparative Risk, Feb. 1992.

Carnegie Commission on Science, Technology, and Government (1993). *Risk and the Environment, Improving Regulatory Decision Making,* Carnegie Corporation of New York, New York.

Graham, J. D., et al. (1988). *In Search of Safety: Chemicals and Cancer Risk,* Harvard University Press, Cambridge, pp. 179–219.

Habicht, H. (1992). Speech to Resources for the Future's conference, "Setting National Environmental Priorities," November 15, 1992, Annapolis, MD, quoted in *Comp. Risk Bull.,* 12, Dec. 1992.

Hornstein, D. T. (1992). Reclaiming environmental law: A normative critique of comparative risk analysis, *Columbia Law Rev.,* 92, 562–633.

Landy, M. K., et al. (1990). *The Environmental Protection Agency: Asking the Wrong Questions,* Oxford University Press, New York.

Minard, R. A., et al. (1993). *State Comparative Risk Projects: A Force for Change,* Northeast Center for Comparative Risk, South Royalton, VT.

National Governors' Association (1993). The Cumulative Impact of Environmental Regulation, policy adopted February 1993, Washington, DC.

Northeast Center for Comparative Risk (1993). *Comp. Risk Bull.,* 11, 7–9.

Reilly, W. K. (1991). Why I propose a national debate on risk, *EPA J,* 2, 2–5.

Ruckelshaus, W. D. (1983). What really threatens the environment? *New York Times,* Jan. 29.

U.S. EPA, Office of Policy, Planning, and Evaluation (1987). *Unfinished Business: A Comparative Assessment of Environmental Problems, Overview Report,* Washington, DC.

U.S. EPA, Region 6 Office of Planning and Analysis (1990). *Comparative Risk Project Overview Report,* Dallas, TX.

U.S. EPA, Science Advisory Board (1990). *Reducing Risk: Setting Priorities and Strategies for Environmental Protection,* EPA publication no. SAB-EC-90-021, Washington, DC.

U.S. EPA, Science Advisory Board (1990). *Reducing Risk: Appendix A: The report of the Ecology and Welfare Subcommittee,* EPA publication no. SAB-EC-90-021A, Washington, DC.

U.S. EPA, Science Advisory Board (1990). *Reducing Risk: Appendix B: The report of the Human Health Subcommittee,* EPA publication no. SAB-EC-90-021B, Washington, DC.

U.S. Senate Bill 2132 (1991). The Environmental Risk Reduction Act proposed by Senator Daniel P. Moynihan, Nov. 27.

Vermont Agency of Natural Resources (1991). *Environment 1991: Risks to Vermont And Vermonters,* Waterbury, VT.

Western Governors' Environmental Policy Council (1993). *Our Lands: New Strategies for Protecting the West: Blueprints for Action,* Western Governors' Association, Denver, CO.

# 42
# The Use of Comparative Risk Judgments in Risk Management[1]

**Carl F. Cranor**
*University of California at Riverside*
*Riverside, California*

## I. INTRODUCTION

When risk managers must make decisions about what risks to address and manage, they must make comparative risk judgments—that is, judgments of which of many risks are most important and which should have priority. A substantial literature explicitly or implicitly appears to assume that risk managers need only examine the magnitude and probability of risks to compare risks and to decide on a course of action. Although there is some truth in this, it can be quite misleading and can lead to public policy effects possibly quite at odds with the public and with a more morally defensible course of action. What is important for public decisions is not only the magnitude and probability of risks, but also a variety of factors that bear on the *acceptability* of risks posed, factors that in many cases are ignored in discussions of these issues.

In what follows, we will explore some morally salient properties of the acceptability of risk; properties that I believe all of us take into account, and that we should take into account implicitly or explicitly, in thinking coherently from a moral point of view about risks that confront us. The features surveyed are not necessarily complete or even always mutually exclusive, but are some of the major facets of the acceptability of risk exposure. Clarifying these features will enable us to think somewhat more clearly about the acceptability of risks and to avoid some obvious as well as some more subtle mistakes. This also suggests what is important and valid in public perceptions of risk, as well as indicating the importance of such considerations to the management of toxic substances such as carcinogens.

Moreover, other literature fails to distinguish between risks that are *permissible* for individuals to take in their own lives and those that they are *required* to live with as a matter of public policy. Both failures results from insufficient attention to the normative components of the acceptability of risk exposure.

## II.  A PARTIAL MATRIX OF THE ACCEPTABILITY OF RISKS

Risk assessment is concerned with the evaluation of risks to human beings. A risk is the chance, or the probability, of some loss or harm—the chance of mishap.[2,3] (In what follows we focus mostly on only life-threatening risks.) In discussing risks, we need a term that is neutral between risks being *imposed* on one and risks that one has *taken;* the somewhat awkward phrases *exposure to risks* or *risk exposure* serve that purpose. In addition, we can use *acceptability* to characterize the normative status of exposure to risks, to characterize the risks that are morally justified or defensible from those that are not.[4] For most of the discussion we focus on the acceptability of risk exposure for an individual. Thus, we are concerned with features of risk exposure that, other things being equal, tend to bear on the acceptability of exposure to the risk in question by a representative person. We rely on persons' commonsense pretheoretical notions of acceptability for the risk in question. Occasionally, the discussion is broadened to address more general notions of the moral acceptability of risks to the public. To clarify the acceptability of exposure to risks and to use risk assessment numbers sensitively several distinctions must be addressed.

### A.  Naturally Caused Versus Humanly Caused Risks

The first distinction is that between risks to which people are exposed resulting from natural phenomena and risks that arise because of human activities. In each case, if the risks materialize, human beings suffer injuries, diseases, or premature death. Thus, reducing risks from whatever the cause will reduce human suffering. However, if we distinguish between the causes of each type of risk, those resulting from human activities are, in principle, avoidable if human beings change their activities, whereas risks that arise from natural causes may or may not be so easily avoidable. If we risk injuring or killing one another by driving our cars, these risks are potentially avoidable, even though we may choose not to avoid them, or it may be undesirable to avoid them because the loss of benefits from having automobiles would be too great. By contrast, no matter where one lives, one is exposed to cosmic rays; the higher the altitude at which one lives, the greater the risk of contracting cancer as a result of such exposure. Such risks may be avoidable, but only at considerable cost (e.g., living in lead-lined buildings, possibly wearing lead-lined clothes). Other natural risks (e.g., exposure to malaria-infected mosquitoes breeding in swamps) might be more easily avoided (e.g., by draining the swamps or by moving away).

  This distinction between naturally caused and humanly caused risks does not take us very far morally. Nevertheless, some commentators appear to conflate these two, apparently thinking that merely by comparing the probabilities of harm from the two classes of activities the difference between humanly and naturally caused risks is not worth remarking. Thus, for instance, Morrall remarks that:

> There is an 2-in-100,000 annual risk of cancer from background radiation at sea level, from drinking one beer a day, or from receiving an average number of diagnostic X-rays.[5]

He further states that "other activities, both voluntary and involuntary, also carry cancer risks that are substantially greater relative to those that are targets of regulatory control."[6] Notice that he has compared naturally occurring risks, voluntarily incurred risks from dietary (or enjoyment) considerations, and risks incurred in trying to detect and prevent, if necessary, life-threatening diseases. His description suggests an implicit argument that, since naturally occurring risks are as bad as, or worse than, humanly produced risks, these risks are all in some sense properly *comparable.* Although it might be true these risks have a similar *probability* of producing the same endpoint harm, cancer, their acceptability varies substantially. Diagnostic x-ray studies used to try to detect a life-threatening disease or other substantial disease threats are probably much more acceptable to individuals than similar risks that are incurred from drinking polluted drinking water. An argumentative strategy such as Morrall's is often used to persuade an audience that those risks that are caused by human activities are more acceptable than risks that are naturally caused. It might then be argued that if humanly caused risks are lower than naturally caused ones, then there is no need to worry about the first.

However, the implicit argument is not persuasive. We cannot merely compare the probability of risks associated with naturally and humanly caused risks and rest content that we have dealt adequately with the issue of acceptability of exposure to risks. Humanly caused risks are imposed on a person by institutions or practices that could be changed (or in some cases that imposed by the agent himself or herself, e.g., by smoking). And such risks typically have at least some compensating benefits, whereas naturally caused risks might not. Such benefits may or may not be sufficient to justify the risks; that is a separate matter. Moreover, on the morality of risk exposure, human activities may be judged right or wrong, just or unjust, defensible or not, whereas none of these predicates apply to natural phenomena or apply only in metaphorical or extended senses.

## B. The Magnitude of the Harm, if the Risk Materializes

A second consideration in judging the acceptability of risks is the magnitude of the harm that will befall persons if the risk materializes. Some risks will materialize into death, others into serious irreversible injuries, some into serious, but reversible injuries (e.g., broken ribs or legs), and still others into relatively minor injuries. Such harms may also be mental or physical, but we restrict our discussion to physical and health harms. And, for the most part we consider only risk of death as the harm of concern. This is not to ignore the importance of risks of serious reversible or serious irreversible harms that may befall one.

Clearly the magnitude of a harm, if it materializes, is *a consideration* in judging the acceptability of risk exposure. It is not the only and not necessarily the most important, however. Mountain climbers may appropriately judge that taking life-threatening risks in climbing are more acceptable despite the greater magnitude of injury they pose than the threat of serious disease from pollution. Thus, other factors relevant to acceptability of risk exposure can outweigh the magnitude of the harm posed by the risk.

## C. The Magnitude of Benefits that Accompany Risks

Third, benefits may or may not be produced as a result of risk exposure, but if they are, their magnitude is a relevant consideration in judging the acceptability of risk exposure. Benefits for an individual may be lifesaving (analogous to lifetaking risks), or important, but not lifesaving, or even minor or trivial. The magnitude of benefits accompanying risks both for each individual and for the group affected is important to an overall judgment of acceptability. Thus, some comparison of the magnitude of the harms risked with the magnitude of the benefits realized by the individual affected is pertinent to the acceptance of the risk in question. A similar balancing of benefits and harms to society as a whole is also relevant to the acceptability of social risks, but this is a more complex issue, for there are several different normative views for judging the acceptability of social risks and harms. We return to an aspect of this distributive issue later.

## D. The Probability of Harms and Benefits

The probabilities of harms and benefits from a course of action clearly are important considerations in judging the acceptability of risks. Much of the discussion about comparative risk exposure concerns the relative probabilities that different risks will materialize into harm. Many discussions involving comparative risk judgments appear to stop with a recitation of the probabilities of two different risks of death, and some appear to assume that the risk having the higher probability is the one we should be more concerned about. Although this may be true *when all other features of risk exposures are equal,* the other features are rarely equal for many risk comparisons. Many other facets of risk exposure may also be relevant to judgments of acceptability.

## E.  Voluntary Versus Involuntary Exposure to Risk

A fourth distinction needed for thinking about the acceptability of risks and the use of risk assessment is that between voluntarily and involuntarily incurred risks. Both humanly caused and naturally caused risks may be voluntarily incurred, for one may choose to put oneself next to a volcano that is about to explode and one may choose to walk across a busy freeway or street at rush hour. Voluntarily placing oneself at risk, in the sense of deliberately making decisions that place oneself in danger, does not, however, imply that one is necessarily *aware* of the nature, extent, and magnitude of the risk.[7] Many of us have voluntarily consumed our favorite alcoholic beverage, but were likely unaware that ethanol is a carcinogen or that we were taking some (quite small) chance of contracting cancer as a consequence. We may voluntarily perform an act that has various risks without being aware or at least fully aware of many features of the act or of the risks it presents. Voluntariness in exposure to risk is thus one consideration in assessing the moral acceptability of exposure to risks, but by itself in this limited sense does not possess much moral weight.

## F.  Voluntary and Knowing Exposure to Risks

Fifth, thus, we should distinguish between *voluntarily* and *knowingly* putting oneself at risk from humanly or naturally caused forces and voluntarily but *unknowingly* doing so.[8] These distinctions are often ignored in much of the literature that indiscriminately compares risks—note the foregoing Morrall statement that conflates voluntarily incurred risks such as drinking beer with involuntarily incurred risks from exposure to background radiation at sea level. Either act might have been done knowingly.

Conflating risks that one voluntarily and knowingly incurs with those that one involuntarily incurs blurs an important distinction. Our legal system and most moralities place substantial importance on this distinction and recognize it in the principle *volenti nonfit inuria*—"he who consents cannot receive an injury."[9] The idea behind this aphorism is that he who has voluntarily and knowingly consented to a risk of harm that materializes is not in a position to complain that an injustice has been done to him.[10] What activities count as those to which we might have voluntarily and knowingly assented requires further discussion. Whether, for example, choice of employment, which poses considerable risks to one's health, is one that is either fully voluntary or fully informed is a much more open question and one that requires more discussion. (We return to this in Sec. III.)

Furthermore, most of us would agree that a person might knowingly and voluntarily incur greater objective risks (e.g., in mountain climbing, motorcycling, or boxing) than it is morally justifiable to impose on a person unknowingly and involuntarily (e.g., fugitive emissions from a benzene or vinyl chloride plant, or perchloroethylene or carbon tetrachloride from a dry-cleaning establishment). Thus, from a normative point of view the magnitude and probability of risks are not determinative, especially where one incurs them knowingly and voluntarily.

In an empirical study, Starr argued that the general public voluntarily accepts risks that are three orders of magnitude (1000 times) greater than risk posed by involuntary exposures.[11] Thus, if he is correct, objective probabilities and magnitudes of risks are not considered determinative of the acceptability of risk, even by the general public.

However, just because persons knowingly and voluntarily take greater responsibility for risks than they would accept if they were involuntarily imposed, it does not follow that such elevated risks should become the standard for a whole community. Yet, curiously, some authors seem to suggest this by inviting us to compare the "objective risks" from activities central to particular plans of life, such as mountaineering or skiing, with risks not central to one's plan of life or even with involuntary exposure to risks. Such comparisons, conflating involuntarily incurred, naturally caused, or humanly caused risks with those knowingly and voluntarily assumed, misleads us, commits a kind of moral mistake, and blurs important distinctions.

Compared with the foregoing pair of cases is the contrast between involuntarily incurred, humanly caused risks that materialize to harm one versus voluntarily and knowingly assumed human risks that harm one.[12] When others have imposed risks of harm on one without one's knowledge and the risks materialize into harm, this is much closer to a matter of injustice. (One needs a theory of justice according to which such treatment would indeed be unjust.) Had the victim suffered the same harm as a consequence of knowingly and voluntarily incurring risks of harm, this would not typically be a matter of injustice (perhaps in part because of the *volenti fit inuria* principle cited earlier). None of these arguments is decisive because the issues are quite complicated, but they serve as reminders that risks carry with them quite different moral properties, depending on some of the distinctions just indicated. Merely comparing objective risks expressed in numerical injury or death rates obscures such properties and frustrates understanding.

## 1. The Palpability of Risks

An important species of knowing risk exposure concerns what we might call the *palpability* of the risks in question. By this we mean that the risk is easily perceptible by one of the senses, or by the mind.[13] Exposure to various chemical carcinogens (e.g., trichloroethylene or chloroform in drinking water, or benzene or vinyl chloride in the air) may place one at risk without one being continuously reminded of the risk in question or its consequences for one. Such risks should be contrasted with those for which one is continuously and palpably made aware of the possibility of harm. Some risks are accompanied by obvious reminders of the harm that can materialize (e.g., a stamping machine operator needs little imagination or reminding to know what a stamping machine can do to his arms or legs should they get into the press, and a sawyer is continually reminded that a saw can do to his appendages what it does to timber). The palpability of risks serves to keep the *awareness* of the possibility and magnitude of harm before one, so that one can better exercise caution, care, and control in providing self-protection. Conversely, where risks are not palpable, those exposed need better protections, because they have greater difficulty *detecting* the risks, they may have a lesser awareness of them, and thus realistically they are less able to protect themselves. It is also a mistake to suggest which risks that are palpable and voluntarily incurred should be used to set the standard for regulating involuntarily incurred, nonpalpable risks imposed by the actions of others, yet some suggest such arguments.[14]

## 2. The Appreciation of Risks

Moreover, clear warnings because of the palpability of risks or because of posted notices may not ensure that one is properly fully aware of a risk. Although one has in some sense been put on notice about the possible harm, one may not have the appropriate appreciation of the risk in that one recognizes the properties of the risk and its consequences for one through judgment, perception, or insight.[15] Ordinarily if a risk is palpable, one would also have appreciation of its consequences, but since there is no logical or evidentiary guarantee of this, the two concepts are treated separately. Moreover, the idea of appreciation goes beyond the ideas of either knowledge or the palpability of a risk, since it suggests one has appropriate recognition of the risk for oneself. Thus, one must be both aware of a risk and have proper understanding and appreciation of it to have incurred it knowingly.

We have considered several features of risks that bear to some extent on our judgment of a person's responsibility for harm suffered when risks materialize and on features of risk exposure that would affect the level of risks to which we might think one should be exposed. The more one is palpably aware of, appreciates, and thus knowingly incurs a risk, the less concern we typically would have in preventing one from being exposed to such a risk and the higher the risks we would likely tolerate in our own case or others, other things equal (assuming one is a normal adult human being with at least average intelligence). Moreover, it is certainly permissible for people to incur such risks, but this permissible level of risks surely should not set the required standard of risk exposure for a whole community. The less such features are present, the more important it is to prevent such harms from occurring, especially for humanly caused risks, and the more concern we would have to lower the odds of a person being harmed, for persons in these circumstances can do much less to protect themselves.[16]

## G.  The Avoidability of Risky Courses of Action

The features discussed to this point do not exhaust the properties of risk exposure that bear on its acceptability. We also want to know how avoidable the risks are. To the extent that it is difficult to avoid exposure to risks, this argues for greater protection from them, if it is available and feasible. If one cannot avoid humanly produced air pollution, or can avoid it only at great cost and inconvenience, this argues for better protections from it. At the other extreme when risks are easily avoidable, much less protection may be justified. Thus, risks from mountaineering are easily avoidable through abstention in the activity. A number of facets of risk exposure bear on the issue of avoidability: alternatives open to one, control over the risks, sacrifices incurred in avoiding them, and the centrality of risks to one's life.

### 1.  Alternatives to Risky Courses of Action

The fewer alternatives there are to risky activities and the harder risks are to avoid, other things being equal, the more this calls for preventive and protective measures, if they can be provided. For example, if air is polluted, there are few alternatives to breathing it, thus making a case for removing or reducing the pollution.

The issue of alternatives to a risky course of action does not take us very far. If our drinking water were polluted with carcinogens, many people could easily avoid the risks by drinking bottled water. However, the norms implicit in the *public* nature of a water supply tend to argue for cleaning it up, even if there are some readily available alternatives to drinking it.

Social alternatives to using toxic substances are especially important in judging the risks from exposure to these substances. Are there other substances that serve the same purposes, but without such high risks? Clearly in judging the acceptability of risks imposed on the society at large, we want to know the facets of the acceptability of the particular risky action, but also all facets of the acceptability of all the alternatives to it before we can make some judgment of the overall acceptability of the risk.

### 2.  Degree of Control Over the Risk

We should distinguish between those risks to which we voluntarily and knowingly consent, but over which we do not exercise much continuing control, and those over which we have some considerable control. The point? Risks over which we have considerable control are more avoidable through our own actions than those over which we have less control. For example, one may voluntarily and knowingly incur risks while driving one's car, but can one control such risks to some extent by driving defensively and by using safety devices. There is a spectrum of one's ability to control risks, ranging from those for which one has no control (e.g., when one is in the midst of an earthquake), to those for which one has considerable control over the outcome (e.g., when one is an expert machinist working with dangerous equipment or when one is an expert rock climber on good hard rock). And there is a spectrum of control concerning the extent to which one has put oneself in a position to be exposed to risks. The greater continuing control one has over a risky situation, the less intervention by others may be needed to protect one. Again this is a complicated matter and true only if everything else is equal.

Failure to make these distinctions again betrays an insensitivity to the complexity of the issues involved, perhaps even a kind of moral insensitivity. We might well tolerate ourselves and others having greater exposure to risks when they are knowingly and voluntarily incurred and over which participants have considerable control than we would when similar risks were imposed by others without knowledge, consent, or control, or when the risks were imposed on us knowingly and voluntarily, but over which we might not have much continuing control. Roughly speaking, other things being equal, greater control over risk exposure and over the materializing of risks carries with it greater responsibility for the outcome, for one can do much to protect oneself. To the extent one lacks control over whether risks materialize and, thus, can do less to protect oneself, other things being equal, the greater the need for protection from the risks. The more control one has, the higher the risks a community might tolerate, if it could influence the level of risk exposure. This appears to accord with Starr's results noted earlier.

The upshot of the preceding paragraph is that it is a conceptual and a moral mistake for one to argue that, because people incur greater risks in activities over which they have considerable control than they incur from emissions of carcinogens from industrial plants (risks over which they have little or no control), the risks from carcinogens should not be regulated or should be regulated so that the risks from carcinogens are as high as those to which we have control over. The mistake is for one implicitly to argue that, other things being equal, the risks that one has considerable ability to control set the standard below which there should be no regulation for involuntarily incurred risks.[17]

### 3. Sacrifice Incurred in the Alternatives

Once we have the idea that a complex factor analysis is important to judging the acceptability of a course of action, we see that it is also important to take account of the sacrifices that might be required to avoid a particular risk. The greater the required sacrifice of one's interests to avoid risk, the less acceptable the risk is likely to be. If avoiding a risk would require changing one's life in unacceptable ways, then the risk is less acceptable and less to be used as a standard for comparing other risks. For instance, if one can avoid risks from airborne malathion spraying only by leaving home during the spraying, such a personal cost might seem exceedingly high. Sacrifice is a cost; the greater the sacrifice the greater the cost and, thus, a reason for reducing the risks in the present course of action.

## H. Centrality of Risks to One's Life

The previous points (Sec. G.1–G.3) are related to deeper views about the centrality of risks to one's life plans. Certain moral views place great importance on an individual having the capacity to choose, revise, and act on her or his own conceptions of the good life.[18] Thus, one might with full knowledge have embraced a particular kind of life (e.g., one that centrally involves mountain climbing), and the goals of such a life may be inseparable from risks, risks that are greater than those faced by the general populace. The more that risky activities are central to one's plan of life, and the more that they are part of what makes life worth living, the more acceptable they are to the individual. In such cases, the objective nature of the risk may be less significant in assessing its acceptability to the person or to others. Such people, thus, embrace or at least accept the risks as part of the kind of lives they live. Most moral traditions consider such choices as quite permissible, recognizing these life-enhancing features. Thus, it would be a mistake to compare risks from activities (e.g., mountaineering or scuba diving) that are central to one's life plan with those that are not central and not "chosen" at all (e.g., involuntary exposure to TCE in drinking water or benzene in the air).

Of course, avoiding risks that are central to one's life would require great sacrifice and thus seems inconsistent with the previous point. However, we distinguish between sacrifices required to avoid unwanted risks imposed by others and sacrifices required to avoid risks that are an integral part to what makes our lives worth living.

## I. The Distribution of Risks and Environmental Justice

To this point we have considered individual risks to persons in isolation from other risks and different aspects of their acceptability. However, this has ignored cumulative risks, as well as the distribution of risks in a community. As with previous discussions, we cannot have an extensive assessment of the issue, but some points are in order. First, persons are typically exposed to multiple risks, both those resulting from the everyday activities of life as well as those from substances that might be subject to regulation. Thus, any consideration of the acceptability of risk exposure must take account such cumulative effects, because these may be unduly burdensome for particular individuals or groups in the community. Second, whether they are unacceptably burdensome is a question of justice, a question of whether they are too much for one person or group, and a question of the burdens imposed on an exposed group in the community, compared with the burdens imposed on others in the community. A principle frequently appealed to in order to address such questions, namely, utilitarianism, or its offspring, cost–benefit analysis, has difficulty accounting for such distributive considerations. Utilitarianism and its offspring tend to focus on maximizing overall community welfare; this may, except for very special versions of these views, tend to ignore the distribution of risks and benefits as well as ignoring minimal protections for persons.[19] By contrast, theories of justice tend to account better for both considerations. For example, according to the best contemporary theory of justice, unequal distributions of wealth in basic institutions, such as the economic system, are to be arranged so that they "are the greatest benefit of the least advantaged [representative] person . . . "[20] Thus, this principle suggests that, in the distributions of harms and benefits that affect a person's wealth, including risks, the avoidance of adversely affecting those who are already in the worst off group in the community is an important consideration. That is, further exposure of persons in such groups to greater risks is justified only if they will be better off as a result of such exposure than they otherwise would have been compared with alternative distributions. However, this appears to be a claim difficult to justify, because, as a matter of fact, in the United States, for example, there are already a number of people in many communities who are suffering from poverty, disease, lack of opportunities, and such. Their exposure to additional life-threatening risks would not likely be permissible on such considerations of justice. If this is correct, such a principle, or one similar to it, provides the moral foundation for some of the claims of the environmental justice movement.

Principles, such as Rawls', accommodate both comparative judgments between groups in the community (they are bearing an unjust burden of social life in comparison to others) and judgments that some groups have already been disadvantaged too much by the exigencies of life and social arrangements (they have been burdened too much in comparison with a baseline distribution). Any adequate risk management policy should, thus also take into account these comparative and cumulative effects.

## III.  SOME APPLICATIONS OF THE MATRIX

Once we have some of the foregoing distinctions, the arguments comparing various risks become more sophisticated, more obviously dependent on implicit moral theories and, thus, the arguments about the acceptability of risks become more philosophical, with fundamental ideas dividing those who disagree. Nonetheless, several arguments for certain uses of risk assessment must be evaluated because the moral issues they raise are of considerable moment.

### A.  Some Common Mistakes

#### *1.  The Alar Argument*

Alar is a systemic growth regulator sprayed on apple trees and other plants to make the fruit stay on the plant longer, ripen more slowly, stay firmer longer, have a longer shelf life, and retain color and attractive properties longer. Its metabolites in the body are also, apparently, fairly potent carcinogens.[21] The salient feature about Alar is that many people have argued that substantial benefits come from using it, even though its metabolites appear to be a potent human carcinogen. However, this argument commits a certain kind of mistake or at least begs an important question. The magnitude of the *benefits to individuals* from Alar is relatively minor—using it provides fruit on a more nearly year-round basis, makes its nutritional benefits available longer, prolongs shelf life, keeps fruits firmer looking for a longer time period. The magnitude of the *harm* to individuals threatened by Alar, however, is life-threatening if, in fact Alar, and some of its metabolites are potent carcinogens for human beings, as the EPA and the California Environmental Protection Agency have judged them to be.[22] Alar presents relatively minor benefits to each of millions of people while posing a low probability of the most serious harm to those who ingest it or who work with it in the fields. Summed over many people, Alar appears to have huge benefits, compared with very low probability risks to some. Even though the magnitude of the risk to each individual posed by Alar is not at all comparable with the magnitude of the benefits provided to each person, the cumulative benefits appear to outweigh the possible harms. While this seems to be an obviously acceptable trade-off to some, because of the great discrepancy between the magnitude of the benefits provided and the magnitude of the harms threatened to each person, for most people, I believe, this is not obviously an acceptable risk. Whether it is or not depends on more fundamental moral views, an extensive discussion of which is beyond this paper, but a few remarks are in order.

Some ethical theories would compare such serious risks and minor benefits quite readily and use the minor benefits to many to outweigh life-threatening risks to a few. Utilitarianism would compare the probability of the benefits times the magnitude of the benefits times the number of people benefited with the probability of harm times the magnitude of the harms times the number of people likely to be harmed. Then, this complex cross product would be compared with alternative ways of providing fruits and vegetables to the public. The alternative with the highest net cross product would be the correct course of action.[23] However, many ethical theories attend to considerations that the utilitarian theories ignore or weigh them differently. In particular, such theories attend to the *magnitude* of the benefits and harms *to discrete individuals,* and they pay attention to the *distribution* of the benefits and harms to individuals.[24] Other moral views would emphasize the *incomparability* between the minor benefits to each person of using Alar on the one hand, even though millions are so benefited, versus the great magnitude of harms to each person that might befall a few, on the other. Such views take seriously the importance of each person and tend to be typical of justice theories. The public may well implicitly take account of such considerations in its reaction to the use of Alar in apples and other produce.

The point here, however, is not to argue for one ethical theory or the other, for space does not permit it, but rather to point out that on a fairly straightforward issue, such as the acceptability of risks posed by Alar, fundamental moral issues of the acceptability of risks for individuals and for the community bear on these questions. Consequently, judging the acceptability of risks is not a simple matter of comparison of the probability and the magnitude of benefits and harms times the number of people affected, for this ignores other features of the acceptability of risks to individuals and to the public at large. Any judgment of the acceptability of such risks must take these other features into account. A more elaborate argument on these points will have to be developed elsewhere.

### 2.  *The Chloroform Argument*

The next argument is the "chloroform argument," so named because some suggest that the risks from chloroform, a carcinogen, in drinking water constitute a normative standard against which to judge the acceptability of all risks the government should regulate. Such critics argue that, since chlorine in our drinking water reacts with the organic material in the water to produce chloroform and other trihalomethanes, carcinogens both, and since we incur certain low level risks from these carcinogens, we should not regulate any carcinogens to which we are exposed to lower levels of risk than the risks posed by chloroform and trihalomethanes.[25] In short, the risk of contracting cancer from exposure to chloroform in drinking water[26] sets the appropriate standard for all other exposures to carcinogens.

This is a nonsequitur. Chlorine is added to water to protect human beings from a variety of diseases and possibly death that are posed by organic material and bacteria in water. Furthermore, according to the Environmental Protection Agency's Office of Drinking Water, the risks of death and disease posed by biological materials in water are much greater than the risks of death and disease posed by exposure to chloroform in drinking water.[27] The invalidity in the chloroform argument is this: just because the use of chlorine in water protects us against much greater risks of death and disease than the risks presented by the chloroform and trihalomethanes in water, it does not follow that we should set the levels of risk presented by chloroform to be the standard for all carcinogens to which we might be exposed from whatever source and whatever benefits are derived from them.

By analogy, while it may be permissible for you to break my leg or to risk breaking it when knocking me out of the way of an oncoming train or car (because this probably prevents me from suffering even greater injuries), it does not follow that it is permissible for you to go around breaking people's legs or to risk breaking their legs when this is not a means to prevent them from some probability of suffering substantial harms.

A variation on the chloroform argument might be that, since we have long consented to and lived with cancer risks from chloroform in our drinking water, this shows the level of risks we are prepared to live with, and thus should set the standard appropriate for regulating risks from other carcinogens.

This argument is similarly not persuasive. First, the notion of consent would be misplaced if the community were not aware that it faced certain lifetime risks of contracting cancer. In many cases of industrially produced carcinogens in our food, air, or water, we are not likely to be aware of risks from them, much less that we are palpably reminded of them and appreciate the nature of the risks. However, even if we grant that the community was aware of the nature and extent of such risks, it does not follow that such risk levels should set the standard for other regulatory purposes. Again, if the community had consented to the risks from chloroform *in order to protect itself from even greater harms,* it does not follow that it *has,* or that it *would,* or that it *should* consent to the same level of risks from carcinogens that do not similarly protect it from such substantial harms. Much more by way of argument would have to be offered in each case. Finally, even if the community has consented to risks from carcinogens from certain substances in certain contexts, it does not follow that the level of risk thereby consented to should set the standard for other, disanalogous cases. Thus, even if such a consent argument were a plausible one, which is doubtful because of the probable absence of awareness and appreciation of the nature, extent, and magnitude of the risk, it does not follow that this is a plausible rationale to set the standard for other risks.

### 3. The Peanut Butter Argument

Similar arguments have been used concerning naturally occurring carcinogens that occur in our food. For example, peanuts, peanut butter, corn, and raw mushrooms, all appear to contain carcinogens—some of them possibly more potent than industrial carcinogens that may invade our water or air.[28] Call this the "peanut butter" argument. It is argued that since we are at risk from such carcinogens in our food, this "consent level" of risk should set the standard for exposure to other carcinogens in our environment.

This argument is not plausible. It is even more doubtful in this case than for chloroform that we have *with awareness of the risks involved* legitimately consented to be exposed to such risks. For one thing we are only just now learning of the risks presented by many carcinogens that occur naturally in our foods (if in fact they have such effects when part of a complex food).[29] If these have come as recent scientific discoveries, we can hardly have consented as individuals or as a community to take the risk of contracting cancer from eating these substances. And, even if some scientists are aware of such risks, this information is not appreciated by the public at large. If we now know the public is exposed to several potent carcinogens in its food, consumers could be put on notice so they could avoid such substances and this might make a substantial difference in their behavior. This typically has not been done, however. Moreover, it does not follow that we should use the level of carcinogens in our food to set regulatory levels for other carcinogens. Just because we may be burdened by carcinogens in our foods, it does not follow that we should add to our body burdens because the *individual risks* from humanly produced carcinogens are no higher in magnitude and probability than the individual risks from naturally occurring carcinogens. The *cumulative* effect of adding many such humanly produced carcinogens could be substantial over the long run, and there may be synergistic effects from exposure to many carcinogens.

There are some differences between the chloroform and peanut butter arguments. Chlorine, which produces chloroform in drinking water, protects us from risks of even greater harms than those posed by the chloroform. No such claim can be made on behalf of peanut butter, mushrooms, or charbroiled meats. Any justification for remaining exposed to aflatoxins in peanut butter or corn rests on our traditional use of such foods,[30] on the centrality of the foods to our lives, on their nutritional benefits, or on our consenting to the presence of carcinogens, none of which is particularly weighty. Even the nutritional benefits of any *single* food are probably not decisive, although the *cumulative* nutritional benefits from a number of foods containing naturally occurring carcinogens might be substantial. Thus, the peanut butter argument is not as seriously flawed as the chloroform argument, but it remains unsound.

There is a generalization to the chloroform and peanut butter arguments. Critics suggest that because there are a number of (even many) carcinogens to which we are exposed naturally, through our food and water, we should not have much concern for industrially induced carcinogens, many of which are much less potent substances than the naturally occurring ones.[31] However, just because we are exposed to or have consented to exposure to many carcinogens in the past, it does not follow that we should permit exposure to more carcinogens. Just because we have consented to some bad things in our lives (if in fact we have so *consented,* many times a doubtful assumption), it does not follow we should be exposed to more harmful substances. The argument is not persuasive with reference to harmful drugs, (e.g., alcohol or marijuana); it seems no more persuasive for carcinogens. Moreover, it ignores the cumulative effects of many individual exposures. As a matter of social policy we should seek to minimize the harms to which we are exposed.

### 4.  *Comparative Risk Arguments*

A fourth argument placed in doubt by the matrix of considerations pertinent to the acceptability of risks are "comparative risk arguments." Such arguments are generalizations of the foregoing arguments, but they deserve separate comment because of the generality of the mistake committed. Some authors (e.g., Wilson and Crouch;[32] as well as Morrall, cited earlier) explicitly compare the magnitude and probability of risks that tend to be quite different and suggest that risks of similar magnitude and probability may be comparably acceptable. For instance, in one table,[33] they compare the annual risk from motor vehicle accidents, air pollution in the eastern United States, sea level background radiation, chloroform in drinking water within the EPA limit, police killed in the line of duty, and mountaineering. Enough has been said to illustrate the difficulty with suggesting that the acceptability of these risks is the same or suggesting that they should be compared in some straightforward way on grounds of probability and magnitude.

Although it is true that one can learn something about the relative probabilities of these risks by putting them into a common table where they can be compared, it is quite misleading to suggest their acceptability should be the same. It is important to know the magnitude and comparative probabilities of different risks, for, *if* our principle is that we should prevent the most likely risks of the same magnitude (e.g., death), this would dictate that we compare risks on magnitude and probability only. Moreover, this is quite consistent with a principle to prevent harm from befalling others. However, this is not the only moral consideration relevant in most circumstances. For example, the risk of death from automobile accidents, which is relatively high compared with some others, is a risk over which individuals have considerable control. And we appear to recognize that they have such control because we teach driver training and defensive driving believing that that is important to reducing the chances of an accident. Such control introduces an additional moral consideration. We might do more to prevent such accidents; that is a separate matter. But the simple comparison of the probability of such risks can be quite misleading.

Wilson and Crouch similarly compare morally disanalogous risks by citing the chance of dying from sea level background radiation, a naturally caused risk that we cannot escape, except by adopting extremely expensive protective devices, such as living in lead houses or wearing lead suits, and greatly altering our lifestyle and undergoing great personal sacrifices. And they compare these kinds of risks with the EPA limit of chloroform in drinking water, which results from chlorinating our drinking water to protect us from other life-threatening harms. Finally, they include in the same table the risk of death to a frequent flying professor, whose trips may be critical to his profession and his way of life, and the risk of death from mountaineering, an activity that may well be central to a mountaineer's conception of life.

By implication in comparing these risks, Wilson and Crouch appear to commit several mistakes because the risks exhibit quite diverse levels of acceptability. For one thing, the acceptability of risks is the outcome of a complex weighing of magnitude, probability, avoidability, control over the risks, voluntariness of the risks, knowledge of the risks, distribution of risks, and so forth. In the end, the acceptability of a risk is an on-balance judgment of the relative importance of all of these properties to an individual (where we are talking about an individual making a judgment about the acceptability of these risks) or to the community as a whole in how these are weighed. Thus, to simplify the issues by focusing only on the magnitude of outcome if the risk materialized and the probability of that outcome and even the numbers of people affected is to ignore other substantial factors in the overall judgment of the acceptability of risk. Furthermore, they commit a kind of moral mistake, for they ignore a number of moral considerations that both individuals and the community take into account in making these judgments about the acceptability of risks. In addition, they lump together risks that are morally *permissible* (because they are voluntary and central to one's life and/or those over which persons have considerable control) with involuntarily imposed risks and, at least by juxtaposition, suggest that the permissible risks might set the required level of acceptability of risks for regulation. Moreover, they tend to compare life-threatening risks to individuals with nonlife-saving benefits, thereby begging a question of whether such comparisons are appropriate. Finally, they fail to give sufficient weight to risks that are central to one's life and that it is within one's prerogative to accept.

Some of the same considerations are apropos when we consider some of the risks from substances that are typically subject to regulation. For example, some substances to which we are exposed protect us from other life-threatening entities (e.g., chlorine in drinking water or anticancer drugs), whereas other potential carcinogens do not obviously hold out such promise (e.g., Alar in apples). For the former we tend to tolerate (correctly in my view) greater exposure than for the latter, precisely because of the lifesaving benefits. Thus, it is a difference in the magnitude of the benefits to individuals versus the potential harm to individuals that appears critical here. However, for many substances that are subject to regulation, the matrix discussed in this paper does not necessarily provide a way of discriminating between them. The reason is that virtually all such substances share a variety of risk characteristics that make them similar to each other (discussed in the next section), but quite different from the risk characteristics of many everyday activities (e.g., driving an automobile, being exposed to cosmic rays, dangerous recreational activities, and so forth). Typically, risks from substances subject to regulation as a group are more similar to each other than they are to many of the risks of every day life; that is what makes arguments comparing the risks of regulated substances with those of everyday activities pernicious. In fact, typically the risks posed by substances that are regulated have a number of special characteristics.

## B. Risk Management and What is Special About Carcinogens

When we focus on risks from carcinogens and other toxic substances, the considerations discussed earlier suggest why the management of exposure to such substances requires a more comprehensive approach to the acceptability of risk exposure. Carcinogens (which are used for illustrative purposes) have several properties that make them special, that call for sensitive evaluation of the moral acceptability of the risks they pose, and that suggest the need for special considerations in managing their risks.

Carcinogens are typically invisible, undetectable intruders that can cause catastrophic harms to the individuals affected after a long latency period and that typically, but not invariably, provide modest benefits in return. Moreover, they typically have a low probability of harm. However, for the most part exposure to them is involuntary and unknowing; any risks they pose are not palpable. And most environmental and workplace carcinogens are not easily avoidable, individuals do not have continuing control over the nature or extent of exposure, avoiding them may require great individual sacrifice, and exposure to them is not something that tends to make the exposed individuals' lives worth living.

This cluster of characteristics in conjunction with the foregoing distinctions and analysis tends to make a good case for more stringent preventive measures than for many other risks in our lives. The magnitude of the harm if it materializes to individuals is among the most serious, but the probabilities of such harms materializing are typically quite small. If these are the only considerations pertinent to judging the acceptability of risks posed, governmental agencies should place some such substances low on their list of priorities for attention.

However, carcinogens have numerous other properties that argue for greater attention and more stringent control by risk managers. Exposure to environmental carcinogens is ordinarily neither voluntary nor knowing, since they may be present in tiny amounts in our food, water, or air. Even if members of the public have some idea that carcinogens are present in some media, they are not palpably put on notice about this and, undoubtedly, fail to appreciate the nature and extent of the threat. Lack of palpability and appreciation both argue for more protective measures, since individuals cannot utilize their own senses and resources to protect themselves; nor given the *public* nature of such contaminated media should they be expected to. Because such exposures are typically involuntary, it is wrong to treat such risks as comparable with voluntary risk exposures or in the same way one might "regulate" exposures that are voluntary.

Moreover, such substances in the environment are not easily avoidable, for we typically do not have continuing control over them, avoiding them may require substantial sacrifices (e.g., selling of homes at losses, or giving up a good paying job and moving to a different area of the country), and ordinarily embracing risks from carcinogens are not central to persons' plans of life. Because they are not easily avoidable or avoidable only at great personal cost, these characteristics are a reason for providing greater protections so that exposure does not occur in the first place.

Workplace risks from carcinogens do not have all the properties of environmental risks. In particular it appears that they might be more easily avoidable and that exposure is more nearly voluntary and knowing. Although there is something to this claim, the apparent attractiveness of this argument can be misleading. Workplace exposures are less voluntary than they appear. Whereas some people have wide choices of employment, many do not and those with constrained choices are likely to be the ones in the heavily polluted industries. This deserves substantial investigation, which cannot be pursued here, but substantial subpopulations have little choice in place of employment. And, even if workers could choose their industry, this does not ensure that their knowledge and appreciation of exposure to carcinogenic risks will be very good. Carcinogens tend to be undetectable whether in the environment or in an industrial plant; to the extent this is true, it argues for providing greater protection for employees. Furthermore, as an additional normative claim, even if employees had greater choice and control over their workplaces, and even if the risks were more palpable and workers had greater appreciation of them, they should not face the Hobson's choice between a decent job and their health. Neither should lower costs of our consumer and economic goods be purchased at the price of their health. That is, fewer preventive regulations might lower the cost of goods produced, but it is a debatable issue when such a policy is justifiable. These complex issues are beyond the scope of this short discussion. However, what appears to be a plausible argument to separate environmental from workplace exposure to carcinogens is not obviously persuasive and is, in fact, quite problematic.

Finally, most carcinogens, unlike chloroform produced in chlorinated drinking water, do not save us from more serious harms than they pose. If they do, however, this is a significant consideration that should weigh in the balance in favor of permitting such exposures, provided there are no safer substitutes that do the job better. However, if there are substances or processes (e.g., ozonization vs. chlorine), that will do the same job with lower risks to our health at about the same cost, it is not defensible to use the more dangerous substance or process.

The general point of the remarks in this concluding section is that the acceptability of risk exposure is a complicated on-balance judgment involving many factors. Risk managers should recognize and acknowledge the plurality of considerations that go into such judgments and take them into account in making decisions about which risks have priority and which to manage. It is difficult to give general guidance because of the complexity of the issues and because decisions will have to be made on a case-by-case basis. However, enough should have been said to discourage the use of simple heuristics and comparisons between the ordinary risks of life, such as those incurred in our recreation (e.g., mountaineering or sky diving), or in every day activities (e.g., driving our cars) and the risks of carcinogens in the environment. Moreover, similar cautions apply to risk communication. Although there may be occasions on which it is insightful to call attention to the low probability of a risk by comparing it with ordinary risks of life, the foregoing discussion suggests such communicative strategies can also be quite misleading if the public has a rich and complicated matrix for judging the acceptability of risks. While I have presented the case for these conclusions on normative grounds, Paul Slovic has reached similar conclusions from empirical investigations.

Slovic concludes his paper "Perception of Risk"[34] with the following passage:

Perhaps the most important message from this research is that there is wisdom as well as error in public attitudes and perceptions. Lay people sometimes lack certain information about hazards. However, *their basic conceptualization of risk is much richer than that of the experts and reflects legitimate concerns that are typically omitted from expert risk assessments.* As a result, risk communication and risk management efforts are destined to fail unless they are structured as a two-way process. *Each side, expert and public, has something valid to contribute. Each side must respect the insights and intelligence of the other.*[35]

Thus, the philosophical theses argued for in this paper and the risk perception research done by Slovic appear largely to converge. Some people, largely the experts on risk assessment and risk management, tend to focus on the probability and magnitude of the risks faced by the public, and tend to ignore a much broader conceptualization of legitimate and valid considerations that go into judging the acceptability of risk. The broader matrix for judging the acceptability of risk is quite legitimate. To ignore such considerations is to commit both conceptual and moral mistakes. Thus, in managing risks we must appreciate the legitimate and complex matrix that goes into making these risk judgments and we must make comparative risk judgments with care.

## NOTES

1. An earlier draft of this was read at the UCLA Legal & Moral Philosophy Discussion Group. Ken Dickey provided valuable research assistance in the writing of this paper. Research on this paper was supported by the University of California Toxic Substances Research and Teaching Program and by NSF research grant #DIR-8912782 (1990–93).

2. Rescher, N. *Risk: A Philosophic Introduction to the Theory of Risk Evaluation and Management,* Washington, D.C.: University Press of America, 1983, 5.

3. The assessment of *risks,* where the probability distribution of some harm is known is contrasted with *uncertainty,* where the probabilities of loss or harm are not known. Very often risk assessment is more characterized by the many *uncertainties* in trying to estimate probabilities of harm than by known or narrowly identified *probabilities.*

4. The idea of "acceptable," "morally justified," or "morally defensible" risks is a complex and difficult one. Lack of space prohibits a general account of these issues here. However, one burden of the paper is to draw attention to considerations that bear on the justification of risks. For a discussion of moral

justification see Franbura, W. *Ethics,* 2nd ed., Englewood Cliffs, NJ, Prentice-Hall, 1970, and Feldman, F. *Introductory Ethics,* Englewood Cliffs, NJ, Prentice-Hall, 1978.

5. Morrall, J. F. A review of the record. *Regulation.* November/December, p. 27, 1986.

6. Ibid.

7. The logic of ordinary language is not decisive on this issue; thus, for purposes of clarity I treat the voluntariness of risk exposure as logically distinct from knowing risk exposure.

8. Perhaps voluntarily exposing oneself to a risk implies that one does so knowingly, but I think not as the alcohol example shows, thus at least initially the two concepts should be kept separate for conceptual purposes.

9. *Black's Law Dictionary,* St. Paul, Minnesota: West Publishing, 1968. 1746. A better statement of this might be "to he who consents no injustice is done," or "he who consents has no right to complain." The first is better than Black's definition because clearly a person can be injured, even though he may not be treated unjustly, since he consented. The second alternative is weaker than the first; if a person has consented to his treatment, this may eliminate his legitimate right to complain, but it may not eliminate all claims that he was treated unjustly.

10. Of course, even this characterization of the principle is too simple. One can knowingly and voluntarily be exposed to risks, but do so because of facing constrained choices—one's choice range may not be very broad.

11. Starr, C. *Perspective on Benefit Risk Decision-Making,* Washington DC, National Academy of Sciences, 1972. However, that there has been considerable discussion of this methodology, so we should not regard this work as definitive.

12. Rescher, N. *Risk: A Philosophical Analysis* notes one can be "at risk" without voluntarily and knowingly having "taken a risk."

13. This account is fairly close to the meaning of the term as defined in *Webster's Third International Dictionary of the English Language* (Springfield, Mass.: G. and C. Merriam and Co., 1966), p. 106.

14. Wilson R., Crouch, E. A. Risk assessment and comparisons: An introduction, *Science,* 236, 267–270; The authors create a table in which they compare the estimates of risks of harm from air pollution and from a policeman being killed in the line of duty. The latter activity presents more *palpable* and *voluntary* incurred risk than the former.

15. Ibid.

16. This analysis may appear quite individualistic in the sense of focusing on individual responsibility for exposure to at least some risks. Whereas this is true for voluntary incurred risks, I do not suggest that individuals should bear the burden of avoiding risks that are in the public media—air, water, food, and in the workplace.

17. Wilson and Crouch, Risk assessment and comparisons: An introduction, appear to blur this distinction. They begin "Everyday we take risks and avoid others." This seems to ignore the point that one can be *at risk* (unknowingly and involuntarily) without *taking a risk* (knowingly and voluntarily).

18. Rawls, J. Social unity and primary goods. In *Utilitarism and Beyond,* Cambridge, Cambridge University Press, 1982, 159–187. Rawls, J. A. *Theory of Justice.* Cambridge, MA: Harvard University Press. 1971; and Scheffler, S. *The Rejection of Consequentialism,* Oxford, Clarendon Press, 1982.

19. Cranor, C. F. *Regulating Toxic Substances: A Philosophy of Science and Law.* New York: Oxford University Press; 1993, 163–168.

20. Rawls. *A Theory of Justice.* 1971, 302.

21. Zeise, L., et al., Alar in fruit: Limited regulatory action in the face of uncertain risks. In Gorick and Gesler, ed. *The Analysis, Communication and Perception of Risk,* New York, Plenum Press, 1991, 275–284.

22. Zeise, et al., Alar in fruit.

23. Frankena, W. *Ethics,* New York, Prentice-Hall, 1977.

24. Rawls, J. A. *Theory of Justice,* Cambridge, MA, Harvard University Press, 1971; Scanlon T. M. Contractualism and utilitarianism. In Sen, A. and Williams, B. ed., *Utilitarianism and Beyond,* Cambridge, Cambridge University Press, 1982, 103–128.

25. Dr. Bruce Ames had made this argument before the State of California's Proposition 65 Science

Advisory Panel and in numerous other contexts as well. Ames, B. et al. Ranking possible carcinogenic hazards, *Science* 236:271–280, 1987.

26. Chlorinated drinking water consumed at the rate of 2 L/day over a 40-year lifetime appears to *double* the rate of bladder cancer. Reported by Kenneth Canter, "Bladder Cancer: Association with Water Source, Treatment and Consumption Level," at the California Department of Health Services Symposium "Mechanism of Carcinogenesis and Reproductive Toxicity: Implications for Public Health," Asilomar Conference Center, Pacific Grove, California, March 23–25, 1988.

27. Personal communication from Joseph Cotruvo, U.S. Environmental Protection Agency, Office of Drinking Water, July 1986.

28. Ames, B. Ranking of possible carcinogenic hazards, *Science* 236:273–275, 1987.

29. See Ames, ibid., and Ames, B. Dietary carcinogenics and anticarcinogens, *Science* 232:1256–1264, 1983.

30. Ames, B. Ranking, and Merrill, R. Regulating carcinogens in food: A legislator's guide to the food safety provisions of the Federal Food, Drug and Cosmetics Act. *Michigan Law Rev.* 77:171–250, 1979.

31. Even though this argument is not persuasive as a matter of social policy, from the perspective of an individual there may be some reason not to worry overly much about carcinogens in one's life. There may be so many naturally occurring carcinogens in my foods, in peanut butter, celery, mushrooms, charbroiled foods, fried foods, etc., that I may not reasonably be able to eliminate all of these from one's life. Trying to eliminate them may be nearly impossible. However, even if it were not, the attempt would take so much time and effort and render one's diet so bland that one may not choose to do so. Even from one's point of view, if one acknowledges all the carcinogens in one's diet, one may still prefer not to be exposed to *additional* carcinogens from human sources in the environment.

32. Wilson, R. and Crouch, E. A. C. Risk assessment and comparisons: An introduction, *Science,* 236:267–270, 1987.

33. Wilson, R. and Crouch, E. A. C. ibid., p. 268.

34. Slovic, P. Perception of risks, *Science,* 236:280–285, 1987.

35. Slovic, P. Perception of risks, ibid., p. 285. (emphasis added).

# 43
# Risk Assessment in Monitoring, Compliance, and Enforcement

**Barton P. Simmons**

*California Environmental Protection Agency*
*Berkeley, California*

## I. INTRODUCTION

This chapter discusses the use of risk assessment in monitoring, compliance, and enforcement. These activities are part of the risk management process, and are normally developed after an evaluation of public health, economic, social, and political consequences of regulatory options (NRC, 1983). The typical result is a risk-based limit, established in law or regulation. This chapter will discuss some common elements to any risk-based monitoring, which involves the collection of measurements and comparison with a risk-based limit. The problems associated with this process are discussed, along with examples of current applications.

Often the product of the risk assessment process is a single concentration limit for each medium, such as air, water, or food, usually with no estimate of the associated uncertainty. As risk-derived standards have been lowered, two typical problems have emerged: (1) the goals based on risk assessment are sometimes less than the reliable measurement level, and (2) the variability of measurements near the standard becomes significant, leading to both false-positive and false-negative results. Many solutions have been proposed for these problems, generally based on statistical models. However, these are multidisciplinary problems, with their roots in toxicology, analytical chemistry, and statistics; comprehensive solutions have not been found. This chapter describes these and related problems and discusses potential solutions.

## II. THE IMPACTS OF INADEQUATE MONITORING

### A. Public Health Impacts

#### 1. Mistakes in Setting Priorities

A principal use of environmental data is the establishment of priorities for intervention and mitigation efforts. If the collection of environmental data is flawed, the resulting priorities will be distorted and will result in mitigation of relatively minor risks. A prominent example of the setting of environmental priorities is the formal risk-oriented Hazard Ranking Systems (HRS) in the federal Superfund Program (USEPA, 1991). The HRS scores, which determine placement on the federal National Priorities List, are based on data for toxicity, hydrogeology, and exposure. The calculation of exposure (usually potential exposure) is based on environmental measurements. Evaluations of sites scored with the HRS have found both false-positive (sites with no significant risks and high HRS scores) and false-negative (sites with significant risk and low HRS scores) results (Doty, 1990). False positive calculations allocate resources to relatively minor risks; false-negative ones ignore the relatively important risks. One source of the problem is inequitable design of site investigations. Other things aside, the more one looks for contamination, the more one finds. The relationship of design to false positives and false negatives is discussed in the following.

On a larger scale than hazardous waste site risk assessment is comparative risk assessment, for which priorities can also be distorted by poor monitoring data. Risk assessors have found "... the poor quality of data and the uncertainties about exposure extrapolations as the most problematic aspect of the endeavor" (Hornstein, 1992). Comparative risk assessment are intended to help establish policy based on a quantitative ranking of risks, but inadequate exposure measurements can obscure the differences in risks from disparate sources, or worse, can skew the ranking of risks based on biased exposure assessments.

### 2. Uncertainty

A major effect of inadequate monitoring is the failure to reduce uncertainty about human exposure and risks. The public perception of environmental risks depends, among other factors, on the uncertainty of exposure data. If the affected community has legitimate concerns about the adequacy of potential or actual exposure data, it will be rightfully skeptical about the selection of choices for the mitigation of risk.

One way to reduce the uncertainty of human exposure is to use biological markers, or "biomarkers" of exposure; the assets and limitations of this approach are discussed in a later section.

## B.  Environmental Impacts

Inadequate environmental measurement can misidentify potential ecological risks. Selenium accumulation in the Kesterson drainage area of California was unrecognized because of the inadequacy of measurements in water, sediment, and tissue. The discovery of birth deformities in migratory birds led to better measurement and speciation of selenium (USGS, 1984). Birth deformities in Great Lakes waterfowl did not correlate with total polychlorinated biphenyl (PCB) measurements, but did correlate with the most toxic "coplanar" PCBs. The congener-specific measurement of PCBs is discussed in the section on monitoring mixed chemical exposures.

Because of bioconcentration, the sensitivity required for assessing ecological risks is often greater than that needed for human risk assessment. In addition, sublethal effects can be found for concentrations of metals, such as copper, far below the levels of concern for human health.

## III.  MONITORING DESIGN

## A.  Goals

Monitoring goals are generally established by law for specific programs. For example, the federal Safe Drinking Water Act (SDWA) requires the administrator to establish "maximum contaminant level goals" for any contaminants that "may have any adverse effect on the health of persons and which are known or anticipated to occur in public water systems" (USEPA, 1991a). For U.S. EPA category I drinking water contaminants, the maximum contaminant level goal (MCLG) is set at zero. The ultimate monitoring program would measure down to zero, that is, would detect a single molecule in each sample. A major issue in the design of monitoring programs is that monitoring program goals are established at levels that cannot be reliably measured by existing methods. Various solutions to this problem are discussed in this chapter.

Another example is the California Safe Drinking Water and Toxic Enforcement Act of 1986 (Proposition 65). The regulations adopted pursuant to this act established "no significant risk levels (NSRLs)" for carcinogens based on a $10^{-5}$ incremental cancer risk. Levels for reproductive toxicants are based on 1/1000 of the no observable effect level (NOEL). Since these levels were based on risk only, without consideration of the feasibility of monitoring, conflicts between these levels and monitoring feasibility can occur.

## B. Objectives

The objectives of monitoring are generally (1) detection monitoring or (2) compliance monitoring. Detection monitoring seeks to detect the lowest concentration of a substance in some environmental medium. Compliance monitoring is designed to determine whether a regulatory limit has been exceeded.

### 1. Detection Monitoring

One example of detection monitoring is routine analysis of groundwater near hazardous waste treatment, storage, and disposal facilities that are regulated by the federal Resource Conservation and Recovery Act (RCRA), as amended. The purpose of the monitoring is to detect leaks or other releases into groundwater. For naturally occurring substances, such as metals, nitrate, sulfate, and chloride, the objective is to determine whether there is a statistically significant increase in hydrologically down-gradient wells compared with up-gradient wells. In practice, this is a complex task, since many substances are measured, and a variety of parametric and nonparametric statistical tests may be used. For nonnaturally occurring substances, such as organic solvents, the objective is to detect the first sign of a release. To accomplish this objective requires a good knowledge of local hydrogeology, correct placement and construction of monitoring wells, reliable sampling, and sensitive analytical methods.

### 2. Compliance Monitoring

The objective of compliance monitoring is to determine whether a regulatory limit or other action level has been exceeded. One problematic example is reaching cleanup levels for contaminated solid and groundwater under site cleanup programs, such as the federal Superfund Program. Factors that may be included are

The limits of remedial techniques
Site-specific conditions
The ranges of risk estimates
The quantitation level of available methods
Uncertainty of monitoring results

### 3. Data Quality

The objectives for environmental monitoring programs are often contained in a quality assurance (QA) plan. The purpose of a QA plan is to produce data of known and acceptable quality for the requirements of the project. The quality of monitoring data can be inadvertently affected (e.g., by the use of improper sampling or analysis techniques), or directly affected as the result of fraud. A good QA program will include sufficient quality control so that invalid data can be identified. The EPA requires a QA plan for all major projects (USEPA, 1984). The original EPA QA project plan guidelines (USEPA, 1980) have evolved with an increasing emphasis on data quality objectives (DQOs). Conceptually, the DQOs include a consideration of false-positives (type I error) as well as false negatives (type II error). In practice, false-positive and false-negative values are often considered only for analytical procedures, although greater contributions to errors come from the sampling and the risk-based limit itself. As shown in Fig. 1, the acceptable levels of type I and type II errors can affect the design of a monitoring program.

The design of a monitoring program typically involves the balancing of false-positive with false-negative values. For example, the design of a monitoring program to detect contamination in groundwater can decrease false-negative results by increasing the number of monitoring wells, increasing the frequency of sampling, increasing the number of substances monitored, and choosing analytical methods with low detection limits. However, this is done with some increase in the probability that artifacts in sampling and analysis will produce false-positive values. The costs associated with both errors can be incorporated into the monitoring design. The decrease in false-negative results is also done with increased cost, although some strategies (e.g., composite sampling) can reduce false-negative results without significant increases in monitoring costs, as discussed in the section on sampling strategies.

### 4. *Confirmation Sampling and Analysis*

In principle, one would confirm positive and negative results with the same proportion. In practice, however, the frequency of false-positive results is reduced by including confirmation analysis or confirmation sampling in the monitoring program. For example, if a single sample result is greater than a drinking water limit, confirmation samples will typically be collected and analyzed before a limit is considered exceeded. If confirmation sampling is done only on positive results, the effect is a reduced frequency of false-positive results, but no effect on the frequency of the false-negative ones.

## C.  Environmental Monitoring Versus Biological Exposure Monitoring

Human exposures can be monitored by measuring levels in environmental samples or by monitoring the internal levels with biological exposure monitoring. Biological exposure indices (BEIs) have been established for occupational exposures by the American Conference of Governmental Industrial Hygienists (ACGIH, 1991) and by other organizations (Fiserova-Bergerova, 1990).

Biological monitoring has the advantage of measuring integrated exposure from all sources

|  | Risk Level Exceeded | Risk Level Not Exceeded |
|---|---|---|
| Decision<br>Exceeded | $1-\alpha$ | $\alpha$<br>(Type I) |
| Not<br>Exceeded | $\beta$<br>(Type II) | $1-\beta$ |

|  | Examples |
|---|---|
| False Positive<br>(Type I error) | Environmental variability<br>Inaccurate or imprecise methods |
| False Negative<br>(Type II error) | Insufficient number of samples<br>Insufficient number of sampling locations (e.g., monitoring wells)<br>Insensitive analytical methods |

**Figure 1**  The effects of errors on monitoring design.

(air, food, water, dermal absorption, and such). It has the disadvantage of being more invasive and often requiring medical professionals for design and implementation. Approved human subjects protocols may be required before monitoring, and confidentiality of results is necessary. In contrast with medical surveillance, biological exposure monitoring is intended to measure a chemical, its metabolite, or a reversible biochemical marker or other effect of exposure. Biological markers, or biomarkers, have numerous applications for environmental monitoring (McCarthy, 1990).

## D. Sampling Strategies

Steps in developing sampling strategies include (Keith, 1988)

Establish data quality objectives
Plan sampling
Design quality assurance
Prepare matrix-specific sampling protocols

Although risk-based levels are often based on an external dose, monitoring programs typically measure exposures indirectly. For example, the federal Safe Drinking Water Program generally monitors the water as supplied by the water purveyor, rather than at the tap. Exceptions include lead monitoring, which uses tap monitoring to include contributions from lead pipe, and monitoring at the tap to measure the possible contamination from permeation of plastic pipe by volatile organic compounds (VOCs) (USEPA, 1991a).

Sampling strategies should be appropriate for the standard, the medium being monitored, and the acceptable levels of $\alpha$ and $\beta$, as shown in Fig. 1. For example, if a cleanup of contaminated soil were to be done, the probability of calling clean soil contaminated might be set at $\alpha = 0.10$. The probability of concluding that contaminated soil is clean (false-negative) might be set at $\beta = 0.05$. With these levels of error established, the required number of samples and sampling strategies can be determined.

### 1. Frequency of Sampling

The environmental variability over time will generally determine the frequency of sampling. For example, drinking water monitoring typically requires an initial quarterly monitoring, followed by annual monitoring if no target contaminants are detected (USEPA, 1991a). If contaminants are detected, quarterly monitoring is continued unless the system is "reliably and consistently" under the maximum contaminant level (MCL).

### 2. Composite Sampling

Composite sampling is the technique of combining portions of homogenized primary sample to form a composite that is representative of the original samples. The advantages and disadvantages of composite sampling are listed in Table 1. Since savings in analytical costs can be considerable, this is a driving force in the selection of composite sampling.

**Table 1** Considerations for Composite Sampling

| Advantages | Disadvantages |
| --- | --- |
| Reduces analytical costs | Can dilute "hot spots" |
| Reduces variance per sample | May require reanalysis of primary samples |
| Reduces sampling costs | |

## E.  The Effect of Variability on Monitoring

The major sources of variability in monitoring are the following:

Environmental or industrial process variability
Sampling
Choice of analytical method
Analysis

Environmental or process variability is generally the major source of monitoring variability. Although some compliance programs address only the variability in sampling and analysis, environmental variability should be considered in the design of monitoring (Nicas, 1991). Environmental variability generally follows a lognormal distribution, whereas sampling and analysis errors tend to follow normal distributions.

For example, the EPA has found that the choice of analytical method was a major source of variability in measuring PCBs (USEPA, 1982). The establishment of approved test protocols and environmental laboratory accreditation has reduced the variability caused by the choice of method.

The final source of variability is the analysis itself. Analytical variability is generally estimated by the analysis of replicate samples or replicate spiked samples. Of all sources of uncertainty, this has received the most attention.

So that all of the major sources of uncertainty are known, the study must be designed accordingly. Table 2 shows the kinds of samples that are needed to measure the major sources of uncertainty.

## F.  Analysis

### 1.  Laboratory Accreditation

The EPA requires approval for laboratories that analyze drinking water, but not other environmental media. In addition, many states and other organizations have accreditation or certification programs for categories, such as wastewater, hazardous waste, air, and pesticide residues in food. A national environmental laboratory accreditation program has been proposed. The minimum requirements of accreditation programs typically include the following:

Education and experience of key laboratory personnel
An approved quality assurance plan
Use of approved analytical methods
Acceptable results on performance evaluation samples

However, the use of a laboratory that is accredited for the needed analysis does not provide a guarantee that the results will be reliable.

**Table 2**  Estimating Sources of Variability

| Sources variability | Estimation technique |
| --- | --- |
| Environmental | Samples taken over time or area |
| Sampling | Colocated samples |
| Choice of analytical method | Analysis of split samples by reference method and proposed method |
| Analysis | Analysis of homogenized replicate samples with the same protocol |

**Table 3**  Analytical Methods for PCBs

| Measurement | Example of method | Comments |
|---|---|---|
| Total PCBs screen | EPA method 508A (perchlorination GC-ECD) | Cannot identify Aroclor mixtures |
| Selected individual congeners | EPA method 8270 | Does not identify Aroclor mixtures |
| Aroclor mixtures | EPA methods 8080 or 8081 | Uses pattern identification |
| Congener-specific analysis | Huckins, 1988 | Results can be used with TEFs |

## 2. Selection and Validation of Analytical Methods

Several sources of approved analytical methods exist. For the measurement of occupational exposures, for example, the sampling and analysis are generally described in the same procedure in *NIOSH Methods of Analysis*. Other risk-based monitoring may require the modification of an approved protocol, typically by extending the range to lower concentrations. In a public health or environmental emergency, an existing protocol may require modification and validation. Criteria have been established for the development of methods in a crisis (Conacher, 1990). It is sometimes desirable to validate a method with actual monitoring samples. For example, matrix-specific detection levels and quantitation levels can be established by using actual samples. These site-specific levels will provide more realistic estimates of detection levels because they will incorporate interferences and other "matrix effects" from actual monitoring samples.

All methods are not equal in their performance or results. For example, Table 3 shows some choices available for the analysis of PCBs. As shown, the available methods offer a range of specificity, from total PCB concentration to congener-specific concentrations. The congener-specific measurements can be used with toxicity equivalency factors (TEFs) to calculate toxic equivalents (USEPA, 1991b), as discussed later in this chapter.

## 3. Chemical Speciation

The risk assessment process may produce risk estimates for an exposure that is not easily measured directly. Table 4 lists examples of regulated substances and the corresponding monitoring target.

Some compliance monitoring will require speciation to meaningfully measure the target substance. For example, hexavalent chromium is generally considered to be carcinogenic by federal and state regulations, but trivalent chromium and elemental chromium are not. The measurement of only hexavalent chromium requires sampling and analytical methods that can reliably measure hexavalent chromium, even in the presence of trivalent and ele-

**Table 4**  Risk-Derived Monitoring Targets

| Regulated substance | Monitoring target |
|---|---|
| Asbestos | Specific mineral forms (e.g., chrysotile) |
| Lead | Total lead |
| Nickel subsulfide | Total nickel |
| PCBs | Aroclor mixtures |
| Tetrachlorodibenzo-*p*-dioxin (TCDD) | Congener-specific polychlorinated dibenzo-*p*-dioxins (PCDDs) and polychlorinated dibenzofurans (PCDFs) |

mental chromium. The design of such a speciation methods can be a critical element of a monitoring program.

## 4. Detection Limits

When the concentration of a contaminant is near zero, the reliability of measurement is an issue. At some concentration, the contaminant can be reliably detected. This threshold, or detection level, primarily depends on the type of sample, the sampling method, and the analytical method. The detection level cannot be measured directly, but is generally estimated using some statistical model. The actual detection process depends on the analytical techniques. For example, the detection of a substance using high-performance liquid chromatography (HPLC) is the measurement of a peak within the expected retention time. Detection by gas chromatography–mass spectrometry (GC–MS), on the other hand, involves (1) detection of a peak with the correct retention time, (2) measurement of the key ions of the suspected compound, and (3) ratios of the key ions within an expected range (EPA Method 8270; USEPA, 1986). Thus, the reliability of the detection process is very different in the two techniques. Unfortunately, the common estimates of detection levels ignore the differences in the actual detection criteria and use statistical estimates that assume one measurement (e.g., a single peak measurement).

## 5. Method Detection Limit

The EPA has defined the *method detection limit* (MDL) as: "The minimum concentration of a substance that can be measured and reported with 99% confidence that the analyte concentration is greater than zero." It is calculated by analyzing replicate samples of high-purity water containing the concentration of the analyte of interest near the expected MDL, and calculating the MDL by using the following equation:

$$\text{MDL} = t_{(n-1, 1-\alpha = 0.99)} s$$

MDL = method detection limit
$t$ = Students $t$ value at a 99% confidence level with $n - 1$ degrees of freedom
$s$ = sample standard deviation

This definition of MDL does not include the reliability of identification. For example, gas chromatography with flame ionization detection (GC–FID) and GC–MS may have similar MDLs, but the reliability of identification by GC–MS is much higher; therefore, it has a much lower proportion of false-positive results.

Other definitions of detection levels have been established by the American Chemical Society (ACS, 1980), but a consensus has not yet been established for the definition and use of detection levels. If a regulatory limit is established at the detection limit, there is a significant probability of false-negative results. If, for example, the true concentration of a substance was equal to the detection limit (which is assumed to be the same as the regulatory limit), half of the measurements would fall below the detection limit; that is, the probability of a false-negative value would be 50%. If the detection limit is lower than the regulatory limit, the probability of false-negative results will be less. Monitoring is often designed with regulatory levels that are at twice the DL. A simple gaussian model, illustrated in Fig. 2, shows that if the regulatory limit is at twice the detection limit, the false-positive values ($\alpha$, the probability that a substance will be reported as present when it really is not), are low, and false-negative ones ($\beta$, the probability that a substance is reported absent when it is present at the regulatory limit), are also low.

## 6. Quantitation Limits

At some concentration above the detection level a substance can be reliably quantitated. This level is sometimes called a quantitation level (QL). The *quantitation level* has been generally

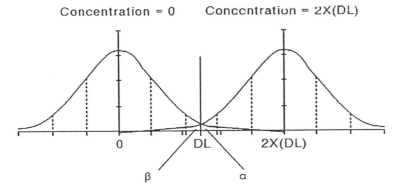

**Figure 2** A gaussian model for the detection limit.

defined as the concentration that can be reported with some specified level of precision. (Other terms which have been used include "limit of quantitation" and "determination limit.") For drinking water monitoring, the EPA has established a "practical quantitation limit (PQL)" as the concentration at which 75% of laboratories participating in an interlaboratory study report results that are within ±55% of the true value (USEPA, 1991a). However, when this procedure would result in a PQL that is greater than a $10^{-4}$ cancer risk, the PQL was established at another level: five times the interlaboratory method detection limit (MDL). Other programs, such as the RCRA hazardous waste management program, routinely calculate PQLs as a multiple of a MDL (USEPA, 1986). For example, Table 5 shows the multipliers for various matrices that are used for guidance in RCRA analysis.

Some programs have explicitly used the quantitation level as a regulatory limit to determine presence or absence of a contaminant. For example, the EPA has used the practical limit of quantitation for PCBs in air, water, wastes, or products to define the "absence of PCBs" (USEPA, 1982). In summary, there is no consensus on the definitions of detection level and quantitation level.

## G. Quality Assurance

### 1. Random Error and Systematic Error

In general, a quality management program seeks to control four sources of data errors: random error, systematic error (bias), blunders, and fraud. The allowable levels of random error and systematic error should be determined by the data quality objectives. Once the allowable levels are established, specific quality control procedures are used to determine whether data meet the specified objectives. For example, the EPA Contract Laboratory Program,

**Table 5** Examples of Guidance PQLs

| Matrix | Factor | PQL for TCE (MDL = 0.12 μg/L) |
|---|---|---|
| Groundwater | 10 | 1.2 μg/L |
| Low-level soil | 10 | 1.2 μg/kg |
| Water-miscible liquid waste | 500 | 60 μg/L |
| High-level soil and sludge | 1250 | 150 μg/kg |
| Non–water-miscible waste | 1250 | 150 μg/kg |

*Source:* USEPA, 1986.

which provides data for the Superfund Program, has a detailed set of quality control procedures and reporting requirements.

## 2. Blunders

Quality control procedures can identify, but not necessary eliminate, the effects of blunders in the field or laboratory. The effect of blunders is greater with a smaller set of samples, such as composite samples, that represent a greater set of original samples.

## 3. Fraud

Unrealistic scheduling, overly detailed contract requirements, and increased use of automated data storage have led to several cases of reporting fraudulent data. One example is "time-traveling," when an analyst falsifies a date and time of analysis to meet holding time requirements. Fraud can be difficult to detect and can have devastating effects on exposure assessments. Draft good automated laboratory procedures have been established in an attempt to improve the security of automated data (USEPA, 1990a).

## 4. Quality Assurance Plans

The goal of quality assurance is to produce data of known and acceptable quality. The USEPA requires quality assurance program plans for any major monitoring program, and quality assurance project plans for site-specific investigations, such as a remedial investigation/feasibility study in the Superfund program.

## 5. Data Validation

In addition to laboratory quality control, a quality assurance program should include data validation, which is generally done by someone who was not involved in sampling or analysis. The results, including field notes, raw laboratory data, and results for quality control samples are reviewed and a judgment is made about whether the data are valid, invalid, or of limited usefulness. One problem that arises in data validation is: Should results be adjusted for bias in the sampling or analytical procedure? To get an unbiased estimate of an exposure dose, the answer is clearly, yes. However, adjusting for bias is not a simple matter; some methods (e.g., NIOSH methods) explicitly include corrections for blank results and recovery bias; some methods (e.g., isotope dilution GC–MS methods) have a "built-in" correction with the use of internal standards; and some methods have no bias correction specified at all. The EPA has proposed that bias correction be done routinely during the data validation process, but this has not become common practice.

## 6. Data Qualifiers

When data are determined to be acceptable and reported, they still may be "flagged" with data qualifiers to indicate the limitations on their usefulness. For example, Table 6 shows examples

**Table 6** Data Qualifiers

| Qualifiers | Explanation |
|---|---|
| U | The substance was not detected. |
| J | Indicates an estimated value; for example, when a concentration is less than its quantitation limit, but more than zero. |
| B | The compound was found in an associated blank as well as in the sample. |
| E | Indicates a result that exceeds the calibration range of the analysis. |

*Source:* USEPA, 1990.

of data qualifiers used in the EPA Contract Laboratory Program. Needless to say, it is important that these qualifiers not be lost when the results are included in a larger data base.

## IV. MONITORING MIXED CHEMICAL EXPOSURES

### A. Mixture Rules

Risk-based limits are usually based on one substance at a time. Other than well-defined mixtures, such as PCBs, monitoring and compliance programs seldom include limits for exposure to chemical mixtures. The American Conference of Governmental Industrial Hygienists (ACGIH) uses a mixture rule for substances that "... act upon the same organ system ..." (ACGIH, 1992):

$$\text{If } \frac{C_1}{T_1} + \frac{C_2}{T_1} + \dots \frac{C_n}{T_n} > 1, \text{ then the limit is exceeded.}$$

$C_i$ = concentration of substance $i$.
$T_i$ = threshold limit of substance $i$.

Most regulatory compliance programs do not address the issue of exposure to chemical mixtures, but consider compliance with regulatory limits one substance at a time.

### B. Well-Defined Mixtures

Monitoring is often done for well-defined mixtures of related substances, such as PCBs, polychlorinated dibenzodioxins–polychlorinated dibenzofurans (PCDDs–PCDFs), or petroleum products. The measurement of petroleum hydrocarbon contamination is problematic. A variety of methods have been established to measure either total petroleum hydrocarbon contamination (e.g., solvent extraction and infrared spectrophotometry; EPA 418), or specific petroleum product contamination (State of California, 1989). Immunoassay procedures have been developed that demonstrate various sensitivities to petroleum hydrocarbon mixtures. However, the measurement technique in such assays should match the risk-based limit. Gasoline contamination, for example, is typically measured by a combination of individual measurements for benzene, toluene, ethylbenzene, and xylenes ("BTEX"), plus total petroleum hydrocarbons calculated as gasoline. The PCBs have been typically measured as Aroclor mixture, based on the composition of the original commercial product. However, if risk assessment is based on specific PCB compounds, or congeners, the analysis must be congener-specific or measure the potency of the mixture using an appropriate assay.

When exposures involve complex mixtures, monitoring and compliance is more complicated. Pattern recognition techniques, such as principal component analysis, have been used to identify sources for mixed chemical exposure (Wold, 1987). The field of source receptor analysis has developed to better understand the sources of airborne chemical mixtures (Gordon, 1988). Other multivariate models such as neural networks may offer even more powerful techniques for monitoring complex mixtures (Jansson, 1991).

## V. COMPLIANCE

### A. Compliance Levels

Risk-derived dose limits have been used to establish compliance levels as shown in Fig. 3. For example, the compliance level (MCL) for chromium in drinking water, based on the

Examples

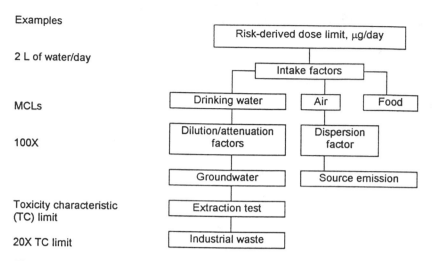

2 L of water/day

MCLs

100X

Toxicity characteristic
(TC) limit

20X TC limit

**Figure 3**  Derivation of compliance limits.

assumption of 2 L of water consumed a day, is 50 µg/L. The hazardous waste limit for the concentration of chromium in an extract from the toxicity characteristic leaching procedure (TCLP) is 100 times the MCL, or 5 mg/L. The total concentration screening level for a solid waste (to decide if extraction by TCLP is necessary) is 20 times the TCLP limit, or 100 mg/kg. In this way, compliance limits have been set to reflect the dilution and/or attenuation that could occur before ingestion of contaminated groundwater.

## B.  Statistical Analysis of Data for Compliance

### 1.  Treatment of Data Below the Detection Limit

Compliance with risk-based limits often involves results below the detection limit. Several techniques have been used for dealing with nondetect values, which can be grouped into (1) substitution techniques, (2) distributional methods, which assume some model for the distribution of results, and (3) robust methods (Helsel, 1990).

As shown in Tables 7 and 8, substitution methods can introduce bias into estimates of the mean, median, or other parameters. Distributional methods can produce unbiased parameters if the data match the assumed distribution. Robust methods have the advantage of not assuming particular distributions. Another approach to "less-than" values is the use of nonparametric tests, which do not require estimates of the mean, standard deviation, or other parameters.

### 2.  Comparison with Regulatory Levels

Groundwater monitoring is required of owners and operators of hazardous waste facilities. The EPA or states have adopted regulations on the statistical analysis of groundwater monitor-

**Table 7**  Estimation Methods for "Less Than" Values

| Estimation method | Example |
|---|---|
| Substitution | One-half the detection limit |
| Distribution | Maximum likelihood estimation |
| Robust | Extrapolation to below the detection limit |

**Table 8** Substitution Techniques for "Less Than" Data

| Value substituted | Bias |
|---|---|
| Zero | Low |
| Detection limit | High |
| DL/2 | Depends on distribution |
| DL/$\sqrt{2}$ | Less bias than DL/2 for lognormal distributions |

ing data using both parametric and nonparametric tests (SWRCB, CCR Title 23, § 2550.7). In "detection monitoring," the objective is to determine statistically significant differences between hydraulically down-gradient and hydraulically up-gradient wells. Since the objective is to determine whether a release has occurred, risk-based regulatory limits are not used. The desire to detect a release at the earliest has placed additional attention on detection levels and quantitation levels.

In compliance monitoring, however, a comparison is made with an established MCL or "alternate concentration limit (ACL)." A permit may require that a MCL or ACL not be exceeded, or alternatively, that the limit not be exceeded more than a specified proportion of measurements. The confidence interval method is a recommended method. If data appear to be lognormally distributed, a log transformation is done, then a confidence interval is created for either the untransformed or log-transformed data:

$$\bar{x} \pm t_{(0.99,\, n-1)} \frac{s}{\sqrt{n}}$$

$\bar{x}$ = mean of values for a sampling period
$t_{(0.99,\, n-1)}$ = $t$ value for $\alpha = 0.01$
$s$ = sample standard of deviation
$n$ = number of samples

## C. Reliability of Compliance Monitoring Data

Most compliance monitoring programs do not deal directly with the uncertainty of monitoring data. The EPA rules for the Safe Drinking Water Act, for example, set limits on the laboratory results for performance evaluation samples as ±40% for concentrations less than 10 µg/L, but do not indicate how this uncertainty is to be used in determining compliance (USEPA, 1992).

Monitoring may involve a choice of approved methods that may differ in precision and accuracy. If the issue of false-positive and false-negative results were not dealt with in the monitoring design, the review of compliance data may reveal these problems.

Analytical methods often include criteria for the quality of results, but these generally do not include criteria for variability from sampling activities. If analytical results do not meet required criteria, corrective action should be taken to identify and solve the problem. Results that do not meet the acceptance criteria are generally unusable.

## VI. ENFORCEMENT

Environmental enforcement has recently moved increasingly to criminal prosecution of corporations and individuals. Since some environmental crimes may have penalties as high as 100,000 dollars/day (Calif. H&SC 25189.5), the challenge of data used in enforcement may be intensive.

Enforcement of environmental standards usually involves regulations, rather than statute, since risk-based limits are normally established by an administrative rule-making body.

## A. Admissibility of Scientific Evidence

If risk-based limits are established in statute or regulation, the scientific basis of the limit is usually not an issue. However, methods that are used to document a violation may be challenged. Criteria for admissibility of scientific evidence have been generally based on *Frye v. United States,* a 1923 federal appellate court decision on the use of polygraph results (*Frye v. United States,* 1924), and subsequent decisions. Typical criteria are (1) a new scientific technique must be generally accepted in the scientific community, (2) a person testifying on the acceptability of the method must be sufficiently qualified as an expert to testify about it, and (3) there must be a demonstration that correct scientific procedures were used in the particular case (*People v. Kelly,* 1976). In 1993, the U.S. Supreme Court, in the case *Daubert v. Merrell Dow Pharmaceuticals,* ruled that, in federal cases, judges should have more latitude in deciding the acceptability of evidence based on its relevance, and reliability (CDOS, 1993).

If sampling and analytical methods are established in regulation, there is little question about the acceptability of methods. For programs that do not have established approved methods, however, the choice of sampling and analysis techniques may be at issue, and may be challenged by expert witnesses.

## B. Weight of Scientific Evidence

Beyond the question of admissibility is the question of what weight will be given to compliance data. This can be argued using several factors, including the reliability of the sampling and testing methods, the quality assurance program, and even the credentials of the witnesses. Expert witness testimony may be used to establish the reliability of sampling and testing methods. Although sampling and analysis guidelines may exist for some regulatory programs, techniques are not limited to those published by regulatory agencies (NEEJ, 1989). As the recent Supreme Court decision is applied, the acceptability of methods may shift from general recognition in the scientific community to reliability as determined at trial.

## REFERENCES

[ACS] American Chemical Society (1980). Guidelines for data acquisition and data quality evaluation in environmental chemistry, *Anal. Chem.,* 52, 2242–2249.

[ACGIH] American Conference of Governmental Industrial Hygienists (1992). *1992–1993 Threshold Limit Values for Chemical Substances and Physical Agents and Biological Exposure Indices.*

[CDOS] *California Daily Opinion Service* (1993). 93 4825 *William Daubert v. Merrell Dow Pharmaceuticals.*

[CalEPA] California Environmental Protection Agency (1992). Safe Drinking Water and Toxic Enforcement Act of 1986 (Prop. 65), Status report, July 1992.

California State Water Resources Control Board, *California Code of Regulations,* Title 23. § 2550.7(e)(8).

Conacher, H. B. S. (1990). Validation of methods used in crisis situations: Task force report, *J. Assoc. Off. Anal. Chem.,* 73, 332–334.

Doty, C. B., and C. C. Travis (1990). Is EPA's National Priorities List correct? *Environ. Sci. Technol.,* 24, 1778–1780.

Draper, W. M., D. Wijekoon, and R. D. Stephens (1991). Speciation and quantitation of Aroclors in hazardous wastes based on PCB congener data, *Chemosphere,* 22, 147–164.

Fiserova-Bergerova, V., and M. Ogata, eds. (1990). *Biological Monitoring of Exposure to Industrial Chemicals,* American Conference of Governmental Industrial Hygienists, Cincinnati.

*Frye v. United States* (1924). *Fed. Rep.*, 293, No. 3968, 1013–1014.

Gordon, G. E. (1988). Receptor models, *Environ. Sci. Technol.*, 22, 1132–1142.

Helsel, D. R. (1990). Less than obvious; statistical treatment of data below the detection limit, *Environ. Sci. Technol.*, 24, 1766–1774.

Hornstein, D. T. (1992). Reclaiming environmental law: A normative critique of comparative risk analysis, *Columbia Law Rev.*, 92, 614.

Huckins, J. A., T. R. Schwartz, J. D. Petty, and J. M. Smith (1988). Determination, fate, and potential significance of PCBs in fish and sediment samples with emphasis on selected AHH-inducing congeners, 17, 1995–2016.

Jansson, P. A. (1991). Neural networks: An overview, *Anal. Chem.*, 63, 357A–362A.

Keith, L. H., ed. (1990). *Principles of Environmental Sampling,* American Chemical Society, Washington DC.

McCarthy, J. F., and L. R. Shugart, eds. (1990). *Biomarkers of Environmental Contamination,* Lewis Publishers, Boca Raton, FL.

[NEEJ] *National Environmental Enforcement Journal* (1989). 4, 15–16.

[NRC] National Research Council (1983). *Risk Assessment in the Federal Government: Managing the Process,* National Academy Press, Washington, DC.

Nicas, M., B. P. Simmons, and R. C. Spear (1991). Environmental versus analytical variability in exposure measurements, *Am. Ind. Hyg. Assoc. J.*, 52, 553–557.

*People v. Kelly* (1976). *Cal. Rep.*, 17 C.3d 24; 130 Cal Rptr 144.549 P.2d 1240, 25–41.

State of California (1989). *Leaking Underground Fuel Tank Field Manual: Guidelines for Site Assessment, Cleanup, and Underground Storage Tank Closure,* October 1989.

[USEPA] Environmental Protection Agency. *Guidance Document on the Statistical Analysis of Ground-Water Monitoring Data at RCRA Facilities.*

[USEPA] Environmental Protection Agency. Office of Monitoring Systems and Quality Assurance, Office of Research and Development (1980). Interim guidelines and specifications for preparing quality assurance project plans, QMAS-005/80, Washington, DC.

[USEPA] Environmental Protection Agency. (1982). *Fed. Regist.*, 47, 204, 46980–46996, Oct. 21.

[USEPA] Environmental Protection Agency. (1984). EPA Order 5360.1, Policy and Program Requirements to Implement the Mandatory Quality Assurance Program, April.

[USEPA] Environmental Protection Agency. (1984a). Appendix B to Part 136—Definition and procedure for the determination of the method detection limit–revision 1.11, *Fed. Regist.*, 49(209):198–199, Oct. 26.

[USEPA] Environmental Protection Agency Office of Solid Waste and Emergency Response (1986). *Test Methods for Evaluating Solid Waste,* 3rd ed., Nov.

[USEPA] Environmental Protection Agency Environmental Monitoring Systems Laboratory (1988). *Methods for the Determination of Organic Compounds in Drinking Water,* EPA/600/4-88/039, Dec.

[USEPA] Environmental Protection Agency (1990). Contract Laboratory Program. Statement of work for organics analysis; multi-media, multi-concentration, No. OLM01.0, Dec.

[USEPA] Environmental Protection Agency Office of Administration and Resources Management (1990a). *Draft Good Automated Laboratory Practices,* Dec 28.

[USEPA] Environmental Protection Agency (1991). Hazard ranking system, 40 *Code of Federal Regulations* § 300, Appendix A.

[USEPA] Environmental Protection Agency (1991a). Drinking water; National Primary Drinking Water Regulations; monitoring for volatile organic chemicals; MCLGs and MCLs for aldicarb, aldicarb sulfoxide, aldicarb sulfone, pentachlorophenol, and barium, *Fed. Regist.*, 56(126, Part XII), 30266, July 1.

[USEPA] Environmental Protection Agency (1991b). *Workshop on toxicity equivalency factors for polychlorinated biphenyl congeners,* EPA/625/3-91/020, June.

[USEPA] Environmental Protection Agency (1992). *Fed. Regist.*, 56 (126, Part XII) 30266, July 1.

[USGS] U.S. Geological Survey (1984). *Selenium Concentrations in Waters Tributary to and in the Vicinity of the Kesterson National Wildlife Refuge, Fresno and Merced Counties, California,* Water Resources Investigations Report 84-4122, May.

Wold, S. (1987). Principal Component analysis, *Chemomet. Intell. Lab. Syst.*, 2, 37–52.

# Index

# About the Editors

**ANNA M. FAN** is Chief of the Pesticide and Environmental Toxicology Section, Office of Environmental Health Hazard Assessment, California Environmental Protection Agency, Berkeley, and Adjunct Professor of Toxicology at San Jose State University, California. The author or coauthor of over 100 professional papers and technical reports, she is a diplomate of the American Board of Toxicology and a member of the Society of Toxicology, among other organizations. She serves on the United States Environmental Protection Agency's Science Advisory Board, Drinking Water Committee, and previously served on the Committee for Groundwater Recharge, Water Science and Technology Board, and National Research Council. Dr. Fan received the B.S. degree (1972) in biological sciences from College of the Holy Names, Oakland, California, the M.S. degree (1974) in biology from the University of San Francisco, California, and the Ph.D. degree (1978) in toxicology from Utah State University, Logan.

**LOUIS W. CHANG** is a Professor in the Departments of Pathology, Pharmacology, and Toxicology, and Director of Graduate Studies in Experimental Pathology at the University of Arkansas for Medical Sciences, Little Rock. Dr. Chang also serves as a Visiting Professor at both Beijing Medical University and the Institute of Occupational Medicine, Chinese Academy of Preventive Medicine, Beijing, and is a Scientific Advisor and Honor Professor at the National Institute for the Control of Pharmaceutical and Biological Products, Beijing, People's Republic of China. Aside from being the author of over 200 scientific articles, he is also the editor of the *Handbook of Neurotoxicology* (with Robert S. Dryer) and *Principles of Neurotoxicology* (both titles, Marcel Dekker, Inc.), *Neurotoxicology: Approaches and Methods,* and *Toxicology of Metals, Volumes 1 and 2*. Dr. Chang is a member of the Society of Toxicology, the American Association of Neuropathologists, the American Association of Pathologists, the Society for Neuroscience, and the International Society of Neuropathology, among others. He has served on the editorial board of numerous scientific journals as well as on the review panel and advisory board of various federal agencies and industries. Dr. Chang received the B.A. degree (1966) in chemistry and biology from the University of Massachusetts at Amherst, the M.S. degree (1969) in neuroanatomy and histochemistry from Tufts University School of Medicine, Boston, Massachusetts, and the Ph.D. degree (1972) in pathology from the University of Wisconsin Medical School, Madison. Dr. Chang also received training in neurocytology from Harvard Medical School, Boston, Massachusetts, and in in vitro and biochemical neurotoxicology from the Brain Research Institute at the University of California, Los Angeles, School of Medicine.